T0177515

OXFORD MEDICAL PUBLICATION

Oxford Desk Reference
Oncology

Second Edition

Oxford Desk Reference
Oncology

Second Edition

Edited by

Thankamma Ajithkumar

Consultant Clinical Oncologist, Cambridge University Hospitals
NHS Foundation Trust, Cambridge, UK

Ann Barrett

Emeritus Professor of Oncology, University of East Anglia, Norwich, UK

Helen Hatcher

Consultant Medical and TYA Oncologist, Cambridge University Hospitals
NHS Foundation Trust, Cambridge, UK

Sarah Jefferies

Consultant Clinical Oncologist, Cambridge University Hospitals
NHS Foundation Trust, Cambridge, UK

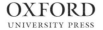

OXFORD
UNIVERSITY PRESS

Great Clarendon Street, Oxford, OX2 6DP,
United Kingdom

Oxford University Press is a department of the University of Oxford.
It furthers the University's objective of excellence in research, scholarship,
and education by publishing worldwide. Oxford is a registered trade mark of
Oxford University Press in the UK and in certain other countries

© Oxford University Press 2021

The moral rights of the authors have been asserted

First Edition published in 2011
Second Edition published in 2021

Impression: 1

Published in the United States of America by Oxford University Press
198 Madison Avenue, New York, NY 10016, United States of America

British Library Cataloguing in Publication Data

Data available

Library of Congress Control Number: 2020941565

ISBN 978–0–19–874544–0

DOI: 10.1093/med/9780198745440.001.0001

Printed in Great Britain by
Bell & Bain Ltd., Glasgow

Oxford University Press makes no representation, express or implied, that the
drug dosages in this book are correct. Readers must therefore always check
the product information and clinical procedures with the most up-to-date
published product information and data sheets provided by the manufacturers
and the most recent codes of conduct and safety regulations. The authors and
the publishers do not accept responsibility or legal liability for any errors in the
text or for the misuse or misapplication of material in this work. Except where
otherwise stated, drug dosages and recommendations are for the non-pregnant
adult who is not breast-feeding

Links to third party websites are provided by Oxford in good faith and
for information only. Oxford disclaims any responsibility for the materials
contained in any third party website referenced in this work.

Dedication

This edition is dedicated to the memory of Kath Walker (1965–2015) and
Nadeera De Silva (1982–2016).

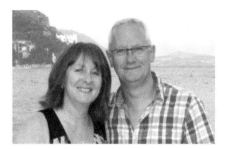

Kath was appointed Head of Radiotherapy when the Radiotherapy Department was facing multiple challenges. She changed the atmosphere, making Addenbrooke's a more desirable place for radiographers to work. She developed and introduced the first assistant radiographers in the UK as well as the research radiographer role. She also introduced ground-breaking technology, which collectively helped the department modernize. Her sudden loss with her partner, Andy Virco, was a tremendous shock. The staff and patients owe Kath a great debt and she is missed by all.

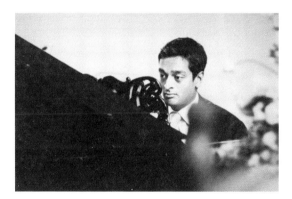

Nadeera was an exceptional clinical oncology trainee who joined the Eastern Region clinical oncology training programme. His excellent knowledge and communication skills led him to undertake a PhD, researching ways to better diagnose cancer in the early stages and to detect relapses from cancer of the oesophagus. He was in his third year of study at Caius College when he died. He is much missed for his academic input and also his musical talents.

Preface

This book forms part of the Oxford Desk Reference series and is designed to bridge the gap between the *Oxford Handbook of Oncology* and the substantial *Oxford Textbook of Oncology*. We hope this book will be on the desk of every oncologist to provide an easily accessible and succinct source of information on the common situations encountered within a normal oncology practice. Many international contributors have ensured this represents global philosophies of cancer management. Up-to-date details of relevant clinical trials are included and useful internet addresses where continuing treatment updates may be found. The editors take responsibility for any mistakes but particular care should be taken to check drug and radiotherapy doses before treating individual patients. We will be glad to receive any feedback on this volume.

Acknowledgements

Any book of this size involves hard work by many contributors and we are grateful to them all. Valuable assistance has been received from Oxford University Press. The editors are grateful for the continuing support and encouragement of colleagues, family, and friends.

Brief contents

Contents

18 Clinical management of cancers—flowcharts *513*

List of abbreviations

±	with *or* without
<	less than
>	greater than
2DRT	two-dimensional therapy
3DCRT	three-dimensional conformal radiotherapy
5-FU	Fluorouracil
aaIPI	age-adjusted IPI
AAO–HNS	American Academy of Otolaryngology–Head and Neck Surgery
ABC	activated B-cell
ABVD	doxorubicin (Adriamycin®), bleomycin, vinblastine, dacarbazine
AC	atypical carcinoid
ACC	adenoid cystic carcinoma
ACCP	American College of Chest Physicians
ACE	angiotensin-converting enzyme
ACLC	anaplastic large cell lymphoma
ACT	adoptive cellular therapy
ACTH	adrenocorticotrophic hormone
AD	autosomal dominant
ADC	antibody-drug conjugate
ADCC	antibody dependent cell-mediated cytotoxicity
ADH	antidiuretic hormone
ADOC	cisplatin, doxorubicin, vincristine, cyclophosphamide
ADT	androgen deprivation therapy
AED	antiepileptic drug
AFP	alpha-fetoprotein
AGES	age, grade, extent, size
AGO	Arbeitsgemeinschaft Gynaekologische Onkologie
AHP	allied health professional
AI	aromatase inhibitor
AIDS	acquired immune deficiency syndrome
AIN	anal intraepithelial neoplasia
AIS	adenocarcinoma in situ
AJCC	American Joint Committee on Cancer
5-ALA	5-aminolevulinic acid
ALIP	abnormal localization of immature precursor
ALK	anaplastic lymphoma kinase
ALL	acute lymphoblastic leukemia
ALP	alkaline phosphatase level
ALPPS	associating liver partition with portal vein ligation for staged hepatectomy
AMES	age, metastasis, extent, size
AML	acute myeloid leukaemia
AOS	Acute Oncology Service
AP	accelerated phase
APBI	accelerated partial breast radiation
APC	adenomatous polyposis coli *or* argon plasma coagulation
APHE	arterial phase hyperenhancement
APL/APML	acute promyelocytic leukaemia
APTT	activated partial thromboplastin time
ARDS	acute respiratory distress syndrome
AS	adenosarcoma
ASCO	American Society of Clinical Oncology
ASCT	autologous stem cell transplantation
ASD	atrial septal defect
ATA	American Thyroid Association
ATG	antithymocyte globulin
ATO	arsenic trioxide
ATP	adenosine triphosphate
ATRA	all-trans retinoic acid
ATRT	atypical teratoid rhabdoid tumour
AUC	area under the concentration curve
AYA	adult and young adult
BAC	bronchioloalveolar carcinoma
BBB	blood–brain barrier
BCC	basal cell carcinoma
BCG	bacillus Calmette–Guérin
BCLC	Barcelona Clinic Liver Cancer
BCNU	carmustine
BCPT	Breast Cancer Prevention Trial
BCR	breakpoint cluster region *or* B-cell receptor
BCS	breast conserving surgery
BCT	breast conservation therapy
beta-hCG	beta-human chorionic gonadotropin
bd	twice daily
BEP	bleomycin, etoposide, cisplatin
BHD	Birt–Hogg–Dube syndrome
BMB	bone marrow biopsy
BMD	bone mineral density
BMT	bone marrow transplant
BOLD	BioCONECT oncology leadership development
BP	blast phase or bisphosphonates

BR	bendamustine plus rituximab
BRCA	Breast Cancer Susceptibility Gene
BSA	body surface area
BSC	best supportive care
BSG	British Society of Gastroenterology
BSO	bilateral salpingo-oophorectomy
BTA	British Thyroid Association
BTK	Bruton's tyrosine kinase
BTP	break through pain
CA	carbohydrate antigen
CAB	combined androgen blockade
CAF	cyclophosphamide, doxorubicin, fluorouracil
CALM	cafe-au-lait macule
CAM	confusion assessment method
CAP	cisplatin, doxorubicin, cyclophosphamide
CAV	cyclophosphamide, doxorubicin, vincristine
CBC	complete blood count
CBF	core binding factor
CBME	ciliary body medulloepithelioma
CBT	cognitive behavioural therapy
CCA	cholangiocarcinoma
CCNU	lomustine
CC-RCC	clear-cell renal cell carcinoma
CCyR	complete cytogenetic response
CDC	complement dependent cytotoxicity
CDKN2A	cyclin dependent kinase inhibitor 2A
CEA	carcinoembryonic antigen
CE-CT	contrast-enhanced computed tomography
CEF	cyclophosphamide, epirubicin, fluorouracil
CEUS	contrast-enhanced ultrasound
CFS	colostomy free survival
CGA	Comprehensive Geriatric Assessment
cHL	classical type of HL
CHART	continuous hyperfractionated accelerated radiotherapy
CHD	carcinoid heart disease
CHM	complete hydatidiform mole
CHOP	cyclophosphamide, hydroxydaunorubicin (doxorubicin), Oncovin® (vincristine), prednisone
CI	confidence interval
CIBP	cancer-induced bone pain
CIN	cervical intraepithelial neoplasia
CIS	carcinoma in situ

CLND	completion lymph node dissection
CLL	chronic lymphocytic leukaemia
CLS	capillary-like space
cm	centimetre(s)
CMF	cyclophosphamide, methotrexate, fluorouracil
CMFVP	cyclophosphamide, methotrexate, fluorouracil, vincristine, prednisone
CML	chronic myeloid leukaemia
CMMRD	constitutional mismatch repair deficiency
CMR	complete metabolic response
CMV	cytomegalovirus
CNS	central nervous system
COMP	cyclophosphamide, vincristine, methotrexate, prednisone
COPAD	cyclophosphamide, vincristine, prednisolone, doxorubicin
COPD	chronic obstructive pulmonary disease
COX	cyclo-oxygenase
CP	critical phase
CPC	choroid plexus carcinoma
CPG	cancer predisposition genes
CPP	choroid plexus papilloma
CR	complete remission
CRASH	Chemotherapy Risk Assessment Scale for High Age Patients
CRC	colorectal cancer
CRF	cancer related fatigue
CRM	continual reassessment method or circumferential resection margin
CRT	chemoradiotherapy
CS	carcinosarcoma or clinical staging
CSF	colony-stimulating factor or cerebrospinal fluid
CSOM	chronic suppurative otitis media
CSRT	craniospinal radiotherapy
CSS	cancer-specific survival
CT	computed tomography or chemotherapy
CTA	clinical trial authorization
CTC	circulating tumour cells
CTCAE	common terminology criteria for adverse events
CT IVU	CT urography
CTL	cytotoxic T lymphocyte
CTLA4	cytotoxic T lymphocyte 4-targeted
CTPA	computed tomography pulmonary angiogram
CTV	clinical target volume
CUP	cancer of unknown primary

CUSA	cavitating ultrasonic aspirator
CVD	cardiovascular disease
CXR	chest X-ray
CyR	cytogenetic response
DAHANCA	Danish Head and Neck Cancer Group
DC	dendritic cells
DCBE	double-contrast barium enema
dCCA	distal
DCIS	ductal carcinoma in situ
DCR	disease control rate
DEC-MRI	dynamic contrast-enhanced magnetic resonance imaging
DES	diethylstilboestrol
DEXA	dual-energy X-ray absorptiometry
DFS	disease-free survival
DHFR	dihydrofolate reductase
DI	diabetes insipidus
DIC	disseminated intravascular coagulation
DIPG	diffuse intrinsic pontine glioma
DIPNECH	diffuse idiopathic pulmonary neuroendocrine cell hyperplasia
DLBCL	diffuse large B-cell lymphoma
DLCL	diffuse large cell lymphoma
DLCO	diffusion lung capacity for carbon monoxide
DLI	donor lymphocyte infusions
DLT	dose limiting toxicity
DNA	deoxyribonucleic acid
DNAR	do not attempt resuscitation
DNMTI	DNA methyl transferase inhibitors
DOAC	direct oral anticoagulant
DOH	Department of Health
DOR	duration of response
DPD	dihydropyrimidine dehydrogenase or 4-deoxypyridoxine
DRC	dexamethasone, rituximab, cyclophosphamide
DRE	digital rectal examination
DSM	Diagnostic and Statistical Manual of Mental Disorder
DSNB	dynamic sentinel node biopsy
DVH	dose–volume histogram
DVT	deep vein thrombosis
DXA	dual X-ray absorptiometry
DXT	deep X-ray
EASL	European Association for Studies of the Liver
EAC	external auditory canal
EBMT	European Group for Blood and Marrow Transplantation

EBRT	external beam radiotherapy
EBUS	endobronchial ultrasound
EBV	Epstein–Barr virus
EC	epirubicin and cyclophosphamide
ECE	extracapsular extension
ECF	epirubicin, cisplatin, and continuous 5-FU
ECOG	Eastern Cooperative Oncology Group
ECPP	extracorporal photophoresis
ECX	epirubicin, cisplatin, capecitabine
ED	extensive disease
EFRT	extended-field radiotherapy
EFS	event-free survival
EFT	Ewing's sarcoma family of tumours
EGC	early gastric cancer
EGCG	epigallocatechin gallate
EGFR	epidermal growth factor receptor
EGGCT	extragonadal germ cell tumours
EHCCA	extrahepatic cholangiocarcinoma
EIAED	enzyme-inducing antiepileptic drug
EIC	endometrial intraepithelial carcinoma
EMA/CO	etoposide, methotrexate, dactinomcin/ cyclophosphamide, vincristine
EMR	endoscopic mucosal resection
EMT	epithelial to mesenchymal transformation
ENT	ear, nose, and throat
EORTC	European Organisation for Research and Treatment of Cancer
EOS	epithelial ovarian cancer
EPO	erythropoietin
EPP	extrapleural pneumonectomy
ER	oestrogen receptor
ERAS	enhanced recovery after surgery
ERC	endoscopic retrograde cholangiography
ERCP	endoscopic retrograde cholangiopancreatography
ERM	embryonal rhabdomyosarcoma
ERSPC	European Randomised Study of Screening for Prostate Cancer
ESA	erythropoiesis stimulating agent
ESD	endoscopic submucosal dissection
ESMO	European Society for Medical Oncology
ESN	endometrial stromal nodule
ESR	erythrocyte sedimentation rate
ESRF	end-stage renal failure
ESS	endometrial stromal sarcoma
ES-SCLC	extensive-stage smallcell lung cancer

EST	Eastern Cooperative Oncology Group	GBM	glioblastoma multiforme
ET	endocrine treatment	GCB	germinal centre B-cell
ETT	epithelioid trophoblastic tumour	G-CSF	granulocyte colony stimulating factor
EUA	examination under anaesthesia	GCT	granulosa cell tumour
EUROPAC	European Registry of Hereditary Pancreatitis and Familial Pancreatic Cancer	GD	gemcitabine and docetaxel
		GDP-NET	gastro-duodeno-pancreatic tumour
		GFR	glomerular filtration rate
EUS	endoscopic ultrasound	GHSG	German Hodgkin Study Group
EUSOMA	European Society of Breast Cancer Specialists	GI	gastrointestinal
		GIST	gastrointestinal stromal tumour
EUTOS	European Treatment and Outcome Study	GM-CSF	granulocyte-macrophage colony stimulating factor
Fab	fragment antigen binding	GnRH	gonadotrophin releasing hormone
FAB	French–American–British	GOG	Gynecologic Oncology Group
FAP	familial adenomatosis polyposis	GOJ	gastro-oesophageal junction
FBC	full blood count	GORD	gastro-oesophageal reflux disease
Fc	crystallizable fragment	GP	general practitioner
FCR	fludarabine, cyclophosphamide, rituximab	GTD	gestational trophoblastic disease
		GTM	gestational trophoblastic neoplasia
FDA	Food and Drug Administration	GTN	gestational trophoblastic neoplasia
FDC	follicular dendritic cells	GTT	gestational trophoblastic tumour
FDG	fluorodeoxyglucose (18F)	GTV	gross target volume or gross tumour volume
FDR	first-degree relatives		
FEV1	forced expiratory volume in 1 second	GVHD	graft-versus-host disease
FFP	fresh frozen plasma or freedom from progression	GWAS	genome wide association studies
		HAART	highly active antiretroviral therapy
FFTF	freedom from treatment failure	HADS	Hospital Anxiety and Depression Scale
FGFR	fibroblast growth factor receptor		
FH	fumarate hydratase	HAL	hexaminolaevulinate
FIGO	International Federation of Gynecology and Obstetrics	HAMA	human anti-murine antibody
		HBIG	hepatis B immune globulin
FISH	fluorescence in situ hybridization	HBOS	hereditary breast/ovarian cancer syndromes
FIT	faecal immunochemical test		
FLAIR	fluid-attenuated inversion recovery	HBV	hepatitis B virus
FLC	free light chain	HCC	hepatocellular cancer
FLCN	folliculin	HCD	heavy-chain disease
FLIPI	Follicular Lymphoma International Prognostic Index	hCG	human chorionic gonadotropin
		HCS	hereditary cancer syndrome
FMTC	familial medullary thyroid cancer	HCV	hepatitis C virus
FN	febrile neutropenia	HDAC	histone deacetylase
FNA	fine needle aspiration	HDCT	high-dose chemotherapy
FNAC	fine needle aspiration cytology	HDR	high-dose rate
FOB	faecal occult blood	HE	hematoxylin-eosin
FOBT	faecal occult blood test	HEPA	high-efficiency particulate air
FOLFIRINOX	fluorouracil, leucovorin, irinotecan, oxaliplatin	HER	human epidermal growth factor receptor
FPC	familial pancreatic cancer	HGD	high grade dysplasia
FRAX	fracture risk assessment tool (WHO)	HGESS	high-grade endometrial stromal sarcoma
FSH	follicle stimulating hormone		
g	gram(s)	HHV	human herpesvirus

HIF	hypoxia-inducible factor		IESS	Intergroup Ewing's Sarcoma Study
HIFU	high intensity frequency ultrasound		IFE	immunofixation electrophoresis
HIT	heparin-induced thrombocytopenia		IFN	interferon
HIV	human immunodeficiency virus		IFOS	ifosfamide
HL	Hodgkin lymphoma		IFRT	involved-field radiotherapy
HLRCC	hereditary leiomyomatosis and renal cell cancer		Ig	immunoglobulin
HNPCC	hereditary non-polyposis colorectal cancer		IGCCCG	International Germ Cell Consensus Classification Group
HNSCC	head and neck squamous cell carcinoma		IGFBPs	insulin-like growth factor binding proteins
HPF	high power field		IgH	immunoglobulin heavy chain
HPRCC	hereditary papillary renal cell carcinoma		IGHV	immunoglobulin heavy-chain variable
HPT-JT	hyperparathyroidism-jaw tumour		IGRT	image-guided radiotherapy
HPV	human papilloma virus		IHC	immunohistochemistry
HR	hazard ratio		IHCCA	intrahepatic cholangiocarcinoma
HR-CTV	high-risk clinical target volume		IJV	internal jugular vein
HRD	homologous recombination deficiency		IL	interleukin
			ILI	isolated limb infusion
HRPC	hormone resistance prostate cancer		ILP	isolated limb perfusion
HRQoL	health-related quality of life		IM	intramuscular
H-RS	Hodgkin and Reed–Sternberg		IMIDs	immunomodulatory drugs
HRT	hormone replacement therapy		IMRT	intensity-modulated radiotherapy
HSCT	haematopoietic stem cell transplantation		IMWG	International Myeloma Working Group
HSIL	high-grade squamous intraepithelial lesion		INR	international normalized ratio
			INRG	International Neuroblastoma Risk Grouping
HSV	herpes simplex virus		INT	intergroup
HTS	high throughput sequencing		IORT	intraoperative radiation therapy
HVA	homovanillic acid		IP	intraperitoneal
IARC	International Agency for Research on Cancer		IPC	indwelling pleural catheter
			IPI	International Prognostic Index
IASLC	International Association for the Study of Lung Cancer		IPMN	intraductal papillary mucinous neoplasm
IBC	inflammatory breast cancer		IPS	International Prognostic Score
IBD	inflammatory bowel disease		IPSID	immunoproliferative small intestine disease
iCCA	intrahepatic			
ICH-GCP	International Conference on Harmonization's Good Clinical Practice		IPSS	International Prognostic Scoring System
			iRAEs	immune-related adverse events
ICP	intracranial pressure		IRB	institutional review board
ICRU	International Commission on Radiation Units and Measurements		IR-CTV	intermediate-risk clinical target volume
			IRIS	immune reconstitution inflammatory syndrome
IDC	interstitial dendritic cells		iRRc	immune related response criteria
IDEA	International Duration Evaluation of Adjuvant Chemotherapy		ISRCTN	international standard randomized controlled trial number
IDRF	image-defined risk factor		IST	immunosuppressive treatment
IDS	interval debulking surgery		ISUP	International Society of Urological Pathology
IE	ifosfamide and etoposide			
IELSG	International Extranodal Lymphoma Study Group		IT	irinotecan and temozolomide
			ITC	isothiocyanate

ITL	intratumoural
ITV	internal tumour volume
IV	intravenous
IVC	inferior vena cava
IVF	in vitro fertilization
IVIG	intravenous immunoglobulin
IVP	intravenous pyelography
J	joule(s)
kg	kilogram(s)
KPS	Karnofsky performance status
KS	Karnofsky score or Kaposi's sarcoma
KSHV	Kaposi's sarcoma herpes virus
L	litre(s)
LA	laparoscopic adrenalectomy
LABC	locally advanced breast cancer
LAVH/BSO	laparoscopically assisted vaginal hysterectomy and bilateral salpingo-oophorectomy
LC	local control or Langerhan's cell
LCC	large cell carcinoma
LCDT	low-dose chest computed tomography
LCH	Langerhan's cell histiocytosis
LCIS	lobular carcinoma in situ
LCNEC	large cell neuroendocrine carcinoma
LCP	Liverpool Care Pathway for the Dying Patient
LD	limited disease
LDCT	low-dose chest computed tomography
LDH	lactate dehydrogenase
LDLT	live donor liver transplantation
LDR	low-dose rate
LEEP	loop electrosurgical excision procedure
LFS	Li–Fraumeni syndrome
LFT	liver function test
LGESS	low-grade endometrial stromal sarcoma
LH	luteinizing hormone
LHRH	luteinizing hormone-releasing hormone
LITT	laser induced thermotherapy
LMS	leiomyosarcoma
LMWH	low-molecular-weight heparin
LOH	loss of heterogeneity
LP	lymphocyte predominant
LPD	lymphoproliferative disorder
LR-CTV	low-risk clinical target volume
LS	Lynch syndrome

LSIL	low-grade squamous intraepithelial lesion
LS-SCLC	limited-stage small cell lung cancer
LUMPO	Liverpool Uveal Melanoma Prognosticator Online
LVI	lymphatic and vascular invasion
LVSI	lymphovascular space invasion
MA	monoclonal antibody
MAB	monoclonal antibody or maximal androgen blockade
MACIS	metastases, age, completeness of resection, invasion, size
MAD	maximal administered dose
MALT	mucosa-associated lymphoid tissue
MAP	MUTYH associated polyposis
MAPK	mitogen-activated protein kinase
MARS	mesothelioma and radical surgery
MASCC	Multinational Association for Supportive Care in Cancer
MBC	male breast cancer or meta-static breast cancer
MBL	monoclonal B-cell lymphocytosis
MBO	malignant bowel obstruction
MC	mixed-cellularity
MCC	Merkel cell carcinoma
mcg	microgram(s)
MCL	Mantle cell lymphomas
MCN	mucinous cystic neoplasms
MC1R	melanocortin 1 receptor
MDAS	Memorial Delirium Assessment Scale
MDR	multidrug resistance
MDS	myelodysplastic syndrome
MDT	multidisciplinary team
MDU	Medical Defence Union
MEA	methotrexate, etoposide, dactinomycin
MEDD	morphine equivalent daily dose
MEN	multiple endocrine neoplasia
MF	mycosis fungoides
MFH	malignant fibrous histiocytoma
MG	myasthenia gravis
MGCT	malignant germ cell tumour
MGMT	methyl guanine methyl transferase
MGUS	monoclonal gammopathy of undetermined significance
MHC	major histocompatibility complex
MHRA	Medical Health Regulatory Agency
MIA	minimally invasive adenocarcinoma
MIBG	metaiodobenzylguanidine
MILND	minimally invasive inguinal lymph node dissection

MIPI	Mantle Cell International Prognostic Index		NHL	non-Hodgkin lymphoma
MIS	Müllerian-inhibiting substance		NICE	National Institute for Health and Clinical Excellence
ml	millilitre(s)		NIFTP	non-invasive follicular thyroid neoplasm with papillary-like nuclear features
MLDS	myeloid leukaemia of Down's syndrome			
MLL	mixed lineage leukemia		NK	natural killer
mm	millimetre(s)		nLPHL	nodular lymphocyte predominant HL
MMC	mitomycin-C		NLST	National Lung Screening Trial
MMR	measles, mumps, rubella *or* mismatch repair		NMDA	N-methyl-D-aspartate
			NND	number needed to diagnose
MMS	Mohs micrographic surgery *or* multimodal screening		NNT	number needed to treat
			NOAEL	no adverse effect level
MOGT	malignant ovarian germ cell tumour		NOS	not otherwise specified
MPE	malignant pleural effusion		NPC	nasopharyngeal carcinoma
MPM	malignant pleural mesothelioma		NS	nodular-sclerosing *or* nerve sparing
MPNST	malignant peripheral nerve sheath tumour		NSAID	non-steroidal anti-inflammatory drug
			NSCLC	non-small cell lung cancer
MRC	Medical Research Council		NSCLC-ND	non-small cell lung carcinoma with neuroendocrine differentiation
MRCP	magnetic resonance cholangiopancreatography			
			NSS	nephron-sparing surgery
MRD	minimal residual disease		NST	no special type
MRI	magnetic resonance imaging		NTCP	normal tissue complication probability
MRS	magnetic resonance spectroscopy			
MSI	microsatellite instability		NUA	non-urachal adenocarcinoma
MRSA	methicillin resistant *Staphylococcus aureus*		NuDESC	Nursing Delirium Screening Scale
			OAR	organs at risk
MS	mass spectrometry		OBD	optimal biological dose
MSI	microsatellite instability		od	once daily
MSS	microsatellite stable		OFS	ovarian function suppression
MSCC	malignant spinal cord compression		OGCT	ovarian germ cell tumour
MSKCC	Memorial Sloan–Kettering Cancer Center		OGD	oesophago-gastro-duodenoscopy
			OLT	orthotopic liver transplantation
MT	malignant teratoma		ONJ	osteonecrosis of jaw
MTC	medullary thyroid cancer		ONS	Office for National Statistics
MTP	mimic muramyl tripeptide		OPG	optic pathway glioma *or* osteoprotegerin
MUD	matched unrelated donor			
nocte	at night		OPSI	overwhelming postsplenectomy infection
NAFLD	non-alcoholic fatty liver disease			
NASH	non-alcoholic steatohepatitis		OR	odds ratio
NaSSA	noradrenaline and specific serotonin antagonist		ORR	objective response rates
			OS	overall survival
NBA	narrow band imaging		OSCCHT	hypercalcaemic
NCCN	National Comprehensive Cancer Network		OTR	organ transplant recipient
			OTT	overall treatment time
NCI	National Cancer Institute		PanIN	pancreatic intraepithelial neoplasia
NCIC CTG	National Cancer Institute of Canada Clinical Trials Group		PAP	prostatic acid phosphatase
			PARP	poly (ADP-ribose) polymerase
NCRI	National Cancer Research Institute		PC	post-chemotherapy
NSCLC	non-small cell lung cancer		pCCA	perihilar
NET	neuroendocrine tumour		PCI	prophylactic cranial irradiation
NF	neurofibromatosis			

pCLE	probe-based confocal laser endomicroscopy		PSA	prostate-specific antigen
PCNSL	primary malignant central nervous system lymphoma		PSC	primary sclerosing cholangitis
			PSCC	pulmonary squamous cell carcinoma
PCPT	Prostate Cancer Prevention Trial		PSTT	placental site trophoblastic tumour
pCR	pathological complete response		PSV	pre-study visits
PCR	polymerase chain reaction		PT	prothrombin time
PCV	procarbazine, CCNU, and vincristine		PTC	percutaneous transhepatic cholangiography or papillary thyroid cancer
PD	pharmacodynamic or progressive disease or programmed death			
			PTCH	patched homologue
PD-1	programmed death receptor 1		PTD	persistent trophoblastic disease
PDAC	pancreatic ductal adenocarcinoma		PTE	pulmonary thromboembolism
PDGF	platelet-derived growth factor		PTHC	percutaneous transhepatic cholangiography
PDGFR	platelet-derived growth factor receptor			
			PTHrP	parathyroid hormone-related peptide
PDL	programmed death ligand		PTL	primary thyroid lymphomas
PDT	photodynamic therapy		PTLD	post-transplant lymphoproliferative disorder
PE	pulmonary embolism			
PEG	percutaneous endoscopic gastrostomy		PTSD	post-traumatic stress disorder
			PTV	planning target volume
PEP	plasma cell dyscrasia, endocrinopathy, polyneuropathy		PUVA	psolarens + UVA
			PVE	portal vein embolization
PET	positron emission tomography		qds	four times daily
PI3K	phosphatidylinositol 3-kinase		QoL	quality of life
PFS	progression-free survival		QUASAR	quick and simple and reliable
PFT	pulmonary function test		RANKL	receptor activator of nuclear factor kappa B ligand
PG	pepsinogen			
PgR	progesterone receptor		Rb	retinoblastoma
PHM	partial hydatidiform mole		RCC	renal cell carcinoma
PICC	peripherally inserted central catheter		RCT	randomized controlled trial
PK	pharmacokinetic		RE	rectal endosonography
PKC	protein kinase C		REAL	revised European and American lymphoma
PLAP	placental alkaline phosphatase			
PLCO	prostate, lung, colorectal, and ovarian		REC	research ethics committee
PLD	pegylated liposomal doxorubicin		RECIST	Response Evaluation Criteria In Solid Tumors
PLWBC	people living with and beyond cancer			
PMR	partial metabolic response		RF	radiofrequency
pNET	pancreatic neuroendocrine tumour		RFA	radiofrequency ablation
PNET	primitive neuroectodermal tumour		RIC	reduced-intensity conditioning
PNH	paroxysmal nocturnal haemoglobinuria		RISS	Revised International Staging System
			RIT	radioimmunotherapy
p.o.	by mouth (per os)		RNA	ribonucleic acid
POEMS	polyneuropathy, organomegaly, endocrinopathy, monoclonal protein, skin changes		RP	radical prostatectomy
			RPLND	retroperitoneal lymph node dissection
PPAP	polymerase proofreading-associated polyposis			
			RPTD	recommended phase 2 dose
PR	partial remission		RR	relative risk
PRN	as required		RRA	radioiodine remnant ablation
PRRT	peptide receptor radionuclide therapy		RSCM	responsible supply chain management
PS	performance status		RT	radiotherapy

RTK	receptor tyrosine kinases
RTOG	Radiation Therapy Oncology Group
RT-PCR	reverse transcriptase polymerase chain reaction
SABR	stereotactic ablative body radiotherapy
SACT	systemic anticancer therapy
SAHA	suberoylanilide hydroxamic acid
SaO$_2$	arterial oxygen saturation
SAR	specific absorption rate
SBA	small bowel adenocarcinoma
SBRT	stereotactic body radiation therapy
SC	subcutaneous
SCC	squamous cell carcinoma
SCF	stem cell factor
SCLC	small cell lung cancer
SCM	sternocleidomastoid
SCN	serous cystic neoplasms
SCPRT	short-course preoperative radiotherapy
SCST	sex cord-stromal tumour
SCT	stem cell transplant
SCTAT	sex cord tumour with annular tubules
SD	stable disease
SDH	succinate dehydrogenase
SDHAF2	succinate dehydrogenase complex assembly factor 2
SDHD	succinate dehydrogenase subunit D
SEER	surveillance, epidemiology, and end results
SEM	self-expanding metallic stent
SERM	selective oestrogen receptor modulator
SFT	solitary fibrous tumour
SIADH	syndrome of inappropriate antidiuretic hormone
SIOG	International Society of Geriatric Oncology
SIR	standardized incidence ratio
SIRT	selective internal radiation therapy
SLCT	Sertoli–Leydig cell tumour
SLL	small lymphocytic lymphoma
SLNB	sentinel lymph node biopsy
SMI	small molecular inhibitor
SMM	smouldering multiple myeloma
SMO	smoothened homologue
SMR	standardized mortality ratio
SNB	sentinel node biopsy
SNHL	sensory neural hearing loss
SNRI	serotonin-noradrenergic reuptake inhibitor

SNUC	sinonasal undifferentiated carcinoma
SOHND	supraomohyoid neck dissection
SO	sarcomatous overgrowth
SPEP	serum protein electrophoresis
sPNETs	supratentorial neuro-ectodermal tumours
SqCC	squamous cell carcinoma
SRE	skeletal-related events
SRS	stereotactic radiosurgery
SRT	stereotactic radiotheapy
SS	Sézary syndrome
SSA	somatostatin analogue
SSI	selective serotonin antagonist
SSRI	selective serotonin reuptake inhibitor
STI	sexually transmitted infection *or* signal transduction inhibitor
STLI	subtotal lymphoid irradiation
STIR	short inversion time inversion recovery
SUV	standardized uptake value
SVC	superior vena cava
SWOG	Southwest Oncology Group
TACE	transarterial chemoembolization
TAE	transarterial embolization
TAH	total abdominal hysterectomy
TAM	transient abnormal myelopoiesis
TAUS	transabdominal ultrasound
TBNA	transbronchial needle aspiration
TC	testicular cancer *or* typical carcinoid *or* topotecan and cyclophosphamide
TCA	tricarboxylic acid cycle
TCC	transitional cell carcinoma
TCGA	The Cancer Genome Atlas project
TCH	docetaxel, carboplatin, trastuzumab
TCP	tumour control probability
tds	three times daily
TDT	terminal deoxynucleotidyl transferase
TEMS	transanal endoscopic microsurgery
TENS	transcutaneous electrical nerve stimulation
TG	thyroglobulin
TGCT	tenosynovial giant cell tumour
TGFB1	transforming growth factor beta 1
TIL	tumour infiltrating lymphocyte
TIN	testicular intraepithelial neoplasia
TIP	paclitaxel, ifosfamide, cisplatin
TK	tyrosine kinase
TKI	tyrosine kinase inhibitors *or* thymidine kinase inhibitor
TLH/BSO	total laparoscopic hysterectomy and bilateral salpingo-oophorectomy

TLS	tumour lysis syndrome		USG	ultrasonography
TME	total mesorectal excision		USO	unilateral salpingo-oophorectomy
TNBC	triple negative breast cancer		USPSTF	United States Preventive Services Task Force
TNF	tumour necrosis factor		USS	ultrasound scan
TNFA	tumour necrosis factor A		UTI	urinary tract infection
TNMB	tumour node, metastasis, blood		UUS	undifferentiated uterine sarcoma
TNM	tumour node metastasis		UV	ultraviolet
TOE	transoesphageal echocardiogram		VAC	vincristine, adriamycin, cyclophosphamide
TORS	trans-oral robotic surgery		VAD	vascular access device
TRAM	transverse rectus abdominis myocutaneous		VAI	vincristine, dactinomycin, ifosfamide
TRM	transplant-related mortality *or* treatment-related mortality		VAIN	vaginal intraepithelial neoplasia
			VALG	Veterans Affairs Lung Study Group
TROG	Trans Tasman Radiation Oncology Group		VATS	video-assisted thoracoscopic surgery
TRUS	transrectal ultrasound		VDC	vincristine, doxorubicin, cyclophosphamide
TSEBT	total skin electron beam therapy			
TSH	thyroid stimulating hormone		VEGF	vascular endothelial growth factor
TTF	time to failure		VeIP	vinblastine, ifosfamide, cisplatin
TTP	time-to-progression		VGPR	very good partial response
TURB	transurethral resection of the bladder		VHL	von Hippel–Lindau
TURBT	transurethral resection of the bladder tumour		VI	vascular invasion
			VIDE	vincristine, ifosfamide, doxorubicin, etoposide
TURP	transurethral resection of the prostate		VIP	vasointestinal peptide *or* etoposide, ifosfamide, cisplatin *or* vasoactive intestinal protein
TWA	thyroxine hormone withdrawal			
TYA	teenager and young adult			
UA	urachal adenocarcinoma		VIN	vulval intraepithelial neoplasia
UC	ulcerative colitis		VMA	vanillylmandelic acid
UES	undifferentiated endometrial sarcoma		VRE	vancomycin-resistant enterococci
UFH	unfractionated heparin		VTE	venous thromboembolism
UICC	International Union against Cancer		VUS	variant of unknown/uncertain significance
UISS	UCLA integrated staging system			
UK	United Kingdom		WAI	whole abdominal irradiation
UKCCCR	UK Coordinating Committee on Cancer Research		WBC	white blood cell
			WBI	whole breast RT
UKCTOCS	UK Collaborative Trial of Ovarian Cancer Screening		WBRT	whole brain radiotherapy
			WCC	white cell count
uPA	urokinase plasminogen activator		WE	wide excision
UPEP	urine protein electrophoresis		WHO	World Health Organization
US	ultrasound		WLE	wide local excision
USA	United States of America			

Contributors

Thankamma Ajithkumar Consultant Clinical Oncologist, Cambridge University Hospitals NHS Foundation Trust, Cambridge, UK
Chapters 1, 2, 4, 10, 14, 16, 18

Anna Bowzyk Al-Naeeb Consultant Clinical Oncologist, Cambridge University Hospital and Bedford Hospital, Cambridge and Bedford, UK
Chapter 13

Christine Ang Queen Elizabeth Hospital, Gateshead Health NHS Foundation Trust, Gateshead, UK
Chapter 9

Gill Barnett Consultant in Clinical Oncology, Cambridge University Hospitals NHS Foundation Trust, Cambridge, UK
Chapter 13

Ann Barrett Emeritus Professor of Oncology, University of East Anglia, Norfolk, UK
Chapters 2, 16

Faisal Basheer Consultant Haematologist, Cambridge University Hospitals NHS Foundation Trust, Cambridge, UK
Chapter 12

Bristi Basu Academic Consultant in Medical Oncology, University of Cambridge, Cambridge, UK
Chapter 2

Charlotte Benson Consultant Medical Oncologist, Royal Marsden Hospital, London, UK
Chapter 11

Mark Beresford Consultant Oncologist and Clinical Lead for Oncology and Haematology, Royal United Hospital Bath, Visiting Chair, University of Bath, Bath, UK
Chapter 8

Tony Branson Consultant Clinical Oncologist, Freeman Hospital, Tyne, UK
Chapter 9

Hannah Buckley Clinical Research Training Fellow, Cancer Research UK Cambridge Institute, Cambridge, UK
Chapters 10, 16

Fatima Cardoso Director/Breast Oncologist, Champalimaud Clinical Centre/Champalimaud Foundation, Lisbon, Portugal
Chapter 6

Ellen Copson Associate Professor in Medical Oncology, University of Southampton, Southampton, UK
Chapter 2

Pippa Corrie Consultant and Associate Lecturer in Medical Oncology, Cambridge University Hospitals NHS Foundation Trust, Cambridge, UK
Chapter 10

Brian Davidson Professor of Surgery, RFHL/UCL, London, UK
Chapter 7

Rhian Davies Consultant Clinical Oncologist, South West Wales Cancer Centre, Swansea, UK
Chapter 5

Claire Dearden Consultant Haematologist, The Royal Marsden NHS Foundation Trust, London, UK
Chapter 12

Helen Dearden Specialist Registrar, Medical Oncology, Leeds Teaching Hospitals Trust, Leeds, UK
Chapter 7

Bryony Eccles Consultant Medical Oncologist, Royal Bournemouth Hospital, Dorset, UK
Chapter 2

Emma Edwards Senior Genetic Counsellor, Westmead Hospital, Westmead, Australia
Chapter 2

Dennis Eichenauer Physician, First Department of Internal Medicine, University Hospital Cologne, Cologne, Germany
Chapter 12

Tim Eisen Professor of Medical Oncology, University of Cambridge, Cambridge, UK Vice President and Global GU Oncology Franchise Head, Roche, UK
Chapter 8

Andreas Engert Professor of Internal Medicine, Hematology, and Oncology Faculty of Medicine and University Hospital of Cologne, University of Cologne, Cologne, Germany
Chapter 12

Edzard Ernst Emeritus Professor, University of Exeter, Cambridge, UK
Chapter 16

Marie Fallon St Columba's Hospice Chair of Palliative Medicine, University of Edinburgh, Edinburgh, UK
Chapter 17

George Follows Consultant Haematologist, Cambridge University Hospitals NHS Foundation Trust, Cambridge, UK
Chapter 12

Ian Geh Consultant Clinical Oncologist, Queen Elizabeth and Heartlands Hospitals, Birmingham, UK
Chapter 7

Paula Ghaneh Professor of Surgery, University of Liverpool, Liverpool, UK
Chapter 7

David Gilligan Consultant Oncologist, Cambridge University Hospitals and Royal Papworth Hospitals, Cambridge, UK
Chapter 15

Raffaele Giusti Consultant Oncologist
Azienda Ospedaliero Universitaria Sant'Andrea—
Sapienza Facoltà di Medicina e Psicologia, Rome, Italy
Chapter 17

Ronald S. Go Chair, Core/Consultative Hematology,
Mayo Clinic, Rochester, USA
Chapter 12

Ioannis Gounaris Medical Director, Merck Serono
Ltd, Feltham, UK
Chapter 15

Debbie Gregory Consultant Clinical Oncologist,
Cambridge University Hospitals NHS Foundation
Trust, Cambridge, UK
Chapter 9

Ewen A. Griffiths Consultant Upper GI Surgeon,
Birmingham University Hospitals NHS Foundation
Trust, Birmingham, UK
Chapter 7

Barry Hancock Emeritus Professor, University of
Sheffield, Sheffield, UK
Chapter 9

Fiona Harris Consultant Clinical Oncologist,
Addenbrookes Hospital, Cambridge, UK
Chapter 4

Helen Hatcher Consultant in TYA and Medical
Oncology, Addenbrooke's Hospital, Cambridge, UK
Chapters 2, 9, 11, 16

Katie Herbert Specialist Registrar, Medical Oncology,
Oxford, University Hospitals NHS Foundation Trust,
Oxford, UK
Chapter 9

M. Hingorani Consultant Clinical Oncologist,
Castle Hill Hospital, Hull, UK
Chapter 7

Gail Horan Consultant Clinical Oncologist,
Addenbrooke's Hospital, Cambridge, and
Queen Elizabeth Hospital, Norfolk, UK
Chapter 8

Nicola Hughes Specialist Registrar, Medical Oncology,
Leeds Teaching Hospitals Trust, Leeds, UK
Chapter 7

Sarah Jefferies Consultant Clinical Oncologist,
Cambridge University Hospitals NHS Foundation
Trust, Cambridge, UK
Chapters 2, 4

Rob Glynne Jones Consultant Clinical Oncologist,
Mount Vernon Centre for Cancer Treatment,
London, UK
Chapter 7

Gaurav Kapur Consultant Clinical Oncologist,
Norfolk and Norwich University Hospitals,
Norfolk, UK
Chapter 13

Yakhub Khan Consultant, University Hospitals
Coventry and Warwickshire NHS Trust, Coventry, UK
Chapter 7

Jorg Kleeff Head of Department and Chair of Visceral
Surgery, Martin Luther University Halle-Wittenberg,
Halle, Germany
Chapter 7

Jason Lester Senior Consultant Clinical Oncologist,
South West Wales Cancer Centre, Swansea, UK
Chapter 5

Suzy Mawdsley Doctor, Mount Vernon Cancer
Centre, Middlesex, UK
Chapter 7

Priyanka Mehta Consultant Haematologist, Spire
Bristol Hospital, Bristol, UK
Chapter 12

Boo Messahel Former Consultant in Paediatic
Oncology, Cambridge University Hospital,
Cambridge, UK
Chapter 14

Raj Naik Consultant Clinical Oncologist and Clinical
Director, Northern Gynaecological Oncology Centre,
Queen Elizabeth Hospital, Gateshead, UK
Chapter 9

John Neoptolemos Professor of Surgery, University
of Heidelberg, Heidelberg, Germany
Chapter 7

Gary Nicolin Paediatric Oncologist, University
Hospital Southampton, Southampton, UK
Chapter 14

Shibani Nicum Consultant Medical Oncologist,
Oxford Cancer Centre, Oxford, UK
Chapter 9

Jonathan Noujaim Consultant Medical Oncologist,
Institut d'hématologie-oncologie, Hôpital
Maisonneuve-Rosemont, Montreal, Canada
Chapter 11

Jan Oldenburg Clinical Oncologist, University of
Oslo, Oslo, Norway
Chapter 8

Dan Palmer Chair of Medical Oncology and
Consultant Medical Oncologist, University of
Liverpool, Liverpool, and The Clatterbridge Cancer
Centre, Birkenhead, UK
Chapter 7

Christine Parkinson Clinical Consultant, Cambridge
University Hospitals NHS Foundation Trust,
Cambridge, UK
Chapter 9

Nicholas Pavlidis Emeritus Professor, University of
Ioannina, Ioannina, Greece
Chapter 16

Barry L. Pizer Consultant Paediatric Oncologist, Alder Hey Children's NHS Foundation Trust, Liverpool, UK
Chapter 14

Sarah Prewett Consultant Clinical Oncologist, Cambridge University Hospitals NHS Foundation Trust, Cambridge, UK
Chapter 9

Roy Rabbie Clinical Research Associate, Cambridge University Hospitals NHS Foundation Trust, Cambridge, UK
Chapter 2

Sophie Raby Clinical Oncology Registrar, The Christie Foundation NHS Trust, Manchester, UK
Chapter 2

Kavita Raj Consultant Haematologist, Guys and St Thomas' and UCLH, London, UK
Chapter 12

Vincent Rajkumar Consultant, Division of Hematology, Department of Internal Medicine, Mayo Clinic, Rochester, USA
Chapter 12

Elie Rassy Oncologist, Department of Medical Oncology, Institut Gustave Roussy, Villejuif, France; Faculty of Medicine, Department of Oncology, Saint Joseph University, Beirut, Lebanon
Chapter 16

Joana M. Ribeiro Breast Oncologist, Champalimaud Clinical Centre/Champalimaud Foundation, Lisbon, Portugal
Chapter 6

Crispin Schneider Specialty Trainee, Royal Free Hospital, London, UK
Chapter 7

David Sebag-Montefiore Professor, University of Leeds, Leeds, UK
Chapter 7

Priyamal Silva Consultant Otolaryngologist, John Radcliffe and Churchill Hospitals, Oxford, UK
Chapter 3

Berta Sousa Breast Oncologist, Champalimaud Clinical Center/Champalimaud Foundation, Lisbon, Portugal
Chapter 6

Amit Sud Academic Clinical Lecturer, The Royal Marsden NHS Foundation Trust, London, UK
Chapter 12

Daniel Swinson Consultant in Medical Oncology, Leeds Cancer Centre, St James's University Hospital, Leeds Teaching Hospitals NHS Trust, Leeds, UK
Chapter 7

Robert Thomas Consultant Oncologist, Addenbrooke's Hospital, Cambridge, UK
Chapter 16

Xavier Thomas Doctor, Department of Hematology, Lyon-Sud Hospital, Pierre-Bénite, France
Chapter 12

Lorenz Trümper Chairman, University Medicine, Göttingen, Germany
Chapter 12

Simona Volovat Medical Oncologist, Champalimaud Clinical Center/Champalimaud Foundation, Lisbon, Portugal
Chapter 6

Matthew C. Winter Consultant in Medical Oncology, Trophoblastic Disease Centre, Weston Park Hospital, Sheffield, UK
Chapter 9

Chapter 1

Clinical approach to suspected cancer

Chapter contents

1.1 Overview

Introduction

The National Institute of Health and Care Excellence (NICE) has recently updated the previous 2005 guidance on referral for suspected cancer (NICE 2015). This guideline provides evidence-based indications for urgent referral from primary to secondary care for further investigations within two weeks of a suspected cancer. It also highlights a number of clinical situations where very urgent (within 48 hours) or immediate referrals (within a few hours) are needed. Indications for the cancer pathway and urgent referrals for various cancers are covered in this chapter.

1.2 Lung cancer

Indications for suspected cancer pathway referral
- Chest X-ray suggestive of lung cancer
- Unexplained haemoptysis in people ≥40 years old

Indications for urgent referral

An urgent referral for a chest X-ray (CXR) within two weeks if there is at least one of the following symptoms in a smoker or two symptoms in people aged 40 years or over:
- Cough
- Breathlessness
- Chest pain
- Fatigue
- Anorexia
- Weight loss
  Urgent CXR is also indicated if there is at least one of the following symptoms in people aged 40 years or over:
- Persistent or recurrent chest infection
- Chest signs consistent with lung cancer
- Supraclavicular lymphadenopathy
- Persistent cervical lymphadenopathy
- Finger clubbing
- Thrombocytosis

1.3 Mesothelioma

Indications for urgent referral

An urgent referral for a chest X-ray within two weeks if there is at least one of the following symptoms in a smoker and/or person who has been exposed to asbestos, or two symptoms in people aged 40 years or over:
- Cough
- Breathlessness
- Chest pain
- Fatigue
- Anorexia
- Weight loss
  An urgent CXR should be considered in people aged 40 years and over with either one of the following:
- Finger clubbing
- Chest signs compatible with pleural disease

1.4 Breast cancer

Indications for urgent referral
- People aged 30 years or over with an unexplained breast lump with or without pain
- People aged 50 years or over with symptoms of discharge, retraction, or any other changes of concern in only one nipple
- People aged 30 years or over with an unexplained axillary lump
- Skin changes suggestive of breast cancer

Indications for non-urgent referral
- Non-urgent referral for women aged <30 years presenting with unexplained breast lump with or without pain
- Indications for emergency referral
- Patients presenting with features of impending or actual spinal cord compression
- Patients presenting with features of brain metastasis

1.5 Urological cancer

Warning features
Warning features of urological cancers include:
- Lower urinary tract symptoms
- Haematuria
- Suspicious lumps
- Bone pain

Indication for emergency referral
- All patients presenting with features of impending or actual spinal cord compression, a presentation common in disseminated prostate cancer, need emergency evaluation (within 24 hours)

Indications for urgent referral
Renal and urinary bladder cancer
Patients presenting with the following features need urgent referral to rule out renal or bladder cancers:
- People aged 45 years or over with either unexplained macroscopic haematuria without urinary tract infection (UTI) or persistent or recurrent macroscopic haematuria after successful treatment of UTI
- People aged 60 years or over with unexplained microscopic haematuria with either dysuria or raised white blood cell (WBC) count
- Clinical or radiological evidence of an abdominal mass suggesting renal or bladder cancer

Prostate cancer
A prostate-specific antigen (PSA) estimation and digital rectal examination (DRE) is indicated when:
- Men present with urinary tract symptoms (such as nocturia, urinary frequency, hesitance, urgency, or retention), erectile dysfunction, or macroscopic haematuria.
- Progressive rise in PSA or raised PSA level above the age-specific reference range
- Symptomatic patients with high PSA (>50)
- Men with hard and irregular prostate on rectal examination

Testicular cancer
Ultrasound of the testis is indicated in men presenting with:
- Non-painful swelling, change of shape, or texture of the testis
- Unexplained and persistent testicular symptoms
- Unexplained persistent lower thoracic/upper lumbar pain in a young man (arising from lymph node enlargement)

Penile cancer
- Ulceration or a mass in the glans or prepuce where a sexually transmitted infection has been ruled out
- Persistent penile lesion after treatment for a sexually transmitted infection

1.6 Nervous system tumours

Warning signs of brain tumours
For primary brain tumours these features include:
- Central nervous system (CNS) symptoms such as:
  - Any progressive neurological deficit
  - Seizure of recent onset
  - New onset of severe headaches for which there is no obvious other explanation
  - Changes in personality or behaviour
  - Cranial nerve palsies
  - Unilateral deafness
- Headaches of recent onset with features of raised intracranial pressure such as vomiting, or positional exacerbation, such as being worse in the morning
- Ataxia and head tilt can be associated with posterior fossa tumours in children

Direct referral to an oncologist
Patients who have previously been treated for cancers at other sites may present with the same symptoms if they develop metastatic disease and direct referral to the oncologist who previously treated them may be appropriate for consideration of palliative radiotherapy.

Indications for urgent referral
Adults with progressive subacute loss of central neurological function need urgent imaging with a magnetic resonance imaging (MRI) scan or computed tomography (CT) scan if MRI is contraindicated.

Children and young adults with new cerebellar or central neurological abnormal functions need very urgent assessment within 48 hours.

Warning features of spinal cord compression
Patients with a history of cancer, especially those with a high risk of bone metastases (e.g. prostate, breast cancer, etc.) and those with primary spinal cord tumours can present with the following features suggestive of spinal cord compression which needs urgent evaluation (within 24 hours):
- Pain in the thoracic or cervical spine region
- Progressive or severe unremitting pain in the lumbo-sacral region
- Spinal pain aggravated by straining
- Nocturnal spinal pain preventing sleep
- Pain associated with weakness, sensory symptoms, or sphincter dysfunction

Patients with known or suspected cancer with the following features suggestive of spinal cord compression need emergency evaluation:
- Radicular pain
- Limb weakness
- Sensory symptoms
- Bladder or bowel dysfunction
- Signs of cauda equina syndrome or spinal cord compression

The aim after emergency evaluation is to start appropriate treatment of spinal cord compression within 24 hours of referral which offers the best chance of maintaining the ability to walk and functional independence.

1.7 Upper gastrointestinal cancer

Indications for urgent referral

- Urgent upper gastrointestinal (GI) endoscopy (within two weeks) is indicated to rule out oesophageal and stomach cancer
- Dysphagia
- Aged 55 years or over with weight loss and upper abdominal pain, reflux, or dyspepsia
- Upper abdominal mass consistent with stomach cancer
- Urgent ultrasound scan is indicated in people with an upper abdominal mass consistent with gall bladder cancer to rule out gall bladder cancer
- Urgent ultrasound scan is indicated in people with an upper abdominal mass consistent with liver enlargement to rule out liver cancer
- Urgent CT scan or ultrasound (if CT not available) is indicated to rule out pancreatic cancer in people aged 60 years or over with weight loss and one of the following:
  - Diarrhoea
  - Abdominal pain
  - Back pain

- Nausea
- Vomiting
- Constipation
- New-onset diabetes
- Patient aged 40 or over with jaundice should be investigated to rule out pancreatic cancer

Patients referred urgently for endoscopy should ideally be free from acid suppression medication, including proton pump inhibitors, for a minimum of two weeks.

Indications for non-urgent referral

People aged 55 or over with the following features should be referred for upper GI endoscopy to rule out oesophageal and stomach cancer:

- Haematemesis
- Upper abdominal pain with low haemoglobin
- Treatment-resistant dyspepsia
- Nausea and vomiting with reflux, dyspepsia, upper abdominal pain, or weight loss
- Raised platelet count with nausea, vomiting, reflux, dyspepsia, upper abdominal pain, or weight loss

1.8 Lower gastrointestinal cancer

Indications for urgent referral

People with the following features should be referred to a colorectal cancer diagnostic service as an urgent case under the two-week standard:

- Aged 40 or over with unexplained weight loss and abdominal pain
- Aged 50 or over with unexplained rectal bleeding
- Aged 50 or over with rectal bleeding and unexplained features of abdominal pain, change in bowel habit, weight loss, or iron-deficiency anaemia
- Aged 60 or over with iron-deficiency anaemia, change in bowel habit, or positive faecal occult blood test
- Rectal or abdominal mass
- Patient with unexplained anal mass or unexplained anal ulceration should be urgently evaluated to rule out anal cancer

Indications for non-urgent referral

Faecal occult blood testing should be offered to people with the following features but without rectal bleeding:

- Aged 50 or over with unexplained abdominal pain or weight loss
- Aged under 60 with change in bowel habit or iron-deficiency anaemia
- Aged 60 or over with anaemia without iron deficiency

Regular colonoscopy is recommended for people in high-risk groups (familial adenomatosis polyposis (FAP), hereditary non-polyposis colorectal cancer (HNPCC), long-standing history of inflammatory bowel disease, previous colorectal cancer, and polyps), but the frequency with which this should be carried out depends on the particular condition.

1.9 Gynaecological cancer

Indications for urgent referral
- Ovarian cancer:
  - Ascites and/or pelvic or abdominal mass
  - Ultrasound suggestive of ovarian cancer
- Endometrial cancer:
  - Women aged 55 or over with post-menopausal bleeding (bleeding 12 months after cessation of menstruation)
  - Consider referral for women aged less than 55 years with post-menopausal bleeding
- Cervix examination is consistent with cervical cancer
- Unexplained vulval lump, ulceration, or bleeding
- Unexplained mass in or at the vaginal introitus

Indications for investigation in primary care
Tests for ovarian cancer
- Women aged 50 or over with symptoms of irritable bowel syndrome within the last few months—measure CA125
- If CA125 ≥35 IU/ml—arrange ultrasound scan of abdomen and pelvis

Direct access ultrasound to rule out endometrial cancer is indicated in the following settings:
- Women aged 55 or over with unexplained vaginal discharge who present with this symptom for the first time or have thrombocytosis or with haematuria
- Women aged 55 or over with haematuria and low haemoglobin, thrombocytosis, or high blood glucose level

Indication for emergency referral
- Patient presenting with acute abdomen

1.10 Haematological cancer

Warning features
A number of features or combinations of features suggest the possibility of a haematological malignancy that requires further investigation. These features are the consequence of bone marrow suppression, or extramedullary haematopoiesis, lymphadenopathy, and hepato- or splenomegaly.
- Features of bone marrow suppression:
  - Fatigue, breathlessness (anaemia)
  - Recurrent infection (white cell abnormality)
  - Bruising and bleeding (low platelets)
- Extramedullary haemopoiesis:
  - Splenomegaly and hypersplenism
- Lymphadenopathy (>1cm) particularly with the following features:
  - Persists for ≥6 weeks
  - Generalized in nature
  - Size >2cm
  - Increasing in size
  - Associated with B symptoms (fever, night sweats, and weight loss)
  - Associated with hepatomegaly, and/or splenomegaly
- General features:
  - B symptoms (fever, drenching night sweats, and weight loss)
  - Generalized itching
  - Bone pain
  - Alcohol-induced pain in lymph nodes

Indications for very urgent referral
Leukaemia
NICE recommends that the following situations in adults, children, and young adults warrant very urgent referral for full blood count (within 48 hours) to rule out leukaemia:
- Pallor
- Persistent fatigue
- Unexplained bruising, unexplained petechiae, or unexplained bleeding
- Unexplained fever
- Unexplained persistent or recurrent infection
- Generalized lymphadenopathy
- Hepatosplenomegaly

Lymphoma in children and young adults
Very urgent referral to rule out lymphoma is recommended for children and young adults with unexplained lymphadenopathy. It is important to take into consideration presence of B symptoms (fever, night sweats, and weight loss), breathlessness, and pruritus during referral.

Myeloma
Very urgent protein electrophoresis and a Bence-Jones protein test is indicated for:
- People aged 60 or over with hypercalcaemia or leukopenia and a presentation that is consistent with possible myeloma
- If plasma viscosity or erythrocyte sedimentation rate (ESR) and presentation are consistent with possible myeloma

Indications for urgent referral
Lymphoma in adults
Adults with unexplained lymphadenopathy should be urgently referred (for an appointment within two weeks). It is important to take into consideration presence of B symptoms (fever, night sweats, and weight loss), breathlessness, alcohol-induced lymph node pain, and pruritus during referral.

Myeloma
If protein electrophoresis or Bence-Jones protein urine test suggest myeloma.

1.11 Head and neck cancer

Indication for emergency referral

All patients presenting with acute shortness of breath suggesting stridor or tracheal obstruction need emergency evaluation (within 24 hours).

Indications for urgent referral

Laryngeal cancer

• People aged 40 or over with persistent unexplained hoarseness or unexplained lump in the neck

Oral cancer

• People with unexplained oral cavity ulceration for more than three weeks or an unexplained persistent lump in the neck
• Lump on the lip or in the oral cavity
• Lesions consistent with erythroplakia or erythro-leukoplakia in the oral cavity

1.12 Thyroid cancer

Indication for emergency referral

Patients presenting with features of stridor due to thyroid swelling need emergency evaluation and management.

Indications for urgent referral

All patients presenting with a thyroid swelling associated with any of the following features should be urgently referred:

• Enlarging solitary nodule
• Unexplained hoarseness
• Associated neck node enlargement
• Those with family history of endocrine tumour(s)
• Prepubertal patients
• Patients aged ≥65 years
• Patients with previous history of neck irradiation

1.13 Bone cancer and sarcoma

Indications for very urgent referral

Indications for very urgent referral (appointment within 48 hours) include:

• Children and young adults with unexplained bone swelling or pain and with an X-ray suggestive of bone sarcoma
• Children and young adults with a lump which on ultrasound is suggestive of soft tissue sarcoma or clinical concern in spite of uncertain ultrasound findings

Indications for urgent X-ray/ultrasound

Any of the warning features noted earlier. These must be clearly stated in the request. People with bone swelling or pain should have X-rays and people with an unexplained enlarging lump should have an ultrasound examination.

Extreme care must be taken to ensure the correct bone(s) and joint are included in the X-ray. A significant number of delays in diagnosis are due to inappropriately reported 'normal' X-rays, either because the incorrect area was imaged or it was viewed without appropriate clinical information or by someone inexperienced in the imaging of bone tumours.

Remember when deciding upon which area to X-ray to consider that the pain may be felt in one part of the bone but referred from another area.

Indications for urgent referral

Any isolated bone lesion or clinically detectable bone mass which is unlikely to be due to another cause. For example, in an elderly man non-isolated lesions are far more likely to be due to metastatic prostate cancer than a primary bone tumour. Conversely in an adolescent man, even with a history of sports injury, an abnormal area on X-ray should always be assessed.

If the centre has significant sarcoma experience, an MRI may be performed in the case of an isolated bone lesion before referral to the surgical sarcoma centre to give more information.

All suspected bone tumours which meet these criteria should be biopsied only at a surgical sarcoma centre. This is to allow planning of future surgery, ensure adequate drainage of the biopsy site, and aim to prevent tumour seeding.

1.14 Skin cancer—melanoma

Warning features
Any change in a pre-existing naevus should be assessed to rule out melanoma. A weighted seven-point checklist is used to assess pigmented lesions. Major features score 2 points each and minor features score 1 point each.
Major features:
- Change in size
- Irregular shape
- Irregular colour

Minor features:
- Largest diameter ≥7mm
- Inflammation
- Change in sensation
- Oozing
- Lesions with a score of ≥3 points are suspicious of melanoma. Low scoring lesions may be monitored for eight weeks unless there is a strong suspicion of melanoma

Indications for urgent referral
All patients with lesions with a strong suspicion of melanoma, and dermoscopy suggesting melanoma, should be referred urgently for further assessment. Excision in the primary care setting is not advised.

1.15 Skin cancer—non-melanoma

Indications for urgent referral
Patients with skin lesions suggesting squamous cell carcinoma (SCC) need urgent evaluation. The following are the indications for urgent referral:
- A non-healing skin lesion of >1cm size with significant palpable induration occurring on the face, scalp, or back of the hand with a progressive increase in size during the previous eight weeks
- All immunocompromised patients who develop new or growing skin lesions
- Patients with a histological diagnosis of SCC
- All patients with suspected Merkel cell carcinoma should also be referred for urgent evaluation and management

Indication for non-urgent referral
Skin lesions that are slow growing and suggestive of basal cell carcinoma need non-urgent referral.

1.16 Further reading and internet resources

Further reading
Barraclough K. New NICE guidance on referral for cancer. *BMJ* 2015; 351:h3640.
Hamilton W, Walter FM, Rubin G, Neal RD. Improving early diagnosis of symptomatic cancer. *Nat Rev Clin Oncol* 2016; 13:740–9.

Internet resources
NICE guideline. Metastatic spinal cord compression in adults: risk assessment, diagnosis and management: http://guidance.nice.org.uk/CG75/NICEGuidance/pdf/English
NICE guideline. Suspected cancer: recognition and referral: http://www.nice.org.uk/guidance/NG12

Chapter 2

Concepts of multidisciplinary management

Chapter contents

2.1 Cancer prevention

Introduction
Carcinogenesis is a multistep process consisting of progressive molecular and cellular changes leading to early invasive cancer and finally to distant metastasis and death. The initiation and progression of cancer usually takes years. Attempts are being made to reverse the molecular and cellular changes at an early stage of cancer initiation or progression. The World Health Organization (WHO) estimates that at least one-third of all cancers are preventable.

Risk and protective factors of cancer

Smoking and cancer
Smoking is the single largest preventable cause of cancer worldwide. It causes 30% of all cancer deaths. Smoking increases the risk of acute myelogenous leukaemia and cancers of the lung, head and neck, oesophagus, stomach, pancreas, cervix, and bladder.

Passive smoking (defined as the inhalation of the smoke coming from the end of a lighted cigarette, pipe, or cigar and the smoke that is exhaled by a smoker) increases the risk of lung cancer by 16%.

Infectious diseases
Infectious agents are responsible for 6% of cancer deaths in developed countries and 26% in developing countries. Preventive measures include vaccination and prevention of infection (Table 2.1.1).

Radiation exposure
Ultraviolet (UV) radiation increases the risk of all types of skin cancers. People at high risk of skin cancer (fair skin, large number of naevi, or family history) should be encouraged to limit time spent in the sun (especially between 10 am and 3 pm), to wear hats, sunglasses, and protective clothing, and to use sunscreen.

Exposure to ionizing radiation increases the risk of haematological cancers and breast and thyroid cancer. A study from Australia suggests that children and teenagers aged 0–19 years, who have had a diagnostic computed tomography (CT) scan, have a significantly increased risk of cancer during adulthood compared with those who did not (RR 1.24; 95% CI 1.20–1.29).

Environmental hazards
Radon is a naturally occurring carcinogen found in soil and rock which can act synergistically with smoking, leading to an increased risk of lung cancer. It has been estimated that approximately one-third of radon-induced lung cancer could be prevented by keeping the radon concentration at home to a level below 4pCi/l.

Immunosuppression
After organ transplantation there is an increased risk of cancer due to immunosuppression and oncogenic viral infections. The most common cancers include non-Hodgkin lymphoma and cancers of the lung, liver, and kidney.

Obesity, diet, and alcohol
Overweight and obesity are linked to cancers of the breast, colorectum, endometrium, pancreas, kidney, and oesophagus. Obesity is also a probable risk factor in gall bladder cancer. Weight loss has been shown to reduce cancer mortality and the risk of endometrial and breast cancers. Dietetic studies have not shown a consistent reduction in the risk of cancer. Alcohol increases the risk of cancers of the mouth, oesophagus, breast, liver, and colorectum.

Physical activity
There is increasing evidence that physical activity is protective, particularly in colorectal and breast cancers. Physical activity probably also decreases the risk of postmenopausal breast cancer and endometrial cancer.

Diabetes
Diabetes increases the risk of and death due to cancers of the liver, pancreas, colorectum, and breast. Cancers of the ovary, endometrium, bladder, and oral cavity are also increased in diabetics. Metformin is reported to decrease the incidence and mortality of breast cancer.

Table 2.1.1 Risk factors of carcinogenesis

Cause	Type of cancer	Preventative measures
Viruses:		
HPV	Cervical, anogenital, and oropharyngeal cancer	HPV vaccine for girls and women aged 9–26 years
HBV and HCV	Liver cancer	Reduced hepatitis B viral load with interferon or nucleoside/tide analogues in patients with chronic HBV infection
		Antiviral therapy in chronic HCV therapy
HIV	Anal cancer, lymphoma, lung cancer, Kaposi's sarcoma, and non-AIDS-defining malignancies	Measures to prevent acquisition of HIV infection and antiretroviral therapy
Bacteria:		
Helicobacter pylori	Stomach cancer and MALT lymphoma	
Parasites:		
Clonorchis sinensis and *Opisthorchis viverrini*	Liver cancer	
Schistosoma haematobium	Bladder cancer	

Hormone replacement therapy (HRT)
In patients with an intact uterus, oestrogen-alone HRT increases the risk of endometrial cancer, and therefore combined HRT is given, as progestin is thought to be protective. HRT has also been shown to increase the risk of breast and ovarian cancer.

Cellular phone
Cellular phones operate at the radiofrequency (RF) level of the electromagnetic spectrum (non-ionizing) and the radio waves have a very low energy (one millionth of an electron volt). Studies (e.g. the INTERPHONE study) so far have not suggested any increased risk of cancer with the use of cellular phones.

Prevention of cancer

Chemoprevention
Chemoprevention is the use of natural or synthetic agents to reverse, suppress, or prevent carcinogenic progression to invasive cancer. Chemoprevention may interrupt multifocal field carcinogenesis (development of multiple areas of genetically distinct clones) and multistep carcinogenesis (progressive changes with accumulation of somatic mutations in a single clone). Since clinical trials of chemopreventive agents take years to assess benefit, intermediate markers (e.g. premalignant lesions) allow a more expeditious evaluation of potential benefits of experimental agents.

Chemoprevention in breast cancer
The Breast Cancer Prevention Trial (BCPT), a placebo-controlled trial of tamoxifen in 13,000 women at high risk of breast cancer has shown that tamoxifen resulted in a 49% reduction in the incidence of invasive breast cancer (P<0.00001). A meta-analysis of chemopreventive studies in breast cancer also showed a reduction in oestrogen receptor (ER) positive but not ER negative tumours. There was also an increase in endometrial cancer (2.5 times greater risk) and thrombotic events especially in women aged ≥50 years. These studies suggest that the benefit of tamoxifen in chemoprevention is not consistent.

The initial results of the NSABP-P2 study, which compared tamoxifen with raloxifene, reported a reduction in the risk of development of invasive cancer by 50% with both drugs. The risk of uterine cancer and thrombotic events were less with raloxifene. Raloxifene did not prevent non-invasive carcinoma whilst tamoxifen decreased the incidence of non-invasive cancer by 50%.

The placebo-controlled NCIC CTG MAP.3 trial has shown that exemestane reduces the risk of breast cancer in women with high-risk features (age ≥60 years, history of atypical ductal or lobular hyperplasia, or carcinoma in situ); however, the long-term safety of aromatase inhibitors (AIs) has not yet been reported.

Chemoprevention in colorectal cancer
Studies have reported potential benefits in terms of reduction in colorectal cancer incidence with selenium (58% reduction in the Nutritional Prevention of Cancer Trial), HRT (a meta-analysis showing 20% reduction in risk), and aspirin (reduction in adenoma and colorectal recurrence).

Chemoprevention in prostate cancer
Studies of 5-alpha reductase inhibitors, finasteride (Prostate Cancer Prevention Trial: PCPT), and dutasteride (REDUCE trial) did not show any favourable risk–benefit profile for the prevention of prostate cancer.

Vaccination
The role of hepatitis B virus (HBV) vaccination in preventing hepatocellular carcinoma is not clearly defined.

Human papilloma virus (HPV) types 16 and 18 together account for about 70% of cervical cancers. Two types of HPV vaccines are available: one protects against HPV 16 and 18 (Cervarix®) and another against HPV 6, 11, 16, and 18 (Gardasil®). A phase 3 study of Cervarix® has shown that it reduces the overall burden of precancerous cervical lesions (CIN2+) by 70% in HPV naïve young girls. Gardasil® also has shown similar benefit. Recent data indicate that Cervarix® also offers cross protection against HPV 31, 33, and 45 which might give an additional 11–16% protection against cervical cancer, including adenocarcinoma. Cervarix® is effective for 6.4 years and Gardasil® for five years.

The current recommendation for HPV vaccination is for girls aged 11–13 years and females up to 26 years old (to catch up with those who missed vaccination or to complete the series). In the UK, cervical cancer screening starts at the age of 25 years.

Boys aged 11–12 years and men up to 21 years (to catch up with those who missed vaccination or to complete the series) are recommended to have HPV vaccination to prevent anal intraepithelial neoplasia in men who have sex with men.

Vitamins and dietary supplements
Based on the hypothesis that oxidative damage to deoxyribonucleic acid (DNA) leads to carcinogenesis, several antioxidants have been evaluated for cancer prevention. Two prospective placebo-controlled studies found that beta carotene supplements increased lung cancer incidence and mortality.

Studies of use of selenium, vitamin C, and vitamin E have not shown a reduction in the incidence of prostate cancer. The Women's Antioxidant Cardiovascular Study showed that supplementation with vitamin C, vitamin E, or beta carotene did not offer any benefit in the primary reduction in total cancer incidence or cancer mortality.

Surgical prevention
One of the common approaches for prevention in high-risk people with genetic disorders is prophylactic surgery such as mastectomy and oophorectomy in BRCA-positive people.

Internet resources
Advisory Committee on Immunization Practices: https://www.cdc.gov/vaccines/acip/
American Cancer Society: http://www.cancer.org
Canadian Task Force on Preventive Health Care: https://canadiantaskforce.ca/
National Cancer Institute: http://www.cancer.gov
NHS immunization information: https://www.nhs.uk/conditions/vaccinations/
World Cancer Research Fund: http://www.wcrf-uk.org
World Cancer Research Fund/American Institute for Cancer Research: Food, Nutrition, Physical Activity and the Prevention of Cancer: a Global Perspective: http://www.dietandcancerreport.org
World Health Organization: http://www.who.org

2.2 Cancer screening

Introduction

The aim of cancer screening is to detect a tumour at a very early stage when treatment is most likely to be effective and to produce thereby a reduction in disease-specific mortality. In the UK only screening programmes for cervical, breast, and bowel cancers are considered to meet these criteria, although there is a continuing search for an effective screening method for lung, prostate, and ovarian cancers.

Cervical cancer screening

In the UK, women are invited for screening between the ages of 25–64: those aged 25–49 every three years and those aged 50–64 every five years to correspond with patterns of sexual activity. With three-yearly screening, 41% of cancers are preventable in those aged <40 years and 69% in those aged 40–54 years. In women aged 55–69 years, three- and five-year screening prevents an equal proportion of cancers (73% each). Studies show that screening women <25 years old is less effective in preventing cancer including advanced stage cancer than screening women aged ≥25 years.

About 80% of eligible patients in fact attend for screening which reduces the long-term death rate by approximately 95%. Approximately four million screening tests are carried out each year in the UK. The introduction of screening has reduced the incidence of invasive cervix cancer by >50%.

Screening is based on cytological examination of cells obtained from the cervix using a curette under direct vision (the Pap smear—Table 2.2.1), liquid-based cytology, or HPV testing (which has a high sensitivity but low specificity). Women who are found to have a low-grade abnormality are tested for HPV with identification of high-risk HPV types. Studies show that HPV testing is more sensitive than cytology (96.1% vs. 53%) and screening intervals can be extended to six years or more.

Of those showing an abnormal result, approximately 0.1% turn out to have cervical cancer, 7% CIN3 or adenocarcinoma in situ, 10.7% CIN2, and 25% CIN1.

Women aged 21–4 years with high-grade squamous intraepithelial lesions (HSIL) undergo colposcopy. Women aged ≥25 years with HSIL have colposcopy or immediate loop electrosurgical excision. Further management depends on colposcopy findings.

Many countries have recently implemented HPV immunization for girls aged 12–13 years. The potential impact on cervical screening of the HPV vaccination programmes will take some time to evaluate.

Breast cancer screening

Currently women between the ages of 50 and 70 years are invited for screening every five years. A study is looking at extending the breast cancer screening to women aged 47–73 years. Nearly two million women per year are screened in the UK. Survival rates for screen-detected cancer are 85% at 15 years. Studies show that breast cancer screening results in a 35% reduction in breast cancer mortality. Digital mammography is gradually replacing film mammography and has particular advantages in detecting cancer in younger patients with denser breast tissue.

The result of the screening is estimated to be one extra survival for every eight women diagnosed with breast cancer. Around one in six women have an abnormality on routine screening and of these 20% have ductal carcinoma in situ (DCIS).

Bowel cancer screening

Bowel cancer screening is based on the detection of faecal occult blood from a stool sample and as well as cancers, polyps will also be detected. Their removal will prevent any risk of subsequent bowel cancer development. In the UK, screening is offered every two years to all men and women aged 60–74, using a faecal immunochemical test (FIT). Screening will reduce the risk of death from bowel cancer by 16%.

Uptake has been around 60% in pilot studies and the overall rate of positive abnormal results was 1.9%. The rate of cancer detection was 1.62 per 1,000 screened. Out of every 1,000 people with a normal result, <1 will be diagnosed with bowel cancer within the next two years.

Prostate cancer screening

There is no national screening programme in the UK yet because there is no evidence that early treatment of small volume disease leads to an improved outcome. There is evidence from a prostate screening trial in Europe of a reduction in mortality by 20% but this was achieved at the cost of a high level of complications from overtreatment in the rest of the group. Forty-eight additional cases of prostate cancer were treated to result in one additional survival. Measurement of prostate-specific antigen (PSA) is not sensitive or specific enough to be routinely recommended. Men with prostate cancer may not have a raised PSA and two out of three men with a raised PSA do not have prostate cancer.

In view of the demand from many men for this test, the UK has introduced a programme of Informed Choice to

Table 2.2.1 Cervical screening

Bethesda classification	Pap	Description	Treatment
Low-grade squamous intraepithelial lesion (LSIL)	CIN1	This carries the lowest risk. Represents mild dysplasia confined to the basal 1/3 of the epithelium. Infection with HPV will typically be cleared by immune response within a year	Observation/colposcopy and biopsy
High-grade squamous intra-epithelial lesion (HSLI)	CIN2	Moderate dysplasia confined to the basal 2/3 of the epithelium	Loop electrosurgical excision procedure (LEEP) cryotherapy or laser
HSLI	CIN3	Severe dysplasia involving >2/3 of the epithelium, or up to full thickness carcinoma in situ	LEEP cryotherapy or laser

help men to decide whether they do wish to be tested and what decisions may then be required, with information given about the benefits and risks of the various treatment options.

Lung cancer screening

Lung cancer screening with annual chest X-rays (CXRs) has been evaluated in the US Prostate, Lung, Colorectal, and Ovarian Cancer Screening Trial but has not shown a benefit. Several trials have evaluated the role of low-dose chest computed tomography (LDCT). While LDCT is more sensitive than a CXR in identifying small asymptomatic lung cancer, both methods have high rates of false positivity. There is global variation in the recommendation for LDCT screening due to cost–benefit implications. Generally, high-risk adults (≥30 pack year history and current smoker or quit within the last 15 years) may benefit from screening.

Ovarian cancer screening

The UK Collaborative Trial of Ovarian Cancer Screening (UKCTOCS) is evaluating the use of CA125 and TVUS for ovarian cancer screening.

Screening women at higher risk

Higher than average risk means having two or more relatives on the same side of the family diagnosed with ovarian cancer or breast cancer at a young age. In this group, early mammography may be replaced with magnetic resonance imaging (MRI) breast screening and regular ultrasound may be undertaken, although prophylactic organ removal may also be advised.

Internet resources

NHS Cancer Screening Programmes: https://www.gov.uk/topic/population-screening-programmes

2.3 Cancer genetics

Introduction

At least 3% of cancers are due to inheritance of alterations in genes that confer a high lifetime risk of certain malignancies and more than 100 cancer predisposition genes (CPGs) have now been identified. These genetic variations can increase both the risk of common cancers, such as breast and colorectal cancer, and very rare tumours. The majority of 'hereditary cancer predisposition syndromes' are due to mutations within a single allele (copy) of a tumour suppressor gene inherited in an autosomal dominant fashion, but autosomal recessive, X-linked, and Y-linked patterns of cancer predispositions are also now recognized.

Mutations in CPGs should not be confused with somatic mutations in tumours which are not inherited.

Mechanisms of inherited cancer

Tumourigenesis involves two classes of genes. Oncogenes act to control cell growth and proliferation under normal circumstances, but once inappropriately activated or overexpressed can promote rapid clonal expansion. Tumour suppressor genes normally inhibit abnormal cell proliferation; reduced expression of these genes can result in uncontrolled cell division.

Most hereditary cancer predisposition syndromes are due to the inheritance of a germline mutation in a tumour suppressor gene. The inherited mutation inactivates one copy of the gene and the subsequent development of a mutation in the remaining 'normal' copy of the gene results in failure of a cell to produce the tumour suppressor protein. Inheritance of two alleles each carrying a mutation within the same tumour suppression gene is extremely rare and often results in a different and more severe phenotype than monoallelic mutation inheritance.

Diagnosis

An underlying hereditary predisposition towards developing a malignancy is typically characterized by:
• Young age at presentation
• Increased incidence of bilateral tumours
• More than one primary tumour site

• Family history of specific cancers

Although most cancer predisposition syndromes are inherited in an autosomal dominant fashion with affected individuals in each generation, penetrance (the likelihood of a mutation carrier developing clinical manifestations of the syndrome) can vary.

Analysis of DNA for mutations in known cancer predisposition genes is performed using DNA derived from a peripheral blood sample. Advances in DNA sequencing technology have resulted in progressive reductions in analysis times. Traditionally, testing for CPG mutations has been performed only following referral to a clinical genetics service. However, increasing demands for testing in short timeframes suggest that this model will not be sustainable in the future. An 'oncogenetic' model of CPG testing, whereby testing in patients with cancer can be performed through the cancer team, with support as required from genetics specialists, has been successfully introduced at several UK centres.

Inherited breast cancer

A positive family history is reported by 20–30% of breast cancer patients. Approximately 5% of all breast cancers are thought to be due to highly penetrant autosomal dominant cancer predisposition syndromes. The two most frequent highly penetrant breast cancer susceptibility genes are BRCA1 and BRCA2. Much rarer syndromes include Li–Fraumeni, Cowden, Peutz–Jeghers, and hereditary diffuse gastric cancer syndromes; these high-risk genes are associated with a lifetime breast cancer risk in the order of 20–100%. It is likely that most familial clusters of breast cancer are the consequence of multiple low-penetrance cancer susceptibility genes acting in conjunction with environmental factors. Several large case–control studies have recently identified variants in DNA repair genes (e.g. CHEK2, ATM, BRIP1, and PALB2), which double the risk of breast cancer. The population prevalence of these variants seems to be only in the order of 1–5%.

Hereditary breast/ovarian cancer syndromes (HBOS)

Clinical features

HBOS are caused by mutations of the BRCA1 or BRCA2 genes and are associated with a lifetime breast cancer risk of 50–85% and an increased lifetime risk of ovarian cancer (40–60% for BRCA1 mutation carriers and 10–25% for BRCA2 mutation carriers).

BRCA1-associated breast tumours typically have a basal-like phenotype being high grade with lymphocytic infiltrate and pushing tumour margins, and ER, progesterone receptor (PR), and human epidermal growth factor receptor 2 (HER2) negative. There is no distinct phenotype associated with BRCA2 tumours although they tend to be high grade and ER positive.

Germline BRCA1 or BRCA2 mutations are detected in 8–18% of patients with ovarian cancer and are predominantly associated with high-grade papillary serous tumours.

BRCA1 mutation carriers additionally have an increased risk of pancreatic cancers whilst male breast cancer, pancreatic, and prostate cancer all occur at an increased frequency in BRCA2 mutation carriers.

Incidence

The population frequency of BRCA1/2 mutation carriers is one in 400, increasing to one in 50 in Ashkenazi Jews.

Inheritance pattern

Autosomal dominant. Biallelic BRCA2 mutations can occur and are associated with Fanconi anaemia type D1 (FANCD1) causing developmental anomalies, a greatly increased risk of childhood cancers, and hypersensitivity to DNA cross-linking agents. Biallelic BRCA1 mutations have recently been described in rare cases and the subtype FANCS has been proposed. However, in most cases biallelic mutations in these genes are likely to be embryonic lethal.

Genetics and pathology

BRCA1 and BRCA2 are located on chromosomes 17 and 13 respectively and are classical tumour suppressor genes. The precise functions of the BRCA1 and BRCA2 gene products remain unclear but these proteins are involved in double-strand DNA break repair and transcription regulation, with additional roles in cell cycle checkpoint control.

Diagnosis

The 2017 National Institute for Health and Care Excellence (NICE) guidelines for the management of familial breast cancer recommend that genetic testing is offered to a patient if their combined BRCA1 and BRCA2 mutation carrier probability is 10% or more. Scoring systems such as Breast and Ovarian Analysis of Disease Incidence and Carrier Estimation Algorithm (BOADICEA) or the Manchester score can be used to calculate a patient's risk of carrying a BRCA1/2 mutation. Tests aimed at mutation finding should first be carried out on an affected family member where possible. However, for some patients with breast or ovarian cancer, even with no family history of cancer, the overall probability of finding a mutation exceeds the 10% threshold based on the tumour subtype and younger onset, e.g. triple negative breast cancer diagnosed under the age of 40.

Screening of the BRCA1/2 genes for mutations can be achieved in two to eight weeks depending on the technology used. Predictive testing for known mutations can be accomplished within a week. Prenatal and preimplantation genetic diagnosis is now available.

Clinical management

Primary prevention

For individuals with known BRCA1 or BRCA2 mutations, prophylactic double mastectomy reduces the risk of breast cancer by up to 90%. More acceptable to many women is prophylactic bilateral oophorectomy which reduces ovarian cancer rates by 95% and also reduces breast cancer risk. The 2013 NICE guidelines for the management of familial breast cancer additionally approved the use of chemoprevention with tamoxifen or raloxifene (the latter for postmenopausal women only and is therefore a suitable option in younger women after oophorectomy) in women with a high risk of breast cancer.

Secondary prevention

Annual MRI offers improved sensitivity for the detection of malignancy in high-risk young women and detects tumours at an earlier stage than mammography. Annual MRI surveillance of all BRCA1/2 mutation carriers aged 30–49 is therefore recommended with annual breast screening by mammography from ages 40–69. All BRCA1/2 carriers should be encouraged to be 'breast aware'. Screening for ovarian cancer remains under investigation.

Treatment of BRCA-associated breast cancer

Comparisons with age-matched controls suggest that local recurrence rates of BRCA-related breast tumours treated by breast-conserving surgery are similar to those of sporadic cancer, providing the BRCA mutation carriers have undergone prophylactic oophorectomy. Risk of contralateral breast cancer remains significantly higher in BRCA mutation carriers than controls (approximately 30% at ten years but risk varies according to age at first diagnosis). Concerns that healthy cells carrying BRCA1/2 mutations are at increased risk of malignant transformation following irradiation have not been verified by clinical studies of contralateral breast cancer rates in patients receiving chest wall radiotherapy.

In vitro studies suggest that BRCA-associated breast tumours are particularly vulnerable to cytotoxic agents that promote cross-linking of DNA but show resistance to the mitotic spindle poisons. The TNT trial (of carboplatin and docetaxol in triple-negative breast cancer) has recently reported superior response rates with carboplatin than docetaxel in metastatic triple negative breast cancers in BRCA mutation carriers. Targeted therapies in the form of poly (ADP-ribose) polymerase (PARP) inhibitors which exploit the underlying DNA repair deficiency in BRCA mutation carriers have a European licence for the treatment of metastatic breast cancer in BRCA mutation carriers and are in trials in the neoadjuvant and adjuvant setting.

BRCA1/2-related serous ovarian cancers are highly sensitive to platinum chemotherapy, and remain sensitive to repeat challenges with platinum chemotherapy, which probably explains the superior survival of BRCA1/2-related serous ovarian cancer compared with BRCA1/2 wild-type serous ovarian cancer. Clinical trials have shown promising activity of the PARP inhibitor olaparib in BRCA1/2 mutation carriers with advanced ovarian cancer and olaparib now has a European licence for this indication.

Hereditary colorectal cancer

Approximately 5% of cases of colorectal cancer (CRC) are due to an underlying hereditary cancer syndrome. Most familial cases are due to either Lynch syndrome (LS), also known as hereditary non-polyposis colon cancer (HNPCC), which accounts for an estimated 2–3% of all colorectal cancers, familial adenomatous polyposis (FAP), which accounts for <1% of all colorectal cancers, and mutYH-associated polyposis (MAP) which is autosomal recessive and has a variable phenotype similar to attenuated FAP and is similarly uncommon—there are several rare genetic syndromes that also predispose to colon cancer (e.g. Peutz–Jeghers and juvenile polyposis syndromes).

Features that suggest a familial colorectal cancer syndrome include:

- Positive family history suggesting autosomal dominant inheritance (most CRC predisposition genes show dominant inheritance but often with incomplete penetrance)
- Early-age onset (<50 years) colorectal cancer or endometrial cancer (LS)
- Two or more primary cancers in the same individual
- Multiple colorectal carcinomas or >10 adenomatous polyps in the same individual
- History of multiple LS-related tumours in the same individual (endometrial, ovarian, gastric, duodenal, and urological malignancies)

Lynch syndrome

Clinical features

LS is an autosomal dominant pattern hereditary cancer syndrome consisting of a high risk of early-onset colorectal cancer with an increased frequency of endometrial, ovarian, gastric, duodenal, and urological malignancies. Pancreatic and brain tumours and sebaceous adenomas/carcinomas are also associated. Characteristically, the colonic tumours are predominantly right sided (70%) and there is an increased rate of synchronous and metachronous tumours.

Incidence

The carrier frequency is one in 1,700. It accounts for 1–3% of CRC.

Genetics and pathology

In up to 70% of patients with LS the underlying genetic defect is a germline mutation in one of the DNA mismatch repair genes MLH1, MSH2, MSH6, and PMS2. In addition, mutations in the EPCAM gene can lead to hypermethylation and silencing of MSH2. Defective mismatch repair promotes malignant transformation by permitting rapid accumulation of mutations in other genes, such as those that regulate the cell cycle. Deficiency of mismatch repair is characterized by the presence in tumour cells of microsatellites (DNA sequences that contain a short motif repeated several times), that have changed in length due to nucleotide insertions or deletions. This feature is termed 'microsatellite instability' (MSI).

The median age at diagnosis of cancer is 44–52 years and, in contrast to FAP, most patients do not have multiple polyps. The lifetime risk of developing CRC depends on gender (men have twice the risk of women) and type of gene mutation, MLH1 and MSH2 mutations carrying a much greater risk than those in MSH6 and PMS2.

The characteristic pathological phenotype includes synchronous or metachronous cancers, right-sided cancers, often with pathological associated features (Crohn-like lymphocytic reaction, tumour infiltrating lymphocytes, mucinous/signet ring histology); immunohistochemistry usually shows loss of the relevant protein and its binding partner and tumour DNA analysis shows microsatellite instability (MSI-H).

Diagnosis

The Revised Bethesda Guidelines (2004) recommend the testing of tumour for MSI if one of the following criteria is met:

- CRC diagnosed in an individual younger than 50 years
- Presence of synchronous, metachronous colorectal, or other LS-associated tumours
- CRC with MSI-H pathological associated features diagnosed in an individual younger than 60 years. (Note: presence of tumour-infiltrating lymphocytes, Crohn-like lymphocytic reaction, mucinous/signet-ring differentiation, or medullary growth pattern)
- CRC or LS-associated tumour diagnosed in at least one first-degree relative younger than 50 years
- CRC or LS-associated tumour diagnosed at any age in two first-degree or second-degree relatives

Presence of MSI-H indicates a probable defect in an MMR gene and in the majority is associated with loss of expression of one of the MMR proteins. Testing for suspected LS is initially performed by immunohistochemistry (IHC) of the tumour specimen for all four MMR proteins using monoclonal antibodies and/or molecular analysis for MSI followed by genetic screening for germline mutations in those showing loss of protein. IHC has the advantage that it can then direct germline testing to a particular gene. In the event of MLH1/PMS2 protein expression loss, further information can be gained from assessing for a somatic BRAF V600E mutation or the presence of MLH1 promotor methylation. If the tumour is MMR deficient and a somatic BRAF mutation is not detected or MLH1 promoter methylation is not identified, testing for germline mutations is indicated.

Universal screening of colorectal tumours for MMR is increasingly being adopted with 2017 NICE diagnostic guidance supporting testing all patients newly diagnosed with colorectal cancer. In familial CRC where three close relatives with early-onset colon cancer are identified, patients should be referred for further genetic assessment even if pathological parameters do not suggest LS.

Primary prevention

The role of prophylactic colectomy in the management of patients with LS remains controversial. Some specialists recommend prophylactic hysterectomy and bilateral salpingo-oophorectomy on completion of child-bearing for female carriers of LS-associated gene mutations. HRT is not contra-indicated in this patient group. Publication of the CaPP2 trial provides evidence that aspirin is effective chemoprevention, reducing risk of CRC, but the data is not robust enough to be adopted yet into national guidelines.

Secondary prevention

Annual colonoscopy screening from the age of 20–25 years is recommended for carriers of LS-associated gene mutations. Regular upper endoscopy screening should also be considered for LS families with a history of gastric cancer and urine cytology for patients with a family history of urological tumours.

Female LS mutation carriers should be screened for ovarian and endometrial tumours by pelvic ultrasonography with annual transvaginal measurements of endometrial thickness and/or endometrial aspirates.

Management of colonic carcinoma

Subtotal colectomy can be offered to LS patients presenting with a colonic carcinoma, because of the high rate of synchronous tumours in these patients.

Familial adenomatous polyposis

Clinical features

FAP is characterized by the development of hundreds of colonic adenomatous polyps often by the age of 20, with a risk of malignant transformation of almost 100%. The average age of diagnosis of colon cancer is 39 years. Patients are also at increased risk of duodenal carcinomas (5–12%), as well as desmoid tumours (15%), papillary thyroid carcinomas (2%), brain (2%), pancreas (1.7%), and hepatoblastomas (1.6%). In the attenuated FAP syndrome, the risk of colon cancer is slightly lower and of later onset, up to 80% by age 70.

Incidence

The carrier frequency is one in 8,000.

Genetics and pathology

Mutations within the adenomatous polyposis coli (APC) tumour suppressor gene on chromosome 5q21 are found in >90% of FAP cases. The APC protein binds numerous proteins including members of the Wnt signalling pathway and cytoskeleton regulators. Loss of the APC protein results in chromosomal instability due to loss of cytoskeleton control and activation of the Wnt pathway which promotes tumourigenesis. The attenuated form of FAP is associated with mutations at either end of the APC gene whereas classic FAP is associated with mutations in the more central regions of the gene.

Diagnosis

A clinical diagnosis of FAP can be made by flexible sigmoidoscopy at an early age. Where the causative gene mutation in the family is known, genetic testing is recommended around the age of 10–12 years to establish a genetic diagnosis in offspring of an affected individual, with the aim of sparing children carrying the wild-type APC gene from invasive colonoscopy surveillance.

Primary prevention

Carriers of APC mutations should undergo surveillance colonoscopy annually starting usually around the age of puberty (ten up to 15 years). Prophylactic colectomy is the only effective management once the number of polyps present are too numerous for safe endoscopic surveillance; typically this procedure is necessary by the age of 20 years. Laparoscopic colectomy is the preferred option in most cases. The COX2 inhibitor celecoxib and non-steroidal anti-inflammatory agent sulindac may both reduce duodenal adenoma formation.

Secondary prevention

Long-term surveillance of the small intestine by upper endoscopy, starting from age 25–30 years, is required as periampullary carcinoma is the commonest cause of death in FAP patients who have undergone prophylactic colectomy. Frequency of examinations is determined by the presence or absence of pathology and varies from annually

to every five years depending on the family history and mutation position. Regular abdominal examination and/or imaging should also be considered if there is a family history of hepatoblastomas in infancy or desmoids.

Management of colonic carcinoma

FAP patients who do develop invasive cancers should be managed in the same way as the general population, although in practice patients frequently opt for a full rather than partial colectomy.

Li–Fraumeni syndrome (LFS)

Clinical features

Classic LFS is a rare cancer susceptibility syndrome characterized by a predominance of soft tissue sarcomas, osteosarcoma, and breast cancer, and an excess of brain tumours, leukaemia, and adrenocortical carcinomas in children and young adults. Many additional tumours have also been reported including lung carcinomas, gastrointestinal and ovarian tumours, lymphomas, and various paediatric tumours.

Inheritance pattern

Autosomal dominant.

Genetics and pathology

Germline mutations of the TP53 gene (chromosome 17), are found in approximately 70% of families meeting the criteria for classic LFS criteria and 40% of families with less stringent Li–Fraumeni-like patterns of disease. The protein product of TP53 is a regulator of the cell cycle and apoptosis. Loss of p53 results in cells with mutated DNA dividing in an uncontrolled fashion to form tumours.

Incidence

The estimated incidence of TP53 germline mutations is 1 in 5,000. Penetrance is at least 50% by age 50.

Diagnosis

TP53 mutations are detected by direct sequencing of the TP53 gene.

Clinical management

NICE guidelines recommend annual MRI breast surveillance for women aged 20–69 years with a known TP53 mutation or who have not had a genetic test but have a greater than 30% probability of being a TP53 carrier.

Exposure to ionizing radiation should be minimized and in the UK mammography is not recommended currently for breast screening in LFS. The use of intensive imaging surveillance of other potential tumour sites is currently under investigation.

The TP53 gene has a key role in cell cycle checkpoint control and DNA repair and apoptosis. LFS is very rare and most of the literature is anecdotal but there are no reports of increased acute toxicity. However, hypothetically at least, DNA-damaging treatments may lead to increased late toxic effects particularly increased future malignancy risk. This should be considered in planning treatments.

Von Hippel–Lindau (VHL) syndrome

Clinical features

VHL is a rare hereditary cancer syndrome consisting of:
- Haemangioblastomas of the retina and central nervous system (CNS) (particularly the cerebellum and spinal cord)

- Phaeochromocytomas
- Clear cell renal carcinomas—frequently bilateral

Inheritance pattern
Autosomal dominant.

Genetics and pathology
The VHL gene is sited on chromosome 3 and is a classic tumour suppressor gene. It encodes a ubiquitin ligase that downregulates hypoxia-inducible mRNAs in the presence of oxygen. Cells lacking pVHL fail to break down the transcription factor complex HIF (hypoxia-inducible factor) which is then able to induce the transcription of genes promoting cell growth, survival, and angiogenesis. Mutations or deletions of the VHL gene are found in virtually all clinically diagnosed VHL families using modern genetic diagnostic methods. Somatic mutations of VHL are also found in most sporadic clear cell renal carcinomas.

Incidence
VHL syndrome is estimated to affect one in 35,000. Twenty to 25% of patients have no previous family history of the disease.

Clinical management
Screening for retinal tumours should begin at the age of five years, with annual blood pressure monitoring and analysis of urinary or plasma catecholamine metabolites. Annual renal imaging should be commenced at approximately 16 years of age. Consideration should also be given to regular screening for CNS tumours using MRI. Regular surveillance using imaging that delivers relatively larger doses of ionizing radiation (e.g. CT scanning) should be avoided if possible in hereditary cancer predisposition syndromes. Prenatal and preimplantation genetic diagnosis is now available for VHL when a mutation has been identified in a family.

Multiple neuroendocrine neoplasia (MEN) syndromes
The MEN syndromes are characterized by the development of multiple benign and malignant tumours of the endocrine glands.

MEN1
Clinical features
- Parathyroid adenomas (up to 95% of cases)
- Pancreatic islet cell tumours (50–75% of cases)
- Pituitary adenomas (25–65% of cases)
- Carcinoid tumours (10% of cases)
- Thyroid tumours
- Benign skin tumours, e.g. multiple angiofibromas

Inheritance
Autosomal dominant.

Genetics and pathology
MEN1 is caused by mutations in the MEN1 gene located on chromosome 11. MEN1 is a tumour suppressor gene which interacts with a number of nuclear proteins including transcription factors.

Incidence
The incidence of MEN1 is one per 30,000.

Diagnosis
Direct mutation detection is now available for the MEN1 gene.

Clinical management
Regular screening of individuals from MEN1 families or known MEN1 mutation carriers should start before the age of ten and should consist of annual serum calcium and prolactin measurements until age 65 as a bare minimum. Consideration should also be given to measurements of pituitary, parathyroid, and pancreatic hormones as well as imaging of the pituitary gland.

MEN2
Clinical features
MEN2A
- Thyroid C cell hyperplasia (up to 100% of cases)
- Medullary thyroid carcinoma (up to 100% of cases)
- Phaeochromocytoma (40% of cases)
- Parathyroid hyperplasia (10–35% of cases)

MEN2B
- Thyroid C cell hyperplasia (up to 100% of cases)
- Medullary thyroid carcinoma (up to 100% of cases)
- Gangliomas (up to 100% of cases)
- Phaeochromocytoma
- Skeletal abnormalities
- Megacolon (due to Hirschsprung's disease)

Familial medullary thyroid cancer (FMTC)
Medullary thyroid cancer (MTC) only, without other endocrine features.

Inheritance
Autosomal dominant.

Genetics and pathology
MEN2A and MEN2B are associated with mutations of the chromosome 10 proto-oncogene RET which codes for a transmembrane receptor tyrosine kinase. It is one of the few cancer predisposition syndromes caused by an activating mutation in a proto-oncogene.

Activating mutations in RET upregulate cell proliferation resulting in tissue hyperplasia with a high rate of malignant transformation. The position of the mutation within the RET gene determines whether the clinical features of MEN2A or MEN2B develop.

Incidence
The incidence of MEN2 is approximately one per 30,000.

Diagnosis
Direct mutation detection is now available for the RET gene.

Clinical management
RET mutation carriers benefit from prophylactic thyroidectomy performed between the ages of three to five years. Screening for phaeochromocytomas with annual 24-hour urine collections for catecholamine concentrations should be performed from adulthood through to the age of 35 years.

Further reading
Burn J, et al. Long-term effect of aspirin on cancer risk in carriers of hereditary colorectal cancer: an analysis from the CAPP2 randomised controlled trial. *Lancet* 2011; 378:2081–7.

Callender GG, Rich TA, Perrier ND. Multiple endocrine neoplasia syndromes. *Surg Clin North Am* 2008; 88(4):863–95.

Foulkes WD. Inherited susceptibility to common cancers. *N Eng J Med* 2008; 359:2143–53.

Garber JE, Offit K. Hereditary cancer predisposition syndromes. *J Clin Oncol* 2005; 23:276–92.

Gonzalez KD, Noltner KA, Buzin CH, et al. Beyond Li Fraumeni syndrome: clinical characteristics of families with p53 germline mutations. *J Clin Oncol* 2009; 27:1250–6.

Guillem JG, Wood WC, Moley JF, et al. ASCO/SSO review of current role of risk-reducing surgery in common hereditary cancer syndromes. *J Clin Oncol* 2006; 24:4642–60.

Haas NB, Nathanson KL. Hereditary renal cancer syndromes. *Adv Chronic Kidney Dis* 2014; 21(1):81–90.

Rahman N. Realising the promise of cancer predisposition genes. *Nature* 2014; 505:302–8.

Stoffel EM, et al. Hereditary colorectal cancer syndromes: ASCO clinical practice guideline endorsement of the familial risk-colorectal cancer: ESMO clinical practice guidelines. *JCO* 2015; 33:209–17.

Tutt A, et al. Carboplatin in BRCA1/2-mutated and triple-negative breast cancer BRCAness subgroups: the TNT Trial. *Nat Med* 2018; 24(5):628–37.

Internet resources

BOADICEA (Breast and Ovarian Analysis of Disease Incidence and Carrier Estimation Algorithm): https://pluto.srl.cam.ac.uk/cgi-bin/bd4/v4beta14/bd.cgi

NCCN clinical practice guidelines in oncology: Colorectal cancer screening: http://www.nccn.org

NCCN clinical practice guidelines in oncology: Genetic/familial high-risk assessment: breast and ovarian: http://www.nccn.org

NICE clinical guideline 164: Familial breast cancer (issue date June 2013): http://www.nice.org.uk

NICE diagnostic guidance 27: Molecular strategies for Lynch syndrome in people with colorectal cancer (issue date February 2018): http://www.nice.org.uk

2.4 Genetic counselling

Introduction

Genetic counselling is the process by which individuals at possible risk of an inherited medical disorder are advised about:

• The natural history of the condition
• Their personal risk of developing or transmitting the condition
• Risk to blood relatives, including current and future children
• The methods available to test for the inherited condition
• The advantages and disadvantages of undergoing testing
• Any management options available if tests confirm that they are carrying the inherited condition
• In the UK, genetic counselling is usually provided by specially trained professionals as part of regional clinical genetics services. It is essential that any individual considering undergoing genetic screening for an inherited cancer predisposition syndrome is given the opportunity to see a genetic counsellor both prior to being tested and on receiving their result

Who should be referred for genetic counselling?

Cancer patients and/or their relatives should be referred to their regional clinical genetics unit for genetic counselling when a suspicion arises that a family or individual history of cancer may be due to an inherited predisposition. Suspicious features include:

• Unusually young age of onset for the type of cancer
• Numerous affected family members with the same type of cancer
• Numerous affected family members with cancers within characteristic groups, e.g. breast and ovarian cancers, colorectal and endometrial tumours
• History of multiple primary cancers in a single individual
• Certain pathological features, e.g. triple negative breast cancer with young onset
• Loss of relevant protein staining by immunohistochemistry on tumour cells

Referral of asymptomatic patients with a strong family history of malignancy permits the potential identification of patients with an underlying CPG mutation who will benefit from primary cancer prevention strategies. Family members who test negative for a known familial CPG mutation can be reassured that they do not require intensive surveillance. Identification of cancer patients with an underlying CPG mutation will permit discussion of secondary cancer prevention strategies, and increasingly can inform the management of the primary malignancy.

The genetic counselling process

Genetic counselling of an individual or family who potentially has a hereditary cancer predisposition syndrome typically consists of a number of key stages:

• Determining the patient's perception and experience
• Explaining the difference between sporadic and inherited cancer risk
• Documenting and verifying the family history of malignancies
• Identifying the most likely underlying genetic fault
• Approximation of personal risk on basis of family history
• Discussing whether genetic testing is appropriate
• Explaining alternative options if genetic testing is uninformative, e.g. available research studies
• Identifying the most appropriate family member to undergo genetic testing (index case)
• Ensuring individuals understand the implications of a positive, negative, and ambiguous genetic result
• Helping to communicate test results to other members of the family

Eliciting the patient issues at the outset is an important step in building rapport and trust and setting up successful communication. The patient's experience of cancer within the family, such as whether people have survived or not and how old the patient was when a parent was affected, can play a huge role in their risk perception.

Taking a family history: key points

- Personal history of cancer including histological details
- Construct a three-generation family tree
- Include both affected and unaffected individuals
- Identify all relatives affected by malignancy including type of cancer and age of diagnosis
- Obtain details of treatments given for cancer
- Confirm whether anyone in the family has previously been assessed by a clinical genetics service, tested, and the result

Accuracy of knowledge about cancer diagnoses in the family varies and it is important when critical decisions are made, for example, when risk-reducing surgery is being considered; whether to have a genetic test and how to interpret the test result; or whether verification of key cancer diagnoses in the family from either medical records, cancer registries, or death certificates is important. Genetic centres seek to confirm the pathology of all reported affected individuals within a family tree. Verification of pathology can be obtained from several sources with pathology laboratory reports being the gold standard.

Oncogenetic model and treatment-focused genetic testing

The traditional clinical genetics model is driven typically by a strong family history of cancer. Until recently, knowledge of an underlying cancer predisposition gene mutation mainly benefited relatives in better quantifying risk and opening options for targeted prevention of cancer. In addition it has been used to inform cancer patients about future new primary cancer risks and to facilitate decisions about risk-reducing surgery; genetic testing did not otherwise alter the immediate management of the presenting malignancy.

However, the advent of targeted therapies such as poly (ADP-ribose) polymerase (PARP) inhibitors which exploit the underlying DNA repair deficiency in BRCA mutation carriers has now changed this paradigm. In treatment-focused genetic testing, testing at the point of cancer diagnosis allows knowledge of a mutation to be incorporated into the management plan of the cancer. An 'oncogenetic' model is becoming more appropriate particularly in cases with no or little family history but presenting with a specific subtype of disease at an early age. Testing is offered to patients presenting with malignancy by the cancer team, with support as required from genetics; this model has been successfully introduced at several sites within the UK. Expansion of this pathway will require additional education and training of oncologists, close collaboration between geneticists and oncologists to ensure correct follow up and family management, and standardization of genetics reporting to assist the clear interpretation of results for patients and families.

Pattern of inheritance

Autosomal dominant

Most of the single high-risk genes that predispose to cancer when a mutation is present are inherited in an autosomal dominant fashion. Gene carriers have a 50% chance of passing the faulty copy on to their offspring. An individual's risk of developing cancer if they are a 'carrier' of a dominantly inherited gene is related to the 'penetrance' of that gene.

Penetrance

- Defines the risk of an individual developing the disease
- CPGs increase with age and vary by gender

Autosomal recessive

A small number of cancer syndromes are inherited in an autosomal recessive fashion, whereby an individual requires two faulty copies of the particular cancer gene to express the condition (one from each parent).

New mutation

A small proportion of patients with a CPG acquire this as a new mutation arising in either egg or sperm. Neither parent carries the mutation, siblings are not at risk of inheriting the mutation but offspring of the new gene carrier will have a 50% risk of inheriting the mutation and the associated cancer risks. Occasionally a mutation arises in the developing embryo and then appears in mosaic form (affecting only some of the cells in an individual). This might be missed in a blood test in a parent but offspring inheriting the mutation will carry it in all cells.

Type of malignancies

Different hereditary cancer predisposition syndromes are caused by mutations in specific genes and are characterized by the co-association of groups of tumours, as detailed in Table 2.4.1.

Risk assessment models

A number of different algorithms exist to predict the probability that an individual/family carries a mutation in a specific cancer predisposition gene based on their family history and and/or pathological details. Examples include models for predicting mutations in Lynch syndrome genes (reviewed by Chen) and the BOADICEA and the Manchester score for familial breast cancer. 2013 NICE guidance for familial breast cancer recommends that women from families with a 10% or greater chance of carrying a mutation such as BRCA1, BRCA2, or TP53 should be considered for genetic testing.

Who should be tested?

Ideally genetic mutation analysis needs to be performed initially in an affected individual. This gives the highest chance of identifying a mutation within a family. The best person to test is generally the youngest affected individual whose pathology matches the type of cancer that fits the pathology seen in the predisposition syndrome being tested for. Testing unaffected individuals poses multiple problems. If a mutation has not been sought within an affected individual, a negative result in an unaffected family member does not necessarily negate the family history, as a mutation may not be identified if testing was performed in an affected member of the family.

When arranging genetic testing, care is taken to ensure that the individual is aware of the possible results and implications of the result and has thought through how they might handle this information. Discussions are also held about informing the wider family.

Genetic testing

Analysis of DNA for mutations in known cancer predisposition genes is performed in a limited number of specialist molecular genetics laboratories using DNA derived from a peripheral blood sample.

Table 2.4.1 Inherited cancer syndromes

Cancer syndrome	Gene	Inheritance	Clinical features and associated cancers/tumours
BAP1-associated tumour predisposition syndrome (BAP1-TPDS)	BAP1	Autosomal dominant (AD)	Uveal/cutaneous melanoma (atypical Spitz tumours: melanocytic BAP1-mutated atypical intradermal tumour), mesothelioma, renal cell carcinoma (RCC), possibly basal cell cancer (BCC), lung cancer, breast/ovarian cancers, meningioma, neuroectodermal tumours, sarcoma
Birt Hogg Dube	FLCN	AD	RCC (chromophobe, clear cell, oncocytoma, hybrid-oncocytic), pulmonary cysts, renal cysts, pneumothoraces, oral lesions, fibrofolliculomas, angiofibromas, trichodiscomas, perifollicular fibromas, multiple epidermoid cysts
Constitutional mismatch repair deficiency (CMMRD)	MMR genes (biallelic)	Autosomal recessive (AR)	Lynch syndrome (LS) related cancers (dx. <25), multiple gastrointestinal polyps, non-Hodgkin lymphoma, glioma, non-pineal supratentorial primitive neuroectodermal tumours (sPNETs), clinical diagnosis. NF1 or features (e.g. cafe-au-lait macule (CALM) or hypopigmented skin areas), pilomatricomas (single or multiple)
Cowden syndrome (PTEN hamartoma syndrome)	PTEN	AD	Breast cancer, follicular thyroid cancer, endometrial cancer, colorectal cancer (CRC), RCC, melanoma, Merkel cell skin cancer, lung cancer, retinal glioma, gastrointestinal hamartomas, ganglioneuromas, Lhermitte–Duclos disease (cerebellar gangliocytoma), macrocephaly, macular pigmentation of the glans penis, mucocutaneous lesions (trichilemmomas), acral keratoses, mucocutanous neuromas, oral papillomas, lipomas, oesophageal glycogenic acanthosis, testicular lipomatosis, atrial septal defect (ASD), intellectual disability (IQ <75), thyroid adenomas, multinodular goitre, benign breast disease, endometrial polyps, vascular anomalies
DICER1 syndrome	DICER1	AD	Pleuropulmonary blastoma, cystic nephroma, Sertoli–Leydig cell tumour (SLCT) of ovary, cervical/bladder/ovarian embryonal rhabdomyosarcoma (ERMs), thyroid cancer, Wilms' tumour, juvenile hamartomatous polyps, pituitary blastoma, pineoblastoma, ciliary body medulloepithelioma (CBME), nasal polyp, anaplastic sarcoma of kidney, medulloblastoma, neuroblastoma, ovarian sex cord stromal tumour, cervix PNET, multinodular goitre, congenital phthisis bulbi
Familial adenomatous polyposis (FAP) including	APC	AD	100+ colorectal adenomas, colorectal cancer, duodenal polyps/cancer, periampullary cancer, gastric fundic gland polyps, CHRPE (bilateral, multifocal)
Gardner syndrome			+ osteomas, desmoid tumours, thyroid cancer (papillary), hepatoblastoma
Turcot syndrome			+ central nervous system (CNS) tumours (medulloblastoma)
Familial melanoma	CDKN2A	AD	Melanoma, pancreatic cancer
Gorlin syndrome (naevoid basal cell carcinoma syndrome)	PTCH1, SUFU	AD	Multiple BCCs, medulloblastoma, ovarian fibromas, cardiac fibroma, odontogenic keratocysts, palmer/plantar pits, macrocephaly, frontal bossing, wedge-shaped vertebrae, bifid ribs, coarse facial features, facial milia ('milk spots'), calcification of falx cerebri, cleft lip/palate, ocular anomalies (including cataracts)
Hereditary breast cancer	PALB2	AD	Breast cancer, possibly pancreatic, ovarian, and male breast cancer
	ATM 7271T>G		Breast cancer, possibly pancreatic cancer
	CHEK2 1100delC		Breast cancer, possibly CRC, thyroid, RCC, testicular germs cell cancer
Hereditary breast and ovarian cancer	BRCA1	AD	Breast cancer, epithelial ovarian/fallopian tube cancer
	BRCA2		Female and male breast cancer, epithelial ovarian/fallopian tube cancer, prostate cancer, pancreatic cancer
Hereditary diffuse gastric cancer	CDH1	AD	Diffuse gastric cancer, lobular breast cancer
Hereditary leiomyomatosis and renal cell cancer (HLRCC)	FH	AD	Uterine/cutaneous leiomyomata, type 2 papillary RCC, renal cysts

(continued)

Table 2.4.1 Continued

Cancer syndrome	Gene	Inheritance	Clinical features and associated cancers/tumours
Hereditary ovarian cancer	BRIP1, RAD51C, RAD51D	AD	Ovarian cancer
Hereditary pancreatitis	PRSS1, SPINK1	AD	Pancreatic cancer, chronic pancreatitis (often childhood)
Hereditary papillary renal cell carcinoma (HPRCC)	MET	AD	Type 1 papillary RCC (multiple, bilateral)
Hereditary paraganglioma-phaeochromocytoma syndrome	SDHA, SDHB, SDHC, SDHD, SDHAF2	AD	Paraganglioma, phaeochromocytoma, RCC (chromophobe), gastrointestinal stromal tumour (GIST), pituitary adenoma
Hereditary retinoblastoma	RB1	AD	Retinoblastoma (infancy/childhood), retinoma, possible risk of sarcoma, melanoma, pineoblastoma
Hyperparathyroidism–jaw tumour (HPT-JT) syndrome	CDC73	AD	Parathyroid carcinoma, ossifying/cemento-ossifying fibroma of maxilla or mandible, renal lesions, hyperparathyroidism
Juvenile polyposis syndrome	SMAD4, BMPR1A	AD	Gastrointestinal (GI) hamartomas, CRC, upper GI cancers, hereditary haemorrhagic telangiectasia
Li–Fraumeni syndrome	TP53	AD	Premenopausal breast cancer, soft tissue sarcoma (childhood), malignant brain tumours, adrenocortical carcinoma (childhood), osteosarcoma (teenage), other cancers (leukaemia, melanoma, stomach, CRC, pancreatic, oesophageal, Wilm's tumour, gonadal germ cell tumours, rhabdomyosarcoma, gastric, RCC, prostate, lung)
Lynch syndrome (HNPCC) including	MLH1, MSH2, MSH6, PMS2	AD	CRC, endometrial cancer, ovarian cancer, GI cancer, pancreatic cancer, urothelial cancers (including, bladder, urethral, ureteric, and renal pelvis)
Muir Torre syndrome			+ sebaceous carcinoma, keratocanthomas
Turcot syndrome			+ brain tumours—gliomas
Multiple endocrine neoplasia type 1	MEN1	AD	Endocrine tumours (parathyroid, pituitary, gastro duodeno-pancreatic (GDP-NETs), carcinoid, adrenocortical, anterior pituitary adenomas, thymic NETs), CNS tumours (meningiomas, ependymomas), leiomyomas, skin tumours (facial angiofibromas, collagenomas), bronchopulmonary NETs, parathyroid hyperplasia, hyperparathyroidism, lipomas
Multiple endocrine neoplasia type 2 and	RET	AD	Type 2A: medullary thyroid cancer (MTC), phaeochromocytoma, parathyroid adenoma, parathyroid hyperplasia, hyperparathyroidisim, cutaneous lichen amyloidosis
			Type 2B: MTC, phaeochromocytoma, mucosal ganglioneuromas, ganglioneuromatosis of GI tract, marfanoid habitus, myelinated corneal nerve fibres
Familial medullary thyroid cancer			MTC
MutYH-associated polyposis (MAP)	MYH	AR	Colorectal adenomas, CRC, extraintestinal malignancies, upper GI cancer
Neurofibromatosis type 1 (NF1)	NF1	AD	Malignant peripheral nerve sheath tumours, gliomas, breast cancer, phaeochromocytoma, GIST, neurofibromas (particularly plexiform neurofibroma), CALM, axillary or inguinal freckling, Lisch nodules, osseous lesions (sphenoid dysplasia or tibial pseudoarthritis)
Neurofibromatosis type 2 (NF2)	NF2	AD	Bilateral vestibular schwannomas, other cranial nerve schwannomas, intracranial/spinal meningiomas, ependymomas, retinal hamartomas, cutaneous tumours, breast cancer (female), CRC, gynaecological, pancreatic, gastric, and small bowel cancers, peripheral neuropathy
Peutz–Jeghers syndrome (PJS)	STK11	AD	Gastrointestinal hamartomatous polyps, GI cancer, breast cancer, sex cord tumours of the ovary with annular tubules (SCTAT), calcifying Sertoli cell (testicular) tumours, cervical cancer (adenoma malignum), mucosal pigmentation
Polymerase proofreading-associated polyposis (PPAP)	POLE, POLD1	AD	CRC, duodenal adenomas, gastric fundic polyps, endometrial cancer
Schwannomatosis	SMARCB1, LZTR1	AD	Non-vestibular schwannomas, peripheral neuropathy

Table 2.4.1 Continued

Cancer syndrome	Gene	Inheritance	Clinical features and associated cancers/tumours
Tuberous sclerosis	TSC1, TSC2	AD	Angiomyolipoma, RCC (clear cell/oncocytoma), skin features (facial angiofibromas, ash leaf patch, shagreen patch), epilepsy, developmental delay, ASD, mental health issues, hyperactivity, sleeping difficulties, other lung, kidney, cardiac, bone, or liver issues
von Hippel–Lindau (VHL)	VHL	AD	Brain/spinal cord hemangioblastomas, renal/pancreatic/ hepatic cysts, RCC (clear cell), phaeochromocytoma, retinal angiomas, endolymphatic sac tumours, epididymal cystadenomas, neuroendocrine tumour (NET)

Full mutation screen

The gold standard for mutation screening is direct sequencing of the entire gene to look for single base changes, small insertions or deletions, and large gene rearrangements. Until recently this has not been commercially viable for very large genes such as BRCA1/2, but molecular genetics laboratories are now routinely moving to next generation sequencing to analyse panels of CPGs. Additional technologies may be required to detect exonic deletions and duplications. A full screen for unknown mutations will take from a few days to several weeks to process depending on the exact technologies used. Clinical interpretation of the implications of clearly deleterious variants in the well characterized genes like BRCA1 and BRCA2 is usually straightforward but may be much more difficult for poorly characterized very rare CPGs.

Predictive testing

Once a causative genetic mutation has been identified within a family, 'predictive testing' can be offered to other family members to establish whether or not they carry the same specific mutation. This is a much faster process than mutation screening and can be offered to individuals both affected and unaffected by cancer. Genetic counselling is critical within these families in giving an individual at risk of having a faulty cancer predisposition gene the opportunity to explore how having this information may impact medically, emotionally, and psychosocially. Individuals at a 50% risk of inheriting a cancer predisposition gene will be counselled about the chance of having the faulty gene, cancer risks associated with this faulty gene, screening recommendations, possible surgical management, implications for current/future offspring, insurance, coping ability, sharing information within the family, and how they think this information will affect them.

Explaining genetic test results

The result of genetic testing is given by a member of staff with whom the patient has built a rapport during pre-test counselling and ongoing support is offered following receipt of the result. Research shows that patients retain little information immediately after being given a 'bad' news result. Discussions are therefore often kept short and simple at this appointment and an early follow-up is arranged to have a more in-depth discussion about future healthcare plans.

Mutation screening

This can result in one of three results:

1. Positive result: a mutation with definite pathogenic potential is identified within the cancer predisposition gene screened. Carriers will be advised of the implications of this result including lifetime risk of malignancies, current recommendations for screening, and other management options including prophylactic surgery.

2. Negative result: no mutation is found within the regions of the gene examined. Patients must be advised that failure to detect a mutation does not always mean that no mutation is present and that further results may become available in the future as genetic testing becomes more sophisticated.

3. Ambiguous result: a DNA sequence variation is identified but it is not clear whether this is pathogenic or not (variant of unknown/uncertain significance (VUS)). The uncertain implications of this result must be communicated carefully to the patient with the advice that further information about their specific DNA alteration may become available in the future. Recommendations for screening and other management strategies should be based upon individual circumstances.

Advantages and disadvantages of mutation screening

- May provide an explanation for the family history
- If positive, allows planning of medical intervention or risk-reducing surgery
- May identify an increased risk of other cancers about which the patient had not previously been concerned
- If negative, may permit reduction of screening
- In some cases, may reassure the patient that there is not a single high-risk genetic factor, but if the family history looks very suspicious it can be difficult to explain that someone may still be at risk despite a 'negative result'
- Genetic testing cannot give all the answers

Predictive testing

This will result in one of two results:

1. Positive result: the tested individual is carrying the same pathogenic mutation previously identified in another family member. Carriers will be advised of the implications of this result including lifetime risk of malignancies, current recommendations for screening, and other management options including risk-reducing surgery.

2. Negative (normal) result: the tested individual has not inherited the pathogenic mutation found in other family member(s). Their risk of developing the malignancy in question is therefore the same as the population risk.

Advantages and disadvantages of predictive testing

Advantages
- Provides definitive answer
- If negative, no additional screening is required

- If positive, allows planning of medical intervention or risk-reducing surgery
- Possible relief that fears were justified
- Ability to warn children

Disadvantages
If negative:
- Feelings of guilt if other close family members are positive
- Readjustment of risk perception
- Increased screening will cease (note: this is not necessarily a negative for all people but is related to readjustment of risk)

If positive:
- Definitive answer versus loss of hope of a normal result
- Emotional consequences (guilt that they may have passed this on to children, concerns about their own risk of cancer now confirmed, anger, fear)
- Surgical options may now need to be considered
- How to inform family
- Possible insurance implications in the future

Confidentiality
Unlike other medical conditions about which individuals seek advice, a referral to clinical genetics may have implications not only for the individual referred, but also for the wider family. A family tree will have information collected on the whole family from one or more individuals, who on their own may not know certain pieces of information. Confidentiality is therefore critical. However, problems with duty to inform can also become an issue if individuals do not want a positive mutation result to be shared within the wider family. This could result in other family members assuming incorrectly that they are not at risk of inheriting a cancer predisposition syndrome and prevent them from seeking genetic testing or appropriate screening themselves.

The General Medical Council and Human Genetics Commission recognize that the doctor's duty of confidentiality to the individual may be breached in exceptional circumstances where the patient refuses consent of disclosure. This may include where failure to disclose may expose others to a risk of death or serious harm.

Further reading
Chen S, Euhus DM, Parmigiani G. Quantitative models for prediction of mutations in Lynch syndrome genes. *Curr Col Ca Rep* 2007; 3:206–11.

Couch FJ, Hart SN, Sharma P, et al. Inherited mutations in 17 breast cancer susceptibility genes among a large triple-negative breast cancer cohort unselected for family history of breast cancer. *J Clin Onc* 2014; 33:304–11.

Douglas FS, O'Dair LC, Robinson M, et al. The accuracy of diagnoses as reported in families with cancer: a retrospective study. *J Med Genet* 1999; 36(4):309–12.

Eerola H, Blomqvist C, Pukkala E, et al. Familial breast cancer in southern Finland: how prevalent are breast cancer families and can we trust the family history reported by patients? *Eur J Cancer* 2000; 36(9):1143–8.

Evans DG, Harkness EF, Plaskocinska I, et al. Pathology update to the Manchester Scoring System based on testing in over 4000 families. *J Med Genet* 2017; 54(10):674–81.

Sijmons RH, Boonstra AE, Reefhuis J, et al. Accuracy of family history of cancer: clinical genetic implications. *Eur J Hum Genet* 2000; 8(3):181–6.

Internet resources
BOADICEA: https://pluto.srl.cam.ac.uk/cgi-bin/bd4/v4beta14/bd.cgi

General Medical Council. Guidance for doctors: Confidentiality (2018): http://www.gmc-uk.org/guidance/ethical_guidance/confidentiality.asp

Human Genetics Commission. Inside information—balancing interests in the use of personal genetic data, London: Human Genetics Commission (2002) p.10: http://www.hgc.gov.uk/UploadDocs/DocPub/Document/insideinformation_summary.pdf

NICE guidance: CG41 Familial breast cancer. Classification, care and managing breast cancer and related risks in people with a family history of breast cancer (last updated 20 November 2019): https://www.nice.org.uk/guidance/cg164

2.5 Principles of cancer diagnosis and management

Introduction
Cancer is the second leading cause of death globally, accounting for 9.6 million deaths in 2018 and one in six deaths is due to cancer. It is estimated that by 2050 more than 27 million cancer cases per year will be diagnosed and result in 17.5 million deaths. In the UK, one in three adults will develop some form of cancer during their lifetime and one in four die from cancer.

Patients presenting to their primary care physician with warning signs of cancer (see Chapter 1) should be referred to a specialist centre for urgent evaluation. In the UK and many parts of the world, cancer treatment is organized around a multidisciplinary team (MDT) which consists of physicians, surgeons, cancer specialists, radiologists, pathologists, and clinical nurse specialists. Many investigations for suspected cancer are done either in 'one-stop' (e.g. for breast cancer) or 'two-stop' clinics (e.g. lung cancer) to expedite diagnosis and treatment.

Investigations for a suspected cancer
Initial investigations are to establish a histological diagnosis of cancer, to assess the extent of local disease, and to look for metastatic disease. Further investigations are done to evaluate suitability for standard or trial treatment and to assess the severity of any comorbid medical conditions.

Diagnostic and staging investigations
Diagnostic investigations are usually undertaken in a logical order beginning with blood tests, including relevant tumour markers, and simple imaging such as CXR as appropriate. After this the diagnostic imaging of choice for particular tumour types is undertaken. Histological confirmation of tumour type is often needed and once the histological diagnosis is established, further investigations are undertaken to stage the cancer, assess degree of comorbidities, and evaluate prognostic factors.

Blood tests

Baseline blood tests include full blood count, and liver and renal function tests. Further blood tests will depend on the type of cancer, e.g. lactate dehydrogenase (LDH) for melanoma and lymphoma, beta2-microglobulin for myeloma.

Serum tumour markers

There are several tumour markers (e.g. beta human chorionic gonadotropin, alpha fetoprotein, PSA, CA125, etc.) currently used for diagnosis, monitoring of treatment, assessing prognosis, and follow-up.

Imaging

Imaging helps to determine the extent of local and distant metastatic spread of disease. A CT scan is the diagnostic imaging of choice for most cancers. Additional information may be gained by MRI scan, isotope scans, and functional imaging depending on the site and type of tumour and proposed management plan.

Endoscopy

Direct visualization of the tumour is important for many tumours in body cavities or hollow organs. Endoscopic ear, nose, and throat (ENT) examination; oesophago-gastro-duodenoscopy (OGD) for cancers in the oesophagus, stomach, and duodenum; colonoscopy for bowel tumours; endoscopic retrograde cholangiopancreatography (ERCP) for pancreatic and gall bladder tumours; and cystoscopy for bladder lesions permit the examining clinician to estimate extent of local disease and assess operability. Careful drawings or photos make this information available to other treating clinicians subsequently.

Histology

Confirmation of the diagnosis can be obtained by cytology from a fine needle aspiration or trucut biopsy. Many tumours subsequently require open biopsy for further characterization and immunohistochemical assessment. Biopsies can be obtained by direct vision, or guided by ultrasound, CT, MRI, or endoscopic visualization.

All patients need a definite histological diagnosis if specific cancer treatment is contemplated. Rarely, treatment can be undertaken with only radiological appearance and tumour markers when they are typical (e.g. choriocarcinoma, germ cell tumours).

Pretreatment assessment

As cancer is often a disease of the elderly, as well as determining all the tumour characteristics, full assessment of the patient's general condition and any comorbidities is essential to determine whether treatment should be undertaken with the aim of cure or for palliation with relief of symptoms and improvement in quality of life. Good palliation may, however, still require optimal use of surgery, radiotherapy, or chemotherapy. Diseases such as cardiovascular impairment, diabetes, and renal dysfunction will affect the tolerance and efficacy of treatment and appropriate history, clinical examination, and investigations should inform treatment decisions. Specialist advice should be sought as appropriate.

Standard internationally agreed scales such as Karnofsky or WHO (see following sections) are used to grade performance status, and baseline assessment of quality of life using agreed criteria is commonly carried out for patients eligible for treatment in a clinical trial.

Staging

The purpose of staging is to assess the extent of disease, choose the appropriate treatment, and to assess the likely outcome. Staging is also important to enable comparison of results between treatment centres.

The TNM staging denotes tumour, node, and metastatic status. T staging is generally based on the size of the tumour (usually according to defined size criteria, e.g. in breast cancer) or depth of invasion in hollow organs (e.g. oesophageal cancer, bladder cancer) or local spread to neighbouring organs or subsites (e.g. supraglottic cancer).

N staging is based on pattern of spread along the lymphatic chain, or number of nodes involved, or size of nodes involved. It may be defined as clinical (from examination or imaging) or pathological (from histology).

M1 denotes distant metastasis. Composite staging involves grouping various T, N, and M combinations into four stages. Each tumour site has a different stage grouping. Other descriptors of TNM staging are shown in Table 2.5.1. Other cancers are staged by slightly different systems such as the International Federation of Gynecology and Obstetrics (FIGO) system which is used for many gynaecological cancers.

Prognostic factors

Many factors influence the prognosis of cancer apart from staging. Two generally important prognostic factors are performance status (PS) (discussed in the 'Decision about the most appropriate treatment' section, p. 24) and significant weight loss ($\geq$10% weight loss in the last three months). A poor PS of WHO 3–4 and significant weight loss suggest poor prognosis for many solid tumours.

Multidisciplinary management

In the UK, all patients with suspected cancer are managed within the MDT. This journey starts from the referral with suspected cancer to the end of the treatment and into follow-up or death. The MDT consists of people from different disciplines who can contribute independently to the diagnostic and treatment decisions about patients. The role of multidisciplinary management is to:

- Standardize the treatment, minimizing the influence of bias and personal anecdotal experience
- Improve continuity of care and avoid delays in the management by choosing the most appropriate investigations and treatment
- Improve communication between health professionals
- Improve recruitment to clinical trials
- Improve educational opportunities

Though there are sufficient data to show that multidisciplinary management has improved the consistency of care, evidence showing an improvement in the treatment outcome is still weak.

If medical litigation should arise as a result of an MDT decision, all those present at the meeting would be personally accountable for the decisions related to their expertise, irrespective of whether they have spoken or not in the meeting.

More work is needed to ensure that the undoubted advantage to the patient and clinician of proper multidisciplinary treatment planning is undertaken in the most relevant and effective way, considering the need for informed input about each individual patient and the time constraints of the involved clinicians.

Table 2.5.1 TNM staging descriptors

Prefix	• c: clinical staging—based on physical examination, imaging, and endoscopy
	• p: pathological staging—after surgery and histopathological examination
	   Some tumours have different c and p staging (e.g. breast cancer) whereas others have only
	   p staging (e.g. colon cancer)
	• y: denotes staging after neoadjuvant therapy
	• r: recurrent tumour: restaging following a disease-free interval
	• a: autopsy staging

Grading (G)	• Gx: cannot be assessed • G1: well differentiated • G2: moderately differentiated • G3: poorly differentiated • G4: undifferentiated
L—lymphatic invasion	• Lx: cannot be assessed • L0: no lymphatic invasion • L1: lymphatic invasion
V—venous invasion	• Vx: cannot be assessed • V1: microscopic invasion • V2: macroscopic invasion
R—residual tumour after surgery	• R0: no residual tumour • R1: microscopic residual tumour • R2: macroscopic residual tumour
Multiple tumours	• Multiple tumours in one organ, the tumour with highest T category should be identified and the multiplicity of the number of tumours is indicated in parentheses, e.g. T1 (m) or T1 • In simultaneous bilateral cancers of paired organs, each tumour is classified independently

Source: data from Wittekind C, Brierley JD, Gospodarowicz MK (eds). *TNM Classification of Malignant Tumours*, 8th edn. 2017. John Wiley & Sons, 2017.

Initial consultation and breaking the news

When patients attend oncology clinics, many of them already have some idea about the details of their cancer and an outline of the further management possibilities. However, most patients are still in shock and may take a long time to come to terms with a diagnosis of cancer. The clinician's role is to help the patient to cope with the situation, to give them clear advice on further management, and to explain the intent of treatment.

Decision about the most appropriate treatment

The decision about the appropriate treatment for an individual patient depends on the type of cancer, stage, fitness of the patient, comorbidities which might necessitate modification of standard treatment, and the patient's preference.

Assessing fitness for treatment is an important part of decision-making. It is mainly based on the PS of the patient, active comorbidities at diagnosis, likely responsiveness of the particular tumour type, and an assessment of the likely tolerance of the patient to any planned treatment.

PS helps to quantify the physical well-being of patients and to determine optimal treatment, make treatment modifications (including dose modification of chemotherapy), and to measure the intensity of supportive care required. It should be clearly documented before and throughout treatment. There are a number of scoring systems but the two most commonly used are Karnofsky PS (KPS) and WHO score (Table 2.5.2). Patients are generally eligible for curative treatment only if PS is 0–1, palliative anticancer treatment when PS is 0–2, and generally no anticancer treatment is given if PS is 3–4. However, in certain situations, when the disease is very responsive to treatment and rapid deterioration is due to the current disease process, modified treatment is considered (e.g. for germ cell tumours, lymphomas, melanoma, etc.). If performance status deteriorates rapidly during anticancer treatment, treatment is either stopped or modified.

A proper assessment of active comorbidities is important in predicting side effects from the proposed cancer treatment. For example, patients with severe chronic obstructive pulmonary disease (COPD) with poor pulmonary function tests (FEV1 <1) are not considered for surgery or radical radiotherapy even if the tumour is very small and potentially curable. Similarly, many chemotherapy drugs have systemic organ effects which need to be taken into account when planning anticancer treatment.

Intent of treatment

With the recent progress in multimodality treatment, the distinction in treatment intent between cure and palliation is becoming increasingly difficult. This is because with multiple lines of treatment a significant number of cancer patients may live for years. However, in most cases, after initial assessment, it is possible to clearly define the intent of treatment. In the rest of the patients a proper assessment of the expected benefit versus cure ratio, and the patient's own views are of major importance in devising a plan for treatment.

Palliation

Relief of symptoms and prolongation of good quality of life determine the choice of treatment for those for whom cure cannot be achieved. Multidisciplinary input by palliative care physicians, oncologists, and surgeons may be appropriate and a clear management plan with

Table 2.5.2 Karnofsky performance status (KPS) and World Health Organization (WHO) score

KPS		WHO (KPS)	
Score (%)	Description	Score	Description
100	Normal, no signs of disease	0 (90–100)	Asymptomatic, fully active and able to carry out all pre-disease activities without restriction
90	Capable of normal activity, a few symptoms or signs of disease	1 (70–90)	Symptomatic, restricted in physically strenuous activity but ambulatory and able to carry out light or sedentary work
80	Normal activity with some difficulty. Some symptoms or signs		
70	Self-caring, not capable of normal activity or work	2 (50–70)	Capable of all self-care but unable to carry out any work activities; <50% in bed during day
60	Needs some help with care, can take care of most personal requirements		
50	Help required often; frequent medical care needed	3 (30–50)	Capable of only limited self-care; >50% in bed during the day
40	Disabled, requires special care and help		
30	Severely disabled, hospital admission needed but no risk of death	4 (10–30)	Completely disabled and cannot do any self-care. Totally confined to bed or chair
20	Very ill, needs urgent admission and requires supportive care		
10	Moribund, rapidly progressive fatal disease		
0	Death	5	Death

Adapted with permission from Oken MM, Creech RH, Tormey DC, et al. Toxicity and response criteria of the Eastern Cooperative Oncology Group. *Am J Clin Oncol* 1982; 5(6):649–55. Copyright © 1982 Wolters Kluwer Health, Inc.

well-defined responsibilities is needed to ensure that the patient is well cared for.

Internet and information overload
Patients who are anxious for more information may search the Internet. If they do not have the knowledge to sift this information appropriately, their anxiety may be increased and their need for medical time paradoxically may therefore be increased. With inappropriate information overload many patients suffer a phase which is like being on an emotional roller coaster. Information sources, such as those available through the national programme in the UK (Macmillan), are helpful but often considered inadequate by patients consciously or subconsciously seeking to know that they will be cured. Valuable additional support is given by specialist nurses and through support and information centres where facilities such as counselling, relaxation, and alternative treatments are valued by many.

Implementing planned treatment
For many early-stage cancers, delay in treatment is proven to compromise the chances of cure (e.g. germ cell tumours) and in tumours with rapid proliferation (e.g. Burkitt's lymphoma which has a doubling time of <24 hours) even a few days delay in initiating treatment can be detrimental. Hence it is important to start curative treatment as soon as possible.

There is good evidence that interruptions in radical radiotherapy treatments for some cancers, such as those in the head and neck, also lead to poorer control rates and adjustment using twice-daily treatments is therefore made if a gap in treatment occurs. It is not clear how important is initial delay for tumours that are not growing very quickly relative to other tumour prognostic factors but with the introduction of cancer treatment time targets as in the UK any risk is minimized.

Follow-up during treatment
Follow-up during treatment is undertaken to assess response to treatment, monitor toxicity, and modify further treatment. Toxicity should be monitored alongside treatment so that patients receiving a three-weekly cycle of chemotherapy will be seen every three weeks before each treatment to modify the dose or adjust supportive treatments. Patients who have had significant toxicities with a previous cycle may be seen in between the cycle dates. Patients undergoing radiotherapy will often be seen at least once weekly throughout their treatment to assess acute toxicities and prescribe supportive measures as necessary.

The optimal timing to assess tumour response to treatment varies depends on the type of cancer treatment. For example, radiotherapy and hormonal agents generally take three to four months to show any response to treatment whereas chemotherapy response is faster (six to nine weeks). Hence, investigations to assess response to treatment should be planned according to the appropriate timescale. However, if there is any clinical suspicion of progression during treatment, prompt investigations are required without waiting for any planned investigations.

Second opinions
A second opinion about treatment options may be sought by the clinician in the case of very rare tumours where there is no local expertise. Formalized referral patterns for specialized surgery have been developed in

the UK (e.g. surgery for osteosarcoma is centralized to a few units). A well-functioning MDT will also fulfil this need for clinicians.

Patients may seek a second opinion if they are unsure of the expertise of the person to whom they have been referred, particularly if they are privately insured or have medical connections. Facilitation of such a request by the person to whom the patient has first been referred can be helpful in enabling them to confidently pursue treatment locally. People giving second opinions have a duty to advise constructively and within any unavoidable constraints. They should avoid undermining other clinicians and work collaboratively.

However, patients in the UK should be clearly informed, when there are national protocols or agreed practices and the diagnosis and treatment are uncontroversial, that a second opinion is unlikely to be useful. Healthcare resources within a publicly funded service must be used in a cost-effective way and seeking second opinions should be limited wherever possible to difficult situations or where patient–doctor relations will preclude good care.

Support during treatment

From the moment of diagnosis of cancer, a person's life is changed forever. It affects not only their physical health but their mental health is also challenged. Different individuals deal with this process in different ways, but each should be offered appropriate support for their needs. This may involve psychological support or something more practical such as directing them to possible sources of financial support. Many people are working at the time of diagnosis and their future employment may be affected depending on their job and employer. Laws exist to protect individuals but those who are self-employed will only be protected if they had pre-existing insurance. Relationships are frequently challenged by the diagnosis of cancer and the journey through treatment and it is not uncommon for couples to separate at this time. Financial worries may continue after treatment is completed as the diagnosis of cancer affects the ability to gain new life insurance or a mortgage. Those living in countries which require health insurance will notice an increase in premiums or difficulty obtaining further health insurance. Holiday planning may be affected by difficulty in getting insurance cover.

Local health providers such as GPs will have a key role in coordinating some of the aftercare for patients and providing additional necessary services such as physiotherapy and occupational therapy.

At the time of diagnosis, an individual should therefore be provided with sources of information to help them through all these areas to facilitate their treatment and return to health. The key areas are:

- Psychosocial support
- Income support
- Macmillan team
- Cancer care in the community

The potential sources of this support can be in the form of documentation of helpful websites or organizations, local cancer support groups, and named key workers such as specialist nurses or Macmillan nurses. It should be emphasized at the start of diagnosis and treatment that it is natural to require the help of others at some point in the journey and that this will help their overall outcome. The special needs of children diagnosed with cancer and their family require expert consideration.

Follow-up after treatment and management of recurrence

Almost all patients who have been treated with curative intent need some regular follow-up to detect an early potentially curable recurrence or a second cancer. The frequency and mode of follow-up depend on the pattern of recurrence of individual cancers, which are dealt with for each cancer in the appropriate chapter. It is still debatable whether early detection of a metastatic recurrence improves overall survival (OS) in most cancers, but continuing care and support of the patient are always important for their overall well-being.

Beyond cure and survivorship

For many patients treatment will be possible and they will succeed in climbing the mountain of diagnosis, treatment, and its complications. However, the long-term impact of this on their lives must not be underestimated and many patients feel at their most lost at the end of treatment or when follow-up is discontinued (see also 'Late effects' in Chapter 16, p. 462). An understanding of this process will help facilitate any further care that is necessary to return them to a functional life.

Internet resources

Macmillan Cancer Support charity: http://www.macmillan.org.uk
TNM staging on UICC site: http://www.uicc.org

2.6 Principles of surgical oncology

Introduction
Surgery accounts for approximately 60% of all cancer cures. It also has a significant role in the prevention, diagnosis, palliation, and rehabilitation of the cancer patient. After extensive curative surgery, the resultant impairment of appearance and function can be corrected to a certain extent by reconstructive surgery (oncoplastic surgery) to restore body image and to enable the patient to return to a normally functioning life.

Role of surgery in diagnosis and staging
Diagnosis
Obtaining a histological diagnosis is an essential step in the management of cancer. The various techniques used to obtain a histological diagnosis include fine needle aspiration (FNA) cytology, core biopsy, incisional biopsy, and excisional biopsy. The choice of a particular technique is based on the location of tumour, anticipated type of tumour, and the reliability of the method to make a definite diagnosis.

The role of FNA is diminishing as it does not yield sufficient material for detailed pathological evaluation.

In needle biopsy, a core of tissue is obtained which helps to visualize architecture as well as to perform immunohistochemical studies. It is useful in the diagnosis of most tumours.

Incisional biopsy involves removal of a small wedge of tissue from a large tumour and is indicated when core biopsy is non-diagnostic and an excision biopsy is inappropriate. A common situation is a suspected sarcoma. Care should be taken when planning any incision biopsy to ensure that the site of biopsy is within the area of definitive surgery and preferably is done by surgeons who will undertake the final surgery. A poorly planned incision biopsy can lead to unnecessary morbid surgery.

Excision biopsy involves removal of the entire mass or skin lesion. It is important to make sure that this procedure does not compromise a later wider excision if necessary. The specimen needs to be oriented in three dimensions and marked for the pathologist to determine surgical margins.

Frozen section is occasionally used perioperatively to confirm the diagnosis when previous histological diagnosis is not available (e.g. solitary lung lesions), to decide need for further surgery (e.g. lymph node dissection), and ensure adequate surgical margins.

Placement of surgical clips during the biopsy is useful in patients who will undergo neoadjuvant chemotherapy (helps to identify the site of primary tumour during later surgery in cases of complete response) and in those who need definitive radiotherapy to a localized area.

Staging
Various surgical procedures such as endoscopy and laparoscopy help to define the extent of disease as well as obtaining histological confirmation of metastatic disease (see later in section).

Role of surgery in treatment
Curative surgery
Surgery plays an important role in achieving a cure when the cancer is confined to the site of origin. A decision regarding curative surgery is made after careful consideration of various patient- and tumour-related characteristics at a multidisciplinary meeting with surgeons, oncologists, radiologists, and pathologists. Patient-related factors which influence the choice of curative surgery include age, performance status, and comorbidities. Tumour-related factors include the chances of long-term benefit and potential surgical risks and complications.

Surgery of the primary tumour
Curative surgery is aimed at removal of the tumour with a clear margin of normal tissue ('R0' resection) with reconstruction of the surgical defect if appropriate. The margin of normal tissue removed depends on the type of malignancy and pattern of local spread. An adequate gross margin helps to ensure an adequate microscopic margin of resection. The tumour should be orientated and marked at the time of surgery so that any positive margins can be identified anatomically should the need for re-excision arise.

Based on the extent of removal of cancer, resections are classified as follows as part of the TNM staging:
- R0: all margins are histologically free of tumour
- R1: microscopic residual disease after resection
- R2: gross residual disease after resection

At the time of surgery, exposure of tumour with the risk of shedding viable tumour cells should be avoided if possible. Certain tumours have a propensity to recur along surgical incision lines or drainage sites, e.g. sarcoma.

Depending on the type of cancer and anatomical site, curative surgery can be:
- Wide excision—the tumour is removed with a margin to account for microscopic spread
- Removal of part of an organ and surrounding tissue at risk of spread (e.g. partial gastrectomy)
- Removal of an entire organ with or without important adjacent structures (e.g. total abdominal hysterectomy with bilateral salpingo-oophorectomy)

Recent advances in multimodality treatment, the use of radiotherapy, chemotherapy, or both has led to the use of less radical procedures with an improvement in quality of life.

Surgery of regional lymph nodes
In some tumours, regional lymph node spread occurs in a predictable fashion. In such situations, the regional lymph nodes in continuity with lymphatics are removed along with the primary tumour. The removal of lymph nodes provides important staging information and if there is nodal involvement often results in a therapeutic gain, in terms of reducing the risk of a regional recurrence and thus preventing further morbidity.

In patients with an unknown or low risk of lymph node involvement, various methods are used to screen for pathological involvement of lymph nodes before extensive lymph node dissection is undertaken. These methods include:
- FNA of enlarged regional lymph nodes
- Node sampling—involves cherry picking of four to five regional lymph nodes (e.g. breast cancer)

- Sentinel node biopsy (SNB)—which is based on the principle that the tumour spreads to a single (sentinel) node before spreading to other nodes in an 'orderly' fashion. Sentinel lymph nodes can be identified by using blue dye or radioisotopes

In many clinical situations, the role of lymph node dissection in OS remains controversial. In practice, patients with positive sentinel lymph nodes undergo a complete node dissection whereas the role of elective lymph node dissection is dependent on the site of cancer, type of cancer, and other prognostic factors. Benefits of nodal dissections in different cancers are discussed in the relevant chapters.

Metastatectomy

Resection of a single metastatic lesion results in better survival for a selected group of patients with certain cancers (see Table 2.6.1). Metastatectomy is also an option for patients with a limited number of metastases (oligometastasis). This approach is especially suitable for a patient with good PS who has limited disease which does not respond well to systemic treatment, has surgically resectable metastatic disease at presentation or recurs with limited disease a long time (at least 12 months) after successful treatment of the primary tumour.

In the absence of proper randomized studies, it is not known whether the observed therapeutic benefit of metastatectomy is real or due to the strict selection process (selection bias). Studies show that resection of isolated or limited liver metastases in colorectal cancer results in 20–40% five-year survival. Pulmonary metastatectomy in sarcomas leads to a five-year survival of 20–30%. An alternative to metastatectomy is the evolving use of radiofrequency (RF) ablation.

Debulking surgery

In certain situations, debulking surgery is useful in improving the ability of other treatments to control the residual tumour (e.g. ovarian cancer) and in some cancers maximal cytoreduction is associated with a better outcome (e.g. ovarian cancer and glioblastoma multiforme (GBM)).

Salvage surgery

Surgery is useful as a salvage measure after primary treatment failure or recurrence after definitive treatment. It is only appropriate for fit patients with a good chance of prolonged survival. Examples include abdomino-perineal resection after chemoradiotherapy for anal cancer, and exenteration in cervical cancer after chemoradiotherapy.

In patients with prior limited surgery or chemoradiotherapy, a second chance of cure is aimed at with salvage surgery. Examples include mastectomy for local recurrence after conservative surgery for breast cancer and neck node dissection for isolated nodal recurrence after chemoradiotherapy for head and neck cancer.

Table 2.6.1 Role of metastatectomy

Liver	Selected patients with colorectal cancer
Lung	Selected patients with colorectal, renal, and testicular cancers and sarcoma
Adrenal	Selected patients with resectable lung cancer and isolated adrenal disease
Brain	Solitary metastasis with controlled/potentially curable systemic disease

Table 2.6.2 Potential indications for risk-reducing surgery

Surgery	Indication
Bilateral mastectomy	BRCA1/2 mutations Familial breast cancer Unilateral breast cancer <40 years
Bilateral oophorectomy	BRCA1/2 mutations Familial ovarian cancer
Total proctocolectomy	FAP or APC mutations HNPCC—germline mutations
Thyroidectomy	RET oncogene mutation MEN2

Palliative and emergency surgery

The aim of palliative surgery is to improve or prevent significant symptoms (e.g. pain, bleeding, and obstruction) which are likely to occur without intervention.

Emergency surgery has a role in life-threatening bleeding, perforation and obstruction of an abdominal viscus, and neurological compression.

Reconstructive (oncoplastic) surgery

Extensive resection often results in the disruption of normal anatomy with subsequent impaired cosmesis and function. Plastic surgical techniques are useful in correcting the anatomical defects and improving cosmesis (e.g. reconstructive breast surgery) and function (e.g. in head and neck surgery).

Risk reduction surgery

Fewer than 5% of patients have a genetic component to their cancer. Increasing understanding of the development of genetically associated cancers has led to prophylactic surgery for some patients. Table 2.6.2 shows the indications for common prophylactic surgeries. Appropriate genetic testing and counselling is, however, an absolute prerequisite before any prophylactic surgery. Women with BRCA1 and BRCA2 mutations have a high risk of breast cancer which is reduced by 90–95% with bilateral mastectomy. However, the decision to undergo prophylactic mastectomy should be made after careful discussion, exploring future quality of life, potential surgical risks, and wishes of the patient. Alternative risk reduction methods such as use of tamoxifen and prophylactic oophorectomy after completion of family should also be considered.

Minimal access and robotic surgery

The role of minimal access and robotic surgery is being increasingly studied in the management of solid tumours.

Laparoscopy has an established role in the staging of many abdominal malignancies. It is useful in identifying peritoneal metastases which are easily missed on anatomical imaging. It is also helpful to correctly stage patients who might otherwise have been overstaged with anatomical imaging. Preoperative laparoscopy has significantly reduced the rates of 'open and close' laparotomies. An example is the use of laparoscopy to detect small peritoneal and liver metastases which reduces the number of 'open and close' laparotomies to <5% in stomach cancer. Laparoscopy has an established role in the staging of oesophageal and stomach cancer. It has a limited role in the staging of pancreatic and liver cancers. Its role in the staging of gynaecological and testicular cancers is evolving.

Laparoscopy has also been evaluated as a treatment option for abdominal malignancies and studies show that laparoscopic surgery results in the same long-term survival as that of open surgery, with no increased risk of abdominal wall recurrence, less surgical morbidity, and faster return to normal function. Laparoscopic surgery is an accepted surgical treatment for gastric, renal, adrenal, and colorectal cancers.

Laparoscopic stapled gastrojejunostomy is a treatment option for the palliation of gastric outlet obstruction in gastric and pancreatic cancer. In intestinal obstruction, a laparoscopic bypass procedure or intestinal stoma creation procedure results in prompt relief of symptoms.

Video-assisted thoracic surgery for stage I lung cancer has been studied recently as an attractive option for the treatment of elderly patients with lung cancer.

Robotic-assisted surgery is being studied in prostate and renal cell cancers. This technique may result in minimal surgical trauma with a better toxicity profile.

Image-guided surgery

Recently, image-guided surgery is being investigated to improve R0 rates. Image guidance is used to distinguish between normal and malignant tissue. Stereotactic neurosurgery uses 3D volumetric reconstructions of advanced MRI images, including blood oxygen level dependent fMRI (BOLD) and tractography to ensure optimal excision of brain tumours with sparing of important functional areas and tracts. Various optimal imaging techniques are under evaluation. Examples include spectroscopic imaging and optical coherence tomography for the intraoperative assessment of breast cancer. Fluorescence imaging is another evolving technique. 5-aminolevulinic acid (5-ALA)-guided resection has an established role in the resection of glioblastoma. Real time fluorescence-guided surgery is being evaluated in other tumours such as hepatocellular carcinoma and hepatic metastases.

Further reading

Azagury DE, Dua MM, Barrese JC, et al. Image guided surgery. *Curr Probl Surg* 2015; 52(12):476–520.

Iqbal H, Pan Q. Image guided surgery in the management of head and neck cancer. *Oral Oncol* 2016; 57:32–9.

Mondal SB, Gao S, Zhu N, et al. Real-time fluorescence image-guided oncologic surgery. *Adv Cancer Res* 2014; 124:171–211.

2.7 Radiotherapy

Role in the treatment of cancer

Radiotherapy is an extremely effective local treatment for cancer and is used in at least 50% of patients in whom cure is achieved. As well as treatment given with the aim of local control and cure, radiotherapy is widely used to palliate symptoms of advanced cancer. It may be given as the sole curative treatment, e.g. for carcinoma of the cervix, as adjuvant therapy after surgery, e.g. for breast cancer, or in combination with chemotherapy, as in head and neck cancer. Recently radiotherapy is being studied as a treatment for oligo-metastatic cancers with a view to improving long-term control or even to achieve a chance of cure.

Mode of action

Radiotherapy uses electromagnetic radiation (X-rays, gamma rays, or electrons) at the high-energy end of the spectrum. The unit of dose is Gy which is defined as 1 joule of energy deposited in 1kg of tissue. Energy deposition in the tissues through which the X-rays pass causes ionization, which in turn produces free radicals, fragments of molecules with an unpaired electron, which interact either directly or indirectly to produce DNA damage. This damage can manifest as single- or double-strand breaks, base damage, DNA or protein cross links, protein–protein cross links, and intra- or interstrand cross links.

One unrepaired double-strand break is enough to kill the cell. Mitotic cell death is the main mechanism of cell death following irradiation. Cells do not generally show evidence of damage until they divide.

The effects of radiation on tissues depend on dose as shown in the diagram for tumour control probability (TCP) and normal tissue complication probability (NTCP) (see Figure 2.7.1). The effects of radiotherapy on normal tissue depend on the volume treated, total dose given, and fractionation schedule used, and whether the tissue has a large functional reserve capacity (parallel organization) such as lung and kidney, or a serial organization like the spinal cord or gut, which means that damage to a small segment only may result in severe injuries such as paralysis. When there is little or no functional reserve, dose is more important than volume.

The ability to give high enough doses to local tumours to destroy them is dependent on fractionation of total dose to exploit underlying biological factors. Recovery of radiation damage between fractions of treatment occurs more readily in normal tissues than in tumour. Between fractions, cells may redistribute into a more radiosensitive phase of the cell cycle, or hypoxic radiation-resistant cells become re-oxygenated and more sensitive as surrounding well-oxygenated cells are killed. The amount of cell kill can also depend on the radiosensitivity of the tumour—for example, lymphomas are very radiosensitive while melanoma is resistant. The overall time in which treatment is given is also important and shorter treatment times allow less repopulation by tumour cells.

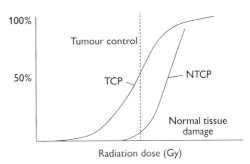

Fig. 2.7.1 TCP and NTCP.

Various fractionation schemes are used. Classically, doses of 60–70Gy in 2Gy/fraction treating five times weekly are used for radical treatments of squamous carcinomas. Different schedules using shorter treatment times (acceleration), several smaller doses per day (hyperfractionation), or fewer large fractions (hypofractionation) can be useful in specific situations.

Types of radiotherapy treatment

Superficial X-rays (orthovoltage)

Low-energy X-rays can be produced by an orthovoltage machine (formerly known as deep X-rays or DXT). The mode of interaction with tissues is by the photoelectric effect rather than by Compton scattering as occurs with high-energy X-rays. This effect depends on the density of tissue and there is therefore maximum absorption of the X-rays in the skin because of their low penetration, and in bone because of its high density. They are therefore used to treat skin tumours, and to palliate metastasis in superficial bones such as the ribs. Erythema of the skin is seen as an acute reaction, and telangiectasia may develop later.

Brachytherapy

Sources of radioactive material may be inserted directly into body cavities such as the uterus and vagina. The dose distribution from such sources gives a conformal treatment, with very high doses close to the surface of the source and rapid fall-off of dose thereafter. Normal tissues are therefore better protected, although great care must be taken to avoid hotspots where high doses in a small area may produce damage (for example, in pelvic treatments) and care must be taken that there are no small bowel loops adjacent to the high-dose region. Originally, radium was used for brachytherapy, but has now been replaced with caesium, cobalt, or iridium. Afterloading techniques, in which hollow source carriers are placed in situ and their position checked before loading with the active source, have helped to reduce doses to personnel. Doses much higher than can be delivered by external beam radiotherapy can be used to control local disease.

Melanoma of the choroid may be treated with iodine-125 or ruthenium-106 plaque brachytherapy. Brachytherapy with iridium wire may be used in conjunction with external beam therapy to deliver a high local dose for some soft tissue sarcomas, to treat recurrent disease in neck nodes, and to give a local boost in breast cancer. Localized prostate cancer may be treated by permanently implanting iodine-125 seeds or with iridium wire loaded temporarily into flexible catheters.

Radio isotopes

These are most commonly used in the treatment of well-differentiated thyroid cancer with iodine-131 which is specifically taken up by the thyroid, thyroid cancer, and its metastases. An initial dose is given to ablate normal thyroid tissue which takes up the isotope most avidly, and this is followed by therapeutic doses to treat the cancer. Strontium-89 and samarium-153 are used for the relief of cancer-induced bone pain, particularly from prostate cancer. Phosphorus-32 can be used in the treatment of polycythaemia rubra vera. Radium-223 (an isotope of radium which has a half-life of 11.4 days) is currently indicated for bone metastases in prostatic cancer.

Megavoltage radiotherapy

Modern linear accelerators accelerate electrons by subjecting them to a series of oscillating electrical potentials in a wave guide. These accelerated electrons can be used directly for therapy, or they can be made to hit a target which produces high-energy X-rays. A series of collimators are used to produce a focused beam which can be further shaped with a series of lead rods in the head of the machine known as a multileaf collimator. Energies in the range of 6–16MV or MeV are commonly used for external beam therapy.

Particle beam therapy

Compared with megavoltage radiotherapy, particle beams offer more precise dose localization and favourable dose–depth distribution, which might theoretically improve the therapeutic ratio of radiotherapy. Proton (the most commonly used particle) beam treatment facilities have rapidly increased globally in the last few years. Protons have a pattern of dose distribution which shows a sharply defined range of energy deposition (the Bragg peak) rather than the attenuation pattern of photons. While this can be favourable for treatment of some tumour types such as skull-based tumours, spinal chondrosarcoma, and some paediatric tumours, a number of studies are also evaluating its role in common tumours. While current studies do not conclusively show superiority of proton beam therapy compared with conventional megavoltage therapy in terms of clinical outcomes, the clinical use of proton beam therapy is likely to increase in the near future, mainly due to widespread availability of these facilities and intense media coverage of the potential theoretical benefits.

Other particle beams currently undergoing evaluation include carbon, helium, neon, and silicon ions.

Radiotherapy techniques

Three-dimensional (3D) conformal radiotherapy delivers high-dose radiotherapy to the tumour target volume with minimal dose to the surrounding normal tissue. It has been further refined with the arrival of advanced computer abilities to develop intensity-modulated radiotherapy (IMRT) and image-guided radiotherapy (IGRT).

IMRT makes it possible to modify the radiation intensity of individual treatments beams during the delivery of radiotherapy, which enables the delivery of different dose levels to different areas within the target volume. While IMRT delivers highly conformal radiotherapy to the target volume with a lesser amount of radiotherapy to critical organs at risk (OARs) compared with conformal radiotherapy, the treatment time can be prolonged, and a larger area of normal issue gets lower doses of radiotherapy. Lower doses of radiotherapy to a larger area of normal tissue are associated with a theoretically increased risk of second malignancies, which can be an issue particularly in children.

IGRT uses images obtained during treatment to check that the actual treatment delivered corresponds to that which was planned by gating it to a specific phase of respiration. Adaptive radiotherapy involves changing treatment on a daily or less frequent basis by comparison of planning scans with images taken during treatment.

Tomographic devices can be used to deliver gated rotational IMRT using a multileaf collimator and a machine-mounted CT scanner. Images taken during treatment are used to gate dose delivery to the correct body slice.

Stereotactic radiotherapy

This technique, using multiple highly collimated (focused) beams, can be used to deliver very high doses to small volumes either as a single dose (called radiosurgery) or with fractionated treatments. A high degree of immobilization with a stereotactic frame is essential (1mm). Stereotactic radiosurgery (SRS) and radiotherapy (SRT) have been developed initially for the management of brain tumours. The principles have recently been adopted to treat diseases at extracranial sites such as lung, liver, spine, etc. The technique is called stereotactic ablative body radiotherapy (SABR).

SABR has an established role in the management of early-stage medically inoperable non-small cell lung cancer. SABR is being studied for prostate and hepatocellular cancer, oligo-metastatic diseases of the lungs and spine, and re-irradiation.

The radiotherapy process

The process of radiotherapy planning can be divided into several phases.

Collection of relevant data

Clinical assessment and decision for radical or palliative treatment, taking into account the extent of disease and any comorbidities, is critical.

Collection of data from appropriate imaging techniques is necessary for target volume definition using internationally standardized criteria. Planning of treatment and estimation of dose distribution relies on electron density measurements and therefore a CT scan is essential. This must be done with the patient in the treatment position using any immobilization devices appropriate.

Techniques for fusing information from CT and MRI scans give the best definition of tumour volume for a number of disease sites and positron emission tomography (PET) scanning may contribute as well.

Several volumes must be defined using the criteria of the International Commission on Radiation Units (ICRU; see Figure 2.7.2). The gross target volume (GTV) is the macroscopic extent of tumour determined from imaging

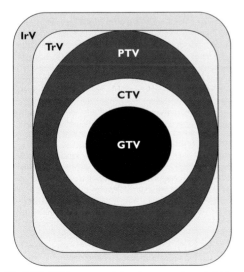

Fig. 2.7.2 ICRU recommendations for target volume definition. IrV irradiated volume; TrV treatment volume.

the entire tumour mass or as defined surgically and pathologically.

The clinical target volume (CTV) includes a margin around the GTV to encompass any subclinical or microscopic disease. A planning target volume (PTV) is then defined to ensure that the CTV remains within the volume that is actually treated each day, taking into account any movement that occurs physiologically, by the patient changing their position, or from errors in setting up the treatment in the same way each day.

These errors can be minimized using immobilization devices to help the patient to maintain the same position for treatment each day. They include the use of arm supports, foot restraints, vacuum bags which can be moulded to support the area being treated, or customized shells made individually using thermoplastic materials (particularly used for head and neck and brain treatments).

Another source of day-to-day variability arises from physiological changes which may be predictable, such as those with respiration, in which case radiation delivery can be gated to a particular phase of respiration to ensure the tumour is always included in the treatment volume. Physiological movements of bowel and bladder are unpredictable and although several studies have explored ways of reducing them, such as by the use of bladder-filling protocols or routine enemas, there is at present no satisfactory solution. Implanted fiducial markers such as gold grains or clips may be helpful in ensuring reproducibility of treatment set up.

Devising an optimal treatment plan/calculation of dose distributions

This is usually done by a physicist or radiation technologist. As the dose from each beam of radiation from the linear accelerator is attenuated as it passes through tissue, the dose in tissues outside the tumour will be greater than that to a deep-seated tumour. Multiple beams are therefore used to deliver a homogeneous dose throughout the tumour while minimizing dose to other normal tissues through which each beam must pass. Conventional plans often use three beams, but intensity modulated radiotherapy may use as many as seven. The distribution of dose may also be modified by insertion of a wedge of absorbing material into the beam so that less dose is delivered through the thick end of the wedge. Beams can be shaped to conform to the tumour using the multileaf collimator in the head of the linear accelerator.

Dose–volume histograms (DVHs) are used to help choose the best plan. A DVH is a plot of the radiation dose against the volume of the structure of interest and the shape and area under the curve is used to ensure that the target volume is covered with a homogeneous dose and that dose to normal structures is within acceptable limits (see Table 2.7.1).

With IMRT, multiple beam segments of variable intensity are defined. These are used to modulate dose and ensure maximum tumour conformality. It also makes it possible to limit dose to normal organs more effectively. As acute side effects are therefore reduced, dose escalation, leading to improved tumour control, may be possible.

Delivery of treatment and verification of accuracy

Radical treatments (other than those for superficial skin tumours where low-energy X-rays are used) are given using a linear accelerator with high energy photons or electrons (6–16MV linear accelerator). The multileaf

Table 2.7.1 Radiation tolerance dose (Gy) for conventional radiotherapy and SABR/SRS

	Conventional radiotherapy (2Gy per fraction)	SABR/SRS	Dose limiting side effects (at a rate of ≤5% at five years)
Brain	Dmax <60	V12 <5–10cc for SRS	Symptomatic necrosis
Brain stem	Dmax <54	Dmax <12.5 for SRS	Necrosis/cranial neuropathy
Bladder	Dmax <65 V65 ≤50%, V70 ≤53%, V80≤15%	–	Grade ≥3 late toxicity
Heart	Pericardium: mean dose <26 and V30 <46% Whole organ: V25 <10%	–	Pericarditis
Kidney	Bilateral whole kidney: mean <15–18 V20 <32%, V28 <20%	–	Renal dysfunction
Lens	10	–	Cataract
Liver	Whole liver GTV: No pre-existing liver disease: mean dose <30–32 Pre-existing liver disease: mean dose <28	Whole liver GTV: 3 fractions <13–15 6 fractions <18–20 Dmax to >700 of normal liver: 15	Hepatitis
Lung	Whole lung: V20 ≤30% and mean dose <20Gy	–	≤20% rate of symptomatic pneumonitis
Oesophagus	Whole organ: mean dose <34	60	Grade ≥3 late toxicity
Optic apparatus	Dmax <55	Dmax <12 (for SRS)	Blindness
Parotid	Bilateral mean dose <25 Unilateral mean dose <20	–	Xerostomia
Rectum	V50 <50%, V60 <35%, V65 <25%, V70 <20%, and V75 <15%	–	Grade ≥2 late toxicity
Small intestine	Individual bowel loops: V15 <120cc Entire peritoneal bag: V45 <195cc	–	Obstruction, perforation
Spinal cord	Dmax <60	Dmax <13 (for one fraction) and <20 (for three fractions)	Myelopathy

collimator is adjusted to conform to the tumour shape in three dimensions. Accuracy of treatment delivery is checked in various ways including measurement of exit doses by in vivo dosimetry using thermoluminescent dosemeters or diodes and analysis of images taken during treatment.

Monitoring treatment effects

Side effects of radiation are classified as early (occurring at <90 days) or late (>90 days). Late effects are much more dependent on dose per fraction, being more severe with high doses per fraction. Overall treatment time affects acute responses, which are increased when treatment times are short and which, in contrast with late effects, are reversible. Unlike the side effects of chemotherapy which are systemic, radiotherapy side effects are local or regional, manifested in the irradiated area only. Acute effects include skin and mucosal damage predominantly. Late effects are the result of vascular damage and fibrosis. They are modified by pre-existing comorbidities such as hypertension or diabetes mellitus, where end-vessel disease may occur.

Other factors which are important include individual radiosensitivity, smoking, age, dose delivered, volume treated, dose per fraction, overall treatment time, type of radiation, concomitant chemotherapy, radiotherapy technique, type of tumour, proximity of any organs at risk, tumour size, tissue type, and structural organization. The effectiveness of any new technique with

combinations of drugs with radiation must be assessed in terms of improved therapeutic ratio and the pattern of relapse, whether within or outside the radiation treatment volume, as well as in overall or disease-free survival.

Tables of maximum tolerated doses to various organs have been devised. The maximum tolerated doses are different for conventional radiotherapy and stereotactic approaches and are shown in Table 2.7.1. Long-term follow-up of patients treated with radiotherapy is important as data on late effects always reflects treatments given some time previously. The use of different combinations of chemotherapy or other novel biological agents may alter the pattern of radiation late effects which are seen and necessitate changes in treatment approach.

Further reading

Folkert MR, Timmerman RD. Stereotactic ablative body radiosurgery (SABR) or stereotactic body radiation therapy (SBRT). *Adv Drug Deliv Rev* 2017; 109:3–14.

International Commission on Radiation Units and Measurements. *Prescribing, Recording and Reporting Photon Beam Therapy*. ICRU Report 50, Bethesda, MD: Nuclear Technology Publishing, 1993.

Marks LB, Yorke ED, Jackson A, et al. Use of normal tissue complication probability models in the clinic. *Int J Radiat Oncol Biol Phys* 2010; 76(Suppl. 3):S10–19.

Mohan R, Grosshans D. Proton therapy—present and future. *Adv Drug Deliv Rev* 2017; 109:26–44.

The Royal College of Radiologists. *Radiotherapy Dose-Fractionation*. London: The Royal College of Radiologists, 2016.

2.8 Systemic therapy

Introduction
Systemic therapy for cancer encompasses a broad range of treatments that are delivered and absorbed systemically. This therefore comprises traditional cytotoxic chemotherapy, hormonal therapies, molecularly targeted agents, and immunotherapies.

Aims of systemic treatment
Curative: Certain tumours display such chemo-sensitivity they are considered curable by conventional cytotoxics alone even when advanced or metastatic (e.g. germ cell neoplasms, high-grade lymphoma, acute leukaemias, and many paediatric malignancies). If chemotherapy is given with curative intent, short-term toxicity is considered more acceptable and as a consequence, intensive support is offered in the event of severe side effects. Long-term toxicities or complications of these 'curative' treatments must be considered in cancer survivors.

Palliative: When cure is not possible, systemic agents may be administered to palliate the adverse effects of the tumour such as pain, weight loss, or local symptoms related to the tumour location and effect on normal structures. As well as improving symptoms and overall quality of life, this approach can improve survival outcomes in some cancer types.

Adjuvant: Adjuvant therapy is administered following a definitive local treatment such as surgery or radiation which removes all clinically apparent disease, in order to eliminate micrometastatic disease and reduce the risk of disease relapse.

Neoadjuvant: Chemotherapy given before definitive surgery or radiotherapy is increasingly being used as a treatment for localized cancers before attempting curative surgery. The aim of this therapy is to treat micrometastases not visible on conventional imaging. It may also reduce the size of the tumour, permitting surgery, or allowing a less radical procedure to be undertaken.

Chemoradiotherapy: Chemotherapy such as fluorouracil can act as a radiosensitiser for radiotherapy such that the combination approach is sometimes more effective than either modality alone. This approach may be used for downstaging bulky tumours that might otherwise have been unresectable.

Chemotherapy
Chemotherapy is now a fundamental component in the systemic treatment of cancer. Classical cytotoxic chemotherapy comprises agents that affect cell division or cause cell death by means of damaging DNA directly or indirectly, and their systemic delivery enables activity at all disease sites, including micrometastatic lesions.

Although chemotherapy can be toxic to non-proliferating cells, it is preferentially cytocidal to actively proliferating cells. Cancer cells may show variable vulnerability due to differential proliferation rates, but they may also be defective in their ability to repair DNA damage, thereby limiting efficient repopulation after cytotoxic injury. Chemotherapy is therefore administered with repeated, regular intervals known as treatment cycles. A gap between cycles is necessary to allow normal tissue to recover and theoretically the administration of successive doses of chemotherapy will kill a constant fraction of cells, rather than a constant number. However, factors such as heterogeneity in tumour cell sensitivity and effective drug delivery with each course can lead to an unpredictable tumour response.

Chemotherapeutic agents may be cell cycle phase specific, killing proliferating cells only during a specific period of the cell cycle. Such drugs include antimetabolites and vinca alkaloids. Alternatively, they can have significant activity in multiple phases and are classified as cell cycle phase non-specific (see Table 2.8.1). These drugs, which include alkylating agents and platinum derivatives, have an equal effect on tumour and normal cells whether they are in the proliferating or resting phase. They have a linear dose–response curve such that the greater the dose of the drug, the greater the fractional kill. An understanding of the mechanism of action is facilitated through an appreciation of the principles of tumour growth and cell cycle kinetics.

Cellular kinetics
The growth and division of cells occurs through the cell cycle. Non-dividing cells are in 'G0' and when actively recruited into the cell cycle they pass through four main phases:
- G1: pre-DNA synthetic phase
- S: DNA synthesis
- G2: post-DNA synthesis
- M: mitosis

The cell then divides and produces two daughter cells which consist of three subpopulations which may all exist simultaneously within tumours:
- Non-dividing and terminally differentiated cells
- Cells that are continually proliferating.
- Cells that are resting but may be recruited into the cell cycle

The cell cycle also includes checkpoints which, when activated, can prevent the cell from moving forward to the next phase if adverse genetic conditions have occurred. These cell cycle checkpoints are often lost in cancers.

Tumour kinetics
Tumour cell kinetics reflect a) the proportion of actively dividing cells (the growth fraction), b) the length of the cell cycle (doubling time), and c) the rate of cell loss. Tumours characteristically follow a sigmoid-shaped growth curve in which tumour-doubling time varies with tumour size. Growth is most rapid during the early period in which

Table 2.8.1 Examples of cell cycle phase-specific drugs

Phase of cell cycle	Class	Characteristic agents
S phase	Antimetabolites	Methotrexate Gemcitabine Fluorouracil Doxorubicin
M phase	Natural products	Vinca alkaloids
G1 phase	Hormone Natural product	Corticosteroids Asparaginase
G2 phase	Natural products	Bleomycin, topotecan

tumour volumes are small. However as tumour mass expands, the ensuing restriction of space, blood supply, and nutrient availability results in a plateauing in the growth curve. Chemotherapeutic agents are most effective during the initial exponential phase of rapid growth when the total cell number is low, and the growth fraction is high. This phenomenon also forms the rationale for the addition of chemotherapy to other anticancer modalities, such as surgery and radiotherapy. These treatments reduce the cell population so that a higher fraction of remaining cells exist within the logarithmic growth phase, therefore potentially rendering them more chemosensitive. Common cytotoxic drugs can be classified according to their mechanism of action (see Table 2.8.2).

Alkylating agents

Alkylating agents disrupt DNA synthesis by forming adducts with DNA bases. They can react with one or both strands of DNA (monofunctional or bifunctional agents). Most alkylating agents are bifunctional, and form cross-links within the DNA double helix, which prevent replication of DNA and transcription of ribonucleic acid (RNA). These links can be formed at any stage of the cell cycle, so alkylating agents are not cell cycle phase specific. Although most of these drugs have similar mechanisms of action, there are differences in the spectrum of activity, pharmacokinetic (PK) parameters, and toxicity. They play a major role in the treatment of breast and ovarian cancer, and the haematological malignancies.

Heavy metals

Platinum agents are used in the treatment of a wide range of cancers, including testicular, lung, breast, bladder, cervical, and ovarian cancers. Following diffusion into cells, chloride ions are lost allowing the compound to form intra- and interstrand DNA cross-links, resulting in inhibition of DNA, RNA, and protein synthesis. These agents include cisplatin and newer generation derivatives carboplatin, and oxaliplatin, which are modified, thus influencing their toxicity profile. For instance, carboplatin has the same platinum moiety as cisplatin, but is bonded to an organic carboxylate group leading to increased water solubility and slower hydrolysis. It is less nephrotoxic and neurotoxic but causes more marked myelosuppression.

Antimetabolites

Antimetabolites are structural analogues of the naturally occurring metabolites involved in DNA and RNA synthesis. They exert their cytotoxic activity either by competing with normal metabolites for the catalytic or regulatory site of a key enzyme or by substituting for a metabolite that is normally incorporated into DNA and RNA. Other antimetabolites inhibit enzymes that are necessary for the synthesis of vital compounds. They exert their effects mostly in the synthetic phase of the cell cycle and have little effect on cells in G0. Consequently, these drugs are most effective in tumours that have a high growth fraction.

The antimetabolites can be divided into:

• Antifolates: e.g. methotrexate, competitively inhibits the enzyme dihydrofolate reductase (DHFR), essential for purine and pyrimidine production and therefore DNA synthesis
• Fluorinated pyrimidines: e.g. fluorouracil (5-FU); prodrugs that are intracellularly activated and whose products inhibit pyrimidine synthesis (inhibition of thymidylate synthase)
• Antipurines: e.g. mercaptopurine; these inhibit purine synthesis and the nucleotide product is incorporated into DNA
• Ribonucleotide reductase inhibitors: e.g. hydroxyurea; reduce availability of all deoxynucleotides
• Cytosine analogues: e.g. gemcitabine; also inhibit ribonucleotide reductase and compete with cytidine triphosphate for incorporation into DNA
• Adenosine analogues: e.g. pentostatin; interact with adenosine deaminase, inhibit both DNA synthesis and repair

Natural products

Drugs possessing antitumour activities have been isolated from natural substances such as plants, fungi, and bacteria. They are separated into the following categories:

Antitumour antibiotics

Drugs that are derived from micro-organisms are termed antitumour antibiotics and include the anthracyclines, bleomycins, mitoxantrone, and mitomycin c. They are useful in treating many solid tumours and haematological malignancies. Several of these drugs interfere with DNA through intercalation, where the drug inserts itself between DNA base pairs. Some antitumour antibiotics have other mechanisms of action, such as inhibition of the enzyme topoisomerase, antimitotic effects, and alteration of cellular membranes. Most of the drugs in this group are not cell cycle specific.

Mitotic inhibitors

The vinca alkaloids (vincristine, vinblastine, vinorelbine) are derived from the periwinkle plant, *Vinca rosea*. They exert their effects by binding to tubulin and preventing polymerization. As polymerized tubulin forms the spindles that retract chromosomes into daughter cells at mitosis, this disrupts the formation of microtubules causing metaphase arrest. In contrast, paclitaxel and docetaxel possess a novel 14-member ring, the taxane, and are

Table 2.8.2 Classification of chemotherapeutic agents according to mechanism of action

Alkylating agents	Antimetabolites	Natural products
Cisplatin	Fluorouracil	Bleomycin
Cyclophosphamide	Methotrexate	Doxorubicin
Melphalan	Cytarabine	Mitomycin C
Chlorambucil	Capecitabine	Vinca alkaloids
Ifosfamide	Gemcitabine	Taxanes

semisynthetic derivatives of extracted precursors from yew plants. They differ from the vinca alkaloids, in that they enhance microtubule formation resulting in production of a stable and non-functional microtubule.

Topoisomerase inhibitors

Topoisomerases are enzymes that break and reseal DNA strands. There are two forms of this enzyme, named topoisomerase I (topo I) and topoisomerase II (topo II). The plant alkaloid camptothecin and its analogues are non-classic enzyme inhibitors of topo I. Inhibitors of topo II include etoposide, and agents from other classes, such as doxorubicin. Topo I binds double-stranded DNA, then cleaves and demotes one strand of duplex DNA. The supercoiled DNA reduction is then used during the process of replication and transcription. Topo II creates transitory double-stranded breakage of DNA, permitting subsequent passage of an intact DNA duplex through the break.

Enzyme

These may deprive cells of critical constituents, for example, asparaginase catalyses the hydrolysis of asparagines to aspartic acid and ammonia and thus deprives selected malignant cells of an amino acid essential to their survival.

Adverse effects of chemotherapy

The processes governing cell proliferation are common to normal and cancer cells; thus both cell populations are susceptible to damage by chemotherapy. The aim of chemotherapy is to achieve maximum tumour cell killing while accepting a certain degree of toxicity to normal tissues. Standardized definitions have been developed for reporting organ toxicities using a graded scale, the Common Terminology Criteria for Adverse Events (CTCAE), also known as 'common toxicity criteria'. Toxicities vary according to the drug, dose, route of administration, and schedule of administration.

The rapidly dividing cells of the bone marrow, gastrointestinal mucosa, hair follicles, and gonads are most sensitive to cytotoxic treatment. Therefore, the most common toxicities include myelosuppression, mucous membrane ulceration or gastrointestinal upset, alopecia, and reduced fertility. Given the potential for significant and possibly long-lasting or life-threatening side effects of chemotherapy, the importance of patient education and adequate monitoring during treatment cannot be overstated.

Adverse effects of cytotoxic chemotherapy can sometimes develop over many months, for example, cardiomyopathy induced by anthracyclines or pulmonary fibrosis associated with bleomycin. With improving cancer survivorship, previously unrecognized late effects are emerging and the risk of developing second cancers is well documented. High-risk groups include young patients cured of Hodgkin lymphoma, acute leukaemia, and germ cell tumours.

Overcoming chemotherapy resistance

The most profound obstacle to long-term efficacy of chemotherapy is the development of resistance. The mechanisms of this may be classified into either intrinsic or acquired resistance. Intrinsic resistance manifests in uncontrolled tumour growth during the treatment regimen, and acquired resistance results in disease progression that emerges after initial efficacy. The position of cells in the cell cycle can influence sensitivity to drugs; so cells in the G0 phase are generally resistant to all drugs active in the S phase. Failure to kill cells may also be a function of insufficient drug concentration. This could be due to:

- Decreased drug-activating enzymes
- Increased drug-inactivating enzymes
- Increased DNA repair
- Mutations in drug targets affecting stoichiometry of interactions.
- Excretion of drug out of the cells

Repeated exposure of a tumour to a single chemotherapy agent may result in cross-resistance to another cytotoxic within the same drug class. This can be due to expression of the multidrug resistance (MDR) gene, which encodes a transmembrane P-glycoprotein that results in an enhanced energy-dependent drug efflux mechanism producing lower intracellular drug concentrations. A high level of MDR expression is reliably correlated with resistance to cytotoxic agents, and tumours that intrinsically express the MDR1 gene before chemotherapy characteristically display poor or short-lived responses.

Novel formulations of chemotherapy

As cancer chemotherapeutic agents are often administered systemically, biological processes such as distribution, metabolism, and elimination can influence drug delivery. Optimizing drug delivery to tumours has been attempted using novel formulations of chemotherapeutic agents, which have altered toxicity profiles, and improved drug administration features. Liposomal formulations incorporating lipid and lipoprotein vesicles can enhance potential for targeting drugs into tumours, as liposomes may aid cancer cell penetration. Liposomal delivery systems also permit encapsulation and stabilization of highly hydrophobic molecules such as doxorubicin (Doxil, Caelyx).

Nanoparticle drugs are composed of therapeutic molecules (e.g. small molecules, nucleic acids) that self-assemble with lipids or polymers into nanostructures, usually 10–100nm diameter. They can be endocytosed or phagocytosed by cells, with resulting cell internalization of the encapsulated drug. Albumin-bound formulations of paclitaxel (nab-paclitaxel) permit higher doses of the drug to be administered with fewer side effects than standard paclitaxel, which requires a toxic excipient, cremophor. This offers practical advantages including a shorter infusion time and avoidance of need for premedication for hypersensitivity reactions.

Prescribing chemotherapy

In the curative setting, reductions in dose intensity are believed to compromise survival outcomes. Dose intensity refers to the total concentration of drug delivered to the patient in a given period, which could be the same whether given as a single administration or in multiple low-dose treatments. Therefore dose intensity is influenced both by delays and reductions in dosing. Chemotherapy dosing is most often calculated based on the body surface area (BSA) of a patient (e.g. in mg/m^2), using a formula originally derived in 1916 by DuBois and DuBois using only eight patients to adjust for basal metabolic rates in extrapolating the human starting dose from animal doses in pre-clinical models. However, BSA dosing is associated with high pharmacokinetic variability as a result of inter-individual variation in clearance and does not indicate optimal drug exposure reliably. Factors such as obesity also raise challenges with this form of dosing. Nevertheless, it is the most common method for dosing cytotoxic agents, mainly for its convenience.

An argument could be made for therapeutic drug monitoring to titrate to a patient's maximum tolerated exposure, measured as 'area under the concentration curve' (AUC), although this is complicated to undertake on an individual basis. For some agents, knowledge of their mechanism of clearance can provide information about optimal exposure. The known toxicity (thrombocytopenia) of the cytotoxic carboplatin was shown by Calvert et al. (see further reading) to bear no relationship to a patient's BSA, but rather to relate to their glomerular filtration rate (GRF), because of the exclusive renal clearance of the drug. Therefore dosing of carboplatin takes into account the GFR of a patient, as well as the desired exposure and is calculated thus: dose = AUC × (GFR + 25).

Hormone therapy

Some tumours have demonstrated sensitivity to hormone manipulation via surgery. For example, prostate cancers may regress after orchidectomy and breast cancers can be controlled by oophorectomy. Systemic therapies have been developed to influence the hormones that may be encouraging tumour growth in hormonally driven cancers, such as prostate, breast, endometrial, and ovarian cancers. For women with oestrogen receptor (ER) and/or progesterone receptor (PR) positive breast cancer, the type of hormone therapy will depend on the menopausal status of the patient. The main therapy for premenopausal ER/PR+ patients is the anti-oestrogen tamoxifen, which binds the oestrogen receptor on cancer cells and competes with endogenously produced oestrogen. Because of its partial agonist action it acts like oestrogen in other tissues such as the uterus and bones and is therefore called a selective oestrogen receptor modulator (SERM). Tamoxifen is taken orally and common side effects include fatigue, hot flushing, vaginal dryness, and mood disturbance. Rare but more serious side effects include increased thromboembolic complications and development of endometrial cancer.

In postmenopausal women, aromatase inhibitors (AIs), e.g. anastrozole or exemestane, have been developed that inhibit the peripheral conversion of androgens to oestrogens. These treatments eliminate oestrogens and therefore can cause osteoporosis, but other side effects include muscle pain and arthralgia, although there is less association with blood clots or endometrial cancers than with tamoxifen.

Hormonal therapies are frequently used in the adjuvant setting and are taken for many years continuously. As a rule, when used to control tumour growth, they are given without chemotherapy, as they result in cell cycle arrest which can abrogate the cytocidal effect of cytotoxic treatment.

Luteinizing hormone-releasing hormone (LHRH) analogues such as goserelin cause a temporary flare of luteinizing hormone (LH) release from the pituitary; thereafter negative feedback inhibition results in LH downregulation and induction of menopause. LHRH analogues are also used in prostate cancer to reduce testosterone concentrations. The temporary surge in testosterone produced following LHRH analogues means that they are often given with a short course of anti-androgens such as bicalutamide (Casodex), or cyproterone acetate in prostate cancer, to limit tumour flare.

Molecularly targeted therapy

The rapid advancements in understanding of the molecular and cellular biology of cancer have resulted in the current generation of molecularly targeted agents which have greatly enhanced the therapeutic armoury of anticancer strategies. These are drugs developed against a specific molecular target, that is not generally present in normal tissues, but which may be mutated or overexpressed in cancerous tissues, to selectively inhibit the target. These drugs are associated with more of a cytostatic, rather than a cytotoxic effect, thereby increasing time to progression via disease stabilization rather than causing tumour shrinkage. For example, fewer than 2% of hepatocellular carcinoma patients treated with sorafenib achieve actual decrease in tumour dimensions or partial response, but the time to progressive disease is significantly longer than with placebo, thus impacting on survival.

Categories of targeted anticancer therapies

Targeted therapies can be broadly divided into small molecule inhibitors and monoclonal antibodies. Small molecule inhibitors (SMI) are low molecular weight (less than 900Da) compounds that can penetrate the cell membrane, blocking receptor signalling and interfering with downstream intracellular targets. They are denoted by the suffix-nib and are typically developed for oral administration. In contrast most monoclonal antibodies (mAbs) cannot penetrate the plasma membrane and target the extracellular components of these signalling pathways, such as ligands and receptor-binding sites. They are denoted by the suffix-mab and typically require intravenous or subcutaneous administration. General differences between small molecule inhibitors and monoclonal antibodies include:

- SMIs are normally taken orally; mAbs are administered intravenously
- SMI achieve less specific targeting than mAbs
- Unlike mAbs, most SMIs are metabolized by cytochrome P450 enzymes, which may result in interactions with certain medications, such as warfarin, St John's wort, and some antifungal agents and antibiotics
- mAbs have half-lives ranging from days to weeks, and are usually administered once every one to four weeks; most SMIs have half-lives of only hours and require daily dosing

Tables 2.8.3 and 2.8.4 give an overview of commonly used agents in these classes

Small molecule inhibitors

Small molecule inhibitors generally target pathways that are continuously activated in cancer cells. The most common class are tyrosine kinase inhibitors, which target enzymes that phosphorylate tyrosine amino acid residues in proteins resulting in a cascade of enzymatic and biochemical reactions that influence signalling cell growth, proliferation, and migration.

Table 2.8.3 Examples of targeted therapies

Agent	Mechanism of action	Approved indications
Afatinib	Protein kinase inhibitor that also irreversibly inhibits human epidermal growth factor receptor 2 (Her2) and epidermal growth factor receptor (EGFR) kinases. Also targets T790M mutations which generally do not respond to the other tyrosine kinase inhibitors	Non-small cell lung cancer (with EGFR exon 19 deletions or exon 21 substitution (L858R) mutations)
Axitinib	Potent and selective inhibitor of vascular endothelial growth factor receptors (VEGFR) 1, 2, and 3	Renal cell carcinoma
Bortezomib	Interferes with the action of large enzyme complexes called proteasomes causing cancer cells to undergo cell cycle arrest and apoptosis	Multiple myeloma Mantle cell lymphoma
Cabozantinib	A potent inhibitor of MET, vascular endothelial growth factor receptor 2 (VEGFR2), and RET	Medullary thyroid cancer Renal cell carcinoma
Crizotinib	Multitargeted small molecule tyrosine kinase inhibitor, which had been originally developed as an inhibitor of the mesenchymal epithelial transition growth factor (c-MET); it is also a potent inhibitor of ALK phosphorylation and signal transduction	Non-small cell lung cancer (with ALK fusion or ROS1 gene alteration)
Dabrafenib	Inhibits the activity of BRAF, an intracellular protein kinase of the RAF kinase family that drives cell proliferation and can be mutated in melanoma cells	Melanoma (with BRAF V600 mutation)
Dasatinib	Multi targeted tyrosine kinase inhibitor; targets most imatinib-resistant BCR-ABL mutations. Kinase inhibition halts proliferation of leukaemia cells. Also inhibits SRC family, c-KIT, EPHA2, and PDGF receptor	Chronic myelogenous leukaemia (Philadelphia chromosome positive) Acute lymphoblastic leukaemia (Philadelphia chromosome positive)
Erlotinib	Inhibits overall EGFR-TK activity. Active competitive inhibition of adenosine triphosphate inhibits downstream signal transduction of ligand-dependent EGFR activation	Non-small cell lung cancer (with EGFR exon 19 deletions or exon 21 substitution (L858R) mutations)
Everolimus	Derivative of rapamycin (sirolimus) and works similarly to rapamycin as an mTOR (mammalian target of rapamycin) inhibitor. Everolimus' effect is solely on the mTORC1 protein and not on the mTORC2 protein	Pancreatic, gastrointestinal, or lung origin neuroendocrine tumour Renal cell carcinoma Breast cancer (HR+, HER2−)
Gefitinib	Inhibits the tyrosine kinase activity of the epidermal growth factor receptor (EGFR). Tyrosine kinase activity appears to be vitally important to cell proliferation and survival	Non-small cell lung cancer (with EGFR exon 19 deletions or exon 21 substitution (L858R) mutations)
Imatinib	Inhibits BCR-ABL tyrosine kinase, the constitutive abnormal gene product of the Philadelphia chromosome in chronic myeloid leukaemia (CML). This in turn blocks proliferation in Philadelphia chromosome positive CML. Also inhibits tyrosine kinase for platelet-derived growth factor (PDGF), stem cell factor (SCF), c-KIT, and cellular events mediated by PDGF and SCF	GI stromal tumour (KIT+) Dermatofibrosarcoma protuberans Multiple hematological malignancies including Philadelphia chromosome-positive ALL and CML
Lapatinib	Inhibits several tyrosine kinases, including the tyrosine kinase activity of EGFR and HER2, blocking phosphorylation and activation of downstream second messengers (Erk1/2 and Akt) and regulating proliferation and survival in EGFR and HER2 expressing tumours	Breast cancer (HER2+)
Olaparib	Inhibitor of poly (ADP-ribose) polymerase (PARP) enzymes, including PARP1, PARP2, and PARP3. PARP enzymes are involved in normal cellular homeostasis, such as DNA transcription, cell cycle regulation, and DNA repair	Ovarian cancer (with BRCA mutation)
Nilotinib	Inhibits the tyrosine kinase activity of the BCR-ABL protein. Nilotinib fits into the ATP-binding site of the BCR-ABL protein with higher affinity than imatinib, overriding resistance caused by mutations	Chronic myelogenous leukaemia (Philadelphia chromosome positive)
Pazopanib	Second-generation multitargeted tyrosine kinase inhibitor against vascular endothelial growth factor receptor-1, -2, and -3, platelet-derived growth factor receptor-alpha, platelet-derived growth factor receptor-beta, and c-kit. These receptor targets are part of the angiogenesis pathway that facilitates the formation of tumour blood vessel for tumour survival and growth	Renal cell carcinoma

(continued)

Table 2.8.3 Continued

Agent	Mechanism of action	Approved indications
Rucaparib	An inhibitor of poly (ADP-ribose) polymerase (PARP) enzymes, including PARP-1, PARP-2, and PARP-3, which play a role in DNA repair. Rucaparib-induced cytotoxicity involves inhibition of PARP enzymatic activity and increased formation of PARP-DNA complexes resulting in DNA damage, apoptosis, and cell death	Ovarian cancer (with BRCA mutation)
Sorafenib	Inhibits Raf kinases (CRAF, BRAF, and mutant BRAF) and cell surface kinase receptors (VEGFR-2, VEGFR-3, PDGFR-beta, cKIT, and FMS-like tyrosine kinase-3 [FLT-3]), thereby inhibiting tumour growth and angiogenesis	Hepatocellular carcinoma Renal cell carcinoma Thyroid carcinoma
Sunitinib	Multitargeted receptor tyrosine kinase inhibitor, whose targets include; PDGFRα and PDGFRβ, VEGFR1, VEGFR2 and VEGFR3, FLT3, colony-stimulating factor type 1, and glial cell line derived neurotrophic factor receptor (RET)	Renal cell carcinoma GIST not responding to imatinib
Trametinib	Highly selective reversible allosteric inhibitor of MEK1 and MEK2 activity. It is an ATP non-competitive inhibitor that binds MEK adjacent to the ATP binding site in common with other MEK allosteric inhibitors	Melanoma (with BRAF V600 mutation)
Vemurafenib	Inhibitor of mutated BRAF-serine-threonine kinase. It is especially potent against the BRAF V600E mutation. This mutation involves the substitution of glutamic acid for valine at codon 600. The BRAF oncogene, most of which have the V600E mutation, activates mitogen-activated kinase (MAPK) pathway which results in cell growth, proliferation, and metastasis. Vemurafenib blocks these downstream processes to inhibit tumour growth and eventually trigger apoptosis	Melanoma (with BRAF V600 mutation)

Table 2.8.4 Examples of monoclonal antibodies

Agent	Mechanism of action	Approved indications
Bevacizumab	Binds to vascular endothelial growth factor (VEGF) preventing it from interacting with its receptors on endothelial cells, thereby inhibiting new blood vessel growth and potentially cancer growth	Cervical cancer Colorectal cancer Glioblastoma Non-small cell lung cancer Ovarian cancer Peritoneal cancer Renal cell carcinoma
Cetuximab	Binds specifically to EGFR and competitively inhibits the binding of EGF and other ligands. Binding to the EGFR blocks phosphorylation and activation of receptor-associated kinases. EGFR signal transduction results in KRAS wild-type activation; cells with KRAS mutations appear to be unaffected by EGFR inhibition	Colorectal cancer (KRAS wild type) Squamous cell cancer of the head and neck
Denosumab	Binds to RANKL, a transmembrane or soluble protein essential for the formation, function, and survival of osteoclasts, the cells responsible for bone resorption. Prevents RANKL from activating its receptor, RANK, on the surface of osteoclasts and their precursors	Prevention of skeletal-related events in patients with bone metastases from solid tumours Increased bone mass in patients at high risk for fracture including androgen deprivation therapy (ADT) for non-metastatic prostate cancer or adjuvant aromatase inhibitor therapy (AI) for breast cancer Unresectable giant cell tumour of bone in adults and skeletally mature adolescents
Ipilimumab	Fully human IgG1κ antibody that binds to CTLA-4 (cytotoxic T lymphocyte-associated antigen-4), a molecule on T cells that is indicated for unresectable or metastatic melanoma. The absence or presence of CTLA-4 can augment or suppress the immune system's T cell response in fighting disease. Ipilimumab is designed to block the activity of CTLA-4, thereby sustaining an active immune response in its attack on cancer cells. The proposed mechanism of action is indirect and may be through T cell-mediated antitumour immune responses	Melanoma

Table 2.8.4 Continued

Agent	Mechanism of action	Approved indications
Nivolumab	Human immunoglobulin G4 (IgG4) monoclonal antibody that binds to the PD-1 receptor and blocks its interaction with PD-L1 and PD-L2, releasing PD-1 pathway-mediated inhibition of the immune response, including the anti-tumour immune response. Binding of the PD-1 ligands, PD-L1 and PD-L2, to the PD-1 receptor found on T cells, inhibits T cell proliferation and cytokine production. Upregulation of PD-1 ligands occurs in some tumours and signalling through this pathway can contribute to inhibition of active T cell immune surveillance of tumours	Head and neck squamous cell carcinoma Hodgkin's lymphoma Melanoma Non-small cell lung cancer Renal cell carcinoma Urothelial carcinoma
Pembrolizumab	Pembrolizumab is an antibody drug that targets the cell surface receptor programmed cell death protein 1 (PD-1) found on T cells. By preventing the binding of its ligands (PD-L1 and PD-L2), pembrolizumab induces an antitumour immune response. Upregulation of PD-1 ligands is a mechanism for tumours to evade antitumour immune response; when PD-1 binds its ligand, the T cell receives an inhibitory signal leading to T cell anergy and blockade of antitumour immune response. Instead of directly targeting tumour tissue to induce tumour cell death, pembrolizumab acts as a checkpoint inhibitor to stimulate immune responses to eliminate cancer cells	Melanoma Non-small cell lung cancer (PD-L1+) Head and neck squamous cell carcinoma
Pertuzumab	Binds to the extracellular domain II of HER2. Its mechanism of action is complementary to trastuzumab, inhibiting ligand-dependent HER2–HER3 dimerization and reducing signalling via intracellular pathways such as phosphatidylinositol 3-kinase (PI3K/Akt)	Breast cancer (HER2+)
Rituximab	Recognizes the CD20 molecule found on B cells. On binding, activates complement-dependent B cell cytotoxicity, mediating cell killing through an antibody-dependent cellular toxicity	Non-Hodgkin's lymphoma
Tositumomab	Recognises the CD20 molecule. Some of the antibodies are linked to a radioactive iodine. The radioactive component delivers radioactive energy to CD20 expressing B cells. In addition, the binding of tositumomab to the CD20-expressing B cells triggers the immune system to destroy these cells	Non-Hodgkin's lymphoma
Trastuzumab	Binds to the extracellular domain of the human epidermal growth factor receptor (HER2). The likely mechanism of action involves binding HER2 on the surface of tumour cells that express high levels of HER2 thereby preventing HER2 from sending growth-promoting signals inhibiting proliferation of cells which overexpress HER2 protein	Breast cancer (HER2+) Gastric cancer (HER2+)

Receptor tyrosine kinases (RTKs) are cell-surface receptors for growth factors, cytokines, and hormones, which modulate transmission of signals from the cell surface, via the cytoplasm to the nucleus, as for example, EGFR, HER2, and VEGF receptors. Common to this class is a substrate binding domain, an ATP binding domain, and a catalytic or kinase domain. The first major success of a tyrosine kinase inhibitor was imatinib mesylate (Gleevec®), a competitive inhibitor of several cellular Abl-kinases, including the BCR-ABL kinase fusion protein which is the result of a reciprocal translocation between chromosomes 9 and 22 in the great majority of cases of chronic myeloid leukaemia (CML). Imatinib can prevent constitutive signalling from the BCR-ABL fusion product by inhibiting phosphorylation and activation of downstream proteins of the tyrosine kinases associated with the active Abl gene. Characteristically, resistance to imatinib in CML patients arises through a mutation in the BCR-ABL gene that results in altered protein conformation so that it no longer binds the drug. As is the

case with many small molecule inhibitors, imatinib shows inhibitory activity against other RTKs, including KIT. It therefore has established activity in patients with gastrointestinal stromal tumours (GIST), which shows frequent gain of function mutations in the c-kit proto-oncogene.

Multitargeted TKIs have affinity for RTK on tumour cells and supporting cells and thereby represent a potentially attractive approach for targeting multiple signalling pathways for a given cancer. Sorafenib and sunitinib are oral multikinase inhibitors that inhibit multiple RTKs including VEGFR, PDGFR, and KIT and as a result have anti-angiogenic and antitumour cell activity.

Some small molecule inhibitors interfere with oncoproteins, e.g. vemurafenib is a specific kinase inhibitor of the mutated protein kinase B-RAF V600E, commonly seen in melanoma patients, which is responsible for constitutive activation of the signalling pathway, promoting tumour cell proliferation and preventing apoptosis. The phosphoinositide 3 (PI3) kinase/AKT/mTOR pathway has regulatory effects on cell proliferation and survival and its dysregulation in diverse cancers can be targeted at multiple levels using different kinase inhibitors, for instance, to mutated, amplified, or over-expressed PI3 kinase, AKT, and mTOR. mTOR (which comprises mTORC1 and mTORC2 complexes) can also be targeted by allosteric rapalogues, such as everolimus, which preferentially binds to only mTORC1 rather than affecting kinase activity of both mTORC 1 and mTORC2, and therefore displays differing effects on downstream targets, and negative feedback pathways.

Greater understanding of biological targets offers exciting potential to generate therapies that may impact on patient outcomes. Novel systemic drugs are being developed that target diverse pathways and processes of:

- Cell cycle regulation, including cyclin-dependent kinase, survivin, and agents that target mitosis (aurora kinases)
- Apoptotic pathways, including death receptor pathways
- Signalling pathways, including RAS and its downstream effectors, insulin growth factor receptors, and Src family kinases
- Epigenetic agents, including histone deacetylase inhibitors
- Senescence
- Telomerase instability
- Ubiquitin-proteosome system
- Developmental pathway inhibitors, such as Notch and Hedgehog pathway inhibitors

Monoclonal antibodies
Although the relative lack of specificity of small molecules may be advantageous if simultaneous targeting of several similar signalling pathways is desirable, this is best avoided if cross-reactivity is detrimental, in which case antibody therapeutics have emerged as an excellent alternative with important advantages. Classical antibodies show very different pharmacokinetics in terms of tissue penetration, tumour retention, and blood clearance due to the size of their traditional IgG format. This IgG scaffold consists of a variable fragment with specific antigen binding properties (Fab), and a crystallizable fragment (Fc), which is the constant domain that mediates effector function such as complement fixation. Use of antibodies therefore creates more possibilities for by-stander (depleting) effects on neighbouring tumour cells from immune-effector interactions, rather than purely blocking ligand or target receptor.

The properties of antibodies have been exploited as therapeutic and diagnostic reagents in oncology for many years. Originally polyclonal antibodies from the serum of immunized animals were the only source of antibodies, and this resulted in serious immune reactions to recognition of foreign proteins in humans, thus limiting their clinical use. An important step in antibody applications came with the use of hybridoma technology. Köhler and Milstein discovered that antibodies derived from single B cells could be produced in culture by fusion of an immortal myeloma cell line with an immune B lymphoblast expressing the single antibody gene from immunized mice, generating a single monoclonal antibody (mAb) species. For this discovery they were awarded a Nobel prize in 1984. As those antibodies were of murine origin, they eventually resulted in human anti-murine antibody (HAMA) responses and immunorejection. Therefore recombinant DNA technology was used to reduce immunogenicity, through generation of chimaeric antibodies that comprised murine antigen-specific variable regions and constant domains of human origin. Further

refinement of this strategy to improve compatibility with human immune systems occurred with the engineering of humanized antibodies, which bear only the murine hypervariable regions within a fully human IgG scaffold. Fully human antibodies are now being developed from human antibodies using recombinant phage display technology or the use of transgenic mice engineered to produce the human antibody gene repertoire. The type of antibody can often be identified by the suffix of the drug name: -momab (murine), -ximab (chimaeric), -zumab (humanized), or -mumab (human).

Given the modular structure of mAbs, smaller fragments may be utilized, with differing pharmacokinetic properties and these may be used as a drug delivery system or antibody–drug conjugate (ADC). ADCs employ a cytotoxic pro-drug conjugated to the mAb, which when engulfed by cancer cells bearing the relevant target releases the toxic payload. This technology may therefore reduce some of the more systemic toxicity of chemotherapies. In 2013, trastuzumab emtansine (T-DM1), which is trastuzumab linked to DM1, was approved for treatment of HER2-positive metastatic breast cancer.

Adverse effects of molecularly targeted agents
Molecularly targeted therapies have a recognized association with important adverse effects, some of which are target-related, others which are more therapeutic class related.

Monoclonal antibodies can precipitate acute hypersensitivity reactions due to immunogenicity at the time of infusion. This may vary in severity from mild skin reactions, pyrexia, and influenza-like responses to much rarer, frank anaphylaxis, systemic inflammatory response syndrome, and life-threatening cytokine release syndrome. Close monitoring during infusions is required, but most such acute reactions are readily controlled with slowing or interruption of the infusion and appropriate symptom management.

Some of the toxicities observed may be target-specific. Epidermal growth factor receptor (EGFR) is also present in normal epithelial tissue and inhibition of this pathway can lead to significant dermatological and gastrointestinal toxicities. Similarly targeting of vascular endothelial growth factor (VEGF) limits cancer growth by preventing angiogenesis (the formation of new blood vessels). However, VEGF is also present on normal endothelial cells and inhibiting VEGF has effects on normal blood vessels including bleeding, thrombosis, and hypertension. Protein phosphorylation by tyrosine kinases is an important regulator of cellular communication in normal and stem cell populations and targeting TKIs can also affect non-cancerous populations. Short-term side effects may include haematological effects such as anaemia, thrombocytopenia, and neutropenia as well as vomiting and diarrhoea.

The future of molecularly targeted agents
Molecularly targeted therapies have expanded the concept of individualized cancer treatment, because activity may be envisaged in only a subpopulation of cancers with a particular molecular change, and be ineffective in the absence of such a target. The selective pressure of targeted therapy leads to expression of pre-existing mutations in receptor tyrosine kinases, the activation of bypass signalling pathways and other resistance mechanisms. Thus tumour responses are relatively brief and are associated with only a modest improvement in OS. Forthcoming challenges will be in overcoming resistance to existing drugs either with next-generation drugs, or

through rational combination approaches of different targeted drugs to address redundancy and feedback mechanisms, or with cytotoxics.

Immunotherapy

Principles of immunotherapy

The goal of cancer immunotherapy is to harness the power of the immune system to recognize and attack tumour cells. The monoclonal antibody therapies offer a form of passive immunotherapy, whereby the immune system constituents manufactured outside of the patient are administered to them as an anticancer treatment. An active immunotherapy strategy encompasses therapeutic manipulations of the immune system to stimulate the host's intrinsic immune response to cancer, using agents such as cytokines, vaccines, transfected agents, and cellular or humoral therapies. The promise of cancer immunotherapy has adopted a centre-stage position in systemic therapy management with recognition of excellent activity from the new generation of immune checkpoint inhibitors. The role for immunotherapy is now recognized in tumours beyond melanoma and renal cancer, which are traditionally associated with immunological control, and are now part of standard therapy across a range of malignancies including head and neck, non-small and small cell lung, gastric and oesophageal, hepatocellular, bladder, and breast cancers amongst others.

Immune checkpoint inhibitors

Immune checkpoint inhibitors target regulatory pathways in T cells to enhance antitumour immune responses. In this way, rather than activate the immune system to attack particular targets on tumour cells, the goal of therapy is to remove inhibitory pathways that block effective antitumour T cell responses. CTLA4 is a gene that has very high homology to CD28 and has been shown to downregulate T cell responses. Thus, activation of T cells results in induction of expression of CTLA4 which accumulates in the T cell, reaching a level where it eventually blocks costimulation and abrogates an activated T cell response. The antibody against CTLA4 ipilimumab was the first therapy shown to improve OS in a randomized trial with metastatic melanoma. Importantly, durable responses have been observed with analyses indicating survival of over ten years in a subset of patients.

The programmed cell death-1 (PD-1) receptor expressed by activated T cells has been shown to be another key immune checkpoint inhibitor with a negative regulatory role when engaged by its ligands PD-L1 and PD-L2. The predominant ligand, PD-L1, is expressed on many tumour cells and binds to PD-1 on activated cytotoxic T cells and natural killer cells in the tumour microenvironment, thereby inducing T cell dysfunction. As a result, T cells have a decreased ability to produce cytokines, or proliferate or cause tumour lysis. Two fully humanized immunoglobulin mAbs against PD-1 (pembrolizumab and nivolumab) were approved in 2011 for the treatment of melanoma. Nivolumab was also recently approved by the US Food and Drug Administration (FDA) for patients with previously treated advanced or metastatic non-small cell lung cancer and promising early phase results have been achieved across multiple tumour types. It has also recently been shown that tumours with exceptionally high numbers of somatic mutations may respond better to immune checkpoint inhibitors. This has led to accelerated approvals for the use of immunotherapy in microsatellite instability-high (MSI-H) or mismatch repair deficient (dMMR) colorectal cancers (Le et al. 2017),

as well as in mutational burden-high (≥10 mutations/megabase) tumours that have progressed on standard therapies (Marabelle et al. 2020).

Given the numerous checkpoints that exist and the multiple mechanisms used by tumours to escape the immune system, targeting distinct checkpoints using combination approaches is an attractive therapeutic strategy. Anti-CTLA4 can lead to enhanced priming and activation of antigen-specific T cells and potentially clearance of regulatory T cells from the tumour microenvironment. The blocking of PD-L1 or PD-1 can also remove the inhibition of cancer cell killing by T cells and good responses were observed in patients with melanoma. Combining a CTLA4 targeted therapy (ipilimumab) with a PD-1 targeted inhibitor (nivolumab), appears to enhance the immune activity in patients more than either therapy alone. These observations have encouraged researchers to further investigate combination therapies.

Cancer vaccines

A successful cancer vaccine activates a patient's immune response towards tumour cells or prevents the development of cancer in certain high-risk individuals. Theoretically this may result in long-term disease control or even eradication. A vaccine typically comprises a tumour antigen in an immunogenic formulation which activates host cytotoxic T lymphocytes (CTLs) and B cells. B cells may then secrete specific antibody receptors to cause lysis or phagocytosis of cells that display recognizable antigens. CTLs use their T cell receptor to specifically recognize peptides bound to the major histocompatibility complex (MHC), releasing cytotoxic molecules and cytokines that will kill the cell and stimulate activation of nearby immune cells. The most successful cancer vaccine approach to date is preventative vaccination against human papilloma virus, which prevents virus-induced cervical cancer, Gardasil®. In 2010 the FDA approved Provenge® (sipuleucel-T), a dendritic cell-based vaccine for the treatment of metastatic prostate cancer. This is a preparation of the patient's own peripheral blood cells, loaded ex vivo with prostatic acid phosphatase (PAP), a prostate-specific antigen, and granulocyte-macrophage colony-stimulating factor (GM-CSF). The GM-CSF stimulates maturation of antigen presenting cells into mature dendritic cells. Following ex vivo activation, the mature APCs pre-loaded with PAP are re-infused into the patient where they stimulate T cells to trigger an immune response against the tumour.

Adoptive T cell therapy

The adoptive T cell therapy strategy combines the antigen-binding property of monoclonal antibodies with the lytic capacity and self-renewal of T cells. Autologous T cells with either a natural or genetically engineered reactivity to a patient's cancer can be transferred back to the patient. This process involves the ex vivo expansion and transfer of autologous lymphocytes with antitumour activity via antigen-specific T cell populations, leading to an enhanced antitumour immune response as a result of cytokine release and tumour cell lysis. Clinical trials have revealed promising results in patients with CD19-positive haematological malignancies and also in the treatment of metastatic melanoma. This highly individualized approach has been limited due to the need for specialized cell culture equipment and the requirements of intensive cell preparations.

Cytokines

Cytokines are soluble proteins that mediate the interactions between cells and their extracellular environment, either in a cell autonomous or non-cell autonomous manner. The first interleukin (IL) discovered, IL-2, a lymphokine produced by activated T cells, was shown to have potent immunomodulatory and antitumour activity in a number of murine tumour models. Recombinant IL-2 has been explored in patients with renal cell carcinoma and melanoma; however, its use is limited by severe toxicity and modest efficacy.

The interferons (IFNs) alpha, beta, and gamma are a family of related proteins produced by the immune system in response to viral infection, whose effects include antiviral activity, antiproliferative properties, inhibition of angiogenesis, regulation of cell differentiation, enhancement of MHC antigen expression, and immunomodulatory activities. They have been used to treat haematological malignancies or melanoma. The most frequent adverse effects are flu-like symptoms.

Non-specific immunomodulating agents are substances that stimulate or indirectly augment the immune system by secondary responses such as increased production of cytokines and include bacillus Calmette–Guérin (BCG) and levamisole. BCG is used in the treatment of patients with superficial bladder cancer. It activates macrophages, T and B lymphocytes, and NK cells, and can also induce local immunological responses via ILs. Levamisole was used with 5-FU chemotherapy in the treatment of colorectal cancer, although more effective 5-FU modulators have taken its place.

Toxicity of immunotherapy

One of the challenges associated with the use of immunotherapy is the management of autoimmune side effects called immune-related adverse events. These are caused by a breakdown of immune self-tolerance and non-specific immunostimulation may affect bystander organs resulting in diarrhoea, hepatitis, dermatitis, and

endocrine disorders. The management strategy typically involves interruption of monoclonal antibody therapy, close clinical monitoring, early symptomatic relief, and if appropriate, the timely use of corticosteroids to prevent rapid deterioration. It appears that the rate of serious immune-related adverse events is lower with PD-1 blockade than with CTLA4 blockade and this is possibly because the PD-1/PD-L1 pathway acts more peripherally than the CTLA4/B7-1 pathway, which may operate in the lymphatic system.

Combining immunotherapy with conventional cancer treatments

One strategy to maximize the effectiveness of immunotherapy is to look for synergistic combinations that could not only reduce tumour load, but also abrogate immune tolerance and enhance antitumour immune responses. Combining immunotherapy with conventional cancer treatments may be more likely to produce durable tumour eradication. There is growing evidence that the immune system may synergize with radiation, which enhances many of the steps needed for the generation of antigen-specific immune response, including inflammatory tumour cell death, dendritic cell activation, antigen cross presentation, and cytotoxic T cell activation. Thus combining radiation with immunotherapy could increase radiosensitization and improve local and distant tumour control.

Each patient's immune system is unique based on both genetic and environmental factors, and given inter- and intra-tumour heterogeneity, efficacious cancer immunotherapy is likely to require personalization of treatment in the future. Intense efforts are ongoing to develop predictive biomarkers to identify patients who may benefit from a selected immunotherapeutic strategy, and to overcome issues of toxicity.

2.9 Clinical trials

Introduction

Well-conducted, systematic clinical trials ensure a reliable evidence base with which to guide the development of oncological treatments. They often involve considerable expense, time commitment, and resources. This section aims to give an overview of current and emerging trial designs as well as some key points to consider in planning a trial.

Phase 1 trials

Phase 1 trials are the first step in translating pre-clinical research into clinical practice and aim to determine the safety and tolerability of a new drug or combination of agents. They are generally set up on the basis of scientific rationale and unmet medical need. The drugs tested in these early phase trials may be first-in-human and first-in-class single agents, combinations of novel and approved drugs, or combinations of approved drugs together or with radiotherapy. The primary objective of phase I trials is to determine the recommended phase 2 dose (RPTD) and schedule of a drug. This is generally done by establishing the maximal tolerated dose (MTD) which is set when the proportion of patients within a cohort experiencing a dose limiting toxicity (DLT)) reaches a

predetermined target threshold. There is inconsistency in the definition of MTD depending on geography, e.g. in Europe and Japan, the MTD is the lowest dose at which 33% or more of patients experience a DLT, so defines a dose level above the recommended dose; in the USA the MTD is defined as the dose level below that causing DLT in 33% or more patients and is therefore the same as recommended dose. Given the confusion arising from differing MTD definitions, there is increasing use of the term maximal administered dose (MAD) and the RPTD is taken as one dose level below the MAD. Other objectives of phase I trials are to describe the toxicity profile of new agents, assess pharmacokinetic profiles ('what the body does to the drug' in terms of absorption, distribution, metabolism, and excretion), assess pharmacodynamic effects in tumour or surrogate tissues ('what the drug does to the tumour or body'), and to identify early evidence of antitumour activity. Trials typically involve small numbers of patients with advanced cancers who have received multiple prior lines of therapy.

Phase 1 trials are open-label, single arm and generally start at a tenth of the lethal dose in 10% (LD10) of animals (usually rodents), or one-third of the lowest dose that causes any toxicity or the 'no adverse effect level'

(NOAEL) in large animals, determined from pre-clinical studies. There are multiple different phase 1 designs, which can be broadly classified as either rule- or model-based. The distinction between these designs centres on the dose–toxicity curve. In rule-based designs, a fixed proportional relationship between increasing cytotoxicity and clinical toxicity, efficacy, and drug dose is assumed. The most frequently used is the '3+3' design in which a cohort of three patients receives an initial drug dose based on pre-clinical data. If 0 of three patients experience a DLT, the next cohort of three patients is given a pre-specified increment in dose. If one of three patients experience a DLT, the cohort is expanded to include an additional three patients. If either two of three or more patients experience a DLT, the trial may be stopped or dose reduction considered. Disadvantages to the rule-based approach include exposing too many patients to subtherapeutic doses from slow dose escalation, a risk of severe toxicity in the later cohorts, and the dose increment being limited by the observed toxicity from only the previous cohort.

A modification to try to circumvent these limitations is the accelerated titration model. In this, larger dose increments of 40–100% with a cohort of a single patient allow faster dose escalation. When moderate toxicities are observed, accelerated titration stops and cohorts are expanded (similar to the 3+3 design). As the designs have single patient cohorts and also allow for intra-patient dose escalation, fewer patients are exposed to subtherapeutic doses.

Model-based 'adaptive' designs allow for reassessment of the dose–toxicity curve based on accumulating trial toxicity data, as well as an initial estimate of the curve from pre-clinical data. The dose increment is assigned by calculating the probability of observing a prespecified target toxicity. The most widely used model is the continual reassessment method (CRM), where a prior probability of toxicity at a particular dose is calculated based on historical and/or pre-clinical data. Once started, toxicity data from the trial accumulates and (using Bayesian statistical approaches) updates the initial estimates, hence adjusting the shape of the dose–toxicity curve and informing the next dose to be given. This continues until the target probability of a DLT occurring is reached and the MAD established. Model-based designs tend to treat fewer patients at suboptimal doses and be more efficient. However, they potentially expose more patients to doses exceeding the MTD, although there are modified designs to limit this. They also have been considered to be more complex, requiring expert statistical input, and are cost intensive.

Overall within phase 1 trials, there has been a broadening of their remit, away from simply finding the maximally tolerated dose, to establish drugs that merit further evaluation. In addition to toxicity-based endpoints the biological activity on the target or pathway of the drug, functional imaging, or drug pharmacokinetics can be monitored to guide dose escalation and determine the eventual RPTD. In the case of molecularly targeted agents and immunotherapies, the optimal biological dose (OBD) may not necessarily be the MTD based on the observed toxicities. In addition, many of the chronic toxicities that develop in the setting of long-term administration may be not be accounted for in traditional phase I trial MTD endpoints, which tend to be geared towards adverse events occurring in the first cycle. A proposed 'pharmacological audit trail' incorporates criteria to help demonstrate proof of concept and reinforce data from pre-clinical studies within phase 1 evaluation. The framework comprises assessment of target expression, drug concentrations in plasma and tumour, target engagement, pathway modulation, biological effects, and evidence of clinical activity. This however may require collection of tumour tissue serially or use of surrogate tissues such as platelet-rich plasma, skin, or hair follicles. Earlier phase 0 'proof of concept' trials may also support the intention of defining the drug–target interaction and pharmacokinetics of a range of potential agents in a small number (10–15) of patients, often with single or very limited dosing. They have no therapeutic or dose-finding intent and aim to expedite progression of drugs that show evidence of target modulation by the intervention into phase 1 trials, minimizing the risk of drug failure in subsequent phases.

Phase 2 trials

The aim of phase 2 trials is an initial assessment of drug efficacy (usually by response criteria), and toxicity, and thereby to determine whether the drug merits further development in phase 3 trials. Therefore these studies enrol larger numbers of patients (around 50–200), usually with a single cancer type, for which there may be a strong scientific rationale, or evidence of efficacy in the earlier phase setting. They may incorporate either a single or two-stage design. In a two-stage design the first stage aims to recruit a small number of patients to screen out any inefficacious drugs. If the target RR is not observed, the trial is stopped without proceeding to the second stage, limiting the total number of patients exposed to the drug. In the second stage, two or more agents may be compared to identify whether efficacy justifies later phase evaluation. Single-stage designs tend to be used when drugs used within a combination are already known to have activity.

Ideally a balance should be set between treating as few patients as possible with a potentially inefficacious treatment and the need to accrue enough patients to assess response. Sample size is usually calculated prospectively based on determining the probability of observing a true response rate that incorporates:

1. The probability of the response exceeding that of the standard therapy, allowing for a small false positive rate (less than α, the type 1 error rate). The null hypothesis is rejected.

2. The probability of the response being high enough to warrant further investigation, allowing for a small false negative rate (less than β, the type 2 error rate). The alternative hypothesis is accepted.

In comparison to later phase 3 trials, phase 2 trials usually allow for a lower power and therefore higher type 2 error (β). Although phase 2 trials are usually open-label and single-arm there are an increasing number of randomized phase 2 trials. In contrast to phase 3 trials, the aim of randomization to treatment and standard arms is not as a comparative statistical measure, but rather to assess whether the enrollment of a small number of highly selected patients may be influencing the response rate.

Phase 3 trials

Phase 3 trials aim to compare the efficacy of a newly developed drug or regimen with the current 'standard of care' treatment and unlike earlier phase trials they are powered to detect a statistical difference between cohorts. Therefore these studies usually involve hundreds or thousands of patients with a specified tumour type, often from multiple trial centres. There are many different trial designs, which are not necessarily mutually exclusive, some of which are summarized in Table 2.9.1.

The 'gold standard' is the randomized controlled trial (RCT). Randomization balances differences in population characteristics occurring by chance between arms, thus minimizing selection bias. Stratification of factors that may be associated with the outcome of interest helps to ensure comparable treatment arms and adjusts for confounding factors. Before the start of the trial, the treatment effect to be determined is decided upon as either superior, equivalent, or non-inferior relative to the control arm. The objective of equivalence trials is to find no clinically significant difference between treatments. Non-inferiority trials aim to prove that the experimental drug is not significantly worse than the existing one in terms of efficacy (it may well have other benefits such as less toxicity or expense). Disadvantages of RCTs may include difficulties with recruiting large numbers of patients, the generalizability of results if subjects are not necessarily representative of the general patient population, and the acceptability of randomization process to patients and clinicians.

Phase 4 trials

These late phase studies are undertaken with the objective of 'post-marketing' long-term surveillance, which may include identification of rare adverse events, evaluation of subgroups, and to determine if the observed benefit from the trial translates into a clinical benefit within the general population.

Novel concepts in trial design

With an increasing number of molecularly targeted and immunotherapy agents, and awareness of the heterogeneity of response to drugs, molecular biomarkers are increasingly being developed concurrently within trials. In 'enrichment' trial design, patients are tested for and non-randomly assigned to trial subgroups based on the presence of a biomarker. This approach increases the power of the trial, can quickly validate a predictive biomarker and potentially reduces exposure to a drug where it may not be effective. However, it may limit the generalizability of the results, especially if it is assumed that biomarker-negative patients will not benefit.

Two different biomarker enrichment strategies are so-called 'basket' and 'umbrella' trials. Basket trial designs attempt to match a molecularly targeted agent with activity against a mutated signalling pathway in a histology-independent manner to patients with a rare activating mutation in multiple different cancer types. An example of this is the phase 2 VE-BASKET trial which evaluated the B-Raf enzyme inhibitor vemurafenib, in patients with a variety of non-melanoma tumours harbouring B-Raf V600E mutations. Outside of melanoma these mutations show a low prevalence and therefore the basket trial design theoretically sped up evaluation of a new targeted drug with potential therapeutic potential in multiple cancers. In contrast umbrella trials aim to test multiple different drugs according to biomarker status within a single cancer type. These multiple sub-trials stem from a central infrastructure and can share a control arm thus decreasing costs and increasing throughput. Both basket and umbrella trials are reliant on good pre-clinical data linking the target biomarker and drug of interest.

Recently trials have adopted adaptive designs to incorporate new potential biomarkers, indications, or combinations with new drugs as they become available, ensuring they remain contemporary—a so-called 'seamless design' approach. An example of this is the first-in-human trial of pembrolizumab (Keynote-001 trial by Merck Sharp & Dohme Corp. NCT01295827) which initially opened as a 3+3 dose-escalation study, but underwent multiple amendments to the original protocol resulting in two dozen expansion cohorts in different tumour types, evaluating efficacy with biomarker variability, testing lower doses in different indications, and accounting for variable prior therapies (Kang et al. 2017).

Trial endpoints

Endpoints within trials can be separated into those that directly impact on the patient's quality or quantity of life (patient-based endpoints) and those that act as a surrogate for this (tumour-based endpoints). Some of the most commonly used endpoints are summarized in Table 2.9.2.

There is debate on whether response or progression-free survival (PFS) represent meaningful surrogates of patient-based endpoints. PFS has only been validated as a surrogate for OS for a few cancers in particular settings and many trials demonstrate an increase in PFS that does not translate into an increased OS. Hypotheses

Table 2.9.1 A summary of different trial designs

Trial design	Description
Parallel	Each patient on the trial is randomized to a single treatment arm
Cross-over	Each patient receives different treatments at different time points. Patients act as their own control (there is no intra-patient variability) and the washout period of the drug needs to be incorporated into timing. It can only be used for diseases which are likely to be stable over a long time period
Factorial	Patients are randomized twice such that single cohort can be used to evaluate a number of treatments within a single trial
Adaptive	Characteristics of the trial (e.g. sample size or randomization probabilities) can be modified based on interim or accumulating data
Group sequential	Several pre-planned interim analyses allow the trial to be stopped on the basis of efficacy and/or futility
Discontinuation	Patients who respond to a treatment are randomized to either continuation or discontinuation of treatment
Seamless	Combines study phases into a single adaptive study, which can be adjusted following interim assessments of the data

Table 2.9.2 Clinical trial endpoints

	Endpoint	Definition	Pros	Cons
Patient-based endpoints	OS	Time from randomization or the start of treatment to death (irrespective of cause)	Gold standard measure with direct patient benefit	Long follow-up period may be required Large numbers of patients required to reach adequate power
	Quality of life	The effect of illness on physical and psychological functioning	Provides a measure of direct patient benefit even with short study duration	Subjective measure Risk of incomplete data (e.g. patients may miss visits) Lack of standardization in terms of analysis and presentation of results
	Cancer-specific survival	Time from randomization to death from primary (index) cancer	Only accounts for deaths due to the underlying cancer	Difficult to ascertain specific cause of death Does not account for deaths attributable to treatment
Tumour-based surrogate endpoints	Progression-free survival (PFS)	Time between randomization and tumour progression or patient death from any cause in the metastatic setting	Smaller size and shorter time duration needed Identifies benefit earlier Not affected by crossover trial design or post-trial therapies	Only statistically validated as a surrogate in a few cancer settings Risk of assessment bias (progression is determined on timing of clinical and/or radiological assessments) Risk of evaluation bias
	Disease-free survival (DFS) (also known as relapse free survival)	Time between randomization and tumour relapse (or death from any cause) following treatment with curative intent	Smaller size and shorter time duration needed	Not statistically validated surrogate Subject to bias (as for PFS)
	TTP	Time to disease progression (deaths before progression excluded)	Small sample size and short time duration	Not statistically validated as a surrogate. Subject to bias Affected by censoring data
	ORR	Proportion of patients with either a partial or complete response according to standardized RECIST criteria	Reflects a direct biological effect	Does not include stable disease (SD) or incorporate differences in response kinetics Criticized as being an arbitrary divide between cut-offs for progressive disease (PD), SD, and partial response (PR) Variability in measurement of response and intra-observer bias

Box 2.9.1 Steps in setting up a trial

1 Hypothesis and literature review to ensure originality, relevance, and necessity of the trial. There should be evidence to support the control arm and the effect size proposed.

2 First draft of the protocol, which should include objectives, background and rationale, subject selection criteria, treatment plan, study procedures, evaluation of response, and statistical section.

3 Pilot study may be considered to provide information on feasibility of recruitment, set-up, and variability in endpoints, thereby identifying and preventing flaws in trial design that could potentially later render a trial useless. Early consultation with a statistician and clinical trials unit is recommended.

4 Funding and insurance. The most appropriate funding body is approached for a grant application. The sponsor is the individual or organization responsible for the funding, clinical governance, and management of the trial and holds legal responsibility. This may be a pharmaceutical company, university, or academic institution. National Health Service (NHS) research and development departments provide trial oversight, risk management, and often act as the sponsor for United Kingdom (UK) trials. Sometimes the sponsor may employ a contract research organization (CRO) to aid in the logistics and conduct of trials. They will assign a chief investigator (CI) who holds overall responsibility for design, conduct, analysis, and reporting of the trial.

5 Ethics approval. Clinical trials involving research on human subjects must be reviewed and monitored by an Institutional Review Board (IRB) or Research Ethics Committee (REC), which is an independent committee of physicians, nurses, statisticians, patient advocates, and pharmacists. They will review trials to assess if they are conducted according to the International Conference on Harmonization's Good Clinical Practice (ICH-GCP) guideline, which provides an international standard on the conduct of clinical trials. The REC will consider factors including the scientific value of the study, the selection process, the risk: benefit ratio, consent, and the suitability of the applicants.

6 Regulatory authorization. For clinical trial approval, a Clinical Trial Authorization (CTA) application must be submitted to regulatory bodies in each member state, e.g. in the UK, the Medical Health Regulatory Agency (MHRA) is the national competent authority, which authorises clinical trials involving medicinal products. For EU multinational clinical trials there is a Voluntary Harmonisation Procedure that permits sponsors to obtain a harmonized assessment of their CTA application by all the National Competent Authorities involved, avoiding the need for multiple applications in each country.

7 Register the trial. All UK medicinal product trials require a European Clinical Trials database number and should ideally be registered within an international standard randomized controlled trial number (ISRCTN) database such as ClinicalTrials.gov.

8 Pre-study visits (PSV) are conducted to ascertain capacity and capability of institutions to recruit to the given protocol, followed by Clinical Trial Agreement which is an agreement between the Sponsor and the participating Institutions.

9 Site initiation visit to ensure the trial team are set-up appropriately to recruit first patient so the site may be activated.

accounting for this discrepancy include the possibility that an initial change in tumour size may not impact on OS, and that interpretation of results may be confounded by multiple post-trial therapies. In addition, these response-based endpoints do not take into account possible evolutionary change of the tumour following the intervention, which may influence survival.

Given the fact that many molecularly targeted agents may have a more cytostatic mechanism of action, endpoints that incorporate stable disease (SD) such as disease control rate (DCR) (number of patients showing response or SD for a set period of time) and duration of response (DOR) may be more meaningful than conventional endpoints. With the rise in use of immunotherapies in oncology management, it has emerged that responses to these agents may differ from those seen as a result of traditional cytotoxic responses. Responses may be delayed and indeed they may manifest with an initial increase in the size of the lesion as a result of immune-cell infiltration rather than tumour growth. Therefore immune-related response criteria (iRRc) have been devised to account for these different patterns of activity.

Efficient drug development through clinical trials is contingent on timely acquisition of evidence for an effective drug regimen to ascertain whether it should be moved forward in testing and ultimately into clinical practice. Considerable thought should therefore be given to the best trial design and endpoints to achieve this aim. Before recruiting the first patient in a trial, there are a number of logistical practicalities to consider. The key steps to consider are listed in Table 2.9.2 but do not necessarily take place in this order. Timing of this process should not be underestimated, and a trial may take many months or even years to initiate. However, careful attention to the clinical trial design will provide robust go/no-go signals and minimize the risk of expensive failures at a late stage of drug development (Box 2.9.1).

Further reading

Calvert AH, Newell DR, Gumbrell LA, O'Reilly S, Burnell M, Boxall FE, et al. Carboplatin dosage: prospective evaluation of a simple formula based on renal function. *J Clin Oncol* 1989; 7:1748–56.

Freidlin B, Korn EL. Biomarker enrichment strategies: matching trial design to biomarker credentials. *Nat Rev Clin Oncol* 2014; 11(2):81–90.

Kang SP, Gergich K, Lubiniecki GM, de Alwis DP, Chen C, Tice MAB, Rubin EH. Pembrolizumab KEYNOTE-001: an adaptive study leading to accelerated approval for two indications and a companion diagnostic. *Ann Oncol* 2017; 28(6):1388–98.

Köhler G, Milstein C. Continuous cultures of fused cells secreting antibody of predefined specificity. *Nature* 1975; 256(5517):495–7.

Le DT, Durham JN, Smith KN, et al. Mismatch repair deficiency predicts response of solid tumors to PD-1 blockade. *Science* 2017; 357(6349):409–13.

Marabelle A, Fakih M, Lopez J, et al. Association of tumour mutational burden with outcomes in patients with advanced solid tumours treated with pembrolizumab: prospective biomarker analysis of the multicohort, open-label, phase 2 KEYNOTE-158 study. *Lancet Oncol* 2020—available at https://doi.org/10.1016/S1470-2045(20)30445-9.

Merck Sharp & Dohme Corp. 'Study of Pembrolizumab (MK-3475) in Participants With Progressive Locally Advanced or Metastatic Carcinoma, Melanoma, or Non-small Cell Lung Carcinoma (P07990/MK-3475-001/KEYNOTE-001) (KEYNOTE-001)' ClinicalTrials.gov Identifier: NCT01295827.

Redig AJ, Jänne PA. Basket trials and the evolution of clinical trial design in an era of genomic medicine. *J Clin Oncol* 2015; 33(9):975–7.

Internet resources

MRC guidelines for GCP in clinical trials: https://www.hra.nhs.uk/planning-and-improving-research/policies-standards-legislation/good-clinical-practice/

National Institute of Health Research: Clinical trials toolkit: http://www.ct-toolkit.ac.uk

New Oncology Clinical Trial Designs: What works and what doesn't: http://www.ajmc.com/journals/evidence-based-oncology/ 2015/the-american-society-of-clinical-oncology-annual-meeting-2015/new-oncology-clinical-trial-designs-what-works-and-what-doesnt

Chapter 3

Tumours of the head and neck

Chapter contents

3.1 Principles of management for cancer of the head and neck

Introduction

The head and neck region encompasses anatomical sites below the brain and above the clavicles, excluding skin and thyroid. The sites most commonly involved with cancer are the oral cavity, larynx, and pharynx. Since 1990, the incidence of oropharyngeal cancer has significantly increased in England. The incidence of oral cavity cancer has increased slightly, whilst the incidence of laryngeal cancer has decreased. Overall five-year survival rates for head and neck cancer have improved only slightly over the past two decades remaining at just over 50%. This reflects the population who present with this disease in terms of age and comorbidity (typically about 15% intercurrent death rates at five years), as well as the tendency to develop second primaries and metastases. The poor long-term survival rates may also reflect the fact that 60% of patients with head and neck cancer have advanced disease at the time of presentation (stage III/IV disease). The dominant treatment failure in head and neck cancer is loco-regional relapse and this remains the main focus for clinicians involved in the management of these patients.

About 90% of head and neck cancers are squamous cell carcinomas, with the remainder being lymphoma, salivary cancers, mucosal melanomas, and sarcomas. Histology is most diverse in the nasal passages and salivary glands. Management of head and neck squamous cell carcinomas (HNSCC) depends largely on clinical parameters, in particular the stage of the tumour. The tumour node metastasis (TNM) staging system as laid out by the International Union against Cancer (UICC) describes the anatomical extent of the tumour. T describes the two-dimensional size of the primary tumour, and is dependent on the subsite within the head and neck from which the primary tumour is arising. N defines the presence of any regional nodal disease and again represents a two-dimensional measurement of nodal size as well as number of nodes. M denotes the presence of any distant metastases. Classification of tumours by the TNM system allows a fairly precise description of the anatomical extent of the disease. Since there are four degrees of T, three degrees of N, and two degrees of M, there are 24 TNM categories; these can be condensed into four stage groups (I–IV), which aim to classify them into homogeneous clusters with similar survival rates which are distinctive for each anatomical subsite. In reality, identically staged tumours often have different survival rates due to diversity in biological characteristics of the tumour and variable patient performance status (PS).

Aetiology and risk factors

Tobacco is an independent risk factor for HNSCC. Smoking during radiotherapy has been related to an increased risk of osteoradionecrosis, hospitalization during treatment, and cancer relapse. Patients who smoke are also at higher risk for complications related to anaesthesia and impaired wound healing after reconstructive surgery. Therefore, smoking cessation prior to treatment should always be advised. Alcohol is another independent risk factor and has a synergistic effect with tobacco. Nasopharyngeal cancers are associated with an Epstein–Barr virus (EBV) infection (90% of cases in the UK). Malignant transformation can occur in 12% of patients with oral dysplasia (mean 4.3 years) and 14% in those with laryngeal dysplasia (mean 5.8 years). Fanconi anaemia patients are at high risk for head and neck cancer and should be managed with quarterly screening and an aggressive biopsy policy. Ataxia telangiectasia, Bloom's syndrome, and Li–Fraumeni syndrome are other inherited conditions with increased risk for HNSCC. Occupational risk factors (asbestos, pesticides, etc.), previous irradiation, low socioeconomic status, and certain preservatives and salty foods have also been related to head and neck cancers.

The causative relationship between human papilloma virus (HPV) infection and oropharyngeal squamous cell carcinoma has been well established. HPV-associated disease is more commonly seen in the tonsil and base of tongue of young male non-smokers. HPV prevalence in oropharyngeal tumours has increased significantly over time (40.5% in studies that recruited patients before 2000 versus 64.3% during the period 2000–4 versus 72.2% during the period 2005–9). More than 90% of HPV-related HNSCC are caused by strain 16 of the virus. The best method to detect the virus in the tumour is yet to be defined. DNA or RNA in situ hybridization can be used to confirm HPV positivity. When immunohistochemistry is used, a strong nuclear and cytoplasmic p16 staining in more than 70% of tumour cells is required to label a tumour HPV positive. Better responses in radiotherapy and chemotherapy have been observed among HPV-positive oropharyngeal cancer patients compared with HPV-negative ones. HPV 16 has been confirmed as a prognostic marker for improved disease-free and overall survival, but not yet as a predictive marker. Ongoing trials are investigating the de-intensification of treatment in HPV-positive oropharyngeal cancers.

Early stage disease

Early head and neck cancer (stage I–II) is generally managed with single modality therapy. The choice of surgery or radiotherapy is determined by the location of the tumour and the likely morbidity, i.e. anticipated structural, functional, and cosmetic preservation. Consideration should also be given as to how easy it would be to identify a recurrence. Salvage surgery usually has to be radical with no option for conservation of normal tissues and may be associated with a poor outcome. There are also significant risks associated with surgery in the salvage setting. The probability of eradicating tumour with radiotherapy is related to tumour volume; for T1 tumours, the primary local control rate is 85–95% and for T2, 70–85%. Surgery is the most frequent approach for early stage oral cancers.

Indications for postoperative radiotherapy include involved surgical margins, extracapsular nodal spread, pT3-4 primary tumour, pN2-3 nodal disease, involved level 4 or 5 nodes, perineural invasion, lymphovascular invasion, and high grade (salivary gland tumours). Concomitant chemotherapy (cisplatin preferred) should be added to postoperative radiotherapy in the presence of involved surgical margins and/or extracapsular nodal spread.

Locally advanced disease

The management of locally advanced disease requires a multidisciplinary approach since the choice of radical treatment involves different combinations of surgery, radiotherapy and systemic treatment. The two commonest approaches are: 1) surgery with postoperative (chemo) radiotherapy, and 2) curative radio-chemotherapy. A nodal dissection can precede curative radio-chemotherapy in some cases (e.g. large cystic neck node). Decisions are often based on clinical intuition and experience, taking into account tumour stage, PS, and of course the wishes of the patient. The main determinants are the likelihood of tumour control and the functional outcome. However, the significance of getting this decision wrong is monumental. A patient who develops a local recurrence following treatment with chemoradiation may be unfit for salvage surgery, and even when resection is possible, the functional and survival outcome is poorer than for primary surgery. On the other hand, the use of surgery to treat a tumour which might have been cured with chemoradiation exposes a patient to the potential morbid effects of surgery. Hence, the ability of the multidisciplinary team (MDT) to ensure the patient receives the most appropriate treatment is crucial.

Surgery

Surgical techniques have advanced significantly over the last two decades and are developing to be as minimally invasive as possible. Laser and trans-oral robotic surgery (TORS) are minimal access techniques that avoid the morbidity associated with previously described radical approaches and are also associated with improved functional outcomes. These have applications in the diagnosis and staging of HNSCC patients (tonsillectomies and base of tongue mucosectomies) and offer organ-preservation surgery for tumours of the oral cavity, pharynx, and larynx. Endoscopic surgery for malignant sinonasal and anterior skull base tumours is being used more frequently and image-guided surgery can be helpful with tumours located at complex anatomical sites in the head and neck region. Neck dissection techniques have also evolved, moving from radical to modified radical and selective dissections. Sentinel lymph node biopsy can replace elective neck dissection in patients with early oral cavity cancer (T1–T2, N0), unless there is a need for synchronous cervical access. Finally, there are now more options for reconstructive surgery than there were in the past.

Radiotherapy

Planning and delivery

Radiation therapy has evolved over the past years from two-dimensional therapy (2DRT) to three-dimensional conformal radiotherapy (3DCRT), which aims to spare surrounding normal tissue whilst delivering radiation to the tumoural target, and more recently to intensity-modulated radiotherapy (IMRT) which is an advanced form of treatment delivery that not only delivers conformally shaped beams but also produces non-uniform beam intensities (fluency profiles). The dosimetric advantages of IMRT can essentially be ascribed to better conformation of dose to target volume or use of differential doses to areas at different risks of harbouring tumour deposits (see Figure 3.1.1). Additional benefits include

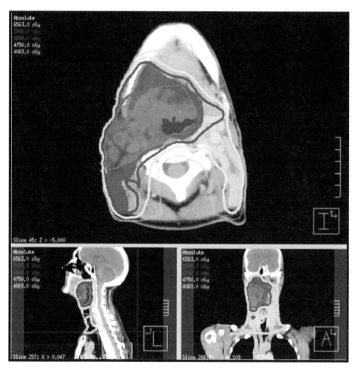

Fig. 3.1.1 IMRT dose plan for patient with oropharyngeal tumour (see also colour plate).

the avoidance of matching field junctions as well as the ease of set-up using a single isocentre. The potential clinical advantages relate to reducing normal tissue toxicity or escalating dose to macroscopic disease. Other forms of IMRT are RapidArc, VMAT, and tomotherapy. Stereotactic body radiation therapy (SBRT) and proton therapy do not have an established role in the management of HNSCC. Brachytherapy is recommended by GEC-ESTRO as a boost after external beam irradiation, a complementary treatment with surgery, a salvage therapy for limited-extent local recurrences, or as radical treatment for small tumours of the oral cavity·

Expert assessment of patients is critical to the interpretation of radiological images in defining target volumes on radiotherapy computer planning systems. A discussion between the radiation oncologist and a radiologist (in postoperative cases a surgeon and pathologist as well) is often important to define the exact anatomical sites at risk. The following target volumes are defined according to the International Commission on Radiation Units and Measurements (ICRU) guidelines: gross tumour volume (GTV); primary tumour (GTV-T); involved lymph nodes (GTV-N); and clinical target volume (CTV). A high-risk CTV (primary tumour and positive nodes with a margin), an intermediate-risk CTV (areas or nodal levels at high risk), and a low-risk CTV (nodal regions at low risk) are often produced depending on primary site and disease extent. In postoperative radiotherapy, CTV can include any gross residual disease with a margin (1–2cm), the tumour bed with a margin (1–2cm), and any areas or nodal levels at risk for recurrence. The Danish Head and Neck Cancer Group (DAHANCA), European Organisation for Research and Treatment of Cancer (EORTC), Hong Kong Nasopharyneal Cancer Study Group (HKNPCSG), National Cancer Institute of Canada Clinical Trials Group (NCIC CTG), National Cancer Research Institute (NCRI), Radiation Therapy Oncology Group (RTOG), and Trans Tasman Radiation Oncology Group (TROG) consensus guidelines are used for contouring nodal CTV. More atlases have now been developed to aid with target definition, e.g. for contouring cranial nerves to the base of skull as part of CTV in adenoid cystic carcinomas with perineural invasion. Planning target volume (PTV): takes into account potential organ and patient movement which for immobilized patients with head and neck tumours usually entails a transaxial margin of 3–5mm around CTV. Organs at risk (OARs): the organs listed in Table 3.1.1 need to be outlined so that every effort is made to ensure they receive a reduced dose. For example, the parotids should be spared to reduce the risk of long-term xerostomia and the COSTAR study uses cochlea-sparing IMRT. Planning risk volume (PRV): an isotropic margin of 3–5mm can be added to some serial OARs (e.g. spinal cord, brainstem) in a similar way that a margin is added to CTV for PTV. Most cases should be planned with IMRT with the exception of T1 N0 M0 glottic tumours and palliative treatments where 3DCRT is sufficient. Image-guided radiation therapy (IGRT) is used in conjunction with IMRT with an aim to reduce set-up errors and to account for target volume changes during treatment such as tumour shrinkage and patient weight loss (adaptive radiotherapy).

Dose and fractionation

The effectiveness of a radiotherapy 'dose' is related to various fractionation parameters including overall

Table 3.1.1 Organs at risk (OARs) and dose constraints

OAR	Endpoint	Dose (Gy)
Spinal cord	Myelopathy	Dmax <50
Brainstem	Permanent neuropathy or necrosis	Dmax <54 D1–10 cc ≤59 Dmax <64 (point dose <1cc)
Brain	Symptomatic necrosis	Dmax <60
Cochlea	Sensory neural hearing loss (SNHL)	Mean dose ≤45
Optic nerve/chiasm	Optic neuropathy	Dmax <55
Lens	Cataract	Dmax <10
Eyes/retina	Retinopathy	Dmax <50 Mean dose <35
Lacrimal gland	Dry eye syndrome	Dmax <35
Parotid	Long-term salivary function reduced to <25% of pre-RT level	Bilateral parotids—mean dose <25 Unilateral parotid—mean dose <20
Larynx	1- Vocal dysfunction 2- Aspiration 3- Oedema	1- Dmax <66 2- Mean dose <50 3- Mean dose <44
Pharynx (constrictor muscles)	Dysphagia, aspiration	Mean dose <50
Submandibular gland	Xerostomia	Mean dose <39
Mandible and TMJ	Osteoradionecrosis	Dmax <70

Source: data from Marks LB, et al. Quantitative analysis of normal tissue effects in the clinic (QUANTEC): An introduction to the scientific issues. *Int J Radiat Oncol Biol Phys* 2010; 76(3) (Suppl.):S3–9. 2010, Elsevier Inc.

treatment time and fraction size, as much as the total dose. 'Conventional' fractionation is defined as 2Gy per day, five days a week. Numerous different doses for IMRT can be encountered in the literature. In 2016, the Royal College of Radiologists published guidelines for dose and fractionation and suggests 70Gy in 35 fractions over seven weeks for high-risk PTV, 63Gy in 35 fractions over seven weeks for intermediate-risk PTV and 56–7Gy in 35 fractions over seven weeks to low-risk PTV for definitive head and neck cancer treatment. The moderate acceleration with hypofractionation used in the PARSPORT study has been adopted by many UK centres (65Gy in 30 fractions over six weeks to the high-risk PTV and 54Gy in 30 fractions over six weeks to the low-risk PTV). For treatment of an intermediate-risk PTV, 60Gy in 30 fractions over six weeks is prescribed. For T1/T2 N0 M0 glottic carcinomas, a marked acceleration with a hypofractionation schedule is preferred (55Gy in 20 fractions over four weeks or 63Gy in 28 fractions over 5.5 weeks). For T1 N0 M0 glottic tumours only, 50Gy in 16 fractions over three weeks can be given. For postoperative radiotherapy, 60–66Gy in 30–33 fractions is the standard dose. For palliative radiotherapy, different fractionation regimens are used depending on tumour location, prognosis, PS, etc. Some of the commonly accepted schedules that apply to the majority of head and neck subsites are 36–39Gy in 12–13 fractions over 2.5 weeks, 40Gy in ten fractions over four weeks 'split course', 30Gy in ten fractions over two weeks, 20Gy in five fractions over one week, and 8–10Gy single fraction. Reirradiation with a curative intent can be an option for carefully selected patients who are not candidates for surgical salvage. Doses of ≥60Gy with conventional or altered fractionation, with or without chemotherapy are commonly used.

Other modifications to conventional fractionations include hyperfractionation (use of >5 smaller fractions per week while maintaining a conventional overall treatment time to deliver an increased total dose) and modest acceleration (use of >5 fractions per week while maintaining a conventional total dose delivered in a shorter overall treatment time). The rationale behind hyperfractionation is to manipulate the two parameters which most influence late effects of radiotherapy, i.e. total dose and fraction size. By reducing fraction size, total dose can be increased to improve tumour control without exacerbating late effects. An example of pure hyperfractionation is the regimen of 80.5Gy in 70 fractions over seven weeks. The radiobiological rationale of modest acceleration is to manipulate the two parameters which most influence local control of squamous cancer, i.e. total dose and overall treatment time; reducing treatment time combats accelerated repopulation of tumour clonogens as a potential cause of treatment failure. An example is the DAHANCA regimen of six fractions per week, reducing treatment time by about a week which showed an improvement in five-year local control of 10% with only a transient increase in acute toxicity. Marked acceleration plus hyperfractionation using the continuous hyperfractionated accelerated radiotherapy (CHART) regimen (54Gy in 36 fractions of 1.5Gy over 12 days) showed similar loco-regional control and survival, but fewer severe late side effects than conventional radiotherapy. A meta-analysis of hyperfractionated or accelerated radiotherapy in head and neck cancer showed an overall absolute survival benefit with altered fractionation of 3.4% at five years. The benefit was higher with hyperfractionated radiotherapy (8% at five years) compared with accelerated radiotherapy (2% with accelerated fractionation without total dose reduction and 1.7% with total dose reduction at five years).

Hyperfractionated or accelerated radiotherapy alone are more efficacious than conventional radiotherapy alone but a few randomized studies failed to show superiority of either of the altered radiotherapy fractionations, used alone or combined with chemotherapy compared with the conventional radiotherapy with synchronous chemotherapy approach. A radiotherapy schedule with synchronous chemotherapy remains the standard of care in locally advanced head and neck cancer.

Systemic treatments
Curative
The addition of concomitant chemotherapy to radiotherapy offers a five-year absolute benefit of 6.5%. This benefit decreases with the increasing age of patients (p = 0.003, test for trend). Three-weekly cisplatin at 100mg/m^2 is the standard of care although in clinical practice weekly cisplatin at 40 mg/m^2 is often used. The value of chemoradiotherapy in these patients can be hindered by the increased and prohibitive toxicity of the treatment, which may be enhanced by any associated comorbidities. This has led to interest in novel non-cytotoxic targeted therapies such as cetuximab, an epidermal growth factor receptor (EGFR) inhibitor. A randomized controlled trial showed that synchronous cetuximab improves survival when compared with radiotherapy alone. The De-ESCALaTE study randomizes HPV-positive oropharyngeal cancer patients between radiotherapy with concomitant cisplatin and radiotherapy with concomitant cetuximab and results are awaited. Induction chemotherapy followed by radio-chemotherapy has failed to show improved outcomes in several randomized trials and a meta-analysis. However, it is sometimes considered for highly selective cases of clinically fit patients with very advanced loco-regional disease. If induction chemotherapy before radiotherapy is deemed appropriate, the three-drug combination of docetaxel, cisplatin, and fluorouracil (5-FU) (TPF) improves survival relative to the previous standard of cisplatin and 5-FU (PF). Immunotherapy has shown activity in metastatic disease and several clinical trials have been designed to investigate its role in the curative setting.

Palliative treatment
Palliative chemotherapy provides a modest benefit overall in advanced HNSCC with objective response rates of 20–40%. Cisplatin, 5-FU, carboplatin, taxanes, capecitabine, methotrexate, gemcitabine, and combinations of these drugs have been traditionally used. The EXTREME study showed that patients with untreated recurrent/metastatic head and neck cancer who received cetuximab with cisplatin and fluorouracil showed improved overall survival (10.1 months vs. 7.4 months) and 46% increase in progression-free survival (5.6 months vs. 3.3 months) compared with patients who received chemotherapy alone. Toxicity was increased in the cetuximab group but treatment-related deaths are increased in the chemotherapy group. Head and neck cancer provides an ideal situation for the study of novel agents as its accessibility permits scrutiny of both tumour control and normal tissue effects.

Recent advances in immunotherapy are starting to find application in the HNSCC field. Tumour cells escape the immune system response by exploiting inhibitory checkpoint pathways that suppress anti tumour T cell activity. Novel immunotherapeutic strategies focus on using antibodies to block immune checkpoints, such as PD-1 and CTLA4, from binding to their ligands, such as CD80, CD84, PD-L1, and PD-L2. Nivolumab, an anti-PD-1 monoclonal antibody, exhibited a longer overall survival than treatment with standard, single-agent therapy in patients with platinum-refractory, recurrent HNSCC. Similarly, pembrolizumab, a humanized anti-PD-1 antibody, showed significant antitumour activity in PD-L1-positive recurrent or metastatic HNSCC.

Principles of patient management

In the management of patients with head and neck cancer, there are at least 'ten commandments' or considerations which need to be addressed before treatment:

1. Performance status: weight loss; associated comorbidities (all central to management plan)
2. Smoking status: smoking cessation programme; smoking during radiotherapy reduces local tumour control and increases late toxicity
3. Dental status: post-radiotherapy extraction may precipitate osteoradionecrosis
4. Nutritional status: consider elective gastrostomy in patients where oral intake is likely to become impaired, or is already poor
5. Bite block tongue depressor for radiotherapy for oral/nasal cancer
6. Routine blood tests: consider transfusion if moderate anaemia; caution in patients with deranged renal/liver function receiving cytotoxic therapy
7. Imaging of chest: to exclude synchronous lung primary—or metastases, particularly if N2/3 disease
8. Alcohol intake needs to be stopped/moderated if possible during radiotherapy
9. Close scrutiny of concomitant medications
10. Fully informed consent

Further reading

Bernier J, Cooper JS, Pajak TF, et al. Defining risk levels in locally advanced head and neck cancers: a comparative analysis of concurrent postoperative radiation plus chemotherapy trials of the EORTC (#22931) and RTOG (# 9501). Head Neck 2005; 27(10):843–50.

Blanchard P, Bourhis J, Lacas B, et al. Meta-analysis of chemotherapy in head and neck cancer, induction chemotherapy project, collaborative group. Taxane-cisplatin-fluorouracil as induction chemotherapy in locally advanced head and neck cancers: an individual patient data meta-analysis of the meta-analysis of chemotherapy in head and neck cancer group. J Clin Oncol 2013; 31(23):2854–60.

Bonner JA, Harari PM, Giralt J, et al. Radiotherapy plus cetuximab for locoregionally advanced head and neck cancer: 5-year survival data from a phase 3 randomised trial, and relation between cetuximab-induced rash and survival. Lancet Oncol 2010; 11(1):21–8.

Bourhis J, Overgaard J, Audry H, et al. Hyperfractionated or accelerated radiotherapy in head and neck cancer: a meta-analysis. Lancet 2006; 368:843.

Budach W, Bölke E, Kammers K, et al. Induction chemotherapy followed by concurrent radio-chemotherapy versus concurrent radio-chemotherapy alone as treatment of locally advanced squamous cell carcinoma of the head and neck (HNSCC):

A meta-analysis of randomized trials. Radiother Oncol 2016; 118(2):238–43.

de Bree R, Leemans CR. Recent advances in surgery for head and neck cancer. Curr Opin Oncol 2010; 22(3):186–93.

Economopoulou P, Agelaki S, Perisanidis C, et al. The promise of immunotherapy in head and neck squamous cell carcinoma. Ann Oncol 2016; 27(9):1675–85.

Ferris RL, Blumenschein G Jr, Fayette J, et al. Nivolumab for recurrent squamous-cell carcinoma of the head and neck. N Engl J Med 2016; 375(19):1856–67.

Grégoire V, Ang K, Budach W, et al. Delineation of the neck node levels for head and neck tumors: a 2013 update. DAHANCA, EORTC, HKNPCSG, NCIC CTG, NCRI, RTOG, TROG consensus guidelines. Radiother Oncol 2014; 110(1):172–81.

Horiot JC, Le Fur R, N'Guyen T, et al. Hyperfractionation versus conventional fractionation in oropharyngeal carcinoma: final analysis of a randomized trial of the EORTC cooperative group of radiotherapy. Radiother Oncol 1992; 25:231–41.

Ko HC, Gupta V, Mourad WF, et al. A contouring guide for head and neck cancers with perineural invasion. Pract Radiat Oncol 2014; 4(6):e247–58.

Marks LB, Yorke ED, Jackson A, et al. The use of normal tissue complication probability (NTCP) models in the clinic. Int J Radiat Oncol Biol Phys 2010; 76(30):S10–19.

Mazeron JJ, Ardiet JM, Haie-Méder C, et al. GEC-ESTRO recommendations for brachytherapy for head and neck squamous cell carcinomas. Radiother Oncol 2009; 91(2):150–6.

Mehanna H, Beech T, Nicholson T, et al. Prevalence of human papillomavirus in oropharyngeal and non-oropharyngeal head and neck cancer—systematic review and meta-analysis of trends by time and region. Head Neck 2013; 35(5):747–55.

National Institute for Health and Clinical Excellence (NICE). Cancer of the upper aerodigestive tract: assessment and management in people aged 16 and over. NICE Guideline 36. Full guideline February 2016 (online). London: NICE 2016—available at: http://www.nice.org.uk/.

Nutting CM, Morden JP, Harrington KJ, et al. Parotid-sparing intensity modulated versus conventional radiotherapy in head and neck cancer (PARSPORT): a phase 3 multicentre randomised controlled trial. Lancet Oncol 2011;12:127–36.

Overgaard J, Hansen HS, Specht L, et al. Five compared with six fractions per week of conventional radiotherapy of squamous-cell carcinoma of head and neck: DAHANCA 6 and 7 randomised controlled trial. Lancet 2003; 362:933–40. Erratum in: Lancet 2003; 362:1588.

Paleri V, Roland NJ (eds). Head and Neck Cancer: United Kingdom National Multidisciplinary Guidelines. J Laryng Otol 2016; 130 (Suppl. S2):S1–224.

Pignon JP, le Maitre A, Maillard E, et al. Meta-analysis of chemotherapy in head and neck cancer (MACH-NC): an update on 93 randomised trials and 17,346 patients. Radiother Oncol 2009; 92:4–14.

Seiwert TY, Burtness B, Mehra R, et al. Safety and clinical activity of pembrolizumab for treatment of recurrent or metastatic squamous cell carcinoma of the head and neck (KEYNOTE-012): an open-label, multicentre, phase 1b trial. Lancet Oncol 2016; 7(7):956–65.

The Royal College of Radiologists (RCR). Publications and Guidance. Radiotherapy Dose-Fractionation. Head and Neck Cancers (online). 2nd edition. London: The Royal College of Radiologists 2016 Dec—available at: http://www.rcr.ac.uk/.

Vermorken JB, Mesia R, Rivera F, et al. Platinum based chemotherapy plus cetuximab in head and neck cancer. N Eng J Med 2008; 359:1116–27.

3.2 Tumours of the eye, orbit, and ear

Tumours of the eye

Malignant tumours of the eyelids include basal cell carcinoma (BCC) and squamous cell carcinoma (SCC). The more common BCC accounts for 90% of tumours of the eyelid and often occurs as a result of sun damage to the skin. Typically it affects the lower eyelids, followed by the canthal area, and less frequently the upper lid. SCCs account for <10% of malignant eyelid tumours, but are capable of metastases. Within the eyelid, the meibomian glands in the tarsal plate, and the sweat and sebaceous appendages adjacent to the cilia, can give rise to adenocarcinomas, which may present as slowly expanding nodules.

SCC is the commonest malignancy affecting the conjunctiva. Lymphocytic proliferative disorders can also affect the conjunctiva. Melanocytic lesions of the conjunctiva have varying degrees of malignant potential.

Clinical features

BCCs often develop as a small indurated, well-demarcated nodule which may have some degree of pigmentation. The overlying skin may break down with resultant painless ulceration. As with other cutaneous BCCs they are usually locally invasive, but rarely metastasize. SCCs may also present in a similar fashion, which may make them difficult to distinguish. Conjunctival SCCs may present as a fleshy vascular mass at the limbus; melanomas may present as a raised pigmented or non-pigmented area on the conjunctiva.

Management

Punch biopsy will confirm diagnosis in diffuse eyelid tumours. Treatment usually comprises complete surgical excision with frozen section control of margins for localized tumours. Dependent on the extent of surgical excision, reconstruction of the eyelids may be required, using sliding skin flaps, rotational flaps, and free skin grafts.

Conjunctival tumours are similarly treated with complete surgical excision with frozen section to confirm margins, with cryotherapy to the tumour bed. Reconstruction may involve grafting of the area. In radiosensitive tumours such as lymphoma, external beam radiotherapy, or plaque brachytherapy can be used.

Tumours of the globe

Malignant melanoma is the most common primary intraocular tumour in adults, commonly affecting adults in the fifth and sixth decades of life. There is no significant difference in the incidences between genders; however, it is more common in Caucasians than non-Caucasians. It may arise from any portion of the uveal tract but commonly affects the choroid, then the ciliary body, and least often the iris. Usually slow to grow and metastasize, it generally affects one eye only and may develop spontaneously or from a mole within the eye. Development of distant metastases rather than local failure determines survival. Common metastatic sites include the liver, lung, and bones.

Retinoblastoma is the most common type of malignant intraocular tumours found in children, though it occurs with lower frequency than malignant melanomas. There is no gender or racial predilection. Retinoblastomas may be hereditary or develop sporadically. The less common hereditary type is usually present at birth and has its clinical onset near one year of age. In both types, the condition is almost always expressed by the age of five years and is bilateral in 30–50% of patients. Although hereditary retinoblastomas are not always present in family histories, any occurrence of bilateral retinoblastoma should be considered indicative of hereditary origin. Other tumours include intraocular lymphomas. These are typically a diffuse large B cell non-Hodgkin lymphoma arising in immunocompromised individuals, although the incidence in both immunocompetent and immunocompromised individuals is rising.

Diagnosis

This is often based on the clinical assessment of the patient. However, ultrasonography can aid diagnosis and staging of disease. Fine needle biopsies, although not usually required, may be helpful in difficult diagnostic cases.

Malignant melanoma

Malignant melanomas are often detected incidentally, when the patient seeks medical help following deterioration in vision. These tumours often cause an exudative detachment of the retina. The displacement of the retina may move the lens forward, creating a pupillary block and angle-closure glaucoma with a resultant painful eye.

Retinoblastoma

Retinoblastomas may present in the first week of life, and are usually evident by the age of two, manifesting as a white mass visible in the pupil as a result of tumour growing forward into the vitreous, and obstructing the retina, with the red pupillary reflex replaced by a white reflex (leucocoria). Other presentations include strabismus, glaucoma with a painful red eye, poor vision, and enlargement of the globe.

Management

The main aim in the management of these patients is clearance of disease, attempting to preserve useful vision, whilst also taking into consideration the morbidity of any treatment. Management decisions will depend on the stage of the disease, and should be made in a multidisciplinary forum. The choice of treatment of malignant melanoma remains controversial in many respects. Enucleation has been the favoured approach in the past; however, various vision-sparing approaches have been shown to confer similar loco-regional control rates. These include plaque brachytherapy, external beam irradiation, and block excision with most patients retaining some useful vision. Proton beam therapy in specialized centres is an effective treatment and should be considered for medium-sized choroidal melanoma.

Tumours of the orbit

Malignant tumours of the orbit have no gender predilection and may present at any age. They may be derived from mesenchymal elements within the orbit, the lacrimal glands, the reticuloendothelial system, the optic nerve, and rarely may even be a manifestation of the anaplastic degeneration of a hamartoma and choristoma.

Rhabdomyosarcoma is the most common malignant orbital tumour in childhood, arising from the mesenchymal tissue within the orbit, usually presenting in the first or second decades of life. The tumour spreads rapidly, but can be detected by a biopsy taken through the eyelid.

Adenoid cystic carcinomas can arise within the lacrimal gland of the eye, and are aggressive tumours capable of local invasion and metastases. They usually present in adult life.

Clinical features
Typical symptoms are of rapidly developing proptosis, as a result of the mass effect; however, other symptoms may occur, including pain, diplopia, and decreased vision. Lid dysfunction or lagopthalmos may result in exposure keratitis and corneal ulceration.

Management
Treatment is usually in the form of exenteration of the eye, with adjuvant radiotherapy. Occasionally dependent on histology and stage there may be options for surgery whilst preserving vision although it is important not to compromise oncological outcome.

Tumours of the ear
The most common malignancies of the external ear are cutaneous BCCs and SCCs, the greatest risk factor being chronic long-term exposure to sun, specifically with UVB radiation (see Figure 3.2.1 for an example of SCC of the pinna). Other risks include fair skin pigmentation. These malignancies tend to be locally invasive with low incidences of metastases. Unlike BCCs, SCCs occur far less commonly, but are much more aggressive, with risk of loco-regional spread. They occur more commonly in males. As well as exposure to UV radiation, other risks include advancing age, immunosuppression, and non-healing ulcers. In the pinna, BCCs are about four times more common than SCCs; however, in the external auditory canal the ratio is reversed, with SCCs being more common than BCCs.

Malignant melanomas may affect the ear, typically the helix and antihelix. The external ear accounts for about 10% of all head and neck melanomas. These tumours are aggressive, and can spread to regional lymph nodes early in the course of disease. Adenoid cystic tumours can also affect the external auditory canal. They have a low tendency for regional spread, but may demonstrate perineural spread.

Clinical features
Patients often present with an ulcerated area typically occurring on the posterior surface of the pinna, or in the pre-auricular area. Lesions may be painless, but are prone to bleeding. Occasionally, depending on the pathology, the patients may have disease in neck nodes.

Investigations
Tissue diagnosis is easily obtained via a punch biopsy which can be taken in clinic. In squamous tumours, spread to adjacent structures such as the temporal bone can be identified with magnetic resonance imaging (MRI) scanning, facilitating proper planning of surgery.

Management
For small cutaneous tumours of the pinna, local excision with an adequate margin of at least 4mm may be performed. Mohs surgery may also be used, which involves complete micrographic excision of the tumour, with the use of intraoperative histopathology to assess the margins. For those patients not fit for surgery, radiotherapy may be used. Definitive radiotherapy for pinna cancer often utilizes electrons with covered lead behind the pinna.

In those tumours arising from the external canal (or middle ear), treatment needs to be more aggressive. This is often because of their high chance of local recurrence if less aggressive treatment is used. It is increasingly suggested that these tumours be treated primarily by a lateral or subtotal temporal bone resection, dependent on the stage, combined with a parotidectomy as well as a neck dissection. Following temporal bone resection, local or free flap reconstruction may be used to repair any residual defect. Even in early stage tumours of the external auditory canal (EAC), local resection of the EAC is often not sufficient and a more aggressive approach may be warranted. The most important survival factor is removal of the primary tumour with histologically clear margins; this combined with adjuvant radiotherapy has been proven to improve local control rates. Prognosis is dependent on the stage of the tumour and the histological subtype. In these cases, depending on stage of disease and treatment protocols, five-year survival rates range from 10% for advanced disease to 83% for early disease.

Tumours of the middle ear
Malignant tumours of the middle ear are extremely uncommon, and histologically are usually SCCs.

Other rare tumours include metastatic tumours (usually adenocarcinomas) and rhabdomyosarcomas. Chronic otitis media and cholesteatoma have been implicated as aetiological factors. Chronic suppurative otitis media (CSOM) and the resulting chronic inflammation may lead to squamous metaplasia. The disease is often advanced at time of presentation.

Clinical features
Benign pathologies such as CSOM or cholesteatoma may present with overlapping symptoms. As a consequence, there may be delays in diagnosis, as the patient may have been treated as for an infective pathology. Features that

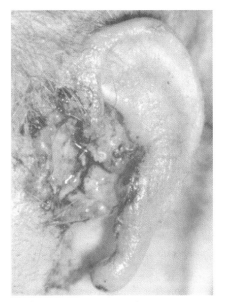

Fig. 3.2.1 Squamous cell carcinoma of the pinna.

should raise the index of suspicion include the presence of significant pain, which may appear out of proportion to the clinical findings, and bleeding.

Investigations
Biopsy of any suspicious tissue identified through a tympanic membrane perforation or at the time of mastoid surgery, should be submitted for pathological analysis.

Imaging in the form of high-resolution computed tomography (CT) scanning will aid in staging the disease and planning the treatment.

Management
Effective treatment of these tumours is by radical surgery with the aim of tumour-free resection margins, with postoperative radiotherapy. This once again usually involves some form of temporal bone resection dependent on the stage, as well as parotidectomy and neck dissection. Due to late presentation and proximity to important vascular structures in the middle ear, there may not be an option for cure. Radical radiotherapy is effective for small tumours and must encompass the full extent of the disease whilst sparing the contralateral parotid.

3.3 Salivary gland cancers

Introduction
Salivary gland malignancies are uncommon with an incidence of about one per 100,000 per year. They present a diverse group, often posing diagnostic and management challenges. The majority typically occur in the sixth decade of life with an equal sex incidence. Unlike other cancers within the head and neck, which are usually related to smoking and alcohol consumption, the aetiology in salivary malignancies is less clear. History of previous irradiation has been shown to increase the risk of tumour development, as demonstrated in patients who received radiotherapy for benign conditions, as well as in studies of atomic bomb survivors. Other purported risks include chemical exposure to silica dust and kerosene and a possible link between EBV and undifferentiated carcinomas.

Anatomy
Salivary glands within the head and neck can be classified into major and minor glands. The major glands refer to the paired parotid, submandibular, and sublingual. The minor glands refer to the 600–1,000 predominantly mucous secreting glands located throughout the upper aerodigestive tract submucosa (i.e. mouth, lip, pharynx, larynx, parapharyngeal space).

Pathology
In 1991, the World Health Organization (WHO) classified salivary tumours into carcinomas, non-epithelial tumours, lymphomas, metastatic tumours, and unclassified tumours. The classification (18 types) is based on the clinical characteristics, histological features, and immunohistochemical staining. Histologically, salivary gland tumours represent the most heterogeneous group of tumours of any tissue in the body.

Approximately 20% of parotid tumours are malignant. In the submandibular gland this rises to approximately 50% and within the sublingual and minor glands approximately 80% are malignant. The most common malignant major and minor salivary gland tumours are the mucoepidermoid carcinomas, which comprise about 10% of all salivary gland neoplasms and approximately 30% of malignant salivary gland neoplasms. This neoplasm occurs most commonly in the parotid gland.

In order of decreasing frequency, the commonest histological types are:

Mucoepidermoid > adenoid cystic > adenocarcinoma > acinic cell carcinomas > SCC, undifferentiated carcinomas, and carcinoma ex pleomorphic adenoma (all <1%).

A division into low and high aggressiveness can be made:

Low
- Acinic
- Adenocarcinoma (some)
- Mucoepidermoid (some)

High
- Squamous
- Undifferentiated
- Carcinoma ex pleomorphic adenoma
- Adenocarcinoma (some)
- Mucoepidermoid (some)

Clinical features
Major glands
Most patients present with an incidental painless swelling of the affected gland. Occasionally deep lobe tumours of the parotid may present as an oropharyngeal mass with no external abnormality.

Features suggestive of malignancy but not exclusive include: pain, nerve palsies (usually the facial nerve in parotid tumours, although the hypoglossal and lingual nerves can be affected in sublingual and submandibular tumours), presence of associated lymphadenopathy, fixation of the tumour to deep structures or overlying skin, and rapid growth.

Minor glands
Presentation will depend on the site, but tumours are often painless submucosal swellings, which may ulcerate following trauma.

Investigations
Clinical examination of these patients must include a thorough assessment of the salivary mass, peroral examination with assessment of the salivary duct orifice, oropharyngeal examination to check for parapharyngeal involvement, facial nerve assessment, and palpation for cervical lymphadenopathy.

Fine needle aspiration cytology (FNAC)
Tumours are usually accessible for cytological assessment, with the risk of tumour seeding being negligible.

However, analysis can prove challenging for the cytologist and depends on local experience. In those tumours which are cystic, aspiration of fluid may prove to be undiagnostic, and unhelpful. As a general rule, if the fine needle aspiration (FNA) is in contradiction to other findings, clinical judgement should prevail.

Imaging

Diagnostic imaging is useful in certain situations. In those tumours arising from the parapharyngeal space, it may help to identify the site of origin. For malignant tumours, it may also help in determining the anatomical extent of the tumour, relationship to other structures, and lymph node status. CT and MRI are complementary modalities.

Management

The main aim of any treatment is complete removal of the tumour, with an adequate margin of normal tissue, whilst ensuring minimal morbidity. Surgery is the mainstay of treatment, which depending on the site may result in significant morbidity.

Major salivary glands

Advanced parotid cancers require a total parotidectomy, with sacrifice of the facial nerve if this is involved. Sacrifice of the nerve is known to impact the patient significantly and therefore if this is anticipated, options for facial nerve reanimation either dynamic or static should be offered. If the deep lobe of the parotid is affected with parapharyngeal space involvement, this area needs to be dissected. This can be approached via a cervicoparotid approach or a paramedian mandibulotomy. Dependent on local experience, TORS may be considered in small parapharyngeal space tumours, with resultant reduced morbidity. In tumours of the submandibular or sublingual glands, excision of the gland is performed in combination with clearance of the nodes at level I. Once again, sacrifice of the hypoglossal or lingual nerves may be required if these are involved.

Minor salivary glands

In minor salivary gland tumours, wide surgical excision is recommended, which depending on the site and size may imply extensive resection.

Those tumours of the paranasal sinuses or nasal cavity may require a partial or total maxillectomy with possible orbital exenteration, and craniofacial resection if there is cranial extension. Tumours arising from the larynx or trachea may be amenable to conservation surgical procedures.

Neck disease

Clinically palpable neck disease is treated by a neck dissection. In carefully selected patients, a selective dissection may be adequate, whilst those with extensive disease require a modified radical neck dissection with attempts to preserve non-lymphatic structures such as the accessory nerve. In the node negative neck, the risk of occult regional disease is low, and therefore elective neck dissection is not routinely warranted. For cancers of

<4cm, five-year survival is >50%. Occult neck disease is uncommon and distant metastases rare. However in patients with high-grade aggressive tumours this may not be the case, and a selective neck dissection of those levels at greatest risk should be carried out.

Radiotherapy

The use of radiotherapy in the adjuvant setting has been shown to improve loco-regional control rates. Indications for postoperative radiotherapy, target volumes, and dose/fractionation are described in detail in 'Radiotherapy' (p. 50). High-risk CTV should encompass the salivary gland bed and neck levels with extracapsular spread. The intermediate or low-risk CTV could include levels 1b–5 in the case of involved nodes after neck surgery. In adenoid cystic tumours with perineural invasion the cranial nerve needs to be included in CTV in its entire route to the base of skull. There is evidence that postoperative radiotherapy increases overall survival in advanced stage disease, though no randomized trials have been performed to demonstrate this. There is no good evidence to support the use of concomitant chemotherapy with radiotherapy. In patients with contraindications to surgery, radiotherapy can be used with enduring local control in at least two-thirds of cases.

Prognosis

Many salivary gland malignancies have an indolent clinical course, warranting long-term follow-up. Overall survival at five years is 60–75% with local control in T1/T2 tumours of 90% and T3/T4 tumours of >50% if postoperative radiotherapy is used.

Outcomes following treatment are dependent on the specific histological subtype. High-grade tumours carry a poorer prognosis, often presenting with loco-regional advanced disease. Other poor prognostic factors include presence of neck nodes, perineural involvement, and involvement of extrasalivary tissue. Overall up to 30% of salivary cancers demonstrate distant metastases at five years. In adenoid cystic tumours, there is a marked propensity for local recurrence which often occurs many years after primary treatment. Systemic spread is also common in adenoid cystic carcinoma with lung being the commonest site.

Pleomorphic adenoma

This is a common benign tumour of the parotid gland usually arising in the superficial lobe and often arising in close proximity to the facial nerve. Treatment is by surgical removal with excellent local control rates of up to 98%. Causes of local recurrence include extension of 'pseudopods' of tumour beyond an incomplete capsule, rupture of capsule during dissection, or tumour adherent to facial nerve.

Postoperative radiotherapy is usually indicated after ≥3 local recurrences, in cases of malignant transformation, and when it is not possible to obtain adequate surgical margins. Standard dose is 50Gy in 25 fractions over five weeks and CTV typically includes the parotid bed with a 1cm margin.

3.4 Nose, nasal cavity, and paranasal sinuses

Introduction

Malignant lesions of this region are diverse and rare. They account for approximately 3% of all head and neck cancers. There is a slight male preponderance, with peak incidences in the fifth to sixth decades of life. Tumours of the nasal cavity are equally divided between benign and malignant types, while most paranasal sinus tumours are malignant. Approximately 50% of sinonasal tumours arise from the maxillary sinus, the remainder arising from the ethmoids (25%) and nasal cavity (25%). In large tumours the site of origin is often difficult to identify.

Pathology

SCC is the most common histological type, accounting for >50% of cancers. The remainder include adenocarcinoma, adenoid cystic carcinoma, malignant melanoma, olfactory neuroblastoma, and undifferentiated sinonasal carcinoma. Other malignancies include a variety of lymphomas, plasmacytoma, and sarcomas.

The glands within the sinonasal tract can give rise to adenoid cystic tumours. These are clinically locally aggressive and usually typified by perineural spread making local control difficult to achieve. Distant metastases and local recurrence may manifest in a delayed fashion several years after primary treatment.

Melanomas comprise <1% of sinonasal malignancies, originating from the neural crest-derived melanocytes present in the submucosa and mucosa, particularly the septum and lateral nasal wall. The aetiology of these tumours is unclear; however, smoking may play a role in metaplastic activation of pre-existing melanocytes. They tend to be more aggressive than their cutaneous equivalent.

Olfactory neuroblastomas arise from the neural crest stem cells, the precursors of the olfactory cells. There is a bimodal age distribution, with a peak in the younger population in the first and second decades and a second peak in the fifth and sixth decades. Tumours are usually locally aggressive involving the cribiform plate and tending to invade adjacent structures such as the orbit and anterior cranial fossa.

Sinonasal undifferentiated carcinomas (SNUCs) are highly aggressive locally invasive tumours thought to be part of the spectrum of neuroendocrine tumours. They frequently involve the nasal cavity and multiple sinuses, and carry a poor prognosis as a result of their local invasion, with mean survival times of <12 months. Prognosis has improved with greater use of chemotherapy.

Metastatic deposits from other locations are rare; however, the most common tumour described is metastatic renal cell carcinoma, which may be its only clinical manifestation.

Aetiology

Whilst smoking and alcohol are recognized risk factors in the pathogenesis of other head and neck cancers, this is not the case with sinonasal tumours. Occupational exposure to nickel and chrome dust have been associated with development of SCCs.

The association between hardwood workers and adenocarcinomas is well documented. The commonest site is within the superior nasal cavity and ethmoidal sinuses. There are three basic histological types: papillary, sessile, and alveolar-mucoid. It is the papillary form which is associated with wood workers, and carries the better prognosis. The other two are more aggressive and carry a poorer prognosis. Adenocarcinomas account for 40–68% of ethmoidal malignancies.

Presentation

These tumours often mimic benign inflammatory conditions in the early stages, often resulting in advanced disease at presentation. An appreciation of the complex anatomy in this region is helpful in understanding the various ways in which these tumours may present.

Symptoms will usually depend on the site of origin, although this is often difficult to identify when the presentation is late. Initial presentation is often insidious. Nasal cavity tumours may present with epistaxis and nasal obstruction. Ethmoidal tumours may present with eye signs, such as proptosis, diplopia, or epiphora if there is breach of the lamina papyracea. Antral tumours may present with a unilateral cheek swelling if the anterior antral wall is breached. Other symptoms may include trismus, oroantral fistulas, and problems wearing dentures. Unlike paranasal sinus tumours, those of the nasal cavity tend to be diagnosed earlier, because of the development of earlier obstructive symptoms. Five per cent of patients may have a neck node on presentation, which portends a poor prognosis.

Patients presenting with unilateral symptoms should be investigated thoroughly as this is suggestive of tumour.

Investigations

A thorough history and examination of these patients should be performed; anterior rhinoscopy and flexible or rigid nasal endoscopy should be performed to thoroughly assess the nasal cavity and nasopharynx and any mass within. Ocular examination should check for diplopia, visual acuity, and pupillary response as well as signs of proptosis. Peroral examination may identify abnormalities of the hard palate and upper alveolus from a maxillary tumour. Neurological examination should concentrate on the cranial nerves I–VI, which may be involved in sinonasal tumours.

Imaging allows delineation of the extent of disease, mapping the extent of any bony or skull base erosion, and facilitating surgical planning. MRI scanning is superior to CT scanning in determining anterior skull base and orbital involvement and differentiating between tumour and adjacent soft tissue. It is also best for assessing for perineural involvement although the use of CT scanning may be complementary with demonstration of invasion of fine bony structures.

Biopsy of the lesion is warranted to obtain tissue to confirm the diagnosis. This is usually easily performed endoscopically. On occasion if accessible, biopsy may be performed in the clinic setting; however, it is important to ensure the tumour is not highly vascular, or indeed contiguous with intracranial contents. The use of radiological imaging before biopsy should reduce the risk of inadvertent surprises.

Management

The management of such patients is often complex and any decisions should be made within a multidisciplinary forum. Factors to consider include: tumour and patient-related factors, tumour histology and stage, the associated treatment morbidity and risks associated with surgical treatment, and ultimately the patient's wishes.

Treatment for most sinonasal malignancies generally involves dual modality treatment with total surgical excision combined with postoperative radiotherapy. The details of the surgical excision are dependent on the site and size of the tumour and the ease of access.

For tumours limited to the lateral nasal wall, nasal cavity, and ethmoid sinuses, a lateral rhinotomy approach may allow adequate access for excision. In the case of maxillary tumours, a total maxillectomy may be required with suitable reconstruction of any residual defect, which may involve microvascular-free tissue transfer.

In those tumours involving the cribiform plate, a craniofacial resection is required, and may also involve orbital exenteration if the tumour has breached the periosteum of the orbit to involve the orbital fat.

In addition to these open approaches, it is important to consider if the tumour may be amenable to an endoscopic excision or indeed combined open/endoscopic approach to limit morbidity.

Clinically positive neck disease is generally managed surgically with a neck dissection, usually with attempts at preservation of non-lymphatic structures such as the accessory nerve, if not involved with tumour. Treatment of the N0 neck is contentious, with some centres only advocating neck dissection if the primary tumour involves sites with increased risk for regional spread such as the nasopharynx, or soft palate.

In those patients where surgical resection of the primary tumour is not considered appropriate, radiotherapy can be used. Principles of radiotherapy planning and dose/fractionation are explained in 'Dose and factionation' (p. 50). Differing acceptable approaches of target delineation are often encountered among departments. The 'compartment-related clinical target volume' approach is one example. In postoperative radiotherapy, the high-dose CTV consists of the GTV with a 5–15mm margin. The intermediate-dose CTV includes the high-dose CTV if present, the preoperative tumour bed with a 5–15mm margin and the entire compartment of all paranasal sinuses involved by the edges of the surgical resection. The cribriform plate can be included for tumours affecting the olfactory region or the ethmoid sinus. If the original tumour has invaded areas that do not provide barriers to its spread such as the parapharyngeal space, orbit, or brain, the intermediate-dose CTV includes either the entire space or the 5–15mm margin already generated around the preoperative tumour bed. Elective nodal irradiation to the ipsilateral level 1b and 2 can be considered in patients with T2–4 or squamous cell or undifferentiated carcinoma of the maxillary sinus and surgically untreated neck. The prophylactic-dose CTV can also be extended along the maxillary division of the trigeminal nerve to the foramen rotundum in cases of adenoid cystic carcinoma or extensive perineural invasion.

Prognosis

The combined treatment of surgery with postoperative radiotherapy markedly improves survival rates, with figures for five-year survival rates of 30–50% being quoted. The difficulties with local control are also linked to the complex anatomy of this region, the often advanced disease at initial presentation, and the histological subtype.

3.5 Nasopharynx

Introduction

The majority (80–95%) of all malignant nasopharyngeal tumours arise from the epithelium and should be considered variants of SCC. The WHO has classified nasopharyngeal carcinoma (NPC) into three subtypes on the basis of light microscopy findings:

- Type 1: keratinizing SCC
- Type 2: non-keratinizing SCC
- Type 3: undifferentiated carcinoma

A variety of other malignant tumours develop in the nasopharynx and include lymphomas and sarcomas.

Cancers of the nasopharynx are rare in most countries of the world; however, they are common in South-east Asia, especially in people originally from the Guangdong, Guanxi, and Fujian regions of China. In North America, WHO types 1, 2, and 3 account for 20%, 10%, and 70% of all NPCs, respectively. In Hong Kong, the respective rates are 3%, 9%, and 88%. Typical presentation is in the fourth and fifth decades, although a bimodal peak is seen with a presentation also seen in late adolescence. The male to female ratio is approximately 2–3:1.

Aetiology

There are three main aetiological factors:

- **Environmental:** diets of salty fish, a common staple diet in certain parts of South-east Asia have been associated consistently with an increased risk of NPC.
- **Viral:** latent EBV infection is also endemic in this population, and has been implicated in the transformation of epithelial cells. Viral genomes are detectable in the majority of NPC tumours from high incidence areas.
- **Genetic:** predisposition for NPC may also exist, as evidenced in the almost 100-fold increase in incidence in a relatively homogeneous genetic group of southern Chinese individuals compared with the incidence in a comparable group of white persons.

Studies have also demonstrated a significantly increased risk of NPC, in particular type I tumours, in long-term smokers.

Clinical features

Tumours typically arise from the fossa of Rosenmüller behind the Eustachian tube cushion, with clinical presentation dependent on the pathway taken. The majority of patients have a metastatic neck node at presentation (70%). Other common symptoms include epistaxis, nasal obstruction, or referred otalgia.

Anterior spread via the Eustachian tube may result in a unilateral middle ear effusion, with the patient complaining of otalgia, or reduced hearing.

Posterolaterally, parapharyngeal spread can occur through the pharyngobasilar fascia, resulting in cranial nerve involvement. Involvement of the mandibular division of the trigeminal nerve may result in the initial development of facial pain which usually precedes motor involvement.

Posterior invasion to the skull base can affect the sympathetic plexus resulting in a Horner's syndrome as well as affecting cranial nerves IX–XII. Tumour infiltration may also occur superiorly through the foramen lacerum into the cavernous sinus, affecting cranial nerves III, IV, and VI as well as the upper divisions of the trigeminal nerve.

Investigations

A comprehensive history and examination as well as specific investigations should raise the suspicion of a nasopharyngeal tumour. The submucosal spread of NPC may result in no abnormality being seen on endonasal examination.

Tissue diagnosis is required to confirm the diagnosis, and can be obtained under local or general anaesthesia via endoscopic guidance.

Imaging should be obtained to stage both the primary site as well as any neck disease. The ideal imaging modality is MRI, which is best for demonstrating soft tissue involvement and the extent of any submucosal involvement (Figure 3.5.1).

Management

Radiation therapy is the treatment of choice for T1 N0 M0 disease. Concomitant chemotherapy is indicated for more extensive cancers while some centres also consider maintenance chemotherapy after the radio-chemotherapy or induction chemotherapy prior to it. The high-risk CTV encompasses the primary tumour and involved nodes with a margin (0.5–1cm). The intermediate-risk CTV can include the entire nasopharynx, the clivus, the skull base, the pterygoid fossae, the parapharyngeal space, the inferior sphenoid sinus, and the posterior third of the nasal cavity and maxillary sinuses as well as bilateral high-risk nodes including level 1b (can be omitted in T1/2 N0 M0 cases), levels 2–5, retropharyngeal, and retrostyloid. The inferior neck nodes (e.g. supraclavicular fossa) can be included in the low-risk CTV if uninvolved.

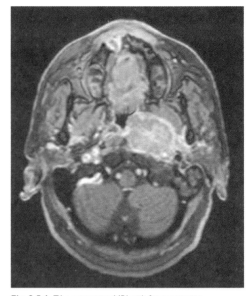

Fig. 3.5.1 T1 postcontrast MRI with fat suppression demonstrating nasopharyngeal carcinoma.

Serious late effects from radiotherapy to the nasopharynx are unusual but may include:

- Xerostomia/dental caries/osteoradionecrosis of jaw
- Fibrosis/stiffness of neck
- Hypopituitarism/hypothyroidism
- Trismus
- Dysphagia/aspiration
- Deafness/vestibular dysfunction
- Carotid artery stenosis/premature cerebrovascular accident
- Temporal lobe epilepsy
- Blindness
- Radiation-induced malignancy
- Spinal cord/brain stem damage

Prognosis

Stage is the most important prognostic factor in terms of survival, with the overall survival rate of 80% for stage I disease dropping down to 30% for stage IV disease. The overall five-year survival has improved to about 60% depending on geography and stage. Adverse prognostic features include cranial nerve palsies, involvement of the skull base, advanced age, male sex, and involvement of the lymph nodes in the supraclavicular fossa. EBV-positive tumours have a better prognosis compared with EBV-negative ones.

3.6 Lip and oral cavity

Introduction

This is the sixth most common cancer worldwide accounting for an estimated 4% of all cancers and approximately 30% of all head and neck cancers, with >20,000 diagnosed in the USA each year. Globally, the highest rates are generally seen within the Indian subcontinent, where the disease accounts for up to 40% of all malignancies, and represents the most common malignancy amongst men.

A recent descriptive epidemiological study of oral cancer from 12 UK cancer registries showed 32,852 oral cancer cases were registered between 1990 and 1999, with a statistically significant increase in incidence over this period. Figures are higher in men than women, in older compared with younger groups, and in northern regions of the UK.

The majority (90%) are SCCs; the remainder include non-Hodgkin lymphoma, minor salivary gland carcinomas, and other rare tumours such as rhabdomyosarcomas. The commonest sites in order of decreasing frequency are lip > lateral border of tongue > anterior floor of mouth > soft palate. Multifocal lesions are not unusual and may be synchronous or metachronous.

Anatomy

The oral cavity extends from the skin–vermilion junctions of the anterior lips to the junction of the hard and soft palates above and to the line of circumvallate papillae below and is divided into the following specific areas:

- Lip
- Anterior two-thirds of tongue
- Buccal mucosa
- Floor of mouth
- Lower gingiva
- Retromolar trigone
- Upper gingiva
- Hard palate

Aetiology and pathology

The major risk factors for the development of oral cancers are smoking and alcohol with at least 80% of oral cancers being attributable to alcohol and tobacco exposure. The effect of alcohol and smoking together is synergistic. As an example of this synergistic effect, the risk of oral cancer with joint consumption of high amounts of alcohol (>5 drinks per day) and cigarettes (>20 per day) is 13-fold greater than expected based upon the independent effects of the same amount of alcohol or tobacco alone. The most significant risk factors for oral cancers among the current non-smoker and non-drinker are previous use of alcohol and tobacco. Other risk factors include the practice of betel nut chewing. Unfortunately, chronic carcinogen exposure creates a field change, which places the entire mucosa at risk. This also increases the chances of developing a second primary.

Other suspected but not confirmed aetiological agents include HPV (subtypes 16 and 18), which have been associated with the development of verrucous squamous carcinomas, poor oral hygiene, and chronic irritation. Premalignant conditions include submucosal fibrosis and lichen planus with reported transformation rates of 0.5–3% and 0.5% respectively.

Clinical features and natural history

The clinical features of oral cavity malignancies can be quite variable. Early cancers may simply present as a white or red patch which is non-ulcerated. Advanced presentation may vary from a predominantly submucosal lesion to an ulcerative, fungating mass. Other presentations include a non-healing painful ulcer, halitosis, difficulty in eating, or ill-fitting dentures. Dental practitioners often make the clinical diagnosis, but unfortunately many patients with oral cancer do not attend for dental checks.

A malignancy may arise within a premalignant lesion such as leucoplakia or erythroplakia. Usually the clinical characteristics of the lesion are sufficient to provide a low threshold to obtain a tissue diagnosis by biopsy. Assessment of patient risk factors may help to stratify further the risk of malignancy and determine fitness for any treatment. Features in the examination which may bode a poor prognosis include the presence of trismus (suggesting pterygoid involvement), cranial nerve involvement, including hypoglossal, facial nerve function, gag and palatal elevation, and the presence of palpable neck nodes.

Management

Early cancers (stages I and II) of the lip and oral cavity are highly curable by surgery or by radiation therapy, and the choice of treatment is dictated by the anticipated functional and cosmetic results of treatment and by the availability of the particular expertise required of the surgeon or radiation oncologist for the individual patient. The presence of a positive margin or a tumour depth >5mm significantly increases the risk of local recurrence and suggests that combined modality treatment may be beneficial. The use of the CO_2 laser has been shown to be effective in the treatment of carefully selected early stage tumours. Brachytherapy, either alone or with a neck dissection, has a role in oral cavity carcinomas. The success of brachytherapy techniques is in part dependent on the experience of the implant team.

Advanced cancers (stages III and IV) of the lip and oral cavity present a wide spectrum of challenges for the surgeon and radiation oncologist. In the majority of patients with stage III or IV tumours, treatment is often a combination of surgery and radiation therapy.

One of the most important advances in head and neck surgery which has greatly transformed the surgical management of advanced disease in this subsite has been the safe and effective use of single-stage free tissue transfer for reconstruction. This includes the use of bone flaps from areas such as the fibula, iliac crest, and scapula, and soft tissue from the radial forearm, trapezius, and anterolateral thigh. The availability of such techniques has made a dramatic impact on the functional outcome of such patients. Factors determining choice of surgical treatment include the size, site, and proximity of the tumour to the mandible or maxilla.

The rehabilitation of patients after oral surgery remains a crucial element in determining outcome. Patients need the support of an MDT for rehabilitation of speech, swallow, dentition, and cosmesis.

Radiotherapy

Definitive radiotherapy can be used for small cancers in the oral cavity with excellent local control rates. The dominant role of surgery is related more to the risk of mandibular necrosis associated with radiotherapy. This risk is increased by concomitant chemotherapy, continuation of smoking, and post-treatment dental extraction. Indications dose/fractionation and techniques for postoperative radiotherapy and chemotherapy are described earlier. Radiotherapy should be ipsilateral where possible and high doses to the oral cavity minimized by use of bite block and tongue depressor if appropriate.

Prognosis

Prognosis of these tumours is largely dependent on the stage and specific site of the tumour. Early lip cancers are usually highly curable by surgery or radiotherapy with rates of 90–100%. Similar local control rates can be achieved for small tumours within the oral cavity.

In advanced tumours of the oral cavity, effective control rates can be achieved with dual modality treatment. The choice of treatment is generally dictated by the anticipated functional and cosmetic results of the treatment. Moderately advanced lesions of the retromolar trigone without evidence of spread to cervical lymph nodes are usually curable and have shown local control rates of as much as 90%; such lesions of the hard palate, upper gingiva, and buccal mucosa have a local control rate of as much as 80%. In the absence of clinical evidence of spread to cervical lymph nodes, moderately advanced lesions of the floor of the mouth and anterior tongue are generally curable, with survival rates of as much as 70% and 65%, respectively.

3.7 Oropharynx

Introduction

Oropharyngeal cancers traditionally have affected patients in their fifth through to their seventh decades of life, with a male preponderance (3–5:1). There is however a change to the demographic with a younger cohort of patients presenting due to the HPV-positive tumours.

The majority of tumours are SCC (85%). The high concentration of lymphoid tissue results in a higher incidence of lymphomas compared to other sites within the upper aerodigestive tract. These usually affect the palatine or lingual tonsils (10%) and are typically of the non-Hodgkin type. The remainder of tumours usually originate from minor salivary glands affecting the glands of the soft palate and tongue base. These are usually adenoid cystic carcinomas.

The commonest sites for malignancies within the oropharynx are the tonsil and tongue base; the remainder usually affect the faucial arch and pharyngeal wall.

Anatomy

The oropharynx extends from the soft palate superiorly down to the hyoid inferiorly. It communicates with the oral cavity anteriorly, with the nasopharynx superiorly, and the larynx and hypopharynx inferiorly. The lateral wall is comprised primarily of the tonsils and tonsillar fossa, the anterior and posterior tonsillar pillars, and the lateral pharyngeal wall. Posteriorly, it is bound by the pharyngeal wall mucosa, which extends from the superior to the inferior limits described previously. Subdivisions of the oropharynx include the tongue base (including the pharyngoepiglottic and glossoepiglottic folds and the vallecula), the faucial arch (including the soft palate, uvula, and anterior tonsillar pillar), the tonsil and tonsillar fossa, and the pharyngeal wall (including the posterior tonsillar pillar, the lateral and posterior pharyngeal walls).

Pathology

As with other head and neck squamous cancers, the most significant risk factors are smoking and alcohol consumption. Other risk factors include poor diet, low in fruits and vegetables, the chewing of betel quid, commonly practised in various parts of Asia, and infection with HPV, in particular subtype 16. HPV infection is an aetiological factor for a subset of tumours that arise predominantly from the lingual and palatine tonsils. Analogously, oral HPV infection has been associated with sexual behaviour, in particular with number of oral sex partners.

Clinical features and natural history

Initial presenting symptoms of oropharyngeal cancers are often vague and non-specific; consequently, the majority of patients who present most often have locally advanced disease at the time of diagnosis.

Presenting symptoms may include sore throat, odynophagia, muffled speech, and referred otalgia mediated though the glossopharyngeal nerve. Twenty per cent of patients may present with a neck lump as the only symptom. Whilst most neck metastases present as firm solid masses in the expected designated levels, there are certain cancers including those of the oropharynx that may present with a cystic neck mass. These are often erroneously misdiagnosed and treated as a branchial cyst, emphasizing the importance of an adequate diagnostic work-up prior to deciding on appropriate management.

Investigations

All patients should have a thorough history taken, eliciting potential risk factors and symptoms, as well as a careful examination of the upper aerodigestive tract and neck. This should also include a flexible nasal endoscopic examination.

An MRI scan will aid in delineating the extent of the disease both locally and regionally in the neck, allowing staging to be performed. Additionally, the chest should be imaged, to check for second primaries and distant disease.

In the case of a clinically palpable neck lump, an FNA should be undertaken. Where there is less obvious neck disease, this may be performed under imaging guidance such as ultrasound or CT.

Assessment of the primary, under general anaesthesia, should be performed to stage the extent of the primary disease and aid surgical planning, with a biopsy being performed to confirm the diagnosis.

Management

As with all head and neck tumours, management decisions should be made in a multidisciplinary forum, with all the information required to hand, allowing the most appropriate treatment to be offered to the patient.

The HPV status of a tumour may aid in planning treatment. Generally HPV-positive tumours have a favourable outcome irrespective of treatment modality.

Early stage disease is generally treated with either surgery or chemoradiotherapy with equivalent rates of local control. The functional effects of either treatment modality should be considered in this situation. The use of TORS may allow single modality, low morbidity treatment to be offered with treatment of the neck surgically if there is no extracapsular disease.

In patients with advanced stage disease, the trend has been to adopt a multimodality approach. Radical chemoradiotherapy is often used for bilateral base of tongue cancer; more lateralized lesions may be suitable for radical excision with free-flap reconstruction. Once again surgical and oncological expertise of the MDT may determine the options.

In these patients, access to the tumour is usually not possible via a conventional peroral approach; but may be possible with a TORS approach or indeed via more traditional approaches such as a mandibulotomy or lateral pharyngotomy approaches to the oropharynx.

Radiotherapy techniques and dose/fractionation are described earlier in this chapter.

Prognosis

The Ang Classification divides oropharyngeal cancer patients in three risk groups:

1. Patients with low-risk oropharyngeal cancer are those with HPV-positive cancer who are non-smokers or have a history of smoking of <10 pack-years, or those with HPV-positive cancer who smoke >10 packs/year but have N0–N2a disease.
2. Patients with intermediate-risk oropharyngeal cancer are those with HPV-positive cancers and N2b, N2c, or N3 disease and >10 pack-year history of smoking or those with HPV-negative cancer and non-smokers with small tumours (T1–T3). Patients with high-risk oropharyngeal cancer are those with HPV-negative cancers related to chronic tobacco and alcohol abuse.
3. Overall survival at three years is 93% for low-risk patients, 70.8% for intermediate-risk patients, and 46% for high-risk patients.

Further reading

Ang KK, Harris J, Wheeler R, Weber R, et al. Human papillomavirus and survival of patients with oro-pharyngeal cancer. *N Engl J Med* 2010; 363:24–35.

3.8 Hypopharynx

Epidemiology

More than 95% of hypopharyngeal cancers are epithelial in origin, predominantly SCCs. Other types and variants include basaloid squamous carcinomas, spindle cell carcinomas, small cell carcinomas, undifferentiated carcinomas, and carcinomas of the minor salivary glands, which comprise <5%. It is a rare disease with a prevalence of <1 per 100,000 of the population, with approximately 2,500 new cases annually in the USA. Hypopharyngeal cancers are uncommon in the UK with an age standardized incidence rate of 0.63 per 100,000 population Peak incidences usually occur in the fifth and sixth decade, with a greater incidence in men than women (3:1).

Anatomy

The hypopharynx extends from the inferior limit of the oropharynx at the level of the hyoid bone down to the level of the cricoid cartilage. The UICC recognizes three anatomical sites for the purposes of tumour classification:

- Piriform fossa: this extends from the pharyngoepiglottic folds to the upper end of the oesophagus.
- Posterior pharyngeal wall: this extends from the floor of the vallecula down to the inferior border of the cricoid cartilage.
- Postcricoid: this extends from the arytenoid cartilage and connecting folds to the inferior border of the cricoid cartilage, therefore forming the anterior wall of the hypopharynx.

Aetiology

Whilst smoking has been implicated in the development of hypopharyngeal cancer, the association seen in other head and neck sites is not as clear. Alcohol has been shown to be a significant cofactor, and it is likely that it promotes the mutagenic effects of tobacco.

Other predisposing factors include nutritional deficiencies in iron and vitamin C. In the past, links between Plummer–Vinson syndrome and postcricoid tumours in women have been suggested although this is more likely to be associated with excessive use of alcohol and cigarette smoking.

Natural history and patterns of spread

Hypopharyngeal cancers tend to be aggressive and demonstrate a natural history that is characterized by diffuse local spread, early metastasis, and a relatively high rate of distant spread. The majority of patients have advanced disease at presentation, with 60% having loco-regional disease, reflecting the regional lymphatics and the anatomy of the region. The piriform fossa is the most common site of origin (60%) followed by the postcricoid (30%) and the posterior pharyngeal wall (10%); however, advanced presentation may make it difficult to identify the site of origin. The tumours demonstrate multisite involvement within the hypopharynx, often extending into adjacent mucosal areas. Dissemination in the submucosal lymphatics may also lead to a high incidence of 'skip' lesions, with >10% of patients having a second primary in the oesophagus.

Superiorly the tumour may extend into the posterior pharyngeal wall and tongue base. Anteriorly tumour spread may occur into the larynx, breaching the paraglottic space and entering the larynx via the pre-epiglottic space. Vocal cord fixation may occur from involvement of the cricoarytenoid joint and invasion of the posterior cricothyroid muscle, paraglottic space, or the recurrent laryngeal nerve. The thyroid gland may be involved by its proximity to the lateral wall of the hypopharynx, although this is clearly a poor prognostic factor.

The presence of nodal metastasis is also a poor prognostic factor of significant importance, occurring more commonly in hypopharyngeal cancer than in other head and neck subsites. The hypopharynx has the highest incidence of distant metastases at presentation (17–24%) compared with other subsites within the head and neck (10%). The most common site of metastases is the lung (80%) followed by liver and bone. In the presence of distant metastases, survival is dramatically decreased, usually to <1 year.

Clinical features

The principal signs and symptoms include dysphagia, initially for solids then liquids, hoarseness as a result of laryngeal invasion, odynophagia, neck mass, and the sensation of a lump in the throat.

Patients may also complain of referred otalgia, mediated via the auricular branch of the vagus nerve. The hypopharynx may be the site of an occult primary in patients presenting with a metastatic neck node from an unknown primary, and should always be considered in the work-up of such patients.

Management

As with all patients, decisions must be made in a multidisciplinary forum. This is often complicated by the considerable comorbidity these patients have as well as poor social support. The nature of the disease and the various treatment options available and their associated morbidities can complicate management decisions.

In the majority of patients who present with large volume, advanced stage disease, surgery is the preferred option with postoperative radiotherapy. Surgery is radical, and often comprises a total pharyngolaryngectomy with appropriate reconstruction of any residual defects. This may include using myocutaneous pectoralis major flaps, visceral grafts using stomach or small bowel, or the use of tubed anterolateral thigh flaps.

Early stage disease, though rare, can be treated with radiotherapy with salvage surgery used for recurrent disease. The use of neoadjuvant chemotherapy in combination with radiotherapy has been shown to confer comparable survival rates to surgical treatment in patients with advanced hypopharyngeal cancers, offering the patients the option of laryngeal preservation. This also potentially gives the patient the option of salvage surgery in the case of recurrent disease. Concomitant radio-chemotherapy as described earlier is a standard treatment choice when organ preservation strategies are considered. The use of radiotherapy versus surgery in this group has to be weighed against the risks of radionecrosis resulting in an incompetent larynx, as well as the possibility of a tracheostomy and gastrostomy tube feeding.

The principles of chemotherapy and radiotherapy as well as irradiation techniques and dose/fractionation are explained earlier. High-risk CTV can be produced by adding a circumferential margin of 1–2cm and superior/inferior margin of 1.5–2cm to the GTV-T and 1cm to the GTV-N. Intermediate-risk CTV includes involved nodal regions or uninvolved first echelon nodes at high risk. Uninvolved neck nodes that need to be treated with a prophylactic dose are included in the low-risk CTV. In N0 disease, these are usually the levels 2–4 and the retropharyngeal nodes. Postoperative radiotherapy CTV usually includes any gross residual disease (GTV) with a margin (1–2cm), the tumour bed with a margin (1–2cm), and any areas or nodal levels at risk for recurrence.

Prognosis

The main prognostic factors affecting outcome are clinical stage, age of the patient, and PS. Generally hypopharyngeal cancers have a poor prognosis compared with other head and neck subsites, although figures vary between different series, ranging from 18% to 65% for five-year disease-free survival rates. In addition to the risk of developing loco-regional recurrence, the risk of second primaries is also high. Poor prognosis may also be related to the poor comorbid health of the patient group.

3.9 Larynx

Epidemiology

Cancer of the larynx represents the most common malignancy within the head and neck; 90% are SCCs of varying degrees of differentiation. There are approximately 12,500 new cases each year in the USA with 2,200 in the UK. The incidence within the UK is four per 100,000 per year. It is more common in men than women (5:1). Epidemiology is complicated by the difficulty in clinically distinguishing between the various anatomical subsites within the larynx as well as the close relationship to the hypopharynx.

Aetiology

Smoking is strongly associated with the development of laryngeal cancer. The carcinogenic effects of tobacco are due to an interplay between carcinogen-DNA adduct formation, tumour-specific mutations, and cancer risk. It is significantly associated with an increased risk of TP53 mutations. Tobacco initiates a linear dose–response carcinogenic effect in which the duration is more important than the intensity of exposure. Other factors increasing the carcinogenic potential include hand-rolled versus commercially available cigarettes, the use of black versus blond tobacco, and the age of the patients when they started smoking. The carcinogenic potential has also been shown to be dependent on gender, where females with identical smoking histories are more susceptible to developing laryngeal cancer than males.

The risk of laryngeal cancer is increased (1.9–3.3-fold) with alcohol intake; however, alcohol potentiates the effect of tobacco acting synergistically to increase the risks dramatically.

There is a subset of patients in whom infection with HPV may be responsible, in particular types 16 and 18. The association between HPV and laryngeal cancer is weakest compared to other sites within the head and neck. Biologically, HPV-positive tumours appear to have a better prognosis than HPV negative, by virtue of a lower rate of TP53 mutations. Various studies have suggested the association of gastro-oesophageal reflux disease with the development of laryngeal cancer; however, there are often several confounding factors which cloud the issue, including the role of smoking and alcohol.

Natural history and patterns of spread

There is a wide variation in outcome between different subsites of the larynx (loco-regional control: glottis > supraglottis > subglottis). This may reflect in part differences in the regional lymphatics resulting in different rates of metastases as well as the T stage at diagnosis with glottic cancers often presenting with T1 disease.

Clinical features

The clinical features are related to the primary tumour, secondary spread, or the general effects of the cancer.

Hoarseness is the most common symptom, particularly in glottic cancers where it may be an early symptom, due to vocal cord involvement.

Supraglottic tumours generally present later with symptoms of pain, which may be perceived as a sore throat, or may be referred otalgia. Dysphagia or odynophagia may occur due to involvement of the pharynx.

Airway compromise in the form of stridor is usually a late sign, which necessitates urgent referral to an ENT team for further assessment and management (see Box 3.9.1).

The patient may occasionally present with metastatic neck disease, with no obvious symptoms of the primary.

Management

The most important factor used to determine management of laryngeal cancer is stage. Early stage disease (stage I–II) is generally managed with single-modality therapy. The choice of surgery or radiotherapy is determined by the location of the tumour and the likely morbidity, particularly voice quality. The popularization of conservation techniques including trans-oral laser surgery allows the chance of organ-preserving conservation surgery to be offered. In carefully selected patients with early stage disease, or small volume disease, these conservation procedures may be considered and include partial laryngectomy, supracricoid/supraglottic, and various similar procedures. Although broadly categorized, the final procedure is tailored to the individual patient with the goal of achieving control of the cancer, and obtaining a functional outcome of speech and swallowing avoiding a permanent tracheostomy.

Box 3.9.1 Emergency management of stridor

Multidisciplinary team approach:
- Involve ENT/anaesthetist
- Treatment depends on underlying cause

Measures that may buy time include:
- Nebulized adrenaline (5ml of 1:1,000)
- Heliox (helium and oxygen)
- Dexamethasone IV
- Needs early recognition!

The determinants of choice between surgery and radiotherapy are complex and multifactorial. Concomitant radio-chemotherapy is the organ-preservation strategy in loco-regionally advanced laryngeal carcinomas, as described earlier .

Decision making for these patients needs to occur in a multidisciplinary forum, taking into consideration both patient-related factors as well as those related to the primary tumour itself. The team should fully discuss with the patient the advantages and disadvantages of larynx-preservation options compared with treatments that include total laryngectomy.

In patients who present acutely with stridor, endoscopic debulking should be carried out before planning definitive management, although if this is not feasible then a tracheostomy may be required initially.

Radiotherapy

Techniques of radiotherapy and chemotherapy as well as dose and fractionation are described in 'Dose and fractionation' (p. 50). High-risk CTV can be produced by adding a margin (1–2cm) to the GTV-T and 1cm to the GTV-N. The entire larynx is then included in the CTV. Clinicians then decide to include any other adjacent regions at risk of microscopic spread depending on tumour extent. Most patients with T1–T2 lesions of the glottis and clinically negative cervical nodes (N0) do not require routine elective treatment of the neck. Intermediate-risk CTV includes involved nodal regions or uninvolved first echelon nodes at high risk. Low-risk CTV includes uninvolved neck nodes (usually bilateral neck nodal levels 2–4) that need to be treated with a prophylactic dose. Postoperative radiotherapy CTV includes any gross residual disease (GTV) with a margin (1–2cm), the tumour bed with a margin (1–2cm), the stoma (if urgent tracheostomy was performed before surgery or if there is evidence of subglottic extension), and any areas or nodal levels at risk for recurrence (if pN0 they can be included in low-risk CTV).

Prognosis

Following radiotherapy glottis cancers have an initial local control of 90% for T1, 75% for T2, and 60% for selected T3 tumours. In supraglottic tumours the control rates are lower stage for stage, due to the larger tumour volumes. With surgical salvage, five-year cancer-specific survival is 95–100% for T1 and 85–90% for T2 glottic tumours. An important point to reiterate to patients is that smoking during radiotherapy has been shown to decrease the chance of loco-regional control.

Rehabilitation

The psychosocial consequences of a total laryngectomy are well recognized and are related not just to the loss of voice, but also the presence of a permanent tracheostomy. Social isolation, job loss, and depression are common sequelae.

Voice rehabilitation

Patients undergoing a laryngectomy should be seen preoperatively by the speech therapist for counselling, education, and support.

There are three main options available for voice rehabilitation.

1. The use of voice prosthesis with a one-way valve inserted either primarily at the time of the surgery or secondarily after the surgery, uses a fistula created between the trachea and oesophagus to create a voice. When

the stoma is occluded pulmonary air passes through the one-way valve in the tracheoesophageal wall, and causes the pharyngo-oesophageal segment to vibrate. Undoubtedly the best results are obtained with use of a voice prosthesis; however, the patient is dependent on the hospital for maintenance of the prosthesis and management of any associated problems. This clearly needs to be factored into making the appropriate choice of voice rehabilitation for the patient. Appropriate training in the maintenance and use of the valve is required and patients must be advised about the possible aspiration of food, fluids, and secretions.

2. Oesophageal speech uses the swallowing of air to create an artificial voice, with the patient having to learn to separate respiration from phonation. The production of a functional voice may take months to acquire, with success dependent on patient motivation.

3. In those patients where these methods are not successful, then an electrolarynx allows a method of communication albeit less realistic. This battery powered source is held against the neck to produce sound. The advantages are that little effort is required; however, the voice created is artificial and robot like.

3.10 Uncommon tumours of the head and neck

Adenoid cystic carcinomas (ACCs)

ACCs arises in minor salivary glands in 60% of cases (predominantly oral) and major salivary glands in 40%. ACCs account for approximately 1% of all head and neck malignancies, and are characterized by an indolent yet persistent growth with a tendency for local recurrence and distant metastases several years after initial presentation. Patients are generally younger and fitter than those with SCC of the head and neck. There is a female preponderance with peak incidence in the fourth to sixth decades. Tumours typically have a predilection for perineural infiltration. Unlike squamous cell head and neck cancer, ACC often spreads systemically, the commonest metastatic site being the lung. Other sites affected include bone. The primary treatment modality of choice is usually surgical resection followed by adjuvant radiotherapy; however, there is significant work being undertaken examining the use of systemic therapies and biomarkers that may predict clinical outcome.

Mucosal melanoma

Primary mucosal melanoma of the head and neck is a rare disease associated with a very poor prognosis (mean survival of 17% at five years). The commonest sites affected include the nasal cavity, oral cavity, and paranasal sinuses. In contrast to cutaneous melanoma, mucosal disease generally occurs in an older age group typically affecting patients in their sixth to ninth decades. The primary treatment modality has been surgical wide en bloc excision. Adjuvant radiotherapy may improve local tumour control. Definitive radiotherapy may be used in patients with unresectable tumours or in those where the functional/cosmetic deficits would be too severe and may result in comparable survival rates to surgically treated patients. Immunotherapy is increasingly being used.

Sarcomas

Sarcomas of the head and neck are rare, accounting for approximately 10% of all soft tissue sarcomas and approximately 1% of all head and neck tumours. There is typically a male preponderance with presentation usually in the sixth decade with a painless mass. Common sites include the scalp, face, and neck. The majority are high-grade tumours. The risk of distant metastases is related to histological grade and tumour size, the commonest site being the lungs. The treatment modality of

choice is surgical resection, with adjuvant radiotherapy in patients with high-grade tumours, or close/positive margins. Radical radiotherapy is usually reserved for large unresectable tumours. The role of adjuvant chemotherapy is unclear, although studies suggest improvements in local control and distant metastases.

Plasmacytomas

Extramedullary plasmacytoma is a relatively uncommon malignancy that may present in the head and neck. The most common sites include the nasal cavity, paranasal sinuses, and nasopharynx, typically affecting the submucosa. There is a male predilection with patients typically presenting in their sixth to eight decades. Clinical presentation is usually with localized disease. The treatment of choice is radiotherapy. Surgery may be employed in patients with small localized lesions, where complete resection is possible with minimal functional deficit. The chance of local control is high (80–90%).

Paragangliomas

Chemodectomas or paragangliomas are rare, comprising 0.6% of all head and neck tumours. They have a female preponderance, with a slow indolent history. Ten per cent of these patients will have an inherited familial form, warranting appropriate genetic counselling and screening. Tumours may be multicentric in 20% of sporadic cases and 80% of familial cases. Mutations of more than ten different genes have been identified in hereditary paragangliomas of the head and neck region. Examples are the succinate dehydrogenase subunit D (SDHD), the succinate dehydrogenase complex assembly factor 2 (SDHAF2), the SDHC, the SDHB, etc. Almost a third of all patients with sporadic head and neck paragangliomas have a mutation one of the SDH subunit genes (SDHD, SDHB, or SDHC). Malignant paragangliomas are commonly seen in patients with a SDHB mutations. SDHD mutation carriers are at high risk of developing a paraganglioma in the head and neck region (91–98%). Screening is advisable in paraganglioma patients who are younger than 50 years or have malignant, multiple, or familial tumours. Mutation carriers should undergo a clinical and radiological screening (not necessary in children of female SDHD and SDHAF2 carriers). Measurement of catecholamines in plasma or 24-hour urine and imaging can also be considered. Common presentations may include a neck mass with associated dysphonia (vagal paraganglioma). Carotid body tumours occur at the bifurcation of the carotid artery. The jugulotympanic paragangliomas (glomus jugulare) may present as a temporal bone mass involving the middle/external ear or the jugular bulb. Surgical removal remains the treatment of choice. Radiotherapy is effective at halting progression of these tumours though complete radiological resolution is unlikely.

Neuroendocrine tumours

Neuroendocrine tumours encompass a broad spectrum of neoplasms. They are of two types, depending on whether they have a neural or an epithelial origin. Paragangliomas represent those of neural origin, whilst neuroendocrine carcinomas represent those of epithelial origin. Neuroendocrine carcinomas are thought to be derived from endocrine cells of the dispersed neuroendocrine system, although some believe they arise from pluripotential stem cells that are capable of dual epithelial and endocrine differentiation. They are further classified into three subtypes: typical carcinoid tumour (well-differentiated neuroendocrine carcinoma), atypical carcinoid tumour (moderately differentiated neuroendocrine carcinoma), and small cell carcinoma (poorly differentiated neuroendocrine carcinoma). These are rare tumours, tending to occur more commonly in the larynx, where they represent 0.5–1% of epithelial cancers. The laryngeal neuroendocrine tumours have an overall male predilection and the same seems to be true of non-laryngeal neuroendocrine carcinomas of the head and neck. Outside the larynx common sites include the paranasal sinuses. Clinically neuroendocrine tumours of the head and neck are usually locally advanced at the time of presentation. Symptoms at presentation are not diagnostic, and differ according to site and extent of disease. Diagnosis requires recognition of typical neuroendocrine architecture, morphology, and the immunohistochemical confirmation of neuroendocrine differentiation. Differentiation of these tumours from SCCs is essential both for purposes of management and prognosis. The treatment of choice is radical surgery with postoperative radiotherapy

Further reading

Boedeker CC, Hensen EF, Neumann HP, et al. Genetics of hereditary head and neck paragangliomas. *Head Neck* 2014; 36(6):907–16.

Bradley PJ. Adenoid cystic carcinoma of the head and neck: a review. *Curr Opin Otolaryngol Head Neck Surg* 2004; 12(2):127–32.

Dodd RL, Slevin NJ. Salivary gland adenoid cystic carcinoma: A review of chemotherapy and molecular therapies. *Oral Oncol* 2006; 42:759–69.

Mendenhall WM, Mendenhall CM, Mendenhall NP. Solitary plasmacytoma of bone and soft tissues. *Am J Otolaryngol* 2003; 24(6):395–9.

Mendenhall WM, Mendenhall CM, Werning JW, et al. Adult head and neck soft tissue sarcomas. *Head Neck* 2005; 27(10):916–22.

Wagner M, Morris CG, Werning JW, et al. Mucosal melanoma of the head and neck. *Am J Clin Oncol* 2008; 31(1):43–8.

3.11 Management of neck nodes

Anatomy of neck nodes

This can be related to cross-sectional imaging taking into account specific radiological landmarks easily identifiable on CT or MRI slices. Cross-sectional imaging is essential in the work-up of head and neck cancer patients allowing assessment of both the primary tumour site as well as the extent of any nodal disease. MRI scanning tends to be the primary imaging modality of choice for tumours above the hyoid bone, whilst CT and MRI are equivalent below this level. In many sites (e.g. paranasal sinuses) CT and MRI are complementary.

Advances in the use of functional imaging techniques such as positron emission tomography (PET) FDG (fludeoxyglucose (18F); Figure 3.11.1 and Table 3.11.1) or CT-PET may provide greater information in specific situations such as patients with unknown primary disease, or in patients with suspected recurrence.

Management of neck nodes in known primary tumour

The N0 neck

The presence of neck disease is a significant prognostic marker of outcome, with a reduction in cure rate by up to 50%. There is some contention as to whether elective neck treatment for potential microscopic disease (clinical stage N0) improves survival among patients with T1–4 lesions with no clinically apparent nodal metastases. Radiation therapy and neck dissection are seemingly equally effective at eradicating subclinical disease. Therefore, management of the neck depends on the management of the primary tumour. If treatment is surgical, an elective neck dissection is frequently performed, resulting in control of subclinical disease in >90% of cases. If the primary treatment is radiotherapy, then radiation therapy can be used. In general, elective neck treatment is advocated for patients with a risk of subclinical disease of greater than 15%, i.e. it is not usually done for T1 N0 cases.

The N positive neck

The management of clinically positive cervical lymph nodes (stage N1–3) is also related to the management of the primary tumour. Small nodes may be treated with radiation therapy alone. When the primary treatment is surgical, a neck dissection represents sufficient treatment for small volume nodal metastasis (stage N1). In this situation, treatment of the neck with a selective neck dissection may be appropriate, the choice of levels being made according to the site of the primary. In patients with advanced nodal disease, treatment of the neck is usually in the form of a modified radical neck dissection, with preservation of various non-lymphatic structures. The use of modified radical neck dissection is not associated with an increased risk of loco-regional failure if the non-lymphatic structures are not affected by disease. Postoperative radiation therapy is added for advanced nodal disease (stage N2 or N3), increasing local control in the neck postoperatively as well as control of subclinical disease on the opposite side of the neck. In cases with extracapsular nodal disease, synchronous chemotherapy is added to postoperative radiotherapy. There

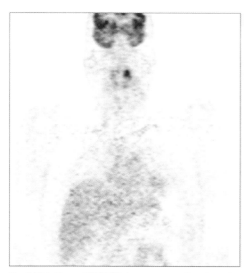

Fig. 3.11.1 Coronal FDG-PET showing increased uptake in the tongue base.

is a view that adding chemotherapy to definitive radiotherapy for N2 disease with a neck dissection in reserve does not prejudice outcome compared with performing a neck dissection *ab initio* with radiological follow-up. In those patients where tumours infiltrate the accessory/ internal jugular vein (IJV) or sternocleidomastoid (SCM), preservation may not be possible, and conversion to a radical neck dissection may be necessary.

Table 3.11.1 The DAHANCA, EORTC, HKNPCSG, NCIC CTG, NCRI, RTOG, and TROG 2013 classification of neck nodes

IA	Submental
IB	Submandibular
IIA	Upper jugular
III	Middle jugular
IVa	Lower jugular
IVb	Medial supraclavicular
Va and b	Posterior triangle
Vc	Lateral supraclavicular
Va	Anterior jugular
VIb	Pre-laryngeal, pre-tracheal, para-tracheal-recurrent laryngeal nerve nodes
VIIa	Retropharyngeal nodes
VIIb	Retrostyloid nodes
VIII	Parotid nodes
IX	Bucco-facial group
Xa	Retro-auricular nodes
Xb	Occipital nodes

Adapted with permission from Grégoire V. et al. Delineation of the neck node levels for head and neck tumors: A 2013 update. DAHANCA, EORTC, HKNPCSG, NCIC CTG, NCRI, RTOG, TROG consensus guidelines. *Radiotherapy Oncol* 2014; 10(1):172–81. Copyright © 2014, Elsevier Ireland Ltd.

Surgery

Radical neck dissection

This is the standard procedure originally described by Crile in 1906, from which other procedures represent a modification. It is defined as an en bloc removal of all the neck nodes from levels I–V, along with the IJV, the SCM, and the accessory nerve.

Modified radical neck dissection

The significant morbidity caused by radical neck dissection has resulted in various modifications, with an attempt to preserve the non-lymphatic structures, namely the accessory, IJV, and SCM, whilst excising the nodal tissue from levels I–V. Conversion to a radical neck dissection may be required in tumours which infiltrate or involve these non-lymphatic structures.

Selective neck dissection

The rationale behind the use of a selective neck dissection is to remove surgically those levels of nodes likely to be affected by metastases, whilst also preserving non-lymphatic structures. There is also a drive to be less radical in the approach to the neck, and treat only those nodal basins which are at risk. The decision on which levels to remove is based on the study of the patterns of lymphatic spread from a particular primary site. Tumours of the oral cavity tend to metastasize to levels I–III, whilst tumours of the oropharynx tend to spread to levels II–IV. There has been a gradual shift in the way neck dissections are described, using the levels removed as the descriptor.

1. Supraomohyoid neck dissection (SOHND): removal of levels I–III—commonly performed in patients with oral cavity tumours, particularly in those with N0 necks. It includes the resection of soft tissue in the submental triangle, as well as the submandibular triangle contents, including the submandibular gland and the fibrofatty tissue along the IJV from the skull base to the omohyoid muscle. The dissected contents include the fascia that covers the medial aspect of the sternocleidomastoid muscle; the muscle itself is laterally retracted and preserved. These neck contents are peeled off from the IJV and from around the accessory nerve, sparing these structures.

2. Lateral neck dissection: removal of levels II–IV—for oropharyngeal, laryngeal, and hypopharyngeal tumours. The lymph nodes are removed from the skull base superiorly down to the clavicle, and from the cutaneous branches of the cervical plexus at the posterior border of the sternocleidomastoid muscle posteriorly to the sternothyroid muscle anteriorly.

3. Posterolateral neck dissection: removal of levels II–V—often used in patients with cutaneous malignancies, consists of an en bloc removal of the lymph nodes in the suboccipital, postauricular, and upper, middle, and lower jugular nodes, with posterior triangle nodes situated superior to the accessory nerve.

4. Anterior compartment neck dissection: removal of nodal tissue from level VI—usually performed in thyroid cancers, with dissection to the level of the hyoid bone superiorly, the suprasternal notch inferiorly, and the carotid sheaths on both sides.

Extended radical neck dissection

In certain patients with very advanced neck disease, other structures not routinely removed in a radical neck dissection may have to be removed to ensure oncological clearance. Such structures may include the prevertebral muscles, the hypoglossal nerve, and the carotid artery.

Radiotherapy

The use of primary radiotherapy in early stage neck disease can give comparable regional control rates with a selective neck dissection alone. Radiotherapy used postoperatively has been shown to confer improved loco-regional control rates.

In selected patients, the use of chemoradiotherapy with surgery to salvage any residual neck disease has the benefit of offering the patient a chance of organ preservation, in terms of speech or swallow. This does however need to be offset against the technical difficulties and increased risks in operating in a field which has previously been irradiated.

Management of neck nodes in unknown primary

Neck nodes from an unknown primary account for 1–2% of head and neck cancer cases where despite thorough clinical, endoscopic, and conventional radiological evaluation, no primary site will be detected. Functional techniques such as PET-FDG may be useful. Treatment of such patients remains controversial.

SCC in upper neck nodes usually arises secondary to a (presumed) head and neck primary, whilst nodes in the supraclavicular fossa tend to be associated with a primary malignancy below the clavicles. In the majority of patients with metastatic cervical lymphadenopathy, a careful assessment will identify the primary site of the cancer. The diagnostic work-up of such a patient includes a comprehensive history and thorough physical examination concentrating on areas most likely to harbour an occult primary such as the tonsil, base of tongue, piriform fossa, and postnasal space. The use of cross-sectional imaging including PET should be performed prior to any surgical interventional (following nodal FNAC).

Management is often a combination of surgery and/or radiotherapy; however, this is dependent on the centre. Most centres adopt a wait and watch policy following neck dissection for N1 disease with no extracapsular spread. However, for the majority of cases, postoperative radiotherapy is advisable and this is given either as wide-field mucosal irradiation or to the ipsilateral neck only. There is no evidence that either of these strategies is superior to the other in terms of impact on overall survival. Wide-field irradiation includes the oropharynx, hypopharynx, larynx, and possibly nasopharynx as well as the neck and is associated with significant morbidity, particularly xerostomia, although the advent of parotid-sparing IMRT has made the effects of wide-field irradiation less morbid. Additionally wide-field irradiation poses the difficulty of re-irradiation if a subsequent primary emerges. The use of HPV status determined from the neck disease would suggest that the primary has arisen from the oropharynx, possibly allowing a more targeted approach, with lesser morbidity.

Further reading

Grégoire V, Ang K, Budach W, et al. Delineation of the neck node levels for head and neck tumors: a 2013 update. DAHANCA, EORTC, HKNPCSG, NCIC CTG, NCRI, RTOG, TROG consensus guidelines. *Radiother Oncol* 2014; 110(1):172–81.

Acknowledgement

The editors thank Dr Dinos Geropantas for editorial updates of this chapter.

Chapter 4

Tumours of the central nervous system

Chapter contents

4.1 Primary brain tumours

Introduction
Tumours of the central nervous system (CNS) are characterized by a remarkable diversity of pathological type and behaviour. Although rare, they affect people of all ages and hence have a disproportionate influence on the number of years of life lost to cancer. After many years of therapeutic stagnation, there have recently been some important improvements in molecular classification, treatment, and outcome.

Classification and grading of CNS tumours
There is no satisfactory staging system for CNS tumours. The brain does not have a lymphatic system. Tumours rarely spread systemically and tumour size is a weak prognostic factor. Hence systems, such as tumour node metastasis (TNM), are of no value for CNS tumours.

The outcome from treatment of CNS neoplasms is determined principally by the underlying pathology and, to some extent, the tumour site:
- Management to date has so far been determined by the tumour grading.
- The most widely accepted grading system is the World Health Organization (WHO) classification of tumours of the CNS. In this system tumours are allocated a grade I–IV based on their pathology.
- Molecular features can provide additional highly relevant prognostic information even within one tumour type and grade. For example, the presence or absence of loss of heterozygosity (LOH) on chromosomes 1p and 19q can have a profound effect on outcome. The 2016 WHO classification includes molecular features.

Benign or malignant?
The terms 'benign' and 'malignant' may be confusing when applied to CNS tumours. Low-grade glial tumours almost never metastasize and show little cellular pleomorphism or mitosis. They are frequently called 'benign'. Usually, however, even these low-grade tumours infiltrate widely into brain parenchyma, which is a cardinal feature of malignancy. It is better that they are labelled by their WHO grade and molecular status, which is a reliable guide to behaviour, rather than the terms benign or malignant.

Truly benign tumours do exist (meningioma, choroid plexus papilloma); however, even these can also appear in intermediate (atypical) and truly malignant forms. Again, the WHO grading system is most useful.

Finally, there is a tendency for many 'low-grade' brain tumours to transform to a more malignant phenotype over time as they acquire additional genetic damage. At this point in their evolution, mixtures of grade can appear in the same tumour specimen. They should be classified by the highest grade and the molecular markers identified in the biopsy sample.

Incidence
The international estimated age-adjusted incidence for all patients with primary malignant brain tumours (not exclusively glioblastoma multiforme (GBM)) is 5.3 per 100,000 population with higher rates in some western developed countries. There are around 4,000 new malignant brain tumours diagnosed per year in the UK.

- Men have a nearly 50% higher risk of CNS tumour than women, particularly of malignant tumours, whereas women have higher rates of non-malignant tumours, particularly meningiomas.
- Mortality rates for malignant tumours are only slightly less (by 20%) than incidence rates, indicating the high lethality of these tumours.
- Whilst brain tumours may occur at any age, the age-specific incidence shows a small peak in early childhood and a rapidly increasing rate in middle age, with a second major peak in the eighth decade.
- The tumour pathology spectrum varies with age. Low-grade glial tumours and medulloblastomas are the most common tumours of childhood whilst the rapidly increasing incidence in middle-aged adults is largely due to malignant tumours particularly glioblastoma.

Aetiology
The great majority of brain tumours are sporadic, and have no known cause. However, an important minority are associated with a variety of genetic syndromes and a few tumours have environmental or occupational links.

Genetic syndromes associated with brain tumour
- Neurofibromatosis I (autosomal dominant (AD) NF1 on 17q11)—neurofibromas, gliomas, sarcomas
- Neurofibromatosis II (AD NF2 on 22q12)—schwannomas (acoustic neuromas), meningiomas, gliomas
- Von Hippel–Lindau syndrome (AD VHL on 3p25–26)—haemangioblastoma
- Cowden's syndrome (AD PTEN/MMAC1 on 10q23)—dysplastic gangliocytoma of cerebellum
- Turcot's syndrome (AD 5q21)—glioblastomas, medulloblastomas
- Tuberous sclerosis (TSC1 on 9q34, TSC2 on16p13)—subependymal giant cell astrocytoma, hamartomas
- Li–Fraumeni syndrome (AD TP53 on 17p13)—gliomas, primitive neuroectodermal tumour (PNETs)
- Basal naevus syndrome (AD PTCH on 9q22)—medulloblastomas

Other aetiological factors
- There is very strong evidence that ionizing radiation is a potent cause of brain tumours, particularly meningioma and gliomas, with a relative risk of approximately 4.6 per Gy for benign meningiomas and 2 per Gy for malignant brain tumours. The latent period is typically ten years but may be as long as 30 years.
- In contradistinction, non-ionizing radiation, particularly exposures in the radiofrequency range including those used by cellular phones, have no proven association with brain tumours.
- There is an increased risk of glioma in higher social class.
- Primary CNS lymphoma is associated with immune suppression either naturally occurring (human immunodeficiency virus (HIV)) or iatrogenic (organ transplants).
- There is an association between breast cancer and meningioma.
- There is an inverse association between atopic disease and glioma.

Referral pathways

Most patients currently who present with symptoms suspicious of a CNS tumour will be referred for imaging of the brain. The discovery of a tumour is then an indication for a referral to a neuro-oncology multidisciplinary team (MDT) or tumour board for discussion of the case (see National Institute of Health and Clinical Excellence (NICE) guidelines in 'Internet resources', p. 95).

Key 'NICE' recommendations

- All patient care should be coordinated through a designated MDT.
- All patients should have face-to-face contact with healthcare professionals to discuss their care at critical points in their care pathway, and be provided with high-quality written information to support this.
- All patients should have a clearly defined key worker.
- Patients should have ready access to specialist care services as appropriate.
- Palliative care specialists should be core members of the neuroscience MDT.

- Cancer networks should ensure that clinical trials on brain tumours carried out by the National Cancer Research Institute (NCRI) are supported.

Where possible, patients with a new diagnosis of brain tumour should be evaluated in the preoperative setting so that a management plan can be formulated by the MDT before surgical intervention. Sometimes this will not be possible and surgical intervention needs to be undertaken urgently. For these cases, protocols agreed by the MDT should be available.

Core membership of the Brain Tumour MDT should comprise: neurosurgeon(s), neuroradiologist(s), neuropathologist(s), neurologist(s), oncologist(s), clinical nurse specialist(s), palliative care physician(s), neuropsychologist(s), specialist allied health professional(s), and MDT coordinator(s).

The patient care plan will frequently begin in the neurosurgical unit but may pass to oncology, neurology, palliative care, and other disciplines. At all times a 'key worker' should be allocated who, for the period of allocation, is the main management reference professional for the patient. This will often be the clinical nurse specialist.

4.2 Clinicopathology of brain tumours

Introduction

Understanding CNS tumour pathology and grading is key to management. There is virtually uniform international acceptance of the WHO classification system shown in abbreviated form here. In the 2016 WHO classification the assessment of molecular alterations has led to further refinement of the classification of some tumours.

The classification is based on the presumed tissue of origin and the grading is based on the predicted biological and clinical behaviour of the tumour.

Molecular status is based on the alterations of specific genes.
- Grade I tumours have low proliferative potential and afford the possibility of cure with surgery alone.
- Grade II lesions have low proliferative potential but are infiltrative and some tumours progress to higher grade lesions.
- Grade III implies cytological evidence of malignancy (nuclear atypia, mitotic activity). Grade 3 lesions that have favourable molecular features may have a better survival.
- Grade IV lesions are histologically highly malignant, often incorporating necrosis and associated with rapid disease progression and often fatal outcome.

WHO Classification System 2016

Astrocytic and oligodendroglial tumours
- Grade II: diffuse astrocytoma, oligodendroglioma
- Grade III: anaplastic astrocytoma, anaplastic oligodendroglioma
- Grade IV: glioblastoma, diffuse midline glioma

Other astrocytic tumours
- Grade I: pilocytic astrocytoma, subependymal giant cell astrocytoma

- Grade II: pleomorphic xanthoastrocytoma
- Grade III: anaplastic pleomorphic xanthoastrocytoma

Ependymal tumours
- Grade I: subependymoma, myxopapillary ependymoma
- Grade II (cellular): ependymoma, ependymoma RELA fusion-positive
- Grade III: ependymoma RELA fusion-positive, anaplastic ependymoma

Other gliomas
- Grade I: angiocentric glioma
- Grade II: choroid glioma of third ventricle

Choroid plexus tumours
- Grade I: choroid plexus papilloma
- Grade II: atypical choroid plexus papilloma
- Grade III: choroid plexus carcinoma

Neuronal and mixed neuronal-glial tumours
- Grade I: gangliocytoma, ganglioglioma, dysembryoplastic neuroepithelial tumour (of childhood), dysplastic gangliocytoma of cerebellum (Lhermitte–Duclos)
- Grade II: central neurocytoma, extracentricular neurocytoma, cerebellar liponeuroma
- Grade III: anaplastic ganglioglioma

Pineal tumours
- Grade I: pineocytoma
- Grade II–III: pineal tumours of intermediate differentiation, papillary tumour of the pineal region
- Grade IV: pineoblastoma

Embryonal tumours
Grade IV: medulloblastoma, atypical teratoid/rhabdoid tumour, embryonal tumour with multilayered rosettes C19MC altered, medulloepithelioma, CNS embryonal

tumour NOS (not otherwise specified), CNS embryonal tumour with rhabdoid features

Tumours of cranial and paraspinal nerves
- Grade I: schwannoma (neurilemmoma, neurinoma), neurofibroma
- Grade II, III, or IV: malignant peripheral nerve sheath tumour

Meningiomas
- Grade I: meningioma (and variants)
- Grade II: atypical meningioma
- Grade III: anaplastic (malignant) meningioma

Mesenchymal (non-meningothelial) tumours
- Grade I: haemangioblastoma, solitary fibrous tumour
- Grade II: haemangiopericytoma
- Grade III: anaplastic haemangiopericytoma

Lymphomas
- Diffuse large B-cell lymphoma, immunodeficiency associated CNS lymphoma, intravascular large B-cell lymphoma, etc.

Germ cell tumours
- Germinoma
- Embryonal carcinoma
- Choriocarcinoma
- Yolk sac tumour
- Teratoma (immature, mature, and with malignant transformation)
- Mixed germ cell tumour

Tumours of the sellar region
- Craniopharyngioma (admantinomatous craniopharyngioma, papillary craniopharyngioma)

Metastatic tumours
- Metastatic spread from primary tumours arising from outside the CNS

Clinical pathological behaviour
In children and young adults there is a marked tendency for tumours to arise in the infratentorial compartment (pilocytic astrocytoma, medulloblastoma) whilst in adults the great majority arise supratentorially.

WHO grade I tumours
- Grow by expansion. Infiltration into brain parenchymal tissue is an unusual feature.
- In general, therefore, grade I tumours are surgically curable.
- Some grade I tumours (e.g. craniopharyngioma) grow into invaginations and tend to recur even after apparent surgical excision. This, however, does not represent true invasion.

WHO grade II gliomas
- These (and all higher grades) demonstrate infiltration as a major feature. Tumour cells tend to migrate along white matter tracks from early in their growth and widespread dissemination is common.
- Migrating tumour cells are clonogenic, hence surgical cure of these tumours is rare.
- Cerebrospinal fluid (CSF) dissemination of glial tumours is unusual and spread beyond the CNS is very

rare. When systemic dissemination occurs, sites of predilection are lung and bone.
- A cardinal feature of gliomas is their transformation from lower grade to higher grade through the acquisition of increasing numbers of genetic mutations.

WHO grades III and IV glioma
- Demonstrate rapid expansive and infiltrative growth.
- Are rarely curable but relapse locally even after aggressive treatment.
- Glioblastomas are highly angiogenic tumours and enhance avidly on scan.
- Glioblastomas are characterized by the formation of regions of necrosis.

Central neurocytoma
- Is an intraventricular tumour predominantly of young adults.
- Is slow growing and may reach a large size before presentation, often with CSF obstruction.

Medulloblastomas
- Are highly malignant tumours that arise in the posterior fossa of children, young adults, and rarely adults.
- Spreads readily throughout the CNS and treatments directed towards the whole neuraxis are appropriate.
- May metastasize outside the CNS particularly if ventricular peritoneal shunts are used to decompress hydrocephalus.

Mesenchymal tumours
- Meningiomas are slow growing benign tumours that arise at any site bearing a meningeal surface.
- High-grade (atypical and malignant) forms occur but are rare.
- Haemangioblastoma, solitary fibrous tumours, and haemangiopericytoma are slow growing tumours that can sometimes be associated with troublesome recurrence and occasional metastases.

Primary CNS lymphomas
- The great majority of primary malignant central nervous system lymphoma (PCNSL) is high-grade diffuse B-cell lymphoma. T-cell lymphoma can occur but is rare.
- They are often multifocal and periventricular and may disseminate through the CSF.
- PCNSL that is not related to immunosuppression has maximal incidence in late middle age. HIV (and other immune suppressed) related PCNSL is more common in younger patients.

Germ cell tumours
- Arise predominantly in the pineal region but also in suprasellar and other midline sites.
- May secrete markers (b-hCG, AFP). Measurement of tumour markers in the blood and CSF is necessary for diagnosis and staging, and may be of use in monitoring disease response.
- Germ cell tumours may disseminate through the CSF.

Molecular biology of brain tumours
Low-grade and intermediate-grade gliomas (WHO grade II and III glioma) have highly variable behaviour which is

not adequately predicted on histological description. The Cancer Genome Atlas Network has performed genome wide analyses in 293 lower grade gliomas and revealed frequent mutations in IDH1 and 2, TP53, ATRX, TERT, CIC, NOTCH1, and FUBP1 genes. The most common copy number alteration was deletion of the chromosome arms 1p and 19q. The analysis revealed three principal groups:

- IDH1 or 2 mutation with 1p19q co-deletion
- IDH1 or 2 mutation with 1p19q intact
- No IDH1 or 2 mutation and 1p19q intact

Further associations were noted. Group 1 also had TERT promoter mutations. Group 2 were enriched for TP53 and ATRX mutations. Group 3 were found to have mutations in keeping with glioblastoma—epidermal growth factor receptor (EGFR), NF1, PTEN, and amplification of EGFR. Similar findings have been published for a study of 1,087 diffuse glioma (II–IV). This identified a further subgroup with only TERT promoter mutations which consisted almost entirely of glioblastomas. For both of these studies survival data needs more time to mature but this illustrates the increased importance of the molecular features of glioma over histological appearance.

Glioblastoma

Glioblastomas are recognized to arise in two distinct patterns.

Primary glioblastoma occurs in older patients with no prior history of tumour. They are characterized by mutations in EGFR, NF1, PTEN, and amplification of EGFR. Secondary glioblastoma appears to arise from a pre-existing low-grade tumour and, as well as carrying LOH of chromosome 10q, there are persisting p53 mutations and mutations in IDH1 and 2.

In both tumour types the methyl guanine-DNA methyl transferase (MGMT) gene has a promoter methylation in approximately 40% of patients. This has prognostic significance.

Oligodendrogliomas

Oligodendrogliomas exhibit LOH on chromosomes 1p and 19q. This molecular finding is required to make a diagnosis of oligodendroglioma and is highly significant with respect to treatment indications and prognosis.

Medulloblastoma

See 'Medulloblastoma' in Chapter 14.3, p.417.

Ependymoma

See 'Ependymoma' in Chapter 14.3, p. 419.

Meningioma

Deletions on chromosome 22 are common and mutations in the neurofibromatosis 2 (NF2) gene are detected in the majority of NF2-associated tumours and in 60% of sporadic meningiomas.

4.3 Presentation and general management of primary brain tumours

Presentation

Brain tumours affect the entire age spectrum. They occur in any part of the brain. Symptoms are caused by excitation, infiltration, or compression of normal CNS tissues. Hence, brain tumours present in a variety of ways although certain recognizable patterns emerge.

Headache

- Is the most common symptom recorded in patients with brain tumours, though it is the main presenting symptom in far fewer.
- Brain tumours are a rare cause of headache in the general population. Guidelines produced by NICE (NG12) have been updated to include guidance on early referral for adults with subacute loss of central neurological function. The recommendation is for urgent direct access for a magnetic resonance imaging (MRI) scan within two weeks of presentation.
- For children and young adults the recommendation is to consider a very urgent referral (for an appointment within 48 hours) for suspected brain or CNS cancer with newly abnormal cerebellar or other central neurological function.

Seizures

- Occur in approximately half of patients with brain tumours over the duration of their disease.
- Seizure is the most common presenting symptom in low-grade glial tumours. Typically, these begin as focal seizures but may become generalized.

- Tumour should be considered in all adults newly presenting with seizure that has no other obvious explanation.
- Tumour is more likely in patients with:
  - Focal seizures
  - Significant postictal focal deficit (excluding confusion)
  - Epilepsy presenting as status epilepticus
  - Associated interictal focal deficit
  - Associated preceding persistent headache of recent onset
  - Seizure frequency accelerating over weeks or months

Progressive neurological deficit

- Suspicion of tumour should be high in a patient presenting with progressive neurological deficit (e.g. progressive weakness, sensory loss, dysphasia, ataxia) developing over days to weeks.
- Some symptoms may be grouped into specific neurological syndromes associated with tumours in particular regions of the brain. Obvious examples are motor or speech dysfunction due to parietal tumours. Less obvious are complex syndromes such as Parinaud's (abnormalities of eye movement and pupil dysfunction) occurring in patients with pineal tumours.

Personality or cognitive change

- Patients frequently present with subtle changes in personality or cognition or a deterioration of performance. A high index of suspicion must be maintained in a person presenting with such features especially if associated with headache.

- Tumours in the elderly may be missed or put down to vascular disturbance. Again, progressive neurological deterioration in an older person may be an indication for evaluation through imaging.

General medical management

Steroids

- The use of steroids is ubiquitous in the care of patients with brain tumours. Their value in reducing intracranial pressure and reversing symptoms is undoubted. However, the side effect profile is severe and many patients are probably left overtreated for long periods.
- Introduce steroid at the maximum dose likely to be useful in a situation and then rapidly titrate the dose downward against the patient's symptoms. The optimal dose is just above that at which deterioration occurs.
- Patients should always be assessed for response. If symptoms do not improve, the steroid should be stopped.
- The most commonly used steroid is dexamethasone in doses between 2mg and 16mg daily. The plasma half-life is long and at low doses dexamethasone can be given once daily. At higher doses it is best divided into two equally spaced doses.
- Prednisolone (x7.5) and hydrocortisone (x30) can also be used but are less satisfactory due to their even greater glucocorticoid side effects.
- It is standard to cover brain surgery with steroids but protocols should be in place to reduce or eliminate the drug as quickly as safely possible after the operation. Even if steroids need to be reintroduced later, say during radiotherapy, a short period off the drugs can be beneficial.
- It is tempting to treat seizures with steroids but this should be resisted except as a very short-term expedient. It should quickly be replaced by modification of the anticonvulsant programme.

Antiepileptic drugs (AEDs)

- Over half of all patients diagnosed with malignant brain tumours will suffer a seizure at some time.
- Almost any patient with a brain tumour who suffers a seizure should be treated with an AED. However, prophylactic use of AED before a seizure has occurred is not recommended.
- Epilepsy in patients with brain tumours can be difficult to control. All such patients should be managed by a specialist in this area.
- Some brain tumour treatments such as chemotherapy and antidepressants impair the effectiveness of AEDs.
- First-line AEDs are successful in suppressing seizure in less than half of patients. Of those that fail, less than half will be controlled with either second-line monotherapy treatments or polypharmacy.
- Many AEDs modify the cytochrome p450 enzyme system of the liver which is responsible for the metabolism of many other drugs including some anticancer agents. If possible for patients with brain tumours in whom treatment with chemotherapy or some

biological therapies is considered, enzyme-inducing AED drugs (EIAEDs) should be avoided.

- Non-enzyme-inducing (or weak) drugs are generally preferred. Lamotrigine (a weak inducer) has good activity but must be introduced slowly. Keppra® (levetiracetam) can be introduced rapidly at therapeutic dose but can produce unwanted mood disturbance in some patients. Valproate is an older but still excellent drug for all types of seizures (particularly if generalized). It may act to alter drug metabolism by suppressing liver activity.
- Of the older enzyme-inducing drugs, both phenytoin and carbamazepine have excellent antiseizure activity and are still used frequently perioperatively. However, their side effect profiles as well as their effects on liver function make them less suitable for patients with brain tumours.

Anticoagulants

The incidence of thromboembolic disease in patients with a brain tumour is dramatic with a 45% reported incidence of deep vein thrombosis (DVT). The prevalence of pulmonary embolus (PE) at autopsy is 8.4%. This is due to coagulins released by the tumour itself, as well as loss of mobility in the patients. There is always anxiety with respect to anticoagulation because of the risk of intratumoural bleed.

- For patients with no prior history of tumour bleed, the balance of risk is in favour of anticoagulation.
- Low-molecular-weight heparins can be used in standard doses. There is currently no evidence to support the use of direct oral anticoagulants (DOACs) in patients with brain tumours, although the risk/benefit ratio could be discussed with patients. Oral anticoagulant may be used on an individual basis.
- For patients with a prior history of bleeding or who are in generally poor health, simple measures such an antithrombotic stockings and analgesia may be more appropriate.

Analgesics

- Pain is a relatively minor problem (numerically) in the brain tumour population. However, raised intracranial pressure and meningeal and blood vessel involvement can be a potent source of pain in a minority of cases. Appropriate analgesics should not be withheld from these patients.
- Use of the conventional WHO cancer analgesic 'ladder' is recommended for pain in patients with brain tumour (see 'Pain management' in Chapter 17, p. 483).

Antidepressants

- True clinical depression is common in patients with brain tumours. Once recognized, treatment with antidepressants and psychotherapy should be considered.
- There is a concern that some antidepressants, particularly tricyclic compounds, might exacerbate seizure. Whilst this is also true to a lesser extent for selective serotonin antagonists (SSIs), these drugs are probably safe if seizures are absent or well controlled. SSIs probably represent the drugs of choice in such patients.
- There is a high incidence of stress and anxiety in this patient group which does not reach the level of true depression. The value of psychological and counselling

support should not be underestimated in this and the depressed population.

Prognostic factors in brain tumours

The outcome for patients with brain tumours depends on a variety of prognostic factors.

Detailed pathology

The importance of a precise pathological and molecular diagnosis has already been emphasized.

Age

In adults there is a direct correlation between increasing age and poorer outcome for almost all brain tumours but particularly for those derived from the neuroepithelium.

Performance status (PS)

As with age, PS is a strong determinant of survival in patients with brain tumours. The PS should be estimated according to a suitable scale (Karnofsky, WHO) as a guide to treatment, before and after optimal general medical treatments have been given (including steroids).

Surgery

There is no satisfactory comparative study that has examined the impact of the extent of surgical excision on survival in any primary brain tumour. However, there is extensive observational evidence that patients who have less residual disease after surgery have a better prognosis. Maximal safe surgical resection if possible is recommended (NICE Guideline NG99).

4.4 Surgical management of primary brain tumours

Surgery has three major roles in brain tumour management:

- **Diagnosis:** a pathological diagnosis is required in virtually all patients in whom subsequent antitumour treatment is contemplated. The brainstem is the only site where risk of morbidity may still prevent biopsy.
- **Symptom control:** relief of pressure symptoms is the most common aim.
- **Cure:** surgery is capable of curing most grade 1 tumours and may contribute to prolongation of survival in others.

Preparation for surgery

- Where possible, the patient should be operated on electively after stabilization of any general medical problems. Drugs affecting coagulation (e.g. non-steroidal anti-inflammatory drugs (NSAIDs)) should be eliminated prior to surgery.
- Steroids are routinely used to improve tolerance to the operative procedure. Daily dexamethasone doses around 16mg are used. This should be reduced as soon as possible after the operation.
- Anticonvulsants need not be given routinely to patients undergoing surgery for brain tumour. For patients already on anticonvulsants, the dose should be optimized to maximize the chance of control in the perioperative period.

Surgical technique

Biopsy

- Closed biopsy is done using image-guided (stereotactic) localization.
- Fusion of functional images with structural magnetic resonance imaging (MRI) or computed tomography (CT) improves localization of the part of the tumour most likely to yield a diagnosis.
- Multiple biopsies taken along a single tract or multiple tracts can be used to maximize diagnostic accuracy.
- Intraoperative diagnosis (frozen section, smear) is essential to ensure adequate tissue has been sampled and to guide subsequent procedures.
- Open biopsy under direct vision may be needed for some lesions where there is surgical risk (bleeding, pressure) or where large quantities of tissue are needed.

Surgical resection

General principles

It is common practice to confirm the diagnosis with an intraoperative frozen section or cytological smear, prior to performing the full resection. The resection itself is typically performed by internal decompression using a mixture of bipolar coagulation, sharp dissection, cautery, ultrasonic aspiration, and, if appropriate, laser vaporization. The aim is always to remove as much of the tumour as is safely possible.

Image-guided stereotactic resection

Obtaining three-dimensional image data and referencing it to a stereotactic frame allows the surgeon to plan an operative approach to minimize injury to neighbouring critical structures. This technique is particularly valuable in technically challenging locations, e.g. perithalamic.

Neuronavigation

- Normal brain anatomy is often distorted by the presence of tumour and its associated oedema making it difficult for the surgeon to resect according to conventional landmarks.
- Neuronavigation systems allow the registration of stored imaging data with 'real time' physical space. There is interaction with a localization device so that the surgeon can use the recent imaging information to guide the resection. Registration is done by either using natural landmarks or external fiducial markers. The system may be 'frame based' or more usually is 'frameless' which gives the surgeon much more freedom of access.
- Real time intraoperative imaging may be based on ultrasound or more powerfully on MRI.
- Intraoperative MRI may be achieved either by moving the patient into the magnet during the surgical procedure or more conveniently by bringing the MR scanner into the operating suite.
- The particular advantage of intraoperative MRI is likely to be in the resection of low-grade tumours where differentiation from normal brain is otherwise difficult.

Cortical mapping 'awake craniotomy'

- Resection of tumours inside or adjacent to functional brain areas may not be safe even if the surgeon remains within obvious tumour boundaries.
- Intraoperative stimulation of cortical and subcortical sites and related tracts allows active areas to be identified and marked. This functional information facilitates avoidance of these areas during resection and allows the surgeon to perform a safer and more extensive tumour removal.
- In 'awake craniotomy' the initial craniotomy and preliminary stimulation is performed with the patient asleep. After arousal, sedative/hypnotic anaesthesia allows the patient to respond to motor and language commands but still provides subsequent amnesia.

Fluorescence-guided surgery

- 5-Aminolevulinic acid (5-ALA) is a metabolite in the haem biosynthesis pathway which elicits accumulation of fluorescent porphyrins within malignant gliomas and can be used for identifying tumour intraoperatively. It is given preoperatively by mouth. The surgeon operates using violet–blue excitation light and appropriate light filters to identify the tumour-bearing fluorescent regions against the dark, normal tissue background. The randomized 5-ALA study demonstrated more frequent complete resections of contrast-enhancing tumour in malignant glioma patients using 5-ALA, translating into prolonged progression-free survival after adjuvant radiotherapy.

Surgery and individual tumours

The scope and role of surgery varies according to tumour type.

WHO grade I tumours

Surgery alone is frequently curative and maximal safe removal should be attempted. However, even if this is incomplete, tumours may fail to progress subsequently and the patients remain well without further intervention. In those where regrowth does occur, second surgery is usually indicated, possibly followed by non-surgical treatment.

WHO grade II gliomas

- If the lesion is amenable to complete (or near complete) macroscopic excision then this group of patients can do well in the longer term without other intervention.
- The value of resection when only a small proportion can be removed is unproven. In these cases, a biopsy followed by non-surgical antitumour treatment may be more appropriate.
- If the patient has relevant symptoms, (pressure, seizure), and the appropriate region of tumour can be safely removed, surgery directed at improving the patient's condition should always be considered.
- Low-grade ependymomas, although technically grade II, should always be considered for resection, which if 'complete' may give long-term control.

WHO grade III and IV gliomas

- It is recommended that patients with high-grade glioma undergo maximal safe resection prior to subsequent non-surgical therapy.

- Patients should not be put at unreasonable risk to achieve resection, however. Where necessary, safety enhancing techniques such as 5-ALA-assisted resection, intraoperative ultrasound, and functional imaging should be considered to improve outcome.
- The brainstem is a surgically challenging region where even biopsy can be associated with high levels of morbidity and mortality. Whilst some exophytic tumours can be biopsied, most cannot and a clinicoradiological diagnosis must suffice.

Medulloblastoma

- There is an association between extent of resection and outcome in medulloblastoma. Maximal safe surgical resection should be attempted for all localized disease.

Lymphoma

- There is no evidence that surgery improves outcome in primary CNS lymphoma. A biopsy sufficient to allow complete pathological typing is all that is required.

Germ cell tumours

- These typically arise in the pineal region—a site where biopsy can be problematic due to access problems and tumour vascularity. Biopsy is necessary, however, except in those cases where tumour marker positivity and imaging make a diagnosis unequivocal even without tissue. Surgical resection may be necessary when troublesome masses remain after non-surgical treatment.

Intraoperative, non-resective approaches

Local chemotherapy

- Gliadel® is chemotherapy (carmustine (BCNU)) impregnated biodegradable polymer wafers. Up to eight are used to line the cavity following surgical excision. BCNU then diffuses into the adjacent tumour-bearing tissue.
- Randomized studies have shown a modest improvement in median survival (approximately eight weeks) in both newly diagnosed and recurrent high-grade gliomas.
- Disadvantages are that it is only applicable to tumours where a >90% resection can be achieved and which do not communicate with the ventricles.
- Treatment is associated with increased postoperative complications such as seizures, brain oedema, problems with wound healing, and intracranial infection.
- Other chemotherapeutic approaches using free intracavitary drugs have not been useful.

Convection enhanced delivery

Using fine interstitial catheters connected to a constant intermediate pressure pump, it is possible to convect large molecules and even viruses through tumours and along white matter tracts following migrating tumour cells. Whilst this technique has been the subject of randomized trials using toxins and antibodies, it has yet to find a place in routine management.

4.5 Radiotherapy for primary brain tumours

Introduction

Radiotherapy is the major life-prolonging treatment for patients with brain tumours.

Indications for radiotherapy

Grade I tumours: radiotherapy has a limited role in these lesions. Although routinely considered in a few tumours (craniopharyngioma), it is usually confined to the setting of recurrent disease that defies complete surgical resection (e.g. pilocytic astrocytoma, meningioma).

Grade II tumours: radiotherapy can produce tumour shrinkage and symptomatic improvement in diffuse gliomas. However, its role in prolonging life is unproven and delayed radiotherapy seems as effective as immediate treatment. Observation for some small, slow growing asymptomatic tumours is acceptable though surveillance in a specialist clinic is required so that timing of intervention can be optimized.

Grade III and IV tumours: all patients with high-grade tumours should be considered for radiation after surgery. Patients of good PS will receive radical treatments, less fit patients may receive short course palliative regimens, and those with very poor PS may receive supportive care only. Virtually all patients with PNETs will receive craniospinal irradiation.

Radiotherapy process

Immobilization and imaging

- Radical radiotherapy planning should use both an MRI and planning CT for tumour delineation and dosimetry. CT is acquired with the patient supine in a custom-made immobilization shell, typically, 3mm slice spacing is used and is acquired post IV contrast. The planning MRI is acquired without immobilization.
- For high-grade gliomas, the most helpful MRI sequence is the T1-weighted post-gadolinium (T1 Gd) sequence. If there is also a low-grade component, a T2-weighted and a fluid-attenuated inversion recovery (FLAIR) sequence should also be obtained.
- For low-grade gliomas, only the FLAIR and T2-weighted sequence is needed. The MRI may be acquired as axial slices or as a three-dimensional volumetric MRI reconstructed into axial slices. The MRI is co-registered with the planning CT and both are accessible as a combined imaging data set on the radiotherapy planning software.

Volume delineation

A standard approach to target volume delineation for grade III and GBM is to define the gross tumour volume (GTV) as the surgical cavity, plus areas of enhancement on the T1 Gd MRI, which represents residual macroscopic disease.

The clinical target volume (CTV) is obtained by applying a uniform (isotropic) expansion to the GTV, most often of 2.0–2.5cm. The CTV should be carefully edited, taking into account anatomical boundaries to tumour spread which include the skull, tentorium, and falx. Areas where spread can be more extensive include the corpus callosum and cerebral peduncles. The CTV to planning target volume (PTV) expansion depends on geometric uncertainties—a 3–5mm margin is most often used.

For WHO grade II gliomas, the GTV is the surgical cavity plus the MRI FLAIR or T2 abnormality. The CTV is obtained by expanding the GTV isotropically by 1 to 1.5cm and then editing this, taking into account

anatomical boundaries, as described above. The CTV to PTV expansion is usually 3–5mm.

Organs at risk should also be outlined (see later) to facilitate the limiting of dose to these structures in subsequent planning.

Radiotherapy planning

- Treatments are planned for a 4–8MV linear accelerator.
- Most treatment plans will require conformal radiotherapy or intensity-modulated radiotherapy planning.
- Dose uniformity should be maintained according to International Commission on Radiation Units and Measurements (ICRU) report 83.
- Dose–volume histograms (DVHs) of target and organs at risk should be calculated to facilitate plan assessment.
- The field arrangement is either checked by verification on the treatment machine or by using image guidance.

Dose prescription

- The dose is prescribed to the isocentre.
- The normal daily dose (for radical treatments) is 2Gy per fraction for high-grade tumours and 1.8Gy or less for low-grade (or benign) lesions.
- An exception is whole neuraxis treatment where radiation delivery is always delivered at <2Gy per fraction.

Timing of radiotherapy

- For high-grade tumours, delays in starting radiotherapy are associated with reduced survival.
- For patients undergoing biopsy only, radiotherapy should begin as soon as possible.
- Following craniotomy there is a need to allow wound healing and reduction of cerebral oedema. Planning here optimally begins at 10–14 days and radiotherapy a week later.
- For low-grade tumours, timing is less critical and longer delays to allow complete healing and to accommodate patient preference are possible.

Radiotherapy delivery and patient assessment

- Patients are normally treated once daily, five days per week.
- Admission to hospital is generally not required.
- Steroid cover may be needed if the tumour has not been resected or large volumes are treated. Doses of dexamethasone vary from 2mg in low-risk situations to 16mg where raised pressure already exists. Attempts should be made to reduce the steroid dose during the course of treatment.
- Patients should be seen at least weekly to monitor treatment, assess symptoms, and modify medication.

Palliative treatments

- Simple planning is possible for patients requiring a purely palliative approach.
- An immobilization mask is still required.
- Opposed beam arrangements or a simple three field beam arrangement can be used.

Stereotactic radiotherapy

Stereotactic radiotherapy (SRT) localizes intracranial structures to an external reference frame for enhanced accuracy.

- For stereotactic treatments immobilization is enhanced by the use of an invasively attached frame or a relocatable frame.
- The CT planning scan is done at 1mm slice spacing.
- Fusion with other imaging modalities (MRI, angiography) is undertaken.
- Delivery is by means of a modified linear accelerator using non-coplanar dynamic arcs, or multiple fixed conformal beams, or alternatively by a multicobalt source gamma knife or by cyberknife.
- SRT is multifraction stereotactically guided radiotherapy and is performed almost exclusively on a linear accelerator.
- Stereotactic radiosurgery (SRS) is single fraction high-dose treatment and can be performed on multiple platforms.

Individual tumour types

- For low-grade gliomas the GTV is the high signal region on T2 or FLAIR MR images. The CTV is created by 'growing' the GTV by 1–2cm. Doses in the range 45–54Gy are prescribed in 1.8Gy fractions.
- For high-grade gliomas, the GTV is taken as the enhancing tumour margin and/or resection bed. The CTV is created by growing the GTV by 2–2.5cm. (This may be reduced in the vicinity of sensitive structures or natural barriers.) The prescribed dose is 60Gy in 30 fractions.
- A palliative treatment for high-grade glioma comprises a pair of opposed fields or simple three field plan to cover the tumour bed plus 2–3cm, prescribed to a dose of 30Gy in six fractions over two weeks (or similar).
- A regimen of particular use in the elderly population comprises a three-dimensional planned volume treated to 40Gy in 15 fractions. This has compared favourably to standard radiotherapy in this population with GBM.
- Planning in medulloblastomas requires craniospinal radiotherapy for phase I which needs careful inclusion of the entire meningeal surface including extension along the cranial nerves. The phase II usually includes the primary site boost (generally the posterior fossa) and a boost to any metastatic deposits.
- Meningiomas rarely invade brain parenchyma so the margin at the brain interface can be small. They may, however, spread along the meninges and these margins should be more generous.
- The CTV for pituitary (and some other benign) tumours is often the GTV plus a small margin as spread beyond the enhancing margin is infrequent. The PTV margin is dependent on the radiotherapy technique used and is typically 1–3mm.
- Radiotherapy for PCNSL is given as a salvage treatment or as consolidation after chemotherapy in younger patients. It is generally given to the whole brain to a dose of 40–45Gy in 1.8–2Gy per fraction. It is not sure whether whole brain radiotherapy (WBRT) can be safely omitted in patients who achieve a complete response to induction chemotherapy and, currently, reduced dose WBRT (23.4–30Gy in 1.8–2Gy per fraction) is being studied in this group of patients. Patients older than 60 years have a high risk of late neurotoxicity with WBRT, especially after high-dose methotrexate and a decision for WBRT should be taken carefully after discussion with the patient.

Normal tissue reactions to radiotherapy
Sparing normal tissue

- Radiation will damage normal tissue in a dose-dependent fashion.
- The concept of 'radiation tolerance' concerns the acceptable level of radiation damage to a tissue in a particular clinical circumstance. Thus a higher tolerance dose is acceptable when treating a high risk, highly malignant tumour than a lower risk tumour with a good prospect of survival.

Radiation tolerance limits of normal tissues

- Radiation injury in the CNS depends on treatment parameters (total dose, dose per fraction, volume irradiated) and patient-related factors (age, vasculopathy, infection). The risks of late side effects according to dose are outlined in detail in the QUANTEC publications. In general, the CNS is a 'late responding tissue' although both early and intermediate effects can also occur.
- Organs at risk that should be considered include: optic chiasm, optic nerves, retina, lacrimal glands, cornea, lens, pituitary, hippocampus, brainstem, spinal cord, and cochlea.

Acute effects

- Symptoms are generally those of acute raised intracranial pressure or a worsening of neurological symptoms caused by the lesion itself.
- Symptoms begin within days or even hours.
- Using conventional dosing, acute effects are rarely troublesome if steroids are appropriately given.

Early delayed (intermediate) effects

- Begin within weeks of completing radiation therapy and may continue for six to ten weeks thereafter.
- The syndrome comprises somnolence, lethargy, and frequently recurrence of the original presenting symptoms and signs.
- Symptoms are usually self-limiting but will respond to steroids. Recovery is the rule.
- The pathogenesis is believed to relate to interruption of myelin synthesis secondary to damage to the oligodendroglial cells.
- A corresponding condition occurs after spinal irradiation and presents with Lhermitte's sign.

Delayed radiation damage

- This is the most sinister form of radiation damage and is uniformly irreversible.
- The onset may be from around three to four months up to many years after the exposure.
- Injury is predominantly to the white matter and is dose and volume dependent. Radiation necrosis is the most severe form of damage.
- The generally accepted tolerance dose for late damage (for malignant tumour) is 60Gy in 30 fractions. In less demanding situations, 50–54Gy in 2Gy fractions is considered the upper limit.
- To minimize late damage, fraction sizes for radical brain treatments should not exceed 2Gy.
- Other late consequences of brain irradiation include hormone (pituitary/hypothalamic) failure, damage to optic tracts, and second malignancy.

4.6 Chemotherapy and new agents for primary brain tumours

Introduction

Cytotoxic chemotherapy of brain tumours is hampered by the intrinsic resistance of many tumours and the poor penetration caused by the blood–brain barrier (BBB). BBB resistance may not exist to the same extent in the vicinity of tumours. The most successful drug treatments for brain tumours have been lipophilic alkylators (nitrosureas) or small molecules (temozolomide). Chemotherapy can be given in a neoadjuvant, adjuvant, concomitant, consolidation, or palliative setting.

Active agents

Nitrosoureas

- The chloroethyl nitrosoureas are highly lipid soluble, non-ionized drugs that rapidly cross the BBB.
- Carmustine (BCNU intravenous), and lomustine (CCNU oral) are the most commonly used drugs in Europe and the USA. They differ in pharmacokinetic properties whilst retaining the same basic chemical activity and toxicity problems. Neither has proved more effective than the other.
- Major adverse effects include delayed and cumulative myelosuppression and lung fibrosis.

Procarbazine

- Procarbazine is an oral agent which is activated in the liver to become an alkylating agent.
- Adverse effects include nausea, vomiting, and myelosuppression.
- It interacts adversely with alcohol and some smoked and preserved foods. Dietary restriction is necessary.

Temozolomide

- Temozolomide is a small molecule that acts as an alkylating agent by adding methyl groups to the O^6 position of guanine in DNA.
- It has high oral bioavailability and is converted spontaneously into the active compound at physiological pH on entering the bloodstream.
- It penetrates readily into brain tumours.
- Methylation by temozolomide is opposed by methyl guanine methyl transferase (MGMT), a ubiquitous enzyme.
- Toxicity includes general myelosuppression, moderate emesis, skin rashes, and selective lymphopenia when given continuously.
- Temozolomide can be used as concomitant treatment with radiotherapy in patients with newly diagnosed glioblastoma followed by adjuvant treatment. It is used as an adjuvant treatment for 12 months for grade III astrocytomas.

Gliadel®

- Gliadel® comprises a biodegradable polymer in wafer form that is impregnated with BCNU.
- A number of these wafers are used to line the cavity left after resecting a brain tumour.
- After wound closure, the polymer slowly breaks down, delivering the BCNU in a more concentrated and protracted fashion than is possible to achieve by systemic delivery.

Epipodophyllotoxins and platinum compounds

Drugs such as VP-16, cisplatin, and carboplatin are valuable for treating non-glial brain tumours such as medulloblastoma and germ cell tumours. They have only minor activity against gliomas and can be used as third-line agents.

Vinca alkaloids

Vinca alkaloids are highly polar molecules with very limited access to the brain. In spite of this vincristine appears regularly in the treatment of brain tumours. Its value is not clear.

Combination chemotherapy

Few drugs are effective as single agents in glioma therapy and hence the potential for combinations is limited. Few have been studied. The combination procarbazine, lomustine (CCNU), and vincristine (PCV) was considered to be a standard first-line treatment in glioma treatment. However, the evidence that it is superior to single agent nitrosourea is very sparse.

Chemotherapy for individual tumours

Gliomas

WHO grade I

- There is no clear role for chemotherapy in WHO grade I tumours in adults.

WHO grade II

- Nitrosoureas and temozolomide can each produce clear symptomatic and radiological response in low-grade gliomas at first diagnosis and relapse.
- 1p19q co-deleted oligodendrogliomas are particularly responsive.
- NICE (2018) evaluated the evidence in relation to the effectiveness of radiotherapy and chemotherapy and concluded that there is a survival benefit for adjuvant PCV for low-grade glioma patients who have residual disease on MRI after surgery.

WHO grades III and IV

- PCV and temozolomide appear to be equieffective in patients with relapsed astrocytoma.
- The objective response rate is around 10% with disease stabilization and symptomatic improvement in around 20–30%.
- Response is better in patients with grade III tumours.
- Temozolomide ($75mg/m^2$) given concurrently with radiation followed by adjuvant monthly treatment ($200mg/m^2$ days one to five) for patients with newly diagnosed glioblastoma produces a survival advantage at two years of 16% sustained at four years when compared with radiation alone (10–26%). Hence this is the treatment of choice for GBM.
- Patients with methylation of the MGMT gene promoter have better prognosis with this regimen than those with unmethylated promoter.
- For 1p19q co-deleted grade III tumours the addition of adjuvant PCV increases overall survival. The value of adjuvant treatment with temozolomide in non-co-deleted grade III tumours has been shown to improve survival and further information is awaited with regard to the role of concomitant temozolomide.
- Gliadel has been shown in a randomized study to prolong survival modestly in patients with newly diagnosed

and relapsed disease who are able to undergo macroscopic tumour removal.

- Ependymomas are highly chemoresistant. The most effective agents are probably platinum compounds.

Medulloblastoma

- Adjuvant chemotherapy with cisplatin, CCNU, and vincristine have become standard treatment for children with medulloblastomas following (reduced dose) radiotherapy.
- This regimen is very toxic for use in most adults but there is evidence of a survival benefit when used, so it is generally given but with close attention to toxicity.
- Effective agents at relapse include carboplatin, epipodophyllotoxins, cyclophosphamide, and temozolomide.
- High-dose alkylating treatment with stem cell rescue has been used in attempts to prolong remission but the results are poor.

Primary CNS lymphoma

- The principal agent used in the treatment of PCNSL is high-dose methotrexate ($>3g/m^2$), which may be combined with other BBB penetrating agents (e.g. Ara-C, BCNU, procarbazine) to improve response. High-dose chemotherapy with autologous stem cell transplantation (HDC-ASCT) is being studied as consolidation after first-line treatment.
- A variety of agents may be effective, particularly alkylating agents (temozolomide, nitrosoureas) in relapsed or refractory PCNSL. Patients less than 60–65 years are considered for HDC-ASCT and high-dose thiotepa-based conditioning regimens are generally preferred over the BEAM (carmustine, etoposide, cytarabine, and melphalan) regimen.

Germ cell tumours

- Agents similar to those used for systemic disease (cisplatin, carboplatin, epipodophyllotoxins, ifosfamide) are used.
- In the primary treatment of germinomas, chemotherapy can be used to reduce the extent of radiotherapy.
- Chemotherapy is an integral part of the treatment for nearly all patients with non-germinomas.
- Chemotherapy alone (without radiation) is not adequate for the curative management of these diseases.

Meningiomas

Chemotherapy has little part to play in the management of meningioma.

Hydroxyurea has a low level of activity and can be useful to stabilize disease in some patients at relapse.

New agents

The greater understanding of the aberrant cellular pathways identified in brain tumours has led to an explosion of interest in novel biological agents directed at correcting them. Few have gained acceptance as single agents but many are in clinical trials as combinations with other similar agents and conventional treatments. Most trials of novel agents are in gliomas.

Antiangiogenesis inhibitors

- Marked neovascularization is a hallmark of glioma.
- Vascular endothelial growth factor (VEGF) has been identified as a potent mediator of angiogenesis, vascular permeability, and tumour growth. VEGF expression is particularly upregulated in glioblastoma and its expression may be a prognostic factor for survival. The expression of VEGF is related to prognosis.
- Bevacizumab has been extensively explored alone or in combination with other agents. To date there has been no convincing evidence of prolonged survival if administered at disease presentation. A recent meta-analysis of three randomized trials showed that the combination of bevacizumab with CCNU improved progression-free survival but not overall survival compared with monotherapies.

Growth factor signalling pathways

- Growth factor signalling pathways are often upregulated in brain tumours and contribute to oncogenesis through autocrine and paracrine mechanisms.
- EGFR is frequently amplified and overexpressed in GBM and is usually accompanied by gene-rearrangements and deletions.
- Although responses to these agents are seen in recurrent gliomas, they have not reached a level to make their routine use worthwhile.
- Trials are ongoing to explore their use in combination with other biological treatments and conventional therapy in newly diagnosed disease.

4.7 Outcome and management of recurrence in primary brain tumours

Outcome

WHO grade I tumours

- The outcome in this group of tumours is good with long-term control or cure in 80–90% and low morbidity.
- Even if a complete resection is not achieved at primary surgery, regrowth may not occur.
- Outcome correlates with the volume of residual tumour.
- When recurrence occurs it is nearly always local.

WHO grade II gliomas

Since the management of these tumours is so variable and prognostic factors so influential, the value of averaged outcome measures is limited. Important positive prognostic variables are:

- Smaller tumour size (<6cm).
- Non-encroachment of the midline.
- Oligodendroglioma rather than astrocytoma.
- Lack of neurological deficit.
- Younger age (<40).
- Median survival is around 5–15 years.
- Most (75%) patients will die of their disease, the majority following malignant transformation.

WHO grades III and IV glioma

- More than 80% of high-grade glioma recur within 2cm of the original tumour or its resection margin.
- Spinal spread can occur but is rare and systemic spread is very rare.

Anaplastic astrocytoma

- The median survival of patients with anaplastic astrocytomas is 2–5 years.
- The same prognostic factors operate as for glioblastoma.
- Recurrence is often accompanied by transformation to glioblastoma.

Anaplastic oligodendroglioma

- Median survival for this group of patients who are treated with radiotherapy and adjuvant temozolomide is >14 years.

Glioblastoma

- Overall median survival remains <1 year for all patients.
- For patients treated with combined chemoradiotherapy median survival is 14.6 months.
- The major prognostic factors are age, PS, and extent of surgery.
- For patients in the best prognostic category, who have methylated MGMT promoter and are treated with chemoradiotherapy, median survival is >2 years.

Medulloblastoma

- Medulloblastoma in adults is a rare disease and survival figures are unreliable. A typical figure is around 70% five-year survival for patients over 18.
- Patients continue to relapse many years after treatment and five-year survival is not synonymous with cure, as shown by the ten-year survival, which is around 50%.
- Good prognostic factors are the absence of metastatic disease, complete resection of primary tumour, and timely completion of craniospinal irradiation.
- Relapse may be local, disseminated through the neuraxis or systemic.
- Lung and bone are sites of preference for systemic spread.

Meningioma

- The prospect of local control depends on:
  - the extent of resection (Table 4.7.1) and hence the site of tumour and the growth pattern
  - the histological grade
- Not all meningiomas regrow even after incomplete removal.
- Recurrence is nearly always local although grade III tumours may metastasize.
- Recurrence following Simpson grade I resection is rare.
- Grade III tumours frequently recur even after surgical excision and radiotherapy.

Primary CNS lymphoma

- Approximately 50% of patients completing treatment with chemotherapy and radiation will live five years.
- Median survival for patients receiving chemotherapy alone is around 30 months.
- Patients not achieving complete remission following chemoradiotherapy have very poor survival.
- Deteriorating cognitive function is very common in patients, particularly those older than 60 years, surviving combined chemoradiotherapy.

Treatment of relapse

WHO grade I tumours

- Treatment of relapse is surgical where possible.
- Treatment with radiotherapy of any residuum following surgery may be justified.

WHO grade II gliomas

- Many patients will have received radiotherapy as part of their initial treatment and many patients will have evidence of malignant transformation at relapse.
- Surgery should be considered particularly if there are pressure symptoms.
- Repeat radiotherapy is an option for some patients.
- The main treatment is likely to be with chemotherapy.
- Chemotherapy regimens will be as for high-grade glioma.

High-grade glioma

- Most patients will have received radiotherapy, and many temozolomide chemotherapy, as initial treatment.
- Further surgery should be considered for patients with pressure symptoms and where resection of all enhancing disease is feasible.
- Chemotherapy should be considered for patients who relapse and who have a reasonable PS (WHO 0–II).
- An MRC study showed no difference in outcome between PCV and five-day temozolomide in chemo-naive patients at relapse.
- For previously (temozolomide) treated patients the options are rechallenge with temozolomide (if initial treatment was beneficial) or PCV.
- Third-line chemotherapy, typically with etoposide and/or carboplatin is rarely of value.
- Chemotherapy should always be considered for patients with anaplastic oligodendroglioma. PCV and temozolomide are equieffective and have response rates up to 90% in co-deleted patients.

Table 4.7.1 Simpson grade of excision of meningioma

Grade	Extent of surgery	Risk of recurrence (%)
I	Gross total resection of tumour, dural attachments, abnormal bone	9
II	Gross total resection of tumour, coagulation of dural attachments	19
III	Gross total resection of tumour without resection or coagulation of dural attachments or extradural extensions	29
IV	Partial resection of tumour	44
V	Simple decompression (biopsy)	

Source: data from Simpson, D. The recurrence of intracranial meningiomas after surgical treatment. *J Neurol Neurosurg Psychiat* 1957; 20(1):22–39. 1957, BMJ Publishing Group Ltd.

Medulloblastoma

- Medulloblastoma recurrence is a sinister event, rarely compatible with survival. Further remission can often be obtained however.
- Surgical resection of 'solitary' recurrences should be considered.
- Recurrences will remain sensitive to a variety of agents including platinum compounds, epipodophyllotoxins, and alkylating agents. Appropriate chemotherapy is the treatment of choice.
- High-dose therapy with stem cell rescue has been tried but its benefit in adults is not established.
- Radiotherapy to isolated metastases can be repeated in some circumstances, particularly to regions not previously irradiated to high dose. Stereotactic localization should be considered.

Meningioma

- The principal treatment for relapsed meningioma is repeat surgery, where possible.
- Radiotherapy can be given for incompletely excised tumours or those where resection is not possible.
- Radiosurgery (SRS) is useful for small recurrences.
- Chemotherapy has little value for relapsed meningioma. Continuous oral hydroxyurea has been used to stabilize disease.

Primary CNS lymphoma

- Approximately one-third of patients are refractory to first-line treatment and half of patients who responded initially will relapse. Those not previously irradiated can receive radiotherapy (typically whole brain) and the reported median overall survival ranges from 11 to 16 months.
- HDC-ASCT is considered for patients younger than 60–65 years with good PS and who have previously responded to chemotherapy. A phase 2 trial reported a median PFS of 41 months with a median overall survival of 58 months for patients who completed the full treatment. The survival was shorter for patients who did not complete the intended treatment.
- Patients who are not suitable for WBRT or HDC-ASCT may be considered for second-line systemic therapy (temozolomide, bendamustine, etc.), though the survival is generally poor.

Palliative care input

Patients with progressive, incurable brain tumours have a number of particular needs that should be addressed by specialists working with this type of patient. Representative specialists should form part of the MDT.

- CNS symptoms such as seizure, headache, nausea, and movement disorder may need input from a specialist neurologist or palliative care physician.
- Appropriate support after loss of motor function or speech should be offered from physiotherapy, occupational therapy, and speech and language therapy.
- Cognitive dysfunction and depression are common in patients with brain tumours. Access to specialist psychological and psychiatric help should be available.
- Loss of function and life expectancy create profound social problems such as loss of employment.

Social care specialists should be available to provide support.

New approaches

Vaccines

Immunotherapy is the subject of intense investigation in GBM with many trials in progress. Some studies have targeted glioblastoma tumour-associated peptides. Rindopepimut is a 14-mer peptide vaccine eliciting responses to EGFRvIII and is currently being evaluated in a phase 3 trial. Another approach being investigated is an autologous dendritic cell plus autologous tumour lysate therapy. Immune checkpoint inhibition is also being investigated. Notably the full complexities of immune/inflammatory reactions in glioblastoma remain to be described and it is not certain that effects in systemic malignancies will translate for glioma.

PARP inhibition

The poly (ADP-ribose) polymerase (PARP) inhibitor olaparib increases the cytotoxicity of radiation by increasing levels of double-strand breaks. Trials are assessing the tolerability and efficacy of adding olaparib to temozolomide and radiotherapy.

Gene therapy

Gene therapy in brain tumours is most commonly delivered by modified viruses although approaches with liposomes and naked DNA have been attempted.

The major killing strategies have been 'suicide' therapy where a gene is selectively inserted into the cancer cells whose product will transform an otherwise innocuous drug into a cellular poison (e.g. the HSV-tk gene sensitizes cells to gancyclovir) and oncolytic viruses that have been disabled such that they are harmless to normal cells but lethal to malignant tissue (e.g. the herpes simplex virus HSV1716).

The first generation of gene therapy agents did not lead to therapeutic advance but second-generation strategies are looking more promising.

Other potential targets

Three intracellular signalling targets are of interest. The PI3K-Akt-mTOR axis is highly contributory to GBM development. Mutations in PIK3CA and other PI3K genes occur in about 60% of GBM. Akt activation occurs in around 85% of glioblastomas. This axis is therefore an attractive therapeutic target particularly as a component of combination therapy approaches. mTORC2 is a central signalling hub in the malignant glioma cell, integrating signals relating to growth factors, cell death, and metabolism and is therefore particularly compelling. Several agents with dual or triple inhibitory activity against mTORC2 and other components of the PI3K axis are in clinical development.

Missed by sequence-based analyses of GBM genomes, fusion between the FGFR and TACC genes was reported in 2012. The protein product was found to be oncogenic. The pan-FGFR inhibitor BGJ398 has entered into phase 2 trial for glioblastoma with FGFR amplification, translocation, or activating mutation. The translocation is present in 5–7% of patients.

Lastly, V600E-mutant BRAF occurs in around 6–10% of adult glioblastoma, enriched in giant cell and epithelioid subtypes. The BRAF inhibitors can be used as therapeutic treatment for this indication.

4.8 Summary of management for primary brain tumours

WHO grade I tumours

- The principal treatment is surgical excision where possible.
- The ambition is total (microscopic) removal.
- Some asymptomatic tumours may be observed.
- Adjunctive treatments are rarely appropriate as part of primary treatment even if excision is incomplete.

WHO grade II gliomas

- The majority of patients present with seizures that should be managed with anticonvulsants.
- Small tumours whose symptoms are controlled can be managed with a policy of imaging and close follow-up.
- Alternatively a macroscopic removal can be attempted.
- Tumours with, or developing, adverse risk factors (tumour of >6cm, encroaching the midline, neurological deficit, or age >40 years) should be offered maximal safe tumour removal followed by adjuvant PCV for those that are IDH mutated.
- All tumours should be tested for LOH 1p and 19q.
- Following resection patients who have residual tumour should be offered radiotherapy and adjuvant PCV.

WHO grades III and IV glioma

Anaplastic astrocytoma

- Patients should be offered maximal safe debulking surgery.
- Postoperative radical radiotherapy is required for nearly all patients.
- Patients should be offered adjuvant temozolomide.

Anaplastic oligodendroglioma

- The same general principles apply as for anaplastic astrocytoma.
- LOH1p,19q should be performed in every case as a guide to prognosis and chemosensitivity.
- Postoperative radiotherapy is required for all patients.
- Patients should be offered adjuvant PCV.

Glioblastoma

- The patient's condition should be optimized (steroids, anticonvulsants, etc.) prior to a management decision. The steroid dose should be optimized throughout the perioperative period through clear protocol guidelines.
- Treatment decisions should be made on the basis of the known major prognostic factors of PS, age, and tumour operability.
- Most patients should be offered maximal safe debulking surgery.
- In some patients biopsy only is possible. Multiple biopsies are desirable with acquisition of sufficient tissue for adequate pathological testing (including molecular studies) and deep freezing.
- Where possible MRI should be done within 48 hours of surgery to assess the extent of resection and to assist radiotherapy planning.
- A decision on subsequent therapy should be made in the postoperative setting.
- The methylation status of the promoter of the MGMT gene should be undertaken.

- Patients <70 years with PS WHO 0–1 should be considered for radical radiotherapy and concomitant/adjuvant chemotherapy.
- For older patients (>70 years) the MGMT status can be used to decide between hypofractionated (three weeks) radiotherapy plus or minus temozolomide treatment; temozolomide treatment alone; or palliative radiotherapy.
- For patients with poor PS (WHO >1) or multifocal disease, shorter course palliative radiotherapy alone is indicated.
- In some patients only supportive/symptomatic care is indicated. Patients >80 years or with PS >3 rarely benefit from disease-modifying treatment.
- In such cases, where the radiological diagnosis is secure, even a biopsy may be withheld.

Medulloblastoma

- Patients with medulloblastoma may present as an emergency with hydrocephalus. In these cases the patients should, where possible, be stabilized prior to definitive surgery.
- If surgical drainage is required, a non-dominant ventriculostomy is preferable to a shunt.
- In all cases where medulloblastoma is suspected, preoperative whole neuraxis imaging (MRI) is mandatory.
- Surgery is performed with the aim of obtaining as complete a resection as possible consistent with good neurological function.
- CSF should be sampled at the time of surgery (or earlier if a drain is placed) to aid staging.
- All patients should be offered whole neuraxis radiotherapy (35Gy) with boosts to primary site and sites of residual bulk disease (20Gy).
- Delays in starting radiotherapy are accompanied by inferior outcomes.

Mesenchymal tumours

- Patients with small asymptomatic meningiomas can be kept under imaging surveillance.
- Patients requiring treatment should be considered for surgery with a view to a maximal removal consistent with good neurological function.
- The outcome of surgery should be recorded in terms of an appropriate reporting system to aid surveillance and management decisions.
- Postoperative treatment should be withheld in the great majority of cases for grade I tumours.
- Incompletely excised grade II tumours should be considered for radiotherapy treatment or followed closely if radiotherapy is not given.
- All grade III tumours should be considered for radiation treatment. If given, the dose and fractionation is as for high-grade glioma.
- Haemangioblastoma and solitary fibrous tumour can usually be managed with surgery alone.
- Haemangiopericytoma should be considered for postoperative radiotherapy.

Primary CNS lymphoma

- The role of surgery is confined to obtaining sufficient material for adequate tissue diagnosis.

- All patients should have whole neuraxis (MRI) imaging, slit lamp ophthalmological examination of the eye for tumour deposits, CSF examination for lymphoma cells, and immune status evaluation, including HIV.
- The value of full lymphoma staging is debated as the pick-up of systemic disease is low. However, it is still performed in many units.
- All patients should be considered for high-dose metho-trexate-based chemotherapy as first-line treatment.
- Patients <60 years should be considered for consolida-tion radiotherapy after discussion of the likely effect on cognitive function.
- Radiation should be withheld in patients >60 achieving remission with chemotherapy.
- Patients not going into remission with first-line chemo-therapy may be considered for palliative radiotherapy or HDC-ASCT.
- Patients aged less than 65 years with an initial chemo-therapy response and good PS should be considered for salvage HDC-ASCT.

Gangliocytoma (and variants)
These are predominantly low-grade tumours, managed by surgical excision.

Central neurocytoma
- An intraventricular tumour predominantly of young adults.
- Although designated WHO grade II, the primary treat-ment is usually with surgery alone.
- Radiation (and even chemotherapy) can be helpful in tumours appearing particularly aggressive on histology or that relapse following surgery.
- Choroid plexus tumours.
- Surgery is the mainstay of treatment for choroid plexus papillomas (CPP) and choroid plexus carcinoma (CPC).
- Complete resection usually achieves cure in CPP. Incompletely removed tumours should be re-operated or observed.

- Craniospinal radiotherapy can have a role in the man-agement of CPC.

Pineocytoma/pineoblastoma
- Form a spectrum of tumours arising from the pineal parenchyma.
- Pathology and behaviour varies from the benign pineocytoma (WHO grade I) to the highly malignant pineoblastoma (WHO grade IV).
- Low-grade tumours are treated with surgery alone.
- High-grade tumours are treated as medulloblastoma.

Germ cell tumours
- A tissue diagnosis may not be necessary if the tumour markers (AFP, hCG) are raised and the history and imaging are indicative.
- Non-secreting germinomas can be managed with whole brain radiotherapy and a ventricular boost or chemotherapy plus ventricular irradiation.
- Secreting germinomas and all teratomas require com-bined (germ cell) chemotherapy and radiotherapy, often to the entire neuraxis.
- Residual masses after treatment are often benign and may be surveilled.

Craniopharyngioma
- Primary treatment is with surgical excision.
- Postoperative radiotherapy should be considered if ex-cision is incomplete.

Chordoma
- Chordomas arise mainly in the region of the clivus al-though they can be found at other midline sites.
- Surgical excision is the first treatment of choice but complete excision is rarely possible.
- Patients should be considered for high-dose localized radiotherapy delivered with protons.
- In situations where it is not possible to deliver protons (metal work), intensity-modulated and image-guided radiotherapy can be used.

4.9 Brain metastases overview

Introduction
- Brain metastasis is an extremely common complication of malignancy occurring in around 25% of all systemic cancers. Metastases are approximately four times as common as primary brain tumours.
- The incidence of brain metastases is increasing because of improved systemic control of those cancers which typically spread to the brain and the increased use of MRI of the brain for staging purposes.
- In adults, the commonest sources of brain metastases are lung cancer, malignant melanoma, and renal and breast cancers.
- The great majority of patients who develop brain me-tastases are considered 'incurable'. However, some with solitary/oligometastases may achieve extended survival following appropriate management.
- Metastases from some rare tumours (particularly germ cell) may form exceptions to the general rule in that

they have a better prognosis even with apparently ad-vanced disease.

Single or solitary?
- Strictly, the term 'single brain metastasis' refers to one isolated lesion within the brain without regard to systemic disease. The term 'solitary brain metas-tasis' describes a single brain lesion that is the only known metastatic site in the body. These terms are often erroneously used interchangeably, even in peer reviewed literature.
- Between 20% and 50% of brain metastases are single at first presentation. Some cancers are more likely to produce single metastases (e.g. breast cancer).
- The term 'oligometastasis' is used to describe a solitary metastasis, or a small number of metastases, that may be amenable to aggressive treatment.

Incidence

- The approximate percentage of patients developing brain metastases over the duration of their disease is:
  - Small cell lung cancer (overall) 30–50%
  - Small cell lung cancer (without prophylaxis) 50–80%
  - Non-small cell lung cancer 33%
  - Breast cancer 18–30%
  - Renal cancer 5–10%
  - Melanoma 10–60%
- The prevalence at postmortem examination in patients dying from their cancer may be more than double that found clinically.
- It is observed that women with HER2-positive breast cancer have a high incidence of brain metastases. This may be related to both a predisposition in these patients and the failure of Herceptin® to pass the BBB.

Presentation

- 80% of brain metastases will be diagnosed later than the primary cancer (metachronous); the remaining 20% are synchronous or precede the primary diagnosis.
- Headache is the most common symptom, especially in patients with multiple brain metastases or posterior fossa lesions.
- 10–20% of patients will have focal or generalized seizures.
- Other symptoms and signs include focal weakness, gait ataxia, speech disturbance, mental change, sensory disturbance, visual impairment, and papilloedema.
- 5–10% may present with an acute neurological syndrome caused by haemorrhage into a metastasis or cerebral infarction due to embolic or compressive occlusion of a vessel. Haemorrhage into a metastasis is particularly common from melanoma.
- A high index of suspicion is required in any patient with a known 'metastasizing' cancer and a change in their neurological symptoms.

Clinicopathology

Metastasis to the brain is the result of haematogenous spread, mostly via the arterial circulation, but also via the vertebral venous system—Batson's plexus.

In the cerebrum, metastases are most commonly found at the junction between the cortex and the white matter where the decreased size of blood vessels acts as a trap for tumour emboli.

They are also common at terminal watershed areas of arterial circulation.

- 80% occur in the cerebral hemispheres
- 15% in the cerebellum
- 5% in the brainstem

Histopathology

Where a metastasis has been resected or biopsied, detailed histopathology is required either to confirm the site of origin, if the primary is known, or to help establish the site if it is not.

- Routine light microscopy will establish malignancy and usually allow classification into a broad histological type.
- Positive immunostaining may identify subgroups of tumour, e.g.:
  - Carcinoma: cytokeratin, EMA (breast cancer: ER, PR, CK-7; lung cancer: CK-7, TTF-1; colon cancer: CK-20)

- Melanoma: HMB-45, s-100, vimentin, NSE
- Germ cell tumour: hCG, AFP
- Lymphoma: CLA
- Sarcoma: vimentin
- Further molecular genetic analysis on the brain metastasis can also add information with regard to diagnosis and potential systemic treatment.

Natural history

- The natural history for patients with untreated symptomatic cerebral metastases is extremely poor. The median survival is four to eight weeks.
- Death is due to progressive loss of neurological function or raised intracranial pressure.
- Treatment with optimal dose steroids relieves symptoms by reducing peritumoural oedema but has little cytotoxic effect. Steroids improve median survival only to eight to 12 weeks.
- The great majority of patients with brain metastases will die an early neurological death, hence the focus of disease management and symptom control centres on the management of the brain metastases even in the presence of systemic disease.

Evaluation of the patient with brain metastasis

The management and outcome of the patient with metastatic disease to the brain is critically dependent on a number of prognostic and predictive factors. Careful evaluation is mandatory in every case.

Brain imaging

- Brain metastases usually show as discrete iso- or hyperdense lesions on CT, or T1 bright lesions on MRI. They arise typically in the junction of grey and white matter of the brain and enhance strongly following the injection of contrast. They may have necrotic regions and are frequently multiple.
- Where a management decision depends on the confirmation of brain metastasis MRI should be structural (T2 weighted, FLAIR, DWI series, and T1 pre and post contrast).
- Double dose contrast, multiplanar imaging, and fine slice thickness can all enhance diagnostic accuracy.
- Gadolinium-enhanced MRI is the appropriate investigation for the detection of meningeal spread.
- Other pathological processes (abscess, inflammation, primary tumour) may mimic metastasis in the patient with known malignancy. Biopsy/surgical resection may be necessary in some cases.

Clinical evaluation

- The outcome in patients treated for brain metastases is strongly dependent on their clinical condition and PS.
- A careful clinical evaluation (history and examination) is required to establish:
  - the presence or absence of active systemic malignancy
  - the PS (e.g. WHO, Karnofsky performance score KPS).

Laboratory and imaging investigations

If a patient is being considered for aggressive treatment to their brain metastasis then a vigorous search for active systemic disease should be made which may include:

- CT chest, abdomen, and pelvis.

- Bone marrow (full blood count, possible aspirate/ trephine).
- Bone (bone profile, isotope bone scan, MRI).
- Tumour markers where appropriate (CEA, CA-125, AFP, hCG).

Diagnostic evaluation for brain metastasis from unknown primary

Brain metastasis from an unknown primary is diagnosed when a metastatic lesion is discovered and after adequate investigation no primary site can be identified. A biopsy/ surgical resection and full pathological examination of the presenting lesion is required in all cases. The pathology may give a clue as to the site of origin and direct further investigation. A thorough work-up (as listed) is required either before or after the biopsy has been done and evaluated.

All cases
- Thorough clinical history.
- Physical examination (may include skin, rectum, breasts, testes, and the oral cavity and nose).

- Full blood count, routine biochemistry.
- CT chest abdomen and pelvis.

Selected cases
- Tumour markers—CEA, CA-125, AFP, hCG.
- Unknown primary—consider PET-CT.
- More detailed radiographic or invasive tests should be restricted to those with organ specific complaints, radiographic abnormalities, or as directed from the pathology. These might include investigation of the:
  - Gastrointestinal tract (contrast studies, endoscopy)
  - Abdomen and pelvis (ultrasound and biopsy of specific organs)
  - Chest (bronchoscopy)
  - Head and neck (head imaging, endoscopy)
  - Bone (nuclear medicine scans)
  - Lymph nodes (biopsy, fine needle aspirate)
  - Skin (biopsy)

4.10 Treatment options for brain metastases

Initial management of the patient with brain metastases

- The great majority of patients with brain metastases will be symptomatic at the time of diagnosis.
- The commonest symptoms are headache, seizure, and neurological dysfunction.
- The mainstay of early management is the administration of steroids, usually dexamethasone.
- The rules for management of steroids are the same as for patients with primary brain tumours (see 'Steroids', p. 75).
- Whilst steroids will frequently reverse many of the symptoms, improvement is often incomplete and short lived. Other specific treatments (anticonvulsants, antiemetics, analgesics) should be administered as required.

Factors to consider in the management of the patients with brain metastases

- The PS of the patient
- The age
- The primary tumour site, type, and molecular profile
- The number and volume of metastases
- The location of metastases
- Extracranial disease
- Leptomeningeal disease
- Resection cavity size
- Patient preference

There are several assessment and prognosis indices that may be used: RTOG RPA, GPA, and DS-GPA.

Systemic treatment

Consider systemic anticancer therapy for people who have brain metastases likely to respond effectively, e.g. germ cell tumours or small cell lung cancer and lung and melanoma metastases where there is an immunotherapy treatment option.

Whole brain radiotherapy (WBRT)

- WBRT for cerebral metastases is established as a treatment for patients with multiple brain metastases.
- Patients with multiple metastases from non-small-cell lung cancer who have a KPS of <70 should not be offered WBRT.
- WBRT does not improve survival for patients with multiple brain metastases but does improve neurological progression so the pros and cons of treatment vs. symptomatic care should be discussed.
- WBRT is normally delivered on a linear accelerator with appropriate immobilization using a pair of unmodified parallel opposed fields.
- Planning is usually by a CT-simulator. Dose prescription is either to midplane or to the isocentre.
- A series of randomized studies in the 1980s established a dose of 30Gy in ten daily fractions as the 'international standard'.
- In poorer prognosis patients (RTOG RPA 2, 3) a dose of 20Gy in five daily fractions appears to produce similar survival and quality-of-life benefits.
- Steroid cover is usually given for patients receiving WBRT. Dexamethasone in doses of 4–16mg is prescribed depending on symptoms. This should be reduced to optimal levels after the radiation is complete.
- Acute side effects of WBRT include transient worsening of neurological symptoms, nausea, vomiting, headache, fever, and hair loss. These will normally resolve or are abrogated by an increase in steroid dose.
- Late effects from the radiation develop 12 months or more after irradiation, and therefore long-term effects have not been an issue numerically because of short survival. However, >10% of patients who survive for >12 months may develop symptoms such as cognitive loss, ataxia, and urinary incontinence.

Neurosurgery

Neurosurgery can be used in patients with multiple brain metastasis to establish a diagnosis (where necessary) or for the relief of symptoms due to pressure or obstruction. Neurosurgery may be particularly useful to relieve symptoms due to disease in the posterior fossa especially if there is obstruction. In these conditions radiotherapy alone may worsen pressure problems.

Radiosurgery

Radiosurgery may be used in patients with multiple brain metastases but there is little evidence that it prolongs survival.

Best supportive care

Some patients in poor clinical condition who have brain metastases should not have them actively treated. The majority of patients who are treated will deteriorate with progressive intracranial disease, often within months. The need for supportive care cannot be overemphasized. Early involvement of the palliative care services, home support, and in social care is vital in order to manage the resulting progressive disability and deteriorating symptoms.

Management of the patient with oligometastasis

Patients with a single brain metastasis have a better prognosis than those with multiple metastases provided other factors are similar. There is evidence that treating the index lesion with either surgery or radiation improves outcome.

Role of surgery

- Surgery should be considered for patients with a single brain metastasis in an accessible location. Multiple studies have shown improved survival when a single brain metastasis was excised before WBRT compared with treatment with WBRT alone.
- Patients showing most benefit were younger (age <65 years) with a KPS score of at least 70, and no evidence of extracranial progression over the previous three months.
- In addition surgery may provide immediate relief of symptoms due to pressure of mass effect or from obstructive hydrocephalus.
- Surgery delivers tissue for pathological assessment.
- The major disadvantages of surgery are the need for an inpatient stay and limitation to accessible intracranial sites. Some patients may have concomitant clinical conditions which may preclude surgery.
- Surgical resection for more than one metastasis has been advocated by some but there are no studies to convincingly demonstrate a survival benefit.
- There is evidence that WBRT following extirpation of a single brain metastasis reduces both intracranial relapse and neurological death in the irradiated patients. A meta-analysis of randomized controlled trials evaluating SRS with or without WBRT for patients with one to four metastases confirmed that the initial omission of WBRT did not impact on distant brain relapse. However, there is no evidence that overall survival is improved so MRI surveillance can be recommended as a primary management post-surgical resection.

- Recent studies have shown improvement in local control with adjuvant stereotactic radiosurgery/radiotherapy to the surgical cavities for people with one to three brain metastases that have been resected.

Role of radiosurgery

- Radiosurgery is the delivery of a single high dose of radiation to a precisely localized target (metastasis) with the view of tissue sterilization. Single doses depend on tumour size and location.
- This is normally delivered using stereotactic localizing techniques (SRS).
- The outcome following treatment for a single metastasis is similar to that following neurosurgery.
- Use of either linear accelerator based systems, gamma knife, or cyberknife yield equal results.
- Consider stereotactic radiosurgery/radiotherapy for people with brain metastases who have:
  - controlled or controllable extracranial disease, and
  - KPS of 70 or more, the number and total volume of metastases can be adequately treated, controlled or controllable extracranial disease

There have been a number of clinical trials assessing local therapy for one to three or four metastases but no randomized clinical studies for greater than four metastases. From the available data patients with two to three metastases have a better outcome than when the number is greater than three. Clinical series have shown a survival advantage for treating metastases that have an overall volume of less than 2cm^3.

Advantages of SRS compared to neurosurgery

- SRS can be delivered to 'brain eloquent' and surgically inaccessible sites.
- SRS does not require inpatient stay.
- SRS allows the simultaneous treatment of multiple metastases in different brain regions and multiple sequential treatments for metachronous metastases.
- No surgical recovery.

Disadvantages compared to microsurgery

- Only metastases with a volume smaller than about 2cm^3 can be treated effectively.
- Pressure symptoms are not relieved and may even be exacerbated by the radiation.
- Particular caution is needed in patients with cerebellar metastases.
- SRS does not provide a tissue diagnosis.
- The strongest evidence for the value of SRS is a large randomized study which compared WBRT with or without SRS in patients with 1–3 metastases. Patients receiving SRS had a significantly longer median survival (6.5 months vs. 4.5 months) and improved PS (43% vs. 27%). However, subgroup analysis showed that the survival advantage was confined to patients with a single metastasis.

Prophylactic cranial irradiation

- Some cancers have a very high rate of intracranial metastasis during their clinical course in spite of systemic treatment. Small-cell lung cancer has a 50–80% cumulative risk of intracranial relapse at two years.

- It has been common practice to offer prophylactic ir-radiation to the brain (prophylactic cranial irradiation (PCI)) to try to prevent their occurrence.
- Meta-analysis data show an overall survival advantage with a relative risk of death of 0.82–0.84, and a re-duction in rate of brain metastases (relative risk 0.46–0.48) when PCI is given.
- The benefits of PCI appear limited to patients achieving a complete response following induction chemotherapy.
- PCI may be associated with later cognitive impairment and it is recommended that dose fractions of 3Gy or less are used. A typical regimen is 25–30Gy in ten fractions.

Management of special cases of brain metastases

- Special management is required for CNS involvement in highly chemosensitive malignancies which offer the prospect of cure even in the case of advanced disease (e.g. germ cell tumours, haematological malignancy).
- Initial treatment will often be with chemotherapy (and sometimes surgery) with subsequent radiation treat-ment for consolidation in some cases.

- High-dose protocols with bone marrow/stem cell rescue have been explored in this situation.

Management of brain metastases after neurosurgery

- Up to 50% of brain metastases will recur locally after a neurosurgical resection.
- Stereotactic radiosurgery to the surgical cavity in the postoperative setting has been shown to reduce this local recurrence rate.

Re-irradiation

- Virtually all patients irradiated for multiple brain me-tastases will relapse intracranially if they survive long enough.
- There is evidence that patients who have bene-fited from WBRT for at least four months may also benefit from re-irradiation. The initial dose used in these studies was usually 30Gy in ten fractions. The retreatment doses were 20–30Gy, usually given in ten fractions.
- The studies reported little evidence of toxicity.

4.11 Outcome and summary for brain metastases

Outcome

Multiple metastases

- In general, patients with multiple metastases from most common cancers have very poor survival prospects even after treatment.

Solitary metastases

- Patients with single brain metastases who are treated aggressively with either surgery or radiotherapy have the longest survival.
- The addition of WBRT does not appear to improve survival though it does reduce intracranial relapse and neurological death.

Summary of management

Patients with multiple brain metastases and unknown primary

- These patients require appropriate staging and evaluation.
- If a tissue diagnosis is not obtained in this process then a biopsy from the brain metastasis is required.
- Once a full diagnosis and staging is established, the pa-tient is treated as having a 'known primary'.

Patients with multiple brain metastases and known primary

- Should undergo systemic staging and general medical work-up appropriate to the overall clinical picture.

Single/oligo brain metastases

- All patients with a single or small volume metastasis who are of good PS (KPS >70) should have a high-quality gadolinium enhanced MRI to confirm the diagnosis.
- All patients should have appropriate staging.
- Patients without systemic disease (or controllable dis-ease) and with good prognosis should be considered for aggressive treatment to the index lesions (surgery or SRS).
- These patients should then be followed up with serial MRI imaging follow-up.
- Postoperative SRS can be considered post neurosur-gical excision.
- Patients with KPS <70 should be considered for WBRT or best supportive care.

Patients with further intracranial relapse following treatment

- If relapse has occurred soon after initial treatment, best supportive care only may be appropriate.
- If there has been benefit from the initial treatment and a period of months or more has elapsed, retreatment with SRS or WBRT may be justified.
- SRS may be performed for new oligometastases ap-pearing after initial treatment with either SRS, surgery, or WBRT provided the patient's condition merits it.

4.12 Spinal cord tumours overview

Introduction

Primary spinal cord tumours account for 2–4% of all primary CNS tumours. They occur within or adjacent to the spinal cord, i.e. they are intra-axial in location. Metastatic lesions can also occur, particularly from lung and breast primaries.

Tumour sites

- Intramedullary tumours arise within the spinal cord. The majority are glial tumours, either ependymomas or astrocytomas. Oligodendrogliomas occur but are rare. Metastases also occur.
- Intradural extramedullary tumours arise within the dura, but outside the spinal cord itself. These are typically meningiomas or nerve sheath tumours.
- Extradural tumours are usually metastatic or primary tumours of bone and cartilage. They most often arise in or adjacent to the vertebral bodies. They are not the subject of this chapter.

Clinicopathology

A similar spectrum of tumours to those in the brain arise in the spine, although the frequency of occurrence is markedly different and some types are absent. The great majority are low grade. High-grade tumours do occur but are rare.

- Gender prevalence is roughly equal though meningiomas are more common in females and ependymomas in males.
- Incidence is greatest in young and middle-aged adults and less common at the extremes of the age spectrum. Astrocytomas occur earlier in life than ependymomas.

Low-grade tumours

Astrocytomas

- Spinal astrocytomas are rare (brain:spine ratio 10:1).
- They arise most commonly in the cervical and cervicothoracic parts of the cord.
- Histologically they divide broadly into pilocytic (WHO grade I) and non-pilocytic (fibrillary, WHO grade II) types, though mixed forms occur.

Ependymomas

- Ependymomas account for >60% of spinal gliomas.
- They are not encapsulated tumours but they are usually well circumscribed and tend not to invade adjacent cord.
- They may occur anywhere along the spinal cord but 50% arise in the conus or filum terminale. They may be intra- or extramedullary. There are two main types:
  - Myxopapillary variant (WHO grade I) has a predilection for the distal spine. It is characterized by perivascular and intracellular mucin. It is slow growing and does not transform to a more malignant phenotype.
  - Cellular variant (WHO grade II) resembles its cerebral counterpart and arises usually in the proximal spine.

Haemangioblastoma

Haemangioblastomas are rare intramedullary tumours that are well circumscribed but not encapsulated. A quarter of patients will have von Hippel–Lindau (VHL) syndrome.

Meningioma (WHO grade I)

- Spinal meningiomas occur mainly in women, the majority in the thoracic spine.
- Most meningiomas are entirely intradural, though a few may be all or partly extradural.
- They tend to be found near the nerve root without involving it directly, hence they often present with myelopathy without radiculopathy.
- They are usually solitary though multiple meningiomas can occur, particularly in association with neurofibromatosis (NF).
- Most spinal meningiomas occur in the thoracic region. Lumbar tumours are rare.

Peripheral nerve sheath tumour (WHO grade I)

- These are categorized as either schwannoma or neurofibroma and constitute 25% of intradural tumours. Schwannomas are the more common and occur maximally in the fourth to sixth decades.
- They more commonly affect the dorsal root and may extend through the dural root sleeve to form a 'dumbbell tumour'.
- Histologically neurofibromas comprise an abundance of fibrous tissue and there is a conspicuous presence of nerve fibres in the stroma. There is fusiform enlargement of the involved nerve and it can be very difficult to separate normal and neoplastic tissue.
- Schwannomas produce masses of elongated cells with dark fusiform nuclei which do not produce enlargement of the nerve but tend to hang from it.

Other low-grade lesions

- There is a plethora of additional uncommon benign tumours which include dermoids, epidermoids, lipomas, teratomas, and neurenteric cysts that are managed with surgery and have excellent outcomes.

High-grade tumours

- WHO grades III and IV astrocytomas account for about 10% of intramedullary astrocytomas. Histologically they appear similar to their brain counterparts. Their clinical course is rapid and CSF dissemination is common.
- Anaplastic ependymomas are rarely found in the spinal cord. When they are they have the usual anaplastic features of necrosis, mitosis, vascular proliferation, cellular pleomorphism, and overlapping of nuclei.
- A very small minority (2.5%) of nerve sheath tumours are or become malignant.

Genetic associations

- As in brain disease, NF1 and NF2 are associated with an increased incidence of cord tumours.

NF1 is particularly (but not exclusively) associated with astrocytoma and NF2 with ependymoma and meningioma.
- In VHL syndrome there is an excess of spinal haemangioblastoma.

Presentation
Tumours of the spine cause symptoms through disruption of normal neural elements and pathways, producing both local and distant effects.
- Pain is the commonest presenting symptom. It usually occurs at the level of the lesion, in the spine itself, or in the appropriate root distribution (radicular pain). It typically causes nocturnal wakening.
- The pain may be exacerbated by straining or coughing.
- Functional loss is caused by direct pressure from the tumour itself and associated oedema. Deficit may also occur through spinal infarction and through invasion into spinal tissue and growth along nerve roots.
- Functional loss is at and below the level of the lesion. For tumours of the thoracic or cervical spine, typical sequelae are spasticity, muscle weakness, loss of balance, sensory loss (pain, light touch, vibration), and difficulties with ambulation. Difficulties with bowel and bladder function may be reported due to loss of sphincter control.
- Tumours of the conus/filum region typically present with low back pain, lower motor neuron leg weakness, and sphincter disturbance.
- A Brown–Séquard syndrome, reflecting effective hemisection of the spinal cord, may occur particularly with slow growing nerve sheath tumours.

Examination
- A full neurological examination is required with particular attention to the extent and distribution of any neurological or muscular abnormalities found.
- A general examination is also needed. Since the majority of tumours in or near the spine are metastatic, a thorough assessment for evidence of other malignant disease is necessary.
- Assessment of ambulatory status must be done as this has prognostic significance.
- In general, expect upper motor neuron signs below the level of the spinal lesion with a combination of upper and lower motor neuron signs at the level of any tumour.
- Presentations can be complex and do not necessarily conform to expectation.
- In the adult, the spinal cord segmental level is approximately two above the bony vertebral level.
- The cord ends in the conus at the level of L1–2. Lesions below this level can only produce lower motor neuron signs.

- Clinical localization of the upper vertebral limit of the symptoms and signs (sensory level) is notoriously difficult and can be unreliable. If done with care, it can be a useful guide to identifying the position of the tumour within the spine. However, it should always be confirmed with imaging.

Differential diagnosis
The symptoms caused by a spinal tumour may be mimicked by a wide variety of conditions. A list of differential diagnoses following clinical examination might include multiple sclerosis, syringomyelia, transverse myelitis, amyotrophic lateral sclerosis, spinal bony disease, Guillain–Barré syndrome, syphilis, nutritional deficiencies, malignant meningitis, ruptured disc, and others.

Investigation
The investigation of spinal cord tumours is almost entirely confined to imaging.

MRI
MRI is the imaging modality of choice in investigating spinal disease, including tumours. T1 (with and without gadolinium enhancement) and T2 sequences are needed in transverse and sagittal presentation.

It is possible to evaluate the internal structure of the cord including oedema, atrophy, haemorrhage, infarct, cyst, and syringomyelia.
- Intramedullary tumours will nearly always show as expansions of the cord and many enhance in spite of low grade. Individual features may help differentiate different tumour types.
- Astrocytomas are hypo- or isointense on T1 and hyperintense in T2. They may be centrally or eccentrically located. They are infiltrative and have an indistinct margin. They tend to enhance more strongly than ependymomas (particularly the pilocytic subtype). High protein cyst inclusions are frequent.
- Ependymomas tend to enhance intensely on MRI, and occur centrally within the cord, expanding it symmetrically as they grow. The spinal cord may be expanded along several segments, and a tumour-associated cyst (i.e. syrinx) is commonly seen.
- Meningiomas tend to be isointense on both T1 and T2 but enhance avidly with gadolinium.
- Nerve sheath tumours and haemangioblastomas are isointense on T1 and hyperintense on T2 imaging. Both enhance avidly on Gd-T1 MRI.

CT scan
CT scan is reserved primarily for patients in whom MRI is contraindicated. The investigation of CT with myelography is then performed. Information from CT on intramedullary tumours is indirect and relies mainly on evidence of architectural change or flow obstruction.

4.13 Management of spinal cord tumours

Management
General management
Spinal cord tumours often present insidiously. At presentation patients may have a combination of pain and disability that needs immediate attention. Appropriate analgesia should be offered. As well as the usual drugs used in neuro-oncology, gabapentin and other nerve stabilizing anticonvulsants may be helpful for neurogenic pain. Steroids may benefit both pain and neurological deficit but their side effects make them inappropriate for long-term use. Early institution of rehabilitation (physiotherapy and functional aids) can help prevent further deterioration and improve the patient's quality of life. As soon as possible definitive treatment should be considered.

Surgery
- Surgery is by far the most important modality in the management of spinal tumours. Although in some cases some may argue for a watch and wait policy until symptoms demand action, this can be dangerous as it might render a previously operable tumour inoperable or allow a deficit to develop that cannot be reversed. In general, therefore, early surgery is advocated if it can be performed safely.
- Most spinal surgery, particularly if intramedullary, is performed through a posterior laminectomy with a midline durotomy. More ventrally positioned lesions (e.g. meningiomas) may need a posterolateral approach. When complete resection of an intramedullary tumour, particularly ependymoma, is considered the myelotomy should extend over the entire rostrocaudal extent of the tumour.
- Unless the intention is simply to obtain a biopsy, a maximal safe removal is usually the intention. This is always undertaken using the operating microscope and often tools such as intraoperative ultrasound and the cavitating ultrasonic aspirator (CUSA).
- In many benign and low-grade tumours it is possible to find a plane of cleavage. For meningiomas it is often necessary to complete the operation with electrocautery of the involved dural base.
- Surgery is covered by the use of corticosteroids to reduce spinal oedema.
- Somatosensory or motor-evoked potential during surgery can be used to evaluate intraoperative spinal function.
- If there has been extensive bony removal a spinal arthrodesis may be necessary.
- Immediately following surgery, neurological deterioration from the preoperative baseline is common. This usually improves back to baseline or better in the following weeks with sensory improvement usually occurring before motor improvement.
- Early specialized rehabilitation following surgery will improve outcome. Antithrombotic prophylaxis should be undertaken. Care must be taken to recognize and manage orthostatic hypotension which can occur following upper thoracic/cervical spinal surgery. Enthusiastic physio- and occupational therapy is helpful in optimizing rehabilitation.

Radiotherapy
- Radiotherapy is usually given with 'radical' intent.
- Patients often require stabilization in a mouldable immobilization device. Stereotactic localization can improve accuracy.
- Patients are scanned with CT in the treatment position. The tumour and planning outlines are constructed from these images and knowledge of the tumour and its pattern of spread.
- Planning usually involves intensity-modulated radiotherapy. It is important to take into account normal organs that might be exposed to radiation from the exit beams.
- For treatments to low-grade tumours, doses of 45–50Gy in 1.8Gy fractions are usual but for highly malignant tumours, doses up to 56Gy may be appropriate. Whilst the risk to the spinal cord from the radiation is increased at these doses, it may be less than previously thought. This risk must be balanced against the risk of under-treating the tumour and the consequences of early regrowth.

Chemotherapy
Chemotherapy has little established role in spinal cord tumours. The same agents used for brain tumours can be tried but responses are few and short-lived.

Management strategies
Low-grade astrocytoma
- Surgery is the initial management of choice with the intention to effect as complete a removal as possible without causing neurological deficit.
- This may be difficult, particularly in the diffuse (fibrillary) tumours as there is not usually a clear plane of cleavage.
- Patients with some degree of deficit may still benefit from surgery but those with complete transection of cord function or who have extensive tumours are not suitable for surgery.
- WHO grade I (pilocytic) tumours: surgery is the treatment of choice. Radiotherapy is not needed whether resection is complete or incomplete.
- WHO grade II tumours: for completely excised lesions radiotherapy can be withheld. For incompletely excised tumours postoperative radiotherapy should be considered.

Ependymoma
- Surgery is the initial treatment of choice. This is often more successful than for astrocytomas because of the presence of a recognizable plane of cleavage. Most patients are cured following gross total resection.
- Myxopapillary ependymoma: for the myxopapillary variant even when excision is subtotal, remission may be prolonged and there is no indication for further treatment (with irradiation).
- Grade II (or III) ependymomas: optimal management consists of gross total resection. Although these are infiltrative tumours, a total or near-total resection can often be achieved. The value of postoperative radiotherapy is controversial though the balance is in favour of offering it only if a total resection has not been achieved. Typical doses are 45–50Gy in 1.8Gy fractions.

Meningioma

- The essential treatment is complete surgical removal.
- Radiotherapy has a limited role but might be considered for patients with more malignant phenotypes (atypical, anaplastic) particularly if resection has been incomplete.
- Patients with multiple meningiomas should be investigated for NF.
- Although the great majority of meningiomas are benign, recurrence rates are relatively high, particularly for en plaque lesions. Regular follow-up with interval imaging is recommended.

Haemangioblastoma

- Patients with spinal haemangioblastoma should be investigated for VHL.
- For sporadic haemangioblastoma and for a first lesion in a patient with VHL, early removal is recommended for both diagnostic and therapeutic purposes.
- For patients with multiple lesions (usually VHL) it is reasonable to observe asymptomatic patients and operate once symptoms occur. If surgery is not indicated or otherwise not possible, radiotherapy can produce symptomatic improvement, particularly for small lesions. Stereotactic localization has been used in some units.

Nerve sheath tumours

The aim of treatment is complete surgical excision which is achievable in the majority of patients.

Other benign tumours

Other benign tumours are managed either by watchful waiting or surgery.

High-grade tumours

- The value of surgery, beyond biopsy, in patients with high-grade glial tumours is not established.
- Radiotherapy can be offered. This usually comprises localized high-dose treatment to the tumour and a generous margin.
- Chemotherapy may be worth considering in rare patients whose tumours carry a majority oligodendroglial component.

Prognostic factors

- Histological type: low-grade tumours, particularly WHO grade I, have a significantly better prognosis than grade II tumours. Ependymomas, grade for grade, have a better prognosis than astrocytomas. High-grade tumours (WHO grade III and IV) have a very poor prognosis.
- Age: youth is associated with better outcomes but this may be due to variations in the distribution of tumour types in different age groups.
- Functional status: there is an association between outcome and functional status before surgery (usually indicated by mobility). Functional deficits present preoperatively are often not reversible.
- Size: tumour size is an important factor, probably because it is associated with operability and functional status. Also, tumour location can dictate the ease with which a surgeon can remove a tumour. Anterior tumours are more difficult to remove.
- Extent of resection: there is clear evidence that if a complete removal of a tumour can be achieved the outcome is much improved.

4.14 Outcome in spinal tumours

Outcome in spinal tumours

Astrocytoma

- Overall, the five-year survival figures for patients with spinal astrocytomas are reported as 50–90%. However, the outcome depends critically on the histology. In a large series treated with surgery alone, patients with grade I tumours had a five-year survival of >90% whilst for those with grade II tumours it was <60% and all the patients with high-grade tumours were dead. Treatment failure is predominantly through local relapse.
- Irrespective of radiotherapy, patients with complete resection and patients with grade I (pilocytic) tumours with or without complete resection have excellent control prospects.

Ependymoma

Spinal ependymomas are associated with a better prognosis than cerebral lesions, particularly when complete resection is possible. In a large series, the ten-year progression-free survival rate for patients with myxopapillary spinal ependymomas was 61.2%. The ten-year overall survival was 92.4%. Recurrence was less likely in patients who had complete surgical resection or postoperative radiotherapy. Recurrence rates are higher for more cellular ependymoma and may occur many years after initial surgery.

Haemangioblastoma

Ninety per cent of patients are either clinically stable or improved after removal of a solitary haemangioblastoma.

Meningioma

- Surgical removal of a spinal meningioma is associated with clinical improvement in >50% of cases. Outcome is worse in patients with en plaque tumours, those in an anterior location and those which are entirely extradural. Older patients do less well.
- The overall recurrence rate is around 10% but rises to 40% for en plaque lesions.

Nerve sheath tumours

Although the majority of patients operated on for nerve sheath tumours will be cured, recurrence rates of 20% are reported. This is especially common in patients with NF2-associated tumours.

Recurrence

- Many patients with truly benign tumours who have done well after surgery can be discharged after a year of follow-up. Patients with meningiomas and those whose tumours were not completely removed should be followed longer.

- Patients with spinal astrocytomas and incompletely excised ependymomas require long-term follow-up.
- Recurrence in all these tumours can occur after many years.
- If a tumour recurs and remains low grade, surgery should again be considered although reoperation is often more difficult than initial surgery.
- Radiotherapy can be considered for some conditions if second surgery is not possible but the value in most cases is not clearly proven. There is a stronger case for radiotherapy following partial removal of a recurrence, particularly in astrocytoma, ependymoma, and meningioma.
- The value of chemotherapy in recurrent disease is very limited. For high-grade lesions, response can sometimes be obtained with nitrosoureas or platinum-based regimens. However, if it occurs, it is generally short-lived.
- Radiotherapy can be considered for patients following surgery for an early recurrence of meningioma.

Late sequelae of treatment
Surgery
- The spinal cord may be damaged during the operation itself, either directly or by interruption of the blood supply. This can lead to neurological deficit. Some contusive injury and peripheral nerve damage is expected in many operations but recovery of function over months is common. With good technique serious damage to the cord is rare.

- Following surgery, adhesions, gliosis, and fibrosis can develop, sometimes leading to pain and functional deficit.

Radiation
- Late radiation damage in the cord may be sudden or insidious in onset with sensory and motor abnormalities (paraplegia or quadriplegia), bowel and bladder sphincter disturbance, and diaphragm dysfunction in high lesions.
- The most serious consequence is complete transection of the cord at the irradiated level.
- The pathology—a combination of vascular lesions with demyelination and malacia—is characteristic of radiation myelopathy. The pathogenesis is obscure with both the vasculature and oligodendrocytes identified as principal targets.
- Imaging may aid diagnosis. MRI performed within eight months of the onset of symptoms shows low signal intensity on the T1-weighted image and high signal intensity on T2-weighted images often with cord swelling. Gadolinium enhancement is common. Late scans show an atrophic cord with normal signal intensity.
- Accepted wisdom has been that spinal cord tolerance at conventional fractionation is 45–50Gy, depending on the clinical situation.
- A dose of 57–60Gy carries a 5% risk of myelitis. There is evidence that re-irradiation of CNS tissue is possible. Some tolerance develops with increasing time from the initial radiation and is virtually complete (50–70%) by two years. However, full tolerance is never regained.
- Some chemotherapeutic drugs can enhance radiation damage in CNS tissue. These include methotrexate, cytosine arabinoside, and the nitrosoureas.

4.15 Further reading and internet resources

Further reading
Ajaz M, Jefferies S, Brazil L, Watts C, Chalmers A. Current and investigational drug strategies for glioblastoma. *Clin Oncol* 2014; 26(7):419–30.

Andrews DW, Scott CB, Sperduto PW, et al. Whole brain radiation therapy with or without stereotactic radiosurgery boost for patients with one to three brain metastases: phase III results of the RTOG 9508 randomised trial. *Lancet* 2004; 363(9422):1665–72.

Baschnagel AM, Meyer KD, Chen PY, et al. Tumor volume as a predictor of survival and local control in patients with brain metastases treated with gamma knife surgery. *J Neurosurg* 2013; 119(5):1139–44.

Bentzen SM, Constine LS, Deasy JO, Eisbruch A, Jackson A, Marks LB, Ten Haken RK, Yorke ED. Quantitative analyses of normal tissue effects in the clinic (QUANTEC): an introduction to the scientific issues. *Int J Radiat Oncol Biol Phys* 2010; 76(3) (Suppl.):S3–9.

Brennan C, Yang TJ, Hilden P, et al. A phase 2 trial of stereotactic radiosurgery boost after surgical resection for brain metastases. *Int J Radiat Oncol Biol Phys* 2014; 88(1):130–6.

Brown PD, Ballman KV, Jaeckle K, et al. Effect of radiosurgery alone vs radiosurgery with whole brain radiation therapy on cognitive function in patients with 1 to 3 brain metastases: a randomized clinical trial. *JAMA* 2016; 316(4):401–09. [Published correction appears in *JAMA* 2018 Aug 7; 320(5):510.]

Brown PD, Ballman KV, Cerhan JH, et al. Postoperative stereotactic radiosurgery compared with whole brain radiotherapy for resected metastatic brain disease (NCCTG N107C/CEC•3): a multicentre, randomised, controlled, phase 3 trial. *Lancet Oncol* 2017; 18(8):1049–60.

Gaspar L, Scott C, Rotman M, et al. Recursive partitioning analysis (RPA) of prognostic factors in three Radiation Therapy Oncology Group (RTOG) brain metastases trials. *Int J Radiat Oncol Biol Phys* 1997; 37(4):745–51.

Hoang-Xuan K, Bessell E, Bromberg J, Hottinger AF, Preusser M, Ruda R, Schlegel U, Siegal T, Soussain C, Abacioglu U, et al. Diagnosis and treatment of primary CNS lymphoma in immunocompetent patients: guidelines from the European Association for Neuro-Oncology. *Lancet Oncol* 2015; 16(7):e322–32.

Jefferies SJ, Harris FP, Price SJ, Collins VP, Watts C. High grade glioma—the arrival of the molecular diagnostic era for patients over the age of 65 years in the UK. *Clin Oncol* 2013; 25(7):391–3.

Louis DN, Perry A, Reifenberger G, von Deimling A, Figarella-Branger D, Cavenee WK, Ohgaki H, Wiestler OD, Kleihues P, Ellison DW. The 2016 World Health Organization classification of tumors of the central nervous system: A summary. *Acta Neuropathol* 2016; 131(6):803–20.

Mahajan A, Ahmed S, McAleer MF, et al. Post-operative stereotactic radiosurgery versus observation for completely resected brain metastases: a single-centre, randomised, controlled, phase 3 trial. [Published correction appears] *Lancet Oncol* 2017; 18(8):e433.

Mulvenna P, Nankivell M, Barton R, et al. Dexamethasone and supportive care with or without whole brain radiotherapy in treating patients with non-small cell lung cancer with brain metastases unsuitable for resection or stereotactic radiotherapy (QUARTZ): results from a phase 3, non-inferiority, randomised trial. *Lancet* 2016; 388(10055):2004–14.

Perry JR, Laperriere N, O'Callaghan CJ, et al. Short-course radiation plus temozolomide in elderly patients with glioblastoma. *N Engl J Med* 2017; 376(11):1027–37.

Sperduto PW, Berkey B, Gaspar LE, Mehta M, Curran W. A new prognostic index and comparison to three other indices for patients with brain metastases: an analysis of 1,960 patients in the RTOG database. *Int J Radiat Oncol Biol Phys* 2008; 70(2):510–14.

Sperduto PW, Yang TJ, Beal K, et al. Estimating Survival in Patients With Lung Cancer and Brain Metastases: An Update of the Graded Prognostic Assessment for Lung Cancer Using Molecular Markers (Lung-molGPA). *JAMA Oncol* 2017; 3(6):827–31.

Stupp R, Mason WP, van den Bent MJ, Weller M, Fisher B, Taphoorn MJ, Belanger K, Brandes AA, Marosi C, Bogdahn U, et al. Radiotherapy plus concomitant and adjuvant temozolomide for glioblastoma. *N Engl J Med* 2005; 352(10):987–96.

van den Bent MJ, Afra D, de Witte O, Ben Hassel M, Schraub S, Hoang-Xuan K, Malmstrom PO, Collette L, Pierart M, Mirimanoff R, et al. Long-term efficacy of early versus delayed radiotherapy for low-grade astrocytoma and oligodendroglioma in adults: the EORTC 22845 randomised trial. *Lancet* 2005; 366(9490):985–90.

van den Bent MJ, Baumert B, Erridge SC, et al. Interim results from the CATNON trial (EORTC study 26053–22054) of treatment with concurrent and adjuvant temozolomide for 1p/19q non-co-deleted anaplastic glioma: a phase 3, randomised, open-label intergroup study. *Lancet* 2017; 390(10103):1645–53.

van den Bent MJ, Brandes AA, Taphoorn MJ, Kros JM, Kouwenhoven MC, Delattre JY, Bernsen HJ, Frenay M, Tijssen CC, Grisold W, et al. Adjuvant procarbazine, lomustine, and vincristine chemotherapy in newly diagnosed anaplastic oligodendroglioma: Long-term follow-up of EORTC brain tumor group study 26951. *J Clin Oncol* 2013; 31(3):344–50.

Weber DC, Wang Y, Miller R, Villa S, Zaucha R, Pica A, Poortmans P, Anacak Y, Ozygit G, Baumert B, et al. Long-term outcome of patients with spinal myxopapillary ependymoma: treatment results from the MD Anderson Cancer Center and institutions from the Rare Cancer Network. *Neuro-oncol* 2015; 17(4):588–95.

Internet resources

National Cancer Research Institute: http://www.ncri.org.uk

National Institute of Health and Clinical Excellence (NICE): https://www.nice.org.uk

NICE Guidelines: https://www.nice.org.uk/guidance/published?type=apg,csg,cg,cov,mpg,ph,sg,sc

Chapter 5

Thoracic tumours

Chapter contents

5.1 Primary tracheal tumours

Introduction

Primary tracheal tumours represent <1% of all respiratory malignancies and can arise from the respiratory epithelium, salivary glands, and mesenchymal structures of the trachea. Most tumours in adults are benign while this is the case in only 30% of tumours in children. Primary tumours in adults are most commonly squamous cell carcinoma followed by adenoid cystic carcinoma.

Squamous cell carcinoma (SCC) is linked to cigarette smoking and more than a third of patients will have either mediastinal or pulmonary metastases at diagnosis. Metachronous or synchronous lesions are common. Up to 40% of tracheal tumours can develop before, concurrently, or after carcinoma of the oropharynx, larynx, or lung. In contrast, adenoid cystic carcinomas (ACC) are not associated with cigarette smoking, tend to spread along both submucosal and perineural planes, and only 10% of patients have regional lymph node or remote metastases at presentation. ACC also progresses slowly, often over several years, which is characteristic even of untreated cases.

Symptoms

Tracheal tumours present with symptoms and signs of upper-airway obstruction, cough, and haemoptysis, or symptoms arising from direct invasion and involvement of continuous structures such as the recurrent laryngeal nerve. Patients with ACCs are more likely to present with long-standing symptoms of wheezing or stridor for months before a definitive diagnosis is made.

Treatment

Evaluation in a specialist centre by a multidisciplinary team (MDT) is of particular importance for these uncommon tumours. Resection should be considered, as a complete surgical resection ensures the best local control and greatest likelihood of cure in almost all patients with tumours of intermediate aggressiveness or/and malignant tumours. Absolute contraindications to surgery that have been cited in the literature include the presence of multiple lymph node metastases, involvement of >50% of tracheal length in adults and 30% in children, mediastinal invasion of unresectable organs, and distant metastases in SCC.

The primary treatment of a non-resectable or node-positive SCC is concurrent chemoradiotherapy with a cisplatin-based regimen and the maximum tolerated dose of radiotherapy. Data are sparse in terms of the optimal radiotherapy dose. For gross residual tumour, >60Gy in 2Gy per fraction is recommended, aiming to give 70Gy if feasible. For postoperative residual disease, 60Gy in 30 fractions is used. Chemotherapy is cisplatin based though there are no prospective studies.

The primary management of tracheal ACC is surgical resection, and patients treated with resection have a 53% five-year overall survival (OS). The role of postoperative radiotherapy is unclear although it is often administered if the operation failed to achieve a clear resection margins in the trachea. In unresectable ACC, radiotherapy (either alone or after debulking) is reported to achieve an OS of 11–30%. There are limited data suggesting that concurrent chemoradiotherapy may achieve good short-term responses. The majority of patients treated without surgery develop local recurrences.

Further reading

Choi EK. A 10-year clinical outcome of radiotherapy as an adjuvant or definitive treatment for primary tracheal adenoid cystic carcinoma. *Radiat Oncol* 2017 4; 12(1):196.

Je HU, Song SY, Kim DK, Kim YH, Jeong SY, Back GM, Choi W, Kim SS, Park SI, Levy A, Omeiri A, Fadel E, Le Péchoux C. Radiotherapy for tracheal-bronchial cystic adenoid carcinomas. *Clin Oncol (R Coll Radiol)* 2018; 30(1):39–46.

Mattioli G, Sarnacki S, Torre M, et al. Tracheal and bronchial tumors. *J Thorac Dis* 2016; 8(12):3781–6.

Sherani K, Vakil A, Dodhia C, Fein A. Malignant tracheal tumors: a review of current diagnostic and management strategies. *Curr Opin Pulm Med* 2015; 21(4):322–6.

5.2 Lung cancer overview

Demographics

Lung cancer is the most common cause of death from cancer worldwide. It is estimated that nearly one in five deaths are due to lung cancer (1.59 million deaths, 19.4% of the total). In the USA and the UK, it is the second commonest cancer in both men and women (not counting skin cancer). It accounts for approximately 13% of all new cancers. The American Cancer Society estimates that 228,150 new cases will be diagnosed in the USA in 2019, and 142,670 deaths will be due to lung cancer. The incidence across countries varies widely.

Aetiology

Smoking is the most important aetiological factor and the risk of dying of lung cancer is <1% in people who have never smoked. Of all smokers, 16% will die from lung cancer by the age of 75, if they do not die earlier from other smoking-related disease. Other forms of tobacco smoke such as second-hand smoke exposure and pipe smoking are also associated with a significant risk of developing lung cancer. Other risk factors are environmental and occupational exposure to asbestos, radon, and wood-burning smoke. Some inflammatory diseases such as pulmonary fibrosis and chronic obstructive pulmonary disease have also been associated with an increase in the incidence of lung cancer.

Smoking cessation

Prevention is the most effective strategy for reducing the burden of lung cancer. The promotion of smoking cessation is essential if lung cancer mortality is to be reduced. Evidence from the UK has shown that legislation prohibiting smoking in enclosed public areas has resulted in a significant reduction in second hand smoke exposure among children, and an increase in the proportion of smokers quitting or trying to quit.

Smoking cessation is also beneficial in patients diagnosed with lung cancer. The National Institute for Health and Clinical Excellence (NICE) lung cancer clinical guidelines recommend patients should be advised to stop smoking as soon as the diagnosis of lung cancer is suspected. This reduces the risk of comorbid disease such as ischaemic heart disease and stroke, and more importantly reduces the risk of developing a second smoking-related malignancy. As continuation of smoking is associated with poorer survival, patients who have undergone a curative treatment should be strongly encouraged to stop smoking and offered pharmacotherapeutic and behavioural therapy. Retrospective evidence suggests morbidity and mortality is reduced in patients who stop smoking prior to surgery for lung cancer. There is also evidence to suggest that smoking cessation is beneficial for patients with advanced disease undergoing treatment.

Smoking cessation remains a formidable challenge for many patients, and American College of Chest Physicians' guidelines recommend offering intensive tobacco cessation programmes, including counselling, behavioural therapy, the use of sustained-release bupropion and nicotine replacement, and telephone follow-up, all of which have been shown to increase successful abstinence significantly.

On a population basis, efforts to decrease smoking work remarkably well, and achieving a major decrease in tobacco deaths in the first half of the 21st century does require many current smokers to stop. In contrast, a big decrease over the next decade or two in the number who start smoking in the population as a whole will only produce a big decrease in deaths around the middle and the second half of the present century.

Screening

There is currently no national lung cancer screening programme in the UK. In the USA, the National Lung Screening Trial (NLST) compared low-dose helical computed tomography (CT) with chest X-ray (CXR) in patients with a 30-pack-year history of smoking. The study showed that participants screened with helical CT scans had a 15–20% lower-risk of death from lung cancer than those screened with CXR. In Europe, there are several ongoing trials of low-dose CT versus no screening in patients at increased risk of lung cancer. One of these is the NELSON trial, which has completed accrual.

Following publication of the NLST trial results, several organizations within the USA have recommended lung cancer screening with low-dose CT, including the National Comprehensive Cancer Network and the American College of Chest Physicians.

Further reading

Barrera R, et al. 2005 Smoking and timing of cessation—impact on pulmonary complications after thoracotomy. *Chest* 2005; 127:1977–83.

Doll R, Peto R, Boreham J, et al. Mortality in relation to smoking: 50 years' observations on male British doctors. *BMJ* 2004; 328:1519–28.

National Lung Screening Trial Research Team: Aberle DR, Adams AM, Berg CD, et al. Reduced lung-cancer mortality with low-dose computed tomographic screening. *N Engl J Med* 2011 Aug 4; 365(5):395–409.

Internet resources

American Cancer Society, Key Statistics for Lung Cancer—available at: http://www.cancer.org/cancer/lungcancer-non-smallcell/detailedguide/non-small-cell-lung-cancer-key-statistics

National Institute of Health and Clinical Excellence (NICE), The diagnosis and treatment of lung cancer (update) April 2011—available at https://www.nice.org.uk/guidance/cg121/evidence/full-guideline-181636957

5.3 Diagnosis and staging of lung cancer

Presentation

The presenting features of lung cancer are often non-specific, and difficult to distinguish from other pulmonary comorbid diseases. Initial assessment should include taking a full clinical history and physical examination. A particular note should be taken of the patient's performance status.

NICE recommend performing an urgent CXR in patients presenting with haemoptysis or persistent (more than three weeks) symptoms of cough, chest/shoulder pain, dyspnoea, weight loss, hoarseness, or signs such as finger clubbing or cervical lymphadenopathy. Other symptoms may relate to sites of metastases, with the commonest sites being the lung, liver, adrenals, bone, and brain.

Simple blood investigations including haemoglobin, bone profile, and liver function tests may suggest the presence of distant metastases.

If initial assessment with CXR (or CT) is suggestive of lung cancer, or there is high clinical suspicion, patients should be offered an urgent referral to a member of a lung cancer MDT, usually a respiratory physician.

Diagnosis and staging

Investigations should be aimed at obtaining histological diagnosis and accurate staging of the disease, which will provide prognostic information and guide decisions on appropriate treatment. Staging is essential for determining the extent of disease. All staging should be according to the International Union against Cancer (UICC) TNM 8 system (Table 5.3.1). The TNM staging system categorizes tumours on the basis of the primary tumour (T), regional nodal status (N), and the presence or absence of metastatic disease (M). The overall tumour stage is established by combining T, N, and M grades (Table 5.3.1). Staging investigations should be performed in a logical fashion in order to minimize unnecessary, expensive, or invasive tests. NICE recommend choosing the investigations that give the most information about diagnosis and staging with least risk to the patient.

Patients should have a CT scan of the thorax and abdomen, which should include the liver and adrenal glands. Intravenous contrast should be used unless contraindicated. A CT scan can provide good anatomical detail, allowing evaluation of the T stage of disease and suitability for resection or radical radiotherapy. Nodal and metastatic disease may also be assessed using CT, but this should not be the sole investigation for N and M staging in patients who are potentially suitable for radical treatment. A short-axis nodal diameter of 10mm or greater is considered suspicious of nodal disease, and a contrast-enhanced CT scan can accurately detect such nodes.

Table 5.3.1 UICC TNM staging (2016) for lung cancer

Primary tumour (T)	
T1	Tumour ≤3cm diameter, surrounded by lung or visceral pleura, without invasion more proximal than lobar bronchus
T1a	Tumour ≤1cm in diameter
T1b	Tumour >1cm but ≤2cm in diameter
T1c	Tumour >2cm but ≤3cm in diameter
T2	Tumour >3cm but ≤5cm, or tumour with any of the following features:
	Involves main bronchus but is not within 2cms of the carina
	Invades visceral pleura
	Associated with atelectasis or obstructive pneumonitis
T2a	Tumour >3cm but ≤4cm
T2b	Tumour >4cm but ≤5cm
T3	Tumour >5cm but ≤5cm or any of the following:
	Directly invades any of the following: chest wall, diaphragm, phrenic nerve, mediastinal pleura, parietal pericardium
	Separate tumour nodules in the same lobe
T4	Tumour of >7cm or any size that invades the mediastinum, heart, great vessels, trachea, recurrent laryngeal nerve, oesophagus, vertebral body, carina, or with separate tumour nodules in a different ipsilateral lobe
Regional lymph nodes (N)	
N0	No regional lymph node metastases
N1	Metastasis in ipsilateral peribronchial and/or ipsilateral hilar lymph nodes and intrapulmonary nodes, including involvement by direct extension
N2	Metastasis in ipsilateral mediastinal and/or subcarinal lymph node(s)
N3	Metastasis in contralateral mediastinal, contralateral hilar, ipsilateral or contralateral scalene, or supraclavicular lymph node(s)
Distant metastasis (M)	
M0	No distant metastasis
M1	Distant metastasis
M1a	Separate tumour nodule(s) in a contralateral lobe; tumour with pleural or pericardial nodules or malignant pleural or pericardial effusion
M1b	Single extrathoracic metastasis in a single organ
M1c	Multiple extrathoracic metastasis in a single or multiple organs

In a patient with widespread metastatic disease, extensive staging is inappropriate, and investigation should be aimed at establishing a pathological diagnosis using the least invasive technique. Appropriate procedures depend on the pattern of disease, but may include ultrasound-guided pleural fluid aspiration, or fine needle aspiration (FNA) of a palpable lymph node. For patients with advanced disease, tissue samples should be sent for genetic analysis to look for the presence of driver mutations (epidermal growth factor receptor (EGFR), anaplastic lymphoma kinase (ALK)) that may influence treatment options.

If there is clinical suspicion of small cell lung cancer (SCLC), then the diagnostic approach should be aimed at establishing a tissue diagnosis as quickly and minimally invasively as possible.

Further staging investigations

A CT- or ultrasound-guided transthoracic needle biopsy may provide histological confirmation in patients with a peripheral primary tumour. In patients where a central tumour is identified, fibreoptic bronchoscopy can be carried out to obtain samples for diagnostic confirmation. The use of real-time endobronchial ultrasound (EBUS) may guide the location of paratracheal and peribronchial lung lesions, increasing the yield of transbronchial needle aspiration (TBNA).

If a curative approach to treatment is being considered, a fluorodeoxyglucose positron emission tomography (FDG-PET) CT scan should be carried out. This provides additional staging information, especially regarding potential nodal involvement and can identify sites of metastatic disease not seen with standard radiological imaging.

In patients who do not have metastatic disease, accurate staging of nodal disease is essential for determining treatment strategy. In patients with peripheral primary tumours, CT and PET-CT may provide confirmation of N0 disease. However, in the presence of radiological evidence of nodal disease, or where there is uncertainty (for example, equivocal FDG uptake on PET), further evaluation with invasive investigations is necessary. EBUS-guided TBNA, endoscopic ultrasound (EUS) guided FNA, or non-ultrasound guided TBNA are possible means of evaluating mediastinal lymphadenopathy. In patients with a high probability of mediastinal lymph node involvement (mediastinal lymph nodes >20mm maximum short axis diameter on CT), a neck ultrasound with sampling of visible lymph nodes should be offered prior to more invasive sampling of the mediastinal nodes.

A magnetic resonance imaging (MRI) (or CT) scan of the brain may identify metastatic disease and should be considered in patients with stage II and III disease who may be eligible for treatment with radical intent. Further staging investigations are directed by clinical presentation. For example, a bone scan may be considered if bone metastases are suspected.

In patients with early stage disease, pathological confirmation may not be possible before definitive treatment. A pre-surgical histological diagnosis is recommended. However, if this is not possible, if the opinion of a lung cancer MDT is that there is a high likelihood of malignancy, this may be sufficient to proceed with a radical approach. Similarly, in patients who are being considered for treatment with stereotactic ablative radiotherapy (SABR), the European Society for Medical Oncology (ESMO) and American College of Clinical Pharmacy (ACCP) guidelines recommend that an attempt should be made at obtaining a pathological diagnosis before treatment. If tissue sampling is considered too high risk, SABR may proceed if there is a high radiological index of suspicion of primary lung malignancy.

Further reading

Rivera MP, Mehta AC, Wahidi MM. *Establishing the Diagnosis of Lung Cancer; Diagnosis and Management of Lung Cancer*, 3rd edn. American College of Chest Physicians Evidence-Based Clinical Practice Guidelines. Also available in *CHEST*® 2013 143(Suppl. 5):e142S–65S.

Vansteenkiste J, Crinò L, Dooms C, et al. 2nd ESMO consensus conference on lung cancer: early-stage non-small-cell lung cancer consensus on diagnosis, treatment and follow-up. *Ann Oncol* 2014; 25:1462–74.

Internet resources

NICE, The diagnosis and treatment of lung cancer (update) April 2011—available at https://www.nice.org.uk/guidance/cg121/evidence/full-guideline-181636957

5.4 Pathology of lung cancer

Introduction

An accurate histological diagnosis of lung cancer subtype is essential in order to formulate a treatment plan and it is no longer sufficient to simply classify cancers as non-small cell lung cancer (NSCLC) or small cell lung cancer (SCLC). Subtypes of NSCLC may differ in their response to chemotherapeutic agents and molecular targeted agents. Consequently, pathology is playing a greater role in determining local and systemic therapy.

The World Health Organization (WHO) classification system is based on morphological features and molecular biology. This broadly divides lung tumours into NSCLC (squamous cell carcinoma, adenocarcinoma, large cell carcinoma, adenosquamous carcinoma, sarcomatoid carcinoma, salivary gland tumours) and neuroendocrine tumours (SCLC, carcinoid).

To address recent advances in molecular biology, pathology, and treatment, a multidisciplinary expert panel published a revision of the classification of lung adenocarcinoma in 2011. Box 5.4.1 outlines the pathological subgroups as defined by WHO 2004 and incorporates the 2011 multidisciplinary reclassification.

Non-small cell lung cancer (NSCLC)

NSCLC includes SCC, adenocarcinoma, and large cell carcinoma (LCC), and broadly any epithelial tumour that lacks a small cell component. SCC typically presents as a central mass but approximately 25% are located peripherally. In the past, this was the predominant histological subtype of lung cancer. More recently however, adenocarcinoma has become more common in many countries, and the incidence in Europe has increased in the last three decades.

The 2004 WHO classification of adenocarcinoma consisted of five subtypes, namely acinar, papillary, bronchioloalveolar carcinoma (BAC), adenocarcinoma with mixed subtypes, and solid carcinoma with mucus formation. In the 2011 reclassification, the terms BAC and mixed subtype adenocarcinoma are no longer used. In addition, new concepts have been introduced such as adenocarcinoma in situ (AIS) and minimally invasive adenocarcinoma (MIA). These are small solitary adenocarcinomas with either pure lepidic growth (AIS) or predominant lepidic growth with <5mm invasion (MIA), tumours that following resection are associated with 100% or near 100% disease-specific survival, respectively. AIS and MIA are usually non-mucinous.

Invasive adenocarcinomas are classified by predominant pattern. Sub-classifications are: lepidic, acinar, papillary, micropapillary, and solid patterns.

LCC accounts for less than 10% of all lung cancers and is defined as an undifferentiated non-SCC that lacks cytological features of SCC and glandular or squamous differentiation. It is a diagnosis of exclusion—tumour cells lack microscopic characteristics that would classify the neoplasm into one of the other lung cancer subtypes. It is differentiated from SCLC by the larger cell size, and a higher cytoplasmic-to-nuclear ratio.

Variants that fall outside the main subtypes are also listed in Box 5.4.1.

Immunohistochemistry

Immunohistochemistry (IHC) can help define subtypes of NSCLC and is also used to differentiate primary lung tumours from secondary metastases. Patterns of positive staining seen in the subgroups are:

- Adenocarcinoma: thyroid transcription factor (TTF-1), mucin, napsin-A, surf-A, surf-B.
- Squamous cell carcinoma: p63, cytokeratin 5/6 (CK5/6), and CK 7.
- Adenosquamous or large cell carcinoma: may have IHC staining patterns of both adenocarcinoma and squamous cell carcinoma.

Negative IHC can help differentiate NSCLC from secondary lung metastases. Examples of these are oestrogen and progesterone receptors (typically positive in

Box 5.4.1 Histological classification of lung cancer

Squamous cell carcinoma
- Papillary
- Clear cell
- Small cell
- Basaloid

Adenocarcinoma
- Preinvasive lesions
  - Atypical adenomatous hyperplasia
  - Adenocarcinoma in situ (≤3cm, formerly BAC)
    - Non-mucinous
    - Mucinous
    - Mixed mucinous/non-mucinous
- Minimally invasive adenocarcinoma (≤3cm lepidic predominant tumour with ≤5mm invasion)
  - Non-mucinous
  - Mucinous
  - Mixed mucinous/non-mucinous
- Invasive adenocarcinoma
  - Lepidic predominant (formerly nonmucinous BAC pattern, with >5mm invasion)
  - Acinar predominant
  - Papillary predominant
  - Micropapillary predominant
  - Solid predominant with mucin production
- Variants of invasive adenocarcinoma
  - Invasive mucinous adenocarcinoma (formerly mucinous BAC)
  - Colloid
  - Fetal (low and high grade)
  - Enteric

Large cell carcinoma
- Large cell neuroendocrine carcinoma
- Combined large cell neuroendocrine carcinoma
- Basaloid carcinoma
- Lymphoepithelioma-like carcinoma
- Clear cell carcinoma
- Large cell carcinoma with rhabdoid phenotype

Adenosquamous carcinoma
Sarcomatoid carcinoma
- Pleomorphic carcinoma
- Spindle cell carcinoma
- Giant cell carcinoma
- Carcinosarcoma
- Pulmonary blastoma

Salivary gland tumours
- Mucoepidermoid carcinoma
- Adenoid cystic carcinoma
- Epithelial-myoepithelial carcinoma

Carcinoid tumour
- Typical carcinoid
- Atypical carcinoid

Small cell carcinoma
- Combined small cell carcinoma

Source: data from Travis WD, et al. International Association for the Study of Lung Cancer/American Thoracic Society/European Respiratory Society international multidisciplinary classification of lung adenocarcinoma. *J Thoracic Oncol* 2011; 6(2): 244–85. 2011, Elsevier Inc.; Travis WD, et al. *Pathology and Genetics of Tumours of the Lung, Pleura, Thymus and Heart*. Lyon: IARC Press, 2004.

adenocarcinoma of the breast) and CK20 (typically positive in adenocarcinoma of the colon).

Targetable driver mutations

In patients with advanced-stage disease, classification of NSCLC by mutation subtype is important for selection of appropriate treatment. Adenocarcinoma or NSCLC not otherwise specified should be tested for EGFR mutations and ALK translocations. The incidence of these mutations varies by sex, ethnicity, and smoking status. The incidence of either mutation in squamous carcinoma is extremely low. However, tumour heterogeneity and potentially subtype misclassification means that testing of other NSCLC subgroups may be considered.

PD-L1

The programmed death receptor 1 (PD-1) protein is a cell-surface receptor on certain lymphocytes that, with its ligand programmed death ligand 1 (PD-L1), helps to downregulate immune responses. Many lung cancers express PD-L1 and evade immune recognition via the PD-1/PD-L1 interaction. Immunotherapy agents targeting the PD-1/PD-L1 pathway are effective in treating lung cancer. PD-L1 immunohistochemistry testing should be considered as standard in helping to select patients for treatment.

Neuroendocrine tumours

Pulmonary neuroendocrine tumours (NETs) of the lung are a distinctive subset that share morphological, immunohistochemical, and ultrastructural features. They comprise a spectrum from the premalignant diffuse idiopathic pulmonary neuroendocrine cell hyperplasia (DIPNECH) through to high-grade small cell carcinoma (Box 5.4.2). Neuroendocrine tumours account for 20–5% of primary thoracic malignancies, the most common of which is small cell carcinoma. Chromogranin, CD56, and synaptophysin are the most helpful neuroendocrine immunohistochemical markers.

Diffuse idiopathic pulmonary neuroendocrine cell hyperplasia

DIPNECH refers to a rare but increasingly diagnosed phenomenon. It is diagnosed in patients found to have widespread peripheral airway neuroendocrine cell hyperplasia and/or multiple tumourlets (cell proliferations that measure <0.5cm in greatest diameter). It is thought to represent a pre-invasive lesion for carcinoid tumours.

Carcinoid tumours

Carcinoid tumours comprise the low grade typical carcinoid (TC) and intermediate grade atypical carcinoid (AC); these represent approximately 1–2% of invasive lung malignancies. They present in the lung periphery in 40% of cases. Endobronchial growth is common in central carcinoids. Tumours are usually round and average 2–3cm in size.

TC is defined as a neuroendocrine tumour with <2 mitoses per $2mm^2$ and lacking necrosis, while AC is defined as a neuroendocrine tumour with either 2–10 mitoses per $2 mm^2$ or necrosis. Most AC will meet both criteria, but occasional AC will have necrosis and <2 mitoses per $2mm^2$. A low proliferation rate (<5%) is seen in TC by Ki67 staining compared with AC where it is usually between 5% and 20%.

Box 5.4.2 Classification of neuroendocrine (NE) tumours

I. Tumours with NE morphology
  A. Typical carcinoid (≥0.5cm)
  B. Atypical carcinoid
  C. Large cell neuroendocrine carcinoma
     Combined large cell neuroendocrine carcinoma
  D. Small cell carcinoma
     Combined small cell carcinoma

II. Non-small-cell carcinomas with NE differentiation

III. Other tumours with NE properties
  A. Pulmonary blastoma
  B. Primitive neuroectodermal tumour
  C. Desmoplastic round cell tumour
  D. Carcinomas with rhabdoid phenotype
  E. Paraganglioma

Adapted with permission from Travis WD. Advances in neuroendocrine lung tumors. *Ann Oncol* 2010; 21 (Suppl 7):vii65–vii71. Copyright © 2010. doi: 10.1093/annonc/mdq380.

Large cell neuroendocrine carcinoma

Large cell neuroendocrine carcinoma (LCNEC) is defined as a NET with a high mitotic rate (>11 per $2mm^2$), and the cytological features of a NSCLC, with associated necrosis. Evidence of neuroendocrine differentiation must be demonstrated by ancillary methods such as immunohistochemistry using a specific marker such as chromogranin or synaptophysin.

Small cell lung cancer

The diagnosis of SCLC is primarily based on characteristic light microscopy appearances. Cells are typically round to fusiform, have scant cytoplasm, are small in size (usually less than the diameter of three small resting lymphocytes) and commonly are associated with necrosis that is often extensive. Nuclei have finely granular chromatin; nucleoli are inconspicuous or absent. The mitotic rate is high, averaging 60–80 per $2mm^2$; however, mitoses may be difficult to identify in small biopsy specimens. The most important stain is good-quality haematoxylin and eosin. The optimal panel of immunohistochemical stains includes a pancytokeratin antibody such as AE1/AE3, CD56, chromogranin and synaptophysin, TTF-1, and Ki67. TTF-1 is positive in 70–80% of SCLCs. Ki67 is helpful in differentiating SCLC from carcinoids as the proliferation is very high (80–100%).

Further reading

Travis WD. Advances in neuroendocrine lung tumors. Symposium article. *Ann Oncol* 2010; 21(Suppl. 7):vii65–vii71.

Travis WD, Brambilla E, Noguchi M, et al. International Association for the Study of Lung Cancer/American Thoracic Society/European Respiratory Society International multidisciplinary classification of lung adenocarcinoma. *J Thoracic Oncol* 2011; 6:244–85.

Travis WD, Muller-Hermelink H-K, Harris CC, et al. *Pathology and Genetics of Tumours of the Lung, Pleura, Thymus and Heart.* Lyon: IARC Press, 2004.

5.5 Treatment of stage I and II non-small cell lung cancer

Background

According to National Cancer Intelligence Network figures, in 2013 in England, 13% of patients were diagnosed with stage I disease and 7% with stage II disease.

Stage I disease is subdivided into stage Ia and Ib. The five-year survival of patients with stage Ia disease is 58–73% and in stage Ib disease the five-year survival is between 43% and 58%. Stage II is also divided into IIa and IIb disease; the five-year survival figures are 36–46% and 25–36% respectively.

Management

A wait-and-see policy is inappropriate for early stage (stage I or II) disease as the five-year OS in untreated stage I NSCLC is 6–14%, and the median survival ranges from 9 to 14 months. It is therefore recommended that surgical resection or other ablative therapies should not be delayed for even small lung tumours.

Surgical resection should be the preferred modality of treatment for fit patients with early stage disease. The role of surgery has not been validated in randomized trials, but historical data from case series support this modality as the standard of care. Patients with early stage disease who are not candidates for or who refuse surgery may be candidates for definitive local radiotherapy. Radiofrequency ablation and cryotherapy are alternatives to radiotherapy but are beyond the scope of this chapter.

Operable early stage disease

Lobectomy is considered the optimal surgical procedure for early stage NSCLC, as local control rates are good and lung function is preserved.

A sublobar resection may involve the removal of one or more anatomical segments (segmentectomy), or a non-anatomical wedge resection. These options may be considered in patients with poor lung function or extensive comorbid disease unable to tolerate lobectomy.

It is likely that local recurrence rates and possibly survival are better with the less extensive sublobar or wedge resection. In the Lung Cancer Study Group trial 801, patients with early stage lung cancer randomized to lobectomy had a trend towards higher survival rates and a significantly lower rate of local recurrence than those randomized to wedge or sublobar resection (1.9% vs. 5.4%).

Video-assisted thoracoscopic surgery (VATS) is a minimally invasive alternative to open thoracotomy for patients undergoing lobectomy that has been reported to decrease surgical morbidity. VATS may allow selected patients with significant medical comorbidities to undergo the more definitive lobectomy procedure rather than a sublobar resection.

The optimal extent of lymph node resection during surgery is uncertain. A meta-analysis concluded that systematic mediastinal nodal dissection was associated with a moderate improvement in survival compared with nodal sampling alone. The European Society of Thoracic Surgeons guidelines recommend systematic lymph node dissection in all cases to ensure complete resection, although it might be that the improved survival seen with systematic mediastinal nodal dissection is as a result of more accurate disease staging.

Inoperable early stage disease

For patients not suitable for or unwilling to undergo surgery, radiotherapy (RT), using either SABR or a more conventional fractionation, is an alternative treatment option. SABR delivers a single or very limited number of high-dose fractions to a small treatment volume with a very high level of accuracy. Prospective phase 2 studies with SABR in patients with small, peripheral, biopsy-proven NSCLC suggest that the local control is approximately 90%. Five-year survival in patients treated with SABR is less impressive than in surgical series, but that may reflect patient selection. Generally, SABR is only suitable for smaller peripheral lung cancers. The UK SABR Consortium Guidelines are a useful guide on selecting appropriate cases for SABR treatment.

For patients with inoperable early stage primary tumours that are not suitable for SABR, definitive standard-fractionation radiation therapy is an appropriate option, although local control rates are at best modest (in the region of 30–40%). There are no data to support the use of concurrent chemotherapy and RT in patients with early stage NSCLC.

Other approaches

Heavy particle radiotherapy with proton beam and carbon ion therapy has been used in patients with stage I NSCLC.

There are inadequate long-term data with radiofrequency ablation (RFA), cryoablation, and microwave ablation in early stage disease and none of these yet have an established role in the routine management of early stage NSCLC.

Adjuvant chemotherapy

Adjuvant platinum-based chemotherapy is recommended for patients with stage II NSCLC following potentially curative surgery.

Adjuvant chemotherapy may also have a role in the treatment of some patients with stage Ib disease and high-risk features (such as lymphovascular invasion) but is not indicated for patients with resected stage Ia disease.

Adjuvant radiotherapy

Generally, postoperative RT (PORT) is not recommended. A meta-analysis showed that PORT was detrimental to patients with early stage completely resected NSCLC and should not be used in the routine treatment of such patients. This analysis included trials that used outdated RT techniques, and the excess deaths in the RT patients may have been due to treatment-related cardiorespiratory toxicity. In patients with positive surgical margins, PORT using modern radiotherapy techniques may be considered to reduce the risk of local recurrence.

Further reading

Haasbeek CJ, Senan S, Smit EF, et al. Critical review of nonsurgical treatment options for stage I non-small cell lung cancer. *Oncologist* 2008; 13:309–19.

Lardinois D, De Leyn P, Van Schil P, et al. ESTS guidelines for intraoperative lymph node staging in non-small cell lung cancer. *Eur J Cardiothorac Surg* 2006; 30:787.

National Cancer Intelligence Network. *Stage Breakdown by CCG 2013*. London: NCIN, 2015.

PORT Meta-analysis Trialists Group. Postoperative radiotherapy for non-small cell lung cancer. *Cochrane Database Syst Rev* 2000; (2):CD002142.

Vansteenkiste J, Crinò L, Dooms C, et al. 2nd ESMO consensus conference on lung cancer: early-stage non-small-cell lung cancer consensus on diagnosis, treatment and follow-up. *Ann Oncol* 2014; 25:1462–74.

Internet resources

Cancer Research UK, Lung Cancer Survival: http://www.cancerresearchuk.org/about-cancer/type/lung-cancer/treatment/statistics-and-outlook-for-lung-cancer

Stereotactic Ablative Body Radiation Therapy (SABR): A Resource, Version 4.0, January 2013—available at https://www.sabr.org.uk/

5.6 Treatment of stage III non-small cell lung cancer

Background

Overall, 19% of newly diagnosed patients with NSCLC will present with stage III disease. Stage III is subdivided into IIIa and IIIb, which have quite different prognoses.

According to Cancer Research UK figures, between 19% and 24% of patients with stage IIIa disease will survive for five years or more after they are diagnosed. For stage IIIb disease, the figure is between 7% and 9%.

Stage III NSCLC represents a heterogeneous group of patients, ranging from those with locally destructive (T3/T4) heavily node positive (N2/N3) inoperable disease, to those with small primary tumours and postoperative microscopic N1/N2 disease. Despite this heterogeneity, the majority of patients with stage III NSCLC will die of metastatic disease. It has been established that improved local control is associated with better outcomes. These two observations have led to a myriad of multimodality treatment schedules being developed, involving a combination of surgery and radiotherapy to effect local control and chemotherapy to control metastatic disease and act as a possible radiosensitiser. There are a bewildering number of combinations of these three modalities published in the literature, and as a consequence this means the optimal treatment of patients with stage III NSCLC remains controversial. In the absence of an established 'gold standard' treatment, randomized trials are diverse in design and often contain unproven treatment schedules in all arms.

Generally, key factors influencing the treatment regimen include the extent of the primary tumour and nodal disease, the ability to achieve a complete surgical resection, and the patient's overall fitness and preferences. Given the range of clinical presentations and complexity of management, the expertise of the MDT managing the patient is probably of more importance to the overall outcome of the patient than the exact multimodality schedule.

Preoperative stage I/II, postoperative stage III

For postoperative patients with microscopic mediastinal lymph node involvement that was not identified preoperatively, cisplatin-based adjuvant chemotherapy should be considered, as this has been shown to increase survival in prospective randomized trials.

The PORT meta-analysis did not demonstrate any clear advantage or detriment for PORT in patients with completely resected N2 disease. In patients with microscopic N2 disease postoperatively, there is no evidence to support the use of PORT.

Potentially operable disease

The role of surgery in stage III NSCLC has yet to be fully established. Surgery for stage III disease often demands technically challenging operations, potentially involving resection of the trachea, superior vena cava, vertebra, and pericardium, and it is essential that any operation is carried out by an experienced thoracic surgeon working as part of a thoracic oncology MDT. Optimal surgical management should aim for complete resection and preserve as much non-involved parenchyma as possible. Complete resection should include systematic mediastinal nodal dissection.

Patients who have undergone primary surgical resection for single station N2 nodal involvement have a better prognosis than patients with multilevel N2 disease, and for this reason surgery is often advocated for this group of patients. The difficulty is that single station N2 is only accurately identifiable postoperatively, which makes rational preoperative patient selection difficult.

Induction chemotherapy/chemoradiotherapy

Although both induction chemotherapy and induction chemoradiotherapy are used in potentially operable stage III NSCLC, there is very little prospective randomized evidence to support either approach. There is one trial of definitive concurrent chemoradiotherapy versus induction concurrent chemoradiotherapy followed by surgery in patients with stage IIIa (N2) disease. Patients had to have potentially resectable disease at randomization. No difference in OS was seen; the received wisdom is that both treatment strategies tested in the trial are reasonable options.

Adjuvant chemotherapy

The standard of care for fit patients with completely resected stage III N2 disease is adjuvant cisplatin-based chemotherapy as it has been shown to prolong survival. A commonly used regimen is four cycles of vinorelbine-cisplatin.

Adjuvant radiotherapy

Prophylactic irradiation of non-involved mediastinal nodes is not recommended. PORT using modern radiotherapy techniques to minimize the dose to normal tissues may be considered in patients who have undergone an incomplete resection, and in selected patients this may be given concurrently with chemotherapy.

Prophylactic cranial irradiation

Patients with stage III NSCLC have a high cumulative risk of developing brain metastases. Several trials have explored prophylactic cranial irradiation (PCI) in patients being treated with radical intent. All trials showed a significant decrease in the incidence of brain metastases with PCI, but no increase in OS. A Cochrane review concluded that currently there is currently no role for PCI in stage III NSCLC outside the clinical trial setting.

Non-surgical management

For patients of good performance status with unresectable stage III NSCLC that can be encompassed within a radical radiotherapy volume, concurrent chemoradiotherapy should be considered the treatment of choice. This group includes both unresectable N2 disease based on bulky/multiple mediastinal nodal involvement and IIIb disease based on unresectable T4 disease or N3 disease.

A Cochrane review of concurrent chemoradiotherapy concluded that trials in this therapy area demonstrate a survival benefit for concurrent chemoradiotherapy over sequential treatment but with increased toxicity compared to radiation alone or sequential chemoradiation, specifically acute oesophagitis.

The absolute survival benefit of concurrent over sequential treatment was estimated to be 10% at two years. The survival benefit was likely to be a result of improved loco-regional control in the concurrent schedules. It is not known what the optimal chemotherapy regimen is to use as part of a concurrent schedule as several have been tested in clinical trials. Most comparative studies of concurrent chemoradiotherapy versus sequential administration have used cisplatin and etoposide or cisplatin and a vinca alkaloid, and it would seem logical to include cisplatin in any schedule. In this situation, cisplatin is used as both a treatment for micrometastatic disease and a radiation sensitizer, increasing the effect of the radiotherapy.

Similarly, the optimal radiotherapy schedule remains uncertain. The accepted paradigm that increased radiotherapy dose delivered to the primary tumour results in increased local control and hence better survival has been challenged following publication of the results of the RTOG 0617 trial. In this trial, patients with stage III NSCLC were randomly assigned to receive either 60Gy (standard dose), or 74Gy (high dose), with or without cetuximab. All patients also received concurrent chemotherapy with paclitaxel and carboplatin. The median OS was 28.7 months for patients who received standard-dose RT and 20.3 months for those who received high-dose RT. It is not yet clear why this apparently counter-intuitive result was seen but increased cardiovascular toxicity secondary to radiotherapy in the high-dose arm might be an explanation.

If concurrent chemoradiotherapy is not possible for any reason, then sequential approaches represent a valid and effective alternative; chemotherapy may be given before (neoadjuvant) or after (adjuvant) a radical radiotherapy schedule.

Conventional radical radiotherapy schedules involve giving one fraction of treatment a day, treating weekdays only, for four to seven weeks. Continuous hyperfractionated accelerated radiotherapy (CHART) involves giving 36 fractions of treatment, three times a day, over 12 consecutive days to a total dose of 54Gy. CHART has been shown in a randomized trial to be more effective than the conventional radiotherapy schedule of 60Gy in 30 fractions (the then standard of care). Survival was significantly improved in patients receiving CHART, particularly squamous cell carcinoma (two-year survival 33% vs. 20%). Despite these impressive results, CHART has not been widely adopted, as it is resource intensive.

Further reading

Andre F, Grunenwald D, Pignon JP, et al. Survival of patients with resected N2 non-small-cell lung cancer: Evidence for a subclassification and implications. *J Clin Oncol* 2000; 18:2981–89.

Bradley JD, Paulus R, Komaki R et al. Standard-dose versus high-dose conformal radiotherapy with concurrent and consolidation carboplatin plus paclitaxel with or without cetuximab for patients with stage IIIA or IIIB non-small-cell lung cancer (RTOG 0617): A randomised, two-by-two factorial phase 3 study. *Lancet Oncol* 2015 Feb; 16(2):187–99.

Burdett S, Rydzewska L, Tierney J, Fisher D, et al. PORT Meta-analysis Trialists Group. Postoperative radiotherapy for non-small cell lung cancer. *Cochrane Database Syst Rev* 2016 Oct 11; 10:CD002142.

Eberhardt WEE, De Ruysscher D, Weder W, et al. 2nd ESMO Consensus Conference in Lung Cancer: locally advanced stage III non-small-cell lung cancer. *Ann Oncol* 2015; 26(8):1573–88.

Ibain KS, Swann RS, Rusch VW, et al. Radiotherapy plus chemotherapy with or without surgical resection for stage III non-small-cell lung cancer: a phase III randomised controlled trial. *Lancet* 2009; 374:379–86.

Lester JF, MacBeth FR, Coles B. Prophylactic cranial irradiation for preventing brain metastases in patients undergoing radical treatment for non-small-cell lung cancer: a Cochrane Review. *Int J Radiat Oncol Biol Phys* 2005 Nov 1; 63(3):690–4.

O'Rourke N, Figuls MR, Bernadó NF, et al. Concurrent chemoradiotherapy in non-small cell lung cancer. *Cochrane Database Syst Rev* 2004;6(6):CD002140.

Saunders M, Dische S, Barrett A, et al. Continuous, hyperfractionated, accelerated radiotherapy (CHART) versus conventional radiotherapy in non-small cell lung cancer: mature data from the randomised multicentre trial. CHART Steering committee. *Radiother Oncol* 1999 Aug; 52(2):137–48.

Vansteenkiste J, Crinò L, Dooms C, et al. 2nd ESMO consensus conference on lung cancer: Early-stage non-small-cell lung cancer consensus on diagnosis, treatment and follow-up. *Ann Oncol* 2014; 25:1462–74.

5.7 Treatment of stage IV non-small cell lung cancer

Background

The aims of treatment for advanced stage IV NSCLC with systemic anticancer therapy (SACT) are to prolong life, improve quality of life (QoL), and control disease-related symptoms.

For many years, first-line platinum doublet chemotherapy was the standard of care for the majority of patients, with second-line docetaxel reserved for the fittest. The discovery that immune checkpoint inhibitor antibodies which disrupt PD-1 and PD-L1-mediated signalling (nivolumab, pembrolizumab, atezolizumab) are effective has meant they are now integrated into treatment pathways in the first- and second-line setting, as monotherapy and in combination with chemotherapy.

Patient factors that influence treatment choices include the presence of other medical conditions, general fitness, cancer symptoms, and patients' wishes. Disease factors that influence treatment include the extent and location of metastatic disease, the histological subtype, PD-L1 status, and the presence or absence of so-called driver mutations.

First-line SACT, absence of driver mutations

PD-L1 ≥50%

Pembrolizumab is now a standard first-line option for patients with advanced disease and a PD-L1 expression of ≥50% with no contraindications to immunotherapy. In the KEYNOTE-024 trial, 305 patients with untreated, advanced NSCLC, and tumour characterized by PD-L1 expression ≥50% without EGFR mutations or ALK translocations were randomized to 200mg pembrolizumab every three weeks (up to two years) or four to six cycles of standard platinum-doublet chemotherapy. OS, safety, and quality of life favoured pembrolizumab.

Any PD-L1 status

For fit patients (PS 0–1) with no absolute contraindications to immunotherapy (such as active autoimmune disease or organ transplantation) new combination treatment regimens have recently been shown to be more effective than conventional platinum-based doublet chemotherapy.

In the KEYNOTE-189 trial, patients with metastatic non-squamous NSCLC, without sensitising EGFR or ALK mutations, were randomized to receive pemetrexed-platinum plus either pembrolizumab 200mg or placebo every three weeks for four cycles, followed by maintenance pemetrexed plus pembrolizumab or placebo for up to 35 cycles. The median OS was significantly longer in the pembrolizumab arm (not reached versus 11.3 months; HR 0.49; 95% CI 0.38–0.64; P<0.001).

In the randomized phase 3 IMpower150 trial, the addition of atezolizumab to paclitaxel-carboplatin plus bevacizumab significantly improved OS in patients with metastatic non-squamous NSCLC, regardless of PD-L1 expression (19.2 months vs. 14.7 months; HR 0.78; 95% CI 0.64–0.96; P=0.02).

In the IMpower132 trial, patients with advanced non-squamous disease were randomized to pemetrexed-platinum plus maintenance pemetrexed +/− atezolizumab given in the induction and maintenance phase. Median progression-free survival (PFS) was improved in the combination arm (5.2 months vs.

7.6 months; HR 0.6; P<0.0001) however, a statistically significant OS advantage has not yet been seen.

KEYNOTE-407 randomized patients with metastatic squamous NSCLC to paclitaxel-carboplatin (or nab-paclitaxel) three-weekly, +/− pembrolizumab/placebo for four cycles, followed by maintenance pembrolizumab/placebo for up to 35 treatments. The combination treatment resulted in improved median OS (15.9 months vs. 11.3 months, HR 0.64, P=0.0008).

The results from the trials looking at adding immunotherapy up front to conventional chemotherapy indicate that for appropriate patients, combination chemo-immunotherapy treatment should be considered the current standard of care.

For patients where immunotherapy is contraindicated, platinum-doublet chemotherapy should be considered. Pemetrexed-platinum is an effective treatment for non-squamous NSCLC, but should not be used in patients with squamous cell carcinoma. A non-inferiority, phase 3, randomized trial compared pemetrexed-cisplatin with gemcitabine-cisplatin in 1,725 patients with advanced NSCLC. OS was better in the pemetrexed arm in adenocarcinoma (12.6 months vs. 10.9 months,) and large cell carcinoma (10.4 months vs. 6.7 months). In contrast, in patients with squamous cell histology, there was a significant improvement in OS with the gemcitabine-based regimen (10.8 months vs. 9.4 months).

Maintenance therapy involves continuing some form of SACT in patients with at least stable disease after completion of platinum-based induction SACT, with the aim of prolonging disease control and improving survival. Pemetrexed has been shown to be effective in the maintenance setting in patients with advanced non-squamous disease.

To date, there are no chemotherapy agents that have shown selective benefit in patients with advanced squamous cell carcinoma. Several platinum-based regimens with a third-generation cytotoxic (paclitaxel, gemcitabine, docetaxel, vinorelbine) have shown comparable efficacy, and can be used where appropriate.

Second-line therapy, absence of driver mutations

Docetaxel has been shown to improve survival in the second-line setting for PS 0–1 patients with advanced NSCLC, irrespective of histological subtype, and up until relatively recently, was the standard of care.

For patients with advanced adenocarcinoma, adding the oral multitargeting anti-angiogenic nintedanib to docetaxel has been shown to improve survival compared with docetaxel alone at the expense of increased toxicity. This added benefit did not hold true for patients with squamous cell carcinoma.

More recently, nivolumab, pembrolizumab, and atezolizumab have all shown improved OS and reduced toxicity compared to docetaxel in the second-line setting. Each has been approved for patients who have not received immunotherapy in the first-line treatment.

In the CHECKMATE 057 trial, patients with non-squamous NSCLC that had progressed during or after platinum-based doublet chemotherapy were randomized to nivolumab or docetaxel. Median OS was significantly longer with nivolumab than with docetaxel (12.2

months vs. 9.4 months, HR 0.73, 95% CI 0.59–0.89, P=0.002), and grade 3/4 toxicity was significantly less. CHECKMATE 017 was a very similar trial in patients with squamous cell carcinoma who had progressive disease during or after platinum-based doublet chemotherapy. Median OS was significantly longer with nivolumab than with docetaxel (9.2 months vs. 6.0 months, HR 0.59, 95% CI 0.44–0.79, P<0.001), and as in the 057 trial, grade 3/4 toxicity was significantly less with nivolumab.

The KEYNOTE-010 trial randomized 1,034 patients with PD-L1 expression of ≥1% to pembrolizumab 2mg/kg, pembrolizumab 10mg/kg or docetaxel. OS was significantly longer with pembrolizumab, with a recently reported two-year survival of 30.1% in the 2mg/kg group compared to 14.5% for docetaxel.

In the OAK trial, 850 patients with advanced NSCLC were randomized to atezolizumab or docetaxel. OS was significantly improved with atezolizumab (HR 0.73, 95% CI 0.62–0.87, P<0.001).

In the second-line setting, nivolumab and atezolizumab are approved irrespective of PD-L1 expression, and pembrolizumab is approved in patients with PD-L1 ≥1%. The optimal second-line treatment for patients who have received immunotherapy in the first-line setting is not known. For patients given first-line pembrolizumab monotherapy, platinum-doublet chemotherapy according to histological subtype would be a reasonable option. For those receiving a chemo-immunotherapy combination, docetaxel alone, or docetaxel plus nintedanib (for fitter patients with adenocarcinoma and no contraindications to vascular endothelial growth factor (VEGF) inhibition) should be considered.

NSCLC with targetable mutations

EGFR mutation-positive disease: first line

Driver mutations in the EGFR gene are found in a subset of lung adenocarcinomas and define cancers in which tumour cell survival is exquisitely dependent on EGFR pathway signalling. These cancers are uniquely susceptible to selective oral EGFR tyrosine kinase inhibitors (TKIs). The commonest sensitizing driver mutations are exon 19 deletions and L858R mutations, which make up approximately 90% of the EGFR driver mutations seen. Multiple randomized phase 3 trials have shown that the first-generation oral EGFR TKIs gefitinib and erlotinib both prolong PFS but not OS compared with chemotherapy and are better tolerated. Two randomized phase 3 trials have shown, that compared to chemotherapy, the second-generation oral EGFR TKI afatinib results in a significantly longer OS in previously untreated patients with the commonest sensitizing mutation, the exon 19 deletion.

Two randomized trials have looked at first- versus second-generation inhibitors. LUX-Lung 7 showed that there was no statistical difference in median OS between afatinib and gefitinib (7.9 months vs. 24.5 months; HR 0.86, 95% CI 0.66–1.12, P=0.258).

ARCHER 1050 reported significant improvement in median PFS (14.7 months vs. 9.2 months; HR 0.59, 95% CI 0.47–0.74, P<0.0001) and median OS (34.1 months vs. 26.8 months; HR 0.76, 95% CI 0.58–0.993, P=0.04) with dacomitinib compared to gefitinib.

Osimertinib is a third-generation EGFR TKI that targets both sensitizing EGFR mutation and the resistant exon 20 T790M mutation. The FLAURA phase 3 study reported a significant improvement in median PFS for osimertinib

compared to first-generation TKIs (18.9 months vs. 10.2 months; HR 0.46, 95% CI 0.37– 0.57, P<0.0001).

EGFR mutation-positive disease: second line

In approximately 50% of patients who develop resistance to first- and second-generation TKIs, the culprit is an acquired exon 20 T790M resistance mutation. AURA3 compared osimertinib with pemetrexed-platinum in patients with proven T790M mutation at time of progression on a first- or second-generation EGFR TKI. Response rate and PFS were both significantly better with osimertinib, which also showed a significantly longer central nervous system (CNS) PFS (11.7 months vs. 5.6 months) in patients with CNS metastases at baseline. All patients with clinical resistance to first- or second-generation EGFR TKIs should be tested for the presence of a T790M mutation and offered osimertinib.

In patients without the T790M resistance mutation, pemetrexed-platinum chemotherapy is a reasonable option. In the IMpower150 trial, patients with EGFR or ALK alterations were included, as long as they had received at least one line of targeted therapy. Outcomes were better in the combination arm (PFS HR 0.59, 95% CI 0.37–0.94; OS HR 0.54, 95% CI 0.29–1.03), indicating this regimen should be considered a treatment option in this group of patients.

ALK-rearranged disease: first line

Crizotinib was the first targeted treatment to show benefit in ALK-rearranged disease. In PROFILE 1014, It showed a significantly longer median PFS (10.9 months vs. 7.0 months; HR 0.45; 95% CI 0.35–0.60; P<0.001) compared to pemetrexed-platinum chemotherapy.

The ASCEND-4 trial compared the second-generation ALK inhibitor ceritinib (750mg once a day on an empty stomach) with pemetrexed-platinum followed by maintenance pemetrexed in squamous NSCLC. Response rate was higher with ceritinib (72.5% vs. 26.7%), as was median PFS (16.6 months vs. 8.1 months, HR 0.55, 95% CI 0.42–0.73, P<0.01). Ceritinib also showed impressive CNS activity, with an intracranial response rate of 72.7% compared to 27.3% with chemotherapy. A high incidence of gastrointestinal toxicity was seen in ASCEND 4; ASCEND 8 looked at 450mg ceritinib taken once daily with food and showed similar exposure and a more favourable safety profile than 750mg taken on an empty stomach. The licensed recommended maximum dose for ceritinib is now 450mg.

In the ALEX trial, patients were randomized to the second-generation ALK inhibitor alectinib or crizotinib. The median PFS with alectinib was 34.8 months compared to 10.9 months with crizotinib. Median PFS was also significantly longer with alectinib (25.7 months vs. 10.4 months). In patients with baseline CNS metastases, median PFS was 27.7 months for alectinib vs. 7.4 months for crizotinib. Grade 3–5 adverse events were less frequent with alectinib. The results from the ALEX and ASCEND trials show that both alectinib and lower-dose ceritinib are effective well tolerated first-line treatments for ALK-rearranged lung cancer and are beneficial in patients with CNS disease.

Crizotinib has relatively poor penetration into the cerebrospinal fluid; taking into account the high propensity of ALK-rearranged lung cancer to metastasize to the brain, alectinib and ceritinib are generally viewed as more effective first-line options.

ALK-rearranged disease: second line
The third-generation ALK inhibitors brigatinib and lorlatinib have a wide coverage of ALK resistance mutations and should be considered in crizotinib-resistant and second-generation resistant populations if available.

Palliative radiotherapy
Radiotherapy is effective at palliating local and metastatic symptoms in patients with advanced NSCLC.

Local disease
Studies suggest that higher dose palliative radiotherapy regimens (30Gy or more) are associated with modest improvements in OS and improvement in lung cancer-associated symptoms, particularly in patients with good PS. This comes at the expense of increased oesophageal toxicity and requires more visits to hospital for treatment. Therefore, in less fit patients, shorter schedules (for example, 20Gy in five fractions, or 8–10Gy single fractions) that still provide good symptomatic relief but with fewer side effects may be used. In poor PS patients without local chest symptoms, palliative radiotherapy is not indicated.

Metastatic disease
As with other solid tumours, palliative radiotherapy is an effective treatment for symptoms related to metastatic disease, particularly bone pain. Shorter fractionation schedules are preferable to more protracted courses of treatment.

In patients with brain metastases, where surgical resection or stereotactic radiotherapy is not appropriate, palliative whole brain radiotherapy should be used with caution. The QUARTZ trial randomized NSCLC patients with brain metastases where surgical resection or stereotactic radiotherapy was not considered appropriate to whole brain radiotherapy or optimal supportive care. Survival in both arms of the trial was poor, and QoL in the radiotherapy arm was significantly worse.

Further reading
Borghaei H, Paz-Ares L, Horn L, et al. Nivolumab versus docetaxel in advanced nonsquamous non-small-cell lung cancer. *N Engl J Med* 2015 Oct 22; 373(17):1627–39.

Brahmer J, Reckamp KL, Baas P, et al. Nivolumab versus docetaxel in advanced squamous-cell non-small-cell lung cancer. *N Engl J Med* 2015 Jul 9; 373(2):123–35.

Camidge DR. Updated efficacy and safety data from the global phase III ALEX study of alectinib (ALC) vs crizotinib (CZ) in untreated advanced ALK NSCLC. *J Clin Oncol* 2018; 35(Suppl.):9064.

Cho BC, Kim DW, Bearz A, et al. ASCEND-8: a randomized phase 1 study of ceritinib, 450 mg or 600 mg, taken with a low-fat meal versus 750 mg in fasted state in patients with anaplastic lymphoma kinase (ALK)-rearranged metastatic non-small cell lung cancer (NSCLC). *J Thorac Oncol* 2017; 12:1357–67.

Ciuleanu T, Brodowicz T, Zielinski C, et al. Maintenance pemetrexed plus best supportive care versus placebo plus best supportive care for non-small-cell lung cancer: a randomised, double-blind, phase 3 study. *Lancet* 2009; 374:1432–40.

D'Addario G, Pintilie M, Leighl NB, et al. Platinum-based versus non-platinum-based chemotherapy in advanced non-small-cell lung cancer: A meta-analysis of the published literature. *J Clin Oncol* 2005; 23:2926–36.

Delbaldo C, Michiels S, Syz N, et al. Benefits of adding a drug to a single-agent or a 2-agent chemotherapy regimen in advanced non-small-cell lung cancer: A meta-analysis. *JAMA* 2006; 292:4405–11.

Gandhi L, Rodriguez-Abreu D, Gadgeel S, et al. Pembrolizumab plus chemotherapy in metastatic non-small-cell lung cancer. *N Engl J Med* 2018; 378:2078–92.

Garassino MC, Martelli O, Broggini M, et al. Erlotinib versus docetaxel as second-line treatment of patients with advanced non-small-cell lung cancer and wild-type EGFR tumours (TAILOR): a randomised controlled trial. *Lancet Oncol* 2013 Sep; 14(10):981–8.

Herbst R, Garon E, Kim D-W, et al. OA03.07 KEYNOTE-010: durable clinical benefit in patients with previously treated, PD-L1-expressing NSCLC who completed pembrolizumab. *J Thoracic Oncol* 2017; 12:S254–S255.

Mok T, Ahn M-J, Han J-Y, et al. CNS response to osimertinib in patients (pts) with T790M-positive advanced NSCLC: data from a randomized phase III trial (AURA3). *J Clin Oncol* 2017; 35:9005.

Mok TS, Wu YL, Ahn MJ, et al. Osimertinib or platinum-pemetrexed in EGFR T790M-positive lung cancer. *N Engl J Med* 2017; 376:629–40.

Mulvenna PM, Nankivell MG, Barton R, et al. Whole brain radiotherapy for brain metastases from non-small lung cancer: Quality of life (QoL) and overall survival (OS) results from the UK Medical Research Council QUARTZ randomised clinical trial (ISRCTN 3826061). *J Clin Oncol* 2015; (Suppl. 33):abstr 8005.

Papadimitrakopoulou V, Cobo M, Bordon R, et al. IMPOWER132: PFS and safety results with 1L atezolizumab + carboplatin/cisplatin + peme-trexed in stage IV non-squamous NSCLC. IASLC 19th World Conference on Lung Cancer 2018:abstr. OA05.07.

Park JO, Kim S-W, Ahn JS, et al. Phase III trial of two versus four additional cycles in patients who are non-progressive after two cycles of platinum-based chemotherapy in non-small-cell lung cancer. *J Clin Oncol* 2007; 25:5233–9.

Paz-Ares LG, de Marinis F, Dediu M, et al. PARAMOUNT: final overall survival results of the phase III study of maintenance pemetrexed versus placebo immediately after induction treatment with pemetrexed plus cisplatin for advanced nonsquamous non-small-cell lung cancer. *J Clin Oncol* 2013; 31:2895–902.

Paz-Ares LG, Luft A, Vicente D, et al. Pembrolizumab plus chemotherapy for squamous non-small-cell lung cancer *N Engl J Med*. 2018 Nov 22; 379(21):2040–51.

Paz-Ares L, Tan EH, O'Byrne K, et al. Afatinib versus gefitinib in patients with EGFR mutation-positive advanced non-small-cell lung cancer: overall survival data from the phase IIb LUX-Lung 7 trial. *Ann Oncol* 2017; 28:270–7.

Reck M, Kaiser R, Mellemgaard A, et al. Docetaxel plus nintedanib versus docetaxel plus placebo in patients with previously treated non-small-cell lung cancer (LUME-Lung 1): a phase 3, double-blind, randomised controlled trial. *Lancet Oncol* 2014 Feb; 15(2):143–55.

Reck M, Rodriguez-Abreu D, Robinson AG, et al. Pembrolizumab versus chemotherapy for PD-L1-positive non-small-cell lung cancer. *N Engl J Med* 2016; 375:1823–33.

Rittmeyer A, Barlesi F, Waterkamp D, et al. Atezolizumab versus docetaxel in patients with previously treated non-small-cell lung cancer (OAK): a phase 3, open-label, multicentre randomised controlled trial. *Lancet* 2017; 389:255–65.

Scagliotti GV, Parikh P, von Pawel J, et al. Phase III study comparing cisplatin plus gemcitabine with cisplatin plus pemetrexed in chemotherapy-naive patients with advanced-stage non-small-cell lung cancer. *J Clin Oncol* 2008 Jul 20; 26(21):3543–51.

Shaw AT, Kim DW, Nakagawa K, et al. Crizotinib versus chemotherapy in advanced alk-positive lung cancer. *Lancet Oncol* 2015; 16:141–51.

Shepherd FA, Dancey J, Ramlau R, et al. Prospective randomized trial of docetaxel versus best supportive care in patients with non-small-cell lung cancer previously treated with platinum-based chemotherapy. *J Clin Oncol* 2000; 18:2095–103.

Shepherd FA, Rodrigues Pereira J, Ciuleanu T, et al. Erlotinib in previously treated non-small-cell lung cancer. *NEJM* 2005; 353:123–32.

Socinski MA, Jotte RM, Cappuzzo F, et al. Atezolizumab for first-line treatment of metastatic nonsquamous NSCLC. *N Engl J Med* 2018; 378:2288–301.

Solomon BJ, Mok T, Kim DW, et al. First-line crizotinib versus chemotherapy in ALK-positive lung cancer. *N Engl J Med* 2014; 371:2167–77.

Soria JC, Tan DSW, Chiari R, et al. First-line ceritinib versus platinum-based chemotherapy in advanced ALK-rearranged non-small-cell lung cancer (ASCEND-4): a randomised, open-label, phase 3 study. *Lancet* 2017; 389:917–29.

Stevens R, Macbeth F, Toy E, et al. Palliative radiotherapy regimens for patients with thoracic symptoms from non-small cell lung cancer. *Cochrane Database Syst Rev* 2015 Jan 14; 1:CD002143.

Wu YL, Cheng Y, Zhou X, et al. Dacomitinib versus gefitinib as first-line treatment for patients with EGFR-mutation-positive non-small-cell lung cancer (ARCHER 1050): a randomised, open-label, phase 3 trial. *Lancet Oncol* 2017; 18:1454–66.

Yang JC, Wu YL, Schuler M, et al. Afatinib versus cisplatin-based chemotherapy for EGFR mutation-positive lung adenocarcinoma (LUX-Lung 3 and LUX-Lung 6): Analysis of overall survival data from two randomised, phase 3 trials. *Lancet Oncol* 2015 Feb; 16(2):141–51.

Internet resources

NICE. Lung cancer: diagnosis and management. Clinical guideline. 21 April 2011—available at http://nice.org.uk/guidance/cg121

5.8 Small cell lung cancer

Clinical presentation

SCLC typically arises in the central airways, and often presents with bulky mediastinal disease. Symptoms include cough, dyspnoea, and weight loss. Over two-thirds of patients present with extensive disease (ED); spread is common to liver, adrenal glands, bone, and brain. Less commonly, presentation can include para-neoplastic syndromes such as Eaton–Lambert syndrome and syndrome of inappropriate antidiuretic hormone (SIADH).

Staging

The latest UICC TNM version 8 recommends staging SCLC in the same way as NSCLC. However, in routine practice, a modification of the two-stage Veterans Affairs Lung Study Group (VALG) system continues to be used because of its simplicity and clinical application. Broadly, limited disease (LD) is defined as tumour confined to the ipsilateral hemithorax and regional lymph nodes able to be included in a single tolerable radiotherapy field. This approximates to TNM stages I–IIIB. In addition, T1/2 N0/1 M0 disease, previously described as very limited disease represents a separate cohort with a better prognosis. ED comprises all patients with more advanced disease.

Very limited disease (T1/2 N0/1 M0)

The evidence-based treatment of patients with LD-SCLC and a good performance status (WHO PS 0–1) is concurrent chemoradiotherapy, followed by PCI. There is no good evidence to support use of surgery in patients who present with LD-SCLC. However, in cases where adequate mediastinal lymph node staging reveals no evidence of metastases, a surgical approach may be justified. This should be followed postoperatively by four cycles of adjuvant platinum–etoposide chemotherapy, and PCI if appropriate. In the case of unforeseen mediastinal nodal disease, postoperative radiotherapy should be considered in addition to chemotherapy and PCI.

Limited disease SCLC

Patients with LD and a good performance status should be treated with concurrent chemoradiotherapy with cisplatin–etoposide. In cases where a good treatment response is seen, this should be followed by PCI in appropriate patients. The addition of thoracic radiotherapy to chemotherapy improves survival, and cisplatin-containing regimens are preferred. The optimal timing and dose-fractionation of radiotherapy has been extensively studied. The Intergroup 0096 trial randomized patients to receive 45Gy of concurrent thoracic radiotherapy given either twice daily over three weeks or once daily over five weeks. All patients received four 21-day cycles of cisplatin–etoposide, and radiation commenced with the start of chemotherapy. The five-year OS favoured twice-daily radiation (26% vs. 16%), and the rate of local failure was lower with twice-daily radiation (52% vs. 36%). The most important toxicity observed with twice-daily radiation was grade 3 or higher oesophagitis, which was seen in 27% of patients receiving twice-daily radiotherapy versus 11% with once-daily radiotherapy. Therefore, a twice-daily 1.5Gy in 30-fraction regimen should be considered in patients who are willing to accept the increased risk of oesophagitis.

The CONVERT trial has compared 66Gy in 33 once-daily fractions with 45Gy in 30 twice-daily fractions. Survival outcomes did not differ between the arms, and toxicity was similar and lower than expected with both regimens.

The optimal radiotherapy target volume remains to be defined. In historical trials, treatment fields routinely included the whole mediastinum even if radiologically lymph nodes were uninvolved, because the risk of nodal spread in SCLC is high. Elective nodal irradiation (ENI) increases treatment-related toxicity, particularly oesophagitis. In the era of conformal radiotherapy this approach has been questioned and involved-field radiotherapy is increasingly being used. Omission of ENI reduces radiotherapy volumes, treatment-related toxicity, and may allow dose escalation. However, there may be a risk of nodal relapse. PET-CT might allow the safe omission of ENI, but this approach has not been tested in large prospective randomized trials.

PCI is part of the standard of care for patients with LD-SCLC as the magnitude of survival benefit with PCI is similar to that achieved using thoracic radiotherapy in LD-SCLC. For patients who respond to chemotherapy, PCI decreases the cumulative incidence of brain metastases from 58.6% (controls) to 33.3%, which in turn is

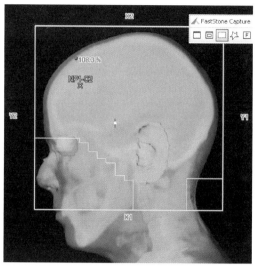

Fig. 5.8.1 Standard radiotherapy portals fields used for delivery of prophylactic cranial radiotherapy. The lens and oral cavity are shielded to reduce toxicity (see also colour plate).

accompanied by an improvement in three-year OS from 15.3% to 20.7%. Currently, the standard dose used for prophylactic cranial radiotherapy is 25Gy in ten once-daily fractions of 2.5Gy. In patients who are over 65 years old or have significant vascular disease, PCI is associated with an increased risk of neurocognitive toxicity (Figure 5.8.1).

Extensive disease SCLC

Treatment of ED-SCLC is palliative. The standard treatment for patients with ED-SCLC and a good performance score (WHO PS 0–1) is sequential chemotherapy with a platinum-based regimen, followed by PCI in appropriate responding patients. A meta-analysis has shown improved OS in patients receiving a platinum-containing regimen compared with other chemotherapy combinations. A second meta-analysis reported an OS benefit in favour of etoposide alone or in combination with cisplatin compared with regimens that did not contain either of these drugs. These results led to cisplatin-etoposide becoming the standard treatment. Evidence suggests cisplatin may be substituted by carboplatin with no significant difference in efficacy. Cisplatin is associated with significant renal and neurological toxicity and is only appropriate for PS 0–1 patients with limited comorbidities. Carboplatin is associated with greater haematological toxicity but is better tolerated overall and is therefore suitable for less fit patients. To date, no chemotherapy doublet has been shown to be superior to cisplatin-etoposide in a Western population. The response rates to first-line chemotherapy range from 70% to 85%, with complete response rates of 20–30%. There is no evidence that treating beyond four to six cycles of chemotherapy is beneficial.

PCI significantly decreases the incidence of symptomatic brain metastases from 40.4% to 14.6% at one year and increases OS. PCI is associated with adverse effects such as fatigue and hair loss and should only be considered in fit patients. The commonest regimen used is 20Gy in five fractions.

The CREST trial showed that thoracic radiotherapy given after chemotherapy in responding patients is associated with a longer PFS and a significant increase in two-year survival from 3% to 13%. Therefore, palliative thoracic radiotherapy should be considered in addition to PCI in appropriate patients who have responded to chemotherapy.

Second-line treatment

Despite response rates to first-line chemotherapy, which range from 70% to 85%, with complete response rates of 20–30%, virtually all patients relapse. Response to second-line chemotherapy is poor. Patients with refractory disease have a very poor outcome and the role of further chemotherapy is uncertain. These patients should be offered entry into a clinical trial or treated with best supportive care. Those who relapse within three months of first-line chemotherapy have a second-line response rate of <10%. Patients with a >3-month interval from completion of first-line chemotherapy have a response rate of about 20%.

Commonly, anthracycline-based regimens have been used, including cyclophosphamide, doxorubicin, and vincristine (CAV). A trial of intravenous topotecan versus CAV showed topotecan was at least as effective as CAV and resulted in improvement in control of several symptoms. Subsequently, oral and intravenous topotecan were shown to be equally effective. ESMO recommend oral or intravenous topotecan, with CAV as an alternative option. In patients who have had a durable response to first-line chemotherapy, re-challenge with the first-line regimen would be a reasonable option.

Follow-up

In patients with LD who have completed potentially curative treatment, the recommendation is for three to six monthly CT scans for two years, with lengthening of intervals thereafter. In patients who have completed treatment for ED, ESMO guidelines suggests regular follow-up with two to three monthly CT scans in patients who would potentially be suitable for further therapy.

Further reading

Auperin A, Arriagada R, Pignon JP, et al. Prophylactic cranial irradiation for patients with small-cell lung cancer in complete remission. Prophylactic Cranial Irradiation Overview Collaborative Group. *N Engl J Med* 1999; 341:476–84.

Eckardt JR, von Pawel J, Pujol JL, et al. Phase III study of oral compared with intravenous topotecan as second-line therapy in small-cell lung cancer. *Clin Oncol* 2007; 25:2086–92.

Früh M, De Ruysscher D, Popat S, et al. Small-cell lung cancer (SCLC): ESMO clinical practice guidelines for diagnosis, treatment and follow-up. *Ann Oncol* 2013; 24 (Suppl. 6):vi99–vi105.

Goldstraw P, Crowley J, Chansky K, et al. The IASLC lung cancer staging project: proposals for the revision of the TNM stage groups in the forthcoming (seventh) edition of the TNM classification of malignant tumours. *J Thorac Oncol* 2007; 2:706.

Mascaux C, Paesmans M, Berghmans T, et al. A systematic review of the role of etoposide and cisplatin in the chemotherapy of small cell lung cancer with methodology assessment and meta-analysis. *Lung Cancer* 2000; 30:23–6.

Pujol JL, Carestia L, Daurès JP. Is there a case for cisplatin in the treatment of small-cell lung cancer? A meta-analysis of randomized trials of a cisplatin-containing regimen versus a regimen without this alkylating agent. *Br J Cancer* 2000; 83(1):8–15.

Slotman B, Faivre-Finn C, Kramer G, et al. Prophylactic cranial irradiation in extensive small-cell lung cancer. *N Eng J Med* 2007; 357:644–72.

Slotman BJ, van Tinteren H, Praag JO, et al Use of thoracic radiotherapy for extensive stage small-cell lung cancer: a phase 3 randomised controlled trial. *Lancet* 2015 Jan 3; 385(9962):36–42.

Sorensen M. Primary surgery revisited in very limited small cell lung cancer: does it have a role? A commentary. *Lung Cancer* 2006; 52:263–4.

Turrisi AT 3rd, Kim K, Blum R, et al. Twice-daily compared with once-daily thoracic radiotherapy in limited small-cell lung cancer treated concurrently with cisplatin and etoposide. *N Engl J Med* 1999; 340:265–71.

von Pawel J, Schiller JH, Shepherd FA, et al . Topotecan versus cyclophosphamide, doxorubicin, and vincristine for the treatment of recurrent small-cell lung cancer. *J Clin Oncol* 1999; 17(2):658–67.

5.9 Bronchial carcinoid

Introduction

Bronchial carcinoid tumours account for approximately 1–2% of all lung malignancies and are characterized by neuroendocrine differentiation and relatively indolent clinical behaviour. Typical carcinoid tumours, which are low grade with a low mitotic rate, are about four times more common than atypical carcinoid tumours that are considered intermediate grade. It is unclear whether smoking is a risk factor.

Clinical features

The majority of tumours arise in the proximal airways, and symptoms are as a result of airway obstruction/irritation. Symptoms include cough, wheeze, haemoptysis, chest pain, or recurrent infections.

About 25% of cases present in the periphery as an asymptomatic solitary pulmonary nodule. Clinical syndromes related to peptide production—a feature of neuroendocrine tumours (NETs) arising in other organs—are relatively rare in bronchial carcinoid. Carcinoid syndrome is caused by release of vasoactive substances such as serotonin, and presents with flushing, diarrhoea, and bronchospasm. Bronchial carcinoid tumours produce less serotonin than do midgut NETs for example, and that accounts for the lower rate of carcinoid syndrome. As a result, elevated plasma or urinary hormone levels are rarely detected. In localized disease, which comprises almost all cases of typical bronchial carcinoid, carcinoid syndrome is occurs rarely. Very rarely, biopsy or manipulation of an actively secreting bronchial carcinoid can induce a carcinoid crisis due to massive systemic release of bioactive mediators, which can be fatal.

The most frequent site of metastases is the liver. Other sites include bone, adrenal glands, and brain. Metastases occur much more frequently with atypical carcinoids than with typical carcinoids.

Staging

Pulmonary carcinoid tumours are staged using the same TNM classification that is used for lung cancer.

Treatment

For patients with localized disease, surgical resection is the treatment of choice. In typical carcinoid where the lesion is entirely endobronchial, transbronchoscopic resection may be an alternative option that has the advantage of sparing lung parenchyma. Currently, there is no evidence to support the routine use of adjuvant chemotherapy or radiotherapy in patients with resected carcinoid tumours.

Metastatic disease

Metastatic bronchial carcinoid is a rare disease, and there are no prospective randomized trials to guide treatment. Most treatment schedules are based on data extrapolated from trials in other primary NETs, or from treatment of SCLC.

Somatostatin analogues are rarely used, as the incidence of carcinoid syndrome with bronchial carcinoid is low, even in the presence of metastatic disease. Chemotherapy regimens used to treat SCLC are sometimes used for metastatic carcinoid, but response rates are lower than those seen in SCLC.

In the phase 3 RADIANT 4 trial, 302 patients with advanced, non-functional lung or gastrointestinal tract NETs were randomized to receive the oral mTOR inhibitor everolimus or placebo. Everolimus was associated with a significant improvement in median PFS (11 months vs. 3.9 months). Among the 90 patients in the trial who had lung NETs, the hazard ratio for PFS was 0.5 (95% CI 0.28–0.88), suggesting everolimus may have a role to play in the management of metastatic lung carcinoid tumours.

Prognosis

Typical carcinoid tumours have a good prognosis with a five-year survival of 87–90% following surgical resection. However, distant metastases may occur many years after surgery, and many clinical guidelines recommend prolonged follow-up as a consequence. Atypical carcinoid tumours have a poorer prognosis and a five-year survival of 44–78%.

Further reading

Yao JC, Fazio N, Singh S, et al. Everolimus for the treatment of advanced, non-functional neuroendocrine tumours of the lung or gastrointestinal tract (RADIANT-4): a randomised, placebo-controlled, phase 3 study. *Lancet* 2015; 387(10022):968–77.

5.10 Large cell neuroendocrine carcinoma

Introduction

Large cell neuroendocrine carcinoma (LCNEC) is rare. Diagnosis is based on high-grade features and the presence of both neuroendocrine morphology as well as immunohistochemical evidence of neuroendocrine markers. The presentation and natural history of LCNEC are similar to SCLC, apart from the observation that primary LCNECs are more commonly located peripherally rather than centrally and a greater proportion present with early stage disease.

Treatment

LCNEC is rare; there are no prospective randomized clinical trials that define the optimum treatment approach. Generally, treatment recommendations are based upon extrapolation from the treatment of NSCLC and SCLC. For patients with localized disease, surgical resection should be undertaken if appropriate. Adjuvant chemotherapy should be considered given the poor prognosis of LCNEC, and generally, SCLC platinum-based chemotherapy regimens are recommended. Unlike in SCLC,

PCI is not recommended for patients treated with radical intent. A recent published series reported 25% of radically treated patients had developed brain metastases after a median follow-up of nearly two years, which is comparable to NSCLC patients in general where PCI is not routinely given.

For patients with stage III disease, it is reasonable to use concurrent chemoradiotherapy where appropriate. For patients with stage IV disease, consider a SCLC regimen.

Prognosis

Survival is worse for LCNEC compared to NSCLC, and slightly better than that of SCLC. Overall, five-year survival for LCNEC is in the region of 15–57%.

Further reading

Glisson BS, Moran CA. Large-cell neuroendocrine carcinoma: controversies in diagnosis and treatment. *J Natl Compr Canc Netw* 2011 Oct; 9(10):1122–9.

Rieber J, Schmitt J, Warth A, et al. Outcome and prognostic factors of multimodal therapy for pulmonary large-cell neuroendocrine carcinomas. *Eur J Med Res* 2015; 20(1):64.

5.11 Malignant pleural mesothelioma

Introduction

Malignant pleural mesothelioma (MPM) is an incurable malignancy affecting the pleural membranes. Malignant peritoneal mesothelioma is a much rarer condition and is beyond the scope of this chapter. MPM incidence is strongly related to age, with the highest incidence rates being in older people. In the UK, nearly half of cases are diagnosed in patients over the age of 75. Age-specific incidence rates peak in the 80–84 age group for males and in the 75–79 age group for females. Incidence rates are higher for males than females aged 50 and over, and this gap is widest at age 80–84, when the male : female ratio is about 9:1. Most MPM cases are caused by previous exposure to asbestos. Mesothelioma incidence rates correlate with the rise and fall of asbestos exposure in the UK, which peaked in the early 1960s and then rapidly decreased. There is an average latency period of over 40 years between asbestos exposure and the development of symptoms from mesothelioma, meaning that the peak in incidence in the UK may not yet have been reached. The burden of this disease in the developing world is likely to increase due to continued exposure in these populations to asbestos in recent decades.

Aetiology

In industrialized countries over 90% of MPM cases are related to previous asbestos exposure. The different asbestos fibre types have varying malignant potential. Amphibole (amosite and crocidolite) asbestos fibres are significantly more potent than chrysotile, and crocidolite is more dangerous than amosite. There are rare other causes which include the naturally occurring non-asbestos fibre erionite (seen only in the Central Anatolia Region in Turkey), and therapeutic radiation.

Clinical features

Dyspnoea and chest wall pain are the most common presenting symptoms of MPM. Other frequently occurring symptoms include fatigue, anorexia, weight loss, fever, and sweats. Some patients may also be asymptomatic, and diagnosis is made following discovery of an incidental pleural effusion. Metastatic disease is uncommon at presentation and occurs late in the course of the illness.

Pathology

There are several distinct histological variations of MPM that may mimic numerous other tumour types,

---

Box 5.11.1 WHO histological classification of tumours of the pleura

Mesothelial tumours
- Diffuse malignant mesothelioma
- Epithelioid mesothelioma
- Sarcomatoid mesothelioma
- Desmoplastic mesothelioma
- Biphasic mesothelioma
- Localized malignant mesothelioma
- Other tumours of mesothelial origin
- Well differentiated papillary mesothelioma
- Adenomatoid tumour

Lymphoproliferative disorders
- Primary effusion lymphoma
- Pyothorax-associated lymphoma

Mesenchymal tumours
- Epithelioid hemangioendothelioma
- Angiosarcoma
- Synovial sarcoma
- Monophasic
- Biphasic
- Solitary fibrous tumour
- Calcifying tumour of the pleura
- Desmoplastic round cell tumour

Source: data from Travis WD, et al. *Pathology and Genetics of Tumours of the Lung, Pleura, Thymus and Heart.* Lyon: IARC Press, 2004.

---

and immunohistochemistry can be a useful tool, particularly in distinguishing mesothelioma from pulmonary adenocarcinoma. A combination of at least two positive mesothelial markers with at least two negative epithelial markers is optimal. Useful mesothelial markers include cytokeratin 5/6, calretinin, WT1, and N-cadherin. Epithelial markers include CEA, CD15, Ber EP4, MOC 31, and TTF-1. However, immunohistochemical findings need to be interpreted in the light of the histological appearance and clinical findings. Desmoplastic mesothelioma is the accepted term for a subtype of highly aggressive sarcomatoid mesothelioma, but there is no universal agreement on the nomenclature of other subtypes, particularly the variants of epithelioid mesothelioma. Recognition of these variants is important for diagnosis, but because they have no clear prognostic significance and do not currently have any therapeutic implication, it is accepted practice to report epithelioid and sarcomatoid mesotheliomas with no further subclassification than shown in Box 5.11.1 .

Investigation and staging
MPM often presents as a pleural effusion on a CXR. CT scanning may show evidence of asbestos-related pleural plaques, circumferential pleural thickening, and contraction of the ipsilateral hemithorax. MPM is usually diagnosed via CT-guided pleural biopsy, or biopsy via VATS. Pleural cytology is not usually sufficient to make a diagnosis. PET is increasingly being used in patients deemed suitable for a surgical approach and detects previously

unidentified metastatic disease in approximately 10% of patients. Neither PET nor CT accurately characterises mediastinal lymph node status, and mediastinoscopy is seen as an important staging investigation preoperatively. The tumour staging of malignant pleural mesothelioma is as follows:
- T1: lesion limited to the ipsilateral parietal pleura
- T2: lesion limited to the ipsilateral pleura with involvement of diaphragmatic muscle or extending to lung parenchyma
- T3: locally advanced resectable tumour
- T4: locally advanced unresectable tumour

(*Source*: data from Brierley JD, Gospodarowicz MK, Wittekind C (eds). *TNM Classification of Malignant Tumours*, 8th edn. 2017, John Wiley & Sons.)

Nodal staging depends on the extent of nodal involvement: N1: ipsilateral hilar nodes, N2: ipsilateral mediastinal, subcarinal, or internal mammary nodes, and N3: contralateral nodes.

Chemotherapy
Most systemic therapy trials in mesothelioma have been small phase 2 trials, usually with commercially available agents. These trials have often suffered from significant design flaws, including loosely defined eligibility criteria with insufficient attention paid to tumour stage, prognostic factors, and vague response criteria.

In 2003, Vogelzang et al. reported the results of a large, randomized phase 3 trial that compared cisplatin alone to cisplatin-pemetrexed in patients with unresectable MPM. The combination chemotherapy was well tolerated and was associated with a significantly better PFS and OS. This was the first such trial to show a significant difference in outcomes for one chemotherapy regimen over another, and cisplatin-pemetrexed subsequently became the standard of care for patients with MPM.

More recently, In the randomized phase 3 MAPS trial the addition of bevacizumab to cisplatin-pemetrexed has been shown to be more efficacious than chemotherapy alone (median OS 18.8 months vs. 16.1 months). To date, there are no licensed agents for the second-line systemic treatment of MPM. Anecdotally, single-agent vinorelbine is used in fitter patients in the second-line setting based on extrapolation of the results from the MSO 1 trial.

Surgery
Encouraging results from large case series have been reported for extrapleural pneumonectomy (EPP), in which the lung and ipsilateral parietal pleura, pericardium, and hemidiaphragm are resected. In some institutions, this procedure, within a multimodal treatment regimen, remains the standard of care in the management of patients with resectable MPM despite no randomized evidence to support this approach.

The Mesothelioma and Radical Surgery (MARS) trial was designed to establish the role of EPP in patients with MPM. An initial feasibility study randomized 50 patients to EPP or no EPP to assess patient acceptability. Patients were eligible for randomization to EPP plus postoperative radiotherapy or no EPP if they had completed preoperative chemotherapy and still had operable disease. Median survival was 14.4 months for the EPP group and 19.5 months for the no EPP group. In addition, median quality of life scores were lower in the EPP group than the no EPP group. This trial was not powered to detect a survival difference between the two arms, but nevertheless, in the absence of any other randomized data, has been viewed by many as an indication to stop offering EPP to patients with MPM. The role of less invasive surgery using radical pleurectomy and decortication is currently being examined in the recently opened MARS 2 trial.

Radiotherapy

Drain site radiotherapy
Prophylactic radiotherapy has been advocated as a way to prevent tumour seeding at the site of a diagnostic or therapeutic intervention for MPM. However, the small randomized trials carried out in this therapy area have yielded conflicting results.

Palliative radiotherapy
There is some evidence to suggest palliative radiotherapy may provide effective pain control in some patients with MPM. Prospective trials in this area have reported that up to 65% of patients derived significant pain relief from palliative radiotherapy for chest wall pain.

Hemithorax radiotherapy
No randomized data exist to support the use of hemithorax radiotherapy after radical surgery, although there are a large number of publications describing its use as an integral part of multimodality therapy.

Symptomatic management
Pleural effusions may cause troublesome dyspnoea, and there are several approaches that can be used to improve symptoms and quality of life.

Pleurodesis
Pleurodesis obliterates the pleural space by causing adhesions between the visceral and parietal pleurae. Complete drainage of the pleural effusion by chest drain or VATS is followed by introduction of talc (or other irritative agent) into the pleural space.

Indwelling pleural catheters
Patients with entrapped lung and a significant effusion can get symptomatic relief from a tunnelled indwelling pleural catheter (IPC) even though the lung does not expand. Currently, there is no randomized evidence to support the use of IPC over pleurodesis, but the procedure is increasingly being used as it seems to be well tolerated and provides effective palliation.

VATS pleurectomy
Video-assisted thoracoscopic subtotal (VATS) pleurectomy may also have a role in the palliative management of pleural effusions in patients with MPM. In the randomized MesoVATS trial, VATS pleurectomy provided better control of pleural effusion at one and six months, but not at three and 12 months compared with pleurodesis. VATS pleurectomy has not been directly compared with the use of IPCs.

Further reading
Muers MF, Rudd RM, O'Brien ME, Qian W, Hodson A, Parmar MK, Girling DJ. BTS randomised feasibility study of active symptom control with or without chemotherapy in malignant pleural mesothelioma: ISRCTN 54469112. *Thorax* 2004; 59(2):144–8.

Price A. What is the role of radiotherapy in malignant pleural mesothelioma? *Oncologist* 2011 Mar; 16(3):359–65.

Rintoul RC, Ritchie AJ, Edwards JG, et al. Efficacy and cost of video-assisted thoracoscopic partial pleurectomy versus talc pleurodesis in patients with malignant pleural mesothelioma (MesoVATS): an open-label, randomised, controlled trial. *Lancet* 2014; 384(9948):1118.

Treasure T, Lang-Lazdunski L, Waller D, et al. Extra-pleural pneumonectomy versus no extra-pleural pneumonectomy for patients with malignant pleural mesothelioma: clinical outcomes of the mesothelioma and radical surgery (MARS) randomised feasibility study. *Lancet Oncol* 2011 Aug; 12(8):763–72.

Vogelzang NJ, Rusthoven JJ, Symanowski J, et al. Phase III study of pemetrexed in combination with cisplatin versus cisplatin alone in patients with malignant pleural mesothelioma. *J Clin Oncol* 2003 Jul 15; 21(14):2636–44.

Zalcman G, Mazieres J, Margery J, et al. Bevacizumab for newly diagnosed pleural mesothelioma in the Mesothelioma Avastin Cisplatin Pemetrexed Study (MAPS): a randomised, controlled, open-label, phase 3 trial. *Lancet* 2016; 387(10026);1405–14.

Internet resources
Cancer Research UK. Mesothelioma incidence statistics—available at http://www.cancerresearchuk.org/health-professional/cancer-statistics/statistics-by-cancer-type/mesothelioma/incidence#heading-Two

5.12 Thymic tumours

Introduction
Thymoma and thymic carcinoma are the most common tumours of the anterior mediastinum in adults, but are rare, accounting for less than 1% of primary neoplasms. Thymoma typically occurs in adults aged 40–70 years, and they are rarely seen in children. They comprise a spectrum of tumours, of low to moderate malignant potential. Approximately one-third of patients present with symptoms of local compression from the primary tumour, such as pain, shortness of breath, and superior vena cava obstruction; in a third of patients, the tumour is identified as an incidental finding. One-third of patients have symptoms caused by an associated autoimmune condition, usually myasthenia gravis. The presence of myasthenia gravis does not adversely influence survival in thymoma. By contrast, thymic carcinoma is rarely associated with autoimmune disease.

Staging
The Masaoka classification is used for the clinical staging of patients with thymic tumours, and is based on the anatomic extent of disease at the time of surgery:

- I: completely encapsulated
- IIA: microscopic invasion through the capsule into surrounding fatty tissue
- IIB: macroscopic invasion through the capsule
- IIIA: macroscopic invasion into pericardium or lung without great vessel invasion
- IIIB: macroscopic invasion into pericardium or lung with great vessel invasion

- IVA: extensive pleural or pericardial involvement
- IVB: distant (extrathoracic) metastases

Histology

The WHO histological classification subdivides thymic tumours into six different subtypes, as outlined below:

A: spindle cell thymoma—tumour composed of neoplastic thymic epithelial cells with spindle/oval shape.

AB: mixed thymoma—tumour with spindle/oval shaped cell and foci of lymphocytes.

B1: lymphocyte-rich thymoma—resembles the normal functional thymus with many lymphocytes and healthy thymic cells.

B2: cortical thymoma: with many lymphocytes but thymic cells do not appear healthy.

B3: atypical thymoma or well-differentiated thymic carcinoma—a few lymphocytes with abnormal thymic cells.

C: thymic carcinoma—exhibiting clear-cut cytological atypia and cytoarchitectural features not specific to the thymus.

Diagnosis

The definitive diagnostic approach varies according to stage. In patients where a thymic tumour is suspected, and the disease is potentially resectable, surgery is often undertaken without prior histological confirmation, as needle biopsy may result in tumour dissemination. The role of PET-CT is yet to be defined in thymic tumours, but there is some evidence that 18F-FDG uptake may predict the grade of malignancy.

Management

The management of thymic tumours is complex and requires a multidisciplinary approach by a team experienced in managing these cases. Surgery is the mainstay of treatment. Before surgery, patients should be evaluated for signs and symptoms of myasthenia gravis. Thymic resection may lead to myasthenic crisis and respiratory failure in patients with pre-existing untreated myasthenia gravis.

Stage I

By definition, stage I thymic tumours are encapsulated, and non-invasive, and are almost always resected completely. Five-year survival rates approach 100%, and recurrence rates are low. There is no benefit from adjuvant treatment. Late recurrences that are limited to the mediastinum or thorax can be treated by repeated re-excision.

Stage II

The gold standard treatment is complete resection. Generally, adjuvant radiotherapy is not recommended. It may be considered for patients at high risk for local recurrence, for example, close surgical margins, WHO type B, capsular invasion. Adjuvant chemotherapy is not recommended. Five-year survival is 86–95%.

Stage III–IV resectable

Neoadjuvant chemotherapy is often used in an attempt to increase the opportunity for resection. However, this approach is unproven, and the optimal chemotherapy regimen is unknown. In resectable disease, most international guidelines recommend adjuvant radiotherapy. Adjuvant chemotherapy may be considered, but again there is a lack of robust evidence to support this approach. Five-year survival is 56–69% (Figure 5.12.1).

Stage III–IV unresectable

Where radical surgery is not possible, chemotherapy and radiotherapy are often used, either alone sequentially or in combination. If a patient has a good response to initial therapy, surgery should be considered, with the aim of complete removal of the tumour. In cases where surgery is carried out, adjuvant radiotherapy should be considered, if not already given in the pre-operative setting. Five-year survival is 11–50% (Figure 5.12.2).

Chemotherapy

Generally, thymomas are considered to be chemosensitive. Active single agents include cisplatin, etoposide, ifosfamide, doxorubicin, and cyclophosphamide. Published studies are non-randomized and include small patient numbers.

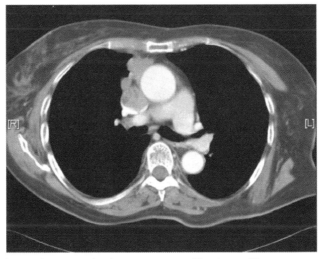

Fig 5.12.1 CT image showing a thymoma invading the superior vena cava (Masaoka stage III).

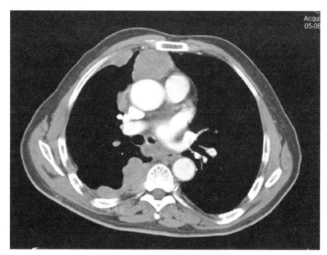

Fig 5.12.2 CT image showing a thymoma with diffuse pleural metastases (Masaoka stage IV).

Reported response rates for combination chemotherapy regimens range from 22% to over 90%. Examples of regimens used include cisplatin, doxorubicin, cyclophosphamide (CAP) and cisplatin, doxorubicin, vincristine, cyclophosphamide (ADOC). Newer agents such as sunitinib and the mTOR inhibitors tacrolimus and sirolimus have shown activity but require further evaluation and are currently not the standard of care.

Radiotherapy

There are no prospective randomized trials to guide treatment. In the preoperative setting, a dose of 40–45Gy can be administered in once-daily fractions of 1.8–2.0Gy. The dose used for postoperative radiation is generally 50Gy, while doses of up to 60Gy are used for patients with incompletely excised tumours and those with inoperable tumours. There is little good evidence to support irradiation of uninvolved mediastinal or supraclavicular nodal regions, nor for hemithorax radiotherapy to prevent pleural metastases.

Further reading

Scorsetti M, Leo F, Trama A, et al. Thymoma and thymic carcinomas. *Crit Rev Oncol Hematol* 2016; 99:332–50.

Breast cancer

Chapter contents

6.1 Breast cancer overview

Epidemiology

Breast cancer (BC) is the most frequent cancer in women, with an incidence that varies worldwide, being highest in North America and Europe (92 cases per 100,000) and lowest in sub-Saharan Africa and Asia (27 cases per 100,000). These geographic variations are related to environmental factors, ethnicity, and level of industrialization, explaining the rising incidence in Japan, India, and China.

Although mortality rates have been decreasing in the last 50 years, it remains the leading cause of death in women in less developed countries (14% of total cancer mortality (source: GLOBOCAN)). In these countries, 50–65% of cases are diagnosed at an advanced stage (stage III or IV), compared to 10–15% of patients in Western countries.

The five-year survival for breast cancer patients reaches 80% in most developed countries, compared with 60% in Algeria, South Africa, Jordan, and Mongolia.

Male breast cancer remains a rare disease, with an incidence of 1% of all breast cancer diagnoses and 1% of all cancers in males.

Aetiology and risk factors

Hormonal and reproductive risk factors

Oestrogen exposure and high endogenous oestrogen levels increase the risk for breast cancer; therefore, women with early menarche and late menopause are more likely to develop the disease.

Nulliparity and increased age at first pregnancy are linked to an increased risk. Studies on infertility have been controversial, showing both a protective or detrimental effect on breast cancer risk.

The use of exogenous hormones (hormone replacement therapy or HRT) is associated with an increase of breast cancer risk by 2.3% in menopausal women, even though a meta-analysis of prospective studies failed to show statistical significance. Current guidelines recommend an individualized approach and HRT is not recommended for patients with risk factors for breast cancer. Patients should be screened for breast cancer before starting treatment.

Some studies link in-utero exposure to diethylstilboestrol (DES), elevated androgen levels, or diabetes to breast cancer, but it has not been yet consistently demonstrated.

Genetic risk factors

Based on Surveillance, Epidemiology, and End Results (SEER) data, there is a 4% risk of contralateral breast cancer in women with a personal history of ductal carcinoma in situ (DCIS) or invasive breast cancer, and a relative risk of two to three for women with one or two first-degree relatives with breast cancer. Regardless of family history, patients with triple negative breast cancer (TNBC), male breast cancer, and ovarian/primary peritoneal cancers should raise suspicion of an inherited susceptibility.

Specific genetic mutations (BRCA1, BRCA2, p53, ATM, and PTEN) are linked to 5–6% of all breast cancers. The prevalence of the BRCA gene mutation is higher in the Ashkenazi Jewish population, and in Iceland, The Netherlands, northern countries, Germany, France, and south-eastern European countries, providing a cumulative risk of 55–60% for breast cancer and 16–59% for ovarian cancer, with a higher lifetime risk for BRCA1 mutations carriers. Male carriers have an increased risk of breast, prostate, pancreatic, and colorectal cancer.

It has been estimated that a mutation in CHEK2 increases the risk of breast cancer by between 1.5- and three-fold.

TP53 mutation (Li–Fraumeni syndrome), PTEN mutation (Cowden syndrome), CDH1 mutation (hereditary diffuse gastric cancer syndrome), and STK11 mutation (Peutz–Jeghers syndrome) account for a small proportion of inherited breast cancer, the link between MMR genes mutation (Lynch syndrome) and breast cancer being controversial.

Lifestyle risk factors

A 2013 meta-analysis of 110 studies showed a small but significant increased risk with alcohol intake.

Active or passive smoking has also been associated with a modest increase in breast cancer risk.

International Agency for Research on Cancer (IARC)/ World Health Organization (WHO) recognized night-shift work to be a risk factor for breast cancer, due to the suppression of nocturnal melatonin production.

Radiation exposure

Exposure to ionizing radiation at a young age, i.e. prior to 45 years (atomic bomb/nuclear plant, cancer treatments) carries a 13–20% risk of developing breast cancer.

Protective factors

Breastfeeding and physical activity protect from breast cancer, the latter providing protection especially in postmenopausal women.

The role of other protective factors such as a Mediterranean diet, phytoestrogens, antioxidants, or calcium/vitamin D intake is still controversial.

Screening

Breast cancer screening recommendations vary depending on the risk factors and include clinical examination, mammography, and magnetic resonance imaging (MRI).

Screening with clinical examination

For women between 20 and 40 years old, breast self-examination is recommended especially for high-risk patients, clinical examination being recommended every one to three years, or immediately if the patient identifies a suspicious nodule.

Screening with mammography

Mammography screening seems to be mostly beneficial on mortality reduction for women between 50 and 69 years old and biannual screening is recommended.

The effect in the 40 and 49-year old age group is controversial and, for these women, shared decision-making and risk factors should be taken into consideration and, if needed, annual screening undertaken.

Screening with breast MRI

Breast MRI and mammography are recommended for high-risk patients, for whom annual screening should start at age 35 or ten years earlier than the youngest case in the family:

- Known BRCA, TP53, or PTEN mutation carriers
- First-degree relatives with BRCA mutation
- Radiation to the chest in childhood

Paget's disease

Paget's disease is a condition of the areolar region of the breast that, in 80% of cases, is associated with an in situ or invasive breast cancer.

Clinical presentation is an ulcerated lesion of the nipple that spreads to the areolar region, sometimes associated with a clear exudate or blood discharge, rarely with nipple retraction and commonly associated with burning sensation or pruritus.

Mammography abnormalities can be present in about 50% of cases, including suspicious microcalcifications, mass, or architectural distortion. In patients with mammographically occult lesions, breast MRI can be more sensitive.

Skin biopsy is needed for diagnosis, identifying intraepithelial adenocarcinoma cells (Paget cells) in the epidermis.

Treatment is usually breast-conserving therapy followed by whole breast radiation therapy, though some patients may need mastectomy especially for multifocal disease. The management of the axilla depends on the features of the underlying disease.

Prognosis depends on the underlying malignancy and the presence of positive axillary lymph nodes.

Further reading

National Comprehensive Cancer Network (NCCN). Clinical Practice Guidelines. Breast cancer screening and diagnosis 2015.

Senkus E, Kyriakides S, Ohno S, Penault-Llorca F, Poortmans P, Rutgers E, et al. Primary breast cancer: ESMO Clinical Practice Guidelines for diagnosis, treatment and follow-up. *Ann Oncol* 2015 Sep; 26 (Suppl. 5):v8–30—available at http://www.ncbi.nlm.nih.gov/pubmed/26314782

6.2 Clinical presentation, diagnosis, and staging of breast cancer

Clinical findings

Most breast cancers are diagnosed during screening but, in some cases, various signs and symptoms may be present (Table 6.2.1).

Diagnosis

In case of suspected breast cancer, further steps for diagnosis include: clinical examination, breast imaging, and biopsy.

Clinical examination

A proper examination includes:

- In the sitting and supine positions both breasts and axillary/supraclavicular regions should be examined for masses. A description of the mass/lymph node size, location, mobility, and associated skin changes should be documented to assess the clinical tumour stage.
- A complete clinical examination should be performed to identify signs of metastatic disease.

Breast imaging

- Mammography evaluation identifies most breast cancers and is part of the initial diagnostic work-up when

there is a suspicion of malignancy. It generally identifies two major categories of abnormality:
  - A soft tissue mass or distortions in breast architecture (90% represent invasive cancer)
  - Clustered microcalcifications can be detected mammographically in 60% of breast cancers, representing intraductal calcifications (0.1mm to 1mm). They are more frequent in DCIS of comedo histology
- The mammographic findings are graded using the BI-RADS system, and managed accordingly:
  - Score 0 (incomplete): needs additional evaluations
  - Score 1–2 (negative or benign): routine screening
  - Score 3 (probably benign): close follow-up
  - Score 4–5 (suspicious or high probability of cancer): biopsy
  - Score 6 (malignancy): excision
- Ultrasonography (US) is generally used as a complimentary investigation to evaluate the breast or the axilla.
- Breast US is used to differentiate between a solid and a cystic mass that was previously identified either by mammography or clinical examination; to identify the possibility of performing a US-guided biopsy and to

Table 6.2.1 Signs and symptoms of breast cancer

Signs	Symptoms
Breast mass (hard, lack of mobility)	Breast pain
Axillary/supraclavicular adenopathy (hard, lack of mobility)	Asthenia
Skin changes (erythema, thickening, 'peau d'orange', local heat, ulceration, or skin/nipple retraction)	Weight loss
	Abdominal pain
Signs of metastatic disease (jaundice, increased liver, cutaneous metastasis, etc.)	Nausea
	Dyspnoea, cough
	Symptoms of raised intracranial hypertension
	Bone pain/fracture

measure and mark (with clips or carbon) a breast lesion before neoadjuvant treatment.

- Axillary US is used to identify and characterize suspicious axillary lymph nodes, or to guide biopsies of suspicious areas.
- Breast MRI has a sensitivity of identifying breast carcinoma of 88–100% and specificity of 70%. It has a 98% sensitivity for identifying high-grade DCIS, but with low specificity. The recommendations for its use are limited and include:
  - High-risk patients
  - Lobular cancers
  - Multifocal breast tumours
  - Positive axillary lymph nodes without an identified breast mass
  - Paget's disease with a negative mammogram
  - In selected cases, it can be used before reconstructive surgery to evaluate the contralateral breast
  - Before and after neoadjuvant treatment and to evaluate the response to systemic treatment

Biopsy

When there is a high suspicion of malignancy, either clinically or on mammography, a biopsy must be done to confirm or disprove the diagnosis. Several methods can be used:

- Fine needle biopsy—is less used as it cannot differentiate between histological types.
- Core needle biopsy—is performed using image- or palpation-guidance, using a larger diameter device, able to extract tissue for pathology and immunohistochemistry assessments. Depending on tumour visibility, stereotactic-, US-, or MRI-guided biopsies can be performed. During the procedure, a marker (clips or carbon) should be placed in the region of the lesion, in case surgery is required and or there is a complete response to neoadjuvant treatment.

Pathology diagnosis

Most breast cancers are carcinomas as they arise from the epithelial cells. However, there are multiple histological types, which present different clinical behaviours.

- DCIS—is characterized by a proliferation of the epithelial cells in the ductal system of the breast, without invasion of the surrounding tissue.
- Infiltrating ductal carcinoma—is the most common type of breast cancer (70–80%), divided into three grades (well, moderately, and poorly differentiated) based on cytological and microscopic features.
- Infiltrating lobular carcinoma—comprise up to 10% of invasive carcinomas, mostly oestrogen receptor positive (ER+), bilateral, or multicentric. Patients with CDH1 mutation appear to have a higher risk of developing lobular breast carcinoma. It is usually associated with a less aggressive biology.
- Other histological types include:
  - Tubular carcinoma
  - Mucinous carcinoma
  - Medullary carcinoma
  - Tubulolobular carcinoma
  - Micropapillary carcinoma
  - Metaplastic carcinoma
  - Adenoid cystic carcinoma

Staging

The preoperative clinical staging of breast cancer relies on clinical examination and measurements, breast imaging (mammography, breast, and axillary ultrasound, breast MRI) and also on evaluation of distant metastasis using abdominal echography, chest X-ray (CXR) or computed tomography scan (Table 6.2.2).

Recently, the American Joint Committee on Cancer (AJCC) has incorporated evidence-based biological factors such as tumour grade, proliferation rate, oestrogen and progesterone receptor expression, human epidermal growth factor 2 (HER2) expression, and gene expression profiling, deriving a prognostic stage aiming to improve accuracy in the staging classification (Table 6.2.3).

Risk assessment

In the early stage setting the risk of local and distant recurrence of the disease will determine treatment strategy. All cases should be discussed in a multidisciplinary meeting before any treatment. Several prognostic and predictive factors are used to stratify patients.

Pathological factors

- Tumour size—is an independent prognostic factor. Patients with T3 tumours have a 60% five-year survival according to the SEER database, compared with 90% in T1. Inflammatory breast cancers also carry a worse prognosis. Moreover, size is correlated with the extent of axillary invasion.
- Axillary nodal status—is one of the strongest and most independent negative prognostic factors for recurrence in early stage breast cancer. The five-year survival is >80.2% in N0 patients, compared with 73% for 1–3 positive nodes, 45.7% for 4–12 positive nodes, and 28.4% in those with >13 nodes involved.
- Tumour grade—according to the Elston–Ellis grading system, breast tumours can be stratified into three groups (from 1, well differentiated to 3, poorly differentiated) taking into account the mitotic index, tubule formation, and nuclear pleomorphism. Grade 3 tumours have a four times higher risk of recurrence compared with grade 1.
- Lymphatic and vascular invasion (LVI)—especially when associated with a high-grade tumour, LVI is an independently negative risk factor for local recurrence, although it has limited clinical utility.
- Ki67—higher Ki67 (>20%) expression is associated with increased tumour proliferation and higher risk of relapse and breast cancer death (HR=2.5) regardless of ER status. However, its use as a prognostic index is controversial, due to methodological issues, including cut-off definition, and heterogeneity of the laboratory procedures that lack analytical validity.
- Oestrogen/progesterone status—ER/PR+ breast cancers are associated with better prognosis, and are also predictive of response to endocrine treatment. The five-year disease-free survival (DFS) women with ER+ tumours is reported to be 74% compared with 66% in ER– and overall survival (OS) 92% compared with 82%. The American Society of Clinical Oncology (ASCO)/College of American Pathologists (CAP) guidelines define ER/PR positivity if found in >1% of

Table 6.2.2 Breast cancer staging (clinical and pathological)

T (tumour)—clinical and pathological		
Tis	Carcinoma in situ	
T1	Tumour <20mm	
	T1a—tumour between 1–5mm	
	T1b—tumour between 5–10mm	
	T1c—tumour between 10–20mm	
T2	Tumour between 20–50mm	
T3	Tumour >50mm	
T4	Tumour of any size with direct extension to the chest wall and/or to the skin	
	T4a—extension to chest wall, not including only pectoralis muscle adherence/invasion	
	T4b—ulceration and/or ipsilateral satellite nodules and/or oedema (including peau d'orange) of the skin	
	T4c—both T4a and T4b	
	T4d—inflammatory carcinoma	
N (lymph nodes)—clinical		**Pathological**
N1	Movable ipsilateral metastasis in level I, II axillary lymph nodes (ALN)	Micrometastases/metastases in 1–3 ALN and/or in internal mammary nodes, with metastases detected by sentinel lymph node biopsy (SLNB) but not clinically detected as follows:
		pN1a—1–3 ALNs, at least one deposit >2mm
		pN1b—ipsilateral internal mammary nodes involved
		pN1c—pN1a and pN1b combined
N2	Clinically fixed metastases in ipsilateral level I, II ALN, or ipsilateral internal mammary nodes without clinically evident ALN	Metastases in 4–9 ALN or in internal mammary lymph nodes in the absence of ALN
	N2a—fixed ipsilateral level I, II ALN	pN2a—4–9 ALN
	N2b—ipsilateral internal mammary nodes and no clinical ALN	pN2b—internal mammary lymph nodes and no axillary ALN
N3	Metastases in ipsilateral infraclavicular (level III axillary) lymph node(s), +/− level I, II ALN/ ipsilateral internal mammary lymph node(s) in the presence of clinically evident level I, II axillary lymph node metastasis; or metastasis in ipsilateral supraclavicular lymph nodes, with or without axillary or internal mammary lymph node involvement	Metastases in ≥10 ALN/infraclavicular lymph nodes/ ipsilateral internal mammary lymph nodes in the presence of ≥1 positive level I, II ALN; or in >3 axillary lymph nodes and internal mammary lymph nodes, with micrometastases or macrometastases detected by SLNB but not clinically detected/in ipsilateral supraclavicular lymph nodes
	N3a—ipsilateral infraclavicular lymph nodes	pN3a—≥10 ALN/infraclavicular nodes
	N3b—ipsilateral internal mammary and axillary lymph nodes	pN3b—ipsilateral internal mammary lymph nodes in the presence of ≥1 positive ALN/>3 ALN and in internal mammary lymph nodes
	N3c—ipsilateral supraclavicular lymph nodes	pN3c—ipsilateral supraclavicular lymph nodes
Stage	**TNM**	
0	TisN0M0	
IA	T1N0M0	
IB	T0-1N1M0	
IIA	TxN1M0, T1N1M0, T2N0M0	
IIB	T2N1M0, T3N0M0	
IIIA	Tx–2N2M0, T2–3N1–2M0	

Source: data from Amin MB, Edge S, Greene F, et al. (eds). *AJCC Cancer Staging Manua, 8th edn.* Springer International Publishing. 2017, American College of Surgeons.

the tumour cells. High positivity for these markers is also predictive of lesser sensitivity to chemotherapy.

• HER2/neu—the overexpression of HER2 is found in about 20–30% of breast cancers and represents a more aggressive biology with higher risk of recurrence and mortality compared with other BC subtypes, especially before the era of anti-HER2 agents. It is a predictive marker of response to these agents.

• Urokinase plasminogen activator (uPA)—is a protease linked to cancer invasion and distant metastasis.

Table 6.2.3 AJCC prognostic staging system—8th edition (Breast)

T is	N is	M is	G is	HER2 is	ER is	PR is	Prognostic stage group	Anatomic stage group
Multigene panel—oncotype Dx RS <11 or mammaprint/PAM50/endopredict/BCI								
T1–2	N0	M0	1–3	negative	positive	any	IA	IA/IB/IIA
T2	N1	M0	1	negative	positive	positive	IB	IIB
T2	N1	M0	2	positive	positive	positive	IB	IIB
T0–2	N2	M0	1–2	positive	positive	positive	IB	IIIA
T3	N1–2	M0	1	positive	positive	positive	IB	IIIA
T3	N1–2	M0	2	positive	positive	positive	IB	IIIA
T1	N0	M0	1	negative	negative	negative	IIA	IA
T1	N0	M0	2	negative	negative	negative	IIA	IA
T1	N0	M0	3	negative	positive	negative	IIA	IA
T1	N0	M0	3	negative	negative	positive	IIA	IA
T1	N0	M0	3	negative	negative	negative	IIA	IA
T0–2	N2	M0	1	negative	positive	positive	IIA	IIIA
T0–1	N1	M0	2	negative	negative	negative	IIIA	IIA
T2	N0	M0	2	negative	negative	negative	IIIA	IIA
T2	N0	M0	3	negative	positive	negative	IIIA	IIA
T2	N0	M0	3	negative	positive	any	IIIA	IIA
any	N3	M0	1	negative	positive	positive	IIIA	IIIC
T2	N1	M0	1–2	negative	negative	negative	IIIB	IIB
T2	N1	M0	3	negative	positive	negative	IIIB	IIB
T2	N1	M0	3	negative	negative	any	IIIC	IIB
T0–2	N2	M0	2	negative	negative	negative	IIIC	IIIA
T0–2	N2	M0	3	negative	positive	negative	IIIC	IIIA
T0–2	N2	M0	3	negative	negative	any	IIIC	IIIA
T3	N1–2	M0	2	negative	negative	negative	IIIC	IIIA
T3	N1–2	M0	3	negative	positive	negative	IIIC	IIIA
T3	N1–2	M0	3	negative	negative	any	IIIC	IIIA

Source: data from Amin MB, edge S, Greene F, et al. (eds). *AJCC Cancer Staging Manual,* 8th edn. Springer International Publishing. 2017, American College of Surgeons.

High levels of uPA have been associated with reduced survival, offering possible prognostic and predictive information, especially in N0 patients. Its clinical use is currently limited, as there is no standardized assessment method.

Other factors

• Circulating tumour cells (CTCs)—have been associated with a worse prognosis and a higher risk of relapse, but they are not routinely used in clinical practice yet.

• p53 mutations—are found in about 20–30% of breast cancer tumours, frequently associated with more aggressive features. Its clinical utility is not proved and testing should be limited to patients with hereditary breast cancer through referral to a genetic clinic. Tumour markers like carcinoembryonic antigen (CEA) and CA15-3 have a limited role due to their low sensitivity and specificity, although they may correlate with tumour burden. However, their use in evaluating treatment response if initially elevated is quite helpful.

- Other—the role of other markers such as microsatellite instability, E-cadherin, and tissue inhibitors of metalloproteinases are still controversial.

Prognostic predictive tools

Various multivariate prediction models have been created to help clinicians estimate individual risk of recurrence. Adjuvant Online or PREDICT are tools that can assist healthcare professionals in assessing the risks and benefits from adjuvant treatment after surgery for early breast cancer patients. Its risk assessments are based on information regarding patient's age, comorbidities, and tumour information about pathology characteristics. The risk estimates are derived from results of clinical trials gathered into a mathematical model. The performance of this model is, however, inadequate and new tools were recently developed based on genomic analysis of breast tumours, recognized as molecular breast cancer signatures.

Molecular characterization of breast cancer

The limited performance of the classical clinicopathological factors in assessment of risk in breast cancer such as tumour size, lymph node invasion, tumour grade, ER, and HER2, led to a search for additional prognostic and predictive tools.

Genomic analysis is available now and gathers information from multiple genes related to ER activity, proliferation, and others, into a multivariate molecular model that can be prognostic and/or predictive.

The seminal work by Sorlie and Perou et al. that evaluated gene expression by cDNA microarray studies, recognized four major intrinsic subtypes of breast cancer with different clinical outcomes: Luminal A, Luminal B, HER2 overexpression, and basal-like tumours.

This classification reflects different biology of the subtypes based on heterogeneity at the molecular level. This includes variation in growth rate, activity of different signalling pathways, and type of cells that compose the tumour (basal or luminal epithelial cells, endothelial cells, mesenchymal and lymphocyte derived).

Additionally, The Cancer Genome Atlas project (TCGA), a large study on single genome sequencing, identified the presence of specific gene mutations in the different subtypes (TP53, PI3KCA, PTEN, AKT1, etc.). The molecular subtypes offer prognostic and predictive information regarding systemic treatment for each group.

A correlation was found between the classification derived by genomic assays and the classic variables that combine ER, PR, HER2, grade, and Ki67 levels and has been used clinically as a surrogate for the molecular classification.

Luminal A

It is the most frequent subtype, characterized by Luminal expression: high expression of hormone receptors or oestrogen regulated genes (ER, PR), GATA-binding protein 3 (GATA3), Bcl-2, forkhead box protein 1 (FOXA1), myeloblastosis gene (MYB), X-nox binding protein-1 (XBP1), and CK 18/8. In terms of conventional pathology this translates into grade 1, highly positive ER/PR+, absence of HER2 expression, and low proliferation rate (Ki67 < 15%). This subtype is very responsive to endocrine treatment, has low sensitivity to chemotherapy, and presents a good long-term prognosis.

Luminal B

It is a Luminal type tumour but compared to Luminal A, Luminal B tumours have lower expression levels of ER or of oestrogen regulated genes, lower or no progesterone receptor (i.e. lower Luminal expression), higher levels of proliferation related genes, higher grade, and activation of growth factor receptor signalling pathways, such as IGF-1R and PI3K/AKT/mTOR. There is an increased expression of proliferation genes such as cyclin B1 or MKI67.

The most frequent somatic mutations in breast tumours are TP53 and PI3KCA. Luminal B tumours have a higher percentage of TP53 mutations (29%) compared with the A subtype, which is closer to the frequency seen in more aggressive subtypes such as basal-like and HER2+. On the other hand, PI3KCA mutations are more frequent in Luminal A subtype (45%) and are indicative of a less aggressive biology. As a result, Luminal B tumours have a poorer clinical outcome with worse response to endocrine treatment compared with Luminal A and increased sensitivity to chemotherapy. Conventional pathology surrogates include: ER positivity, PR positive or negative, HER2 negativity or positivity, and Ki67 higher than 15%. However, it can be difficult to obtain clinically reproducible Ki67 levels unless high or low levels are present. For intermediate levels, genomic assays are needed to better define prognosis and likely benefit from chemotherapy, i.e. to differentiate between Luminal A versus B disease if there are intermediate or uncertain Ki67 levels.

HER2 enriched

HER2 positivity is found in 20–30% of breast tumours and the main characteristic in the expression of high levels of HER2 is amplification of the Erb-B2 cluster genes. In TCGA two subgroups have been identified: HER2 enriched (about 50%) and Luminal. The first has strong EGFR and HER2 signalling activation and high sensitivity to HER2 targeted therapy. They were also associated with high frequency of TP53 mutations (75%), amplification CCND1, CDK4 gain, MDM2, FGFR, and EGFR amplification. The Luminal subtype has enriched expression of Luminal cluster genes (GATA3, BCL2, ESR1, GATA3 mutations). Mutations of HER2, EGFR, and HER3 are rarely seen in this subtype, where PI3KCA mutation (39%) is more frequently seen. At the pathological level they usually lack ER expression but can also be ER+, have high grade, and high Ki67 levels. The biology of this disease is aggressive, but improved survival has been seen with anti-HER2 therapy to which these tumours are very sensitive. They also benefit from chemotherapy.

Triple negative breast cancers (TNBC)

These are characterized by expression of basal (myoepithelial) cells, i.e. CK5, 6 and 17 and high-level expression of proliferation genes. TP53 mutations are seen in 80%. They represent 15% of breast tumours and pathology reveals lack of ER, PR, HER2 receptors, and high grade. However, gene expression analysis reveals heterogeneity between TNBC, and divides them into six subtypes, offering a better insight into biological features and clinical behaviour, as well as offering potential treatment targets for future research. These molecular subtypes include:

- Basal-like (BL1 and BL2): express CK5/6, p-cadherin, CD44, and EGFR; they frequently have p53 and BRCA1 mutations. Potential benefit for PARP inhibitors or platinum agents needs to be explored in this setting. BL1 tumours seem to respond better to chemotherapy and have a higher pathological complete response (pCR) rate but further prospective studies are needed.

- Immunomodulatory: presents alterations in the immune system transduction pathways.
- Mesenchymal and mesenchymal stem-like: are associated with a claudin low subtype, overexpressing epithelial-mesenchymal transition and immune response markers, and lacking expression of E-cadherin. It seems to be associated with better clinical outcome.
- Luminal androgen receptor (AR)—frequently harbour PI3KCA mutations: are AR positive and have a lower response to chemotherapy.

The prognostic impact of the intrinsic subtypes has been demonstrated in large retrospective studies and several assays are currently available to classify breast tumours molecularly. They are already in clinical use for patients for whom the benefit of chemotherapy is not certain when estimated by the classical variables, i.e. ER+ disease, N0 or N+ with up to three nodes involved, grade 2, and with an intermediate Ki67 level. The most used genomic assays are as follows.

MammaPrint-70®

This prognostic assay measures the mRNA expression of 70 genes and classifies tumours into low- or high-risk groups. It has been tested in large retrospective studies of ER+, N0/+ disease. It is in use clinically in the United States and Europe for risk evaluation in women under 61, early stage (I/II), ER+, N0/+ disease (up to three lymph nodes invaded). The MINDACT trial proved the clinical utility of MammaPrint in selected early BC patients who can be safely spared adjuvant chemotherapy (about 46% of clinically characterized high-risk patients can avoid chemotherapy if their MammaPrint risk is low). It was the first genomic test with level 1A evidence for a chemotherapy decision.

Oncotype DX®

This widely used prognostic microarray assay, evaluates the expression of 21 genes. It was tested in large retrospective studies of ER+ patients, N0, or N+. The result of the assay is summarized in a score that categorizes patients into low risk (score <18), intermediate risk (score 18 to 30), and high risk (score >30) for relapse. The benefit of chemotherapy is seen only if there is a high-risk score and is uncertain for intermediate risk. In the prospective study TAILORx 1,626 women with low-risk oncotype DX score received endocrine treatment only, and had an excellent five-year DFS of 93.8% and OS of 98%. Patients with intermediate risk were randomized to receive chemotherapy or not, plus ET. The study met its primary endpoint of ET non-inferiority in the intermediate-risk group with similar nine-year DFS between the two groups (83.3% vs. 84.3%).

Prosigna®

This assay uses mRNA expression of 50 genes (PAM-50) and was approved in the United States and Europe in 2013. It generates a score of high, intermediate, and low risk (PAM50 ROR score). This assay is predictive for both early and late recurrences (>5 years), which is important to select patients for extended adjuvant treatment.

EndoPredict®

This is an RNA-based multigene test that assesses the risk of recurrence in ER+/HER2–/N+ patients who have undergone adjuvant endocrine therapy. It classifies patients into low or high risk of recurrence if treated with ET alone, based on EPClin scores that combine nodal status and tumour size with the molecular results. This score was assessed in retrospective analysis from two randomized phase 3 trials (ABCSG6 and ABCSG8). Additional data from the GEICAM 9906 trial showed that EndoPredict could be an independent prognostic tool in ER+/HER2–/N+ pre- and postmenopausal patients who underwent adjuvant chemotherapy and sequential endocrine therapy. It seems to be predictive of late recurrence.

Further reading

Amin MB, Edge S, Greene F, Byrd DR, Brookland RK, Washington MK, Gershenwald JE, Compton CC, Hess KR, et al. (eds). *AJCC Cancer Staging Manual*, 8th edn. Springer International Publishing: American Joint Commission on Cancer, 2017.

Coates AS, Winer EP, Goldhirsch A, Gelber RD, Gnant M. Tailoring therapies—improving the management of early breast cancer: St Gallen International Expert Consensus on the Primary Therapy of Early Breast Cancer 2015. *Ann Oncol* 2015; 26:1533–46.

Győrffy B, Hatzis C, Sanft T, Hofstatter E, Aktas B, Pusztai L. Multigene prognostic tests in breast cancer: past, present, future. *Breast Cancer Research: BCR* 2015; 17(1):11.

Piccart M, Rutgers E, van't Veer L, et al. Primary analysis of the EORTC 10041/ BIG 3-04 MINDACT study: a prospective, randomized study evaluating the clinical utility of the 70-gene signature (MammaPrint) combined with common clinical-pathological criteria for selection of patients for adjuvant chemotherapy in breast cancer with 0 to 3 positive nodes. Presented at AACR Annual Meeting 2016, New Orleans; 16–20 April 2016. Abstract CT-039.

Senkus E, Kyriakides S, Ohno S, Penault-Llorca F, Poortmans P, Rutgers E, et al. Primary breast cancer: ESMO Clinical Practice Guidelines for diagnosis, treatment and follow-up. *Ann Oncol* 2015 Sep; 26 (Suppl. 5):v8–30—available at http://www.ncbi.nlm.nih.gov/pubmed/26314782

The Cancer Genome Atlas Network. Comprehensive molecular portraits of human breast tumors. *Nature* 2012; 490(7418):61–70.

Internet resources

Predict Breast Cancer: https://breast.predict.nhs.uk/

6.3 Management of breast cancer: Carcinoma in situ

Ductal carcinoma in situ (DCIS)

DCIS represents a heterogeneous group of low- to high-grade lesions that arise from the proliferation of epithelial cells from the breast ducts. Its detection has increased with screening by mammography and peaks at age 60–74 years but fewer than 20% of screen-detected breast cancers are DCIS. The risk of death or metastatic disease in DCIS patients is <1% and the main reason for treatment is to reduce the risk of invasive breast cancer.

With an appropriate treatment approach, these patients have an excellent prognosis; the 20-year mortality is 3.3%, according to the SEER database.

Associated risk factors are breast density, family history, and/or genetics (BRCA1/2 genes) and nulliparity.

Diagnosis

DCIS is often asymptomatic and is found during routine mammography, but it can also be associated with Paget's disease and nipple discharge, or felt as a small lump in the breast. The risk factors for DCIS are similar to those of invasive carcinoma.

Mammography findings include microcalcifications in >90% of the cases. The role of breast MRI is debatable, due to its low specificity. It may be used to identify multicentric disease or lesions in the contralateral breast. A meta-analysis has shown that breast MRI is not associated with improvement in surgical outcomes.

Pathology

The diagnosis should be confirmed by biopsy (stereotactic or core-biopsy). The pathology report classifies DCIS according to architectural pattern (solid, papillary, micropapillary, cribriform, comedo), tumour grade (low, intermediate, or high grade), and the presence or absence of comedo necrosis. The report should also include status of margins, ER status, and tumour size. Although HER2 overexpression may be associated with an increased risk of recurrence, it should not be routinely tested and anti-HER2 therapy is not indicated.

Surgery

Either mastectomy or breast conserving surgery (BCS) are surgical options for patients with DCIS, with good long-term clinical outcomes.

- Mastectomy gives a five-year DFS of 95% and a ten-year OS of 86%. However, it is associated with higher morbidity compared with BCS and should be only considered if there is extensive disease, low probability of free margins, or multicentric disease. The benefit of contralateral prophylactic mastectomy for high-risk DCIS has not been clearly assessed. Reconstructive surgery should be performed.
- Breast conserving surgery has a better cosmetic outcome and lower morbidity if negative margins (no ink/invasive carcinoma/DCIS on specimen, according to St. Gallen guidelines) are achieved.
- Sentinel lymph node biopsy (SLNB) is not generally recommended for DCIS, except for those cases associated with invasive or microinvasive disease. Only 10–15% of initial DCIS have invasive cancer in the mastectomy specimen, which may require axillary staging. As SLNB is not feasible after mastectomy, it should be considered in high-grade DCIS, large tumour size, aggressive histology, or if the patient will undergo a mastectomy.

Radiation therapy (RT)

Randomized trials such as NSABP-17, EORTC 10853, and UKCCCR have shown that RT after BCS is safe and reduces the risk of all recurrences (DCIS and invasive carcinoma recurrence) in up to 50% when compared with no RT treatment, with no impact on non-breast cancer mortality. However, treating all women with RT after BCT may not be beneficial when the risk of local recurrence is low. The debate on whether RT can be omitted in patients with low-risk disease with negative margins is ongoing.

Chemoprevention

The role of chemoprevention in DCIS is to reduce risk of invasive carcinoma in the contralateral breast. Tamoxifen (20mg/day) or letrozole (2.5mg/day) have shown benefit in reducing the risk.

- Endocrine treatment based on menopausal status is an option after surgery for most women, especially those without bilateral mastectomy.
- The protective role of hormone therapy in ER negative patients is still unknown.
- Endocrine treatment for five years reduces the risk of DCIS and invasive carcinoma, without influencing mortality (NSABP B-24/B-35 trials).
- Treatment with a low dose of tamoxifen (5mg per day/5 years) after surgery halved the risk of disease recurrence and new disease and did not cause more serious adverse in the phase 3 TAM-01 trial. It represents a new treatment option for these patients.

Lobular carcinoma in situ (LCIS)

LCIS is considered to be a benign lesion arising from the terminal duct-lobular units of the breast, providing an additional risk for invasive cancer in both ipsilateral and contralateral breasts. It is mostly diagnosed in premenopausal women and is frequently multifocal or bilateral.

Diagnosis and pathology

It is usually discovered in a biopsy specimen and may be associated with other benign or malignant lesions. Using imaging techniques, LCIS may be suggested by microcalcifications, architectural distortion, or, in rare cases, a mass. Whether breast MRI can provide a more accurate diagnosis of LCIS is still debatable, as its specificity is limited, especially in young women.

Most tumours are associated with ER overexpression, suggesting a hormonal influence in its development. Moreover, molecular features and genetic alterations, similar to the luminal subtype, can be identified.

Treatment

Although in most cases surveillance or chemoprevention is indicated, in the presence of additional risk factors, surgical treatment is recommended. In 30–40% of cases, DCIS can be associated.

In the presence of invasive carcinoma, BCS is an option, as current data have failed to demonstrate an increased risk with a conservative approach. Aggressive surgical treatment such as bilateral mastectomy is not recommended.

Chemoprevention for five years with endocrine therapy (tamoxifen or aromatase inhibitors) is recommended in patients with LCIS, according to menopausal status.

Further reading

Coates AS, Winer EP, Goldhirsch A, Gelber RD, Gnant M. Tailoring therapies—improving the management of early breast cancer: St Gallen International Expert Consensus on the Primary Therapy of Early Breast Cancer 2015. *Ann Oncol* 2015; 26:1533–46.

Virnig B, Tuttle T, Shamliyan T, Kane R. Ductal carcinoma in situ of the breast: a systematic review on incidence, treatment and outcomes. *J Natl Cancer Inst* 2010; 102(3):170–8.

6.4 Loco-regional treatment of invasive breast cancer: Surgery

Introduction

Surgery is a mandatory treatment for early breast cancer and BCS associated with breast RT is the gold standard, as this approach offers similar survival benefits to mastectomy but with better quality of life. Moreover, improved responses after neoadjuvant treatments have widened the possibility for breast conserving surgery, especially in specialized centres.

Surgery of the breast

Breast conserving surgery

For BCS, randomized trials have proved that adjuvant RT of the breast is mandatory to achieve similar OS and DFS benefits to mastectomy.

Contraindications for BCS include:
- Contraindication for RT
- Positive margins (ink/invasive carcinoma/DCIS on the specimen) after multiple re-excisions

Previous RT to the chest wall, an active connective tissue disorder (lupus, scleroderma, etc.), and tumours >5cm represent relative contraindications.

Multifocal disease no longer represents a contraindication for BCS, according to the 14th St. Gallen and SSO-ASRO Consensus.

Margins

Negative margins must be achieved with BCS. National Comprehensive Cancer Network (NCCN), St. Gallen, and SSO-ASRO consider negative margins as no ink present on tumour.

Positive margins are associated with a two-fold increased risk of recurrence, even with adjuvant treatment such as a RT boost, endocrine therapy, or chemotherapy, as suggested by the EORTC 22881 trial. These patients require re-excision or mastectomy.

Mastectomy

This includes the complete removal of the breast and may be a radical, modified radical, simple, nipple-areolar, or skin-sparing mastectomy according to the technique and the preservation of the pectoral muscle or the nipple-areolar complex.

Choice of mastectomy technique depends on whether patients will have immediate reconstruction or whether the intent is prophylactic or curative. Mostly, patients who present contraindications for BCS or inflammatory breast cancer will undergo mastectomy.

Breast reconstructive surgery can be performed with the primary surgery, or it can be delayed, and includes two options:
- Prosthetic reconstruction
- Autologous reconstruction using either a pediculated flap (latissimus dorsi) or a free flap (transverse rectus abdominis myocutaneous (TRAM))

Inflammatory breast cancer is a contraindication for immediate reconstruction.

Surgery of the axilla

The surgical approach to the axilla depends on staging. For cN0 patients—SLNB should be performed:
- If SLNB is negative—axillary lymph node dissection (ALND) is not indicated. Recurrence rates in patients with negative SLNB who do not proceed to ALND are variable between 2% and 10%, but no negative long-term survival impact has been seen, especially in small, low-grade tumours.
- If SLNB is positive (>3 axillary lymph nodes)—ALND is indicated for axillary staging.
- If SLNB is positive for micrometastasis(<2mm)—both American and European guidelines suggest a case-by-case approach, as there are few data available on which to base a recommendation. If there is only one micrometastasis the approach is the same as for the negative axilla.
- If SLNB is positive for macrometastases—St. Gallen Consensus recommends avoiding ALND if there are less than two macrometastatic lymph nodes. In some cases of positive SLNB ALND can be avoided (ACOSOG Z0011 and IBCSG 23-01 trials). In these studies of over 3,000 patients, with cT–2 tumours, cN0, mostly ER+ (82%), with up to two positive sentinel lymph nodes, ALND was omitted with no impact on overall and DFS. All these patients received level I axillary RT as part of the breast irradiation treatment. The AMAROS trial also supports this approach as patients with T1–2 tumours, positive sentinel lymph nodes, and a clinically negative axilla had similar loco-regional recurrence benefits from axillary RT versus ALND and ALND+RT, with less morbidity.

For cN+ patients—pathological confirmation is needed, using ultrasound-guided fine needle aspiration (FNA), to determine whether ALND is indicated. ALND is necessary in patients with positive sentinel lymph nodes after downstaging with neoadjuvant chemotherapy. However, in patients with fewer than three examined lymph nodes, there is a risk of a false negative result.

Patients with occult primary breast cancers with positive axillary lymph nodes may undergo ALND and whole breast irradiation (WBI) rather than mastectomy and ALND, according to a 2016 meta-analysis.

Oncoplastic surgery

There is an increased need for trained doctors in oncoplastic surgery, as the techniques aim to merge principles of both oncological and plastic surgery, offering a natural appearance of the breast with a good oncological outcome. This approach is suitable for women with a large tumour mass compared to the breast volume or for those whose tumour localization requires repositioning of the nipple-areolar complex.

Further reading

Cardoso F, Costa A, Norton L, Senkus E, Aapro M, André F, et al. ESO-ESMO 2nd international consensus guidelines for advanced breast cancer (ABC2). *Ann Oncol* 2014; 25(10):1871–88.

Coates A, et al. Tailoring therapies—improving the management of early breast cancer: St Gallen International Expert Consensus on the Primary Therapy of Early Breast Cancer 2015. *Ann Oncol* 2015; 26:1533–46.

Donker M, et al. Radiotherapy or surgery of the axilla after a positive sentinel node in breast cancer (EORTC 10981-22023 AMAROS): A randomised, multicentre, open-label, phase 3 non-inferiority trial. *Lancet Oncol* 2014; 15(12):1303–10.

Giuliano AE, et al. Axillary dissection vs no axillary dissection in women with invasive breast cancer and sentinel node metastasis. *JAMA* 2011; 305(6):569–75.

Moran MS, Schnitt SJ, Giuliano AE, et al. Society of Surgical Oncology-American Society for Radiation Oncology consensus guideline on margins for breast-conserving surgery with whole-breast irradiation in stages I and II invasive breast cancer. *Int J Radiat Oncol Biol Phys* 2014; 8:553–64.

6.5 Loco-regional treatment of invasive breast cancer: Radiation therapy

Introduction

RT has an important role in decreasing loco-regional recurrence rates and the long-term risk of death from breast cancer.

RT treatment can include:

- Breast or chest wall
- Axillary region
- Other regions (infraclavicular, supraclavicular, or internal mammary region)

Indications for adjuvant RT

- Breast conserving surgery: the benefit of whole breast RT (WBI) has been proved in a meta-analysis of the Early Breast Cancer Trialists' Collaborative Group (EBCTCG), with a reduction in loco-regional recurrence (RR=0.52) and in the 15-year risk of breast cancer death (RR=0.82). The St. Gallen group favoured axillary and internal mammary RT only for patients with node-positive disease (positive SLNB/capsular invasion) for whom ALND was not performed. According to NCCN guidelines any benefit is debatable in older patients (>70 years) with stage I, ER+ disease who would benefit from endocrine treatment.

- Mastectomy: if patients have T3–4N0–1 tumours, more than four invaded lymph nodes, or positive margins after resection. Both the St. Gallen consensus and NCCN agree that for patients with one to three positive nodes disease there is a benefit for recurrence and survival with RT, data reinforced by a 2014 EBCCTG meta-analysis.

- Patients with locally advanced breast cancer who undergo neoadjuvant treatment: the indication for adjuvant RT should be made based on the initial stage and risk factors and not on the tumour response to neoadjuvant treatment.

Breast RT techniques

- WBI—is used after BCS and, in node positive patients (or those with capsular invasion) for whom ALND was not performed, it includes axillary RT. The total dose varies between 45 and 50Gy in 1.8–2Gy fractions, over 4.5 to five weeks. Hypofractionated (40–42.5Gy in three weeks) regimens have proved to have the same benefit, according to the START trials.

- Accelerated partial breast radiation (APBI)—delivers a higher dose to a limited tissue volume in a shorter period of time in patients with BCS. Although this approach may be considered for T–2N0 patients in terms of long-term effectiveness and safety, the ASTRO consensus does not recommend it yet outside a clinical trial. Options for delivering APBI are external RT (3D or intensity-modulated radiotherapy (IMRT)), brachytherapy or intraoperative RT, but several studies (ELIOT and TARGIT-A) have reported an increased risk of recurrence.

- Chest wall RT—is indicated after mastectomy in patients with T3–4 tumours, positive lymph nodes, or positive margins after surgery, to reduce the risk of local recurrence and breast cancer-related death.

For patients with positive lymph nodes, RT treatment plans differ according to the extent of the disease and may include the supraclavicular area, internal mammary region, and axilla. In patients with one to three positive lymph nodes, RT improves DFS and OS in patients with BCS (EORTC 22922/10925, AMAROS, and NCIC-CTG MA.20 trials). After mastectomy, RT may decrease the local recurrence risk but, because of increased morbidity, an individualized approach should be taken, especially in patients with ALND. The inclusion of internal mammary nodes in the radiation field should be discussed on a case-by-case basis, according to tumour localization, size, and stage.

In patients with positive margins after BCS or a residual mass after mastectomy, a 10–14Gy RT boost to the tumour bed may be indicated (Table 6.5.1).

Indications for axillary RT

- Extracapsular invasion on a case-by-case basis
- Positive axilla, without ALND

Table 6.5.1 Radiotherapy (RT) complications

Acute complications	Late complications
Redness and soreness of skin	Lymphoedema, reduced arm mobility, and strength (if ALND was performed)
Swelling of breast area	Skin and soft tissue fibrosis/necrosis
Fatigue	Pneumonitis and cardiac failure (rare)
Hyperpigmentation	Second cancers (rare)

Further reading

Cardoso F, Senkus E, Costa A, Papadopoulos E, et al. 4th ESO–ESMO International Consensus Guidelines for Advanced Breast Cancer (ABC 4). *Ann Oncol* 2018 August; 29(8):1634–57—available at https://doi.org/10.1093/annonc/mdy192

Curigliano G, Burstein H J, Winer E P, Gnant M, et al. De-escalating and escalating treatments for early-stage breast cancer: the St. Gallen International Expert Consensus Conference on the Primary Therapy of Early Breast Cancer 2017, *Ann Oncol* 2017 August; 28(8):1700–12—available at https://doi.org/10.1093/annonc/mdx308

Goldhirsch A, Winer E, Coates A, Recht A, et al. Effect of radiotherapy after mastectomy and axillary surgery on 10-year recurrence and 20-year breast cancer mortality: meta-analysis of individual patient data for 8135 women in 22 randomised trials. *Lancet* 2014; 383(9935):2127–35.

6.6 Systemic treatment for early breast cancer

Introduction

Breast cancer survival has continually been increasing over recent years due to improvements in cancer diagnosis and treatment such as adjuvant systemic treatments. These include endocrine treatment (ET), chemotherapy (CT), and anti-HER2 therapy, which may be given as a neoadjuvant or adjuvant approach. The first strategy, besides having the effect of decreasing breast cancer relapse and mortality, aims to increase rates of breast conservative surgery by downstaging the tumour, and to assess in vivo tumour response to treatment.

Treatment decisions are based on the presence of well-established prognostic markers for breast cancer recurrence and mortality such as: axillary lymph node involvement, lympho-vascular invasion, tumour size, and proliferation rate, measured by tumour grade and Ki67. Hormonal receptor status and HER2 status, in addition to their prognostic information, are also predictive factors of response to endocrine treatment and HER2 treatment. uPA and PAT-1 are prognostic factors with level 1 evidence but not used routinely due to logistical constraints. Furthermore, multi-parameter molecular marker assays have allowed us to understand the heterogeneity among breast cancers. Nowadays treatment decisions are also tailored to a molecular classification provided by these tests. Different assays have been validated as previously discussed: Oncotype DX®, MammaPrint®, PAM-50 ROR® score, EndoPredict®, and the Breast Cancer Index® are prognostic for years one to five; Enopredict and PAM-50 have demonstrated prognostic information beyond five years of follow-up.

Individual factor such as age, comorbidities, patient preferences, and general health status should also be taken into account in the decision process. The complexity of adjuvant systemic treatment for breast cancer has led to the development of tools and guidelines to help physicians to better decide treatment based on individual patient risk, the most frequently used being the St. Gallen Early Breast Cancer Consensus Guidelines and NCCN guidelines. Adjuvant Online is an informatics tool developed based on SEER data and the Oxford Overview, and presents estimates of the risk of cancer-related mortality or relapse based on patient age, comorbidities, and tumour characteristics. Together with the PREDICT tool, it was developed to help clinicians in treatment decisions but can over- or underestimate risk of certain features, and is still undergoing further development and validation for better accuracy.

In summary, the decision to use systemic adjuvant therapy requires considering and balancing risk for disease recurrence with local therapy alone, the magnitude of benefit from applying adjuvant therapy, toxicity of the therapy, and comorbidity. The decision-making process requires collaboration between the healthcare team and patient.

Treatment of Luminal breast cancer

Luminal tumours represent approximately two-thirds of all breast cancers and are characterized by ER positivity. At the gene-expression profiling level, these tumours may be differentiated into Luminal A and B types with Luminal B tumours having a more aggressive biology. ET is indicated in both Luminal types, but chemotherapy has shown lower efficacy in the low proliferative subset Luminal A.

Adjuvant endocrine treatment

ET is the mainstay treatment for Luminal tumours and is indicated for all patients with hormone receptor-positive disease. ET treatment works by blocking the oestrogen stimulus to breast cancer cells. Ovarian ablation was the first ET treatment used starting in the 1950s, but subsequently pharmacological methods have been developed.

Tamoxifen

The EBCTCG in an individual patient-level meta-analysis of multiple adjuvant trials, showed that, in ER+ patients, five years of tamoxifen significantly reduced recurrence rates and mortality by about a third throughout the first 15 years (RR 0.71 during years 0–4, 0.66 during years 5–9, and 0.68 during years 10–14; P<0.0001). This benefit was independent of PR status, lymph node status, use of CT, and menopausal status. Because the risk of recurrence in hormone-receptor-positive disease persists after the first decade, extended tamoxifen treatment beyond five years has been assessed in three large prospective trials (NSABP-B14, aTTom trial, and ATLAS trial). These results, together with data from the overview, have shown benefit for extended tamoxifen in terms of decrease in cancer recurrence, DFS, and OS. In the ATLAS trial, the ten-years cancer-specific mortality was 2.8% lower in the extended treatment group (event rate ratio 0.83, 95% CI 0.72–0.96).

Tamoxifen is a selective oestrogen receptor modulator (SERM), one of a group of drugs that interact with oestrogen receptors and have oestrogen agonist activity in some tissues and oestrogen antagonist activity in others. In breast cancer cells, tamoxifen binds to the E domain of the oestrogen receptor working as an antagonist. However, in bones and uterus it has a partial agonist function contributing to a risk of uterine cancer but having a protective effect against loss of bone mineral density. Benefit must be balanced with side effects in extended treatment because this is associated with a small increased incidence of ovarian cancer. There is also a higher risk of thromboembolic disease.

Aromatase inhibitors (AIs)

AIs inhibit the enzyme aromatase that converts androgens to oestrogen. The three drugs available are anastrozole, letrozole, and exemestane, and current evidence does not suggest any difference in efficacy or toxicity between them. AIs alone should not be used in women with functioning ovaries because the decrease in oestradiol levels will cause release of increased amounts of gonadotropins, which will stimulate follicular growth and oestradiol production through a feedback mechanism.

AIs have been investigated in a number of trials of postmenopausal patients. The inclusion of AIs in ET treatment (alone or with a switch strategy) is associated with a modest benefit in DFS and OS and current guidelines support the use of AIs either as an upfront strategy, sequential after two to three years of tamoxifen (TAM), or as extended therapy after 4.5–6 years of TAM. Recently the EBCTCG meta-analysis compared five years of AIs with five years of TAM, showing that AIs are associated with an absolute 2.9% decrease in recurrence (9.6% for AI vs. 12.6% for tamoxifen; 2P< 0.00001) and an absolute 1.1% decrease in breast cancer mortality (4.8% for AI vs. 5.9% for tamoxifen; 2P = 0.1). In trials where there was a switch strategy, the recurrence risk favoured AIs when treatments were changed but not thereafter. The absolute difference in breast cancer mortality was 0.7% five years after diagnosis and 1.7% eight years after diagnosis. Both tamoxifen and the AIs have similar side effects (hot flushes, vaginal dryness, and night sweats). AIs are associated with increased rates of osteoporosis, fractures, and musculoskeletal complaints whereas taxoxifen is associated with increased rates of thromboembolic events or uterine cancer.

Endocrine therapy in premenopausal women

Tamoxifen is the mainstay of treatment for premenopausal patients. Extended treatment for a duration of ten years should be considered if there is node-positive disease or in the presence of any other adverse prognostic factors.

Recent results of ovarian function suppression (OFS) trials have helped to better tailor this treatment as well as the inclusion of AIs combined with OFS. Two trials, SOFT and TEXT, compared the combination of OFS (luteinizing hormone-releasing hormone (LHRH) agonists, oophorectomy, or ovarian irradiation) with either tamoxifen or AIs (exemestane), and the SOFT trial included an arm of tamoxifen alone. The joint SOFT/TEXT analysis comparing tamoxifen with AIs has shown a decrease in recurrence for the AIs arm, but with no impact on OS. Statistical analysis has taken into account two risk groups of patients—a lower risk group (older women, node negative, T ≤2cm, lower grade) and high risk (younger–median age 40, larger T, higher grade, nodal involvement, those who received chemotherapy but remained premenopausal). The higher risk group achieved more benefit from OFS either with tamoxifen or AIs with significant improvement in DFS and distant recurrence. Recent ASCO guidelines and St. Gallen consensus recommend OFS based on the classification of patients into high or lower risk. If there is an indication for chemotherapy (involvement of four or more axillary nodes or adverse pathology features such as

Table 6.6.1 Side effects (SE) of tamoxifen (TAM) and aromatase inhibitors (AIs)

	Tamoxifen	Aromatase inhibitors
Common SE	Hot flushes	
	Vaginal dryness	
	Night sweats	
Particular SE	Risk of uterine cancer	Osteoporosis
	Thromboembolism	Bone fracture
		Musculoskeletal syndrome (pain, stiffness)
		Vaginal atrophy
		Sexual dysfunction

grade 3, high Ki67, and high score on a molecular assay) or there are persisting premenopausal oestrogen levels after adjuvant chemotherapy, OFS and ET may be considered with either tamoxifen or AI. Low-risk patients do not benefit from this strategy. Given the long natural history of endocrine-responsive breast cancer, longer follow-up of all trials will be critical to ascertain benefit and document unexpected late toxicities, if any. The duration of OFS based on these trials should be five years. However, OFS is associated with a greater risk of menopausal symptoms and decrease in bone mineral density as well as side effects on sexual function. Exemestane was associated with increased osteoporosis, fractures, musculoskeletal symptoms, vaginal dryness, decreased libido, and dyspareunia. Currently there are no predictive markers to tailor ET treatment.

Endocrine therapy for postmenopausal women

Treatment options for postmenopausal women include either tamoxifen or an AI or a sequence of the two, given for five or ten years. The tolerability profile should be taken in account when selecting patients for ET (see Table 6.6.1).

Patient preferences should be taken in account to improve tolerability and adherence to treatment. Longer durations of treatment improve on outcomes seen with tamoxifen alone, but also carry risks of ongoing side effects. There are no data for the safety or efficacy of AI therapy beyond a total duration of five years though clinical experience does not suggest emerging toxicity concerns. Although predictors of recurrence in ER positive breast cancer are well defined (T size, nodal stage at presentation, tumour grade, measures of proliferation such as Ki67, quantitative degrees of ER/PR expression, and molecular diagnostic profiles), there is a need for predictive markers of efficacy of specific drugs and length of treatment.

Adjuvant chemotherapy (CT)

The benefit from adjuvant CT for patients with BC was seen in large randomized trials and meta-analysis from the EBCTCG. First-generation CT regimens such as cyclophosphamide, methotrexate, fluorouracil (CMF), four cycles of AC, and four cycles of FEC50 reduce the risk of recurrence and overall mortality by 20–25% (survival benefit of 5.0%) compared with no CT.

- Anthracyclines are better than CMF if higher cumulative doses are used and given for at least six cycles.

- The incorporation of taxanes has also resulted in improvement of DFS and OS, the most effective regimens being those that incorporate anthracyclines and taxanes (reduction of overall mortality of 36%). In the EBCTCG 2012 meta-analysis the benefit for the incorporation of a taxane into an anthracycline CT regimen was seen independently of age, nodal status, tumour size, tumour grade, or ER status.
- Sequential chemotherapy with anthracyclines and taxanes should be used in preference to use in combination, due to similar efficacy rates and a better toxicity profile.
- Dose-dense regimens were developed after the introduction of granulocyte-colony-stimulating factors based on the rationale that increasing the dose intensity of cytotoxic therapy by shortening the intervals between cycles could enhance efficacy. The pivotal trial CALGB9741 testing twice-weekly AC followed by paclitaxel showed significant improvement in DFS and OS in patients with node-positive disease. Similar results were reproduced in subsequent trials. In the 2019 EBCTCG meta-analysis dose-dense regimens moderately reduced the ten-year risk of recurrence and death from breast cancer without increasing mortality from other causes. Proportional reductions in recurrence with dose-intense chemotherapy were similar and highly significant (P<0.0001) in ER-positive and ER-negative disease and did not differ significantly by other patient or tumour characteristics.
- Luminal A-like disease is less responsive to CT so the indications for CT in this setting should not be based on T size, or involvement of 1–3 lymph nodes. Current consensus guidelines recommend CT in this subset when four or more nodes are involved, and first-generation regimens may be considered.
- In Luminal B-like disease the decision to give adjuvant CT is based on the estimated risk of relapse and degree of endocrine responsiveness. Guidelines consider the relative indications to be: grade 3 disease, low hormone receptor staining, high Ki67, node positive disease, and extensive lymphovascular invasion. Although CT is more active in this subset the optimal regimen and duration of treatment is unknown. Current recommendations support an anthracycline and taxane regimen, and four cycles only may be considered if there is a low burden of disease. It is also unknown in which Luminal B patients CT can be omitted and consensus guidelines only consider it if scores are low on Oncotype DX, MammaPrint, PAM-50 ROR score, or EndoPredict.

Treatment of triple negative breast cancer (TNBC)

TNBC accounts for approximately 10–17% of all breast cancer and may be responsible for a higher proportion of cases in developing countries. They are associated with shorter survival and more aggressive biology compared with the other subtypes, having a peak risk for recurrence between the first and third years and mortality rates higher in the first five years after diagnosis and treatment. The definition of TNBC is the absence of expression of oestrogen, progesterone, and HER2 receptors. As a result, the only available adjuvant treatment is chemotherapy. The standard treatment approach includes a regimen of anthracyclines and taxanes, preferably administered as a dose-dense approach. Although TNBC have

an increased sensitivity to CT with a high rate of pCR (17–58%), some tumours present intrinsic treatment resistance. There are also data suggesting that the subgroup of triple negative cancers that have a high proportion of tumour infiltrating lymphocytes (TILs), have a better overall prognosis due to increased sensitivity to CT.

At the molecular level, the majority of these tumours are basal-like, but there is molecular heterogeneity among TNBC with studies showing that 71% of TNBC are basal-like and 77% of basal-like tumours are TNBC. There have been attempts at genomic subclassifications, but the clinical significance of these remains unclear. There is ongoing research concerning the subgroup of tumours that have a defect in homologous recombination, a feature of BRCA1-associated triple negative cancers. The efficacy of PARP inhibitors in BRCA1/2 mutated patients is currently being investigated in clinical trials in the neoadjuvant and adjuvant settings (PrECOG 0105 trial, OlympiA, NCT02032823), and several studies are attempting to determine if these tumours are more sensitive to platinum-based therapy. The addition of platinum agents (cisplatin/carboplatin) in the neoadjuvant setting achieved pCR of up to 60% (GeparSixto, PrECOG 0105, CALGB 40603 trials). A systematic review and meta-analysis (Annals Oncology, F Poggio 2018) that included nine RCTs (N = 2,109) showed that platinum-based neoadjuvant chemotherapy significantly increased pCR rate from 37.0% to 52.1% (OR 1.96, 95% CI 1.46–2.62, P<0.001). However, no significant difference in event-free survival (HR 0.72, 95% CI 0.49–1.06, P=0.094) and OS (HR 0.86, 95% CI 0.46–1.63, P=0.651) was observed (N=748) and significant higher risk of grade 3 and 4 hematological adverse effects was observed with platinum-based neoadjuvant chemotherapy. Confirmatory phase 3 trials are needed to have accurate data on treatment response and survival.

For ER negative, early stage breast cancer patients who undergo neoadjuvant/adjuvant treatment, BCY2 guidelines recommend the use of GnRH agonists to prevent chemotherapy-induced ovarian failure/infertility based on a recent randomized phase 3 trial (POEMS). In this study, patients were randomized to receive cyclophosphamide containing CT regimens plus LHRH analogues versus CT alone. There was a decrease of ovarian failure rate at two years from 22% to 8%.

Treatment of HER2 positive breast cancer

Overexpression of HER2 occurs in 20% of breast cancers. Anti-HER2 therapy proved to be effective in early breast cancer when added to chemotherapy and is recommended for the majority of patients with positive disease, except for those with clinical congestive heart failure or significantly compromised left ventricular ejection fraction, who should be evaluated on a case-by-case basis. The first agent in clinical use was trastuzumab which is a monoclonal antibody directed against the extracellular domain of HER2.

Adjuvant anti-HER2 therapy

In the adjuvant setting, the addition of trastuzumab to CT decreased breast cancer recurrence by 50%, based on several large randomized trials. A joint analysis of NSABP B-31 and NCCTG N9831 trials has consistently showed an increased OS (HR = 0.63; 95% CI 0.54–0.73; P = 0.001) and DFS (HR = 0.60; 95% CI 0.53–0.68; P = 0.001). The results appear to be independent of ER hormonal status. Guidelines recommend the use of adjuvant CT in HER2+ disease, node positive and node negative with tumour size >0.5cm. The use of trastuzumab earlier, concurrently with the taxane part of the CT regimen, is the current standard, and more effective than the sequential approach (based on NCCTG N9831). The docetaxel, carboplatin, and trastuzumab (TCH) regimen has been shown to be inferior to conventional chemotherapy but is an option if there are concerns about cardiac toxicity. A single arm trial of weekly paclitaxel x 12 and trastuzumab showed a three-year rate of survival free from invasive disease of 98.7%. Only 0.5% of symptomatic congestive heart failure was seen and recent guidelines consider this an acceptable regimen for T1a-bN0M0. Cardiac toxicity associated with trastuzumab is the most worrying side effect, and is increased if concurrent approaches are used with CT including anthracyclines and taxanes. The higher reported grade III/IV congestive heart failure and cardiac-related death was 4.1% from the NSABP B-31 trial.

The duration of anti-HER2 therapy was investigated in the HERA trial, comparing one year vs. two years and the PHARE trial, comparing six months vs. one year of treatment. The HERA trial did not find a difference in DFS between the two arms (HR = 0.99, 95% CI 0.85–1.14), while the PHARE trial failed to show non-inferiority for the six months treatment duration.

Therefore, currently anti-HER2 therapy for one year is recommended.

In the adjuvant setting, dual HER2 blockade was tested in two RCTs. In the ALTTO Trial patients were randomized between trastuzumab versus lapatinib versus sequential treatment versus the combination of the two. The addition of lapatinib to trastuzumab did not improve the five-year DFS or OS (four-years HR = 0.8, 95% CI 0.62–1.03) and lapatinib was associated with a significant increase in adverse events (diarrhoea, hepatobiliary, and rash). In the APHINITY trial addition of pertuzumab to trastuzumab and chemotherapy was evaluated. The primary endpoint, three-year invasive-disease-free survival, was 94.1% in the pertuzumab group and 93.2% in the placebo group (HR 0.81, 95% CI 0.66–1.00; P=0.045) in favour of pertuzumab. Analysis of a high-risk population defined by positive axillary lymph node involvement or negative HR status showed an 1.8% and 2.4%, respectively, absolute benefit in DFS that was not statistically significant. The use of adjuvant pertuzumab should be restricted to high-risk populations.

Neoadjuvant anti-HER2 therapy
In the neoadjuvant setting the HER2 dual blockade has shown a significant increase in pCR rates. The dual blockade (trastuzumab and pertuzumab) has already been approved by the US Food and Drug Administration (FDA) and European Medicine Agency, based on the results of the NeoSphere and TRYPHAENA trials. Long-term outcomes for the NeoSphere trial reveal a three-year PFS of 90% (dual blockade) versus 86% (HR = 0.69, 95% CI 0.34–1.40). Lapatinib in association with trastuzumab was investigated in NeoALLTO, CHER-LOB, TBCRC006, and NSABP-B41 trials, suggesting superiority of the dual blockade. Long-term follow-up from all of these studies is needed to understand the impact of a higher pCR on long-term outcome.

Postneoadjuvant anti-HER2 therapy
Patients with HER2 + EBC (early breast cancer) who have residual invasive disease after neoadjuvant chemotherapy and HER2-targeted therapy have a high risk of recurrence and death. The phase 3 KATHERINE trial compared ado-trastuzumab emtansine (T-DM1; Kadcyla) versus trastuzumab (Herceptin) as adjuvant therapy in patients with HER2+ EBC with residual invasive disease after receiving neoadjuvant chemotherapy and trastuzumab. The use of T-DM1 was associated with a highly clinical and statistically valid benefit—invasive DFS—and was significantly higher in the T-DM1 group (HR 0.50; 95% CI 0.39–0.64; P<0.001). Safety data was consistent with the known side effects of T-DM1. One death in a patient without disease recurrence occurred due to intracranial haemorrhage after a fall associated with T-DM1-induced thrombocytopenia.

Bisphosphonates in the adjuvant setting
Oral and intravenous bisphosphonates have been tested in the adjuvant setting, aiming to prevent bone density loss. An unexpected decrease in relapse was seen in these trials and led to the investigation of these drugs with adjuvant intent in several studies that included clondronate and zoledronic acid. The recent EBCTCG meta-analysis of these studies has shown a 17% reduction in the risk of breast cancer death and a 34% reduction in risk of bone recurrence, which was highly significant, but this effect was only seen in postmenopausal women, and no advantage was seen in the premenopausal setting, for which this treatment is not recommended. The incidence of breast cancer in elderly patients has been rising. Evidence shows a similar efficacy of systemic treatment in this population compared with other groups. The challenge in older patients is to manage toxicity which is higher and balance benefit against comorbidities to minimize both under- and overtreatment. More trials are needed in this population as it is usually an under-represented group in most breast cancer trials. Treatment decisions should not be influenced exclusively by age, and a comprehensive geriatric assessment should be done in order to decide the best course of treatment. Endocrine treatment is preferred whenever indicated and the chemotherapy decision should be based on comorbidities and toxicity profile. The preferred regimens in the adjuvant setting are doxorubicin and cyclophosphamide or docetaxel and cyclophosphamide, because capecitabine alone proved to be inferior to standard chemotherapy in elderly patients (CALGB 49907 trial).

Very young patients
Patients under 40 years old are more likely to develop more aggressive cancers (HER2-positive, TNBC), with a worse prognosis. However, the treatment decision should not be based on age alone, rather on the biology of the tumour, comorbidities, and additional risk factors. Another important factor is the long-term toxicity profile of the treatment, and fertility issues should be addressed. Information provided from retrospective studies on pregnancy after breast cancer suggest no detrimental effect on breast cancer outcome and, for this reason, pregnancy should not be discouraged. However, prospective data are still awaited from the POSITIVE trial that is currently recruiting.

Systemic therapy in pregnant patients
During the second or third trimester, chemotherapy may be used for breast cancer treatment based on tumour biology and other prognostic factors. Anthracyclines and cyclophosphamide, as well as taxanes (especially weekly paclitaxel), can be safely administered. No endocrine

therapy or anti-HER2 treatments (trastuzumab) should be given during pregnancy due to the high risk of teratogenicity.

Further reading

Amant F, et al. Breast cancer in pregnancy: Recommendations of an international consensus meeting, *Eur J Cancer* 2010 Dec; 46(18):3158–68.

Bedard PL, Cardoso F. Can some patients avoid adjuvant chemotherapy for early-stage breast cancer? *Nat Rev Clin Oncol* 2011 May; 8(5):272–9.

Biganzoli L, et al. Management of elderly patients with breast cancer: updated recommendations of the International Society of Geriatric Oncology (SIOG) and European Society of Breast Cancer Specialists (EUSOMA). *Lancet Oncol* 2012 April; 13(4):e148–60.

Biganzoli L, Wildiers H, Oakman C, et al. Management of elderly patients with breast cancer: updated recommendations of the International Society of Geriatric Oncology (SIOG) and European Society of Breast Cancer Specialists (EUSOMA). *Lancet Oncol* 2012 April 13;13(4):e148–60.

Cardoso F, van't Veer LJ, Bogaerts J, et al. 70-Gene Signature as an Aid to Treatment Decisions in Early-Stage Breast Cancer. *N Engl J Med* 2016; 375(8):717–29.

Coates AS, Winer EP, Goldhirsch A, Gelber RD, Gnant M. Tailoring therapies—improving the management of early breast cancer: St Gallen International Expert Consensus on the Primary Therapy of Early Breast Cancer. *Ann Oncol* 2015; 26(8):1533–46.

Denduluri N, et al. Selection of Optimal Adjuvant Chemotherapy Regimens for Early Breast Cancer and Adjuvant Targeted Therapy for Human Epidermal Growth Factor Receptor 2-Positive Breast Cancers: An American Society of Clinical Oncology Guideline Adaptation of the Cancer Car. *J Clin Oncol* 2018; 36(23):2433–43.

EBCTCG. Adjuvant bisphosphonate treatment in early breast cancer: meta-analyses of individual patient data from randomised trials. *Lancet* 2015; 386:1353–61.

EBCTCG. Long-term outcomes for neoadjuvant versus adjuvant chemotherapy in early breast cancer: meta-analysis of individual patient data from ten randomised trials *Lancet Oncol* 2018 January 1; 19(1):27–39.

EBCTCG. 20-year risks of breast-cancer recurrence after stopping endocrine therapy at 5 years. *N Engl J Med* 2017 November 9; 377(19):1836–46.

Gradishar WJ, Robert CH, Anderson BO, Fred V-C, Balassanian R, Blair SL, et al. NCCN Guidelines Version 2. 2016 Breast Cancer Panel Members.

Henry NL, et al. Role of Patient and Disease Factors in Adjuvant Systemic Therapy Decision Making for Early-Stage, Operable Breast Cancer: American Society of Clinical Oncology Endorsement of Cancer Care Ontario Guideline Recommendations. *J Clin Oncol* 2016 Jul 1;34(19):2303–11.

Paluch-Shimon S, Pagani O, Partridge AH, Bar-Meir E, Cardoso F, et al. Second international consensus guidelines for breast cancer in young women (BCY2). *Breast* 2016 April; 26:87–99.

Paluch-Shimon S, Pagani O, Partridge AH, Abulkhair O, Cardoso M-J, Dent RA, Gelmon K, et al. ESO-ESMO 3rd international consensus guidelines for breast cancer in young women (BCY3). *Breast* 2017 Oct; 35:203–17.

Peto R, Davies C, Godwin J, Gray R, Pan HC, Clarke M, et al. Comparisons between different polychemotherapy regimens for early breast cancer: meta-analyses of long-term outcome among 100,000 women in 123 randomised trials. *Lancet* 2012; 379(9814):432–44.

Schiavon G, Smith IE. Status of adjuvant endocrine therapy for breast cancer. *Breast Cancer Res* (online) 2014; 16(2):206.

Senkus E, Kyriakides S, Ohno S, Penault-Llorca F, Poortmans P, et al. Primary breast cancer: ESMO Clinical Practice Guidelines for diagnosis, treatment and follow-up. *Ann Oncol* (online) 2015 Sep (cited 2016 Jun 1); 26(Suppl 5):v8–30.

Sparano JA, Gray RJ, Makower DF, et al. Adjuvant Chemotherapy Guided by a 21-Gene Expression Assay in Breast Cancer. *N Engl J Med* 2018 Jul 12; 379(2):111–21.

6.7 Management of locally advanced breast cancer

Definition/pathology

Locally advanced breast cancer (LABC) includes a subset of stage IIB (T3N0) and stage III disease. These patients either have large tumours, extensive lymph-node involvement, or inoperable tumours without metastasis. The five-year survival in this stage is around 50% according to SEER data and a multimodal approach of neoadjuvant chemotherapy, surgery, and radiation therapy is indicated. LABC also includes inflammatory breast cancer (IBC), as a more aggressive and rare entity.

The histology and biology of LABC is similar to early breast cancer, with the inclusion of IBC as a special category. IBC is more aggressive, frequently high grade, ER negative, and more commonly HER2+ or basal-like, associated with overexpression of angiogenic markers (VEGF, VEGFR), E-cadherin, and TP53 mutations.

A complete clinical, laboratory, and imaging evaluation is recommended by ABC2 guidelines as well a good quality biopsy to assess ER, PR, HER2, Ki67, and tumour grade to guide the choice of systemic treatment.

Primary systemic treatment according to BC subtype

Neoadjuvant systemic therapy

Six to eight cycles of anthracycline and taxane-based sequential regimens are the current standard as this regimen leads to a higher pCR rate and improved OS. Sequential administration is less toxic according to the BCIRG-005 study. Several combinations have been studied to try to increase pCR rate in various subgroups, but none has yet shown an impact on long-term outcomes.

- In HER2 negative patients—the addition of carboplatin increased pCR rate in the TNBC subgroup (pCR=50%) in GeparSixto and CALGB 40603; the last trial also shows an increased pCR with the addition of bevacizumab, but at the cost of higher toxicity.

- In high-risk ER negative patients—dose-dense chemotherapy with a conventional chemotherapy schedule can provide a better OS and DFS according to a 2010 meta-analysis.

- In HER2 positive patients—this subgroup achieves high pCR rates, especially ER-negative patients. The benefit from trastuzumab added to taxane-based chemotherapy has shown an increased pCR (30–51.3%) in NOAH, NeoALTTO, and GeparQuattro trials, leading to its approval for use in the neoadjuvant setting. Adding pertuzumab to trastuzumab has shown an additional improved response (46%) in the NelSphere trial. Neither the association of trastuzumab to lapatinib, nor lapatinib alone has proved to achieve a statistically significantly better response in this subset of patients (GeparQuinto and TBCRC 006 trials). Bevacizumab has been tested with chemotherapy (NSABP B40 and CALGB 40603 trials) or in association with trastuzumab (BEVERLY-2 trial), and though it showed improved pCR (35–60%), increased toxicity was reported and no long-term outcome benefit has been proven. Moreover, it has not proved beneficial in IBC patients.

- In ER positive patients—Luminal breast cancer may have a lower pCR and response to CT and neoadjuvant ET may be an option in older patients with slow growing ER+ tumours. The Neo-tAnGo trial has suggested an improved pCR after taxanes (in TEC regimen) in an ER+ population. Neoadjuvant ET has shown lower pCR rates (2–10%) in premenopausal women. In postmenopausal women, aromatase inhibitors (letrozole and anastrozole) offer an increased response rate compared with tamoxifen according to the ACOSOG Z1031 trial so AIs are recommended in the ET neoadjuvant setting, and may be considered in 'Luminal-A' postmenopausal patients, for four to eight months, or until maximal response.
- Whether pCR is a clear marker for improved long-term survival is debatable. Lower pCR rates do not always indicate worse disease and OS, particularly in the ER+ population and lobular tumours. This is mainly related to the tumour biology. Furthermore, most neoadjuvant trials have defined it differently. Adjuvant capecitabine, in residual HER-2 negative, after neoadjuvant chemotherapy (with anthracyclines, taxanes, or both), has shown a improvement in five-year OS (89.2% vs.

83.6%, P=0.01) in one randomized study including 910 patients (CREATE-X trial), in particular in triple negative breast cancer.
- Clinical trials enrollment—for patients who progress with standard NACT with anthracyclines and taxanes. Outside clinical trials, management should be as for metastatic disease (see section 6.8, 'Management of recurrent and metastatic breast cancer').

Surgery according to BC subtype

Mastectomy with ALND is an option for patients with a large residual tumour, for those with a minimal response to treatment, with or without reconstruction.

Inflammatory BC must be treated with mastectomy without reconstruction even if pCR is obtained, due to the very high risk of relapse.

The management of the axilla has been studied in SENTINA and ACOSOG Z1071 trials, suggesting that SNLB after neoadjuvant treatment gives an increased rate of false-negative results. According to the AMAROS trial, patients with cN2, cN3 should undergo ALND after neoadjuvant treatment regardless of response.

Radiation therapy according to BC subtype

Incorporating RT into the multimodal treatment of LABC reduces the loco-regional recurrence risk, as suggested by an ECOG and two Danish trials and also by an EBCTCG meta-analysis. RT should be performed four to six weeks after surgery with a dose between 40 and 42.5Gy to the chest wall/breast in post-mastectomy patients and with a boost for BCS patients.

RT should always be administered independently of the response to neoadjuvant chemotherapy.

Further reading

Cardoso F, Senkus E, Costa A, Papadopoulos E, Aapro M, et al. 4th ESO–ESMO International Consensus Guidelines for Advanced Breast Cancer (ABC 4). *Ann Oncol* August 2018; 29(8):1634–57—available at https://doi.org/10.1093/annonc/mdy192

6.8 Management of recurrent and metastatic breast cancer (MBC)

Loco-regional recurrence: general considerations and initial work-up

Large tumours with extensive lymph-node involvement, positive margins, high grade, aggressive subtype not treated with adjuvant radiation therapy have an increased risk of local recurrence.

The diagnosis is suggested by clinical examination (inflammatory changes of the breast, a new mass in the axilla or supraclavicular fossae, nodules in the chest wall/scar) and these patients should be further evaluated by blood tests and imaging (computed tomography, MRI, PET-CT, bone scan) for distant metastases. A biopsy should be done to confirm the recurrence and to tailor treatment decisions.

Breast recurrence after BCS

The surgical standard is mastectomy (especially in BRCA carriers), but breast re-excision followed by RT

(especially if no prior RT was given) may be feasible in some patients. If surgery is not possible, and there is failure to respond to systemic treatment, RT alone may be given for loco-regional control. For those without ALND, axillary re-staging is indicated. Regarding systemic treatment, patients with loco-regional recurrence may receive chemotherapy (CALOR study), or endocrine treatment (if the disease progresses during ET, a change of agent is needed), or an anti-HER2 agent for one year.

Isolated chest wall recurrence after mastectomy

Surgical resection if possible, with axillary evaluation (especially if cN+) is the preferred option. RT can improve local control, especially in those without prior irradiation. However, the approach for previously irradiated patients is less clear and retreatment with a lower dose may be considered but must be decided case-by-case due to potential toxicity.

Regional axilla and/or supraclavicular recurrence

- Axillary recurrence management depends on the previous approach. ALND may be indicated in patients with initially negative SLNB. However, for those who underwent initial ALND, surgical resection may be possible for isolated recurrence. The role of RT is less clear, but it may be considered in oligometastatic disease or if the axilla is the only site of recurrence.
- Patients undergoing supraclavicular recurrence management seem to have a less favourable prognosis compared with patients with isolated axillary recurrence and the optimal approach has not yet been established. In addition to local therapy with RT if possible, ABC2 guidelines recommend systemic treatment according to the profile of the tumour, DFS interval, and patient comorbidities.

Metastatic breast cancer: systemic treatment according to BC subtype

Although five-year survival rates have increased for MBC due to progress in treatment, they have not exceeded 25% and median OS is still two to three years. The goal for these patients remains prolongation of survival with a good quality of life. For MBC patients, a multidisciplinary team should be involved in the management of the disease and treatment should be guided by tumour characteristics, relapse-free interval, metastatic sites, and patient factors such as menopausal status as well as patient preference.

An initial work-up including clinical examination, complete blood-test panel and imaging (computed tomography, MRI, PET-CT, bone scan, and a re-biopsy with reassessment of biology may influence treatment decisions (Table 6.8.1).

Table 6.8.1 Treatment options for MBC

Status	Premenopausal	Postmenopausal
ER+ HER2–	Ovarian ablation/ suppression with: tamoxifen (TAM) or AIs +/– CDKi	Aromatase inhibitors (AIs)
		TAM
		CDKi + Ais (*)
		Fulvestrant
		Everolimus + AIs/TAM
ER+/– HER2+	Chemotherapy + Trastuzumab +/– Pertuzumab	
	+ Lapatinib	
	TDM-1	
	Trastuzumab + TAM (**)	
	Trastuzumab + AIs (**)	
	Lapatinib + AIs (**)	
ER– HER2–	Chemotherapy (single agent preferred):	
	Taxanes	
	Gemcitabine	
	Anthracyclines	
	Vinorelbine	
	Capecitabine	
	Eribulin	
	Platinum agents	
	Etoposide	
	Metronomic CM	

* Only approved in the USA.

** For ER+ disease, ET should be offered in association with an anti-HER2 agent.

ER positive and HER2 negative

In these patients, endocrine treatment is preferred even in the presence of visceral metastases, unless there is organ dysfunction or rapid progression. The majority of these patients will be HER2 negative and treatment options will be dependent on the menopausal status.

- For premenopausal patients, the preferred option is tamoxifen in combination with ovarian suppression (goserelin, ovarian ablation/oophorectomy). AIs are also an option in association with OFS, especially if TAM was used in the adjuvant setting. Fulvestrant + ovarian ablation/suppression can be used at progression. In case of progression after first-line TAM, and where there are no criteria for CT, ovarian ablation is recommended with an AI.
- For postmenopausal patients, AIs have proven superior to tamoxifen according to a meta-analysis in 2006 in terms of OS and no difference has emerged between the three AIs. Other options in first-line treatment include fulvestrant and tamoxifen (depending on what was used in the adjuvant setting). The FALCON trial, a randomized phase 3 trial comparing first-line fulvestrant to anastrazol showed improved outcome with fulvestrant mostly in patients with bone-only disease. The combination of CDK 4/6 inhibitors and letrozole was approved as first-line treatment based on a phase 2 PALOMA-1/TRIO-18 trial that showed a PFS of 20.2 months and an OS of 37.5 months. Further phase 3 trials showed improved PFS with CDKi based on PALOMA 2/MONALEESA 2 and MONARCH 3 trials.
- For second-line treatment, options include changing to another AI, tamoxifen, fulvestrant alone, or in combination with CDKi (based on the significant improvement in PFS shown in the PALOMA-3/MONALEESA 3 and MONARCH 2 trials) and everolimus + endocrine therapy. The addition of everolimus to both AIs exemestane, (as in Bolero-2 trial) and tamoxifen (TAMRAD trial) has shown an increased time to progression (8.46 months vs. 4.5 months) after progression with first-line treatment, but not statistically significant OS benefit (31 months vs. 26.6 months).

HER2 positive disease

The choice of anti-HER2 treatment in the metastatic setting depends on whether the patient has been previously treated with adjuvant anti-HER2.

Previously untreated

- Trastuzumab in association with a taxane has been considered for many years the standard first-line treatment (based on trials showing an increased OS of 25–31 months (HO648g trial, M77001 trial, HERTAX trial). However, the combination with vinorelbine has been shown to have the same efficacy and less toxicity (TRAVIATA and HERNATA trials). Due to increased cardiac toxicity, the combination of anti-HER2 and anthracyclines is generally avoided. However, liposomal doxorubicin has shown cardiac safety in several phase 2 and 1 trials, in combination with trastuzumab.
- Trastuzumab and pertuzumab in combination with a taxane have given seven months gain in PFS (18.5 months) and 15.7 months in OS (56.5 months) in the Cleopatra study and is now recommended in first-line treatment, mainly in this setting of previously untreated patients.

- The superiority of trastuzumab + chemotherapy vs. lapatinib + chemotherapy in terms of PFS and tolerance has been shown in the NCIC CTG MA.31and Cerebel studies of first-line treatment.

Previously treated with adjuvant trastuzumab
The combination of CT with an anti-HER2 agent (monotherapy or dual blockade) is the preferred choice. Options include the combination of CT (capecitabine, taxanes, or vinorelbine) with trastuzumab or docetaxel + pertuzumab + trastuzumab.

If there is progression with first-line treatment and beyond:

- TDM-1 has showed an improved PFS and OS after trastuzumab (EMILIA trial) and is the preferred second-line treatment, even though it can be used if progression after more than two lines of treatment.
- Trastuzumab beyond progression is supported by retrospective and prospective trials (Hermine study and GBC 26/BIG 03-05 trial).
- The combination of lapatinib and transtuzumab without chemotherapy has shown an improved PFS (in the EGF104900 trial).
- Lapatinib in association with capecitabine is a valid option after progression after trastuzumab regimens. However, two randomized phase 3 trials (MA.31 and Cerebel) have proven the superiority of trastuzumab and chemotherapy to lapatinib and chemotherapy.
- The addition of everolimus to trastuzumab and vinorelbine after progression with trastuzumab and a taxane has been studied (BOLERO-3 trial) and has shown a small increase in PFS, but the toxicity was significant and there was no benefit in OS.
- In postmenopausal women, with ER+ and HER2 positive disease, three trials assessed first-line treatment with AIs (letrozole/anastrozole) plus trastuzumab, or letrozol plus lapatinib, showing a significant increase in PFS even though there was no impact on OS. There are no studies comparing this strategy with CT and anti-HER2 agents. Because the combination with CT has resulted in better PFS and OS results, the use of ET is indicated in selected cases with low burden disease, indolent biology, and comorbidities that favour a good tolerability profile.

Triple negative

Although TNBC is a heterogeneous disease, it is frequently characterized by a poor response to treatment, rapid recurrence, and an unfavourable prognosis. For these patients, CT is the main treatment. Combination CT is used if there is a need for rapid symptom control or extensive visceral metastasis, while single-agent chemotherapy is the preferred option in other cases. There is no standardized sequence, the choice being influenced by tumour burden, toxicity profile, patient's performance status (PS) and preferences, and previous therapies and their response to them (Table 6.8.2).

Antiangiogenic targeted therapies (bevacizumab) in combination with a taxane have been studied in TNBC (Beatrice and Ribbon-2 trials). However, since it only slightly improves PFS (by approximately three months) without influencing survival data and is associated with increased toxicity and substantial cost, approval has been withdrawn in the United States.

A subgroup of TNBC patients is BRCA1/2-associated. A possible sensitivity to platinum agents has

Table 6.8.2 Chemotherapy regimens for MBC

Single-agent chemotherapy	Combination chemotherapy
Taxanes (docetaxel, paclitaxel, nab-paclitaxel)	**Anthracycline containing regimens:**
Anthracyclines (doxorubicin, epirubicin, caelyx)	AC
	AT
Capecitabine	**Non-anthracycline**
Gemcitabine	**containing regimens:**
Vinorelbine	Gemcitabine + taxane
Etoposide	Capecitabine + docetaxel
Eribulin	CMF
	Metronomic chemotherapy
	Cisplatin + 5-FU

been suggested (TBCRC009 trial) in advanced breast cancer. PARP-inhibitors have recently demonstrated efficacy in this setting, namely olaparib and talazoparib. Olaparib was approved for the treatment of HER2 negative metastatic breast cancer in patients with germline BRCA mutation based on the results of the OlympiaD study, a phase 3 trial comparing the PARP-inhibitor to standard treatment when no more than two previous chemotherapy regimens were used. An improvement of PFS was shown together with a better tolerability profile, but it is important to notice that most patients included were platinum naïve. Similar results were obtained in the phase 3 EMBRACA study, where the drug used was talazoparib, where again only 16% patients were platinum exposed.

Evaluating treatment response

In the metastatic setting, treatment is continued until progression or unmanageable toxicity. If there is complete response, it is not clear if treatment should be continued or interrupted but if treatment is well tolerated it should be continued. Response should be evaluated periodically using clinical examination, laboratory findings, and imaging methods.

- Clinical examination—can assess treatment response (decrease/increase in size of metastases) and the presence of symptoms.
- Laboratory tests—can evaluate medullary, hepatic, renal toxicity to treatment, as well as tumour marker evolution.
- Imaging evaluation—is indicated and the specific study will depend on the metastatic sites. Computed tomography/MRI are good tests to evaluate soft tissue and bone disease, and RECIST criteria are used to define response to treatment. PET-CT can offer additional information about the metabolic activity of the tumour and is a good option, although more expensive.

Specific metastatic sites
Brain metastases

The risk of developing brain metastases depends upon the tumour subtype, being more frequent with HER2 positive and TNBC and less frequent in Luminal-A subtype. It confers a very unfavourable prognosis, especially if PS is poor or symptoms and comorbidities are present.

For patients with limited brain disease (<3 tumours <3cm), surgery with or without whole brain radiation therapy (WBRT) or stereotactic radiosurgery (SRS) should be considered. Treatment modalities are:

- Surgery—improves symptoms and local control in patients with less than four, small, accessible metastases. Postoperative WBRT improves local control, without having an impact on survival and is associated with neurological toxicity.
- SRS—may be an option in patients with good PS, stable extra-cranial disease, and limited brain disease that is not accessible to surgery and can deliver high doses in a limited number of fractions. Although there is no prospective data comparing SRS and surgery, a meta-analysis suggests similar efficacy.
- WBRT—improves local control and survival in patients treated by surgery or SRS, and it may be used as a definitive treatment in those with symptomatic multiple lesions, poor PS, or comorbidities. WBRT with 30–45Gy is an option, especially when more than four lesions are present.
- Systemic treatment—can be used in treating disseminated disease noting that although the blood–brain barrier (BBB) is generally impenetrable by large molecules, the presence of metastases, surgery, or radiation therapy alters BBB's structural features, allowing such molecules to pass.
- In HER2 positive patients, trastuzumab does not pass the intact BBB, but in metastatic patients studies have shown an improved survival with trastuzumab. Some phase 2 studies have shown a response with lapatinib and capecitabine (LANDSCAPE trial). However, in the CEREBEL study, lapatinib was not more effective than trastuzumab and capecitabine.
- Several chemotherapeutic agents have been described to have activity against brain metastases (cyclophosphamide, doxorubicin, methotrexate, or fluorouracil), but data are limited.

In addition to local treatment, management of brain oedema and symptom management must be initiated immediately.

Bone metastases

Bone is the most common metastatic site in patients with breast cancer, especially with ER+ disease. Disease confined to bone usually has a good response to systemic treatment and a slow evolution. Complications include fracture, nerve, or spinal cord compression and hypercalcemia.

Treatment methods include:

- Radiation therapy—to manage symptoms and preserve skeletal function and integrity, both external beam RT (EBRT) and stereotactic body RT (SBRT) may be used. ASTRO and European guidelines support single dose EBRT (8Gy) to manage bone pain. Although there are no randomized trials comparing SBRT with conventional RT, preliminary data consider it a non-invasive treatment option for selected patients with spinal metastases, especially those with oligometastatic disease. Reports show an improvement in pain control, but with a possible increased risk in vertebral compression fracture, depending on the administered dose, the proportion of the vertebrae that is irradiated and its localization.
- Surgery—laminectomy is less used now due to similar benefits from RT and an increased risk of failure. However, improvements in surgical techniques favour tumour resection followed by surgical spinal reconstruction or minimally invasive approaches such as vertebroplasty and kyphoplasty, as they may offer a better functional outcome for patients with an unstable spine compared with RT alone. Surgery must be followed by RT for better disease control.
- Bisphosphonates—are a class of bone-targeted agents that can improve bone pain, reduce skeletal-related events (SREs), and treat malignant hypercalcemia. Current recommendations are to use zoledronic acid as it is more effective than clodronate. The CALGB 70604 study has shown that there is no difference in SREs if zoledronic acid is administered every 12 weeks or every four weeks, and it is equally effective. Regarding treatment duration, several studies have continued using it beyond 24 months, although there are limited data concerning the additional benefit from this approach.
- Denosumab—is a monoclonal antibody against RANKL that has been successfully studied in bone metastases. Several reviews have showed reduced SREs with denosumab, a similar adverse events profile but with no impact on survival. Current guidelines consider it an option for metastatic disease. Clinicians should pay attention to possible side effects of bone modifying agents, such as osteonecrosis of the jaw and dose adjustments should be made according to the glomerular filtration rate.
- Systemic treatment—should be given in virtually all cases depending on tumour biology (chemotherapy versus ET).

Local treatment of primary tumour

The issue of local treatment in the metastatic setting, especially in patients with de novo metastatic disease, has been addressed by several retrospective and prospective studies.

Patients who would be eligible for this approach have oligometastatic, slow progressing disease. In these cases, a more aggressive multimodal treatment with 'curative' intent might provide long-term DFS and survival benefit, while maintaining a good quality of life.

The biological rationale for treating the primary tumour in the metastatic setting is debatable, as most hypotheses have been tested only in animal models.

Nevertheless, the results of multivariate analyses of various studies show that there may be a survival benefit in younger, fit patients, with slow growing tumours and low tumour burden.

In this setting, both ABC2 and NCCN guidelines opt for a case-by-case approach, suggesting that in some selected patients, treatment with 'curative' intent may be appropriate. However, in these situations, the quality of the surgery must be similar to that for early stage disease, as only in these circumstances may benefit be seen.

Further reading

Cardoso F, Senkus E, Costa A, Papadopoulos E, Aapro M, et al. 4th ESO–ESMO International Consensus Guidelines for advanced breast cancer (ABC 4). *Ann Oncol* 2018; 29(8):1634–57—available at: https://doi.org/10.1093/annonc/mdy192

Giordano SH, et al. Systemic therapy for patients with advanced human epidermal growth factor receptor 2-positive breast cancer: American Society of Clinical Oncology Clinical Practice Guideline. *J Clin Oncol* 2014 Jul 1; 32(19):2078–99.

Gradishar WJ, Anderson BO, Balassanian R, et al. Breast cancer, version 4.2017, NCCN Clinical Practice Guidelines in oncology. *J Natl Compr Canc Netw* 2018 March;16(3):310–20.

Ramakrishna N, et al. Recommendations on disease management for patients with advanced human epidermal growth factor receptor 2-positive breast cancer and brain metastases: American Society of Clinical Oncology Clinical Practice Guideline. *J Clin Oncol* 2014 Jul 1; 32(19):2100–08.

Reinert T, Barrios CH. Overall survival and progression free survival with endocrine therapy for hormone receptor-positive, HER2-negative advanced breast cancer: review. *Therap Adv Med Oncol* 2017 November; 9(11):693–709.

Rugo HS, et al. Endocrine therapy for hormone receptor-positive metastatic breast cancer: American Society of Clinical Oncology Guideline. *J Clin Oncol* 2016 September 1; 34(25):3069–103.

6.9 Male breast cancer

Introduction

Male breast cancer (male BC) accounts for 1% of all breast cancers and 0.1% of male cancer deaths. The incidence rates, as for female BC, are higher in North America and Europe and lower in Asia. In Africa high incidence rates have been reported in Uganda (5%) and Zambia (15%), where an endemic infectious disease has been speculated to be the cause (by leading to liver damage and hyperoestrogenism).

Risk factors

Risk factors for male BC include the following:

- Genetic/familial factors: 15–20% of male BC have a family history of breast or ovarian cancer. A family history of breast cancer increases the risk of male breast cancer by 2.5 times. BRCA2 mutation is the most common mutation found. BRCA1 is less common (occurring in 4–40% of hereditary male BC). Genetic testing should be recommended for all men with BC.

- Klinefelter's syndrome incurs a 20–50 times higher risk of male BC. Other relevant genetic mutations are androgen gene mutation, PTEN mutation (Cowden syndrome), CHEK 2 mutation (Li–Fraumeni syndrome), and Lynch syndrome.

- Endocrine factors: lower testosterone and hyperoestrogenism are a cause for male BC (undescended testis, orchiectomy, and lifestyle factors,). Lifestyle factors include obesity, alcoholism, or exogenous oestrogen intake. Cirrhosis and gynecomastia are also linked to male BC.

- Prior radiotherapy for unilateral gynaecomastia and thymic enlargement also increases the risk of male BC (1.6–1.9-fold).

- Occupational exposure to high temperatures (e.g. steel works, blast furnaces) is thought to increase the risk of male BC.

Clinical findings and diagnosis

Mean age at diagnosis is older in men compared with women—68.4 years old.

Tumours are normally found by palpation of a painless mass (50–97%). Nipple retraction occurs in 10–51%, local pain in 4–20%, nipple ulceration in 4–17%, nipple discharge in 1–12%, and nipple bleeding in 2–9%. Compared with women, a later stage is found at diagnosis with 48% of node positive disease.

Investigations should be as previously discussed. Microcalcifications in mammography are less common in male compared to female BC.

Pathology and prognosis

The International Male BC Programme has been developed to improve understanding of the biology and define better treatment strategies. The majority of male BC are ER and PR positive (~90%), PR positive (~80%), and androgen receptor (AR) positive (88%). Only 9% are HER-2 positive and less than 1% TNBC. 80% are infiltrating ductal carcinoma, 5% papillary, and 1% lobular. The recent International Male BC Programme evaluated Ki67 values, and only 25% had >20%, confirming that most male BCs are of Luminal A-like subtype. This is in accordance with studies evaluating the intrinsic subtype of BC by genomic assays in which 83–98% belong to the Luminal A type tumours.

Recent results report a median OS of 10.4 (95% CI 8.84–11.77) years in node negative disease; 8.36 years (95% CI 7.11–9.35) in node positive disease and 2.63 (95% CI 2.01–3.71) years in metastatic disease.

Treatment

Due to the lack of prospective and randomized data for this population, treatment strategies are based on extrapolation from female BC guidelines. Surgery is recommended for localized disease and includes BCS or mastectomy with sentinel node biopsy or ALND.

Radiation therapy should follow the same guidelines as for female BC. There are some data recommending RT after mastectomy if there is large tumour size, extension to the skin, areola, or pectoralis major muscle, axillary lymph-node involvement, retro-areolar location, or involved margins. The benefits of RT should be balanced against cardiotoxicity risk, as risk factors for cardiac disease are more prevalent in the male population.

Tamoxifen is the standard adjuvant treatment in most patients, as ER+ disease is commoner. Adjuvant AIs should not be used without LHRH agonists due to a negative feedback loop.

Data on adjuvant CT in the male population suggest a similar risk reduction for recurrence and death and it is indicated for high-risk disease as defined in previous chapters. There is a trend for increase in its use internationally (30% patients receiving adjuvant anthracycline/taxane-based therapy). There are scarce data on the use of trastuzumab but it is recommended in the HER2 positive population.

Patients with locally advanced cancer should receive neoadjuvant systemic therapy to facilitate complete surgery.

For metastatic disease endocrine therapy with tamoxifen is the mainstay of treatment. The role of AIs is still not clear, and if used should be in combination with LHRH or orchiectomy as 80% of oestrogen in men is produced peripherally and 20% from the testis. When disease progresses on endocrine therapy, CT should be offered following the same guidelines as in women.

Further reading

Cardoso F, Bartlett JMS, Slaets L, van Deurzen CHM, van Leeuwen-Stok E, et al. Characterization of male breast cancer: Results of the EORTC 10085/TBCRC/BIG/NABCG International Male Breast Cancer Program. *Ann Oncol* 2018; 29(2):405–17.

Korde LA, Zujewski JA, Kamin L, Giordano S, Domchek S, et al. Multidisciplinary meeting on male breast cancer: summary and research recommendations. *J Clin Oncol* 2010; 28(12):2114–22.

6.10 BRCA and hereditary breast cancer

Prevalence of BRCA mutations

Less than 20% of breast cancer patients have hereditary susceptibility. The prevalence of BRCA mutations varies in certain ethnic groups (Ashkenazi Jews) and in some geographic areas. The estimated frequency in the general population for BRCA1/2 mutations is 1/800 to 1/1,000 per gene.

A higher prevalence is associated with younger age at diagnosis, family history, TNBC, or male breast cancer and multiple tumours.

Referral for testing

There are several risk assessment models for hereditary cancer syndromes that are used in clinical practice: Gail model, Claus model, BRCAPRO, BOADICEA, and the Tyrer-Cuzick model to assess individual risk. These tools can help stratify risk and tailor screening recommendations.

According to European Society of Medical Oncology (ESMO) and National Comprehensive Cancer Network (NCCN), recommendations for testing include breast cancer patients who have one of the following:

- Breast cancer at a young age (<45 years old), with bilateral tumours or aggressive subtypes (TNBC).
- Personal or family history of breast, ovarian, pancreatic, male breast, or prostate cancer, especially diagnosed at less than 50 years old.
- Diagnosis under 45 years old.
- Bilateral tumour <50 years old
  - TNBC diagnosed under 50 years old
  - Diagnosis under 50 years old and one or more relatives with breast, pancreatic, or prostate (Gleason >7) cancer
  - Diagnosed at any age with one or more relatives with breast cancer under 50 years old
  - Diagnosed at any age with two or more relatives with breast cancer at any age
  - Diagnosed at any age with one or more relatives with invasive ovarian cancer at any age
  - Diagnosed at any age with two or more relatives with pancreatic or prostate cancer at any age
  - Ashkenazi Jewish heritage
  - Close male relative with breast cancer at any age
  - Personal history of invasive epithelial ovarian cancer/male breast cancer at any age
  - Personal history of prostate cancer (Gleason >7) and at least one relative diagnosed with breast cancer <50 years old and/or ovarian cancer and/or pancreatic cancer diagnosed at any age
  - Personal history of pancreatic cancer in Ashkenazi Jewish women

Management of asymptomatic carriers

Once a BRCA mutation is identified in an asymptomatic carrier, several options for screening or risk reducing procedures are available.

- Chemoprevention—is considered an option for BRCA carriers who do not opt for prophylactic surgery, according to (ASCO and US Preventive Services Task Force guidelines). Although there are limited data to support the use of SERMs. Both five years of tamoxifen and raloxifene have shown effectiveness in these patients according to a 2013 USPSTF meta-analysis.

- Surveillance—for breast and ovarian cancer is also an option for BRCA carriers who do not wish to proceed with prophylactic surgery. Although there are no data showing that surveillance strategies reduce mortality in BRCA carriers, guidelines recommend starting screening at age 30 years (or earlier if a family member was diagnosed with breast cancer at 25 years or younger):
  - Breast examination should be done twice a year starting at age 25 years and monthly self-examination should begin at age 18 years.
  - Mammography annually is recommended from age 30 years and is currently the standard screening method. Current data suggest increased false-negative results with mammography in BRCA patients, related to a higher breast tissue density.
  - Breast MRI has increased specificity in this population and is recommended annually starting at age 30 years, along with mammography, although it can be associated with an increased false-positive rate. In patients younger than 30 years old, the optimal surveillance strategy is still unknown; some guidelines recommend the use of MRI rather than mammography in this sub-population.

- Surgery—reduces the risk of cancer, although it does not completely eliminate it. Bilateral mastectomy provides a 90% decreased risk in BRCA carriers in both retrospective and prospective studies. Bilateral salpingo-oophorectomy should be considered in patients who do not want/already have children at age 35–40 years, depending on family history. These procedures must be thoroughly discussed with the patient and sufficient time must be given to take a decision.

Special considerations in the treatment of BRCA-associated breast cancer

Cancer patients with the BRCA mutation have a higher risk of ipsilateral and contralateral recurrence.

- Surgery—although BCS has been associated with an increased risk of recurrence in the ipsilateral breast, it does not impact on survival or systemic recurrence compared with mastectomy. However, for these patients, surgery can also incorporate risk-reducing strategies for both breasts.
- Radiation therapy—some authors have suggested an increased radiosensitivity and recurrence risk in BRCA carriers, but this association has not been proved. Radiation therapy recommendations are similar to sporadic breast cancer patients.
- Systemic treatment—several studies suggest that BRCA carriers may have a higher chemosensitivity, especially to DNA-damaging agents. Moreover, a higher pCR with neoadjuvant platinum compounds has been observed. For platinum therapy, response rates seem to be influenced by BRCA germline mutations in the neoadjuvant setting, as in this subgroup, studies have reported pCRs of 70–80%. As a result, the St. Gallen consensus approved the use of platinum agents in patients with mutations. However, there is little clinical evidence due to the low number of included patients.

PARP inhibitors, such as olaparib, are approved in the treatment of BRCA positive metastatic ovarian cancer patients. They are still being evaluated in BC, both early and metastatic.

Current guidelines recommend similar therapeutic approaches as in sporadic BC.

Further reading

Balmaña J, Díez O, Rubio IT, Cardoso F, ESMO Guidelines Working Group on behalf of the EGW. BRCA in breast cancer: ESMO Clinical Practice Guidelines. *Ann Oncol* (online) 2011 September (cited 2016 Jun 2); 2(Suppl. 6):vi31–4.

Paluch-Shimon S, Cardoso F, Sessa C, Balmana J, Cardoso MJ, et al. On behalf of the ESMO Guidelines Committee. Prevention and screening in BRCA mutation carriers and other breast/ovarian hereditary cancer syndromes: ESMO Clinical Practice Guidelines for cancer prevention and screening. *Ann Oncol* 2016; 27(Suppl. 5):v103–10.

Chapter 7

Cancers of the gastrointestinal system

Chapter contents

7.1 Epidemiology of oesophageal cancer

Introduction

Oesophageal cancer is a common cancer in the UK with an annual incidence of 22.8 for men and 8.9 for women per 100,000 and >7,000 new cases per year. The incidence has risen steadily over the last 20 years mainly due to an increase in adenocarcinomas, whereas squamous cell carcinomas (SCCs) have decreased slightly. There is a male to female ratio of 2.5:1 although the incidence of cervical oesophageal cancer is higher in women. Despite advances in treatment, overall survival (OS) remains poor at <15%.

Aetiology and pathology

The majority of oesophageal malignancies are adenocarcinomas, SCCs, or undifferentiated carcinomas. 85% are SCCs. The increase in adenocarcinomas in the Western world over the last 20 years is thought to be associated with gastro-oesophageal reflux disease (GORD) as a consequence of increasing obesity.

The majority of tumours arise within the middle and lower third of the oesophagus with 15% in the upper third. Most adenocarcinomas occur at or immediately above the gastro-oesophageal junction (GOJ). It is often difficult to determine whether an adenocarcinoma extending through the GOJ originated in the oesophagus or in the proximal stomach.

Oesophageal reflux and Barrett's oesophagus are recognized causative factors. Other risk factors include high salt intake, alcohol, smoking, and excessive starchy food such as rice and maize. Chronic thermal injury to oesophageal mucosa from consumption of high temperature beverages and food also increases the risk. A diet rich in fruit and vegetables has been shown to reduce the relative risk. Non-steroidal anti-inflammatory drugs (NSAIDs), which inhibit cyclo-oxygenase (COX), might protect against development of oesophageal cancer, particularly in the setting of Barrett's oesophagus (BEACON Consortium). A number of tumour-related genes including p53, pRb, and bcl-2 may be associated with a potential risk. Polymorphism of certain epidermal growth factor (EGF) genes results in high levels of serum EGF and a potential increased risk of adenocarcinomas.

Clinical features

Most patients present with progressive dysphagia. Difficulty in swallowing liquids is indicative of an advanced stage. Other symptoms include odynophagia, reflux, regurgitation, and vomiting. Generally, patients will have rapid weight loss. Locally advanced disease can cause pain due to invasion of neighbouring structures such as the mediastinum and vertebral bodies. Other signs may include Horner's syndrome, recurrent laryngeal nerve palsy, and a raised hemi-diaphragm. Advanced metastatic disease may result in liver capsule discomfort, painful bony metastases, ascites, or peritoneal deposits.

Screening and surveillance

Even if detected sufficiently early for radical treatment, the probability of cure remains around 30%. In countries where SCC of the oesophagus is endemic, screening may be beneficial. The British Society of Gastroenterology (BSG) (2014) guidelines state that screening in an unselected population of patients with gastro-oesophageal reflux symptoms is not justified. However, endoscopic screening may be considered in patients with chronic GORD symptoms and multiple risk factors (at least three of age 50 years or older, white race, male sex, obesity). High-risk patients with conditions such as tylosis and Plummer–Vinson syndrome are also regularly screened with endoscopy.

In patients with non-dysplastic Barrett's oesophagus this risk is increased ten-fold to ≤1% per annum. Current BSG guidelines do not recommend surveillance for patients with <3cm of Barrett's oesophagus and only gastric metaplasia as these patients have a very low risk of cancer progression. However, patients with Barrett's oesophagus with <3cm and intestinal metaplasia should have an endoscopy every three to five years. Patients with Barrett's length >3cm should be surveyed with endoscopy and biopsy every two to three years.

Patients with Barrett's oesophagus diagnosed with indefinite or low-grade dysplasia should have acid suppression therapy followed by a repeat endoscopy and multiple four quadrant biopsies. If this dysplasia remains stable and low grade, repeat biopsy is recommended every six months or the patient may be referred for radiofrequency ablation. Patients with high-grade dysplasia (HGD) on endoscopic biopsy have a 30–40% risk of having invasive adenocarcinoma. This disease therefore should be aggressively re-biopsied to ensure a cancer has not been missed. Endoscopic techniques such as endoscopic mucosal resection (EMR) and endoscopic submucosal dissection (ESD) can be used to treat small areas of HGD or even a T1a oesophageal cancer. After HGD or early tumour clearance has been achieved, radiofrequency ablation can be performed to clear the residual Barrett's oesophagus and reduce risk of recurrence. Oesophagectomy is now reserved for patients with long segments of multifocal HGD dysplasia or those who have incomplete margins or are at higher risk of lymph node metastases (T1b) after endoscopic resection.

Investigations and staging

Barium swallow

It should not be the first-line investigation, except perhaps when a very proximal oesophageal cancer is suspected and endoscopy may be difficult. Barium swallow is very good for identifying trachea-oesophageal fistulation.

Endoscopy and endoscopic ultrasound

Flexible endoscopy is the cornerstone for diagnosis and subsequent follow-up of oesophageal cancer. It enables the operator to visualize and record the position and extent of the tumour upper limit measured from the incisor teeth and also to obtain tissue for histological diagnosis. Multiple (>8) biopsies should be obtained to allow accurate histological analysis. The main limitation of endoscopy is that only the mucosal surface of the oesophagus can be seen and biopsied.

Endoscopic ultrasound (EUS) allows the operator to see the depth of tumour invasion through the five layers of the oesophageal wall and extension of tumour into adjacent structures such as the pleura. Accurate assessment of any submucosal spread is also possible. EUS is indicated in patients who are candidates for surgery to allow accurate local staging for resectability. It may also be used immediately before endoscopic resection to ensure a tumour is suitable for such treatment, i.e. confined to the mucosal layer.

Assessment of lymph nodes is based on size as well as signal characteristics. EUS-guided fine needle aspiration (FNA) of any suspicious lesions, particularly lymph nodes outside the surgical or RT field, can improve the diagnostic accuracy. For loco-regional staging, EUS is the most accurate means of predicting local tumour (T) stage and lymph node involvement (N stage).

Computed tomography (CT) and magnetic resonance imaging (MRI)

A staging CT scan of the thorax, abdomen, and pelvis is recommended routinely in all patients to demonstrate the size of the primary tumour and its relationship with adjacent organs as well as any enlarged mediastinal, supraclavicular fossa, or perigastric/coeliac lymph nodes. CT is good for assessing direct invasion into the bronchial tree and detecting distant metastases. The use of CT and EUS improves the accuracy of staging.

Whilst MRI avoids ionizing radiation, it offers no additional benefit to a combination of CT and EUS in staging oesophageal cancers. The ST03 observational MRI substudy of the ST03 trial assessed the role of MRI in the selection of patients with lower oesophageal and GOJ adenocarcinomas for surgery, based on the ability of MRI to predict an involved circumferential resection margin (CRM). Data from this trial are awaited.

Positron emission tomography (PET)

18FDG-PET/CT scanning is indicated in patients with oesophageal cancer who are being considered for radical therapy (surgery or definitive chemoradiotherapy (CRT)). It can detect distant metastases not easily identified on CT, as well as incidental primary cancers (such as lung, head and neck, colon, and breast). It is important to correlate PET positive lesions with the corresponding contrasted CT images and ensure that patients are not denied potentially curative treatment on the basis of PET findings alone. The use of PET for loco-regional staging is limited by low specificity and resolution. A further sub-study of the ST03 trial is evaluating the role of PET/CT scan as a surrogate marker for prediction of treatment response and prognosis.

Staging laparoscopy

Laparoscopy allows the visualization and biopsy of small peritoneal or liver metastases which may not have been detected on CT or PET/CT scan. Up to 20% of patients are found to have peritoneal metastases, and futile major surgery can be avoided. This is more useful in lower-third oesophageal and GOJ cancers than upper- and middle-third cancers where the risk of intra-abdominal dissemination is low. Laparoscopy can also assess for T4 status and unresectable disease by direct visualization of the hiatus. Some units perform subphrenic and pelvic cytology on a routine basis as microscopic peritoneal disease has a poor prognosis and rules out curative surgery (Nath et al. 2008). Staging laparoscopy can be combined with surgeon-performed upper gastrointestinal (GI) endoscopy to measure the tumour accurately in relation to the GOJ and other key structures to plan subsequent resectional surgery. This is particularly important in cases of GOJ adenocarcinoma when surgical options include oesophagectomy or extended total gastrectomy depending on tumour location. In patients with

> #### Box 7.1.1 The Siewert classification
>
> Type I: adenocarcinoma of the distal oesophagus, which may infiltrate the oesophagogastric junction from above.
> Type II: true carcinoma of the cardia often referred to as 'junctional carcinoma'.
> Type III: subcardial gastric carcinoma which infiltrates the oesophagogastric junction and distal oesophagus from below.
>
> Reproduced with permission from Siewer JR, Stein HJ. Classification of adenocarcinoma of the oesophagogastric junction. *Brit J Surg* 1998; 85:1457–9. Copyright © 1998, John Wiley & Sons.

severe dysphagia, enteral feeding access with feeding jejunostomy can be performed during the same general anaesthetic.

Bronchoscopy

Many upper- or middle-third oesophageal cancers impinge on the bronchial tree causing compression or direct invasion. This is often visible on CT scan but bronchoscopy may be required to determine whether or not the tumour is potentially operable. Endobronchial ultrasound (EBUS) can also be used for this indication and can sample critical lymph nodes for histological evidence of disease involvement.

Staging

The UICC TNM classification (Tumour, Nodes, Metastases) (2017) can be found in the article '8th edition AJCC/UICC staging of cancers of the esophagus and esophagogastric junction: application to clinical practice' (Rice et al. 2017).

Siewert classification

It is often difficult to distinguish whether adenocarcinomas arising in the vicinity of the oesophagogastric junction have originated at the junction, the stomach, or the lower oesophagus. The Siewert classification aims to standardize how these tumours are described and treated (Box 7.1.1).

In most units type 1 tumours are treated by oesophagectomy and type 3 by total gastrectomy. Treatment of type 2 tumours is controversial and they may be treated by either oesophagectomy or extended total gastrectomy. Selection will depend on surgeon preference and patient fitness for one lung anaesthesia.

Further reading

Nath J, Moorthy K, Taniere P, Hallissey M, Taniere P, Alderson D. Peritoneal lavage cytology in patients with oesophagogastric adenocarcinoma. *Brit J Surg* 2008 Apr 16; 95(6):721–6—available at: https://doi.org/10.1002/bjs.6107

Rice TW, Patil DT, Blackstone EH. 8th edition AJCC/UICC staging of cancers of the esophagus and esophagogastric junction: application to clinical practice. *Ann Cardiothor Surg* 2017; 6(2):119–30—available at: https://www.ncbi.nlm.nih.gov/pmc/articles/PMC5387145/

Internet resource

NICE guideline [NG83]. Oesophago-gastric cancer: assessment and management in adults. 2018 Jan 24—available at: https://www.nice.org.uk/guidance/ng83

7.2 Treatment of localized disease for oesophageal cancer

Principles of management

Less than half of newly diagnosed patients with oesophageal cancer are curable. All curative treatments are associated with significant morbidities. Patient selection based on stage, physical fitness, and psychological preparedness is therefore important.

The two main curative options are surgical resection or CRT. Cure rates from single modality therapies are poor and attempts to improve survival using multimodality approaches, such as combining surgery with chemotherapy or radiation therapy (RT) or all three, have been made. However, any benefit from multimodality therapy must be weighed against the increased toxicity, particularly in a generally frail and elderly population of patients.

There have been two small trials comparing surgery alone with RT alone. Both trials showed a survival advantage in favour of surgery. A third trial by the MRC failed to accrue.

Surgery

The five-year overall survival (OS) of patients with oesophageal cancer referred for surgery is <10%. Major surgery should be avoided in patients whose disease is unlikely to be surgically curable. The best results are achieved in high volume specialist centres with established multidisciplinary teams (MDTs). These centres can achieve five-year survival rates of 35% with postoperative mortality <5%. Patients with very early cancers may expect a five-year survival of 80%.

The specific surgical approach is dependent on site of the tumour, histology, and the extent of lymphadenectomy intended. The most common procedure for middle- and lower-third cancers is the two-stage Ivor Lewis approach. The first stage consists of laparotomy and mobilization of the stomach, followed by right thoracotomy to remove the tumour and to form an oesophagogastric anastomosis. Modern techniques to perform this operation include either a hybrid approach (a minimal access/laparoscopic gastric mobilization combined with an open thoracotomy) or a fully minimally invasive technique (laparoscopy and thoracoscopy).

Tumours in the upper third of the oesophagus are often resected using a three-phase approach (including a cervical/neck incision) to achieve adequate longitudinal margins. This will also allow more extensive lymph node removal, particularly in the mediastinum and supraclavicular fossa. However, this operation is associated with significant morbidity (including anastomotic leak and vocal cord palsy) and in less fit patients it may be more appropriate to offer a non-surgical treatment such as RT with or without concurrent chemotherapy.

Radiotherapy

Radical RT for oesophageal cancers may cause significant acute and late morbidity and patients need to have a minimum level of fitness to tolerate treatment. Patients selected for RT tend to be less fit and have more advanced disease than those having surgery. RT alone yields a five-year survival of 6%.

Definitive chemoradiotherapy

Definitive CRT is an option for patients who are not fit for surgical resection and its associated morbidity

and mortality. This is especially true for mid- to upper-oesophageal SCC where patients are often smokers with poor respiratory reserve for surgery. Some centres have also reported good outcomes using CRT in adenocarcinomas. The main reason for adding concurrent chemotherapy to RT is to exploit the radio-sensitizing interaction and improve local control. Randomized trials comparing CRT with RT alone in oesophageal cancer have shown improved outcome for CRT.

The Radiation Therapy Oncology Group trial (RTOG 85-01) randomized 123 patients to radical RT (64Gy) or CRT (50Gy) with two cycles of synchronous cisplatin and 5-fluorouracil (FU) followed by a further two cycles. The five-year OS in the randomized and non-randomized CRT arms was 26% and 14% respectively compared with 0% in the RT alone arm. The Eastern Cooperative Oncology Group (EST-1282) also showed a significant improvement in survival for CRT compared with RT alone. Subsequent publications have shown that three-year survival of around 30% can be consistently achieved with definitive CRT. Despite improved outcomes with CRT, loco-regional failure remains a major problem at around 50%. In an attempt to improve local control, the Intergroup trial (INT 0123) explored radiation dose escalation by randomizing 236 patients to high dose (64.8Gy) versus standard dose (50.4Gy) CRT. There was no improvement in loco-regional control or OS. More treatment-related deaths occurred in the high-dose arm (10% vs. 2%), but most of the events occurred prior to receiving dose escalation.

No randomized trials have compared definitive CRT with surgery in resectable oesophageal cancer. Most of the data on CRT are for SCCs, which usually arise in the mid to upper oesophagus and are more likely to be surgically unresectable. Two trials have compared definitive CRT against a trimodality approach (CRT followed by surgery).

The EORTC trial (FFCD 9102) treated 444 patients (90% SCC) with induction CRT (using cisplatin and fluorouracil (5-FU)). A total of 259 patients who had a clinical response were then randomized to surgery or further CRT. OS was similar (median 17.7 months vs. 19.3 months and two-year OS 34% vs. 40% respectively). However, treatment-related mortality was higher in the surgery arm (9% vs. 1%; P=0.002).

The German Oesophageal Cancer Study Group Trial compared induction chemotherapy followed by CRT (40Gy) and surgery with induction chemotherapy followed by CRT alone (65Gy). A total of 172 patients with SCC were randomized. The data showed that although local progression-free survival (PFS) was better in the surgery group (64% vs. 41%; P=0.003), it did not improve OS (median 16.4 months vs. 14.9 months and two years 40% vs. 35% respectively). Treatment-related mortality was higher in the surgery arm (13% vs. 3%; P=0.03).

Most trials of definitive CRT use cisplatin and 5-FU. To improve the effectiveness of CRT, new chemotherapy regimens and drugs are being tested. The UK SCOPE 1 trial investigated the addition of weekly cetuximab (EGFR inhibitor) to standard CRT (50Gy with four cycles of cisplatin/capecitabine). At a median follow-up of 46.2 months, patients receiving cetuximab experienced greater toxicity, poorer compliance to treatment and worse OS (median OS 24.7 months vs. 34.5 months, HR 1.25, P=0.137). However, through the quality assurance programme of the SCOPE 1 trial, the delivery of high-quality RT has resulted in survival rates which are amongst the best published.

In the UK, definitive CRT has become a standard of care for SCC oesophagus.

Preoperative chemotherapy

Only one major trial has shown a statistically significant benefit in survival with preoperative chemotherapy. The Medical Research Council (MRC) OEO2 trial recruited 802 patients to receive either surgery alone or two cycles of preoperative cisplatin and 5-FU (CFU) followed by surgery. The use of chemotherapy improved OS from 34% to 43% at two years (P=0.004). This strategy is now the standard of care in most UK centres. An updated meta-analysis has shown an absolute survival benefit at two years of 5.1% for preoperative chemotherapy relative to surgery alone.

In an attempt to improve outcomes further, the UK OEO5 trial compared two cycles of preoperative CFU with four cycles of epirubicin, cisplatin, and capecitabine (ECX). Although there was some benefit with ECX, in terms of PFS (HR 0.86, CI 0.74–1.01), disease-free survival (DFS) (HR 0.88, CI 0.75–1.03), and tumour regression (Mandard grade <3 15% vs. 32%), this did not translate into a survival benefit (HR for OS 0.95, CI 0.79–1.08, P=0.3017). Chemotherapy-related toxicity was higher with four cycles of ECX compared with two cycles of CFU but surgical morbidity was not increased.

The MRC MAGIC trial evaluated the role of perioperative chemotherapy for patients with gastric, lower oesophageal, and GOJ tumours with three cycles of ECX given before surgery followed by three cycles postoperatively. A significant OS difference of 13% at five years was reported.

In the ST03 trial, perioperative bevacizumab (VEGF inhibitor) in combination with ECX for patients with operable oesophagogastric adenocarcinoma was evaluated. However, patients receiving bevacizumab were found to have a higher risk of surgical complications including anastomotic leak and, therefore, the trial was stopped. The ST03 also conducted a feasibility study evaluating the role of lapatinib in HER2 positive oesophagogastric adenocarcinomas in a perioperative combination treatment regimen. There was no improvement in three-year OS with the addition of bevacizumab (48.1% vs. 50.3%, HR 1.08, P=0.36).

Preoperative chemoradiotherapy

A large number of different preoperative CRT schedules using varying radiation doses and fractionations and varying chemotherapy regimens have been published. Pathological complete response (pCR) rates range from 7% to 56%. In the Dutch CROSS trial, patients with oesophageal and GOJ tumours (366 patients, 75% had adenocarcinoma) were randomly assigned to preoperative treatment with weekly paclitaxel and carboplatin given concurrently with RT 41.4Gy versus surgery alone. The complete (R0) resection rate was higher with CRT (92% vs. 65%). At a median follow-up of 32 months, both the median survival and OS was higher in the CRT group (49.4 months vs. 24.0 months; HR 0.65, CI 0.495–0.871). There was no increase in postoperative complications.

Meta-analyses show a statistically significant improvement in OS, an absolute survival benefit of 8.7% at two years with preoperative CRT followed by surgery compared with surgery alone. This benefit was only seen when chemotherapy was given concurrently with RT (P=0.005) rather than sequentially (P=0.36). However, treatment-related mortality was increased with preoperative CRT (P=0.053). In an attempt to find the optimal CRT regimen, a systematic analysis of 26 trials showed that there is a dose–response relationship between RT and chemotherapy dose and pCR rate. One gram/m^2 of 5-FU was calculated to be equivalent to 1.9Gy of radiation and 100g/m^2 was equivalent to 7.2Gy.

The currently recruiting UK NEOSCOPE trial is attempting to identify an optimum concurrent RT-chemotherapy regimen and is randomizing between oxaliplatin plus capecitabine and carboplatin plus paclitaxel. In addition, the NeoEGIS trial is also recruiting in the UK and randomizing patients between neoadjuvant CRT (CROSS style) and perioperative chemotherapy (MAGIC regimen includes Epirubicin, Cisplatin and 5-Flourouracil/Capecitabine) prior to oesophagectomy in patients with oesophageal adenocarcincoma.

Postoperative treatment

There is no definite role for adjuvant treatment after surgery for oesophageal cancer. One trial showed a five-year OS advantage with adjuvant RT (35% vs. 13%), but confined only to stage III disease. A meta-analysis suggested a survival benefit with adjuvant CRT but the numbers were too small to make a definitive conclusion.

7.3 Treatment of advanced disease for oesophageal cancer

Principles of management

Over two-thirds of oesophageal cancer patients present with advanced, incurable disease. In addition, a significant number of patients who initially undergo radical treatment will relapse. Palliative treatment aims to improve symptoms and quality of life. The main symptom encountered in advanced oesophageal cancer is dysphagia and palliation is aimed at improving swallowing. The most appropriate option is dependent on local tumour extent as well as the individual patient.

Localized treatments for dysphagia

Dilatation

Dilatation leads to immediate but short-lived (two to four weeks) improvement of dysphagia, but with a significant risk of oesophageal perforation. It is therefore not recommended.

Stenting

The use of self-expanding metallic stents (SEMS) has improved palliation and reduced complication rates. Approximately 66% of patients can eat some solid foods after successful deployment. Early complications are uncommon but late complications occur in 25% of patients and include most commonly recurrent dysphagia due to stent migration or recurrent tumour overgrowth. Most modern stents are removable in case of poor deployment or subsequent migration. Fully covered stents are particularly useful for occluding a trachea-oesophageal fistula.

Oesophageal stents are not recommended in patients whose disease is potentially curable and who may subsequently undergo surgery, as stenting may worsen prognosis, may migrate during neoadjuvant therapy and persistent fibrosis or inflammation makes surgical resection very difficult.

Injection/thermal ablation

Alcohol injection or thermal ablation with *YAG* laser or photodynamic therapy can improve dysphagia. The benefit is often short lived and may need to be repeated regularly. All techniques are also associated with potential morbidity including haemorrhage and perforation in 10–15%.

Radiotherapy

This can be delivered either by conventional external beam radiotherapy (EBRT) or by brachytherapy (insertion of an iridium-192 radioactive source into the oesophagus). Improvement in swallowing will not occur immediately and may sometimes deteriorate initially before improving. EBRT is often given as 30Gy in ten fractions over two weeks or 20Gy in five fractions. Brachytherapy has been shown to be effective using a high-dose rate machine to give 16Gy in two fractions or 18Gy in three fractions over five days. Both techniques can be used with other local therapies to try to maximize symptom control.

Chemotherapy

Chemotherapy for advanced oesophageal and gastric cancer has been shown to improve survival when compared with best supportive care alone. Meta-analysis showed that the benefit was greatest when using a three-drug regimen including 5-FU, an anthracycline, and cisplatin.

The treatment of advanced adenocarcinomas of the oesophagus with chemotherapy is similar to gastric cancers and is discussed in the next chapter.

Further reading

Lordick F, Mariette C, Haustermans K, Obermannová R, Arnold D. ESMO Guidelines Committee. Oesophageal cancer: ESMO Clinical Practice Guidelines for diagnosis, treatment and follow-up. *Ann Oncol* 2016; 27(suppl. 5):v50–7.

Internet resources

Neoadjuvant trial in adenocarcinoma of the oesophagus and oesophagogastric junction international study (Neo-AEGIS): https://clinicaltrials.gov/ct2/show/NCT01726452

7.4 Epidemiology of gastric cancer

Introduction

It is the eighth commonest cancer in the UK with an incidence of 19.8 for men and 8.3 for women per 100,000 (ONS 2014) and approximately 8,200 new cases per year. Although the overall incidence of distal gastric cancers has decreased significantly, there has been an exponential rise in tumours involving the proximal stomach and cardia. The overall five-year survival remains low at around 18%.

Pathology

The term gastric cancer is generally applied to adenocarcinomas which account for approximately 95% of all gastric neoplasms. The Lauren classification divides gastric adenocarcinomas into two different histological variants, intestinal and diffuse. In the intestinal subtype, tumour cells adhere to each other in a tubular or glandular formation, similar to adenocarcinomas arising in other parts of the intestinal tract. In the diffuse subtype, tumour cells lack adhesion molecules and have a more infiltrative appearance with little in the way of tubule or gland formation. The intestinal subtype tends to affect older patients and arise in the distal stomach, whereas the diffuse subtype is more common in younger patients. A variant of the diffuse subtype which extensively infiltrates the stomach wall is known as linitis plastica.

Other malignant tumours which arise in the stomach include lymphomas, GI stromal tumours (GISTs), and carcinoid tumours. The stomach is the most common site for GISTs and extranodal lymphomas.

Aetiology

The risk factors include increasing population weight and high calorific intake associated GORD and chronic reflux disease causing Barrett's oesophagus. Smoking and diets rich in nitrates and salt are associated with an increased risk of developing gastric cancer, whereas fruits and vegetables high in vitamin C and E, and antioxidants are considered to have a protective effect.

Helicobater pylori infection is associated with both intestinal and diffuse subtypes of gastric cancer and MALToma. *H. pylori* eradication is associated with significantly lower rates of gastric cancer (1.6% vs. 2.4%, RR 0.66, 95% CI 0.46–0.95). *H. pylori* eradication is also indicated in patients with gastric MALToma.

Germline mutations in the E-cadherin (CDH1) gene have been found in families with hereditary diffuse gastric cancer. Gastric cancer is associated with other cancer syndromes including hereditary non-polyposis colorectal cancer, familial adenomatous polyposis, and Peutz–Jeghers syndrome. Other risk factors include chronic atrophic gastritis and hypochlorhydria, pernicious anaemia, gastric surgery, Epstein–Barr virus infection, hypertrophic gastropathy, and various immunodeficiency syndromes. Regular use of aspirin and other NSAIDs is associated with a reduced risk of non-cardia gastric adenocarcinomas.

Clinical features

Weight loss and persistent abdominal pain are the most common symptoms. Nausea, anorexia, and early satiety are common features. Dysphagia occurs with tumours involving the proximal stomach or GOJ. Distal tumours can present with symptoms of gastric outlet obstruction. Iron deficiency anaemia due to occult GI bleeding is not uncommon, whilst approximately 20% present with haematemesis or melaena.

Up to 50% of patients present with symptoms of metastatic disease. Clinical signs indicating advanced disease include a palpable epigastric mass, an enlarged stomach with succussion splash, hepatomegaly, obstructive jaundice, and cachexia. Presence of ascites is usually indicative of peritoneal carcinomatosis. Virchow's node (left supraclavicular adenopathy) occurs with distant lymphatic spread. Peritoneal spread may result in a Sister Mary Joseph nodule (periumbilical metastasis), Krukenberg tumour (ovarian metastasis), and Blumer's shelf (mass in the anterior rectal wall on rectal examination). Associated paraneoplastic syndromes include dermatomyositis, acanthosis nigricans, sudden appearance of diffuse seborrhoeic keratoses (sign of Leser–Trélat), circinate erythemas, and microangiopathic haemolytic anaemia are occasionally described. Patients may also present with symptoms and clinical features suggestive of bone, lung, and central nervous system (CNS) metastases.

Screening

The role of screening asymptomatic individuals for gastric cancer is not entirely proven. Although endoscopy increases the rate of detection of gastric cancer compared with barium studies as a tool for mass population screening it is limited by cost and availability of experienced operators. More recently, there is more interest in the use of serological markers (e.g. serum pepsinogen, *H. pylori* antibody, etc.) to identify patients at risk of developing gastric cancer.

In the UK, the national screening committee has not recommended routine screening, but have suggested a more pragmatic approach, for example, following up patients with gastric ulcers with repeated biopsies until complete healing. For patients with hereditary diffuse

gastric cancer (CDH1 mutation/E-caderin defects), annual chromo-endoscopic surveillance should be performed in regional centres using an agreed protocol. In mutation positive individuals, prophylactic total gastrectomy at a regional centre should be strongly considered. The systematic histological study of prophylactic gastrectomies almost universally shows pre-invasive lesions including in situ signet ring carcinoma.

Diagnosis and staging

Endoscopy

Flexible oesophago-gastro-duodenoscopy (OGD) is the diagnostic procedure of choice. It permits direct visualization and biopsy of any suspicious lesions. The sensitivity of OGD is about 98% when multiple (at least seven) biopsies are taken from a suspicious lesion. Newer techniques, such as chromoendoscopy or narrow band imaging (NBI), may enhance the detection of subtle lesions or dysplasia. However, the diagnosis of the diffuse-type gastric cancer may be difficult endoscopically as the overlying mucosa may appear normal. Subtle endoscopic signs of this include poor gastric distention. Multiple biopsies in the same area, to try to reach the submucosal layer, can reveal useful histology or in some cases EUS and deeper targeted FNA samples may be required to establish a diagnosis.

Barium studies

Double-contrast barium studies are now rarely performed and may be useful when endoscopy is not feasible or in the diagnosis of diffuse-type gastric cancer (linitis plastica with 'leather bottle' appearance).

CT

Contrast enhanced multislice CT scan following gastric distension with 600–800ml of water should be performed routinely in the staging of gastric cancer. However, up to 30% of peritoneal metastases will not be detectable on CT scan and its accuracy for staging early cancers is poor.

Endoscopic ultrasound

EUS provides a more accurate prediction of depth of tumour invasion, particularly in early cancers. In a systematic review the sensitivity and specificity for EUS in distinguishing T1 from T2 tumours was 85% and 90%, respectively, and distinguishing T1/2 from T3/4 tumours was 86% and 90%, respectively (Mocellin et al. 2015). The accuracy for lymph node staging is only slightly better compared with CT (Kelly et al. 2001); however, EUS-guided FNA of suspicious lymph nodes can improve the accuracy of EUS. EUS is indicated in the assessment of early gastric lesions to see whether they are suitable for endoscopic resection. It is also useful in patients who are suspected to have T4 invasion, most commonly to the diaphragmatic crura, left lobe of liver, spleen, or pancreas.

FDG-PET

Although PET is more sensitive than CT in detecting distant metastasis, it is not routinely used in the staging of gastric cancer due to limitations of spatial resolution in distinguishing between primary tumour and level 1–2 lymph nodes, and lack of unified criteria in how to interpret PET for management decisions. FDG-PET does have a role in staging proximal/junctional type gastric cancers, especially of intestinal type, to exclude metastatic disease before radical surgical resection.

Laparoscopy and peritoneal cytology

Up to 20–30% of gastric cancer patients will have peritoneal metastases which are not detected on CT. Positive identification of such lesions will prevent the patient undergoing a futile laparotomy and resection. Laparoscopy is recommended in all patients with gastric cancer and gastro-oesophageal cancer where there appears to be a gastric component. Peritoneal cytologically positive disease should not be routinely treated with resection surgery; however, some units do offer neoadjuvant chemotherapy and repeat cytological assessment. If the staging becomes cytologically negative after chemotherapy, resection can be offered with reasonable survival outcomes.

Staging

The current UICC staging is shown in 'Stage grouping'.

T: primary tumour

- TX: primary tumour cannot be assessed
- T0: no evidence of primary tumour
- Tis: carcinoma in situ: intraepithelial tumour without invasion of the lamina propria
- T1a: tumour invades lamina propria or muscularis mucosae
- T1b: tumour invades submucosa
- T2: tumour invades muscularis propria
- T3: tumour penetrates subserosal connective tissue
- T4a: tumour invades serosa (visceral peritoneum)
- T4b: tumour invades adjacent structures

N: regional lymph nodes

- NX: regional lymph nodes cannot be assessed
- N0: no regional lymph node metastasis
- N1: metastasis in 1–2 regional lymph nodes
- N2: metastasis in 3–6 regional lymph nodes
- N3: metastasis in >7 regional lymph nodes
- N3a: metastasis in 7–15 lymph nodes
- N3b: metastasis in >16 lymph nodes

M: distant metastasis

- MX: distant metastasis cannot be assessed
- M0: no distant metastasis
- M1: distant metastasis

Stage grouping

- Stage 0: TisN0M0
- Stage IA: T1N0M0
- Stage IB:
  - T1N1M0
  - T2N0M0
- Stage IIA:
  - T3N0M0
  - T2N1M0
  - T1N2M0
- Stage IIB
  - T4aN0M0

- T3N1M0
- T2N2M0
- Stage IIIA:
  - T4aN1M0
  - T3N2M0
  - T2N3M0
- Stage IIIB:
  - T4bN0/1M0
  - T4aN2M0
  - T3N3M0
- Stage IIIC:
  - T4bN2/3M0
  - T4aN3M0
- Stage IV:
  - Any T any N M1

(Reproduced with permission from Brierley JD, Gospodarowicz MK, Wittekind C (eds). *TNM Classification of Malignant Tumours*, 8th edn. Copyright © 2017, John Wiley & Sons.)

Prognosis

Important prognostic factors in resectable gastric cancer include depth of invasion, number of lymph nodes involved, and positive resection margins. In the UK five-year survival rates remain low at approximately 15%. Estimated five-year survival by stage is:

- Stage 1: 70%
- Stage 2: 40%
- Stage 3: 20%
- Stage 4: <5%

Further reading

Fitzgerald RC, Hardwick R, Huntsman D, et al. Hereditary diffuse gastric cancer: updated consensus guidelines for clinical management and directions for future research. *J Med Genet* 2010; 47(7):436–44.

Kelly S, et al. A systematic review of the staging performance of endoscopic ultrasound in gastro-oesophageal carcinoma. *Gut* 2001; 49:534–9.

Mocellin S, Pasquali S. Diagnostic accuracy of endoscopic ultrasonography (EUS) for the preoperative locoregional staging of primary gastric cancer. *Cochrane Datab Syst Rev* 2015 Feb 6; (2):CD009944—available at: https://www.ncbi.nlm.nih.gov/pubmed/25914908

NICE guideline [NG83]. Oesophago-gastric cancer: assessment and management in adults. 2018 Jan 24—available at: https://www.nice.org.uk/guidance/ng83

Smyth EC, Verheij M, Allum W, Cunningham D, Cervantes A, Arnold D. ESMO Guidelines Committee. Gastric cancer: ESMO Clinical Practice Guidelines for diagnosis, treatment and follow-up. *Ann Oncol* 2016; 27(suppl. 5):v38–49.

Internet resources

Cancer Research UK: http://info.cancerresearchuk.org

The UK NSC Recommendation on Stomach Cancer Screening in Adults (currently under review): https://legacyscreening.phe.org.uk/stomachcancer

7.5 Treatment of localized disease for gastric cancer

Principles of treatment
Surgical resection offers the only curative treatment option for gastric cancer but is only appropriate in <50% of newly diagnosed patients. Cure rates from surgical resection as a single modality treatment range from 13% to 50%. Multimodality treatment results in a modest survival benefit but at the cost of increased toxicity.

Early gastric cancer (EGC)
EGC is tumour that is limited to the gastric mucosa or submucosa irrespective of nodal involvement. It is associated with a favourable prognosis compared with cancers that invade beyond the submucosa. Following resection, five-year survival rates of >90% have been reported.

The risk of lymph node metastasis in EGC is 10–15% and depends on the size of tumour, histological subtype, and presence of submucosal invasion. If untreated, up to two-thirds of patients with EGC may progress to advanced cancer over five years. Patients with a low risk of nodal involvement may be considered for less radical treatment options such as EMR. Five-year survival rates of 84% have been reported with EMR. Limitations of EMR include risk of incomplete tumour resection and tumour/lymph node understaging despite optimal work-up.

H. pylori is classified as a group I carcinogen for gastric cancer. The evidence for *H. pylori* eradication in reducing the incidence of gastric cancer remains controversial. In a Japanese randomized trial, 554 patients with EGC treated endoscopically received *H. pylori* eradication or no eradication. At three-year follow-up, the OR for development of metachronous gastric cancer was 0.353 (95% CI 0.161–0.775) in favour of eradication. Further studies are required to confirm these findings.

Surgery
The aim of surgical resection is to achieve complete removal of the tumour and involved lymph nodes. Guidelines from ESMO recommend recovery of a minimum of 14 lymph nodes.

The size and location of the primary tumour determine the extent of gastric resection. Three randomized trials have compared distal versus total gastrectomy for distal gastric cancer. The largest involved 648 patients and showed no difference in five-year survival. Total gastrectomy has higher operative risks and patients have a poorer quality of life after surgery. It should therefore be offered to patients who are fit enough for radical surgery and in those who require removal of the whole stomach for oncological reasons. Tumours involving the proximal stomach or the GOJ (Siewert types II and III) require total gastrectomy. Tumours involving the body of the stomach, especially of diffuse type, should be considered for total gastrectomy. Frozen section histology of the margins can be obtained intraoperatively to ensure R0 resection. Distal gastrectomy reduces morbidity, results in better function, and is the preferred surgical option when the primary tumour can be completely resected. Regardless of what type of gastrectomy is performed, surgical technique should focus on achieving negative proximal and distal margins and ensuring an adequate lymphadenectomy. Minimal access/laparoscopic gastrectomy has been developed to improve outcomes of patients undergoing surgery. The early postoperative morbidity and mortality are similar to the results of open surgery, but length of hospital stay is shorter. Laparoscopic gastrectomy is increasingly offered by specialist units in the UK; however, its uptake is still less than 10% of procedures and the long-term outcomes have not been adequately assessed in randomized trials.

Lymphatic drainage of the stomach is extensive and multidirectional. D1 lymphadenectomy involves dissection of the perigastric lymph nodes within 5cm of the primary tumour. D2 lymphadenectomy involves dissection of lymph nodes along the major vessels (coeliac axis, hepatic artery, and splenic artery) and in the splenic hilum in addition to D1 lymphadenectomy. D3 lymphadenectomy includes the porta hepatis and para-aortic lymph nodes in addition to D2 lymphadenectomy. The recommended extent of lymph node dissection remains controversial.

Although results of prospective surgical series suggested significant survival advantage of D2 lymphadenectomy over D1, the MRC and Dutch Gastric Cancer Group randomized trials showed no difference in OS. Patients undergoing D2 resection had higher surgical morbidity and mortality. This was attributed to the pancreatico-splenectomy component of the D2 arm. A subset analysis of patients undergoing D2 lymphadenectomy without pancreatico-splenectomy suggested improved survival compared with D1. However, the quality assurance of both trials has been questioned. Non-compliance with D2 dissection in the Dutch Gastric Cancer Trial may have obscured a survival benefit of radical D2 lymphadenectomy. The Japanese Clinical Oncology Group trial compared D2 with D3 lymphadenectomy. There was no difference in five-year survival (69% vs. 70%) or recurrence-free survival. Surgical complications were more common in the D3 arm.

The UK recommendation is to perform D2 lymphadenectomy without pancreatico-splenectomy in patients considered to be sufficiently fit to tolerate this procedure.

Gastric cancer surgery is associated with significant morbidity and mortality. Patients should be treated in high volume regional specialist centres to improve outcomes. In addition, patients need intensive support to minimize the physical and psychosocial morbidity associated with gastrectomy to enhance recovery.

Chemotherapy
Despite undergoing surgical resection for gastric cancer, most patients remain at high risk of recurrence. Multiple trials and meta-analyses of the role of adjuvant chemotherapy suggest some survival improvement. A Japanese randomized trial using S-1 (an oral fluoropyrimidine prodrug combined with a 4-deoxypyridoxine (DPD) antagonist and potassium oxonate which reduces GI toxicity) showed survival improvement compared with surgery alone, 72% vs. 61% at five years. The CLASSIC trial comparing oxaliplatin/capecitabine with no treatment showed a 15% improvement in three-year DFS (HR 0.56, 95% CI 0.44–0.72; P<0.0001) and marginal OS benefit using adjuvant capecitabine and oxaliplatin (78% vs. 69%, HR 0.66, 95% CI 0.51–0.85) (Noh et al. 2014).

An alternative strategy is to use preoperative (neoadjuvant) therapies. The potential advantages include improving curative resection rates, earlier treatment of micro-metastases and better treatment compliance. The UK MRC MAGIC trial compared three cycles of preoperative ECF (epirubicin, cisplatin, and continuous infusional 5-FU) followed by a further three cycles postoperatively with surgery alone for resectable gastric and lower oesophageal cancers. Five-year survival was significantly better in patients receiving chemotherapy (36% vs. 23%; HR for death 0.75; P=0.009). Results of the MAGIC trial are supported by a French trial comparing perioperative cisplatin and 5-FU versus surgery alone, demonstrating improved five-year survival (38% vs. 24%, P=0.02).

The FLOT-4 trial comparing perioperative (three cycles of preoperative and three cycles of postoperative docetaxel, oxaliplatin, and 5-FU) FLOT with ECF/ECX in ≥cT2 or cN+ gastric and GOJ adenocarcinomas demonstrated further improved OS (median 50 months vs. 35 months, HR 0.77), with benefits seen in all subgroups. This is likely to become the reference perioperative chemotherapy regimen in gastric and GOJ adenocarcinomas.

Adjuvant chemoradiotherapy

The role of postoperative radiotherapy was explored following high rates of loco-regional failure. The Intergroup trial 0116 randomized 556 patients to postoperative chemotherapy, and CRT versus surgery alone. Patients received 5-FU and leucovorin before, during, and after RT (45Gy in 25 fractions). The three-year survival rate was better in the CRT arm (50% vs. 41%; P=0.005). However, this trial has been criticized in a number of areas. Firstly, over 50% of patients entered had suboptimal lymph node removal. Secondly, the acute toxicity of this treatment was significant. The ARTIST trial randomized 458 patients with completely resected gastric cancer and D2 lymph node dissection to postoperative CRT with capecitabine versus chemotherapy alone with cisplatin and capecitabine and showed no improvement in DFS with the addition of radiotherapy. However, on subgroup analysis of patients with pathological lymph node involvement, adjuvant CRT improved DFS (P=0.0365).

A meta-analysis of trials comparing adjuvant CRT versus chemotherapy alone has shown improved five-year DFS (OR 1.56, 95% CI 1.09–2.24) and reduced loco-regional recurrence rate (OR 0.46, 95% CI 0.32–0.67) but no improvement in OS (OR = 1.32, 95% CI 0.92–1.88) (Dai et al. 2015). Adjuvant CRT is currently not a standard treatment in the UK and Europe.

Ongoing clinical trials are evaluating optimization of chemotherapy regimens, role of radiotherapy, and timing of therapies (preoperative, postoperative, or both).

The ARTIST-II trial is comparing adjuvant chemotherapy versus CRT in lymph node positive completely resected gastric cancer. The intervention arm of TOPGEAR trial is investigating whether the addition of CRT is superior to chemotherapy alone in the preoperative setting in improving pCR and OS (see 'Internet resources' at end of this section).

Targeted therapies

Targeted therapies include monoclonal antibodies and small molecules targeting intracellular signalling cascades which promote cancer cell proliferation. Data on targeted therapies for gastric cancer are limited to phase I trials. The role of perioperative bevacizumab in combination with ECX chemotherapy for patients with operable oesophagogastric adenocarcinoma was evaluated in the UK NCRN ST03 trial. An elevated postoperative anastomotic leak rate in the bevacizumab group in those undergoing oesophago-gastrectomy (9% ECX, 23% ECX+B) resulted in recruitment being closed to such patients towards the end of the trial. Neither the response rate nor the OS improved with addition of bevacizumab.

Further reading

Al-Batran SE, et al. Perioperative chemotherapy with fluorouracil plus leucovorin, oxaliplatin, and docetaxel versus fluorouracil or capecitabine plus cisplatin and epirubicin for locally advanced, resectable gastric or gastro-oesophageal junction adenocarcinoma (FLOT4): a randomised, phase 2/3 trial. *Lancet* 2019; 393(10184):1948–57.

Dai Q, Jiang L, Lin RJ, Wei KK, et al. Adjuvant chemoradiotherapy versus chemotherapy for gastric cancer: a meta-analysis of randomized controlled trials. *J Surg Oncol* 2015; 111(3):277–84.

Noh SH, Park SR, Yang HK, Chung HC, Chung IJ, et al. Adjuvant capecitabine plus oxaliplatin for gastric cancer after D2 gastrectomy (CLASSIC): 5-year follow-up of an open-label, randomised phase 3 trial. CLASSIC trial investigators. *Lancet Oncol* 2014; (12):1389–96.

Smyth EC, Verheij M, Allum W, Cunningham D, Cervantes A, Arnold D. ESMO Guidelines Committee. Gastric cancer: ESMO Clinical Practice Guidelines for diagnosis, treatment and follow-up. *Ann Oncol* 2016; 27 (suppl. 5):v38–49.

Van Cutsem E, Sagaert X, Topal B, Haustermans K, Prenen H. Gastric cancer. *Lancet* 2016; 388:2654–64.

Internet resource

US National Institute of Health: http://www.clinicaltrials.gov

7.6 Treatment of advanced disease for gastric cancer

Principles of management

The majority of patients with gastric cancer either present with metastatic disease or will develop recurrent disease following resection. Management of advanced disease is a significant challenge in the treatment of gastric cancer.

Endoscopic treatment

Tumours at the cardia and GOJ often cause dysphagia and regurgitation, whilst distal tumours can cause gastric outlet obstruction. Patients present with vomiting, dehydration, epigastric pain and discomfort, poor oral intake, and weight loss or cachexia. They are often in a poor clinical state due to malnourishment and have

a severely reduced quality of life. Consequently, expected survival in these patients is short (three to four months) and therefore management should be focused on palliation of symptoms and treatments to improve quality of life (QoL). Endoscopic stent placement can be effective in relieving symptoms and improving QoL. Technical success rates from endoscopic stenting range from 86% to 100%. Fluoroscopic visualization of the stent position is important to ensure accurate placement. In tumours causing gastric outlet obstruction, endoscopic stent placement appears as effective as gastric bypass in relieving symptoms. However, 15–40% may require further intervention due to recurrent symptoms

Up to 20% of patients will develop frank GI bleeding. Endoscopic laser photocoagulation or argon plasma coagulation can be effective in palliating tumour-related haemorrhage. If this is not effective, radiological embolization or palliative radiotherapy should be considered.

Surgery

Indications for surgical intervention include gastric outlet obstruction and occasionally uncontrollable haemorrhage. Options include bypass surgery (gastrojejunostomy) or palliative gastrectomy. Surgical bypass is often not possible due to the poor condition of these patients and associated comorbid disease may preclude general anaesthesia. Palliative gastrojejunostomy, even if performed laparoscopically, has a high complication rate and may result in a prolonged hospital stay due to gastroparesis.

Palliative gastrectomy is unusually performed in clinical practice as most patients can be adequately palliated using other modalities. However, there is increasing evidence that palliative surgery can provide a prognostic and symptomatic benefit, particularly in combination with chemotherapy and/or radiotherapy. Laparoscopic approaches may result in lower morbidity and more rapid recovery.

Radiotherapy

EBRT can be useful in palliating local symptoms such as haemorrhage, dysphagia, and pain. It is also useful in treating painful metastatic disease. In a retrospective review of 115 patients with gastric cancer treated with palliative radiotherapy for symptoms of bleeding, dysphagia, and pain, control was achieved in 81%, 53%, and 45% respectively, dose ranged from 8Gy in a single fraction to 40Gy in 16 fractions, and effective palliation was achieved with short radiotherapy schedules.

Chemotherapy and targeted therapies

Before deciding to embark on palliative chemotherapy treatment, the patient's ability to tolerate treatment must be assessed. A significant proportion will not be sufficiently fit for chemotherapy.

The use of chemotherapy has been shown to improve OS as well as QoL when compared with best supportive care (BSC) in multiple randomized trials. A recently published systematic review demonstrated the superiority of combination chemotherapy compared with monotherapy and chemotherapy compared with BSC; the survival benefit of combination chemotherapy was estimated to be around six months.

In the UK the combination of epirubicin, cisplatin, and continuous 5-FU (ECF) has been the reference regimen following results of two randomized trials. The main disadvantage of this regimen is that an indwelling venous catheter is required to deliver the 5-FU and this is associated with infection and thromboembolic risk. Capecitabine (X), an oral pro-drug of 5-FU, has been successfully integrated into the ECX regimen as a direct substitute for infusional 5-FU. The REAL-2 trial demonstrated equivalence of capecitabine to 5-FU when combined with either cisplatin or oxaliplatin (O) in terms of efficacy and toxicity. In a subset analysis there was suggestion of prolonged survival with EOX when compared with ECF.

Other chemotherapy agents have been shown to be active in gastric cancer including the taxanes and irinotecan. A US/European randomized trial showed that the addition of docetaxel to cisplatin and 5-FU (DCF) was superior to cisplatin and 5-FU in terms of OS and response rate; however, this was at the expense of greater grade 3/4 toxicity. A randomized trial compared the combination of S-1 with cisplatin versus S-1 alone and showed improved survival and response rates in Japanese patients using the combination, but again this was more toxic.

Recently there have been a number of randomized trials for patients who progress on first-line treatment. Docetaxel, irinotecan, paclitaxel, and cisplatin have been trialled but only few demonstrated statistically significant differences. However, OS was statistically significantly improved for all interventions compared to best supportive care. Patients responding to second-line chemotherapy experience symptomatic benefit and may survive longer compared with non-responders.

Targeted therapies have demonstrated only modest benefit in advanced gastric cancer. A phase 2 trial reported response rates of 65% for a combination of bevacizumab with irinotecan and cisplatin. Addition of panitumumab to EOX did not improve the OS as shown by the REAL 3 trial

A phase 3 international study of trastuzumab in patients with HER2-positive gastric cancer showed a 26% reduction in risk of death in comparison with those who received chemotherapy alone. OS was increased by 2.7 months. There was no increase in cardiac morbidity.

Ramucirumab, a VGEF receptor antagonist has been evaluated with or without paclitaxel in a phase 3 randomized trial in patients previously treated for advanced gastric cancer. The combination treatment increased OS (9.6 months vs. 7.4 months, HR 0.8, 95% CI 0.67–0.96, P=0.017).

Best supportive care

Simple measures including adequate analgesia and steroids can improve a patient's quality of life. Access to hospice care and other relevant specialists, where appropriate, should be made easily accessible in accordance with National Service Framework guidelines.

Further reading

Smyth EC, Verheij M, Allum W, Cunningham D, Cervantes A, Arnold D. ESMO Guidelines Committee. Gastric cancer: ESMO Clinical Practice Guidelines for diagnosis, treatment and follow-up. *Ann Oncol* 2016; 27(suppl. 5):v38–49.

Internet resources

Department of Health: http://www.dh.gov.uk

National Service Cancer Research and Treatment: Guidance and Regulation: http://www.nhs.uk/nhsengland/NSF/pages/Cancer.aspx

7.7 Hepatocellular cancer

Epidemiology
Hepatocellular cancer (HCC) is the most common form of primary liver cancer with an age adjusted global incidence of 10.1 per 100,000 person years. It is the sixth most common neoplasm in the world and is the third leading cause of cancer mortality with as many as 746,000 deaths annually. There is a wide geographical variation in the incidence of new HCC cases with the disease predominantly affecting men rather than women.

Aetiology
The majority (70–90%) of HCC arises on the background of chronic liver disease.

Populations at risk of HCC include:
- Hepatitis B virus (HBV) infection: around 5% of the word population has a chronic HBV infection, 75% of those infected are Asian. HBV at present accounts for over 50% of all cases of HCC. The five-year cumulative risk of HCC among cirrhotic patients ranges from 5% to 30%. There is evidence that vaccination against HBV is of benefit. Nationwide vaccination of infants in Taiwan reduced the incidence of HCC from 0.922–0.23 per 100,000
- HCV infection: main risk factor in Europe, the USA, and Japan alongside high alcohol consumption
- High alcohol consumption
- Non-alcoholic fatty liver disease (NAFLD)
- Obesity
- Diabetes mellitus
- Genetic haemochromatosis

Surveillance
Currently there are no screening programmes for HCC; conversely HCC surveillance has been adopted widely. The two most common tests used for surveillance are serum alpha-fetoprotein (AFP) and ultrasonography.

AFP is the most widely used serological test for HCC. Using the most effective diagnostic range (10–20ng/ml), sensitivity and specificity for HCC diagnosis is approximately 60% and 80% respectively. Unfortunately diagnostic accuracy is worse if AFP level monitoring is used for surveillance.

Ultrasonography is highly dependent on operator experience and nodule size. Allowing for these variations sensitivity is 60–90% and specificity >90%. Nodules with a median size above 1.6cm can be reliably diagnosed in non-cirrhotic livers. The main difficulty for use of ultrasound is differentiating regenerative and dysplastic nodules from HCC on the background of liver cirrhosis. CT and MRI are most useful for confirming the diagnosis.

Surveillance for HCC
Surveillance in Europe is recommended for the at risk groups listed below:
- Liver cirrhosis of any aetiology Child–Pugh stage A and B
- Liver cirrhosis Child–Pugh stage C if awaiting liver transplantation
- Non-cirrhotic HBV carriers with active hepatitis or family history of HCC
- Non-cirrhotic patients with chronic HCV infection and advanced liver fibrosis, stage F3

Surveillance interval
It is challenging to confidently diagnose liver lesions of <1cm as HCC. Therefore, based on median doubling times of 110–170 days, surveillance is usually performed every six months. Three-monthly surveillance detects more small nodules but does not improve survival whereas annual surveillance has inferior results compare with a bi-annual regime.

Pathology
HCC usually develops following a multistep pathway starting with a cycle of cell necrosis and proliferation that is triggered by liver cell injury due to hepatotoxic factors (e.g. HBV).

This cycle leads to the formation of hyperplastic nodules surrounded by proliferating collagen fibres. These hyperplastic nodules transform into dysplastic nodules and eventually develop into HCC (Figure 7.7.1).

Metastases are most frequently found in the lungs. Other locations with decreasing frequency are abdominal lymph nodes, bones, and brain.

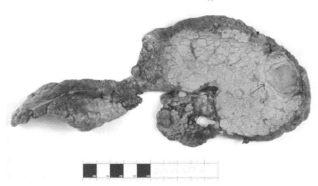

Fig. 7.7.1 Multifocal HCC on the background of cirrhotic liver.

Clinical features

The clinical findings depend on the stage of the tumour and the function of the liver. Large HCC may present with abdominal pain associated with malaise, weight loss, asthenia, anorexia, and fever. Spontaneous haemorrhage and rupture of HCC occurs in 5–15% of patients. Portal vein invasion by HCC may present with upper GI bleeding from varices or the acute development of ascites due to portal hypertension. Invasion of the hepatic veins or inferior vena cava may cause thrombosis or tumour embolization which can result in pulmonary embolism. A small number of patients may present with obstructive jaundice or haemobilia due to infiltration of the bile duct. Only large and superficial tumours are palpable.

Patients with chronic liver disease may have clinical signs secondary to the liver disease such as jaundice, parotid enlargement, spider naevi or cutaneous bruising, palmar erythema, clubbing, ascites, splenomegaly, caput medusa, pedal oedema, or testicular atrophy. Paraneoplastic syndromes may occur and include hypercalcaemia and hypoglycaemia. HCC on the background of a normal liver often presents with a large palpable mass but this does not preclude curative treatment.

Diagnosis

The tests used to diagnose HCC include radiology, biopsy, and AFP serology. In the setting of a patient with known chronic liver disease a mass found incidentally or on screening ultrasound has a high likelihood of being HCC. The sequence of tests used to diagnose HCC depends on the size of the lesion. Two commonly used diagnostic algorithms have been published by the European Association for Studies of the Liver (EASL) and the Barcelona Clinic for Liver Cancer (BCLC). For the purpose of this chapter the EASL approach will be further described (Figure 7.7.2).

In cirrhotic patients, nodules found on ultrasound surveillance that are <1cm should be followed with ultrasound at intervals of four months. If there has been no growth over a period of one year, the routine surveillance interval of six months can be reinstated.

Nodules >1cm found on ultrasound surveillance should be evaluated with a three-phase CT or a MRI scan. If the appearances are typical of HCC (arterial phase hypervascularity with washout in the portal venous or delayed venous phase (Figure 7.7.3) the lesion should be treated as HCC. Contrast enhanced ultrasound is unable to reliably distinguish between HCC and intrahepatic

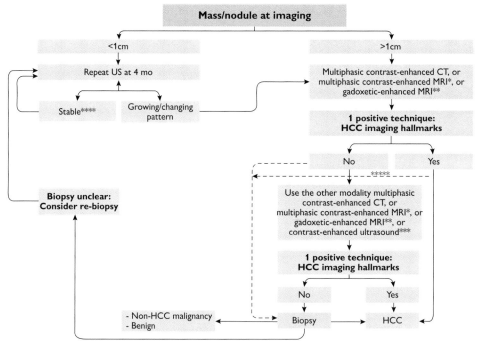

Fig 7.7.2 Diagnostic algorithm and recall policy for liver nodules found on surveillance of liver cirrhosis patients.
*Using extracellular MR contrast agents or gadobenate dimeglumine.
**Using the following diagnostic criteria: arterial phase hyperenhancement (APHE) and washout on the portal venous phase.
***Using the following diagnostic criteria: arterial phase hyperenhancement (APHE) and mild washout after 60 seconds.
****Lesion <1cm stable for 12 months (three controls after four months) can be shifted back to regular six months surveillance.
*****Optional for centre-based programmes.
Reproduced with permission from EASL Clinical Practice Guidelines. Management of hepatocellular carcinoma. *J Hepatol* 2018; 69(1):182–36.

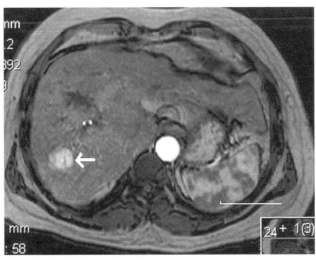

Fig. 7.7.3 MRI showing a typical HCC appearance characterized by a hypervascular lesion in the arterial phase.

cholangiocarcinoma and is therefore no longer recommended as a diagnostic technique for HCC.

For a lesion detected within a non-cirrhotic liver, typical radiological findings in combination with an increased AFP level are diagnostic of HCC. A liver biopsy is justified if radiology and AFP serology are inconclusive and the lesion is not suitable for surgical resection but could be amenable to an alternative therapeutic approach. It should be noted however that the false negative rate for liver biopsies can reach up to 30% due to sampling error or absence of discriminatory histopathological features of HCC. Because liver biopsy is associated with a 1.6% risk of clinically significant bleeding and a 2.7% risk of tumour needle tract seeding, it is only justified if the outcome has an impact on patient management.

Staging systems
BCLC staging system (Figure 7.7.4) identifies those with early HCC who may benefit from curative therapies and those at intermediate or advanced disease stage who may benefit from palliative therapy or should be considered for inclusion into clinical trials of new therapies.

The BCLC system establishes a prognosis in accordance with the five stages that are linked to first-line treatment recommendation. If the recommended option is not feasible because of an individual patient's condition, the treatment approach for the next disease stage should be considered. Accordingly, patients in BCLC stage A may benefit from transarterial chemoembolization, BCLC B patients from sorafenib, and some patients in BCLC stage C with contraindications for sorafenib could enter research trials to assess new agents. Liver function should be assessed using standard criteria, e.g. MELD score or Child–Pugh classification.

Prognosis
A significant number of HCC patients die from non-malignancy related causes such as hepatic failure and upper GI bleeding. Patients with BCLC stage 0 (very

early stage HCC; tumours <2 cm, Child–Pugh A, and performance status (PS) 0) and patients with stage A (early stage HCC; single or up to three nodules <3cm, Child–Pugh A–B, and PS 0) are candidates for radical therapies (resection, transplantation, or percutaneous ablation) and depending on treatment modality, have a median OS exceeding five years. Patients with BCLB stage B (intermediate stage; multinodular tumours, Child–Pugh A–B, PS 0) who undergo transarterial chemoembolization (TACE) have a median survival of more than 30 months. Patients with BCLC stage C (advanced stage disease; Child–Pugh A–B, PS 1–2, vascular invasion, extrahepatic disease) are currently considered for palliative systemic therapy (e.g. sorafenib) or within a palliative trial. They have a median survival of more than 12 months. Best supportive therapy is the recommended treatment option for BCLC stage D patients (terminal stage; any tumour stage, Child–Pugh C, PS 3–4) who have a median survival time of approximately three months.

Principles of management
To achieve the best outcome, the careful selection of candidates for each treatment option and the expert application of these treatments are necessary. Therapies that are known to offer a high rate of complete responses and thus a potential for cure are:
- Liver resection
- Liver transplantation
- Tumour ablation

Among non-curative therapies TACE, transarterial embolization (TAE), and the tyrosine kinase inhibitor sorafenib have been shown to improve survival. Selective internal radiation therapy (SIRT) may provide comparable outcomes to TACE and is particularly useful in patients with portal vein thrombosis. Systemic chemotherapy has marginal activity, frequent toxicity, and no survival benefit.

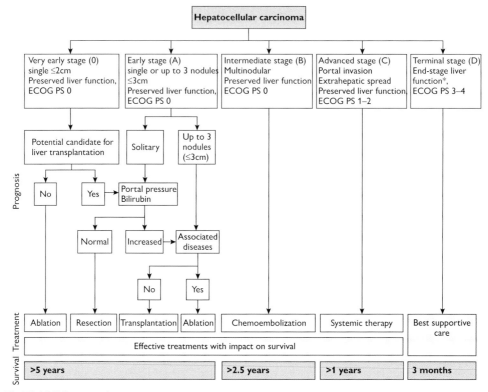

Fig. 7.7.4 BCLC staging and treatment strategy.
* Patients with end-stage cirrhosis due to heavily impaired liver function (Child–Pugh stage C or earlier stages with predictors of poor prognosis or high a MELD (model of end-stage liver disease) score) should be considered for liver transplantation.
Reproduced with permission from Forner A, Reig M, Bruix J. Hepatocellular carcinoma. *Lancet Oncol* 2018; 391(10127):1301–14. Copyright © 2018, Elsevier Inc.

Surgical resection

Non-cirrhotic liver

This is the treatment of choice for HCC in non-cirrhotic patients. With a five-year survival of >50% no other treatment equals these results. Percutaneous ablation is not usually feasible in this group because the cancers at time of diagnosis tend to be larger than in cirrhotic patients. Liver transplantation does not improve the outcome for this group and is associated with a higher early mortality and the risks of life-long immunosuppression.

Cirrhotic liver

Criteria for liver resection for HCC in cirrhosis are:
* No jaundice
* No portal hypertension (ascites, varices, hepatic vein pressure gradient >10mmHg)
* No extrahepatic disease.

The size and site of the tumour dictates the extent of resection required. The main risk of resection with a cirrhotic liver is postoperative liver failure due to inadequate functional residual liver parenchyma. Risk of vascular invasion and dissemination also increase with the size of the HCC, although some tumours attain a large size without vascular invasion and their resection is associated with a good outcome. Although still controversial, resection of large or multiple HCC or resection in patients with impaired liver function, can be justified in well

selected patients. Patients with HCC on the background of cirrhosis should be carefully selected for resection to diminish the risk of postoperative liver failure and mortality. A normal preoperative level of bilirubin and portal pressure are the best predictors of excellent outcomes after surgery and an overall five-year survival of 70% can be achieved with this approach in early stage HCC. Surgical techniques and patient selection have improved and surgery-related mortality is currently <3%.

Novel operative approaches

Laparoscopic liver resection can reduce postoperative morbidity and length of stay while being non-inferior in long-term oncological outcomes compared to open resection. In a single centre series, robotic resection of HCC has been shown to be safe and provide similar outcomes and advantages to laparoscopic liver resection, albeit at the cost of longer operating times. Preoperative planning using three-dimensional liver models created from preoperative CT scan data is utilized in some units and has been shown to be particularly beneficial for complex hepatic resections (Figure 7.7.5). Preoperative portal venous embolization can achieve hypertrophy of the future liver remnant. It is safe, reduces the frequency of postoperative liver failure, and may render some large or centrally placed tumours amenable to resection. Another technique that can improve resection rates of marginally resectable HCC, at the cost of increased

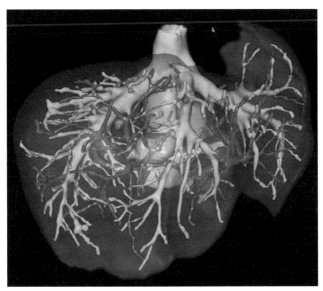

Fig. 7.7.5 A 3D model of the liver is reconstructed using preoperative CT data. On the model liver vasculature, bile ducts and the position of tumour nodules can be appreciated which aids in deciding on the optimal resection strategy (see also colour plate). (Visualization was performed with the Visual Patient™ planning software.)

procedure related morbidity and mortality, is the 'associating liver partition with portal vein ligation for staged hepatectomy' (ALPPS) approach. In the first stage, the portal vein is ligated and the liver parenchyma transected to induce liver hypertrophy. Completion hepatectomy is performed in a second stage within one to two weeks of the first procedure.

Risk of recurrence

Tumour recurrence is approximately 70% at five years and includes true recurrence which usually arises within two years of resection and de novo tumours arising in the cirrhotic liver. Risk factors for true recurrence are:

• Poorly differentiated HCC
• Microvascular invasion
• Multifocal HCC
• Satellite lesions

There is no accepted adjuvant or neoadjuvant therapy option that can reduce recurrence rates. Recurrence is usually multifocal. A solitary recurrence may be considered for repeat liver resection. The only accepted treatment to reduce recurrence is liver transplantation. Salvage liver transplantation has been used for recurrence following resection but is of limited applicability because most recurrences appear early, are due to tumour dissemination and have an aggressive biological pattern.

Liver transplantation

This removes the HCC and replaces the cirrhotic liver. The shortage of donor organs has prompted the application of strict selection criteria. Indications for liver transplantation for HCC (Milan criteria) are:

• Solitary HCC <5cm
• Up to three HCC all <3cm

The five-year survival of these patients following transplantation exceeds 70%. As only 10% of HCC patients meet these strict criteria there is considerable interest in extending the criteria to include selected patients with larger tumours. Most groups have reported a five-year survival of over 50% in patients transplanted using extended criteria. The 'up-to-seven' rule (sum of largest tumour diameter (cm) and number of lesions in addition to largest tumour ≤7) has been validated in an independent series. The lack of sufficient organ donors is the major limitation and waiting for a suitable organ may allow the tumours to grow beyond criteria for transplantation. In Europe and the USA fewer than a third of patients on the waiting list ultimately receive a liver transplant. Considering patients with more advanced tumours for liver transplantation will increase the waiting list drop-out rate and translate into poorer post-transplant survival unless selection criteria are improved and effective methods of preventing disease progression are established. In the UK patients with the following criteria are eligible for transplantation listing: single tumour ≤5cm, up to five tumours ≤3cm, or single tumour >5 and ≤7cm with no evidence of progression over a six-month period. For the latter category loco-regional bridging therapy may be given during the observation period. Absolute contra-indications for transplantation are AFP level >10,000IU/ml, extraperitoneal disease, tumour rupture, and macroscopic vascular invasion. A French study found evidence that the cut-off for the AFP level may need to be decreased further to <1,000ng/ml (1,090IU/ml) because it was associated with an increased risk of tumour recurrence. In the patient population studied, histopathological tumour features such as macrovascular invasion, tumour size, and grade of differentiation did significantly correspond with AFP levels.

The results of this study raise the question whether tumour differentiation, if known from a previous biopsy, should be included into transplantation listing criteria. Salvage transplantation following HCC recurrence after initial liver resection or percutaneous ablation is advocated by some authors in an attempt to reduce the number of patients listed for transplantation. Histopathological evaluation of the resection specimen may indicate the individual risk of cancer recurrence. Patients identified as high risk for recurrence may benefit from immediate listing for liver transplantation.

Loco-regional therapy as a bridge to transplantation or downstaging of HCC

To avoid tumour progression in patients on the transplant waiting list, treatments such as liver resection, ablation therapy, stereotactic ablative body radiotherapy, or transarterial embolization can be used. Robust evidence for the clinical effectiveness of this bridging strategy, however, is lacking. Based on observational and cost-effectiveness studies, EASL guidelines recommend percutaneous ablation or TACE if liver transplant waiting times exceed six months.

A number of centres employ these treatments to 'downstage' HCC in patients who do not fulfil the Milan criteria on initial presentation, to make them eligible for liver transplantation. Further research to evaluate the benefit of downstaging is required and therefore it is not currently endorsed in international guidelines.

Priority listing for transplantation for HCC

In the USA patients with HCC are prioritized for organ allocation to prevent tumour progression during the waiting period for transplantation. The most effective approach to reduce the drop-out rate on the orthotopic liver transplantation (OLT) waiting list is to expand the number of available donor livers.

Despite efforts to improve the available donor pool by utilization of live donors, marginal cadaveric donors, and non-heart-beating donor livers, waiting list drop-out rates have not significantly improved. Alternative strategies to increase the number of donor livers are use of domino transplants (e.g. amyloidosis), livers from hepatitis viral carriers, split liver transplantation, and normothermic organ or regional perfusion.

Live donor liver transplant for HCC

A decrease in numbers of deceased liver organ donations in Europe has been partially substituted by an increase in live donor liver transplantation (LDLT), which in Asia makes up the majority of all liver donations. The outcome after LDLT is similar to that of cadaveric donation, although some authors report an increased HCC recurrence rate potentially secondary to proliferative stimuli. LDLT, however, is a complex intervention and in the best hands has a donor complication rate of up to 40% and donor mortality risk of 0.3–0.5%. Live donor transplantation can be done without the delays of cadaveric transplantation and therefore has been increasingly advocated as an alternative to cadaveric transplantation if waiting list time exceeds six months. Because of ethical implications live donor transplantation for HCC remains controversial. Live donation is minimal in the UK but increasing utilization of non-heart-beating liver donors is partially replacing the falling numbers of brain-dead liver donors.

Management after resection or transplant

Effective therapy is available for HBV to prevent or treat viral graft re-infection using lamivudine and hepatitis B immune globulin. Prevention of HCV graft re-infection has been revolutionized in recent years with the emergence of direct acting antiviral agents. In contrast to previous regimes of interferon and ribavirin, these agents have a better efficacy, tolerability, and safety profile. Antiviral therapy is also effective in preventing disease progression in HCV patients with established liver cirrhosis and it has been shown that de novo HCC formation is reduced in patients who achieve a sustained viral response. There is data suggesting that HCC recurrence risk in HCV patients with cirrhosis is reduced if they respond to interferon therapy but it remains to be shown if this is also true for therapy with direct acting antivirals (Singal et al. 2019). Immunosuppression may increase the risk of HCC recurrence as a result of decreased immune surveillance. Calcineurin inhibitors have been associated with an increase in tumour recurrence, whereas sirolimus inhibits tumour growth and angiogenesis. The results of a multinational RCT evaluating whether its use reduces recurrence of HCC post-transplant has indicated that DFS and OS are improved with sirolimus immunosuppression in the first three to five years. Long-term follow-up data however shows that this benefit does not extend beyond five years (Geissler et al. 2016).

Liver transplant and HCC

- Liver transplantation is an effective option for patients with HCC corresponding to the Milan criteria: solitary tumour <5cm or up to three nodules <3cm. Modest expansion of these criteria, e.g. using the up-to-seven rule requires further prospective validation.
- Loco-regional tumour therapy or living donor transplantation should be considered if the transplant waiting time exceeds six months.

Percutaneous ablation

Alongside surgical resection, this is considered the best treatment option for patients with early stage HCC who are not suitable for transplantation. For single tumours ≤3cm size outcomes following ablation come close to that of resection and choice of therapy should be governed by patient age, comorbidities, and tumour location. In larger (≥3cm) tumours the failure rate following ablation increases and therefore surgical resection either alone or in combination with ablation should be given preference. Ablation therapy cannot provide information on histopathological tumour features. Therefore, patients with high-risk factors for recurrence cannot benefit from early listing for liver transplantation. Destruction of tumour cells can be achieved by:

- Injection of chemical substances (ethanol, acetic acid, boiling saline)
- Thermal ablation (radiofrequency (RF), microwave, laser, cryotherapy).
- Irreversible electroporation

Thermal ablation is now the first-line choice for ablation because it is more effective than ethanol injection in tumours larger than 2cm. Some groups propose ethanol injection as a safer alternative if tumours are located close to vulnerable structures (e.g. bowel, gallbladder) which may be injured by thermal ablation. More recently however irreversible electroporation has gained increasing popularity for ablation of tumours in proximity to major vascular structures or bile ducts. Several groups have successfully applied this modality to tumours that had contraindications to other thermal ablation methods (Sutter et al. 2017). RF ablation is less effective in tumours located close to vessels and a subcapsular tumour location increases the risk of peritoneal seeding. Further research is required to elucidate if newer ablation modalities such as microwave ablation, irreversible electroporation therapy, or computer assisted image guidance ablation can provide improved outcomes. Recurrences are thought to be due to microscopic satellites not included in the ablation zone. In Child–Pugh A patients a 50–75% survival at five years has been achieved in some studies which parallels the outcome following surgical resection for early stage HCC. A meta-analysis comparing RF ablation with surgical resection in small HCC found comparable one- and three-year OS and one-year disease-free survival in both groups with a higher procedural morbidity in the surgical resection group. The OS at five years and disease-free survival at three and five years, however, was superior in patients undergoing surgical resection.

Authors' tip: Ablation therapy for HCC
- Local ablation is a safe and effective treatment for small single HCC.
- Trials comparing local ablation and surgery for HCC suggest similar one-year outcomes but better long-term survival with resection.
- Thermal ablation is currently the first-line modality for ablation therapy.

Non-curative treatment
TACE has been established as the first-line option for patients in BCLC category B. Patients with lobar or segmental portal vein occlusion from thrombosis or tumour infiltration, advanced stage liver disease (Child–Pugh class B or C), or vascular invasion are poor candidates as they have a risk of developing postembolization liver failure. Side effects of TACE include nausea, vomiting, bone marrow depression, alopecia, renal failure, and postembolization syndrome. The latter occurs in >50% of patients and consists of fever, abdominal pain, and ileus which is usually self-limiting.

TACE induces extensive tumour necrosis in >50% of patients, however fewer than 2% of treated patients achieve a complete response. Tumour regrowth is common and repeat TACE is often required. Initial studies showed a median patient survival of up to 20 months following TACE. Use of drug-eluting beads facilitates accumulation of maximal chemotherapeutic agent concentration within the tumour while minimizing systemic effects, thereby improving the tolerance profile. Stricter patient selection and technical refinement in the most recent studies has increased median patient survival following TACE beyond 30–40 months.

Some authors claim that embolization without chemotherapeutic agents has the same efficacy as TACE (Brown et al. 2016). Selective intra-arterial radiotherapy (SIRT) also known as radioembolization, employs high-dose, low-penetration radioactive agents delivered via the hepatic artery. In contrast to TACE, portal vein thrombosis is not a contraindication for SIRT and the survival benefit observed in cohort studies has been comparable to TACE. Ongoing randomized controlled trials (RCTs) will help in characterizing the patient population that is most likely to benefit from SIRT.

Systemic therapy
Sorafenib, an oral multikinase inhibitor with antiangiogenic and antiproliferative effects was the first available effective systemic therapy agent for the treatment of patients with advanced HCC (BCLC stage C). Two RCTs have demonstrated a good safety profile and 30% improvement in median survival time for patients receiving sorafenib. No clear recommendations exist for patients with impaired liver function but two cohort studies have indicated a similar safety profile in Child–Pugh class A and B. Regorafenib blocks similar kinases to sorafenib but has more activity against vascular endothelial growth factor, c-KIT, and TIE2-receptors. The RESORCE trial compared regorafenib versus placebo in 573 patients who had progressed during sorafenib treatment. An improved median OS of 10.6 vs. 7.8 months was found for the treatment and control group, respectively. Due to these results regorafenib is now recommended by the National Institute for Health and Clinical Excellence (NICE) as second-line treatment for advanced HCC. Levantenib is a multikinase inhibitor which compared with sorafenib has more pronounced activity against fibroblast growth factor receptors. Results from the REFLECT trial indicate that levantenib may have better antitumour activity than sorafenib and is non-inferior as a first-line treatment. Conventional systemic chemotherapy has had a limited role because of low response rates, high toxicity, and no clear impact on survival. Multiple other treatment modalities have been trialled including octreotide, interferon, external radiation, tamoxifen, or antiandrogenic therapy, but none have been shown to improve survival.

Palliative therapy for HCC
- TACE is recommended for cirrhotic patients with large or multifocal HCC in the absence of extrahepatic disease.
- Systemic therapy with sorafenib is the most widely used first-line treatment for patients in category BCLC C.
- Further evidence about the clinical benefit of SIRT is needed before its role in the treatment of advanced HCC can be defined.

Future developments in the treatment of HCC
The treatment of HCC has evolved rapidly over the last ten years and now there are effective treatment options available at any disease stage. With regards to the near future, immunotherapy is a treatment strategy that has shown promising early results. The Checkmate 459 trial comparing nivulomab, a programmed cell death protein-1 immune checkpoint inhibitor versus sorafenib in the treatment of advanced HCC, is expected to complete in 2020. Other ongoing studies that may have an impact on the prevention of HCC and its treatment are evaluating direct acting antiviral agents in HCV; SIRT as a locoregional treatment alternative to TACE; minimal invasive resection of tumours; and the optimal selection of HCC patients for liver transplantation.

Further reading
Brown KT, Do RK, Gonen M, et al. Randomized trial of hepatic artery embolization for hepatocellular carcinoma using

doxorubicin-eluting microspheres compared with embolization with microspheres alone. *J Clin Oncol* 2016 Jun10; 34(17):2046–53.

European Association for the Study of the Liver. EASL Clinical Practice Guidelines: Management of hepatocellular carcinoma. *J Hepatol* 2018; 69(1):182–236.

Forner A, Reig M, Bruix J. Hepatocellular carcinoma. *Lancet* 2018 March 31; 391(10127):1301–14.

Geissler EK, Schnitzbauer AA, Zulke C, et al. Sirolimus use in liver transplant recipients with hepatocellular carcinoma: a

randomized, multicenter, open-label phase 3 trial. *Transplantation* 2016; 100:116–25.

Singal AG, Rich NE, Mehta N, Branch AD, Pillai A, et al. Direct-acting antiviral therapy for hepatitis C virus infection is associated with increased survival in patients with a history of hepatocellular carcinoma. *Gastroenterology* 2019; 157(5):1253–63.

Sutter O, Calvo J, et al. Safety and efficiency of irreversible electroporation for the treatment of hepatocellular carcinoma not amenable to thermal ablation techniques. *Radiology* 2017; 284(3):877–86.

7.8 Biliary tract tumours overview

Epidemiology

Cholangiocarcinoma (CCA) accounts for approximately 3% of all GI cancers and is the second most common hepatic malignancy after HCC. There is a slight male predominance. Most patients with CCA are older than 65 years.

On the basis of anatomical distribution, CCA has been classified as intrahepatic (iCCA), perihilar (pCCA), or distal (dCCA) with the latter two historically being described as extrahepatic CCA (Figure 7.8.1). Tumour locations proximal (in the direction of bile flow) to second order bile ducts are classified as intrahepatic (10–20%), between second order bile ducts and the insertion of the cystic duct as perihilar (50–60%), and between insertion of the cystic duct and papilla of Vater as distal CCA (20–30%). Klatskin tumour is a term used for perihilar CCA. Several studies reported an increased incidence of iCCA and a concomitant decline in the incidence of pCCA and dCCA in Japan, Australia, the USA, and Europe. Whether this is a true increase in disease incidence or whether this is related to a change in classification, reporting, or other factors remains widely debated.

Aetiology

Most cases of CCA are sporadic. Less than 30% of patients have risk factors which include:

- Primary sclerosing cholangitis
- Liver fluke infestation
- Hepatolithiasis
- Congenital biliary cysts
- Chronic viral hepatitis
- Toxic damage, e.g. thorotrast

Pathology

There are distinct histological classifications for the individual types of CCA. Regardless of CCA type, a desmoplastic reaction secondary to rapid proliferation of tumour associated stroma cells is characteristic for this tumour.

Intrahepatic CCA

Intrahepatic CCA have been macroscopically classified into a mass-forming, periductal infiltrating, and intraductal growth type. The mass-forming type is most commonly encountered and tends to infiltrate the hepatic parenchyma via the portal venous system. The periductal type has the worst prognosis and spreads longitudinally along bile ducts within the Glissonian sheath. Papillary growth towards the ductal lumen similar to a tumour thrombus is

the main characteristic of the intraductal type, which has the best prognosis.

Perihilar CCA

Macroscopically these can be divided into exophytic or intraductal types. Exophytic tumours can display a nodular or periductal infiltrating growth with the latter being the most common subtype. As periductal tumours increase in size they tend to form mass lesions. Intraductal tumours can be further subdivided into intraductal growing, mucin producing, papilloma, and cystic types. The papillary projections of this tumour are long and friable; tumour debris or mucin produced by these lesions can cause intermittent bile duct obstruction that may be mistaken clinically for stone disease. Papillary tumours grow along the mucosal surface and produce multiple metastatic deposits along the adjacent bile ducts.

Distal CCA

Recognized precursor lesions are intraductal papillary neoplasms and biliary intraepithelial neoplasia. With increasing tumour size, concentric thickening eventually produces complete obliteration of the duct lumen. Malignant strictures resulting from pCCA or dCCA can be difficult to distinguish from inflammatory strictures.

Histology

Over 90% of CCAs are adenocarcinomas which are graded from 1 to 4 according to the percentage of glandular components. Rarer forms of CCA are: mucinous cystic neoplasm, squamous cell carcinoma, small cell carcinoma, carcinoids, and signet cell carcinoma. Kaposi sarcoma and lymphomas have been described in patients with acquired immune deficiency syndrome (AIDS). Mixed hepatocellular-cholangiocarcinoma is a hybrid tumour that consists of HCC and CCA cells. The Ras-MAPK pathway is one of the major signalling networks and was demonstrated to contribute to carcinogenesis by promoting inflammation and proliferation in one study that correlated genetic signatures with clinicopathological traits of CCA patients.

Clinical features

The presentation of CCA largely depends on the anatomical site of the tumour. Intrahepatic CCA typically presents as a mass lesion detected incidentally by abdominal imaging or with non-specific symptoms such as cachexia, fatigue, and abdominal pain. In contrast, pCCA and dCCA usually present with jaundice, pruritus, weight loss, and abdominal pain. Cholangitis on first presentation is uncommon, unless previous biliary instrumentation has been performed.

Patients with primary sclerosing cholangitis (PSC) are at a high risk for developing CCA. The diagnosis of malignancy in these patients is clinically challenging as the presentation and cholangiographic findings of biliary tract strictures in PSC are similar to those of CCA. The new development of jaundice and a dominant bile duct stricture in an individual with previously stable PSC should raise the suspicion of malignancy.

Diagnosis

Serum tumour markers

Serum CA19-9 is usually increased, but is not diagnostic of CCA. It is usually elevated with obstructive jaundice independently of cause and with several other GI malignancies. Concentrations of over 1,000U/ml are often associated with advanced disease. In PSC, sensitivity, specificity, and positive predictive value for CA19-9 in the diagnosis of CCA are 79%, 98%, and 57% respectively, if a cut-off value of 129U/ml is chosen. It is important to note that patients who are Lewis-antigen negative (7% of general population) have undetectable CA19-9 levels.

Ultrasonography

This is used as a first-line test in patients presenting with abnormal liver function tests, jaundice, or abdominal pain. Ultrasonography can differentiate obstructive from non-obstructive jaundice, detect a mass lesion in intrahepatic CCA, exclude gallstones, and confirm ascites in patients with advanced disease. Further imaging is always needed to further evaluate and fully stage the disease.

Computed tomography

CT is commonly used to evaluate patients with suspected CCA (Figure 7.8.1c) and has a sensitivity of about 80% for all forms of CCA. The location of the lesion, extent of local spread, vascular involvement, atrophy of liver, and metastases may be determined. For iCCA the typical appearance is that of a rim enhancement in the arterial phase followed by a centripetal enhancement in delayed phases. CT and MRI performance is equivalent in the detection of intrahepatic lesions and satellite lesions. Due to better visualization of vascular involvement however, CT is superior to MRI for predicting resectability in patients with iCCA. For completion of staging CT of the chest and pelvis have to be performed as well.

Magnetic resonance imaging

MRI can be treated as a valuable adjunct or alternative to CT. It can determine the local extent of tumour, relationship to blood vessels, extent of hepatic atrophy, lymph node involvement, and intrahepatic or distant metastases (Figure 7.8.1a). In pCCA and dCCA, MRI combined with MR cholangiography (MRCP) has a greater diagnostic accuracy than CT in the detection of biliary neoplastic lesions (Figure 7.8.1b). Frequently CT is used in addition to MRI to assess for vascular involvement (Rizvi et al. 2018). Sensitivity and accuracy in this scenario is approximately 89% and 76%, respectively, and resectability, of pCCA can be predicted with up to 95% accuracy. MRCP is at least equivalent and possibly superior to diagnostic, endoscopic retrograde cholangiopancreatography (ERCP) in the evaluation of biliary obstruction, because it carries virtually no procedure related morbidity and offers advantages in terms of cost effectiveness and quality of life.

(a)

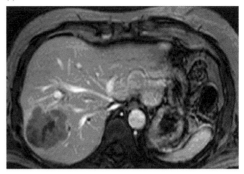

(b)

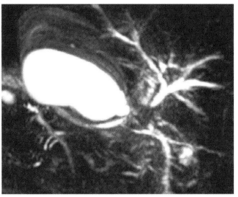

(c)

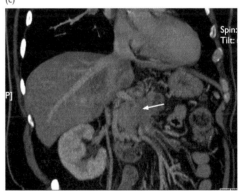

Fig. 7.8.1 (a) MRI showing an intrahepatic CCA, (b) MRCP showing a perihilar CCA, and (c) CT showing a distal CCA.

Endoscopic retrograde cholangiography (ERC) and percutaneous transhepatic cholangiography (PTC)

These are methods of obtaining access to the biliary tract to determine the extent of bile duct involvement by cancer, to allow drain insertion for resolution of jaundice, and to obtain samples for culture, biliary cytology, or histology. Staging and an assessment of a patient's suitability for resection should be completed before considering biliary tract drainage by ERC or PTC. PTC can aid in accessing strictures where ERC has failed. To enable chemotherapy administration, enhance patient comfort, and physiological bile flow, internal stents placed via PTC are preferable to external drainage.

Positron emission tomography

The use of PET in the diagnosis of CCA is limited. Depending on pathological type of CCA, sensitivity is 18–80% for iCCA and about 55% for pCCA and dCCA. PET usually adds little to the diagnostic algorithm and should only be considered if there is a strong suspicion of undetected distant metastasis.

Cytology and biopsy

For patients with resectable disease there is no indication for a preoperative biopsy. Obtaining a tissue diagnosis in suspected CCA is vital if staging suggests unresectable or metastatic disease. Cytological samples can be obtained from bile juice aspirated through a drainage catheter or brush cytology collected during ERCP or PTC. Due to the desmoplastic and paucicellular nature of CCA, conventional cytology has a poor sensitivity of 43% but specificity has been reported as high as 97%. Fluorescence in situ hybridization (FISH) is based on the analysis of quantitative chromosomal anomalies (e.g. polysomy) and has been shown to increase the sensitivity of brush cytology from 21% to 58%. FISH may detect CCA lesions in PSC up to 2.7 years before the tumour becomes apparent on imaging studies.

Endoscopic ultrasound (EUS) with fine needle aspiration

EUS enables visualization of the distal biliary tree, hilar lesions, gallbladder, hilar lymph nodes, and vasculature. EUS-FNA may allow a tissue diagnosis in distal biliary lesions and assessment of hilar lymphadenopathy for the diagnosis of advanced pCCA. However, the negative predictive value is low and negative cytology does not therefore exclude malignancy. Some centres advice against EUS-FNA in patients who are candidates for liver transplantation because of the risk of needle tract seeding.

Laparoscopy ± laparoscopic ultrasound

This is useful in identifying patients with liver or peritoneal metastases in whom an unnecessary laparotomy can be avoided.

Emerging technologies

Advances in endoscopic technologies hold promise for improving the diagnosis and staging of cholangiocarcinoma. Examples of such technologies include endoscopic cholangioscopy and probe-based confocal laser endomicroscopy (pCLE). Cholangioscopy is useful to distinguish benign from malignant strictures compared with ERCP alone. When employed during ERCP, pCLE allows direct microscopic examination of pancreatobiliary strictures on a cellular level. There has been increasing interest in utilizing bile samples obtained via ERCP or PTC for diagnostic purposes. The analysis of microRNAs and extracellular vesicles for example has shown promising early results with an increased sensitivity compared to standard bile cytology (Rivzi et al. 2018).

Summary of imaging recommendations

- All patients suspected of pCCA or dCCA should have a combined MRI and MRCP.
- Triple phase CT of the liver should be used for local assessment of iCCA and in any pCCA or dCCA where there is concern about vascular involvement.
- CT of the chest, abdomen, and pelvis should be used to screen for distant metastases.

- Invasive cholangiography should be reserved for tissue diagnosis or therapeutic decompression where there is cholangitis, or stent insertion in unresectable cases.
- The diagnostic techniques are complementary and sometimes several are necessary as part of a surgical assessment.

Staging

Bismuth–Corlette classification

The Bismuth and Corlette classification for pCCA (1975) stratifies patients based on the location and the extent of involvement of the biliary tree by cancer (Figure 7.8.2) (Box 7.8.1).

Prognosis

A complete surgical resection with histologically negative resection margins (R0 resection) is the main curative option for CCA. Five-year survival following R0 resection of iCCA, pCCA, and dCCA is 22–44%, 11–44%, and 27–37%, respectively. For intrahepatic tumours, good prognostic factors are single tumours, R0 resection, and absence of vascular invasion or lymph node involvement. Histology, R0 resection, and lymph node status are prognostic factors for survival following resection of pCCA. Involved resection margins are the single most important predictor of recurrence in dCCA.

Liver transplantation

A multicentre study from the USA which enrolled patients with unresectable localized pCCA, a tumour size ≤3cm, and no lymph node or vascular involvement for liver transplantation has demonstrated five-year recurrence-free survival and five-year OS of 65% and 70%, respectively.

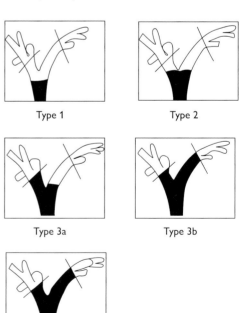

Type 1   Type 2

Type 3a   Type 3b

Type 4

Fig. 7.8.2 Bismuth–Corlette staging system.

Box 7.8.1 Bismuth–Corlette classification

- Type 1: bile duct cancers proximal to the bifurcation.
- Type 2: cancer involves the hepatic duct confluence but neither the right nor left hepatic ducts.
- Type 3: cancer occluding the hepatic duct confluence and extending into the right (type 3A) or left (type 3B) hepatic ducts.
- Type 4: cancers of the hepatic duct confluence which extend into both the right and left hepatic ducts or with multi-focal duct involvement.

Source: data from Bismuth H, Corlette MG. Intrahepatic cholangioenteric anastomosis in carcinoma of the hilus of the liver. *Surg Gynecol Obstet* 1975; 140:170–6.

Liver transplantation was only carried out in patients who responded well to a combination of neoadjuvant chemotherapy and radiochemotherapy. The majority of patients came from one centre but other centres had similar survival rates (Darwish Murad et al. 2012). With CCA developing secondary to PSC, liver transplantation rather than resection is an attractive option as the liver function may be poor, the cancer may be multifocal, and recurrence after resection is common due to the neoplastic field changes. A high preoperative drop-out rate due to the extensive neoadjuvant regimen and increased surgical morbidity and mortality in patients who proceed to transplantation have been the main problems associated with this approach. These issues may partially explain why many transplant centres have been unable to replicate the results of this study.

The results of liver transplantation for iCCA have historically been disappointing with high recurrence rates and poor long-term survival. A retrospective multicentre study published in 2016, however, showed a five-year OS rate of 65% in 15 patients who were found to have an incidental early stage iCCA of ≤2cm on a background of liver cirrhosis. These results may indicate that early iCCA may be effectively treated by liver transplantation or at the least that incidentally found iCCA during liver transplantation work-up may not necessarily be an absolute contraindication to liver transplantation.

Palliative therapy and median survival
- Stenting: four to six months
- Chemotherapy: up to 12 months
- TACE or SIRT: up to 12–22 months (iCCA only)

Role of surgery and resectability

The aim of treatment for patients with cholangiocarcinoma is to perform a complete resection of the cancer with histologically negative resection margins (R0 resection) (Figure 7.8.3). With the exception of liver transplantation in a highly selective population, this offers the only hope of cure. The emerging trend in the surgical approach to pCCA is to combine an extended liver resection and lymphadenectomy with excision of the extrahepatic bile duct. This radical approach has been shown to decrease recurrence and improve survival in perihilar lesions without a significant increase in postoperative morbidity and mortality. Achieving clear resection margins is technically demanding in pCCA as the bile duct bifurcation is close to the vascular inflow of the liver and microscopic seeding into the adjacent caudate lobe (liver segment I) is common which is why its excision is advisable. Portal vein and hepatic artery resection and reconstruction may facilitate achieving clear resection margins and may improve survival in selected cases. Evidence of locoregional lymph node involvement is no longer an absolute contraindication to resection. Compared to patients with N0 status, the survival rate is lower but better than with non-surgical treatment.

Portal vein embolization (PVE) is being increasingly used preoperatively to ensure there is an adequate functioning liver remnant following resection. The technique of ALPPS (associating liver partition and portal vein ligation for staged hepatectomy) promotes rapid liver regeneration and was introduced as a salvage procedure for patients deemed at the time of surgery to have inadequate residual liver remnant. The procedure produces a very rapid liver hypertrophy but carries a high risk of morbidity and mortality and requires further evaluation for the treatment of CCA. For iCCA the extent of liver resection is guided by the anatomical location of the tumour. A pancreatoduodenectomy is usually indicated for the resection of dCCA. The survival data of our unit is comparable to outcomes published in the world literature (Figure 7.8.4).

Extent of surgery
- Intrahepatic cholangiocarcinoma is treated by resection of the involved liver segments.
- Surgical treatment strategy for pCCA is guided by the expanded Bismuth–Corlette classification.
- To achieve good outcomes, an aggressive approach including extended hepatectomy and vascular reconstruction may be required.
- Therefore, treatment of pCCA should be performed in specialized centres.
- Microscopic seeding to the caudate lobe (segment 1) is well recognized, justifying its resection in the majority of pCCA.
- Distal cholangiocarcinomas are managed by pancreatoduodenectomy as with ampullary or pancreatic head cancers.

Criteria of unresectability
- Bilateral involvement of the second-order bile ducts
- Bilateral, contralateral, or distal (e.g. coeliac trunk) vascular involvement
- Presence of metastatic disease
- Portal vein occlusion with collaterals
- Distant lymph node metastases
- Insufficient future liver remnant
- Poor clinical status and comorbidities

Adjuvant treatment

The BILCAP trial studied adjuvant capecitabine versus observation in patients with CCA or gallbladder cancer who underwent R0 or R1 resection. Per protocol analysis showed an improved median OS of 53 vs. 36 months for patients randomized to adjuvant capecitabine (Primrose et al. 2019).

A smaller trial published in the same year investigated adjuvant gemcitabine and oxaliplatin in a similar setting. In this study no survival advantage was found for patients receiving adjuvant chemotherapy (Edeline et al. 2019). Despite these contradicting results, the BILCAP study

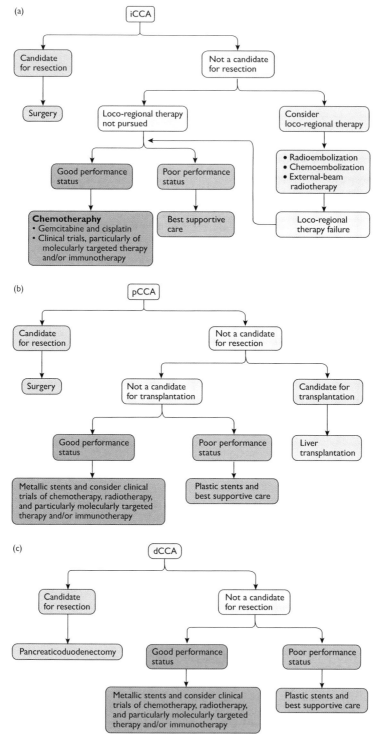

Fig. 7.8.3 Management algorithms according to CCA locations. Please note that liver transplantation for pCCA is only practiced at a very limited number of centres.
Reproduced with permission from Rizvi S, et al. Cholangiocarcinoma—evolving concepts and therapeutic strategies. *Nat Rev Clin Oncol* 2017; 15(2):95–111. Copyright © 2017, Springer Nature Limited.

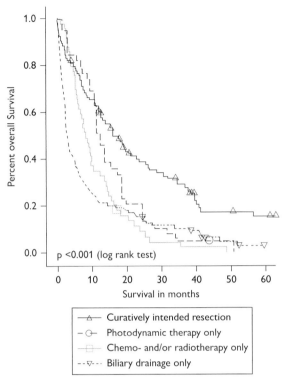

Fig. 7.8.4 Survival with various treatment options (Royal Free Hospital and University College Hospital, London data). Source: Reproduced with permission from Matull WR, et al. R0 but not R1/R2 resection is associated with better survival than palliative photodynamic therapy in biliary tract cancer. *Liver Intl* 2011; 31(1):99–107. Copyright © 2011, John Wiley & Sons.

currently defines the standard of care in the UK for this patient cohort.

Neoadjuvant treatment involving chemoradiation or chemotherapy has been proposed as a method of improving outcome or for downstaging unresectable disease, but evidence is not robust. Therefore, neoadjuvant therapy may be considered within a clinical trial.

Management of unresectable tumours

Treatment of biliary obstruction

The aim of palliation is the relief of jaundice and related pruritis, prevention of cholangitis and hepatic dysfunction, and improvement of QoL. This can be achieved endoscopically or surgically. These techniques are equally effective in resolving jaundice. However non-surgical procedures offer significantly lower morbidity, mortality, and cost. The optimal use of palliative stents depends on the life expectancy of the patient and location of the tumour in the biliary tree. In Bismuth type I and distal CCA, placement of a single biliary stent is adequate. With perihilar tumours, bilateral stents may provide better drainage and improved survival.

Expanding uncovered metal, covered metal, and plastic stents have advantages and disadvantages. Once employed, uncovered metallic stents cannot be removed and therefore tissue confirmation of cancer is mandatory before placement. For distal tumours, metal stents

provide a longer patency and are more cost-effective for patients expected to survive ≥4 months. Patency of hilar plastic stents is <4 weeks and they are at high risk of distal migration and are not therefore recommended for long-term palliation. Covered metal stents can be removed endoscopically, have similar patency rates to uncovered metal stents, but have a higher risk of stent migration, acute cholecystitis, and pancreatitis. To achieve adequate biliary drainage involves a combination of endoscopic and percutaneous approaches in one-third of patients.

Loco-regional therapy

Like HCC, unresectable iCCA may be amenable to loco-regional therapy. However, high-quality evidence is currently not available. RFA of iCCA is safe and achieves an overall three-year survival of 30–50%. This treatment modality appears to be more beneficial in smaller lesions.

In a retrospective case matched study TACE was associated with an improved OS time of 12 months versus three months when compared to best supportive treatment. Transarterial radioembolization using yttrium-90 microspheres was of particular benefit in patients with good PS (ECOG 0) whose median survival improved to 29 months.

Loco-regional therapies have not been shown to be of benefit for patients with pCCA or dCCa. Intraoperative radio- or brachytherapy did not improve survival over established treatment modalities. There is no proven benefit for photodynamic therapy and in fact there are some concerns that it may be harmful.

Radiotherapy

In the past radiotherapy was not recommended for routine use in an adjuvant or palliative setting. More recently the increased sophistication of cross-sectional imaging has enabled more precise targeting of lesions and dosing of radiotherapy. Intensity-modulated and three-dimensional conformal radiotherapy enable sparing of non-malignant tissue whereas charged particle beams (proton or carbon) may achieve similar benefits because of their improved physical dose-deposition profile when compared to conventional X-ray beams. Stereotactic body radiation therapy has been proposed as an effective method for delivering high-dose ablative radiotherapy to CCA patients. Several single arm phase 2 studies indicate a potential role for adjuvant radiotherapy with concurrent chemotherapy for resected CCA, especially in patients with R1 resections or N1 status. For unresectable iCCA, a number of single centre studies have demonstrated median survival of 22.5–30 months which is superior to outcomes following palliative chemotherapy. Unfortunately, these promising results have not been replicated for unresectable pCCA or dCCA. Although the results of one RCT investigating radiochemotherapy in unresectable iCCA are awaited (NCT02200042), there is need for more high-quality data to define the role of radiotherapy in the treatment of CCA (Rivzi et al. 2018).

In patients with unresectable CCA who are not candidates for liver transplantation, combination chemotherapy with gemcitabine and cisplatin is the current standard of care. An OS and progression-free survival of 11.7 months and eight months, respectively, was observed in the ABC-02 trial. Therapeutic or preventive biliary stenting should be performed before starting systemic chemotherapy.

Molecularly targeted agents

There are a large number of agents that target specific mutations in CCA and a complete summary is beyond the scope of this chapter. Given later are examples of molecular therapeutics with specific consideration given to agents that have been evaluated in phase 2 trials and beyond. In analogy to advances in the systemic treatment of HCC, tyrosine kinase inhibitors are being investigated for the treatment of CCA. One example for tyrosine kinase inhibitors currently evaluated in phase 2 trials is NVP-BGJ398 which on analysis of preliminary results was shown to have a disease control rate of 82% (NCT02150967). Depending on the location, between 11% and 25% of CCA harbour KRAS mutations, which are associated with poor survival. Selumetinib inhibits KRAS related downstream activation of the MAPK pathway and has demonstrated a median OS of 9.8 months in patients with metastatic biliary tract cancer. Although the OS is lower than the 11.7 months in the ABC-02 trial, further research may be warranted to explore its efficacy in tumours with increased sensitivity to MAPK inhibition or as a second-line treatment option. Genetic profiling studies have indicated that mutations in epigenetic regulators are common in CCA. A study investigating AG-120, an inhibitor of IDH1, has shown a partial response in one patient and stable disease in 11 out of 20 patients with CCA. The ClarIDHy study,

a multicentre RCT investigating AG-120 (ivosidenib) in 185 CCA patients with mutations in IDH1 reported significant improved PFS with ivosidenib compared with placebo. Aberrant mesothelin expression, a cell surface protein found on mesothelial cells, is another potential therapy target. The antibody–drug conjugate anetumab ravtansine has activity against mesothelin and is currently being investigated in a phase I trial recruiting patients with advanced stage CCA (Rivzi et al. 2018).

Immunotherapy

Many cancer types develop mechanisms to protect against antitumour immune response. Some of these mechanisms include changes to the tumour microenvironment, loss of MHC expression, or expression of immune checkpoint proteins. Although it remains to be elucidated how CCA mounts an immune escape, there has been widespread interest in evaluating immunotherapy of CCA.

Immune checkpoint inhibitors targeting cytotoxic T-lymphocyte associated antigen 4 and programmed cell death protein 1 (PD-1) have shown anti-tumour activity in a subset of patients across a wide spectrum of solid tumour types. The majority of clinical data on immune checkpoint inhibitors in CCA has been published on PD-1. To identify patients that will benefit from PD-1 therapy it is crucial to study biomarkers and genetic aberrations that are associated with a treatment response. Expression of PD-1 ligand (PD-L1) has been observed in non-small cell lung cancer and melanoma patients who were sensitive to PD-1 monotherapy. It is estimated that PD-L1 is present in 9–72% of CCA specimens but it remains to be seen if expression of this marker correlates with treatment response to PD-1 inhibitors. Genetic aberrations that may indicate sensitivity to PD-1 directed therapy are mismatch repair (MMR) deficiency and/or microsatellite instability (MSI). The anti-PD-1 antibody pembrolizumab has been approved by the US Food and Drug Administration (FDA) for treatment of unresectable or metastatic solid tumours with MMR deficiency or a high MSI content, which have progressed on therapy and have no alternative treatment option. The FDA approval is irrespective of histology and does include CCA.

Clinical data on immunotherapy in CCA is limited at this stage. In the KEYNOTE-028 basket trial 20 CCA patients with PD-L1 expressions on ≥1% of cells received pembrolizumab. Partial response was observed in three patients and another three patients had stable disease. At the time of publication the median progression-free survival in patients with partial response had not been reached yet, indicating a durable treatment effect. Grade 3 toxicities were observed in 16.7% of patients and there was no grade≥4 toxicity. The follow-up KEYNOTE-158 basket trial will include 100 biliary tract cancer patients who will receive up to two years treatment with pembrolizumab. In MMR-deficient CCA patients, preliminary results with pembrolizumab have also been promising. In four treated patients, three had stable disease and one patient had a complete response. In analogy to the KEYNOTE-028 findings, the median progression-free survival was not reached at the time of reporting (Rivzi et al. 2018).

The available data although limited is suggesting that patient selection is crucial for effective immunotherapy. It has therefore been postulated that biomarkers research is an essential step in advancing immunotherapy of CCA and other cancer types.

Further reading

Darwish Murad S, Kim WR, Therneau T, et al. Predictors of pretransplant dropout and posttransplant recurrence in patients with perihilar cholangiocarcinoma. *Hepatology* 2012; 56:972–81.

Edeline J, Benabdelghani M, Bertaut A, Watelet J, Hammel P, et al. Gemcitabine and oxaliplatin chemotherapy or surveillance in resected biliary tract cancer (PRODIGE 12-ACCORD 18-UNICANCER GI): a randomized phase III study. *J Clin Oncol* 2019 Mar 10; 37(8):658–67.

Primrose JN, Fox RP, Palmer DH, Malik HZ, et al. Capecitabine compared with observation in resected biliary tract cancer (BILCAP): a randomised, controlled, multicentre, phase 3 study. *Lancet Oncol* 2019 May 1; 20(5):663–73.

Rizvi S, Khan SA, Hallemeier CL, Kelley RK, Gores GJ. Cholangiocarcinoma—evolving concepts and therapeutic strategies. *Nat Rev Clin Oncol* 2018 Feb; 15(2):95–111.

Valle JW, Borbath I, Khan SA, Huguet F, Gruenberger T, Arnold D. ESMO Guidelines Committee. Biliary cancer: ESMO Clinical Practice Guidelines for diagnosis, treatment and follow-up. *Ann Oncol* 2016 Sep; 27(suppl. 5):v28–37.

7.9 Pancreatic cancer overview

Epidemiology

Pancreatic ductal adenocarcinoma is the commonest cancer affecting the exocrine pancreas. It is the fifth cause of cancer death in the UK. In 2013 there were 9,408 new cases in the UK, with similar numbers in men and women. In 2015, there were an estimated 367,000 new cases of pancreatic cancer and 359,000 deaths worldwide. The peak incidence is in the 65–75-year age group with 60% of patients being >65 years of age.

Aetiology

Major risk factors include:
- Tobacco smoking
- Chronic pancreatitis
- Hereditary pancreatitis
- Blood groups (B>AB>A; reference=O)
- Increasing age
- Diabetes mellitus
- Increased BMI/low physical activity
- Genetic (familial pancreatic cancer; cancer family syndromes)

Weaker associations include:
- Increased consumption of red and processed meat
- High intake of (saturated) fats
- Low intake of vegetables and fruits

Familial pancreatic cancer (FPC) and cancer family syndromes

A variety of familial cancer syndromes are associated with an increased risk of pancreatic cancer; these account for approximately 10% of cases (see Table 7.9.1). In the absence of a syndrome there is familial clustering of pancreatic cancer but a gene responsible for a large proportion of these cases has not been identified. Diagnostic criteria are:
- Two or more first-degree relatives with pancreatic ductal adenocarcinoma

or
- Two or more second-degree relatives with pancreatic cancer, one of whom has early-onset pancreatic cancer (age <50 years at diagnosis)

Overall, the observed to expected rate of pancreatic cancer is significantly raised by nine-fold, rising specifically from four-fold in families with one first-degree relative, to 6.4-fold where there are two affected relatives to 32.0-fold with three relatives with pancreatic cancer.

Secondary screening

The European Registry of Hereditary Pancreatitis and Familial Pancreatic Cancer (EUROPAC) has been established to provide a database of these families for long-term follow-up, and to develop a screening programme in the future.

Screening in pancreatic cancer

- Primary screening for pancreatic cancer in the general population is not feasible at present.
- Secondary screening for all patients with an increased inherited risk of pancreatic cancer who should be referred to a specialist centre for clinical advice, genetic counselling, and, where appropriate, genetic testing.
- Modalities for screening are CT and MRI with EUS for FPC and cancer syndromes but not hereditary pancreatitis (fibrosis and calcification may mask an early cancer).

Pathology

Pancreatic ductal adenocarcinoma (PDAC) is the most common malignant tumour of the pancreas. The variants are:
- Mucinous non-cystic carcinoma
- Signet ring cell carcinoma
- Adenosquamous carcinoma
- Undifferentiated (anaplastic) carcinoma
- Undifferentiated carcinoma with osteoclast-like giant cells
- Mixed ductal endocrine carcinoma

Characteristically, there is an intense desmoplastic reaction in the stroma surrounding these tumours. In about 5% of cases it is not possible to distinguish the tissue of origin from pancreatic, ampullary, duodenum, and bile duct and the term 'non-specific periampullary cancer' is often applied.

PDAC develops through an adenoma-carcinoma sequence of epithelial preneoplastic lesions called (low to high grade) pancreatic intra-epithelial neoplasia (PanIN).

Other pancreatic tumours include intraductal pancreatic mucinous neoplasms (IPMNs), which may be premalignant. Side-branch IPMNs are present in 2–5% of the adult population. Main duct IPMNs have a much greater risk of progression. Mucinous cystic neoplasm and solid-pseudopapillary neoplasm are also premalignant. Pancreatoblastomas are malignant and are mostly found in children.

Clinical features

Tumours of the head of the pancreas tend to present with obstructive jaundice or less commonly with acute pancreatitis, but the onset is usually insidious. Tumours of the body and tail tend to present even later and are associated with a worse prognosis.

Symptoms
- Painless jaundice
- Pruritus secondary to jaundice
- Vague dyspepsia or abdominal discomfort or pain
- Fatigue
- Weight loss/cachexia
- Back pain
- Anorexia
- Constipation (reduced food intake)
- Steatorrhea (fatty stools)
- Late-onset diabetes mellitus without risk factors for diabetes
- Acute pancreatitis of unknown cause
- Chronic pancreatitis
- Acute cholangitis
- Vomiting from duodenal obstruction

Signs
- Jaundice
- Scratch marks secondary to jaundice
- Cachexia
- Multiple bruises (ecchymoses) secondary to impaired clotting
- Hepatomegaly
- Palpable gallbladder: Courvoisier's sign
- Ascites
- Anaemia
- Abdominal mass
- Metastasis at the umbilicus: Sister Joseph's sign
- Migratory thrombophlebitis
- Venous gangrene of lower limbs

Diagnosis
Blood tests
Look for anaemia, check clotting profile, liver function tests, and serum proteins.

Tumour markers
Serum CA19-9 is the most commonly used marker.
- Sensitivity 75% and specificity of 78%. Better than carcinoembryonic antigen (CEA) and other markers.
- False positives with obstructive jaundice, chronic pancreatitis, and ascites.
- Useful to assess response and identify tumour recurrence.
- Negative in 5% of the population.

Non-invasive imaging
Transabdominal ultrasound (TAUS)
This may be the initial investigation and can detect dilated biliary and pancreatic ducts (double duct sign), tumours >2cm in size, and liver metastases. There is enhanced sensitivity with contrast media. It is not useful in early disease and obese patients. It should not be relied upon to exclude a diagnosis of pancreatic cancer.

Contrast-enhanced CT
CT is the gold standard for diagnosis and staging, especially for vascular involvement (see Figure 7.9.1). Diagnostic accuracy rates are more than 90% for pancreatic cancer. Accuracy for an unresectable lesion is in general higher than accuracy for a resectable lesion.

Table 7.9.1 Familial pancreatic cancer and pancreatic cancer predisposing genes

Syndrome (gene)	Relative risk
Peutz–Jeghers (STK11)	132
Familial atypical multiple mole melanoma, FAMMM (CDKN2A, 16)	22–38
Lynch syndrome, hereditary non-polyposis colon cancer, HNPCC (mismatch repair genes: MLH1, MSH2, MHS6, and PMS2)	0–8.6
Breast and ovarian cancer syndrome (BRCA1)	3.5
Breast and ovarian cancer syndrome (BRCA2)	0–2.3
Li–Fraumeni syndrome (p53)	Increased (low)
Ataxia telangiectasia (ATM)	Increased (low)
Familial pancreatic cancer (no single gene)	6–32
Cystic fibrosis (CFTR)	~5
Hereditary pancreatitis (PRSS1)	up to 67

False negatives may be due to small liver metastases and peritoneal deposits.

MRI
This has a similar diagnostic accuracy to CT, and better for the diagnosis of liver lesions. It is useful for patients who are allergic to intravenous contrast.

Magnetic resonance cholangiopancreatography (MRCP)
MRCP may enhance diagnosis by revealing a double duct sign and is important for diagnosing and assessing cystic tumours.

Positron emission tomography and PET-CT
This may increase the diagnostic accuracy and staging compared with CT alone.

Invasive diagnostic imaging
Endoluminal ultrasonography (EUS)
This is highly sensitive in the detection of small tumours (see Figure 7.9.2) and small lesions can be biopsied (FNA) for increased accuracy in diagnosing malignant lesions (not seen on CT). The diagnostic accuracy of EUS with FNA carries a sensitivity and specificity of >90% and approximately 100%, respectively. It is poor for diagnosing distant metastases and distant nodal involvement.

Endoscopic retrograde cholangiopancreatography (ERCP)
ERCP should not be used for diagnostic imaging; it is only used for the insertion of stents to relieve jaundice and to obtain a biopsy or brush cytology.

Percutaneous transhepatic cholangiography (PTHC)
This is used for the relief of jaundice when ERCP has failed or is not possible. It can also be used to obtain brushings or biopsy for diagnosis.

Laparoscopy and laparoscopic staging
Laparoscopy with laparoscopic ultrasound enables intra-operative scanning of the liver and pancreas to be performed and is highly predictive of resectability, altering the management of up to a third of patients already assessed as resectable by dual-phase multidetector CT. Selective

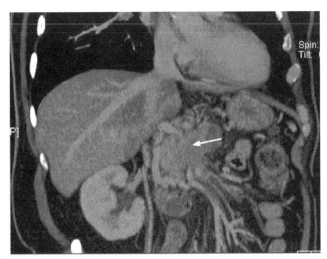

Fig. 7.9.1 Coronal section of multidetector CT scan demonstrating pancreatic tumour encasing the portal vein (white arrow). This patient has unresectable disease.

laparoscopy based on the serum level of CA19-9 is a more efficient strategy, reducing the proportion of patients under-going laparoscopic ultrasound while increasing the yield.

The TNM classification for pancreatic cancer (UICC 8th edition 2017)

T: primary tumour
- TX: primary tumour cannot be assessed
- T0: no evidence of primary tumour
- Tis: carcinoma in situ
- T1: tumour 2cm or less in greatest dimension

- T2: tumour more than 2cm but ≤4cm in greatest dimension
- T3: tumour >4cm in greatest dimension
- T4: tumour involves coeliac axis or superior mesenteric artery (unresectable primary tumour)

N: regional lymph nodes
- NX: regional lymph nodes cannot be assessed
- N0: no regional lymph node metastasis
- N1–3: lymph node metastasis
- N2 to ≥4: lymph node metastasis

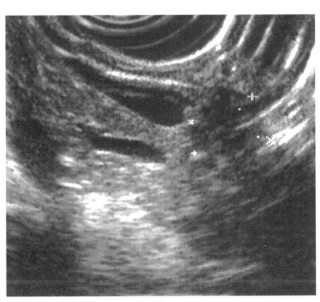

Fig. 7.9.2. Endoluminal ultrasound demonstrating a small pancreatic cancer (between two crosses).

M: distant metastasis
- M0: no distant metastasis
- M1: distant metastasis

Stage grouping
- Stage 0: TisN0M0
- Stage IA: T1N0M0
- Stage IB: T2N0M0
- Stage IIA: T3N0M0
- Stage IIB: T1, T2, T3N1M0
- Stage III: T4, any N, M0
- Stage IV: any T, any N, M1

(Reproduced with permission from Brierley JD, Gospodarowicz MK, Wittekind C (eds). *TNM Classification of Malignant Tumours*, 8th edn. Copyright © 2017, John Wiley & Sons.)

Prognosis
Due to late presentation only a minority (10–20%) of patients can undergo potentially curative surgery, which increases median survival to 15–25 months. Five-year survival ranges from 15% to 25%. Metastatic pancreatic cancer has a median survival of 5–9 months and 6–11 months for locally advanced disease.

The prognostic factors can be categorized into tumour-related, patient-related, and treatment-related groups.

Tumour-related factors
- Stage of tumour: patients with locally advanced disease have a better prognosis than those with metastatic disease.
- T stage: Tis/T1/T2 tumours have better prognosis.
- Grade of tumour differentiation: well-differentiated tumours have a better prognosis.
- Lymph node involvement, lymph node ratio >2 and lymph node 8a involvement indicates poor prognosis.
- Location (head lesions better than body and tail).
- Presence of perineural invasion is associated with decreased survival.
- Resection margins involvement is associated with decreased survival (a positive resection margin is defined as cancer cells within 1mm of any margin).
- CA19.9>400U/ml is a marker for poor prognosis.
- Molecular markers, e.g. Kras mutation, Smad4 mutation/deletion, EGF/TGF-alpha, MUC4, MMPs, and many more.
- Other markers, e.g. leucocytosis, elevated C-reactive protein level, high platelet/lymphocyte ratio indicate poor outcome.

Patient-related factors
- Poor PS/ASA is associated with decreased survival.
- Age ≥70 years is associated with a worse outcome.
- Presence of severe pain is a poor prognostic factor in advanced disease.

Treatment-related factors
- Treatment centre with expertise and high case load.
- Relief of jaundice and gastric outlet obstruction in advanced disease.
- Systemic (adjuvant, palliative) chemotherapy.

7.10 Treatment of resectable pancreatic cancer

Definition of resectability
Once a diagnosis of pancreatic cancer has been made, the patient will be assessed for fitness to undergo resection and the tumour will be staged. Resection can be considered in case of:
- No liver, peritoneal, or other distant metastases.
- Absence of portal hypertension and cirrhosis.
- No severe comorbidity to exclude surgery.

Tumours are classified as resectable, borderline resectable, or locally advanced, unresectable. Borderline resectable disease is defined as:
- Infiltration/encasement of the superior mesenteric vein or portal vein, but resection and reconstruction of the vessel seems technically feasible.
- Encasement of the gastroduodenal artery as well as a short involvement or direct contact of the hepatic artery without extension of the tumour to the coeliac trunk.
- Encasement of the superior mesenteric artery, but a maximum infiltration of 180 degrees of circumference.

Anything beyond those criteria is considered locally advanced, unresectable.

Principles of management
These are broadly to:
- Treat patients in a centre of expertise with a high case load.
- Consider preoperative biliary drainage in jaundiced patients.
- Resect all tumour to achieve R0 resection.
- Reduce/manage postoperative complications.
- Offer adjuvant chemotherapy for all patients.

Preoperative biliary drainage
- Stents are used mainly to facilitate logistical planning of staging and treatment.
- Covered metal stents should be used and placed endoscopically if possible.

Surgical management
- The aim of surgery is to achieve an R0 resection (clear microscopic resection margins).
- Nevertheless, 30–60% of resections are R1: complete clearance of macroscopic tumour with positive microscopic resection margins.
- R2 resections are associated with increased morbidity/mortality with no survival advantage, and should be avoided.

Tumours of the head of pancreas
The standard operation for tumours of the head of pancreas is the Kausch–Whipple partial pancreato-duodenectomy. The most commonly used approach at the present time is the pylorus-preserving partial

pancreato-duodenectomy. There is no difference in long-term outcome between these two approaches. Pancreato-jejunostomy, hepatico-jejunostomy, and duodeno-jejunostomy are performed for reconstruction. Reconstruction using pancreato-gastrostomy rather than a pancreato-jejunostomy has similar outcomes, and there may be no advantage for the routine use of pancreatic stents.

- There is no survival advantage for extended radical lymphadenectomy in pancreatic cancer.
- Resection of the portal or superior mesenteric vein may be necessary to achieve an R0 resection and can be done with acceptable morbidity.
- Arterial resections increase morbidity and mortality and should be carried out in highly selected cases only.
- Multivisceral resections increase morbidity but might be necessary to achieve R0 resection.

Tumours of the body and tail of pancreas
A left pancreatectomy is performed, which includes splenectomy and en bloc removal of the hilar lymph nodes.

Morbidity and mortality
- The overall mortality for major pancreatic resections is <5% in major centres.
- Postoperative morbidity is around 40%.

Management of complications
Intra-abdominal abscess
This occurs in 1–12% of patients. The usual cause is anastomotic leak at the pancreas, bile duct, or enteric anastomosis. CT is indicated and the preferred management is CT-guided percutaneous drainage.

Haemorrhage
Postoperative haemorrhage occurs in 2–5% of patients. Bleeding within 24 hours is due to insufficient intraoperative haemostasis or bleeding from an anastomosis. Free intraperitoneal haemorrhage requires immediate reoperation. Management of anastomotic bleeding can be initially conservative and/or endoscopic. Secondary haemorrhage (one to three weeks after surgery) is commonly related to an anastomotic leak and secondary erosion of the retroperitoneal vasculature, or a pseudoaneurysm with a high mortality rate. Investigations include CT scan, endoscopy, and selective angiography with embolization. Bleeding from the pancreatic anastomosis may require completion total pancreatectomy or refashioning of the anastomosis.

Fistula after pancreatoduo-denectomy
The incidence ranges from 2% to 24%. The mortality risk from a major pancreatic fistula may be as high as 28%; the cause of death is retroperitoneal sepsis and haemorrhage. Most leaks, however, can be managed conservatively with little upset to the patient.

Delayed gastric emptying
The incidence ranges from 14% to 70%. The problem resolves with conservative treatment and may require intravenous prokinetic therapy with erythromycin.

Role of somatostatin analogues
Postoperative complications may be reduced by the prophylactic use of somatostatin analogues given just before the start of the operation for seven days.

Role of neoadjuvant and adjuvant treatment
Radical resection alone will result in a five-year survival rate of around 10%. Nearly all patients develop metastatic disease, most commonly of the liver and peritoneum but also the lungs, and this may occur with or without local recurrence.

Neoadjuvant therapy
Indications are to:
- Convert borderline resectable or locally advanced, unresectable tumours to resectability.
- Be used with adjuvant therapy to improve OS.

  Combined evidence suggest that around one-third of borderline resectable and few unresectable tumours become resectable following neoadjuvant therapy, with a similar outcome to upfront resectable tumours. There is no conclusive evidence for the value of neoadjuvant therapy in resectable tumours.
- Most reported protocols have used CRT but it is not necessarily superior to chemotherapy alone.
- FOLFIRINOX (5-FU, leucovorin, irinotecan, and oxaliplatin) or gemcitabine-based regimens are currently studied in the neoadjuvant setting.
- There is a lack of high-quality trial data.
- Neoadjuvant therapy should only be assessed as part of a clinical trial.

Adjuvant therapy
Adjuvant chemotherapy
The results from several large randomized trials (including ESPAC-1, -3, and -4 trials and the Unicancer GI PRODIGE 24 trial) show that adjuvant systemic chemotherapy will increase median survival from 17 to 20 months with resection alone to 23–24 months with either 5-FU and folinic acid or gemcitabine, to 28 months with gemcitabine plus capecitabine, to 54 months with modified FOLFIRINOX.
- The survival benefit is maintained irrespective of the type of operation used and whether or not patients develop postoperative complications.

Adjuvant chemoradiotherapy
- No benefit has been observed from adjuvant CRT alone or in combination with chemotherapy in large randomized trials.

Key points
- Adjuvant chemotherapy significantly improves survival.
- Modified FOLFIRINOX is more effective than gemcitabine but associated with higher toxicity. Effective alternatives include gemcitabine plus capecitabine, and 5-FU/folinic acid or gemcitabine monotherapy.
- Adjuvant chemoradiation has not been shown to improve survival.
- Neoadjuvant treatments should only be administered as part of a controlled clinical trial.

7.11 Treatment of unresectable and metastatic pancreatic cancer

Unresectable cancer

Approximately 80–90% of patients will present with unresectable disease. The treatment of patients who have unresectable pancreatic cancer due to localized advanced disease and/or metastases consists of symptom control and palliative therapy.

Pain relief

Intractable pain is a major problem.
- Necessitates use of high dose opiates.
- Additional approaches include intraoperative, percutaneous CT-guided, or EUS neurolytic coeliac plexus block and bilateral or unilateral thoracoscopic splanchnicectomy.

Jaundice and duodenal obstruction

Jaundice is best relieved using ERCP and a biliary stent.
- PTC-endoscopy approach is used only if ERCP is not technically possible.
- Main complications are acute cholangitis, bleeding, and peritonitis.
- Self-expanding covered metal stents should be used.
- Endoscopically-placed expandable metal stents are deployed for duodenal obstruction (occurs in approximately 15%).
- The success rate is around 85%. Complications include: perforation, fistula, bleeding, and recurrent obstruction due to stent migration or fracture.
- Surgical bypass (open and laparoscopic) can be used to relieve jaundice using a Roux-en-Y loop hepatojejunostomy, and duodenal obstruction by gastrojejunostomy, especially in younger patients.

Weight loss

- This is initially due to pancreatic exocrine insufficiency owing to obstruction of the main pancreatic duct as well as exclusion of bile acids because of obstruction of the main bile duct.
- Fat maldigestion may also contribute to abdominal pain and bloating.
- Relief of biliary obstruction and pancreatic enzyme supplementation will alleviate these symptoms.
- Cachexia may be a marked feature of the later stages of pancreatic cancer, and there is no good treatment.

Systemic chemotherapy

- See following section for metastatic disease treatment options.

Chemoradiation

This was the preferred option in the past. However, a RCT comparing CRT and chemotherapy failed to show a survival benefit for the addition of radiation.

Local ablative therapies

There are several techniques for local treatment available:
- Radiofrequency ablation
- Irreversible electroporation
- Stereotactic body radiation therapy
- High-intensity focused ultrasound
  These techniques are feasible and safe but should only be evaluated as part of a clinical trial.

Metastatic disease

Principles of management

These include the relief of pain, jaundice, and reduction of weight loss as outlined previously.

Treatment options

Systemic chemotherapy

Pancreatic ductal adenocarcinoma is highly resistant to conventional methods of cytotoxic treatment and radiotherapy. Few chemotherapeutic agents have been shown to have reproducible response rates of >10%.
- The nucleoside analogue gemcitabine replaced 5-FU as the preferred drug in 1997 and the following decade.
- In 2011, FOLFIRINOX was shown to be superior to gemcitabine (median survival 11.1 months vs. 6.8 months). Toxicities remain a problem; the combination is reserved for patients with good PS.
- In 2012, the combination of gemcitabine and albumin-bound paclitaxel was shown to be superior to gemcitabine (median survival 8.5 months vs. 6.7 months). It is tolerated also by patients with slightly worse PS.

Second-line therapy:
- Following gemcitabine, 5-FU and oxaliplatin or 5-FU and liposomal irinotecan may be used.
- Following 5-fluorouracil-based therapy, gemcitabine alone or gemcitabine plus albumin-bound paclitaxel are used.

> **Key points**
> - Chemotherapy improves survival and QoL in patients with advanced pancreatic cancer.
> - FOLFIRINOX for patients with excellent PS.
> - Gemcitabine and albumin-bound paclitaxel for patients with a slightly worse PS.
> - Gemcitabine monotherapy for patients with poor PS.
> - Second-line therapy for fit patients.

Novel approaches

These include defining subgroups of pancreatic cancer patients, e.g. patients with tumours that exhibit defects in DNA repair who might benefit from cisplatin or poly (ADP-ribose) polymerase (PARP) inhibitor-based therapy. Innovative approaches include:
- Targeted pathway blockage, e.g. IGF1-R (MM-141), JAK/STAT (ruxolitinib, momelotinib), and others.
- Stroma modulation by PEGPH20 or hedgehog inhibitors.
- Immunotherapy, e.g. by immune checkpoint blockade (PD1, PD-L1 antibodies).
- Vaccination with agents such as GVAX, oncolytic virus therapy, and others.

Further reading

Kleeff J, Korc M, Apte M, La Vecchia C, Johnson CD, Biankin AV, Neale RE, Tempero M, Tuveson DA, Hruban RH, Neoptolemos JP. Pancreatic cancer. *Nat Rev Dis Primers* 2016 Apr 21; 2:16022.

Neoptolemos JP, Kleeff J, Michl P, Costello E, Greenhalf W, Palmer DH. Therapeutic developments in pancreatic cancer: current and future perspectives. *Nat Rev Gastroenterol Hepatol* 2018 Jun; 15(6):333–48.

Internet resources

Cancer Research UK: http://info.cancerresearchuk.org/cancerstats/
EUROPAC: http://www.europac-org.eu/
GLOBOCAN: http://globocan.iarc.fr
NICE guidance NG857 February 2018: http://www.nice.org.uk
Useful sites for pancreatic cancer and clinical trials include:
National Cancer Institute: http://www.cancer.gov/clinicaltrials
Liverpool Clinical Trials Centre: http://www.lctu.org.uk/
Pancreatic Cancer Research Fund: http://www.pancreaticcancer.org.uk/

7.12 Uncommon pancreatic tumours

Cystic tumours of the pancreas

These are detected with increasing frequency and can be challenging in terms of diagnosis and management. The most common primary pancreatic cystic neoplasms are:

- Serous cystic neoplasms (SCN) which predominantly affect elderly women and are found mostly in the head of the pancreas.
- Mucinous cystic neoplasms (MCN) are found almost exclusively in women, mostly in their 40s and 50s and mostly in the body and tail of the pancreas. The cyst does not communicate with the main duct.
- Intraductal papillary mucinous neoplasms (IPMNs). These affect more men than women, may involve part or the whole of the pancreatic ductal system, affect patients in their 60s, and represent the most common cystic tumour of the pancreas. IPMNs are classified as arising either from the main duct (MD-IPMN) or side branch ducts (SB-IPMN). Further gastric, intestinal, pancreatobiliary, and oncocytic subtypes have been described.

The most common differential diagnoses include:

- Non-neoplastic cystic lesions e.g. pancreatic pseudocysts
- Papillary cystic neoplasm e.g. solid pseudopapillary neoplasm
- Cystic pancreatic neuroendocrine tumours

Diagnosis

This is by CT/MRI scan, EUS, FNA cystic fluid (cytology and tumour markers CEA/CA-19.9).

Management

- Confirmed serous cystic neoplasm. These are benign and a conservative approach without follow-up imaging is justified. Occasionally they may cause symptoms because of size and fibrotic reaction necessitating resection.
- MCN should be resected if the patient is fit for surgery owing to the high malignant potential.
- All main duct IPMNs should be resected if the patient is fit for surgery. A total pancreatectomy is usually required.
- Patients with side branch IPMN require an individualized approach according to the revised Sendai consensus. SB-IPMN with high-risk stigmata or defined EUS/FNA findings require resection if the patient is fit for surgery. For all other patients surveillance is tailored according to cyst size and worrisome features.

SB-IPMN: high-risk stigmata

- Obstructive jaundice with cystic lesion of the pancreatic head
- Enhancing solid component within cyst
- Main pancreatic duct >10mm

SB-IPMN: EUS/FNA findings indicating resection

- Definite mural nodule
- Main duct features suspicious for involvement
- Cytology suspicious or positive for malignancy

SB-IPMN: worrisome features

- Cyst >3cm
- Thickened/enhancing cyst walls
- Main duct size 5–9mm
- Non-enhancing mural nodule
- Abrupt change in calibre of the main duct with distal atrophy

Pancreatic lymphoma

By definition, pancreatic lymphoma is restricted to the pancreas and draining lymph nodes; it is extremely rare.

Treatment is similar to extranodal lymphomas in other sites and depends on histological subtype and stage of the disease. The standard of care is chemotherapy with or without radiotherapy. Patients who had resection for an undiagnosed lymphoma may need chemotherapy.

Metastases to the pancreas

The pancreas is a site for metastases from cancers arising from different primary sites. Sometimes these metastases are isolated, in which case radical resection is the treatment of choice.

Pancreatic neuroendocrine tumours (PNETs)

These represent about 2–10% of all pancreatic tumours. The aetiology is poorly understood. There are inherited diseases associated with pancreatic endocrine tumours (Table 7.12.1). These patients should undergo screening

Table 7.12.1 Inherited diseases associated with pancreatic endocrine tumours (PNETs)

Condition	Comment
Multiple endocrine neoplasia type 1 (MEN-1)	Autosomal dominant
	Pituitary adenomas, primary hyperparathyroidism, PNET (often multiple)
	Mutation of MEN-1 gene
	Around 55% have PNET
Von Hippel– Lindau	Autosomal dominant
	Mutation of VHL tumour suppressor gene
	Around 16% have PNET
Type 1 neurofibromatosis (NF1)	Autosomal dominant
	Mutation of tumour suppressor gene NF1
Tuberous sclerosis	Mutation of TSC1 or TSC2 genes

to identify early tumours which are treatable with agents used as for neuroendocrine tumours in other sites.

Further reading
Battula N, Srinivasan P, Prachalias A, et al. Primary pancreatic lymphoma: diagnostic and therapeutic dilemma. *Pancreas* 2006; 33(2):192–4.

Tanaka M, Fernández-del Castillo C, Adsay V, et al. International consensus guidelines 2012 for the management of IPMN and MCN of the pancreas. *Pancreatology* 2012; 12(3):183–97.

Internet resources
ENETS: http://www.enets.org/
http://www.pancreaticcancer.org.uk/types

7.13 Tumours of the small intestine

Epidemiology

The small intestine constitutes 75% of the length of the GI tract but is the site of only 2–3% of malignant GI cancers. The median age at presentation for small bowel adenocarcinoma (SBA) is in the mid-60s; Higher rates of incidence are seen in the Maori people of New Zealand and among ethnic Hawaiians, with low rates in India, Romania, and other parts of Eastern Europe.

Pathology

There are four main types of small intestinal tumours:
- Adenocarcinomas (45%)
- Neuroendocrine tumours (NETs) (30%)
- Sarcomas (10%) (majority are GI stromal tumours (GISTs), 20% occur in the small bowel)
- Lymphomas (15%)

The majority of SBAs occur in the duodenum or jejunum with a minority occurring in the ileum. NETs and lymphoma commonly arise in the terminal ileum. Sarcomas are more evenly distributed although more common in the ileum. Metastatic lesions are more common than primary tumours and may occur from direct invasion or by intraperitoneal seeding (colon, ovary, endometrial, and stomach cancers), or by haematogenous spread (melanoma, breast, lung cancer, and hepatocellular carcinoma).

Aetiology

Several findings suggest that SBA arise as a result of a malignant transformation in adenomatous polyps in a similar manner to the adenoma-carcinoma sequence of large bowel adenocarcinoma. SBA is the major cause of death in such patients post colectomy. Other risk factors for SBA include:
- Crohn's disease
- Coeliac disease
- Neurofibromatosis
- Urinary diversions (i.e. ileal conduits)

Coeliac disease and tropical sprue have been associated with lymphoma, most commonly enteropathy-associated T cell as opposed to B cell type, they tend to involve more proximal small bowel, and are associated with a worse prognosis.

GISTs are believed to originate from precursor cells of the interstitial cells of Cajal. These are intermediates between the GI autonomic nervous system cells and smooth muscle cells regulating GI motility. Mutually exclusive mutations in c-kit or platelet-derived growth factor receptor A (PDGFR-A) receptor tyrosine kinase proteins are seen in ~95% of newly presenting GISTs. These mutations are somatic. They cause functional change in c-kit and platelet-derived growth factor receptor A (PDGFR-A) proteins leading to ligand-independent activation and are early key 'hits' in GIST tumourogenesis and excellent targets for treatment. Ninety-five per cent of GISTs are sporadic. A minority are associated with three tumour syndromes: neurofibromatosis type 1 (NF1), Carney triad, and familial GIST syndrome. GISTs that occur in NF1 have a high predilection for the small bowel and are normally clinically indolent. GISTs in Carney triad occur in the stomach together with paraganglioma, pulmonary chondroma, or both. These also have a relatively indolent behaviour.

Clinical features

The presenting symptoms of SBA depend on site and size. These include:
- Non-specific symptoms: abdominal pain, anaemia, nausea, bleeding and weight loss, palpable mass
- Obstructive jaundice
- Surgical emergencies: intussusception, perforation

Tumours in the duodenum frequently present with pain and gastric outlet syndrome. Periampullary tumours often present with jaundice. More distal tumours may present with small bowel obstruction. Occult bleeding is common but frank haemorrhage rare. Adenocarcinoma of the small and large bowel have a similar pattern of spread; common sites include regional lymph nodes, liver, lung, and the abdominal cavity. Because of late presentation many patients have metastatic disease at diagnosis.

Lymphomas commonly present with acute and/or chronic abdominal pain relating to bowel obstruction or less often perforation. Patients often have a history of weight loss and fatigue. A mass may be palpable and blood tests may reveal anaemia. Mediterranean-type lymphoma presents with a triad of fatigue, malabsorption, and clubbing. Enteropathy-associated lymphoma is also associated with malabsorption.

The most common presentation of GISTs is GI bleeding that may be insidious or haemorrhagic. Patients may present with an acute abdomen due to tumour rupture, bowel obstruction, or appendicitis-like pain. Smaller GISTs are often incidental findings at surgery. Patients with advanced disease may present with symptoms arising from metastases in the abdominal cavity and liver.

Diagnosis

The initial investigations will often be dictated by the presenting symptoms. They may include:

- Small bowel follow-through
- Plain X-rays
- Abdominal ultrasound
- CT scan
- EUS
- Endoscopy and capsule endoscopy

CT scan of the chest, abdomen, and pelvis may help delineate the primary tumour and provide staging information. Different tumour types have characteristic appearances on CT. Larger carcinoid tumours may be seen with fixation, separation, and angulation of bowel loops, and often calcification at the centre of a desmoplastic reaction giving a 'starburst' appearance. Diffuse segmental thickening of a length of small intestine is suggestive of lymphoma. GISTs are often well-circumscribed submucosal masses. Diagnosis of GIST should be based on both tumour morphology and immunohistochemistry. In all GISTs mutation analysis is recommended as it is predictive for response to treatment and prognostic for the course of the disease. In tumours which are c-kit negative, DOG-1 immunohistochemistry is recommended.

A tissue diagnosis is necessary prior to planning non-surgical treatment. For proximal tumours this may be obtained by an upper GI endoscopy. Occasionally tumour masses may be amenable to CT-guided biopsies—otherwise a diagnostic laparoscopy or laparotomy is required.

Staging

Adenocarcinomas are staged using the AJCC TNM system which is similar to cancers of the large intestine.

Lymphomas are staged using the Ann Arbor staging system (see 'Clinical features, diagnosis, and staging for Hodgkin lymphoma' in Chapter 12, p. 332). The most powerful and widely applied criteria for evaluating the biological potential of GIST are tumour size and mitotic activity. Using these criteria, tumours can be classified as very low risk, low risk, intermediate risk, and high risk (Miettinen and Lasota 2006). In addition to this, tumour rupture is an adverse prognostic factor.

Principles of treatment

When disease is localized a radical surgical resection with removal of all visible disease and regional lymph nodes should be undertaken. When there is evidence of metastatic disease the aim of treatment is to minimize symptoms and prolong life expectancy. Clear communication with the patient and relatives is paramount so that the physician understands the patient's expectations and the patient understands the possible gains and potential treatment related toxicity and inconvenience.

Surgery

Surgery is performed to obtain a histological diagnosis, to palliate symptoms, and to attempt to cure. A potentially curative approach necessitates complete resection of the primary tumour, often en bloc with adjacent organs and a radical lymph node dissection. Anatomical constraints permit this more often in distal than in proximal small intestine tumours. As a result, curative surgery is performed more frequently for distal tumours, 52% versus 90% in one large series. Failure to achieve a complete resection results in median survival of 10–14 months, similar to patients with inoperable disease.

Both National Comprehensive Cancer Network (NCCN) and European Society of Medical Oncology (ESMO) guidelines agree that GISTs >2cm should be surgically excised/biopsied. The standard approach to smaller lesions is EUS assessment then annual follow-up.

Systemic therapy

Small bowel adenocarcinoma

Chemotherapy is commonly used for metastatic SBA. The approach and choice of chemotherapy is largely extrapolated from the management of large intestinal cancer and currently there is no standard chemotherapeutic regime. There are a few reported phase 2 clinical trials but no randomized data. The largest trial of palliative chemotherapy used a combination of 5-FU, doxorubicin, and mitomycin C, and had a response rate of 18% but with an unacceptably high toxicity. Single institution experiences have reported similar response rates with less toxicity using single-agent 5-FU or a combination of 5-FU and platinum agents in the first-line setting and irinotecan and 5-FU in the second-line setting. More recently a small phase 2 study of oxaliplatin and capecitabine reported a higher response rate of 50% and median survival of 20.3 months.

In current practice, adjuvant chemotherapy for SBA is not standard of care. The BALLAD trial aims to answer the question of whether adjuvant chemotherapy improves disease-free survival and OS over observation alone postoperatively for stages I–III SBA. It will also compare different chemotherapy regimes to see if the addition of oxaliplatin to single agent fluoropyrimidines is of benefit.

Small bowel lymphoma

Ann Arbour stage I and II B-cell non-Hodgkin lymphoma (NHL) are treated surgically with or without chemotherapy. Stage III and IV disease are treated with primary chemotherapy with or without surgical debulking. Chemotherapy regimens are similar to nodal NHL. Low-grade NHL may be managed conservatively in the absence of symptoms.

Sarcoma

GIST: imatinib is a competitive inhibitor of multiple tyrosine kinase inhibitors including c-kit and PDGFR. In metastatic GIST imatinib 400mg once a day is the standard of care (except in patients with kit exon 9 mutations where a higher dose of 800mg per day is considered). Large clinical trials report excellent response rates with disease control seen in ~85% of patients, and median PFS and OS of 20–24 months and 57 months, respectively. Imatinib can be continued whilst tolerated until evidence of disease progression. Treatment interruption has been shown to result in rapid progression of disease but the majority are salvaged by restarting therapy promptly.

After disease progression on imatinib, the options of either dose escalation of imatinib to 800mg daily (currently not NICE approved in the UK) or treatment with the tyrosine kinase inhibitor sunitinib can be considered. Following a phase 3 trial comparing sunitinib to placebo, which showed a significant improvement of PFS (27.3 weeks vs. 6.4 weeks), sunitinib became NICE approved for second-line use.

The multikinase inhibitor regorafinib can be applied for via the cancer drug fund for third-line use. The phase 3 GRID trial comparing regorafinib to placebo after failure of both imatinib and sunitinib reports PFS of 4.8 months vs. 0.9 months.

Adjuvant imatinib given for 36 months post resection in high-risk patients has been shown to improve five-year recurrence-free survival to 65.6% and five-year OS to 92%.

Imatinib may be considered in locally advanced inoperable disease, allowing a large or locally invasive GIST to become resectable.

Non-GIST sarcomas: doxorubicin with or without ifosfamide remains the chemotherapy choice, as well as other regimens in specific sarcoma subtypes.

Response evaluation

CT scans are commonly used to monitor disease response to treatment. In GIST the Choi criteria define response as the change in tumour size or a decrease in tumour density on contrast-enhanced CT. The evaluation of imatinib response requires an experienced MDT. When used corrected, Choi criteria more accurately assess prognosis than RECIST-type response.

Prognosis

Prognosis relates primarily to the stage of disease at diagnosis and to the type of tumour.

SBA frequently present with advanced disease and unfortunately carries a poor prognosis at all stages. Five-year OS rates are 50–60% in stage I, 40–50% in stage II, and 25–35% in stage III disease. If distant metastases are present this is further reduced to <5%.

Most series of small intestinal lymphomas include lymphoma of the stomach. For early stage disease, ten-year survival rates range from 60% to 86% but are worse for advanced disease.

The prognosis of metastatic small bowel GISTs depends on their response to therapy and is highly influenced by mutation type. From the 2010 LFG registry the median OS was 6.4 years with some patients continuing with disease controlled on treatment with imatinib for over ten years.

Further reading

Casali PG, Abecassis N, Bauer S, et al. Gastrointestinal stromal tumours: ESMO-EURACAN Clinical Practice Guidelines for diagnosis, treatment and follow-up. *Ann Oncol* 2018; 29(Suppl. 4):iv68–78.

Miettinen M, Lasota J. Gastrointestinal stromal tumors: pathology and prognosis at different sites. *Semin Diagn Pathol* 2006; 23(2):70–83.

Puccini A, Battaglin F, Lenz HJ. Management of advanced small bowel cancer. *Curr Treat Options Oncol* 2018; 19(12):69.

Reynolds I, Healy P, Mcnamara DA. Malignant tumours of the small intestine. *Surgeon* 2014; 12(5):263–70.

7.14 Colorectal cancer overview

Introduction

Colorectal cancer (CRC) is the third most common cancer diagnosed in men and in women in the UK—and comprises 12% of all cancers diagnosed. Around two-thirds of the cancers arise in the colon and one-third in the rectum. However, the sigmoid colon and rectum account for half of the cases.

Epidemiology

From 2015–17, there were around 42,317 new cases of bowel cancer in the UK compared to 36,109 new cases in 2004. In the last decade bowel cancer incidence rates have increased by less than a tenth (7%) in the UK. Around 16,272 people died of bowel cancer in 2015–17, that is similar to 16,092 deaths from colorectal cancers reported in 2005. In the last decade CRC mortality has reduced by 12%.

Aetiology

Multiple factors play an aetiological role in the development of colorectal cancer. The majority (approximately two-thirds) of the tumours arise sporadically without any obvious predisposing factor. The remaining develop on the background of an increased familial risk (positive family history, hereditary CRC syndromes), and rarely on the background of inflammatory bowel disease.

Colorectal polyps

- In approximately 80% of cases invasive cancer arises on the background of adenomatous polyp formation.

- Colorectal polyps are classified histologically as non-neoplastic (hyperplastic, inflammatory, hamartomatous) or neoplastic (adenomatous).

- Adenomatous polyps may be tubular (85%), tubulovillous (15%), or villous (5%).

- The mean age of adenoma diagnosis is ten years earlier than with carcinoma.

- Malignant potential of adenomatous polyps increases with size (>1cm), higher degrees of dysplasia, and increasing percentage of villous tissue within polyp.

- The risk of cancer development is approximately 4% after five years and 14% after ten years. Villous adenomas have significantly higher risk (15–25% overall, but higher with size >2cm).

- Risk factors that increase the probability of future malignant progression include male gender, presence of multiple/metachronous polyps, and positive family history of CRC.

- The progression of adenoma-carcinoma sequence is characterized by the development of functional abnormalities in several genes that regulate important cellular functions, including proliferation and apoptosis. These processes promote development of an invasive phenotype.

Undefined familial colorectal cancer

- Approximately 15–20% of patients present with a positive family history of CRC in the absence of a well-defined genetic abnormality.

- Presence of one affected first-degree relative is associated with a two-fold higher risk of CRC that doubles with two or more relatives. Risk is further enhanced with an affected younger relative (<45 years) and a family history of colon, rather than rectal cancer.
- Inherited susceptibility is most likely due to genetic instability from low penetrance/recessive mutations in genes regulating DNA repair and other important cellular functions.
- Previous observational studies have suggested that increased risk may be due to combined effect of genetic susceptibility and environmental factors.

Hereditary colorectal cancer syndromes (HCS)
See 'Cancer genetics' in Chapter 2, p. 12.

Inflammatory bowel disease
Inflammatory bowel disease (IBD) is associated with an increased risk of CRC. The overall prevalence of CRC in patients with ulcerative colitis (UC) is approximately 3.7%. Patients with Crohn's disease who have associated colitis also have a similar risk of developing CRC.

Risk factors for CRC in IBD patients
- Duration of colitis is the most important factor. The cumulative incidence of CRC in UC patients is 2.5% after 20 years, 7.6% after 30 years, and 10.8% after 40 years of follow-up.
- Extent of colonic involvement. A study of over 3,000 UC patients in Sweden demonstrated a standardized incidence ratio (SIR) of 1.7 in patients with proctitis compared to 2.8 in left-sided colitis, and 14.8 in patients with pancolitis.
- Family history of colorectal cancer.
- Primary sclerosing cholangitis.

Screening
Screening can potentially reduce CRC mortality rates by 15%. Since 90% of sporadic CRCs occur in people >50 years, most current screening programmes target the specific population subgroup ranging from 50 to 69 years. Earlier age of screening is recommended for high-risk individuals with other associated factors (e.g. familial, IBD, etc.).

UK CRC screening initiative
In the UK NHS Bowel Cancer Screening Programme, people aged 60–74 are invited to carry out a faecal occult blood test (FOBT) once every two years. Additional one-off endoscopy screening is gradually being introduced in England and is offered to people at the age of 55 years.

Screening protocols
These include faecal occult blood (FOB), faecal immunochemical testing (FIT), faecal DNS test, endoscopic (sigmoidoscopy and colonoscopy), and radiological assessment (e.g. double-contrast barium enema, CT colonography).

Faecal occult blood test
Guaiac-based FOBT detects the pseudoperoxidase activity of the iron-containing prosthetic subgroup haem. Different commercial kits are available for home-based use (e.g. Haemoccult®). Patients with a positive test require further assessment such as colonoscopy or barium enema.

Commonly used protocols recommend testing on three different days to improve sensitivity and prevent sampling error. A single-office FOB is less sensitive, detecting only 58% of cancers compared to those detected after a three-card test. Sensitivity of a single unrehydrated FOB for cancer is approximately 40%; its specificity seems to range from 96% to 98%. Test sensitivity may also be increased to 50–60%.

Three randomized studies have demonstrated a significant reduction in CRC-associated mortality rates following the use of FOB in the general population. The Minnesota trial, that employed a three-card rehydrated test, showed a 33% and 21% cumulative reduction in mortality at 18 years of follow-up after annual and biennial screening, respectively. Similarly, two European studies (UK and Denmark) have shown a 15–18% reduction in mortality following the use of a biennial three-card unrehydrated FOB screening protocol.

One of the important caveats of using FOB as an initial screening tool is the presence of false-positives leading to the performance of unnecessary colonoscopies. Similarly, a false-negative result may be falsely reassuring.

Faecal immunochemical test
Standard guaiac-based FOBT has relatively poor sensitivity and specificity which is further disadvantaged by dietary modulation from ingestion of red meat and certain peroxidase-containing vegetables. In contrast, FIT is based on the detection of the globin moiety which is more sensitive and not affected by dietary habits. It also does not detect upper GI bleeding (as the globin is digested).

Several observational studies have reported improved sensitivity with the use of FIT. In a comparison study, FIT identified 50% more cancers and 256% more high-risk adenomas than guaiac-based FOBT. This has led to many organizations around the world endorsing the use of FIT for screening purposes, despite the lack of randomized evidence.

At the currently employed analytical threshold, FIT is associated with lower specificity (significantly higher false-positives) that will limit its usefulness in public screening programmes. It has been previously reported that 47 false-positive results would be required to detect one extra case of invasive CRC, and 2.2 false-positive results would be required to detect one extra advanced adenoma.

In an attempt to reduce the number of false-positives and improve the future applicability of FIT, the Scottish Bowel Screening Centre proposed a two-tier reflex screening algorithm in which positive FOBT is followed by FIT prior to colonoscopy. In an observational study of 1,124 individuals following this algorithm approximately 40% with a positive FIT were found to have cancer or high-risk polyps compared to <5% with negative FIT. Since 2017, FIT has replaced FOB as the screening test in the Scottish Bowel Screening programme.

Faecal DNA test
A prospective, multicentre study of stool DNA analysis—using a multitarget DNA testing panel—in 4,404 participants demonstrated a 52% sensitivity for cancer detection. Other small observational studies have shown 62–91% sensitivity for cancer detection with rates independent of cancer stage and site. While, the optimal screening interval for stool DNA testing remains undefined, guidelines recommend testing once in three years.

Sigmoidoscopy

Randomized trials have shown that sigmoidoscopic screening leads to reduced incidence and mortality of colorectal cancer. In the UK Flexible sigmoidoscopy screening trial, in which people aged 55–64 years were randomized to a single flexible sigmoidoscopy or to a control group, the incidence of CRC was reduced by 26% and the mortality by 30%. Similar results were reported in an Italian trial.

Previous randomized studies have shown that the addition of sigmoidoscopy to FOB doubles the detection rate of significant adenomas and cancer. United States Preventive Services Task Force (USPSTF) screening guidelines recommended that flexible sigmoidoscopy should be performed every three to five years.

Colonoscopy

Colonoscopy has been reported to have a sensitivity of >90% for cancer and large adenomas and 75% for smaller adenomas (<1cm). The role of colonoscopy as a screening procedure has not been addressed in a randomized trial, but two randomized trials are ongoing in Europe.

The US National Polyp Study reported that approximately 75–90% of cancers can be prevented by regular colonoscopies. An update of this study suggested a 52% reduction in CRC mortality.

Colonoscopy is widely accepted as the gold standard for the diagnosis of CRC. However, it does not merit a similar status for CRC screening—except in high-risk patients—due to lack of randomized evidence, invasive nature, associated complications (e.g. perforation), poor adherence, and limited availability.

USPSTF guidelines recommend that colonoscopy should be performed every ten years.

Double-contrast barium enema (DCBE)

There are no studies that have assessed the role of DCBE in reducing the incidence and death from CRC cancer. With the widespread use of endoscopy and CT scan, the use of DCBE has declined and it is no longer recommended as a screening method.

CT colonography

CT colonography is now regarded as an acceptable non-invasive substitute for colonoscopy in the diagnosis of CRC even though there are no randomized trials. USPSTF recommends screening using CT colonoscopy every five years.

Screening in high-risk individuals

First-degree relatives of individuals diagnosed with CRC or adenomatous polyps at <50 years should have colonoscopy starting at 40 years or ten years earlier than the age of previous diagnosis, whichever came first. Subsequent examinations should be repeated at five years.

Patients suspected of hereditary CRC syndromes should have first colonoscopy around the second to third decade and then every one to three years.

First colonoscopy in patients with IBD is recommended at eight to ten years after diagnosis and should be repeated every one to three years.

Prevention

NSAIDs—by virtue of their ability to inhibit COX-2 enzyme—have undergone extensive investigation for their possible role in preventing adenoma formation and subsequent CRC development.

In a prospective cohort of 662,424 patients enrolled in the ACS Cancer Prevention Study II, risk of colon cancer death decreased about 40% with the use of aspirin. Similarly, two randomized trials confirmed that aspirin reduces risk of colorectal adenomas. However, in the Physicians Health Study of 22,000 men aged 40–84 years, there was no reduction in invasive cancer or adenoma development. The UK ADD-ASPIRIN trial evaluates the effect of aspirin on recurrence and survival after primary treatment for non-metastatic solid tumours including CRC (NCT02804815).

Meta-analyses have shown an approximately 20% reduction in risk of CRC with the use of HRT and oral contraceptives. Recently, the UK Royal College of General Practitioners Oral Contraceptive study has reported a reduced incidence of CRC (incidence rate ratio 0.81; 95% CI 0.66–0.99) with oral contraceptives. However, the protective effect of HRT has been questioned.

7.15 Clinical features, diagnosis, and staging of colorectal cancer

Clinical features

Approximately 5–20% of cancers are asymptomatic and diagnosed during screening. 3–21% of cancers (predominantly left-sided) present as an emergency with symptoms of obstruction and perforation and carry a worse prognosis. Remaining cancers often present in the primary care setting with symptoms that may be difficult to distinguish from benign causes.

Rectal bleeding

Rectal bleeding is an important presenting symptom of CRC (in 20–58% of patients). However, it is also observed in 14–33% of the general population and is mostly from benign causes. Bleeding observed in presence of one or more of the following features should be urgently referred for further investigations.

- Increasing age (>50 years).
- Change in bowel habit and abdominal pain.
- Positive FOB.
- Passage of dark blood mixed with stools.
- Isolated rectal bleeding without anal symptoms. Presence of anal symptoms (soreness, lump, pruritus) may indicate other benign causes (fissure, haemorrhoids). However, it is important to note that rectal tumours also present with local symptoms (pain, tenesmus, pruritus).

Change in bowel habit

Many patients (39–85%) with CRC will experience change in bowel habit. Prevalence of bowel irregularity (constipation or diarrhoea) ranges from 10% to 25% in the general population. The following clinical features increase the probability of underlying CRC.

- Recent change in bowel habit, especially in older patients.
- History of passage of blood or mucus should be urgently referred for specialist opinion.
- History of new onset diarrhoea (increased frequency or looseness).

Abdominal pain
- Prevalence of CRC in patients presenting with unexplained abdominal pain is 1%.
- Abdominal pain in a patient with CRC may be sign of impending obstruction.
- Colicky abdominal pain combined with other obstructive symptoms (abdominal distension, nausea, and vomiting) should be urgently investigated.

Other symptoms
- Chronic blood loss: iron-deficiency anaemia, tiredness, lassitude; more frequently observed in right-sided tumours.
- Abdominal mass: sign of advanced disease; right iliac fossa mass classically observed in caecal carcinoma.
- Rectal mass: digital rectal examination (DRE) may reveal a palpable mass in low/mid rectal tumours.
- Weight loss, loss of appetite: suggestive of advanced/metastatic disease.

Emergency presentation
- Up to 20% of tumours may present as an emergency with obstruction or perforation/peritonitis.
- Worse prognosis.
- 60% of these patients would have seen the GP previously with one or more symptoms suggestive of CRC.
- Abdominal pain, weight loss, diarrhoea, and anaemia are more common in this group.

Features of hereditary colorectal syndrome-associated CRC
Diagnosis of one of the hereditary colorectal syndrome (HCS) should be suspected in presence of one or more of the following:
- Early age of onset (<40 years).
- Presence of multiple (>10) polyps.
- Synchronous or metachronous cancers (CRC or other associated).
- Positive family history for one or more of these features.

Features of CRC in inflammatory bowel disease
- Affects younger patients.
- Higher proportion of invasive tumours arising from flat non-polypoidal lesions.
- Higher frequency of tumours with mucinous and signet ring histology.
- Multifocality with higher rate of two or more synchronous primaries.

Diagnosis
History and physical examination
- Detailed history of onset and duration of local and systemic symptoms.
- Identify patients at risk of obstruction.
- Family history to identify patients with familial predisposition and hereditary CRC syndromes. Clinical suspicion of genetic susceptibility may have important implications for other members of the family.
- Complete physical examination including DRE.

Flexible sigmoidoscopy
- First most appropriate investigation for most patients.
- Diagnostic reach of 60cm (assess lesions in rectum, sigmoid, and descending colon).
- Patients with rectal bleeding or change in bowel habit have a 0.2% risk of possible bowel neoplasm after negative flexible sigmoidoscopy (FS).
- Diagnostic assessment of rectal lesions should include evaluation of the length, position (distance from anal verge), and mobility of the primary tumour.
- Low risk of complications and is relatively easy and quick to perform.

Colonoscopy
- Employed to assess the colon beyond the reach of the sigmoidoscope.
- Performed following a negative FS in patients with persistent bowel symptoms, especially abdominal pain and weight loss.
- Important procedure to exclude other synchronous lesions.
- Initial investigation in patients with history suggestive of right-sided lesions (anaemia, tiredness, abdominal pain).
- Average risk of perforation is 0.1–0.2%. However, this may be as low as 0.02% with endoscopists performing at least three procedures per week or 100–200 per annum. Furthermore, increasing experience is associated with higher completion rates.

Barium enema
- Less risk of complications, but also reduced diagnostic sensitivity compared to colonoscopy.
- Least preferred choice of patients compared to FS, colonoscopy, and CT colonography.
- Use of barium enema in the diagnosis of CRC has significantly declined following the optimization and widespread availability of endoscopic procedures.

CT colonography
CT colonography (virtual colonoscopy) has greater accuracy than barium enema and is possibly as sensitive as colonoscopy for detection of larger polyps. However, endoscopy is needed to obtain histology. A meta-analysis of data from 14 studies with a total of 1,324 patients demonstrated an overall specificity of 95% for the detection of polyps 10mm or larger. In a review of 4,086 asymptomatic patients, the use of CT colonography was associated with sensitivities of 82.9% and 87.9% and specificities of 91.4% and 97.6% for adenomas ≥6mm and ≥10mm, respectively.

Endoscopic-guided biopsy
Patients should have endoscopic-guided biopsy to establish a diagnosis of CRC cancer. Most CRC are adenocarcinomas exhibiting CK20 positivity. Other histological variants include mucinous, squamous, signet-ring-cell, and neuroendocrine carcinomas.

Transabdominal ultrasonography (USG)
Transabdominal ultrasound is not routinely employed in diagnosis of CRC, but recent advances have prompted new interest in this technology that may be used in association with other investigations to improve diagnostic accuracy. In a recent study, the use of ultrasound was

associated with an overall T staging accuracy of 64% which increased to 89% when a three-tier approach was used (Tis/TI, T2, and T3/4). From the 98 biopsy proven cancers, ultrasonography detected all except two lesions at splenic flexure.

Staging
Laboratory tests
Full blood count, liver function tests, urea and electrolytes, tumour markers (CEA).

Local staging of rectal tumours
MRI scanning
- Patients with rectal tumours should undergo pelvic MRI scan to define the local extent of primary tumour.
- MRI helps in defining the relationship of primary tumour with mesorectal fascia and also identifies the presence of pelvic lymphadenopathy and extramural vascular invasion.
- Distance of less than 1mm between the primary tumour and mesorectal fascia is predictive of potential involvement of CRM (<1mm) following initial surgery.
- The MERCURY study demonstrated the equivalence between the measured extramural spread on imaging and pathology. In patients proceeding to curative resection the correlation between the MRI-predicted clear margins (>1mm from mesorectal fascia) and pathological outcome (R0) was 0.92, with an observed agreement of 84%.

Rectal endosonography (RE)
- Sensitive technique for diagnosis of early rectal lesions. Previous studies have reported diagnostic accuracy of 76–100% (better for primary than nodes).
- RE may be employed to differentiate between various early rectal lesions (Tcis, T1, T2). The depth of submucosa involvement can predict early T1 lesions (superficial one-third of submucosa) which may be amenable to initial local excision.

Exclusion of metastatic disease
- CT of thorax, abdomen, and pelvis is the most commonly performed and preferred investigation to exclude metastatic spread.
- USG may be employed to assess metastatic spread to the liver. USG has low sensitivity (50–76%) compared to CT scan (>90%) for assessment of liver disease. Nearly, half of the patients with a negative USG will be found to have liver metastasis on subsequent investigations. However, the diagnostic accuracy and specificity of USG is high at approximately 90%.
- MRI scan of the liver is performed for patients with liver metastasis considered fit for liver resection.
- There is no definitive evidence to support the routine use of PET/CT in the staging of primary non-metastatic CRC. However, it may be useful in selected cases where initial imaging is inconclusive and the presence of metastatic disease would change management.

Staging classification
- The Duke's classification was originally developed for rectal cancer, and then modified by Astler-Coller for classification of disease extent of both colon and rectal cancer. The Dukes system did not differentiate between T3 and T4 disease. Furthermore, the number of involved nodes was not a parameter for classification of node-positive tumours.

- The tumour, node, metastasis (TNM) staging classification was developed by the American Joint Committee on Cancer (AJCC)/International Union Against Cancer (UICC) and has undergone regular revision. Version 8 is currently used. This subdivides the pN1 category into three substages based on the number of involved nodes and recognizes tumour deposits without lymph node involvement as a specific subcategory (pN1c). The N2 category is also subdivided with pN2a nodes as four to six involved nodes and pN2b as seven or more.
- The College of American Pathologists recommends examination of at least 12 lymph nodes for assessment of nodal status as suboptimal lymph node yield may be associated with high probability of under staging. Furthermore, higher lymph node yield may be associated with improved prognosis even in node-negative tumours (Lykke et al. 2013).

TNM staging of colorectal cancer
- pT   Primary tumour
- pTX   Primary tumour cannot be assessed
- pT0   No evidence of primary tumour
- pT1   Tumour invades submucosa
- pT2   Tumour invades muscularis propria
- pT3   Tumour invades into subserosa or into non-peritonealized pericolic or perirectal tissues
- pT4   Tumour perforates visceral peritoneum and/or directly invades other organs or structures
- pN   Regional lymph nodes
- pNX   Regional lymph nodes cannot be assessed
- pN0   No regional lymph node metastatic disease
- pN1   Metastatic disease in one to three regional lymph nodes
  - pN1a Metastasis in one regional lymph node
  - pN1b Metastases in two to three regional lymph nodes
  - pN1c Tumour deposit(s) i.e. satellites, in the subserosa, or in non-peritonealized pericolic or perirectal soft tissue without regional lymph node metastatic disease
- pN2   Metastatic disease in four or more regional lymph nodes
  - pN2a Metastases in four to six regional lymph nodes
  - pN2b Metastases in seven or more regional lymph nodes
- pM   Distant metastatic disease
- pM1   Distant metastatic disease
  - pM1a Metastasis confined to one organ without peritoneal metastases
  - pM1b Metastases in more than one organ
  - pM1c Metastases to the peritoneum with or without other organ involvement

(Reproduced with permission from Brierley JD, Gospodarowicz MK, Wittekind C (eds.). *TNM Classification of Malignant Tumours*. 8th edn. Copyright © 2017, John Wiley & Sons.)

Further reading
Lykke J, Jess P, Roikjær O. Danish Colorectal Cancer Group. A high lymph node yield in colon cancer is associated with age, tumour stage, tumour sub-site and priority of surgery. Results from a prospective national cohort study. *Int J Color Dis* 2016; 31(7):1299–305.

7.16 Colorectal cancer: Localized disease

Introduction

Surgery is the mainstay of treatment for localized CRC, after complete staging. There is evidence that preoperative antibiotic prophylaxis (usually with a cephalosporin and metronidazole) reduces postoperative infection. Patients also require thromboembolism prophylaxis (usually with low-molecular-weight heparin and graded compression stockings), anaesthetic assessment, and blood cross-match. The use of mechanical bowel preparation is controversial but it is performed less commonly than in the past due to concerns over dehydration.

Technique

Radical excision of a colonic tumour, with the appropriate vascular pedicle and accompanying lymph nodes, is the standard approach to gaining local control and acquiring important prognostic information about nodal spread. Occasionally, a more limited procedure may be required in an unfit patient, or one with incurable disease, where relief of obstruction is the main purpose of the procedure.

The arterial supply to the segment of bowel to be resected determines the length of bowel removed. Ideally 5cm of normal bowel will be taken proximal and distal to the tumour.

Colon cancer

Elective procedures

Right hemicolectomy

Tumours of the caecum, ascending colon, and proximal transverse colon are removed by a right hemicolectomy. This involves division of the ileo-colic artery, right colic artery, and right branches of the middle colic artery. If the main branch of the middle colic artery is also taken then the remainder of the transverse colon is removed (an 'extended right hemicolectomy'). Included in the specimen will be the distal 10cm of the ileum.

Left hemicolectomy

Tumours of the descending and upper sigmoid colon are removed using a left hemicolectomy. This involves resection of the inferior mesenteric artery near its origin on the aorta.

The ideal procedure for tumours at the splenic flexure is less certain, since this is at the boundary between vessels supplied from the superior mesenteric and inferior mesenteric arteries. There is also heterogeneity between individuals as to the predominant feeder blood vessel. Technique is therefore individualized based on anatomy and the need to have well-vascularized bowel ends for the anastomosis.

Rectal cancer

Sphincter preservation and surgical approaches

Tumours of the distal sigmoid and mid to upper rectum are usually removed by an anterior resection. Lower rectal tumours also require removal of the anal canal (known as an abdomino-perineal resection), which then necessitates a permanent stoma. To avoid this, there has been a trend for lower anastomoses, joining the colon ever closer to the anal canal. These procedures require considerable skill and can be limited by increased complication rates (such as anastomotic leakage) and relatively poor functional results unless performed by experienced

surgeons. It is important that such procedures are oncologically sound and do not unnecessarily increase the risk of residual disease.

Development of total mesorectal excision (TME)

For many years the results of surgery alone were poor in rectal cancer. Local recurrence rates were >20%. With the growing realization that involvement of the CRM was predictive for local recurrence, the concept of TME developed. This procedure removes not just the rectum but also the surrounding envelope of fatty tissue (mesorectum). Evidence that this improves surgical results comes directly from individual surgical series, population-based studies, and within the context of recently published, randomized-controlled trials. Current rates of local recurrence for surgery alone are often <10%.

Temporary stomas

Many patients having surgery for rectal cancer will require a temporary stoma. This allows the new pelvic anastomosis to heal and reduces the sequelae of any anastomotic leak.

Quality of life

There is an increasing appreciation that treatments for rectal cancer can adversely affect patients' QoL. Bowel function is frequently abnormal following rectal surgery and this dysfunction can be increased further by adjuvant radiotherapy. Sexual function can also be affected (with radiotherapy and/or surgery potentially causing erectile dysfunction, low sperm counts, early menopause), dyspareunia, vaginal stenosis, and vaginal dryness. Combined with the adverse effect of a stoma on body image, many patients are starting to ask if less aggressive approaches can be taken to avoid the morbidity of treatment. One approach is to adopt a non-surgical or less aggressive surgical approach for early rectal cancers. Using a combination of endoscopic resection, external beam (chemo) radiotherapy and contact radiotherapy (applied directly to the rectum per-anally) some patients are spared a stoma. However, no direct comparison with the 'gold-standard' surgical techniques has been made and clinical trials are required to determine the benefits and risks.

Surgery for early stage disease

As screening for CRC increases in the UK, an increasing number of tumours are being discovered at an earlier stage of their development. Frequently, premalignant polyps are also identified. Many of these lesions can now be removed endoscopically using a variety of dissection techniques.

Benign polyps or very early T1 lesions can be removed by EMR, where saline is infiltrated into the base of a lesion (to raise it away from underlying layers) and it is then resected with diathermy or a hot loop. This technique can be applied around the whole colon at colonoscopy.

Transanal endoscopic microsurgery (TEMS) is another way of removing lesions up to 20cm from the anal verge. It uses a specially designed 40mm diameter operating rectoscope with a three-dimensional, magnified optical system. Unlike EMR, TEMS allows a full-thickness excision to be performed. Nevertheless, it is an insufficient treatment on its own for all but the earliest rectal cancers because it fails to remove local lymph nodes and local recurrence rates are higher than with classical approaches.

Anastomotic technique

Anastomoses can be formed using a variety of stapling devices or by hand-sewing. For a long time surgeons had individual preferences, but recent evidence suggests that staples produce fewer leaks and are otherwise very similar.

Laparoscopic and robotic-assisted surgery

Laparoscopic surgery has become standard for many major abdominal procedures including colorectal surgery. With appropriate expertise on laparoscopic surgery, there are no significant differences in terms of DFS rate, local recurrence rate, mortality, morbidity, anastomotic leakage, resection margins, or recovered lymph nodes compared with open colectomy. The important short-term benefits include less blood loss, quicker return to normal diet, less pain, less narcotic use, and shorter average stays in hospital. In the longer term, incisional hernias and adhesions are also reduced. Laparoscopic colectomy is therefore safe particularly for left colon cancer provided there is no previous major abdominal surgery leading to adhesions, tumour is not locally advanced, and there are no complications such as obstruction or performation. In right colon cancer, since anastomosis is hand sewn, laparotomy is required.

Robotic-assisted rectal surgery has technical advantages compared with laproscopic surgery, but is still under evaluation. The ROLARR trial which compared robotic-assisted with laparoscopic surgery did not show any significantly reduced risk of conversion to open laparotomy (8.1% vs. 12.2%, P=0.16).

Emergency procedures

In the UK, about 20% of patients with colon cancer present as an emergency. Commonly, this is with an obstructed bowel, but bleeding and perforation can also be responsible. Ideally such patients should be treated in a unit where they can be seen and operated on by a specialist colorectal surgeon. Following resuscitation and initial investigations to establish the cause of the problem (which may include plain films, CT, endoscopy, or water-soluble enemas) different options exist for treatment.

Surgical

Obstruction

The bowel is initially decompressed before proceeding. Right-sided obstruction is then usually dealt with by a right hemicolectomy. Treatment option for left-sided lesions is a two-stage procedure using Hartmann's operation to bring out an end proximal colostomy with closure of the distal segment. The stoma may then be closed later if appropriate. Alternatively, some surgeons attempt one-stage procedures with anastomosis following resection (mainly for colonic tumours).

Perforation

Caecal perforation, due to a distal tumour, is usually treated by right hemicolectomy. When the cancer itself perforates, the resection can be technically demanding. For left-sided lesions a Hartmann's procedure is usually required.

Stenting

Emergency surgery has a high perioperative mortality rate, often reflecting the advanced stage of disease, electrolyte disturbances, poor nutritional state, and unprepared bowel that can be present. The use of endoscopically or radiographically placed self-expanding metal stents is of interest—as either primary treatment, for those unfit for surgery, or as a 'bridge to surgery' for those whose condition could be improved if the obstruction was relieved. Subsequent elective resection can then more safely include primary anastomosis.

The potential complications include perforation, pain, bleeding, re-obstruction, and distal migration. The reported risk of perforation is less than 5%, but much higher in patients receiving the anti-angiogenic agent, bevacizumab. Therefore, patients receiving bevacizumab are not considered for stenting.

Postoperative care

Following surgery, postoperative care has traditionally been similar to that of other patients undergoing abdominal surgery. Analgesia has usually been provided with opiates, in a patient-driven system, for the first few days. Intravenous fluids have been used initially but oral intake has been gradually increased as normal bowel function returns (audible bowel sounds and passage of flatus). Patients have slowly been mobilized when they feel able to.

Enhanced recovery after surgery (ERAS) protocol after elective colorectal operation has significantly reduced in-patient stay and morbidity with faster recovery. The elements of ERAS include optimizing a patient's status preoperatively (education, nutrition, control of risk factors); efficient discharge planning; avoidance of mechanical bowel preparation and complete fasting preoperatively (risk of dehydration); optimized anaesthesia (including postoperative epidural analgesia); early feeding and mobilization; and multidisciplinary involvement (e.g. physiotherapy, social worker, dietician).

Further reading

Jayne D, Pigazzi A, Marshall H, et al. Effect of robotic-assisted vs. conventional laparoscopic surgery on risk of conversion to open laparotomy among patients undergoing resection for rectal cancer: The ROLARR Randomized Clinical Trial. *JAMA* 2017; 318 (16):1569–80.

7.17 Adjuvant treatment for colorectal cancer

Introduction
Many of the patients who receive adjuvant therapy do not benefit, either because they are cured already or because the treatment fails. Nevertheless, even a small effect in a common disease translates into many hundreds or thousands of lives saved. When counselling individual patients it is therefore important to outline some of these uncertainties, and to carefully evaluate any comorbid factors, which may increase the risks of treatment.

Chemotherapy in colorectal cancer
Chemotherapy, based on 5-FU, is widely used as an adjuvant treatment in colon cancer. Single agent 5-FU improves absolute survival by 3–5% in stage II and 10–15% in stage III colon cancer. The addition of oxaliplatin with 5-FU improves absolute survival by an additional 4–5% in stage III colon cancer.

Why 5-FU-based chemotherapy?
In 1989 and 1990 two large randomized trials clearly showed a survival benefit for 12 months of 5-FU plus levamisole over observation alone. Subsequent trials assessed the value of combining 5-FU with folinic acid (FA) (which potentiates its effect on the target enzyme thymidylate synthase) and examined the importance of levamisole (an antihelminthic with immunostimulatory properties that had been proposed to enhance the effect of 5-FU). Studies were also performed addressing the optimum duration of therapy. In summary, these trials concluded that treatment with six months of chemotherapy with 5-FU/FA was equivalent to 12 months of 5-FU/levamisole, and superior to six months of 5-FU/levamisole. Furthermore, combining 5-FU/FA with levamisole gave no extra benefit.

Particularly influential in the UK was the Quick and Simple and Reliable (QUASAR) study. In this large study, patients were given chemotherapy either as a weekly bolus or for five consecutive days every four weeks (the so-called 'Mayo regimen'). Although not randomly allocated, the weekly schedule appeared much less toxic, with equivalent efficacy. This very large trial encouraged widespread adoption of the weekly regimen in the UK.

In the last few years a variety of trials have combined 5-FU/FA with other chemotherapy agents in an attempt to increase the impact of adjuvant chemotherapy. Despite enhanced responses in metastatic disease the combination of 5-FU and irinotecan has so far shown no benefit; the CALGB-89803 trial was prematurely closed due to increased mortality in patients receiving irinotecan, whilst the PETACC-3 trial did not show any significant advantage for the irinotecan combination in terms of DFS.

More importantly, three large randomized trials (MOSAIC, NSABP-C07, and XELOXA) have now shown a benefit in combining oxaliplatin with fluoropyrimidine regimens in the adjuvant setting. The MOSAIC and NASBP-C07 studies compared FU/FA with or without oxaliplatin. Both studies have shown improved disease-free survival rates with the oxaliplatin combination, at the expense of increased toxicity.

Furthermore, in the MOSAIC study, the addition of oxaliplatin significantly improved ten-year OS for stage III disease (67% vs. 59%, P=0.016) but not for stage II disease.

Intravenous 5-FU can be inconvenient and indwelling lines for infusional therapy are also vulnerable to complications such as infection or thrombosis. In a randomized phase 3 trial (XELOXA), capecitabine, an oral fluoropyrimidine, in combination with oxaliplatin (XELOX) was compared with standard FU/FA in patients with stage III colon cancer. At a median follow-up of 74 months, the seven-year DFS (63% vs. 56%, P=0.004) and seven-year OS (73% vs. 67%, P=0.04) were significantly superior with the oxaliplatin-capecitabine combination. The XELOX combination also resulted in less treatment-related side effects compared with FU/FA.

Toxicity
Some of the side effects 5-FU can cause are fatigue, nausea, vomiting, diarrhoea, stomatitis, plantar-palmar erythema, epistaxis, and sore eyes. Alopecia and significant myelosuppression are uncommon. The severity and site-specific side effects are dependent on the regimen used. Capecitabine tends to mimic infusional 5-FU, with plantar-palmar erythema and diarrhoea being particularly common. A rare complication is angina, which may be related to coronary artery spasm and is commoner in those receiving continuous infusions of 5-FU or capecitabine. This does not necessarily occur in patients with known coronary artery disease, although there is some evidence that this slightly increases the risk.

A small proportion of people are deficient for the enzyme dihydropyrimidine dehydrogenase (DPD), which is important in metabolizing 5-FU. Such individuals will be otherwise healthy but have extremely severe and early toxicity with standard doses of 5-FU and often require emergency admission to the oncology centre. If these toxicities can be successfully managed, it is sometimes possible to recommence treatment with a 50% dose reduction after careful consideration of the balance of benefit and risk.

Oxaliplatin in combination with 5-FU/FA increases toxicity. In the MOSAIC trial, significant neutropenia was much commoner in the combined arm (41.1% vs. 4.7%), but was complicated by infection/fever in only 1.8%. However, perhaps the biggest problem in the clinic is the increased incidence of sensory neuropathy with oxaliplatin, which can be clinically significant and long-lasting. This was sufficiently severe to interfere with function in 12.4% of patients receiving combined treatment in MOSAIC, although for the majority this resolved in the subsequent months (down to 0.7% after four years' median follow-up). Therefore, if patients develop clinically significant neurotoxicity, oxaliplatin should be stopped and fluoropyramidine continued.

Patient selection
While the standard adjuvant chemotherapy for stage III disease is a doublet of oxaliplatin and a fluoropyramidine (FOLFOX or XELOX), patient selection continues to be challenging. A pooled analysis and subgroup analysis of the MOSAIC study suggest that patients aged ≥70 years may not benefit from the addition of oxaliplatin to fluoropyramidines. A number of nomograms (e.g. MAYO clinic, MSKCC) are now available to quantify the individual risk of recurrence and OS, which may guide clinical decision-making (see 'Internet resources, p. 184).

For patients who are not fit for the doublet regimen, six months of infusional FU/FA or capecitabine remains the standard treatment.

Another area of considerable debate is the role of chemotherapy in stage II colorectal cancer. Such patients already have a reasonable prognosis and their benefit from chemotherapy is likely to be small. Indeed, one large UK study of adjuvant 5-FU-based chemotherapy (QUASAR) demonstrated only a modest absolute survival benefit at five years (3.6% assuming a recurrence rate of 20% without chemotherapy).

Although not directly addressed by this study, it is known that some stage II tumours have a worse prognosis, such as those presenting with perforation, obstruction, extramural vascular invasion, peritoneal involvement, or poorly differentiated histology. In the MOSAIC trial for patients with stage II disease there was no statistical difference in DFS or OS with FOLFOX compared with FU/LA. However, there was a suggestion of absolute improvement in DFS by 7% and OS by 2% in patients with stage II disease with high-risk factors. The NSABP C-07 study did not show any significant survival benefit in patients with stage II disease. Nevertheless, many clinicians would target this group of patients for adjuvant chemotherapy, on the basis that their absolute risk of relapse is higher and therefore the likely benefit is greater. A careful discussion is required in patients with stage II disease with any of the following high-risk factors: poorly differentiated tumour, vascular, lymphatic, or perineural invasion, pT4 disease, tumour presentation with obstruction or perforation, and fewer than 12 lymph nodes sampled.

After resection of a primary rectal cancer, many patients are referred for chemotherapy with a defunctioning stoma. Despite their obvious desire to have a reversal as soon as possible this is commonly deferred until after chemotherapy. This is to allow chemotherapy to start as soon as possible after surgery, as most clinical trials have required chemotherapy to commence within six to eight weeks. There is inadequate evidence to define the benefit from chemotherapy at later time points or for interrupting chemotherapy to allow reversal.

Can current treatments be improved?
Adjuvant chemotherapy could be improved if:
- It was better tolerated.
- It was more effective.
- There was better selection of patients based on molecular predictive factors.

The increasing use of capecitabine in adjuvant therapy is one approach to improving the acceptability of chemotherapy for patients (by avoiding the need for intravenous access and indwelling line complications) but it is not without toxicity. For some patients, diarrhoea and plantar-palmar erythema may be greater than that seen with weekly 5-FU/LV (leucovorin). Furthermore, agents such as oxaliplatin continue to require intravenous access, meaning that some of the convenience is lost when contemplating combination approaches. Nevertheless, for patients who are not candidates for oxaliplatin, single agent capecitabine is better tolerated treatment with a similar DFS compared with FU/LA (levulinic acid) (the X-ACT trial).

Much of the toxicity with conventional six-month regimens could be reduced by treating for a shorter period. An interesting approach would be to determine if less chemotherapy had equivalent efficacy. A number of randomized trials (e.g. SCOT, TOSCA, IDEA) evaluated three versus six months of adjuvant chemotherapy for resected colon cancer. A preliminary analysis of the pooled data from six trials in the International Duration Evaluation of Adjuvant Chemotherapy (IDEA) collaboration suggests that three months of adjuvant chemotherapy may be effective for early disease (T1–3, N1) whereas high-risk disease (T4, N2) may require six months of adjuvant therapy. For three months of adjuvant chemotherapy, XELOX (capecitabine plus oxaliplatin) appears to be a better choice than FOLFOX.

Increasing effectiveness
In advanced CRC, a range of targeted biological agents have been shown to enhance the benefits of conventional chemotherapy. Of particular interest are antibodies specific to the epidermal growth factor receptor (EGFR) and vascular endothelial growth factor (VEGF), which are both important for the growth and spread of CRC. Cetuximab and panitumumab are licensed products (in metastatic disease) targeting EGFR, whilst bevacizumab targets VEGF. Despite relatively modest improvements in outcome in metastatic disease, randomized trials have so far failed to demonstrate a survival benefit with the addition of these agents to conventional adjuvant chemotherapy. The NSABP C-08, AVANT, and the QUASAR trials evaluated the addition of bevacizumab to conventional chemotherapy whereas the N0147 and the European PETACC8 trials evaluated the role of cetuximab.

Risk classification using molecular predictive markers
Various different molecular markers have been examined as potential predictive factors for response to adjuvant treatment. These include thymidylate synthase gene overexpression, microsatellite instability (MSI), mismatch repair (MMR), enzyme deficiency (dMMR), 18q deletion, KRAS, BRAF, and TP53 mutations and deleted in colorectal cancer (DCC) gene. Patients with stage II disease without high-risk features and a high MSI/dMMR have a favourable prognosis and are therefore unlikely to benefit from adjuvant chemotherapy. Studies suggest that dMMR colon cancers are resistant to fluoropyrimidine and patients with stage III disease with high levels of MSI/dMMR are considered for a regimen with an oxaliplatin-containing regimen. The clinical application of gene-expression profiling, including 12-gene recurrence score (Oncotype-Dx Colon Cancer Assay) is not yet defined.

Rectal cancer
The largest evidence base supporting the use of chemotherapy exists in patients with colon cancer and its applicability to patients with rectal cancer remains controversial. Nevertheless, in the UK, it is common to use the same criteria to select patients, irrespective of the primary site within the large bowel.

Radiotherapy
Radiotherapy is the use of ionizing radiation to eliminate cancer cells. It is used almost exclusively for the treatment of rectal cancer, rather than colon cancer, since small bowel toxicity and the mobility of much of the colon limits treatments outside the pelvis. Local pelvic recurrence is also a particularly unpleasant feature of rectal cancer which is ideally prevented if possible.

Indications

There are three main indications for adjuvant radiation in rectal cancer:

- Reducing the risk of local recurrence in patients with resectable rectal cancer.
- Shrinking locally advanced rectal cancer to facilitate successful resection.
- Using radiation to shrink or 'downsize' resectable disease to achieve sphincter-preserving surgery.
- Reducing local recurrence in resectable disease.

Many early trials tested the value of adding radiotherapy to surgery. Two meta-analyses of these early studies, and a recent Cochrane review demonstrated unequivocal evidence that adjuvant radiation reduced the risk of local recurrence in resectable rectal cancer.

As well as a dose effect, analysis of these data also demonstrated that preoperative treatment seemed more effective than postoperative radiotherapy. Only one of these overviews demonstrated an improvement in OS, although both reported improvements in cancer-specific mortality.

The evolution of short-course preoperative radiotherapy (SCPRT)

To avoid unnecessary delays before surgery, many early studies used large (5Gy) fraction sizes in short duration treatments. It was clear that these were well-tolerated as long as the radiotherapy was carefully planned, to spare excessive doses to normal tissues. The Swedish Rectal Cancer Trial was particularly influential since it showed an improvement in OS when 25Gy in five fractions SCPRT was added to surgery. Meanwhile, TME surgery has dramatically improved the outcome of surgery alone. It could therefore be hypothesized that radiotherapy in these early studies was simply compensating for inadequate surgery. To establish the role of SCPRT in the TME era, the Dutch Colorectal Cancer Study Group and the Medical Research Council (MRC) CR07 trials were both designed to compare SCPRT with selective postoperative approaches, based on CRM status (radiotherapy alone in the Dutch study, CRT in CR07).

Results from the Dutch trial and the CR07 study showed a reduction in local recurrence with routine SCPRT. CR07 also demonstrated a 6% improvement in three-year DFS but without any improvement in OS. Overall, the proportional reduction in local recurrence appeared very similar to the pre-TME era, but the absolute reduction was smaller due to the better surgical outcomes.

SCPRT followed by immediate surgery (<10 days from the start of radiotherapy) does have some well-established, long-term complications, including permanent sterility for men and premenopausal women. There is also an increased incidence of erectile dysfunction and impaired bowel function, although rates of pelvic fractures and bowel obstruction do not appear to be increased.

The recently reported Stockholm III trial compared SCPRT followed by surgery within one week with SCPRT followed by surgery after four to eight weeks or long course RT (50Gy in 25 fractions) followed by surgery after four to eight weeks in patients with 'intermediate risk' operable rectal cancer. At a minimum of two-year follow-up, there was no difference in oncological outcome among the three treatment arms. However, the

risk of surgical complications was less with SCPRT with delayed surgery, suggesting a useful alternative. It is therefore important to weigh up the pros and cons of SCPRT in different groups of patients. Many clinicians would not treat patients with stage I disease but opinions vary on where the threshold should be set for more advanced tumours.

Conventionally fractionated radiation schedules

An alternative approach to SCPRT is to use a longer course of radiation with a lower (more conventional) dose per fraction. This is an approach favoured in much of mainland Europe and North America. Most current long-course schedules use 45–50.4Gy over 5–5.5 weeks using 1.8–2Gy per fraction. As with SCPRT, there is evidence for improved local control using this strategy but no trial evidence for improved survival.

While randomized trials and a meta-analysis have suggested that concomitant chemotherapy with long-course radiotherapy (CRT), improves local control, there was no improvement in DFS or OS. As yet it is not clear what the advantage of preoperative CRT may be over SCPRT, although the former is clearly more expensive and resource intensive. One trial from Poland compared these strategies and this study was powered to detect differences in sphincter-preservation rather than local recurrence or survival. Unsurprisingly, CRT followed by a four to six week wait, led to greater tumour downstaging, pathological complete response rates (pCR: 16% vs. 1%), and CRM negative resections, but was also associated with higher rates of acute toxicity. Nevertheless, there was no significant difference seen in the rate of sphincter-preserving surgery and, interestingly, no statistical difference in local recurrence or late toxicity. A second trial (Trans-Tasman Radiation Oncology Group 0.1.04 trial) also reported a similar increase in pCR (15% vs. 1%) with CRT but without differences in recurrences or survival.

The choice of preoperative radiotherapy treatment approaches

A clear recommendation on the appropriate preoperative treatment approach for non-metastatic rectal cancer is not possible. Generally, patients with MRI predicted CRM of ≤1mm at TME are considered for CRT whereas SCPRT or CRT may be used in other patients.

Postoperative chemoradiotherapy approach

Giving radiotherapy after surgery enables targeting of higher risk individuals on the basis of surgical pathology. However, treatment is more toxic because of adherent small bowel in the pelvis and hypoxia in the tumour bed may compromise effectiveness. Although early trials showed improved local control the results were less impressive when compared with preoperative techniques. Nevertheless, adjuvant chemoradiotherapy had been the standard of care for operable rectal cancer in North America until the publication of the results of the German CAO/ARO/AI0 94 trial. This trial compared pre- and postoperative CRT. All patients had TME and the same regimen of CRT either preoperatively or postoperatively. At a median follow-up of 46 months the preoperative approach resulted in lower local recurrence rates (6% vs. 12%) and reduced complications (both acute and late). The benefit of a lower recurrence rate persisted at ten years (7% vs. 10%) and the DFS and OS were similar for both treatments. This study combined with the preoperative superiority of CRT over long-course radiotherapy alone appears to have decisively changed the treatment paradigm in rectal cancer to a pre-operative approach. Patients with rectal cancer who have not received preoperative radiotherapy should be considered for postoperative CRT if there are unexpected high-risk features such as CRM positivity, incomplete mesorectal resection, perforation in the tumour area, extranodal disease, etc.

Radiotherapy for locally advanced rectal cancer

Locally advanced disease can be defined clinically or on the basis of imaging. Transrectal ultrasound is considered a gold standard for assessing transmural tumour extent and MRI the best way of demonstrating the relationship of the tumour to the mesorectal fascia (the intended 'CRM' for a mesorectal excision).

Given the difficulty of surgery alone in this group of patients there is limited randomized trial evidence to support the use of radiotherapy. Nevertheless, in recent years, neoadjuvant concurrent CRT has become a standard treatment for locally advanced rectal cancer, because of increased response rates seen in the very large number of phase 2 studies that have been performed. Many have used either infusional 5-FU or bolus 5-FU/LV but no direct comparison has been undertaken and there remains considerable uncertainty as to how to derive the optimum regimen or the most useful endpoint.

Currently, there is considerable interest in the use of other drugs such as capecitabine, oxaliplatin, irinotecan, and the targeted biologicals in chemoradiation schedules. A recent study by the Polish Colorectal study group compared SCPRT and two cycles of FOLFOX with long-course oxaliplatin-based CRT in patients with fixed cT3 or CT4 rectal cancer. This study reported similar R0 resection rate and three-year DFS. However, SCPRT with consolidation chemotherapy led to a better three-year OS (73% vs. 65%, P=0.046) and a lower rate of pre-operative acute toxicities compared with preoperative CRT. However, long-term results are needed to confirm whether SCPRT with consolidation chemotherapy would be more effective than CRT in MRI-predicted CRM-positive rectal cancer.

There is considerable uncertainty as to the benefit of adjuvant chemotherapy following prior neoadjuvant CRT. If it is to be used, should it be given to those who have responded well to CRT (and therefore have chemosensitive disease) or should combination treatment be given to those who have not responded to CRT containing a single agent?

In routine clinical practice, adjuvant chemotherapy may be considered after preoperative chemoradiotherapy/radiotherapy in patients with high-risk yp stage II and yp stage III (pathological staging after preoperative therapy), similar to colon cancer.

Improving sphincter preservation

It remains controversial whether preoperative treatment (usually with CRT) can increase rates of sphincter-preserving surgery in low rectal cancer (i.e. converting a planned abdomino-perineal resection into a low anterior resection). Indeed, a systematic review has found no evidence of increased sphincter preservation following preoperative treatment. The authors argue that surgeons are reluctant to change their initial plan, even after a good response, because of understandable concern over residual microscopic disease at the original site of the tumour. There is also concern about the functional outcome following very low anterior resections. Nevertheless, some series have shown it to be possible, without excessive local recurrence, and the debate continues.

Conservative management of rectal cancer

Recently, there has been an increasing interest in conservative management of early stage rectal cancer especially in elderly patients at high surgical risk. Local radiotherapy using HDR brachytherapy or contact therapy (Papillon technique) is an alternative to surgery in patients with grade 1/2 tumours limited to the submucosa (T1). Similarly, frail patients with T2 tumours measuring less than 4cm may be treated with preoperative CRT or radiotherapy followed by a local excision.

In patients with locally advanced rectal cancer, preoperative CRT leads to a complete clinical response (cCR) in 20–30% and complete pathological response in 10–20%. Some reports suggest that surveillance alone may be an option for the group with cCR and any future relapses may be salvaged with surgery without compromising OS. However, this approach is still experimental and cannot be advised outside a clinical trial setting. The STAR-TEC trial is a randomized three arm trial comparing the standard TME surgery with organ sparing strategies of either long-course CRT or short-course radiotherapy in patients with T1-3bN0 rectal cancer (NCT02945566).

Summary

Deciding on the optimal adjuvant therapy for CRC may be straightforward, but can often be complex. Increasing options are available and patients vary in risk factors for recurrence, preferences for treatment, comorbidities, perception of risk/benefit, and acceptance of toxicity. Many questions remain unanswered which must be addressed by future studies.

Internet resources

Mayo Clinic. Gastroenterology and GI surgery: https://connect.mayoclinic.org/page/gastroenterology-and-gi-surgery/tab/colorectal-cancer/

Memorial Sloan Kettering Cancer Center. Prediction tools: https://www.mskcc.org/cancer-care/types/colon/prediction-tools

7.18 Treatment of advanced colorectal cancer

Introduction

The broad principles of management of advanced CRC are the same. Approximately 22% of patients with CRC present with stage IV disease (~7,000 per year in the UK) and around 25% of patients with early stage CRC develop distant recurrence. In the UK 15,000 people die each year of CRC (10% of cancer-related deaths).

The treatment paradigm is changing rapidly with the evolution of systemic anticancer therapies (SACT), including personalization of therapy based on biomarkers, and increasing use of local or regional approaches. Median survival of over 30 months has been reported in the latest trials of systemic therapy with chemotherapy plus a biomarker-directed targeted therapy, although caution should be exercised before extending this to patients managed in routine practice. Epidemiological data has also shown an improvement in survival over time but one-year survival for unselected patients with stage IV CRC is only 46% and five-year survival is less than 10%.

A sub-set of patients with liver and/or lung only disease can be treated with potentially curative intent.

Molecular subtypes

Understanding of the molecular abnormalities underlying CRC is improving. Mutations in key genes within signalling pathways have been identified but there is considerable heterogeneity between patients and this is a fast evolving field. The best characterized are mutations within the RAS-RAF-MEK-ERK signalling cascade initiated by the EGFR:

- RAS. Activating mutations (mt) in KRAS and NRAS are found in ~40% of patients and confer resistance to anti-EGFR monoclonal antibodies. KRASmt tumours have a poor prognosis compared to wild type (wt).
- BRAF. BRAF V600E mt is found in 8–10% of patients and is strongly associated with sporadic microsatellite instability (MSI) and right-sided tumours. It is a major adverse prognostic factor in advanced CRC.

Other targets of interest include mutations in the PIK3CA-PTEN-AKT pathway which also mediates EGFR signalling; and deficiencies in DNA repair mechanisms, which result in MSI and accumulation of mutations within tumour cells with high immunogenicity. MSI is found in ~5% of advanced CRC, where it is a poor prognostic marker (in contrast to early stage).

Clinical features and investigations

The commonest site of metastasis is the liver followed by lung, distant lymph nodes, peritoneum, and bone. Rarer sites include ovary and brain. There are ~30% of patients that have liver-only metastases at diagnosis.

Adverse clinical prognostic factors include: age, survival is poorer in both young and old patients; number of metastatic sites and extent of disease; presentation with stage IV disease vs. recurrence; right-sided tumours; and poor PS.

Assessment of patients should include their wishes, age, fitness, comorbidities, end organ function, and extent and distribution of disease. Important investigations include bloods to assess end organ function and tumour markers, and CT for initial staging. MRI of the liver to assess operability is used when considering a potentially curative approach; some centres routinely include PET scanning but others restrict this to borderline cases. Histology should be sought for confirmation of diagnosis and assessment of tissue biomarkers, including KRAS, NRAS, and BRAFmt status.

General principles of treatment

The key is to determine the goal of treatment based on assessment of the patient and their disease. Involvement of a multidisciplinary team is essential.

Questions to consider are:

- Suitability for SACT—fitness and patient's wishes?
- Is there potential for treatment with curative intent? If yes, are the metastases (and primary tumour) currently resectable or potentially resectable if downstaged?
- If there is no potential for resection:
  - Does the extent of disease warrant immediate treatment? A watch and wait approach can be considered if the burden of disease is low and this is in accordance with the patient's wishes.
  - Can a staged combination approach be adopted where single agent chemotherapy is initially used ahead of combination chemotherapy? Clinicians should be confident that patients will remain fit for combination chemotherapy if disease continues to progress.
  - If combination chemotherapy is indicated either due to patient wishes, extent of disease or symptoms, a decision should be taken about whether treatment is continued until disease progression/toxicity or used on an intermittent basis with 'treatment holidays'.

Need for palliative intervention for the primary tumour?

Management of advanced CRC is now considered to be a continuum of care, including periods on SACT, treatment breaks, and local therapies to maximize survival while maintaining quality of life.

Systemic therapies include: cytotoxic chemotherapy, fluoropyrimidines (5-FU, capecitabine), oxaliplatin, and irinotecan; anti-angiogenic agents, bevacizumab and aflibercept; and anti-EGFR targeted therapy, cetuximab and panitumumab.

Potentially curative disease

Upfront resectable

Resection of liver and lung metastases is now regarded as standard care for selected patients. There are no RCTs of metastasectomy but multiple case series have shown survival rates higher than reported with SACT.

All patients with liver only or liver predominant disease should be discussed in a hepatobiliary multidisciplinary meeting. In the multicentre EPOC study, an RCT investigating the role of perioperative chemotherapy versus surgery alone, five-year survival was ~50%. Surgical mortality is <5%. Criteria for resectability are continuously expanding. Current consensus is that disease is operable if the metastases can be completely resected with an adequate functional liver remnant (typically 20% of liver volume). In patients presenting with stage IV disease, the primary tumour has to be resectable. Patients with extrahepatic metastases (mainly lung and ovarian) may be considered for surgery providing all sites of disease can be removed, but their likelihood of cure is less. A variety of surgical techniques are used including anatomical and non-anatomical resections and wedge excisions. Portal vein embolization may be utilized to allow hypertrophy of the future liver remnant before surgery. Alternatively, the ALPPS approach may be considered where a two-stage approach is used involving metastasectomies to clear the future liver remnant and ligation of the portal vein to the contralateral lobe resulting in rapid hypertrophy of the remaining perfused lobe. Patients may undergo repeated resections as long as disease remains operable but long-term survival decreases with each round of surgery.

In cases that are initially operable there is no definite survival benefit for the use of preoperative chemotherapy. The EPOC trial reported a strong trend for improved PFS with peri-operative oxaliplatin + 5-FU (FOLFOX), but this did not translate into a survival benefit. A recent RCT in KRASwt CRC (New EPOC) found that addition of cetuximab to FOLFOX reduced PFS and it should not be used in this setting. If patients are chemotherapy naive, offering adjuvant chemotherapy is appropriate. A pooled analysis of two small RCTs has reported a PFS benefit; otherwise, evidence is extrapolated from the use of adjuvant chemotherapy in early stage CRC.

The surgical management of lung metastases has largely been extrapolated from the evidence base for liver resection. One RCT investigating the efficacy of pulmonary metastasectomy is underway (the PulMiCC trial). Successful resection of low volume disease from other anatomical sites has been reported but the evidence base is limited to small case series.

Potentially resectable

A further group of patients with initially unresectable metastases, generally liver only, may become operable following a response to SACT with five-year survival rates of 30–5%.

In these patients, the primary aim of treatment should be to achieve a high response rate to initial SACT. The optimum regimen is not clearly defined but the highest reported response rates have been with the triplet combination FOLFOXIRI (5-FU, oxaliplatin, and irinotecan). This regimen had response rates of >60%, and improved survival, compared to FOLFIRI in two Italian RCTs (including the TRIBE study which included bevacizumab in both arms) with higher rates of diarrhoea, neutropenia, stomatitis, and peripheral neuropathy. Both studies had an upper age limit of 75. This regimen may be considered for younger patients with a high tumour load. An alternative in KRASwt CRC is FOLFIRI plus cetuximab.

Patients receiving conversion therapy should be reassessed frequently and surgery performed as soon as the disease is deemed operable to avoid chemotherapy-induced hepatotoxicity.

Non-resectable disease

For patients with inoperable disease, the intent of treatment is palliative, with the aim of prolonging survival and maintaining quality of life. SACT remains the mainstay of treatment with supportive care for management of symptoms from disease and treatment-related toxicity.

There is a clear improvement in survival with SACT compared to BSC alone. Prior to the introduction of effective chemotherapy, median survival was less than six months. The first benefit was seen with single agent 5-FU, with a meta-analysis of several small studies showing median survival of 12 months and improved quality of life over BSC. Capecitabine, the oral prodrug of 5-FU, has equivalent efficacy and avoids the need for long-term intravenous access but causes more diarrhoea and palmar erythema.

Most patients receive first-line doublet chemotherapy with oxaliplatin or irinotecan plus a fluoropyrimidine. Studies using these regimens now consistently show median survival times of around 14–20 months, in conjunction with advances in multidisciplinary care including surgical palliation, local therapies and supportive care.

Who to treat and when to start?

The ECOG PS scoring system is a useful and easy assessment of a patient's fitness for chemotherapy. Those who score 0–2 are generally suitable (see 'Internet resources', p. 189). Comorbidities also need to be taken into account.

The majority of patients commence chemotherapy immediately even if they are asymptomatic. One RCT and a meta-analysis have addressed this question, and suggested a trend to improved survival with early treatment vs. delay until symptomatic. However, if patients have low volume disease (particularly lung only metastases) it is reasonable to opt for careful surveillance initially, especially if there are comorbidities present that increase the risk of chemotherapy.

Does the patient need initial combination SACT?

A series of RCTs have compared first-line irinotecan or oxaliplatin plus a fluoropyrimidine with single agent chemotherapy, and shown improved response rates, PFS, and OS for combination therapy. In patients with significant symptoms and burden of disease, who are at risk of rapid deterioration and organ dysfunction, this should be the standard approach.

Patients with low volume, minimally symptomatic disease may be considered for initial single agent fluoropyrimidine with addition of oxaliplatin or irinotecan at progression. This is known as a staged combination approach. It is based on the observation that survival in advanced CRC is strongly correlated with exposure to all three of fluoropyrimidines, irinotecan, and oxaliplatin during treatment but that the sequence or combination in which they are given seems to be less important. It has the advantage of delaying exposure to more toxic agents thus reducing overall toxicity. It has been investigated in two large RCTs (FOCUS and CAIRO), which both showed no detriment to survival with sequential staged therapy. Median survival in these studies was lower than expected (14–17 months) and the proportion of patients who were exposed to all three active agents was low. However, it should be noted that patients with potentially resectable disease were excluded from these trials and there was no upper limit of alkaline phosphatase in the eligibility criteria.

Which first-line combination chemotherapy backbone?

Doublet regimens are standard. They have similar efficacy and the main factor in choosing which regimen to use are the differing toxicity profiles. Irinotecan can be safely combined with infusional 5-FU (FOLFIRI) but there may be increased risk of severe diarrhoea with capecitabine. Oxaliplatin can be combined with both 5-FU (FOLFOX) and capecitabine (XELOX). Oxaliplatin causes a cumulative peripheral sensory neuropathy, which can be debilitating particularly in diabetic patients, and neutropenia (although without increase in infections). Irinotecan causes more frequent hair loss. Rates of diarrhoea are similar. Irinotecan can cause severe diarrhoea and strict education regarding the use of loperamide to control such symptoms is vital. The lack of a cumulative toxicity supports FOLFIRI as the preferred first-line regimen. Liver dysfunction contraindicates irinotecan and severe renal impairment contraindicates oxaliplatin and capecitabine. Other factors influencing choice are: whether patients received oxaliplatin during adjuvant therapy and the time interval from that; and planned combination with a biological agent.

What is the evidence for using a biological agent in first-line SACT?
Both the anti-VEGF monoclonal antibody (MAB) bevacizumab and the anti-EGFR MABs cetuximab and panitumumab, have evidence of efficacy in the first-line setting but there are conflicting findings from clinical trials about their benefit, with additional toxicity and significant increase in treatment cost.

Bevacizumab
Addition of bevacizumab improved survival from 16 to 20 months in the landmark RCT by Hurwitz et al, which used a suboptimal irinotecan/5-FU regimen, but a subsequent study with FOLFOX (NO16966) showed only a PFS benefit. In the second-line setting, the ES3200 and VELOUR trials found a modest benefit for the addition of anti-VEGF MABs to chemotherapy; analyses from these studies suggest treatment should be continued until progression to achieve maximum benefit and, thus, anti-VEGF therapy should not be given with planned treatment breaks. An interesting approach for frailer and/or elderly patients where combination chemotherapy is a less attractive option is to use bevacizumab with single agent fluoropyrimidines. The AVEX trial randomized patients aged over 70 to capecitabine +/− bevacizumab with a four-month improvement in PFS in the combination arm.

Anti-EGFR agents
Several large RCTs have looked at the benefit of using cetuximab and panitumumab in the first-line setting. None of the trials were biomarker selective but retrospective subgroup analyses by RAS mutation status have been performed. The COIN trial and the CRYSTAL trial both looked at the addition of cetuximab to FOLFOX and FOLFIRI, respectively. The CRYSTAL trial showed a 3.5-month improvement in survival with FOLFIRI + cetuximab for patients with KRASwt disease but this benefit was not replicated in COIN (or a third trial, NORDIC VII). The PRIME trial showed a six-month improvement in survival with panitumumab + FOLFOX in patients who were both KRAS and NRASwt after extended RAS testing but a treatment disbenefit in patients with RASmt disease.

All patients being considered for anti-EGFR therapy need extended RAS testing of their tumour before commencing therapy.

Patients with RASwt disease should have an informed discussion about the evidence for anti-EGFR therapy versus the risks and the need for continued treatment to progression to obtain maximum benefit. No phase 3 trials of intermittent anti-EGFR therapy have been conducted. Toxicity includes skin rash, increased diarrhoea, infusion-related reactions, and hypomagnesaemia.

Choice of first-line bevacizumab or cetuximab in KRASwt disease
The most recent large phase 3 RCTs have investigated the optimum first-line biological therapy in KRASwt CRC. The FIRE-3 trial compared cetuximab or bevacizumab in combination with FOLFIRI. The results of this trial are intriguing. The primary outcome measure was objective response rate. There was no significant difference in ORR or PFS but the trial did demonstrate a 3.7-month improvement in OS with cetuximab (from 25 to 28.7 months), and a greater benefit in the subgroup of extended RASwt patients. The reasons for this are not clear and may be related to differences in post-progression therapies between the treatment arms or a true biological effect. A similar effect has been seen in the phase 2 PEAK trial of FOLFOX + panitumumab or bevacizumab but not in the CALGB/SWOG 80405 trial which showed no difference between cetuximab or bevacizumab when presented at the ASCO Annual Meeting in 2014.

Intermittent or continuous chemotherapy?
Patients receiving combination chemotherapy (without a biological) have the option of continuous treatment until progression or cumulative toxicity, or to be treated using an intermittent strategy, where chemotherapy is given for a defined period of time (usually 12–16 weeks) then stopped and re-introduced at progression.

Intermittent treatment has been investigated in a number of RCTs which have taken a variety of approaches including complete treatment breaks (the COIN, OPTIMOX-2, and GISCAD trials) or stepping down to single agent fluoropyrimidine +/− biological therapy (OPTIMOX, CONcePT, TTD-MACRO, CAIRO3, and COINB trials). The largest study was the COIN trial, which reported similar median survival for patients treated with intermittent versus continuous FOLFOX, with improved quality of life and reduced cumulative toxicity. However, a pre-planned subgroup analysis found a detriment to survival in patients with a high baseline platelet count. This finding requires verification in other studies but suggests that intermittent treatment is not appropriate for all patients. Intermittent treatment should be considered an option for many patients but disease-related factors need to be taken into account, and an informed discussion had with each patient. If an intermittent approach is used, patients should be carefully monitored off treatment with regular clinical assessment and CT scanning so that treatment can be restarted promptly on progression.

Using biomarker-directed targeted therapies during the treatment break is an attractive strategy and is being investigated in the FOCUS4 and MODUL trials.

How should we treat older and poor performance status patients?
Decision-making in older and frailer patients requires careful consideration of potential benefit from chemotherapy and risk of toxicity, particularly in the context of multiple comorbidities. Treatment decisions should not be based on age alone, as fit elderly patients and those with poor PS due to CRC alone derive the same benefit from chemotherapy as younger patients. The FOCUS2 study showed that these patients can be safely treated with reduced dose combination chemotherapy and that is the preferred approach in patients with a significant

volume of disease or symptoms. Single agent 5-FU or capecitabine may be used in patients with significant co-morbidities or low volume disease. The AVEX trial suggests a role for capecitabine + bevacizumab, although the potential for bevacizumab toxicity must be considered.

Is there a role for local or regional therapies?

Selected patients with inoperable metastases may still benefit from local ablative or regional therapies.

A variety of tumour ablative techniques are available including cryo-ablation, radiofrequency ablation (RFA), microwave ablation and more recently electroporation. The procedure can be done using local anaesthesia or with the patient under general anaesthesia, either percutaneously or during open or laparoscopic surgery. A probe is advanced into each targeted lesion under imaging guidance. RFA and microwave ablation use heat and have NICE approval (IPG553). They become less effective when tumours exceed 3cm in size or when there is an adjacent large vessel due to a 'heat sink' effect. The CLOCC trial explored the use of RFA in the setting of inoperable liver metastases. Initially the trial was designed as a phase 3 study but was amended to a phase 2 following slow accrual. Long-term follow-up was presented in 2015 showing a survival benefit for the use of RFA. Other prospective data comparing different techniques is lacking.

SIRT aims to deliver open source radiotherapy to liver tumours and has been used for patients with inoperable CRC liver predominant metastases. The technique takes advantage of the differential vascular supply between the liver parenchyma and liver tumours. The former is predominantly perfused by the portal vein and the latter by the hepatic artery thus permitting a relatively selective treatment via injection of SIRT through the hepatic artery. Two products are available; sirspheres which are resin beads coated with yttrium-90 (Y90) and theraspheres which are Y90 impregnated glass beads. Small randomized studies support the use of sirspheres in the third-line setting. More recently three large scale RCTs have been completed for patients with liver predominant metastatic CRC in the first-line setting combining sirspheres with chemotherapy. The initial SIRFLOX results were presented in 2015 and showed an eight-month liver PFS benefit. Further results for the FOXFIRE and Global FOXFIRE studies are awaited and a combined analysis is planned to observe the impact on OS. The EPOCH TS trial is exploring the use of theraspheres in the second-line setting and is currently recruiting patients.

Second-line treatment and beyond?

Following progression on combination SACT, fit patients commonly receive further lines of treatment.

For second-line therapy, patients should switch to the alternative doublet (FOLFOX to FOLFIRI and vice versa) so that they receive all active cytotoxic agents. Response rates in these circumstances are low although disease stabilization is common, usually lasting for a short number of months. There is evidence for addition of biologicals to doublet chemotherapy in the second-line setting. However, all improvements in PFS and survival have been modest. In KRASwt CRC, cetuximab and panitumumab increase PFS but not OS. The anti-VEGF MABs, bevacizumab and aflibercept have shown a survival benefit of 1.5–2 months.

On further progression, if a long period has elapsed since first-line chemotherapy, rechallenge with the initial regimen may temporarily achieve disease control.

In chemotherapy refractory patients, several agents have shown improvements in survival versus BSC: cetuximab and panitumumab in KRASwt CRC; regorafenib, a multi-targeted tyrosine kinase inhibitor; and TAS-102, a new oral cytotoxic.

Management of the primary tumour

In patients undergoing potentially curative treatment, the primary should be managed as for early stage CRC.

In patients with inoperable metastatic disease, surgery may be performed for palliation of symptoms, including obstruction and bleeding. Impending obstruction requires intervention prior to palliative chemotherapy as outcomes are worse following acute obstruction during treatment. Persistent anaemia requiring blood transfusion may warrant a limited resection. Surgical options include resection with a stoma, an anastomosis, colo-colonic/ileocolonic bypass, or a defunctioning stoma alone (which allows fastest recovery and earlier chemotherapy). An alternative to surgery for an obstructing cancer is stenting, which may avoid need for an operation, decrease stoma formation, and allow earlier chemotherapy. Strictures on the right side and those at or close to the colonic flexures are difficult to stent. Stenting low rectal cancer carries a high risk of tenesmus. Some studies have found increased perforation rates but results of the phase 3 CREST trial, presented at the 2016 ASCO Annual Meeting, support stenting as a safe and effective approach. For advanced rectal cancer, palliative radiotherapy can help pelvic symptoms such as bleeding, tenesmus, and pain.

Future developments

The current focus of clinical research in advanced CRC is developing biomarker-targeted SACT. Molecular subtypes with different prognoses (e.g. BRAFmt) and potential targets for therapy are being defined but there is significant heterogeneity between patients. Multiple pathogenic mutations and processes are now recognized but many occur at low frequency (e.g. sporadic MSI in ~5%; ALK mutations in <2.5%). This presents a challenge for clinical trial design.

A major current study is the UK-based FOCUS4 trial, which is a novel adaptive, biomarker-driven, multi-arm multi-stage RCT that allows simultaneous testing of multiple drugs in biomarker-defined cohorts. Patients receive 16 weeks of doublet chemotherapy and tumour molecular profiling is performed. Patients with response or stable disease at 16 weeks are randomized to a targeted therapy versus placebo depending on their tumour biomarkers, and first-line chemotherapy is restarted at progression. Patients who do not fit into the current biomarker-defined cohorts may be randomized between capecitabine versus a treatment break. The initial planned molecular cohorts were: BRAFmt; PIK3CAmt; KRAS/NRASmt; and all wt with PTEN expression. A key aspect of the design is that it allows new drugs and cohorts to be added in response to emerging data, e.g. the finding that MSI CRC appears to be a target for immunotherapy with evidence for activity of anti-PD1 therapy. Up-to-date information on the latest cohorts can be found via the FOCUS4 trial website (see 'Internet resources', p. 189).

Conclusion

A steady improvement in outcomes of advanced CRC has been achieved in recent years through a combination of multidisciplinary management and developments in SACT. Future developments will focus on increased understanding of molecular subtypes and biomarker-directed personalized therapy.

Further reading

Hurwitz H, Fehrenbacher L, Novotny W, Cartwright T, Hainsworth J, et al. Bevacizumab plus irinotecan, fluorouracil, and leucovorin for metastatic colorectal cancer. *N Engl J Med* 2004 Jun 3; 350(23):2335–42.

Wiggers T, Jeekel J, Arends JW, Brinkhorst AP, Kluck HM, et al. No-touch isolation technique in colon cancer: a controlled prospective trial. *Br J Surg* 1988; 75(5):409–15.

Internet resources

Cancer Research UK Bowel Cancer Statistics: http://www.cancerresearchuk.org/health-professional/cancer-statistics/statistics-by-cancer-type/bowel-cancer

FOCUS4 trial website: http://www.focus4trial.org

7.19 Prognosis, follow-up, and management of recurrence of colorectal cancer

Prognosis

Approximately one-third of patients undergoing curative surgery will relapse. Relapse most often presents within three years, but rarely can occur up to ten years after resection. Patients can develop local recurrence or may relapse at distant sites with liver and lungs representing the most common sites. Although the majority of patients who relapse are incurable, approximately one-third of patients with isolated local or distant recurrences are alive at five years.

Prognosis after surgery for CRC is primarily determined by the following factors.

Key prognostic factors

1 The five-year survival for Europe was 57% for colon and 56% for rectal cancer in the Eurocare 5 study. Survival related to the stage at diagnosis based on T and N stage with early stage disease was 90%, 50% for spread to lymph nodes, and 10–20% for metastatic disease.

2 Vascular invasion: presence of tumour cells beneath the endothelium of unmuscularized veins and small vessels influences the rates of local and distant relapse. Vascular invasion is an independent adverse prognostic factor (Wiggers et al. 1988).

3 Residual tumour: presence of residual microscopic (R1) or macroscopic (R2) disease is associated with high rates of local and distant relapse. Presence of tumour within 1mm of the CRM (R1) adversely affects the clinical outcome following surgery (TME) for rectal cancer (Quirke et al. 1986).

4 Serum CEA: high preoperative CEA levels are associated with increased rates of recurrence possibly related to the higher incidence of micrometastases in these patients (Compton et al. 2000).

Other prognostic factors

Tumour grading
- Higher tumour grades (poor glandular differentiation, atypia, mitotic figures) are associated with worse prognosis.
- The American College of Pathologists has recommended a two-tiered grading system (high vs. low) based on glandular differentiation as the sole criterion (greater than or less than 50% gland formation).

Tumour border and 'budding'
- Presence of an irregular infiltrating border without any associated stromal reaction is a negative prognostic factor.
- Similarly, a concentrated presence of tumour cells in front of the advancing infiltrative edge ('budding') is associated with an adverse prognosis.
- Absence of tumour budding has been correlated with the presence of intratumoural (ITL) and peritumoural lymphocytes, indicating a possible immune-mediated destruction of 'buds' which may lead to an improved prognosis.

Perineural invasion
- Perineural invasion is quantified by the depth and number of foci of malignant cells per field.
- Perineural invasion has been reported to carry important prognostic significance following neodjuvant CRT.

Nodal micrometastasis
- Tumour deposits of less than 0.2mm detected by detailed histological assessment or immunohistochemistry (IHC).
- However, the prognostic significance of sole nodal micrometastasis remains unclear, unless associated with foci of neovascularization or attainment of a certain size.
- The TNM version 7 staging protocol does not recognize nodal micrometastasis of less than 0.2mm to be an independent prognostic factor. It is recommended that tumour deposits of greater than 0.2mm, but less than 2mm, should be used to classify nodal status but designated as pN (mi).

Tumour immunity
- Increased number of tumour-infiltrating lymphocytes (TIL) is associated with an improved overall and recurrence-free survival. In addition, there is a possible inverse correlation with tumour stage.
- Favourable response is primarily mediated by CD8+ TILs expressing cytotoxic proteins (granzyme B, perforin).
- Maximum protective effect was observed in tumours with lymphocyte infiltrate at both the centre and invasive margin.

Microsatellite instability

- A recent meta-analysis of 7,000 patients showed that tumours with microsatellite instability (MSI) were associated with superior survival compared to microsatellite stable (MSS) cancers. Subsequently, it was shown that this may be related to an increased number of ITL.
- However, MSS tumours may derive a higher survival benefit from 5-FU based adjuvant chemotherapy.

Loss of heterozygosity (18q deletions and TP53)

- Chromosomal loss at 18q is observed in up to 70% of CRCs.
- 18q deletion affects the function of DCC gene which plays a crucial role in the late phase of colorectal carcinogenesis.
- Previous studies have shown that stage II and III cancers with 18q deletions have a worse prognosis.
- TP53 is mutated in 50% of CRCs. However, the association with clinical outcome remains unclear. The TP53-CRC collaborative study showed that patients with Dukes C disease and wt-TP53 status probably derive a higher survival benefit from adjuvant chemotherapy.

Protein marker profiling (EGFR, VEGF, and ki-RAS)

- Although several proteins (e.g. β-catenin, TGFβ, bcl-2, Bax) have been investigated, the most consistent prognostic correlation has been observed for VEGF and EGFR.
- EGFR and VEGF expression can be detected in up to 75% of tumours and has been linked to several poor prognostic features, including increased potential for metastatic spread, inferior DFS and OS, and poor response to radiotherapy.
- K-RAS mutations are observed in 20–50% of CRC and most frequently involve the codon 12 or 13. The RASCAL study of more than 3,000 cases demonstrated a significant reduction in DFS and OS in Dukes stage C tumours harbouring K-RAS mutation.
- More recently, it has emerged that only patients with wt-RAS status may derive a useful benefit from anti-EGFR targeted therapies.

Follow-up

- Primary aim is to detect any recurrence (loco-regional or distant) and metachronous tumours at an early asymptomatic stage.
- Patients with isolated local or limited systemic (liver and lung) recurrence may be amenable to surgical resection with curative intent.
- Patients with image-detected recurrences have higher frequency of limited disease that is amenable to curative resection compared to those with symptoms.
- Previous meta-analyses have demonstrated a superior outcome following intensive FU schedules with a survival benefit of 7–10% compared to minimal or no FU.
- In a recent meta-analysis that included 4,055 patients from 11 studies with resected CRC intensive follow-up (history and physical examination with serum, radiological, and endoscopic tests) was associated with a significantly higher probability of detecting asymptomatic disease recurrence (RR 2.59, 95% CI 1.66–4.06), of curative intent surgery at recurrence (RR 1.98, 95% CI 1.51–2.60), and of all-cause (but not disease-specific) survival after tumour relapse (RR 2.13, 95% CI 1.24–3.69).

- In the large UK randomized trial of follow-up strategies (FACS) 1,202 patients with resected CRC were randomly assigned to post-treatment follow-up with CEA 'alone' (every three months for the first two years then every six months for three years, combined with a single CT scan at 18 months), CT alone (every six months for two years, then annually for three years), both tests, or minimal follow-up. After mean follow-up period of 4.4 years, two-thirds of recurrences were detected by a scheduled follow-up investigation. Patients in the intensive surveillance group had a 3–4-fold increased rate of potentially curative recurrence (6.7, 8.0, and 6.6%, respectively for CEA 'alone', CT alone, and combined CEA/CT) compared to 2.3% in minimal FU group. However, there was no significant difference in OS between the different groups (Primrose et al. 2014). A recent update concludes that the any survival benefit is unlikely to exceed 4% and harm cannot be absolutely excluded (Mant et al. 2013). These results are leading to more risk defined follow up strategies with low-risk patients having less intensive follow-up.
- Currently used FU schedules for CRC patients commonly involve a combination of regular clinical reviews, CEA monitoring, interval imaging, and colonoscopy.
  - Clinic reviews: significant geographical variation in review patterns; no evidence that more frequent reviews improve outcome; most commonly patients are reviewed at 3–6 month intervals for first two years followed by 6–12 monthly.
  - CEA: frequently elevated in recurrent disease (especially liver) and often earlier compared to image-detected recurrences; false-negative rate of 40%; false-positive of 10%; usually performed at 6–12 monthly intervals.
  - Liver imaging: in a previous meta-analysis the survival benefit from intensive surveillance was most pronounced in trials that used both CT imaging (every three to 12 months) and frequent measurement of CEA (Renehan et al. 2005).
  - Colonoscopy: patients without a previous colonoscopy should have one within six months of curative surgery; other patients should have it performed at three to five yearly intervals depending on underlying risk; patients with limited life-expectancy are unlikely to benefit from colonoscopy.

Recurrence and management

- Patients with loco-regional and isolated liver and lung recurrences should be appropriately staged to identify those who would benefit from further curative resection. One-third of such patients will be cured and alive at five years.
- PET/CT is useful and should be considered in selected cases. However, there is no evidence to support its routine use in this situation.
- 20–30% of patients with liver relapse will proceed to surgery. In contrast, a relative minority of patients with lung metastases will have localized disease that is amenable to surgical resection.
- Patients with multiple liver lesions are sometimes referred for neoadjuvant combination chemotherapy with the aim of downstaging disease prior to future surgery. NICE recommends the use of oxaliplatin/5-FU regimes in these patients.

- The incidence of loco-regional recurrence following surgery alone for rectal cancer is now 5–10% with the use of either preoperative, short-course pre-operative radiotherapy, or concurrent neoadjuvant chemo radiation for patients at moderate or high risk of local recurrence based on pelvic MRI staging.
- Patients with non-resectable disease at recurrence are incurable and have median survival of 6–9 months without any active treatment. However palliative chemotherapy can have a significant impact in extending OS in this patient group with a wide range of treatment options now available.

Further reading

Compton CC, Fielding LP, Burgart LJ, Conley B, et al. Prognostic factors in colorectal cancer. College of American Pathologists Consensus Statement 1999. *Arch Pathol Lab Med* 2000;124(7):979–94.

Glynne-Jones R, Wyrwicz L, Tiret E, Brown G, Rödel C, Cervantes A, Arnold D. ESMO Guidelines Committee. Rectal cancer: ESMO Clinical Practice Guidelines for diagnosis, treatment and follow-up. *Ann Oncol* 2017; 28(suppl 4): iv22–40.

Mant D, Perera R, Gray A, et al. Effect of 3–5 years of scheduled CEA and CT follow-up to detect recurrence of colorectal cancer: FACS randomized controlled trial. 2013 ASCO Annual Meeting. *J Clin Oncol* 2013; (Suppl.):A3500.

Primrose JN, Perera R, Gray A, et al: Effect of 3 to 5 years of scheduled CEA and CT follow-up to detect recurrence of colorectal cancer: The FACS randomized clinical trial. *JAMA* 2014; 311:263–70.

Quirke P, Dixon MF, Durdey P, Williams NS. Local recurrence of rectal adenocarcinoma due to inadequate surgical resection. Histopathological study of lateral tumour spread and surgical excision. *Lancet* 1986 Nov 1; 2(8514):996–9.

Renehan AG, Egger M, Saunders MP, O'Dwyer ST. Mechanisms of improved survival from intensive followup in colorectal cancer: a hypothesis. *Br J Cancer* 2005; 92:430–3.

Van Cutsem E, Cervantes A, Adam R, et al. ESMO consensus guidelines for the management of patients with metastatic colorectal cancer. *Ann Oncol* 2016; 27(8):1386–422.

Wiggers T, Jeekel J, Arends JW, Brinkhorst AP, Kluck HM, et al. No-touch isolation technique in colon cancer: a controlled prospective trial. *Br J Surg* 1988; 75(5):409–15.

7.20 Anal cancer

Epidemiology

Anal cancer is a rare cancer representing only 4% of all lower GI cancers. The incidence is 1.0–2.5 per 100,000 population in Western countries. In the UK the annual incidence is now approximately 1,200 new cases per year. The median age of onset is 50–64 years. There is a slight predominance in women (1.5–2), with rates increasing more in women over the last ten years.

There is a high incidence of anal cancer in men who have receptive anal sex with men (MSM), estimated at 12–35 per 100,000. There is only a weak association in women (relative risk, RR 1.8). However, the incidence in HIV positive MSM is much higher and some studies have suggested it could be as high as 70–75 per 100,000. The relative risk of invasive squamous cancer in HIV positive women is 6.8 and a similar increase is seen in HIV positive heterosexual males. The relative risk of the precursor lesions for invasive cancer is also higher in HIV positive MSM with a value of 60 compared to 7.8 for HIV positive women.

Other groups of immunosuppressed patients, in particular transplant patients, have an increased risk of developing anal cancer. The relative risk for all anogenital malignancies for this group of patients has been estimated to be up to 20-fold.

Aetiology

Most benign lesions, in particular chronic irritation, do not progress to invasive cancer, although recent data suggest that in inflammatory Crohn's disease there is a higher incidence of SCCA, an earlier age of presentation and a poorer outcome. Listed are the most important risk factors for the development of anal cancer.

Human papilloma virus (HPV)

HPV infection is a virtually endemic sexually transmitted disease, with a lifetime risk of acquiring genital HPV at least once of >80%, which is usually cleared by the immune system. Although sexual contact is a common means of transmission, anal intercourse is not necessary. High risk subtypes (including 16 and 18 amongst others) have been shown to be associated with the development of the premalignant condition, anal intraepithelial neoplasia (AIN) which can progress from low to high grade and in a proportion of patients to invasive cancer. HPV subtype 16 is most commonly associated with anal cancer, being detected in up to 70% of cases in population-based studies. There is a growing recognition that HPV induced tumours, with immunohistochemistry for p16INK4A (p16) used as a surrogate for HPV involvement, fare better with both CRT and surgery as in head and neck cancer. Tumour-infiltrating lymphocyte scores can also be used to stratify p16+ cases even further in terms of the risk of relapse. In contrast, HPV-negative SCCA although uncommon often fail to respond to CRT.

Immunosuppression

Patients who are immunosuppressed either as a result of HIV infection or iatrogenic causes (post-transplant, azathioprine, or corticosteroids) have a higher risk of anal cancer. In the post highly active antiretroviral therapy (HAART) era the incidence of invasive anal cancer has increased. This has led to the suggestion that firstly HIV alone is probably not a causative factor in invasive cancer, as if it were, a decrease in incidence would have been expected as has been the case for other malignancies. Secondly, the increased incidence has been postulated to be due to the fact that individuals are living longer and therefore have more time for pre-invasive lesions to progress to invasive disease.

Vaccination

Vaccination of girls and boys against the nine most common HPV subtypes (HPV16, 18, 31, 4, 11, 33, 45, 52, and 58) is now recommended in the UK from the age of 12 years. A recent meta-analysis indicated that ≥80% of anal cancers could be avoided by vaccination. Evidence from Australia where there is high uptake of vaccination suggests it is having a major impact and precancerous cervical lesions have fallen by 70% in women under 20 years of age and by 50% in women aged 20–24.

Screening using anal cytology and high resolution anoscopy remains controversial and there are currently no screening programmes.

Smoking

Smoking increases the risk of anal cancer by approximately four times, slightly higher for men than women, and may reflect modulation/persistence of HPV infection. Smoking may worsen acute toxicity during treatment and enhance late toxicity, so patients should be advised to quit.

Anatomy of anal canal

The anal canal extends from the perianal region known as the anal verge to the rectal mucosa. It is 3–4cm long. The upper portion commences at the anorectal ring which is formed by the junction of the upper portion of the internal sphincter, the distal portion of the longitudinal muscles, the puborectalis, and the deep portion of the external sphincter. The anal canal terminates at the junction of squamous epithelium and the perianal skin. It is divided into two sections by the dentate line. Below the dentate line the mucosa is lined with squamous epithelium and above by columnar epithelium. This is not an abrupt histological demarcation but rather a transition zone that is 6–12mm in length. The recognized consensus is that all tumours arising between the anorectal ring and the anal verge are classified as anal canal tumours and those arising distal to this as anal margin. Using this definition approximately 15% arise at the margin only and the remainder in the canal.

The lymphatic drainage relates to the dentate line. Below the line, drainage is to the inguinal and femoral nodes and subsequently to the external iliac and common iliac nodes. Above the dentate line drainage is to perirectal and superior rectal, inferior mesenteric, and eventually the para-aortic nodes. However, there are extensive interconnections which explain why patients with distal cancers may have involvement of mesenteric nodes.

Pathology

The most common tumours are squamous, constituting 75% of all cancers. They arise from the whole length of the canal and margin. Those arising below the dentate line are keratinizing whereas those arising above the line are more likely to be non-keratinizing. Basaloid, also known as cloacogenic, are subtypes of non-keratinizing SCC which arise around the dentate line. Despite this distinction, stage rather than subtype is more important in determining prognosis, as all behave in a similar manner. High-grade tumours were considered to confer a worse prognosis, but this is not confirmed on multivariate analysis.

Other pathologies such as adenocarcinoma of the anal canal, probably arising from ducts or glands, are rare and are treated in a similar way to low rectal cancers. Small cell cancers and lymphomas can also occur but are exceptionally rare. At the margin, other skin tumours including basal carcinoma, Kaposi's sarcoma, and malignant melanomas may occur.

Clinical features

The most common presentation is with rectal bleeding and pain. Diagnosis may be delayed as bleeding is often attributed to haemorrhoids. Some patients present with pain and/or the palpation of a rectal mass. Small, early cancers are sometimes diagnosed serendipitously following the removal of anal tags. Patients may also occasionally present with inguinal lymphadenopathy.

Patients presenting with larger (T3/T4) tumours may have symptoms of incontinence associated with anal sphincter disruption. Incontinence might also relate to vaginal infiltration and fistulation. In both of these situations patients require formation of a defunctioning stoma before definitive treatment. Large tumours may also extend into the lower rectum, perineum, and less commonly the prostate and bony pelvis.

Gynaecological assessment should also include cervical smear history and assessment of the vulva and cervix (if no recent smear) in view of the association with HPV-related malignancies.

In most reported series inguinal nodes are found to be involved at presentation in about 15–20% of patients. Pelvic nodal involvement can be determined by CT or MRI, but is less common and if present is usually associated with tumours arising above the dentate line.

Clinical assessment

Digital rectal examination (DRE) is mandatory to examine the anal lesion and any perirectal nodal involvement. In women (particularly with low anteriorly placed tumours) a vaginal examination can identify vaginal septal involvement, mucosal involvement of the vagina itself, or the presence of a fistula.

Diagnosis and staging

A multidisciplinary team (MDT) approach is essential for the optimal management of SCCA. Patients with a new diagnosis of SCCA should be reviewed in the MDT before initial treatment to facilitate decisions regarding a defunctioning stoma, optimizing clinical staging which influences target delineation for CRT and enabling appropriate surgical salvage.

Histopathological diagnosis by biopsy is mandatory. Examination under anaesthetic, documenting the extent of tumour including any involvement of the vagina and palpation of the inguinal nodal regions for the presence of lymphadenopathy may be required.

Staging requires MRI of the pelvis to determine the extent of local disease and CT of the chest and abdomen to exclude distant metastases. FNA of suspicious lymph nodes can be performed, but is of limited exclusion value. Excision biopsy of suspicious nodes is not recommended as it leads to increased morbidity and delays definitive treatment. Sentinel lymph node biopsy (SLNB) may reveal micro-metastatic spread of disease in normal sized lymph nodes, and hence may be more accurate than conventional diagnostic imaging with MRI, and CT, but remains to be validated. The role of PET-CT has been investigated prospectively in small series of patients undergoing CRT treatment. These suggest an increase in the proportion of patients with involved nodes by about 15–20%. At present whether this information directly leads to improved outcome is not clear.

A summary of the current AJCC8 staging is given here:
- Stage I: T1N0M0—tumour of ≤2cm in maximum dimension

- Stage IIA: T2N0M0—tumour of >2cm but ≤5cm
- Stage IIB: T3N0M0—tumour of >5cm
- Stage IIIA:
  - T1–2N1M0—regional lymph node metastases
  - N1a—inguinal, mesorectal, and/or interal iliac nodes
  - N1b—external iliac nodes
  - N1c—N1a+N1b nodes
- Stage IIIB: T4N0M0—tumour of any size invades adjacent organ(s), e.g. vagina, urethra, bladder (involvement of sphincter muscle(s) alone is not classified as T4)
- Stage IIIC: T3–4N1M0
- Stage IV: any T any N M1—distant metastasis

Principles of management

A series of randomized clinical trials have established CRT as definitive treatment for SCCA, and confirmed that CRT with mitomycin-C (MMC) and 5-FU combined with 45–60Gy in 1.8–2Gy fractions to the pelvis is the standard of care.

Surgery

Historically, the treatment of choice for SCCA was abdominal perineal resection (APR) with a permanent colostomy. Local failure rates were 27–47% and OS 50–70% depending on stage and extent of disease. Although no randomized trials have compared surgery with radiotherapy or CRT, the high local control and cure rates coupled with the avoidance of a stoma have led to CRT as the standard of care. APR is now reserved for salvage treatment, or where RT has been previously given. Local excision could be considered for small anal margin tumours <2cm in diameter, where there is no evidence of disease in the anal canal or nodal spread and clear margins can be achieved without compromising function.

Radiotherapy

Several studies investigated the role of radiotherapy alone before CRT was established as the standard of care. Treatment comprised either external beam alone or in combination with a brachytherapy boost.

Local control and survival rates comparable to those seen with CRT have been reported with external beam therapy alone. However, high doses (60Gy or more) are required, potentially resulting in higher rates of toxicity, with around 10% of patients requiring surgery to ameliorate late effects.

The use of brachytherapy to apply a highly focused, high-dose radiation 'boost' to the primary tumour area is feasible in selected patients especially those with more locally advanced disease (T3/T4) where dose escalation may be of benefit. Brachytherapy is a highly conformal treatment which can deliver a radiation boost to a small volume (usually the primary tumour), limiting or sparing the adjacent normal tissues, but it demands skill and operator experience. Local control rates comparable to CRT have been reported in the region of 75–79% with five-year OS rates of up to 64%. Most studies report anal necrosis rates of 10% or more.

RT alone might be considered in patients who are unable to tolerate chemotherapy; however, high doses are required leading to higher rates of significant toxicity.

Combined modality treatment

Following encouraging results of initial non-surgical treatment with RT alone or concurrent CRT, three pivotal randomized control trials investigated the role of 5FU / MMC and CRT.

Radiotherapy versus chemotherapy

The UK Coordinating Committee on Cancer Research (UKCCCR) reported the results of a trial comparing RT alone with CRT. Five hundred and eighty-five patients were randomized to either RT alone, 45Gy over five weeks, or the same dose with the addition of 5-FU (1,000mg/m^2 per day for four days or 750mg/m^2 per day over five days) during the first and last week of RT and mitomycin (12 mg/m^2 on day one only). Response was assessed at six weeks. Good responders received a boost of 15Gy in six fractions using either photons or electrons or a brachytherapy boost of 25Gy at 10Gy per day. The primary endpoint was local failure and secondary endpoint was overall and cause-specific survival. Approximately 50% of patients in each arm had T3/4 disease and 20% were node positive. The local failure was 59% in the RT alone arm and 36% in the CRT arm. There was no OS benefit (58% vs. 65% for CRT) probably due to the effect of salvage surgery; however, the risk of death from anal cancer was reduced in the CRT arm. Of note, early morbidity was higher in the CRT arm; however, reported late morbidity was similar for both arms.

A second similar trial was reported by the European Organization for Research and Treatment of Cancer (EORTC). One hundred and ten patients were randomized to either RT alone (45Gy in five weeks) followed by a boost of 15Gy for complete responders and 20Gy for poor responders six weeks after completion of initial treatment. In the CRT arm, patients received chemotherapy similar to that in the UKCCCR trial. CRT improved local control by 18% with a 32% higher colostomy-free survival rate in the CRT arm. They found no difference in acute toxicity whilst event-free survival (including tumour progression and late toxicity) was better for the CRT arm.

Following publication of these trials, CRT with combination 5-FU and MMC was accepted as the standard treatment for anal cancer.

Which chemotherapy?

MMC was felt to add significant toxicity and Flam and colleagues investigated CRT with 5-FU and MMC or 5-FU alone. RT and chemotherapy doses were similar to those in the UKCCCR and EORTC trials. Evaluation was at four to six weeks with a biopsy and patients with residual disease went on to have a further 9Gy. The addition of MMC resulted in a significantly higher colostomy-free survival rate at four years (71% vs. 59%) and DFS rate (73% vs. 51%). However, these results were balanced by a higher significant toxicity rate (23% vs. 7%) with four deaths in the MMC compared with one in the 5-FU arm. The authors concluded that MMC was an important component of the treatment and remained the standard of care.

The Radiation Therapy Oncology Group (RTOG) reported the results of the RTOG 98-11 trial evaluating the role of cisplatin given both neoadjuvantly and concurrently with RT in place of MMC. Six hundred and eighty-two patients were randomized to either 5-FU (1,000mg/m^2 days 1–4 and 29–32) and MMC 10mg/m^2 days one and 29) combined with 45–59Gy of RT or the same doses of RT preceded by two cycles of 5-FU and cisplatin (75mg/m^2) and two cycles with the RT. No significant difference was found in DFS (60% in MMC group and 54% in cisplatin arm) and OS (75% vs. 70%). However, the colostomy rate was higher in the cisplatin arm: 19%

vs. 10%. Updated results actually showed an advantage in five-year DFS for the standard 5-FU/MMC arm compared with the arm with induction cisplatin and CRT with 5-FU/cisplatin.

The ACT II trial is the largest randomized trial (940 patients) with four arms using a factorial 2x2 design comparing: 1) concurrent cisplatin 5-FU CRT with MMC 5-FU CRT (50.4Gy in both arms); and 2) maintenance chemotherapy post-CRT (two cycles of 5-FU and cisplatin) versus no maintenance chemotherapy. Patients received 5-FU (1,000mg/m^2/day on days 1–4, 29–32) and RT (50Gy in 28 daily fractions), and were randomized to receive a single dose of MMC (12mg/m^2, day 1) or cisplatin (60mg/m^2 on day 1, 29).

The second randomization was between two further courses of chemotherapy as consolidation after CRT (5-FU/cisplatin), or no consolidation. Neither the strategy of CRT with cisplatin versus CRT with MMC, nor two further courses of chemotherapy as consolidation were superior in terms of achieving cCR, reducing tumour relapse, or cancer-specific deaths to the standard arm using MMC/CRT.

The Action Cliniques Coordonées en Cancerologie Digestive ACCORD-03 phase 3 trial randomized 307 patients in a factorial 2x2 trial design between two cycles of induction chemotherapy (ICT) with 5-FU and cisplatin and secondly a radiation dose escalation. The primary end point was colostomy free survival (CFS). Secondary end points included local control (LC), OS, and cancer-specific survival. The trial compared 45Gy in 25 daily fractions plus a 15Gy boost after three weeks' gap with a higher boost dose of 20–25Gy (i.e. 65–70Gy total dose), but found no benefit in CFS at doses above 59Gy. With a mean follow-up of 50 months, results did not show any benefit of ICT compared with standard treatment. The optimal boost dose remains undefined.

Results of phase 3 trials examining induction or maintenance chemotherapy

Current neoadjuvant or induction chemotherapy schedules with combinations of 5-FU and cisplatin (two cycles) before CRT do not benefit the patient and may lead to worse outcomes if toxicity causes a prolonged overall treatment time for the CRT component. Similarly, there is no evidence to support the use of consolidation or maintenance chemotherapy following CRT using 5-FU and cisplatin (two cycles).

Treatment of elderly and HIV positive patients

The randomized trials included patients with good PS and a median age of 55–60 years. Although many elderly patients can tolerate full dose CRT, there remains a group of patients where comorbidity or frailty precludes a radical strategy. Palliative approaches can be used with a single or short fractionated course of RT treating the tumour plus margin only to control bleeding or pain. However, if significant tumour regression is to be achieved, a modified CRT regimen of 30Gy encompassing the tumour and involved nodes combined with 600mg/m^2 of 5-FU on days 1–4 can achieve long-term control in up to 70% of patients.

Data from small series suggest that outcome is similar in HIV positive and HIV negative patients, especially in the era of HAART, but with an increased level of acute and late toxicity. HIV patients were usually excluded from the randomized trials. Hence we have no robust randomized data to guide best practice in immunocompromised

and HIV-positive patients. Prior to HAART, a small series suggested that treatment-related toxicity was higher for patients with CD4 counts <200.

In general, HIV-positive patients should be treated with standard protocols although modification in radiation volume and chemotherapy dose, especially MMC (if haematological abnormalities are present or there is a previous history of significant opportunistic infection), may be necessary. It is important to start HAART before CRT treatment.

Newer techniques of radiotherapy

The use of more sophisticated RT techniques such as intensity-modulated radiotherapy (IMRT) or rapid arc confines radiation doses within the clinical target volumes, at the same time reducing the average and threshold doses for the organs-at-risk (OARs), such as the genitals, femoral head, small bowel, and bladder, compared with conventional three-dimensional conformal RT. IMRT can improve compliance and with a simultaneous integrated boost (SIB) could even allow escalation of radiation doses.

Current trials

PLATO is an integrated protocol comprising three separate trials (ACT 3, 4, and 5). It is designed to investigate the optimal radiotherapy dose for low-, intermediate-, and high-risk cancers. In cancers with margins >1mm no further treatment will be given and for margins <1mm the patient will receive low-dose CRT 41.4Gy in 23 fractions. ACT 3 (T1–2N0, intermediate risk) randomizes between standard CRT 50.4Gy in 28 fractions and 41.4Gy in 23 fractions. ACT 5 is for high-risk cancers. The phase 2 component will randomize between standard CRT 53.2Gy in 28 fractions and two higher doses of CRT 58.8Gy and 61.6Gy in 28 fractions. One of the two higher dose arms will then be selected for the phase 3 component of the study.

Role of postoperative CRT

Some patients will be referred following excision of a lesion which turns out to be a cancer, or following excision of small cancers—most commonly in anal margin tumours. Local excision should be avoided in anal canal tumours as incomplete excision may compromise sphincter function especially when excision is followed by CRT.

Excision is often piecemeal but if a small tumour (<2cm) has been excised locally with close or involved margins a number of approaches have been advocated, including brachytherapy, full dose CRT, RT alone, or modified CRT (30Gy to an involved field only combined with 5-FU on days 1–4 and MMC on day 1). There are however no randomized trials to support any of these approaches. Some consider diameter >2cm, poorly differentiated histology, depth of tumour invasion beyond fat, and perineural invasion as adverse features predicting a higher risk of lymph node metastases.

Toxicity

CRT (particularly if mitomycin C is used) is associated with high risks of G3/G4 haematological toxicity. Acute skin toxicity ranges from erythema to moist desquamation. In some cases the severity can lead to treatment gaps or early discontinuation of treatment. Other dose limiting toxicity includes diarrhoea, proctitis, urinary frequency, dysuria, acute lymphoedema, and pain. Compliance is improved by the use of strong analgesia, creams for skin care, anti-emetics, anti-diarrhoeal agents, advice regarding nutrition, and psychological support. Smoking should be strongly discouraged because it can exacerbate acute toxicity.

Late toxicity includes anal ulceration, stenosis, and necrosis necessitating a colostomy in up to 10% of patients who are otherwise disease free. More common, but poorly documented in the literature, is functional toxicity including urgency, frequency, incontinence, and 'toilet dependency'. Vaginal stenosis and premature ovarian failure can occur, and male patients should be offered sperm banking as permanent azoospermia is likely. There is also a risk of treatment induced second malignancy.

Compliance

Compliance can be jeopardized by the attendant acute GI, genitourinary, dermatological, and haematological toxicities. Extending the overall treatment time and prolonged treatment breaks may impact negatively on local control. In the ACT II trial poor treatment compliance (lower dose and/or prolonged overall treatment time (OTT)) adversely impacted on PFS.

Management of metastatic and recurrent disease

Salvage therapy should be considered for patients with either persistent or recurrent disease, in general with an APR. The definition of persistent disease is controversial. Response is generally assessed initially at six to eight weeks following completion of CRT, but disappearance of the tumour after CRT may take longer than previously expected. The median time to complete regression after CRT is about 12 weeks (range 2–36 weeks). The UKCCCR ACT I trial showed that 77% of patients who had not achieved complete tumour regression at the six-week assessment, eventually achieved a complete response with longer follow-up. However, persistent tumour may continue to regress up to and beyond 26 weeks after the end of CRT, and it is therefore safe to observe responding patients up to the 26-week time-point.

For patients with suspected recurrent disease a small biopsy should be performed followed by restaging (approximately one-third will have synchronous distant failure). For those patients with isolated local failure only around 60% will be able to undergo salvage surgery (usually APR) and the long-term disease control is in the region of 30–50% with a similar OS.

Distant metastases occur in approximately 10% of patients with liver being the commonest site. Combination cisplatin and 5-FU has been widely reported as active. A recent randomized phase 2 internationally conducted trial (InterAAct) showed similar ORR between carboplatin-paclitaxel and cisplatin-5-FU, but with less toxicity and significantly longer survival. The present authors believe that carboplatin-paclitaxel should be considered a new standard of care for advanced anal cancer.

Prognosis

Overall five-year survival is 65% in the USA for males and 70% for females, but has changed little over the past two decades. A worse prognosis for men <50 years old may partly reflect HIV infection and/or male pharmacogenomics. The risk of local failure is substantially higher for patients with T3/T4, >5cm, or node-positive disease. Haemoglobin level at presentation may also influence outcomes. The overall risk of local failure for T1/2N0 patients is 10–15%. The majority of local failures are identified within the first six months after completion of CRT with the remainder found within two to three years. Five-year survival rate for distant disease is 10–15%.

Follow-up

Follow-up is dictated by the pattern of recurrence and the recognition that a proportion of patients can be salvaged with surgery. Most recurrences will occur in the first two years. Therefore it is recommended that patients are seen every three months for the first two years and then six-monthly for year three, and annually to five years. Digital rectal examination and examination of inguinal regions should be performed at each visit and other investigations dictated by symptoms or findings.

The role of regular MRI and CT scanning to detect loco-regional recurrence or metastatic disease is controversial. The current ACT II study, where regular imaging is part of the follow-up protocol will hopefully answer this question. Tumour markers have no current role in follow-up.

Further reading

Brierley JD, Gospodarowicz MK, Wittekind C (eds). *TNM Classification of Malignant Tumours*, 8th ed. Oxford: Wiley-Blackwell, 2016.

Glynne-Jones R, Nilsson PJ, Aschele C, Goh V, Peiffert D, Cervantes A, Arnold D. ESMO; ESSO; ESTRO. Anal cancer: ESMO-ESSO-ESTRO clinical practice guidelines for diagnosis, treatment and follow-up. *Radiother Oncol* 2014; 111(3):330–9.

Chapter 8

Cancers of the genitourinary system

Chapter contents

8.1 Cancer of the kidney

Epidemiology

Renal cell carcinoma (RCC) accounts for approximately 3% of cancer diagnosis worldwide. It has the highest mortality of any urological cancer. With the increased use of radiological investigations in medicine, up to 60% of diagnoses are now made incidentally.

Clear-cell renal cell carcinoma (CC-RCC) is the commonest RCC. CC-RCC has the highest prevalence in Eastern Europe and is the fifth commonest solid tumour in the UK. Incidence of primary CC-RCC rises after the age of 40 years old and there is a 2:1 male to female ratio.

Aetiology

Most renal cancers are sporadic. Tobacco smoking is the best established risk factor, accounting for approximately 25% of disease. Several different genetic mutations are associated with RCC.

Pseudohypoxic syndromes

In these syndromes there is alteration of levels of expression of hypoxia-inducible factors (HIF) which are regulators of oxygen homeostasis. Loss of von Hippel–Lindau (VHL) or fumurate hydratase (FH) (described below) results in a pseudohypoxic state so that cellular response pathways are inappropriately activated.

- VHL syndrome is manifest by germline loss of VHL at chromosome 3p. Multifocal and/or bilateral CC-RCC tumours are well recognized. VHL syndrome is divided into two types: in type 1 there is a low risk of developing phaechromocytoma and in type 2 a higher risk. Type 2 is subdivided into types a and b based on the risk of developing RCC and hemangioblastomas.
- Mitochondrial germline deletions of enzymes involved within the tricarboxylic acid cycle, such as FH and succinate dehydrogenase (SDH), also can lead to CC-RCC with cutaneous/uterine leiomyomas or paragangliomas/abdominal phaechromocytomas, respectively.

Non-pseudohypoxic syndromes

- Birt–Hogg–Dube (BHD) syndrome: 15–30% of BHD patients develop RCCs. It is caused by homozygous deletion of the folliculin (FLCN) gene, and leads to fibrofolliculomas and pleural blebs causing pneumothorax.
- Hereditary leiomyomatosis renal cell carcinoma (HLRCC) leads to type II papillary RCCs (distinguished histologically from the better prognosis type I) which show lymphovascular invasion and can be very aggressive and metastasize rapidly, although they often present as single primary tumours. Cutaneous leiomyomata as well as uterine fibroids are also recognized.
- Hereditary papillary renal cell carcinoma—type 1: germline mutation in c-Met; presents with slow growing primary papillary tumours (with type 1 papillary histology).
- Xp11.2 translocation involving the TFE3 gene on chromosome X is a recognized cytogenetic abnormality leading to the development of CC-RCCs in children and young adults.

Genetics of sporadic CC-RCCs

More than 85% of CC-RCCs are deficient in the expression or function of the tumour suppressor, pVHL, which is found on chromosome 3p. Sporadic CC-RCCs also arise in patients with end-stage renal failure (ESRF) on long-term haemodialysis, but their carcinogenesis may be different, although loss of pVHL is also recognized.

Genetics of sporadic non-CC-RCC tumours

Papillary RCCs are thought to arise mainly through acquired mutations in c-Met.

Pathology

Renal tumours are classified using the World Health Organization (WHO) system (revised in 2013) which defines histopathological tumour subtypes with different clinical behaviours and underlying genetic mutations. RCC arises from the nephron tubular epithelium. More than 90% of tumours are one of the common subtypes: CC (conventional) RCC (80%), papillary RCC (10–15%), chromophobe RCC (5%), renal oncocytoma, and collecting duct tumours (<1%). CC-RCC has the highest rate of metastasis and poorest survival. Papillary and chromophobe carcinomas are less aggressive but can metastasize or transform to high-grade sarcomatoid tumours. Collecting duct tumours are usually aggressive. Oncocytomas and angiomyolipomas usually behave benignly.

Newly recognized RCC histological subtypes include tubulocystic RCC, acquired cystic disease-associated RCC, clear cell (tubulo) papillary RCC, MiT translocation RCC, and HLRCC syndrome-associated RCC.

Grading of RCCs was revised in 2013 on a four-point grading scale by the International Society of Urological Pathology (ISUP).

Benign renal lesions may progress to malignancy.

Clinical features

- 'Incidentalomas' detected at routine ultrasound or computed tomography (CT) scanning are increasing.
- Haematuria is the most common symptom.
- Twenty-five per cent of patients present with metastatic disease and the thorax is the commonest site.
- Less than 10% of primary CC-RCC present with the 'classical triad' of flank pain, haematuria, and fever.
- Bone lesions occur in up to 30% of patients with metastases and are typically osteolytic and painful.
- Soft tissue metastasis may be hypervascular and have an audible bruit.
- Atypical metastatic sites of disease may include the ovaries, the pancreas, and small intestine, with the latter causing problematic gastrointestinal (GI) tract bleeding.
- Para-neoplastic manifestations (common): weight loss and fever (IL-6 mediated); hypercalcaemia (PTHrP); polycythaemia, and hypertension (erythropoietin, EPO).

Diagnosis

Imaging

There are no specific radiological characteristics suggesting RCCs. However, cystic lesions and contrast-enhancement are typical of CC-RCCs, particularly using CT.

- The Bosniak classification (I–IV) of CT-detected renal cysts can be used to predict the likelihood of

Table 8.1.1 Bosniak classification of renal cysts on CT

Bosniak category	Features
I	A simple benign cyst with a hairline thin wall that does not contain septa, calcification, or solid components. It measures as water density and does not enhance with contrast material
II	A benign cyst that might contain a few hairline thin septa. Fine calcification might be present in the wall or septa. Uniformly high-attenuation lesions of <3cm that are sharply marginated and do not enhance
IIF	These cysts might contain more hairline thin septa. Minimal enhancement of a hairline thin septum or wall can be seen and there might be minimal thickening of the septa or wall. The cyst might contain calcification that might be nodular and thick but there is no contrast enhancement. There are no enhancing soft-tissue elements. Totally intrarenal non-enhancing high-attenuation renal lesions of >3cm are also included in this category. These lesions are generally well marginated
III	These lesions are indeterminate cystic masses that have thickened irregular walls or septa in which enhancement can be seen
IV	These lesions are clearly malignant cystic lesions that contain enhancing soft-tissue components

Source: Reproduced with permission from McFarlane J, Warren KS. The Bosniak classification of renal cystic masses. *BJU International* 2005; 95(7):939–42. Copyright © 2005, John Wiley & Sons.

Table 8.1.2 The Mayo primary CC-RCC classification system—Mayo scoring algorithm to predict metastases after radical nephrectomy in patients with clear cell renal cell carcinoma

Feature	Score
Primary tumour status (pathological T stage)	
pT1a	0
pT1b	2
pT2	3
pT3a	4
pT3b	4
pT3c	4
pT4	4
Regional lymph node status (N stage)	
pNx	0
pN0	0
pN1	2
pN2	2
Tumour size (cm)	
<10	0
>10	1
Nuclear grade	
1	0
2	0
3	1
Histological tumour necrosis	
No	0
Yes	1

Source: Reproduced with permission from Bradley C, Leibovich MD, et al. Prediction of progression after radical nephrectomy for patients with clear cell renal cell carcinoma: A stratification tool for prospective clinical trials. *Cancer* 2003; 97(7):1663–71. Copyright © 2003, John Wiley & Sons.

malignancy (Table 8.1.1). Bosniak IV lesions are typically multi-septated, rim-enhancing lesions that invariably correlate with the pathological findings of CC-RCC.
- Pitfall: Bosniak III lesions may occasionally represent necrotic cancers.
- Oncocytomas on CT may have a typical low-attenuation 'naked-eye' appearance.
- Magnetic resonance imaging (MRI) is particularly used in the assessment of the superior extension of tumour-thrombus precavotomy/thrombus resection.
- Transoesophageal echocardiogram (TOE) may also be useful for Mayo level III/IV tumour-thrombus in pre-operative planning.
- The 99Tc-isotope bone scan is not sensitive in the detection of CC-RCC bone metastasis and MRI has a better sensitivity.
- The 19FDG-PET (fluorodeoxyglucose-positron emission tomography) scan has an undefined role at present, but initial studies suggest that it may have a significant impact in the surgical management of disease.

Clinical risk stratification

Non-metastatic disease
The Mayo and UCLA (University of California, Los Angeles) integrated staging system (UISS) nomograms are commonly used (Leibovich et al. 2003). The Mayo system (Table 8.1.2) classifies primary tumours into low-, intermediate-, and high-risk groups. The UISS system stratifies clinical risk into five categories (I–V) based on TNM staging (AJCC 1997), Fuhrman's grade, and Eastern Cooperative Oncology Group (ECOG) performance status (PS). Such nomograms are useful in the allocation of patients into adjuvant trials.

Metastatic disease
The cornerstone of prognostic models in metastatic CC-RCC is the Memorial Sloan–Kettering Cancer Center (MSKCC) prognostic system, which was later modified (Table 8.1.3).
- Good prognosis (no risk factor): median survival 29 months.
- Intermediate prognosis (one to two risk factors): median survival 15 months.
- Poor prognosis (three or more risk factors): median survival 4.5 months.
  It should be noted that with the development of multiple lines of targeted and immunological therapy, much better survival figures can now be expected for fit patients. Many of the datasets are currently immature and will be updated in the next few years. However, as an indicator, patients with poor and intermediate risk disease treated with sunitinib in a recent phase 3 trial had a median overall survival (OS) of 26 months.
  The model has recently been updated to include the mutation status of BAP1, PBRM1, and TP53. There is a considerable volume of work investing the prognostic and predictive value of angiogenic and immunological signatures. However, none of these are currently in general use.

Table 8.1.3 The modified MSKCC prognostic system

Modified MSKCC prognostic markers	Risk factor
Karnofsky score (KS)	<80%
Corrected calcium	>10mg/dL
Haemoglobin	<lower limit of local reference range
Serum LDH	>1.5x upper limit of local reference range
Time to immunotherapy from initial diagnosis of metastasis	<12 months

Source: data from Motzer RJ, Mazumdar M, Bacik J, et al. Survival and prognostic stratification of 670 patients with advanced renal cell carcinoma. *J Clin Oncol* 1999; 17(8):2530–40. 1999, American Society of Clinical Oncology.

Surgical management

Curative surgery

Radical nephrectomy is the initial management of primary RCCs. The roles of nephron-sparing surgery (NSS) and laparoscopic approaches are being developed. NSS is particularly suited to small (<4cm) lesions at the poles or periphery of the kidney, and anatomically isolated from the hilum or collecting-duct system. There are no large randomized studies to date comparing open versus laparoscopic radical nephrectomy. Laparoscopic surgery has a lower complication rate and operative blood loss than open surgery, but a large tumour is an indication for open surgery.

In T3c disease, radical nephrectomy with vena cavotomy and resection of the caval thrombus can provide long-term survival rates up to 68% at five years.

Radiofrequency ablation (RFA), cryoablation, or the developing technique of high intensity frequency ultrasound (HIFU) are alternatives to surgery that are actively being developed. Concerns remain as to the most reliable means of detecting dead tumour tissue treated with either RFA or HIFU.

Role of surgery in metastatic disease

Surgery of primary tumour
The usual indications for radical nephrectomy in metastatic disease are:

- A symptomatic primary tumour usually causing haematuria and/or primary tumour pain.
- Debulking where the large majority of disease (~90%) is in the primary lesion and the patient is very fit.

It should be noted that it is very rare for nephrectomy alone to result in a response in metastatic disease (<0.5%).

Surgery of loco-regional metastasis
The retroperitoneal lymph node (RPLN) is the commonest loco-regional site of metastasis. RPLN metastasis increases the risk of distant metastasis three- to four-fold. Studies show that an isolated RPLN metastasis is as detrimental to OS as a single-site distant metastasis. However, the role of prophylactic RPLN dissection (RPLND) is controversial and has not been shown to improve OS compared with radical nephrectomy alone. In patients with proven RPLN metastases, lymphadenectomy is standard of care.

Surgery of distant metastasis (metastatectomy)
Surgery of distant metastases may be performed with either palliative or potentially curative intent.

Patient selection is paramount when considering potentially curative surgery. Many specialists would observe a patient with an apparently solitary lesion for three to six months before restaging to confirm that no new metastasis had arisen. The role of 18FDG-PET is being evaluated in diagnosing CT-occult disease. Small scale studies suggest that it may alter the initial surgical decision in up to 35% of all CC-RCC cases. Favourable features for a curative metastatectomy include good PS and a PFS of at least one year. Clinical benefit from surgery declines very rapidly if multiple metastases are present.

Resection of pulmonary metastasis is the most common surgical procedure with curative intent. Complete pulmonary metastatectomy may give five-year OS of about 50%. Stereotactic neuro- or gamma-knife radiosurgery may be used in the treatment of isolated brain or spinal cord metastasis. For potentially operable bone metastasis, with curative intent, assessment by an experienced orthopaedic cancer surgeon is mandatory.

Orthopaedic surgery is the commonest palliative surgical intervention and is often used prophylactically to prevent pathological fracture.

8.2 Non-surgical management of cancer of the kidney

Radiotherapy

Radiotherapy is indicated to palliate pain (e.g. bone/soft tissue), bleeding (e.g. lung/GI metastasis), spinal cord compression, and brain metastases. Selective arterial embolization can also be used for inoperable primary tumour or metastases.

Special situations

Thorax

- Symptomatic endobronchial lesions may be treated with cryotherapy or photocoagulation.
- Selective arterial embolization can also be used for inoperable bleeding pulmonary lesions that are not suitable for or refractory to radiotherapy.

Bone

- Bisphosphonate infusions are used in either focal or diffuse bony pain or for hypercalcaemia.
- Osseous selective arterial embolization and RFA can also be used to treat refractory focal bony pain.
- Percutaneous vertebroplasty with methyl methacrylate can be used in cases of vertebral collapse.

Systemic therapy in RCC

CC-RCC has been most extensively studied with multiple large scale phase 3 studies in the past decade. Other RCC subtypes are much less fully studied and treatment is based on phase 2, expanded access programme or anecdotal information. CC-RCC is treated by three main systemic modalities:

- Anti-angiogenic tyrosine kinase inhibitors
- T cell checkpoint inhibitors
- mTOR inhibitors

Adjuvant (postnephrectomy)

Multiple studies have shown no benefit from chemotherapy, cytokines, chemo-immunotherapy, vaccine-based approaches, or postoperative radiation to the renal bed. The results of large phase 3 studies investigating the use of anti-angiogenic tyrosine kinase inhibitors have generally failed to show consistent benefit, although one study (S-TRAC) showed modest benefit in a very high-risk population. Observation remains the standard of care after resection of RCC with curative intent.

Advanced/metastatic CC-RCC

The treatment algorithm for patients with metastatic CC-RCC carcinoma is rapidly evolving (Table 8.2.1). There are now multiple choices in the first and second line and many patients are now receiving third- and fourth-line therapy.

Single agent antiangiogenic multitargeted tyrosine kinase inhibitors (TKIs)

Development of TKIs such as sunitinib, pazopanib, axitinib, sorafenib, and tivozanib represent treatment options in the first- and second-line setting. Increasingly, single agent TKI use in the first-line setting is being restricted to patients with good risk disease and those who will not tolerate immunotherapy. Treatment with tyrosine kinase inhibitors results in significant improvements in progression-free survival, with many patients remaining on treatment either continuously or intermittently for years.

The main molecular target of these agents is vascular endothelial growth factor receptor 2 (VEGFR2).

However, these drugs also inhibit a range of other kinases. These properties give rise to a range of unwanted effects. It is important to remember that these drugs are maintenance agents and patients are likely to be treated for prolonged periods. Careful training of patients in the recognition and early management of sideeffects and the use of prophylactic measures is key to successful maintenance of quality of life (QoL) and compliance on treatment.

Common side effects and their management include:

- Hypertension: maintain blood pressure (BP) at or below 150/90. Use of angiotensin receptor blockers or ACE inhibitors is preferred in many units as non-randomized data suggest they augment the anti-tumour effect of TKIs. Echocardiography, to assess left ventricular (LV) function, is advised in patients with known cardiovascular comorbidities.
- Hand–foot skin reaction: frequent use of moisturizers of all dry skin areas and especially of the hands and feet minimizes or prevents toxicity. Areas of thickened skin may look innocent but are in fact very painful. Topical use of urea-containing creams can lyse areas of thickened skin.
- Stomatitis: avoid strong spirits and stringent mouthwashes. Use low fluoride or children's toothpaste and a soft toothbrush to help maintain a healthy oral mucosa.
- Liver function test (LFT) abnormalities: monitoring of LFTs every fortnight in the first cycle of treatment, especially with pazopanib, is indicated. Drug interruption or even cessation in the face of severe abnormalities is occasionally required.
- Thyroid function should be monitored at least every other cycle of treatment and be treated by standard means.
- Other well-recognized side effects include: fatigue, nausea, rash, diarrhoea, myelosuppression, hoarse voice, hyponatraemia, alopecia, skin and hair discolouration, thromboembolism, and bleeding.
- Drug interactions are well recognized and include warfarin, clarithromycin, and citalopram.
- In general sunitinib produces more clinically significant fatigue and stomatitis. Pazopanib has a higher incidence of LFT abnormalities. Axitinib causes the most marked hypertension and sorafenib produces more alopecia and skin toxicity.
- The suggested treatment schedule for the most commonly used first-line agent, sunitinib, is 50mg once daily orally for 28 days and the cycle is repeated every 42 days. Radiological disease evaluation is usually performed every two cycles.
- Many patients tolerate the first two weeks of the cycle well but find weeks three and four hard going. In these patients an alternative regimen of repeated mini-cycles of 14 days of treatment followed by seven days off treatment is often better tolerated. Phase 2 comparative data suggest the regimens are of equivalent efficacy.

Growth factor pathway inhibitors: mTOR inhibition

In second and later line settings, everolimus has shown modest PFS benefits. The standard dose is 10mg po once daily.

Table 8.2.1 Treatment algorithm for metastatic CC-RCC divided according to MSKCC prognostic criteria

	Good risk	**Intermediate risk**	**Poor risk**
First line	Tyrosine kinase inhibitor (sunitinib, pazopanib, or tivozanib)	Ipilimumab + nivolumab	Ipilimumab + nivolumab
	Pembrolizumab + axitinib	Pembrolizumab + axitinib	Pembrolizumab + axitinib
	Avelumab + axitinib	Avelumab + axitinib	Avelumab + axitinib
		Tyrosine kinase inhibitor (cabozantinib, sunitinib, pazopanib, or tivozanib)	Tyrosine kinase inhibitor if unable to tolerate immunotherapy
Second line	Nivolumab (if not given immunotherapy first line)		
	Cabozantinib or axitinib		
	Lenvatinib + everolimus		

Side effects include anaphylaxis, diarrhoea, intestinal perforation, interstitial pneumonitis (acute and chronic), myelosuppression, hepatic/renal dysfunction, and drug interactions with steroids, non-steroidal anti-inflammatory agents, and macrolide antibiotics.

Everolimus has shown significant survival benefit in combination with the tyrosine kinase inhibitor, lenvatinib.

T cell checkpoint inhibitors

A phase 3 study reported results indicating that use of the programmed death 1-targeted (PD1) T cell checkpoint inhibitor nivolumab in the second-line setting increased OS by 5.4 months to 25 months in an biomarker-unselected population (HR=0.73; P=0.002). This major benefit established nivolumab as a new standard of care in the second-line setting for patients who have not had prior immunotherapy.

In combination with the cytotoxic T lymphocyte 4-targeted (CTLA4) T cell checkpoint inhibitor, ipilimumab, nivolumab resulted in remarkable benefit for patients across all risk groups but particularly for patients with intermediate and poor risk and especially for patients with high-grade sarcomatoid tumours, which have always had a very poor prognosis in the past. 42% of patients achieved a partial response and the median OS for these patients has not yet been published.

The unwanted effects of treatment with T cell checkpoint inhibitors are largely those of uncontrolled activation of the immune system resulting in autoimmune phenomena. These can affect any organ, most commonly causing dermatitis, hepatitis, thyroid dysfunction, pneumonitis, uveitis, and colitis. Rarer, though occasionally dramatic effects include hypophysitis, diabetes, and adrenal failure.

Side effects are largely manageable but experience is needed both to recognize them and initiate timely measures to control them. With single agent PD1 or PD-L1 therapy, the chance of severe side effects is much lower than with combination PD1/CTLA4 therapy.

Combinations of TKI and T cell checkpoint inhibitors

Multiple large studies have been performed investigating combinations of T cell checkpoint inhibitors with tyrosine kinase inhibitors. These are now at the point of entering standard treatment paradigms in the first-line setting. One of the most influential studies to date is a phase 3 study comparing pembrolizumab with axitinib versus sunitinib. This showed an objective response rate of 59% in the pembrolizumab with axitinib arm versus 35% in the sunitinib arm. Survival data are not yet mature, although

the median progression-free survival in the combination arm was over 15 months.

Treatment algorithm for CC-RCC

At the time of writing, immunotherapy is making substantial inroads into the standard of care. The role of single agent TKIs in the first-line setting is now restricted to good-risk patients and those who are unable to tolerate immunotherapy. The role of mTOR inhibitors has been redefined; the combination of lenvatinib with everolimus is an attractive treatment option, although single agent mTOR inhibition is now much less used than previously.

A typical algorithm is presented here but readers should be aware that this is likely to change radically, especially if predictive biomarkers are developed to direct choice of therapy. The development of reliable predictive biomarkers would have a very great impact on the choice and order of therapies for RCC.

Non-CC-RCC

Treatment decisions are based on lower quality data in this setting. However, it is clear that both TKIs and mTOR inhibitors do have activity against non-CC-RCC.

Chemotherapy generally has modest response in RCC (10–15%). In RCC with sarcomatoid features chemotherapy may have some benefit. In one study a combination of gemcitabine with adriamycin produced a response rate of 28%. However, results with combination immunotherapy are impressive for patients with sarcomatoid tumours which tend to be inflamed and consequently tend to respond well to this form of treatment.

Experimental immunotherapies

Much effort in the last 20 years has been concentrated in various immunological trials in CC-RCC (e.g. dendritic cell vaccines). To date, no trial has provided a significant improvement in OS, although anecdotal cases of prolonged complete remissions are well documented. However, further work continues.

Further reading

Escudier B, Porta C, Schmidinger M, Rioux-Leclercq N, Bex A, Khoo V, Grünwald V, Gillessen S, Horwich A. ESMO Guidelines Committee. Renal cell carcinoma: ESMO clinical practice guidelines for diagnosis, treatment and follow-up. *Ann Oncol* 2019; 30(5):706–20.

Leibovich MD, Bradley C, et al. Prediction of progression after radical nephrectomy for patients with clear cell renal cell carcinoma: A stratification tool for prospective clinical trials. *Cancer* 2003; 97(7):1663–71.

8.3 Urothelial and bladder cancer overview

Epidemiology

Bladder cancer is the seventh most common cancer worldwide, accounting for 3.2% of all cancers. There were an estimated 68,810 new cases and 14,100 deaths from bladder cancer in the USA in 2008. Most tumours occur rarely before age 40. In Europe, it is the seventh most common cancer in males and 14 in women. Each year approximately 36,500 deaths due to bladder cancer occur in males and nearly 13,000 in females.

Aetiology

Gene abnormalities resulting in disruption of cell-regulatory processes

- Proto-oncogenes involvement, e.g. Ras p21 proteins
- Tumour suppressor genes involvement, e.g. p53, p21, p27, retinoblastoma gene (pRB), thrombospondin-1
- EGFR 1–2
- VEGFR
- Loss of heterozygosity of chromosome 9

Chemical exposure

- Tobacco smoking
- Occupational exposures, i.e. aromatic amines, aniline dyes, nitrites, nitrates, plastics, tar, coal, asphalt

Chronic irritation

- Infection by *Schistosoma haematobium* (Egypt)
- Catheters
- Irradiation
- Diet
- Volume of liquid intake
- Analgesic abuse of phenacetin

Pathology

Anatomy of urinary bladder and patterns of spread

Primary site

The urinary bladder consists of three layers: the epithelium, the subepithelial connective tissue, the muscularis and the perivesical fat. In males, the bladder is adjacent to the rectum and seminal vesicles posteriorly, the prostate inferiorly, and the pubis and peritoneum anteriorly. In females, the vagina is located posteriorly and the uterus superiorly. The bladder is an extraperitoneal organ.

Regional lymph nodes

- Hypogastric
- Obturator
- Iliac (internal, external, not otherwise specified (NOS))
- Perivesical
- Pelvic (NOS)
- Sacral (lateral, sacral promontory (Gerota's))
- Presacral

Metastatic sites

- Lymph nodes (common iliac nodes are considered M1)
- Lung
- Bone
- Liver

Anatomy of renal pelvis and ureter and patterns of spread

Primary site

The renal pelvis and ureter form a single unit that is continuous with the collecting ducts of the renal pyramids including calyces (major and minor) through the urinary bladder wall as the intramural ureter opening in the trigone of the bladder at the ureteral orifice. The renal pelvis and ureter are composed of three layers: epithelium, subepithelial connective tissue, and muscularis, which is continuous with the connective tissue adventitial layer.

Regional lymph nodes

- Renal hilar
- Paracaval
- Aortic
- Retroperitoneal, NOS
- Regional lymph nodes for the ureter
- Iliac (common, internal (hypogastric), external)
- Paracaval
- Peri-ureteral
- Pelvic, NOS

Metastatic sites

- Lung
- Bone
- Liver

Histology

Urothelial or transitional cell carcinoma (TCC)

TCC begins in cells in the innermost tissue layer of the bladder. Approximately 90% of TCCs occur in the bladder and the remaining 10% develop from the renal pelvis, ureter, and urethra.

Squamous cell carcinoma

This tumour is characterized by keratinization which begins in squamous cells, which are thin, flat cells that may form in the bladder after long-term infection or chronic irritation. SCCs account for 5% of bladder tumours. This type of bladder cancer is frequent in countries where *Schistosoma haematobium* is endemic.

Adenocarcinoma

Adenocarcinoma is characterized by glandular (secretory) cells that may form in the bladder after long-term irritation and inflammation. Other less common bladder cancers include small cell carcinomas, giant cell carcinomas, and lymphoepitheliomas.

Histological grading

Classification of bladder tumours includes cellular characteristics such as grading into low (G1) and high-grade (G2–3). This is most clinically significant in non-invasive tumours.

- Gx: grade cannot be assessed
- G1: well differentiated
- G2: moderately differentiated
- G3/4: differentiated or undifferentiated

Clinical features

Macroscopic haematuria may be painless in 75–95% of patients with ureteral, renal, pelvic, and bladder cancer and should always be followed by imaging of upper tracts, flexible cystoscopy, and further clinical evaluation.

Diagnosis

Symptoms

Painless haematuria, urgency, dysuria, increased frequency, and pelvic pain. Pelvic pain and symptoms related to urinary tract obstruction may be found in more advanced tumours.

Physical examination

Includes rectal and vaginal bimanual palpation. A palpable pelvic mass may be found in patients with locally advanced tumours.

Imaging

MRI and CT scan

Tumours may be seen as filling defects in the bladder. CT urography/intravenous urogram (CT IVU) is used to detect filling defects in the calices, renal pelvis, and ureters, and hydronephrosis, which may indicate the presence of a ureteral tumour. CT scans are used more commonly now than intravenous pyelography (IVP) especially for invasive tumours of the upper tract, and detection of lymph nodes or other potential metastases. Bladder MRI is used as it can delineate the level of involvement of the different muscle layers in the bladder wall. CT chest or chest X-ray (CXR) to stage the chest to exclude metastases is advised.

Ultrasonography

Transabdominal ultrasonography permits characterization of renal masses, detection of hydronephrosis, and visualization of intraluminal filling defects in the bladder.

Urinary cytology and urinary markers

Examination of voided urine or a specimen of bladder-washings for exfoliated cancer cells has high sensitivity in high-grade tumours. It is, therefore, useful when high-grade malignancy or carcinoma in situ (CIS) is present. Positive urinary cytology may indicate urothelial tumour anywhere in the urinary tract including the calyces, ureters, bladder, and proximal urethra. Cytological interpretation is highly dependent upon the pathologist's experience; urinary biomarkers should not be used instead of cystoscopy, except in the context of a clinical trial.

Cystoscopy

The diagnosis of bladder cancer ultimately depends on cystoscopic examination of the bladder and histological evaluation of the resected tissue. In general, cystoscopy is initially an outpatient procedure using flexible instruments. A careful description should include the site, size, number, and appearance (papillary or solid) of the tumours as well as a description of mucosal abnormalities. Use of a bladder diagram is recommended.

Transurethral resection of invasive bladder tumours

The goal of transurethral resection of the bladder tumour (TURBT) is diagnostic, which means that bladder muscle must be included in the biopsies. Small tumours (<1cm) can be resected en bloc, where the specimen contains the complete tumour plus a part of the underlying bladder wall including the bladder muscle. Larger tumours should be resected separately in fractions, which include the exophytic part of the tumour, the underlying bladder wall with the detrusor muscle, and the edges of the resection area. The specimens from different fractions must be referred to the pathologist in separate containers to facilitate correct diagnosis.

Bladder and prostatic urethral biopsy

The involvement of the prostatic urethra and ducts in male patients with bladder tumours has been reported. Although the exact risk is not known, it seems to be higher if tumour is located on the trigone or bladder neck, in the presence of bladder CIS and when there are multiple tumours. In these cases and when cytology is positive or when abnormalities of the prostatic urethra are visible, biopsies of the prostatic urethra are recommended. Special care must be taken with tumours at the bladder neck and trigone in female patients where urethral preservation and an orthotopic neobladder is planned.

Fluorescence cystoscopy

Fluorescence cystoscopy is performed using filtered blue light after intravesical instillation of a photosensitizer, usually 5-aminolaevulinic acid (5-ALA) or hexaminolaevulinate (HAL). It has been confirmed that fluorescence-guided biopsy and resection are more sensitive than conventional procedures in detecting malignant tumours, particularly CIS. However, false-positive results can be induced by inflammation, recent TURB, or intravesical therapy.

Second resection

A second TURBT should always be performed when the initial resection has been incomplete, e.g. when multiple and/or large tumours are present, and especially when the pathologist reports that the specimen does not contain muscle tissue. There is no clear consensus as to the timing of a second TURBT. Most urologists recommend resection at two to six weeks after the initial TURBT. The procedure should include resection of the primary tumour site.

Staging

The UICC TNM classification (2016) for bladder cancer can be found at the American Cancer Society website (see 'Internet resources', p. 204).

Prognosis

Prognostic factors of primary tumours

- Grading
- Stage
- Hydronephrosis
- Anaemia
- Size
- Expression of blood group substances
- Expression of EGFR
- Mutation of p53
- Upregulation of RB
- Other oncogene expression

Prognostic factors for metastatic disease

- PS poor (Eastern Cooperative Oncology Group performance status (ECOG PS) >2).
- Visceral metastasis.
- Abnormal liver function.
- Expression, upregulation, or mutation of known oncogenes (e.g. p53, Rb, P21, etc.) is still under investigation, no consensus has been achieved, and controversial results on p53 have been published.

- Loss of heterozygosity of chromosome 9 is associated with genesis of superficial bladder cancer.
- Loss of heterozygosity of chromosome 17 with mutation of the p53 suppressor gene seems to be associated with evolution of invasive disease and/or metastatic disease.
- Ploidy has been investigated in superficial disease. Aneuploid DNA content is associated with shorter disease-free survival (DFS) and higher chances of progression to higher stage.

Guidelines on assessment of tumour specimens after radical cystectomy
Mandatory evaluations
- Depth of invasion (categories pT2 vs. pT3a, pT3b or pT4)
- Margins, with special attention paid to the radial margin
- Histological subtype
- Extensive lymph node examination (>8)

Optional evaluations
- Bladder wall blood vessel invasion
- Pattern of muscle invasion

Comments
- The incidence of muscle invasive disease has not changed in the last five years.
- Active and passive tobacco smoking continues to be the major risk factor while occupational exposure-related incidence is decreasing.
- The estimated male to female ratio is 3.8:1.
- Currently, treatment decisions cannot be based on molecular markers.

Internet resources
American Cancer Society. Bladder Cancer Stages: https://www.cancer.org/cancer/bladder-cancer/detection-diagnosis-staging/staging.html

8.4 Management of localized and muscle invasive disease of bladder cancer

Surgery
Superficial bladder cancer
Transurethral resection of Ta and T1 bladder tumours
The goal of TURBT in Ta and T1 bladder tumours is diagnostic and also has the scope of removing all visible lesions. The strategy of resection depends on the size of the lesion. Small tumours (<1cm) can be resected en bloc, where the specimen contains the complete tumour plus a part of the underlying bladder wall. Larger tumours should be resected separately in fractions, which include the exophytic part of the tumour, the underlying bladder wall with the detrusor muscle, and the edges of the resection area. Specimens from different fractions must be sent to the pathologist in separate containers to permit correct diagnosis. Cauterization should be avoided during resection to prevent tissue destruction. A complete and correct TURBT is essential to define prognosis.

Cystectomy for non-muscle invasive bladder cancer
Many experts consider that it is reasonable to propose immediate cystectomy to patients with non-muscle invasive tumours which are at highest risk of progression. These subgroups include:
- Multiple and/or large (>3cm) T1G3 and/or recurrent T1G3 tumours
- High-grade T1 tumours associated with bladder or prostatic CIS
- Unusual urothelial histological types
- Lymphovascular invasion

Cystectomy is advocated for patients with non-muscle invasive disease who have failed bacillus Calmette–Guérin (BCG) therapy. Delaying cystectomy in these patients may lead to decreased disease-specific survival.

In all T1 tumours at high risk of progression (such as high-grade, multifocal, with CIS, and large tumour size, as outlined in the non-muscle invasive bladder cancer EAU guidelines), immediate radical cystectomy is an option.

In all T1 patients failing intravesical BCG therapy, cystectomy is the preferred option. A delay in cystectomy increases the risk of progression and cancer-specific death.

Invasive bladder cancer
Radical surgery
- Aim: removal of the tumour-bearing bladder.
- Background: radical cystectomy is the standard treatment for localized muscle invasive bladder cancer in most countries of the western hemisphere.
- Timing: delay in surgery beyond 90 days of primary diagnosis is associated with a significant increase in extravesical disease.
- Indications: radical cystectomy is recommended for patients with muscle-invasive bladder cancer T2–T4a, N0–Nx, M0. Other indications include high-risk and recurrent superficial tumours, BCG-resistant CIS, T1G3, as well as extensive papillary disease that cannot be controlled with TURBT and intravesical therapy alone.
- Technique and extent: standard surgery for urothelial tumours infiltrating the muscularis propria, i.e. clinical stage T2 or greater, is a radical cystectomy with pelvic lymph node dissection. A radical cystectomy involves wide resection of the bladder with all of the perivesical fat and tissue in an attempt to achieve negative margins. Men undergo prostatectomy and women require resection of the uterus, fallopian tubes, ovaries, anterior vaginal wall, and surrounding fascia. A urinary stoma or a continent urinary diversion (bladder substitution or a catheterizable reservoir) is used to redirect urinary flow.

Laparoscopic cystectomy
Laparoscopic cystectomy has been shown to be feasible both in males and females. Cystectomy and subsequent urinary diversion are most often performed by open surgery, but there is increasing use of hand-assisted or robot-assisted laparoscopic surgical techniques.

Urinary diversion after radical cystectomy
An increasing proportion of patients is given a continent reservoir which is usually an orthotopic neobladder which allows patients to void through the urethra. Although continent diversions are more technically demanding, postoperative complications are not, thereby improving QoL after cystectomy.

Urinary diversion or bladder substitution after cystectomy can, however, be performed in several ways:

- Abdominal diversion such as uretero-cutaneostomy, ileal or colonic conduit, and various forms of cutaneous continent pouch.
- Urethral diversion which includes various forms of GI pouches attached to the urethra as a continent, orthotopic urinary diversion (neobladder, orthotopic bladder substitution.
- Rectosigmoid diversions, such as uretero(ileo-)-rectostomy.

Conclusions

- There is limited evidence of which is the best curative treatment for localized bladder neoplasms, either cystectomy or radical radiotherapy with a radiosensitizer.
- Radical cystectomy includes removal of regional lymph nodes, although the extent of removal necessary has not been sufficiently defined.
- Radical cystectomy in both sexes does not necessarily include the removal of the entire urethra in all cases, which may serve as an outlet for an orthotopic bladder substitution.
- Terminal ileum and colon are the intestinal segments of choice for urinary diversions.
- The type of urinary diversion does not affect oncological outcome.

Role of radiotherapy

Primary radiotherapy

- Preoperative radiotherapy for operable muscle-invasive bladder cancer does not increase survival.
- Preoperative radiotherapy for operable muscle-invasive bladder cancer, using a dose of 45–50Gy in fractions of 1.8–2Gy may result in downstaging after four to six weeks, but is not standard treatment.

Radiotherapy

- External beam radiotherapy (EBRT) should be considered as a therapeutic option, ideally as part of a multimodality bladder-preserving approach with a radiosensitizer. (Chemotherapy or nicotinamide and carbogen).
- Radiotherapy can also be used to stop bleeding from the tumour when local control cannot be achieved by transurethral manipulation because of extensive local tumour growth.

Chemoradiotherapy

Multimodality treatment is an alternative in selected well-informed patients.

The algorithm of bladder preserving therapy for muscle-invasive cancer includes maximal TURBT of the bladder tumour, modern EBRT with radiosensitizers given concurrently, and a careful urology-based surveillance programme with prompt cystectomy for persistent or recurrent invasive tumours. Tumour presentations with the highest success rates include: solitary T2 or early T3 tumours <6cm, no tumour-associated hydro-nephrosis,

tumours allowing a visibly complete TURBT, invasive tumours not associated with extensive CIS, and adequate renal function to allow cisplatin administration concurrently with radiation.

Radiosensitizers include: concurrent oral nicotinamide with carbogen inhaled before each radiotherapy fraction, or chemotherapy using mitomycin with fluorouracil (5-FU).

Role of chemotherapy

Neoadjuvant chemotherapy

Advantages include:

- Chemotherapy is delivered when the burden of micro-metastatic disease is expected to be low.
- In vivo chemosensitivity is tested.
- The tolerability of chemotherapy is expected to be better before rather than after cystectomy.
  Disadvantages of neoadjuvant chemotherapy include:
- Differences between clinical and pathological staging.
- Delayed cystectomy might compromise the outcome in patients not sensitive to chemotherapy.
- Side effects of chemotherapy might affect the outcome of surgery and type of urinary diversion.
- In patients with muscle invasive disease, neoadjuvant cisplatin-containing combination chemotherapy improves OS by 5% at five years, based upon meta-analyses of randomized studies, particularly in cystectomy series.
- Neoadjuvant chemotherapy has limitations with regard to patient selection and current chemotherapy combinations.

Adjuvant chemotherapy

The benefits of chemotherapy in the adjuvant setting include:

- Chemotherapy is administered after accurate pathological staging.
- Overtreatment in patients at low risk for micro-metastases is avoided.
- There is no delay in definitive surgical treatment, especially in patients not sensitive to chemotherapy.
  The drawbacks of adjuvant chemotherapy are:
- Assessment of in vivo chemosensitivity of the tumour is not possible.
- There may be delay in administration or intolerance of chemotherapy because of postoperative morbidity.
  There is insufficient evidence on which to base reliably adjuvant chemotherapy treatment decisions. Randomized trials have been underpowered and meta-analyses have not been conclusive. Failure to enrol patients into adjuvant chemotherapy trials after cystectomy has led to this dilemma. Further research and support of clinical trials is required.

Conclusions

Cisplatin-based combination neoadjuvant chemotherapy before cystectomy produces a 5% improvement in survival according to meta-analysis of randomized trials.

There is not enough evidence of benefit for the routine use of adjuvant chemotherapy.

Recommendations

Radical radiotherapy

- Radical radiotherapy is considered for patients with T2–T4a, N0–NX, M0, muscle invasive bladder cancer and unfit for surgery.

- There is limited evidence about whether cystectomy or radiotherapy with a radiosensitizer is the most effective cancer treatment.
- Patients should be counselled about both options, including the impact on sexual and bowel function and the risk of death as a result of treatment.

Radical cystectomy

- Radical cystectomy is recommended for patients with T2–T4a, N0–NX, M0, and high-risk non-muscle invasive bladder cancer as outlined earlier.
- Lymph node dissection should be an integral part of cystectomy, but the optimal extent is not established.
- Preservation of the urethra is reasonable if margins are negative. If there is no bladder substitution, the urethra must be checked regularly.
- Laparoscopic and robot-assisted laparoscopic cystectomy may be an option. Current data, however, have not sufficiently proven its advantages or disadvantages.

Urinary diversion

- Treatment is recommended at centres experienced in major types of diversion techniques and postoperative care.
- Before cystectomy, the patient should be counselled adequately regarding possible alternatives, and the final decision should be based on a consensus between the patient and surgeon.
- An orthotopic bladder substitution should be offered to male and female patients where there are no contraindications and who do not have tumour in the urethra and at the level of urethral dissection.

Intravesical therapy

Intravesical therapy is recommended for Ta, T1 tumours, and CIS, based on the risk for tumour recurrence and progression.

- Low risk tumours (primary, solitary, Ta, low-grade/G1, <3cm, no CIS)—one immediate instillation of chemotherapy. If chemotherapy is given, the drug should be used at its optimal pH and the concentration of the drug maintained during instillation by reducing fluid intake.
- Intermediate risk tumours (all cases between low and high risk tumours)—one immediate instillation of chemotherapy followed by further treatment with chemotherapy for one year or full dose BCG for one year.
- High risk tumours (T1 tumours or high-grade or CIS or multiple, recurrent, and >3cm Ta grade 1–2 tumours)—full dose BCG for one to three years. Immediate radical cystectomy may be offered to the highest risk patients.
- The absolute risks of recurrence and progression do not always indicate the risk at which a certain therapy is optimal. The choice of therapy may be chosen differently according to what risk is acceptable for the individual patient and the urologist. The risk of tumour recurrence after TURB can be predicted using the European Organisation for Research and Treatment of Cancer (EORTC) calculator (available at: http://www.eortc.be/tools/bladdercalculator/).

Neoadjuvant chemotherapy

- Neoadjuvant cisplatin-containing combination chemotherapy should be considered in muscle-invasive bladder cancer (T2–T4a cN0M0) patients before cystectomy.
- Neoadjuvant chemotherapy is not recommended in patients with PS >2 and impaired renal function.

Adjuvant chemotherapy

Consider adjuvant chemotherapy for patients after radical cystectomy with pT3/4 and/or lymph node-positive (N+) disease for whom neoadjuvant chemotherapy was not suitable (because muscle invasion was not shown on biopsies before cystectomy). Ensure the patient has the opportunity to discuss the risks and benefits with an oncologist who treats bladder cancer.

8.5 Management of advanced and metastatic disease of bladder cancer

Principles of management

Metastatic disease

Approximately 30% of patients with urothelial cancer present with muscle-invasive disease. About half will relapse after radical cystectomy, depending on the pathological stage of the primary tumour and the nodal status. Local recurrence accounts for about 30% of relapses, whereas distant metastases are more common. About 10–15% of patients already have metastatic disease at the time of diagnosis. Before the development of effective chemotherapy, patients with metastatic urothelial cancer rarely had a median survival of less than three to six months.

Prognostic factors and treatment decisions

Bladder cancer is a chemosensitive tumour. Response rates differ with respect to patient-related factors and pretreatment disease. Prognostic factors for response and survival have been established. Karnofsky performance status (KPS) of 80 and the presence of visceral metastases are independently prognostic of poor survival after treatment with M-VAC (methotrexate, vinblastine, adriamycin, and cisplatin). These prognostic factors have also been validated in other newer combination chemotherapy regimens. Additional data exist on the prognostic value of elevated alkaline phosphatase and the number of disease sites (>3 or <3). In elderly patients, an ECOG PS 2–3 and a haemoglobin level of <10mg/dl are independent predictors of poor survival. Age itself has no impact on response or toxicity. Besides these prognostic factors, treatment decisions should be based on whether a patient is 'fit' enough to receive a cisplatin-containing combination regimen taking into account renal function (creatinine clearance >50ml/min, PS, comorbidities).

Role of radiotherapy and multimodality treatment for muscle-invasive disease

After a TURBT which is as complete as possible, radiation to the bladder tumour to a dose of 64Gy is considered standard therapy. This is usually given with a radiosensitizer-chemotherapy or nicotinamide and carbogen on each day of radiation. Close cystoscopic surveillance with salvage cystectomy for tumour persistence or for invasive recurrence is required.

Tumour presentations with the highest success rates include: solitary T2 or early T3 tumours <6cm, no tumour-associated hydronephrosis, tumours allowing a macroscopically complete TURBT, and invasive tumours not associated with extensive CIS with adequate renal function to allow cisplatin administration concurrently with radiation.

Palliative radiotherapy
Radiotherapy can also be used to stop bleeding from the tumour when local control cannot be achieved by TURBT because of extensive local tumour growth.

Role of chemotherapy
- Urothelial carcinoma is a chemosensitive tumour.
- PS and the presence or absence of visceral metastases are independent prognostic factors for survival. These factors are at least as important as the type of chemotherapy administered.
- Cisplatin-containing combination chemotherapy can achieve a median survival of up to 14 months, with long-term DFS reported in some 15% of patients with nodal disease and good PS. Patients must have adequate renal function with EGFR >60ml/min/1.73m^2.
- PD-L1 expressing bladder tumours can be offered immunotherapy with PD-L1 inhibitors.
- Carboplatin combination chemotherapy is less effective than cisplatin-based chemotherapy in terms of complete remission and survival.
- Non-platinum combination chemotherapy has produced substantial responses in first- and second-line use, but has not been tested against standard chemotherapy in fit patients, nor in a purely unfit patient group.
- To date, there is no defined standard chemotherapy for 'unfit' patients with advanced or metastatic urothelial cancer.
- Small-sized phase 2 trials provide evidence of moderate response rates for single agents or non-platinum combinations for second-line use.
- Post-chemotherapy surgery after a partial or complete response may contribute to long-term DFS.

Role of surgery
Palliative cystectomy for muscle-invasive bladder carcinoma
For patients with inoperable locally advanced tumours (T4b, invading the pelvic or abdominal wall), radical cystectomy is not usually a therapeutic option. Treatment of these patients remains a clinical challenge but they may be candidates for palliative treatments with radiotherapy or chemotherapy. Inoperable locally advanced tumours may cause debilitating symptoms, including bleeding, pain, dysuria, and urinary obstruction. There are several treatment options for patients with these symptoms. In advanced bladder cancer cases complicated by bleeding, cystectomy with urinary diversion is the most invasive treatment. It carries the greatest morbidity and should be considered only if there are no other options.

Low volume disease and post-chemotherapy surgery
With cisplatin-containing combination chemotherapy, patients with lymph node metastases only, and good PS and adequate renal function, may achieve excellent response rates, including many complete responses, with up to 20% of patients achieving long-term DFS. Stage migration may play a role in this positive prognosis.

Post-chemotherapy surgery may contribute to long-term DFS in selected patients.

Conclusions
- Primary radical cystectomy in T4b bladder cancer may be a palliative option in symptomatic patients where chemotherapy or radiation therapy are not indicated.
- Recent organ-preservation strategies combine TURBT, chemotherapy, and radiation therapy (trimodality therapy). The rationale for performing TURB and radiation with radiosensitizing chemotherapy is to achieve bladder preservation.
- There are no randomized trials comparing radical cystectomy with or without chemotherapy to trimodality organ preservation with chemoradiation therapy.

Palliative care
Palliative radiotherapy
Advanced carcinoma of the bladder with pelvic fixation carries a poor prognosis and no significant differences in results can be shown whether the patient is treated with radical or palliative intent. Patients should be carefully selected, as those in very poor condition or with grossly reduced bladder capacity can have their symptoms aggravated by radiation. Haematuria may be controlled by a short course of irradiation in about 50% of cases. Pelvic pain may be due to a bladder mass or to bone lesions, with or without nerve involvement. If the site of disease is well identified, pain control may be achieved in >50% of cases. Palliation is generally obtained with doses of about 30Gy in two weeks; shorter regimens are generally excluded in order to avoid toxicity. Single fraction treatments with 8Gy or 10Gy to a well circumscribed bladder volume are reported as safe and effective in controlling haematuria. Painful bone metastasis in sites other than the pelvis can be treated effectively with short course radiotherapy.

The evaluation of health-related quality of life (HRQoL)
Evaluation of QoL should consider physical, emotional, and social functioning. Several questionnaires, e.g. FACT (Functional Assessment of Cancer Therapy)-G, EORTC QLQ-C30, and SF (Short Form)-36, have been validated for assessing HRQoL in patients with bladder cancer. A psychometric test such as the FACT-BL should be used for recording bladder cancer morbidity.

Conclusions
- The overall HRQoL after cystectomy remains good in most patients, whichever type of urinary diversion is used. Some data suggests that continent diversions produce better HRQoL.
- Radiation oncologists also report excellent HRQoL as evidenced by urodynamic studies, QoL questionnaires, and late pelvic toxicity analyses.

Recommendations
- For muscle-invasive bladder cancer, there is no evidence that radiotherapy with radiosensitizers is less effective than radical cystectomy.
- Consider neoadjuvant chemotherapy with a cisplatin-containing regimen in patients fit enough and with adequate renal function.

- For patients with metastatic cancer first-line treatment for fit patients is cisplatin-containing combination chemotherapy with GC, M-VAC, preferably with G-CSF, or HD-MVAC with G-CSF.
- Carboplatin and non-platinum combination chemotherapy is not recommended as first-line treatment in patients fit for cisplatin.
- First-line treatment in patients unfit for cisplatin is carboplatin combination chemotherapy or PD-L1 immunotherapy for PD-L1 positive tumours.
- For second-line treatment, consider immunotherapy with PD-L1 inhibitors for PD-L1 expressing tumours or paclitaxel/gemcitabine or carboplatin/paclitaxel for patients with a good PS.
- Morbidity of surgery and QoL should be weighed against other options.
- TURBT alone is not a curative treatment option for most patients with muscle-invasive disease.

- HRQoL in patients with muscle-invasive bladder cancer should be assessed using validated questionnaires.
- Continent urinary diversions should be considered when possible.

Further reading
Bellmunt J, Orsola A, Leow JJ, et al. Bladder cancer: ESMO practice guidelines for diagnosis, treatment and follow-up. *Ann Oncol* 2014; 25(Suppl. 3):iii40–48.
Witjes JA, Comperat E, Cowan NC et al. EAU Guidelines on muscle-invasive and metastatic bladder cancer: Summary of the 2013 guidelines. *Eur Urol* 2014; 65:778–92.

Internet resources
American Urological Association: https://www.auanet.org/
European Association of Urology: http://www.uroweb.org
National Comprehensive Cancer Network: http://www.nccn.org
NICE Bladder Cancer Guidelines 2015 http://www.nice.org.uk/guidance

8.6 Management of non-transitional urothelial cancer

Introduction
More than 90% of all bladder tumours are transitional cell carcinomas. Non-urothelial bladder tumours are rare and account for <5% of all vesical tumours. These include:
- Squamous cell carcinomas 3–5%
- Adenocarcinomas 0.5–2%
- Small cell carcinoma <0.5%
- Sarcomas <0.1%

Other histological types such as melanomas and lymphomas may also be found in the bladder but are extremely rare and account for less than 0.5% of all bladder malignancies.

Squamous cell carcinomas (SCCs)
SCCs are the second most prevalent epithelial tumours of the bladder. They are usually aggressive tumours. The aetiology is chronic bladder inflammation, as for example from use of catheters for neurogenic bladders that rely on intermittent catheterization. A well-recognized pathogenic factor is chronic infection with *Schistosoma haematobium*. SCC accounts for 30% of cancers and is the second most common malignancy in women in countries with endemic schistosomiasis. This is a poor prognosis disease, due to local invasion. Most patients have extravesical tumour extension at the time of diagnosis and death is usually related to locally recurrent disease. Treatment is therefore directed to local control of the disease with radical cystectomy and bilateral pelvic node dissection. Preoperative radiation for invasive (stages T2–3) SCC of the bladder can downstage the disease in up to 40% of patients. Therefore, it may protect patients from pelvic recurrence which is usually the main cause of death. Two growth characteristics of carcinoma of the bilharzial bladder have been observed:
- High mitotic rate with a potential doubling time of six days
- Extensive cell loss factor

Tumours with such growth characteristics are expected to respond to radiation. Nevertheless, early experience with external beam radiation therapy for definitive control of these tumours was disappointing.

Adenocarcinomas
Pure adenocarcinomas of the bladder are the third most common type of epithelial tumour and represent 0.5–2% of all bladder tumours. The definition of vesical adenocarcinoma is still controversial. Pathological variations of tumours include: glandular structures resembling colonic adenocarcinomas (enteric type) and/or tumours that produce intra- (signet cell type) or extracellular mucin (mucinous type). Adenocarcinomas of the urinary bladder can be divided into three different subtypes depending on their origin. Adenocarcinomas may arise from an urachal remnant (urachal adenocarcinoma (UA)), from metaplasia of the bladder urothelium (non-urachal adenocarcinoma (NUA)), or from a metastatic site from another primary tumour such as from the colon, rectum, prostate, stomach, breast, endometrium, or ovary. NUAs arising from ectopic bladder urothelium account for 0.4–3.9% of all bladder tumours, whereas primary UAs account for only 0.17–1.18% of those tumours. Males are more frequently affected than females, with a ratio of approximately 7:3. Although there is no consensus regarding diagnostic criteria for UA, important clinical pathological features include location in the bladder dome, a sharp demarcation between the tumour and surface epithelium, and exclusion of primary adenocarcinoma that may have metastasized to the bladder. Standard treatment for vesical adenocarcinomas is radical cystectomy and bilateral pelvic node dissection, followed by urinary diversion. In rare instances where patients have a well-differentiated UA localized to the bladder dome, partial cystectomy with removal of the urachus and umbilectomy may be considered. The largest series from the USA reported five-year survival rates of 40–50% for patients with UAs. In the series from Siefker-Radtke et al., nodal status and surgical margins were significantly associated with survival. It is noteworthy that 13 of the 16 long-term survivors were treated with en

bloc resections. In this largest published series, no patient had disease confined to the epithelium or urachal ligament at presentation, with most patients showing locally advanced disease. In addition, more than 29% of all cases presented with positive nodal or systemic disease. Local management usually required surgery and radiation therapy. For patients with NUA, radical cystectomy is usually the first-choice treatment. Too few patients have been studied to make it possible to recommend systematic adjuvant treatment after cystectomy. The most effective regimens appear to contain 5-FU and cisplatin (CDDP), suggesting that a regimen for adenocarcinoma of the colon may be more beneficial for UA than the traditional urothelial cancer chemotherapy regimens. Therefore for patients with NUA, radical cystectomy is usually the first treatment choice with radiation therapy.

Further reading
Siefker-Radtke AO, Gee J, Shen Y, et al. Multimodality management of urachal carcinoma: the MD Anderson Cancer Center experience. *J Urol* 2003; 169:1295–8

Internet resources
American Urological Association: http://www.auanet.org
European Association of Urology: http://www.uroweb.org
National Comprehensive Cancer Network: http://www.nccn.org

8.7 Cancer of the ureter and renal pelvis

Introduction
Urothelial tumours of ureters and renal pelvis account for 5% of all urothelial tumours. The majority of tumours of the upper urinary tract are transitional cell carcinomas (TCCs). However, they are rarer than bladder cancers, with approximately 3,000 new diagnoses per year in the USA. Histologically, 90% are TCCs and 10% are SCCs.

Clinical features and investigations
Gross haematuria is the first symptom in >75% of patients. It may be followed or accompanied by colic and flank pain if the tumour itself or blood clots cause obstruction of the ureter. Sometimes patients describe passing blood clots, a symptom which is rare in lower tract bleeding. Urine cytology is not very sensitive for low-grade tumours. However, sensitivity increases for high-grade tumours up to 70%.

Normally, staging is performed using helical CT scans with an iodinated contrast medium. MRI may be performed in patients who are sensitive to contrast. If renal function is poor or compromised, retrograde pyelography is the imaging method of choice. Complete staging in patients with aggressive (> grade I) or advanced (> stage I) disease should include chest CT, and imaging of the abdomen and pelvis for possible hepatic or RPLN metastases. Isotope renal scanning estimates of kidney function should be used to calculate residual function when standard treatment is radical nephrectomy and ureterectomy.

Treatment
Surgery
Surgery is the treatment of choice for patients with TCC of the ureter and renal pelvis of all grades and stages. Patients with low risk disease can be treated with kidney-sparing surgery provided close follow-up is feasible. All the following factors need to be present to categorize as low risk disease: unifocal disease, tumour of <1cm, low-grade cytology, low grade on uterorenoscopic biopsy, and no invasion on multidetector CT urography. Patients whose tumours cannot be removed endoscopically are considered for open surgical approach. All other groups of patients are considered for radical nephroureterectomy, involving complete resection of the kidney, peri-renal fat, Gerota's fascia, and en bloc resection of the ureter to the urinary bladder. When the vena cava or renal veins are involved, thrombus extraction and/or partial vena cava dissection may be needed. Both open surgery and laparoscopic approach can be used. Special attention should be paid because invasive TCC has the capacity to seed, implant, and proliferate if spilled in the abdomen. In patients at high risk of severe renal insufficiency following surgery, physicians should consider other surgical therapies. Percutaneous endoscopic surgery of renal pelvic and calyceal TCC has been developed as a treatment option in selected patients with poor renal function and with medical conditions not permitting open surgery. However, due to the technical complexity and high risk of tumour seeding and the difficulty of resection, vigilant follow-up is required. Recurrence is very common.

Adjuvant combined modality therapy
After nephroureterectomy for invasive TCC of the upper urinary tract, the five-year survival is only 0–30%. Metastatic disease seems more frequent than local relapse and extrapolation from experience in advanced bladder cancer suggests that cisplatin-based chemotherapy may be useful. EBRT has been used as adjuvant therapy but results are not clear cut. Local control may be better, but studies are limited in predicting survival due to the small patient numbers in phase 2 trials. Because of this and the relatively low frequency of disease, data to guide physicians managing local relapse after nephroureterectomy are scanty. If local relapse is bulky and metastases present elsewhere, palliative chemotherapy is the treatment of choice. On the other hand, when relapse appears isolated and the patient is fit, other approaches than systemic chemotherapy may occasionally be considered. The recurrence may be reduced in size with a preoperative radiotherapy dose of 30–45Gy given with sensitizing chemotherapy. An attempt at debulking and possible intraoperative radiation therapy (IORT) directly to the tumour bed or unresectable mass may be considered.

Even though instillation of BCG or chemotherapy in the urinary tract is feasible after kidney sparing surgery, the exact clinical benefit is not known.

Chemotherapy
The biology of upper urinary tract TCC is considered identical to bladder TCC. Chemotherapy regimens are, therefore, the same as those recommended for advanced or metastatic bladder cancer. Standard treatment is cisplatin-based combination therapy using gemcitabine and cisplatin or methotrexate, vinblastine, doxorubicin, and cisplatin. Like bladder cancer, upper urinary tract

TCC is highly responsive to chemotherapy, most often however with a short median duration of response.

Summary
- Tumours of the renal pelvis and the ureter are rare. Accurate diagnosis, surgical recognition, and effective local treatment are difficult.
- Haematuria is the most common symptom.
- Urinary cytology may be somewhat less sensitive than in bladder cancer.
- CT scan with contrast is the most useful imaging tool.

- Surgical treatment with new laparoscopic and robotic techniques has changed the approach to this disease.
- Both chemotherapy and radiation therapy seem to be important in extending survival, yet published data are insufficient to fully support these approaches and carefully planned trials are needed.

Further reading
Roupret M, Babjuk M, Comperat E, et al. European Association of Urology Guidelines on Upper Urinary Tract Urothelial Cell Carcinoma: 2015 update. *Eur Urol* 2015; 68:868–79.

8.8 Prostate cancer overview

Epidemiology
- Prostate cancer accounts for 23% of cancers in European men.
- It is the second most common cancer in men worldwide.
- There has been a large increase in incidence over the past 20 years due to increased detection through prostate-specific antigen (PSA) screening and surgery for benign prostatic disease. In 1985–92, the age-adjusted incidence of prostate cancer in the USA more than doubled due to the introduction of PSA screening.
- In the UK there are 32,000 new diagnoses and 10,000 deaths from prostate cancer each year.
- There is significant geographical variation in incidence, with the highest rates in the USA (125/100,000 population). These rates are twice those in the UK, primarily due to wider availability of PSA screening in asymptomatic men. Black Americans have a particularly high incidence (274/100,000).
- Incidence rates are particularly low in China, India, and Japan.
- The majority of cases occur in the >70 age group and the disease is rare in the <50s.
- As yet there is no evidence that PSA screening reduces mortality rates from prostate cancer.

Aetiology
- Age is the most important risk factor for prostate cancer.
- Postmortem studies have shown that men >80 years of age have a 60–70% incidence of histological evidence of prostate cancer.
- Various environmental risk factors have been proposed, including a high fat diet, anabolic steroids, and oestrogen exposure.
- High circulating testosterone levels are associated with increased risk.
- Genetic risk factors have been identified, including a hereditary prostate cancer gene on chromosome 1p and genetic variation at the insulin-like growth factor-1 locus.
- Recent studies have concentrated on 8q24—single nuclear polymorphisms at multiple loci have been demonstrated to be independent risk factors for prostate cancer.

- Mutation of the vitamin D receptor gene may also lead to increased risk (vitamin D itself may be protective).
- Mutation of the androgen receptor domain may be associated with high-grade disease, extraprostatic extension, and distant metastases.
- Laboratory and observational studies have suggested that selenium, vitamin E, and beta-carotene may be protective. Evidence from prospective studies suggests that benefit is restricted only to those with particularly low dietary intakes or, in the case of vitamin E, to current smokers. There is no strong support for population-wide use of antioxidant supplementation.
- Soy products may be protective, perhaps partly explaining the relatively low incidence of prostate cancer in Asian countries. This may be due to phytooestrogenic components of soy.

Pathology
- The majority (95%) of prostate tumours are adenocarcinoma.
- Cells tend to be uniform with relatively little anaplasia. Lymphatic, vascular, and perineural invasion differentiate from benign prostatic hypertrophy.
- Malignant areas are frequently multifocal and most often involve the posterolateral part of the gland.
- Seventy per cent arise in the peripheral zone of the prostate.
- Rare variations include mucinous, signet-ring, small cell, squamous cell, adenoid cystic, and endometrioid carcinoma. With the exception of mucinous and adenoid cystic carcinomas, prognosis tends to be poor. Squamous cell and endometrioid carcinomas are characterized by a normal PSA and lack of hormone response.
- Transitional cell carcinoma of the prostatic urethra may occur and there are rare reports of secondary spread from other tumours such as melanoma and lung cancer.

Gleason grade
The Gleason grading system, developed in the early 1970s, is used to describe the degree of differentiation and cytological atypia of the malignant cells. Each tumour is graded twice, each out of five to give a total score out of ten—the first grade relates to the most commonly

observed pattern (primary pattern) and the second to the next most common pattern (see Table 8.8.1). This scoring system allows for the heterogeneity and multifocality of prostate cancer. The major pattern has prognostic significance—patients with Gleason 3+4 tend to do better than those with 4+3.

Table 8.8.1 Summary of Gleason grading

1	Well differentiated; uniform gland pattern
2	Well differentiated; glands variable
3	Moderately differentiated; papillary/cribriform features or well-spaced acini
4	Poorly differentiated; cords, sheets, fused cells
5	Very poorly differentiated; minimal gland formation, necrosis

8.9 Clinical features, diagnosis, staging, natural history, screening, and prognosis of prostate cancer

Clinical features

- The majority of prostate cancers are initially detected following a raised serum PSA level, either as a result of investigations into non-specific lower urinary tract symptoms of bladder outflow obstruction such as hesitancy, frequency, nocturia, and terminal dribbling, or increasingly as part of a well-man screening programme.
- Approximately half of patients are completely asymptomatic.
- In symptomatic patients who require a transurethral resection of the prostate (TURP) for presumed benign prostatic hypertrophy, it is not uncommon to discover cancer cells in the prostatic chippings.

Locally advanced cancers can be detected on rectal examination, and occasionally patients may present with symptoms due to local extension such as pain, bleeding, or impotence. Metastases to bone are common and bone pain or pathological fracture can be presenting features, although this is becoming less frequent due to better availability of PSA testing. Occasionally patients will present with weakness or paraesthesia due to spinal cord or nerve root compression from vertebral metastases. Other areas of spread include obturator, perivesical, and para-aortic lymph nodes and rarely liver, lung, or brain metastases. It is unusual for patients to present with symptoms related to metastases in these areas.

Diagnosis

- Initial investigations should include a PSA blood test and digital rectal examination (DRE).
- Patients with raised PSA or suspicious examination may be offered transrectal ultrasound-guided biopsy (TRUS biopsy) of the prostate to obtain histological diagnosis.
- If clinical suspicion of advanced disease is high, with markedly raised PSA levels and evidence of metastases on imaging, then TRUS biopsy is not necessary to confirm the diagnosis.
- Not all men with a raised PSA level require a biopsy. There has been a tendency to over-investigate modestly raised PSA levels, resulting in overdiagnosis of clinically insignificant prostate cancer. The large Prostate Cancer Prevention Trial (PCPT) showed that low-grade prostate cancers were also common in men with normal PSA levels. The aim of histological diagnosis of prostate cancer is to be able to offer treatment to those cancers which might impact on patients' life expectancy. Predictive models have been developed that define the need for biopsy. The PCPT identified variables predictive of prostate cancer including higher PSA level, positive family history of prostate cancer, and abnormal DRE result, whilst a previous negative prostate biopsy was associated with reduced risk. Age and PSA velocity did not appear to be predictive in this study. However other models have identified additional predictive factors such as prostate volume and PSA density.
- There is increased evidence for the use of prostate MRI in diagnosis, with the aim of avoiding invasive biopsies. The UK PROMIS study suggests MRI in men presenting with raised PSA levels might avoid the need for biopsy in 27% and also reduce the rate of overdiagnosis.

TRUS biopsy

TRUS biopsy is a short outpatient procedure performed under local anaesthetic. Typically, 8–12 core biopsies are obtained; four to six from each lobe of the prostate, although current guidance supports a minimum of ten cores for histological assessment.

If the biopsy is negative, then the risk factors should be reviewed, including PSA level, PSA density, DRE findings, patient age, and prostate volume. If there is still concern, repeat biopsy is indicated. Various studies have revealed a 10–25% rate of detection of malignancy on second biopsy, although they differ in which of the PSA parameters are predictive of a positive repeat biopsy.

Prostate-specific antigen

As well as the absolute PSA level, various other PSA parameters have been developed in an attempt to improve the predictive value of the test for diagnosis and monitoring:

- PSA density (PSA/volume of gland)—allows for higher PSA levels in older men with large, hypertrophied glands. A value of 0.1ng/ml/cc is considered normal (e.g. a PSA of 5ng/ml with a 50cc prostate volume).
- Percent-free PSA (fPSA)—is the ratio of how much PSA circulates free compared with the total PSA level, including that attached to blood proteins. The percentage of free PSA is lower in men who have prostate cancer than in men who do not and may be useful in determining which patients with intermediate PSA levels should have a prostate biopsy for diagnosis.

Table 8.9.1 Staging of prostate cancer (2016)

Stage	Description		
I	T1a	Not palpable, confined to prostate	Diagnosed on TURP, <5% of chippings involved, Gleason grade 2–4 only
	T1a		Diagnosed on TURP, <5% of chippings involved, Gleason grade 5
	T1b		Diagnosed on TURP, >5% of chippings involved
	T1c		Diagnosed by needle biopsy in response to a raised PSA
	T2a	Palpable, but confined to prostate	Confined to 1 lobe, <50% involved
II	T2b		Confined to 1 lobe, >50% involved
	T2c		Both lobes palpably involved
III	T3a	Breaches prostate capsule	Extension through the prostate capsule
	T3b		Involvement of one or both seminal vesicles
	T4	Local invasion	Invasion of other nearby structures
IV	Any T N1M0		Spread to regional lymph nodes

Reproduced with permission from Brierley JD, Gospodarowicz MK, Wittekind C (eds). *TNM Classification of Malignant Tumours*, 8th edn. Copyright © 2017, John Wiley & Sons.

There is some controversy over where the cut-off should lie, but fPSA levels of <10% are very suspicious.
- PSA kinetics—give an indication of the rate of tumour growth, and include the PSA doubling time, expressed in months or years, and the PSA velocity, expressed as ng/ml/year (this is commonly utilized in patients on active surveillance. To get an accurate indication of PSA velocity, at least three measurements should be taken over a period of 18 months.

Note that very poorly differentiated cancers may not secrete PSA and are therefore more difficult to diagnose, predict, and monitor.

Staging

If cancer is confirmed, further staging investigations are determined by the grade, volume of disease, and PSA level. These investigations are aimed at diagnosing advanced or metastatic disease, which would preclude radical local treatment options (Table 8.9.1).
- Pelvic MRI to define extracapsular spread, seminal vesicle or lymph node involvement, or local extension of disease should be offered to patients in whom radical treatment is being considered with Gleason 4+3 disease or above, those with PSA levels >20ng/ml, or those with clinical T3 or 4 disease on examination. Diffusion-weighted MRI imaging gives better definition of the location of the tumour within the prostate gland and can be helpful in targeting biopsies. For patients unable to tolerate MRI, CT scanning of the pelvis is a reasonable alternative.
- Bone scan is used to detect metastatic bone disease. Bone scans are sensitive but not specific, with a high

rate of false positives. Any equivocal areas should be examined with plain radiographs and/or cross-sectional imaging. At PSA levels of <10ng/ml, the rate of true positive bone scans is <1%, so this investigation should only be requested in patients with PSA levels >10–15ng/ml.

If there is doubt over lymph node involvement on pelvic imaging, a laparoscopic RPLN biopsy might be considered before proposed radical treatment.

Risk stratification

A commonly used risk stratification for biochemical recurrence of localized disease is into low-, intermediate-, and high-risk based on PSA, Gleason score, and clinical stage (Table 8.9.2). Patients with locally advanced disease (cT3–4 or CN+) are considered as high risk irrespective of PSA level and Gleason score.

The strongest predictors of metastasis are a high PSA, high Gleason score (8–10), and age >70 years. The Partin tables, developed in 1997 by urologists at Johns Hopkins University and updated in 2001 (Han et al. 2001), are used in treatment algorithms to predict the risk of local extension and lymph node spread. The Roach formulae, based on the Partin tables, are simple equations that can be used to predict these risks (Roach 1993).

Roach formulae
- Percentage risk of lymph node involvement 2/3 PSA + 10(Gleason −6)
- Percentage risk of seminal vesicle involvement: PSA + 10(Gleason −6)
- Percentage risk of extracapsular extension: 3/2 PSA + 10(Gleason −3)

Table 8.9.2 Risk stratification

Risk	PSA	Gleason score	Clinical stage
Low	<10ng/ml	<6	T1a–T2a
Intermediate	10–20ng/ml	7	T2b or T2c
High	>20mg/ml	8–10	T3 or T4

Natural history

- The natural history of prostate cancer is very variable and is poorly understood.
- Low-grade tumours tend to follow an indolent course, whilst higher grade tumours present more risk of local extension and metastatic spread.
- For localized low-intermediate Gleason grade disease the first decision to be made is whether to treat radically or to initially plan a period of surveillance, with regular PSA monitoring and rectal examination. Many of these tumours might never progress to a point that they influence life expectancy, particularly in elderly patients.
- Cohort studies of untreated prostate cancer reveal that the majority of tumours follow an indolent course over the first ten years with prostate cancer-specific survival rates of approximately 80%, but by 15–20 years deaths due to prostate cancer become more common (cancer specific survival of approximately 50%).
- For this reason if a patient has a life expectancy of more than ten years due to age or comorbidity, then it is reasonable to defer radical treatment in the first instance.
- For tumours that do spread, local invasion is usually into the seminal vesicles, directly through the capsule of the prostate or, for transitional zone tumours, into the bladder neck. Metastases are most often to bone and pelvic lymph nodes.
- With the wider use of screening, there are more small, low-grade tumours being diagnosed in younger men and the natural history of these tumours in this group of patients is particularly poorly understood.

Screening

- Screening for prostate cancer principally employs PSA testing and/or DRE, with the aim of early detection of malignant disease.
- Various applications have been utilized to suggest the need for further investigation, including absolute PSA level (for example >4ng/ml), age-specific PSA, or per cent-free PSA.
- However, there is no convincing evidence that earlier detection and treatment of prostate cancer leads to improvements in mortality.
- There is potential harm associated with screening. False positive PSA tests have been shown to cause psychological harm for up to a year after the testing. Also many patients with low-risk cancer may end up having aggressive and debilitating treatment for limited or no benefit.
- The American Cancer Society recommends that men make an informed decision with their doctor about whether to be tested for prostate cancer. Screening for prostate cancer is not recommended in men aged 75 years or over.
- These statements are based on cross-sectional and cohort data only. Three large-scale randomized trials have been carried out and the long-term follow-up results are being analyzed.
- The European Randomised Study of Screening for Prostate Cancer (ERSPC) is the largest of these studies aiming to determine whether early detection and treatment of prostate cancer will lead to a reduction in mortality; 180,000 participants from eight European countries are randomized between PSA screening (with or without DRE) or no screening. A third analysis was published in 2014 at 13 years' follow-up. Although it revealed a 21% reduction in prostate cancer mortality in the screening group, the findings were not felt to be sufficient to justify population-based screening due to a number needed to diagnose (NND) of 27 to avert one prostate cancer death.
- The large US screening trial is the prostate, lung, colorectal, and ovarian screening programme (PLCO study), which undertakes annual PSA screening and DRE for five years along with screening tests for the other tumour types. This study recruited 154,000 men and women in 1992–2001, half of whom were allocated screening tests and half received routine care as a control group. This study had relatively few prostate cancer deaths and there was insufficient power to compare death rates for the follow-up period. Also the study was weakened by the fact that over half of patients in the control group actually underwent PSA testing during the study period.
- In the UK, the PROTECT study aims to evaluate the effectiveness, acceptability, and cost-effectiveness of treatments for men with localized prostate cancer and involves >100,000 men. Participants were recruited before diagnosis and underwent a screening programme, with the offer of randomization between active surveillance, radiotherapy, and surgery on detection of an abnormal PSA and diagnosis of prostate cancer. This study is unique in that it evaluates both the utility of screening and the relative benefits of different treatment approaches.

Prognosis

- Figures for survival from prostate cancer vary widely, depending on histology, stage, PSA level, and therapeutic intervention.
- The Partin tables, based on PSA level, Gleason score, and clinical stage, remain the best method of predicting spread and prognosis of prostate cancer.
- For well differentiated tumours, the risk of developing metastases at ten years is <20%.
- Patients with localized disease treated with either radiotherapy or radical surgery have five-year biochemical control rates of 75–85% and ten-year OS rates of 60–70%.
- Patients with metastatic disease can survive for many years, particularly if the tumours are endocrine-responsive and if the metastatic spread is confined to the bones.
- There is some evidence that particular genetic polymorphisms influence prognosis. Polymorphisms affecting alleles of insulin-like growth factor 1 and cytochrome p450 may be associated with a worse outcome. Other polymorphisms (such as transforming growth factor β1 (TGFB1)) may be protective.

Further reading

Han M, Partin AW, Pound CR, Epstein JI, Walsh PC. Long-term biochemical disease-free and cancer-specific survival following anatomic radical retropubic prostatectomy. The 15-year Johns Hopkins experience. *Urol Clin North Am* 2001 Aug;28(3):555–65.

Roach M. Re: The use of prostate specific antigen, clinical stage and Gleason score to predict pathological stage in men with localized prostate cancer. *J Urol* 1993 Dec;150(6):1923–4.

8.10 Treatment of localized disease for prostate cancer

Principles of management

For localized low-intermediate Gleason grade disease the first decision to be made is whether to treat radically or to initially plan a period of surveillance. Patients with high-grade localized disease should be offered radical treatments if fit. Radical treatment options for prostate cancer include radical prostatectomy, EBRT, and brachytherapy (low-dose rate or high-dose rate). Each treatment has its own characteristics and may be suitable for certain types of patients, but reported success rates are similar if patients are chosen appropriately.

Active surveillance

Many patients will have slow-growing disease that might have little or no impact on their life expectancy, and they might therefore be spared the toxicities and inconvenience of radical treatment. Active surveillance implies close monitoring with early curative treatment offered to patients who show signs of progression (Table 8.10.1).

There are no absolute criteria for considering active surveillance, but initial studies used the following parameters: T1–T2b disease, Gleason grade 7, and PSA 15 (with favourable kinetics). The approach is most suited, however, to those with the following characteristics:

- T1b/c disease
- Gleason 3+3
- PSA density of <0.15ng/ml
- Less than 50% of cores involved

A typical surveillance programme consists of three-monthly visits for the first two years, followed by six-monthly visits thereafter, with a DRE and PSA checked at each visit. Repeat transrectal biopsies should be performed at 18 months. Criteria for consideration of radical treatment would be PSA progression (doubling time <2 years), clinical progression, or upgrading of the Gleason score on repeat biopsy. Increasingly MRI scanning is being built in to surveillance programmes in addition to or in place of repeat biopsies, particularly if the tumour is well-visualized on the baseline MRI investigation.

The concept of active surveillance was first reported by a group from Toronto in 2001 (Choo et al. 2001). After a median follow-up of 29 months, more than three-quarters of men remained under surveillance without progressing on to radical treatment. Similar results were confirmed from a UK series from the mid-1990s, where median PSA doubling time was found to be approximately 12 years, suggesting an indolent course of disease in many men. Prospective studies of active surveillance are underway, but preliminary results suggest that only around 20% of patients will require radical

treatment. The PROTECT study randomizes suitable patients between active surveillance, primary surgery, or radiotherapy.

Watchful waiting

The approach of watchful waiting is distinct from active surveillance. Patients deemed unsuitable for radical treatment are watched before being treated with endocrine therapy upon symptomatic progression. It is usually reserved for elderly or unfit patients who are thought unlikely to suffer significant cancer progression during their expected lifespan.

Radical prostatectomy

- Radical prostatectomy is often considered the definitive treatment for localized prostate cancer.
- Perineal, retropubic, or laparoscopic approaches can be considered.
- Of the open techniques, the perineal approach gives better access to the urethra and less blood loss, whilst the retropubic approach allows lymph node staging and better nerve sparing. There have been suggestions that the perineal approach might result in positive surgical margins more commonly than the retropubic approach, but this has not been confirmed.
- Robotic-assisted laparoscopic surgery is becoming increasingly popular. Short-term functional and PSA-related outcomes compare favourably with standard surgical approaches, but long-term data are not yet available.
- Surgical series of prostatectomies for organ confined disease report five-year PSA-free survival rates of 69–84% with ten-year rates of 47–75%.
- Surgery is generally discouraged for T3 disease due to the risk of positive surgical margins and lymph node metastases, although there is a move to recommend surgery followed by immediate adjuvant radiotherapy in this group of patients. It should also be noted that there is a degree of overstaging, particularly with the prediction of seminal vesicle invasion on MRI—approximately 25% of patients thought to be T3 will in fact be T2 and therefore achieve good biochemical control from radical prostatectomy.
- There is a 5–15% risk of significant urinary dysfunction after surgery (stress incontinence, urine leak, or fistulas).
- Nerve-sparing techniques have improved morbidity, with approximately 50% impotence rates, but these are very much surgeon-dependent and not appropriate for patients with high risk of extracapsular disease.

Radical radiotherapy

Radical radiotherapy is an alternative to surgery in localized prostate cancer. There are two small randomized trials comparing surgery and radiotherapy, but these suffer from methodological problems and relatively small numbers of participants. Historical series suggest similar success rates in terms of PSA control.

Radiotherapy techniques

Conformal CT planning has been well established in prostate radiotherapy for many years. Patients are scanned

Table 8.10.1 Active surveillance

Advantages	Disadvantages
Better quality of life	Risk of progression or metastases
Avoids treatment side effects	Anxiety of living with untreated cancer
Cost savings if treatment expensive	Regular follow-up and re-biopsy
	Optimal schedule not established

with an empty rectum (to minimize variation in prostate position) and target volumes are defined on CT. The clinical target volume (CTV) includes the whole prostate and any tumour extension. The seminal vesicles are generally included for intermediate/high-risk patients (based on clinical stage, Gleason grade, and PSA). The CTV is expanded by 1cm in all directions to give the planning target volume (PTV). A second phase of treatment is planned with reduced margins of 0.5cm.

Conformal planning enabled escalation of doses from 64–66Gy in 32–33 fractions to 74–78Gy in 37–39 fractions, whilst remaining within predefined tolerance doses to the rectum and bladder. Various studies have shown that improved local control is achieved with dose escalation. The Medical Research Council RT01 study randomized between 64Gy and 74Gy and found a hazard ratio for biochemical PFS of 0.67 in favour of the escalated group. However, this was achieved at the expense of increased late bowel and bladder toxicity (Dearnley et al. 2007). Similarly an MD Anderson study found significantly better five-year PSA control with 78Gy delivered conformally than with conventional 70Gy dose (Zelefsky et al. 1998). It is not yet known whether there will be any improvements in OS, but doses of 74–78Gy in 2Gy fractions came to be considered the best standard.

Typical rectal tolerance doses are 55.5Gy to no more than 50%, 70Gy to no more than 25%, and 74Gy to no more than 3% of the rectum. Less than 50% of the bladder should receive 67Gy.

Newer techniques such as intensity-modulated radiotherapy (IMRT) enable further sparing of normal tissues, potentially allowing further escalation of the dose to the target volume. IMRT is now the standard technique for delivering radical prostate cancer radiotherapy and in the UK there has been significant resource input at a national level to enable this.

Image-guided radiotherapy (IGRT) involves tracking the target volume and position of the prostate through a course of treatment to ensure that the target remains within the planned volumes. This can be done with regular scanning and soft tissue matching, or more accurately with the insertion of radio-opaque markers into the prostate prior to the treatment starting (fiducial markers). This might enable tighter margins and hence less normal tissue damage, but care should be taken to avoid being too tight and increasing the risk of marginal or local recurrence.

Radiobiological studies have suggested a surprisingly low alpha-beta ratio for prostate cancer (1.2–1.5Gy), which implies that hypofractionated courses of radiotherapy with a high dose per fraction might result in improved cancer control for a similar level of side effects. For this reason, doses such as 57–60Gy in 19–20 fractions over four weeks were investigated. These shortened schedules have the additional advantage of sparing resources and being more convenient for patients. The CHHiP trial compared 74Gy in 37 fractions with two different hypofractionated schedules (60Gy in 20 fractions and 57Gy in 19 fractions). Over 3,000 men were recruited. There were no significant differences in five-year biochemical or disease-free recurrence rates for the 60Gy in 20 fractions regimen when compared with the standard schedule and, although there was a slightly earlier peak in bladder and bowel toxicity with

the shorter schedule, by 18 weeks the side effect profiles were similar. This has now been adopted as the standard across much of the UK.

For patients with poor prognostic risk factors and a high risk of pelvic lymph node involvement (15% on Roach criteria), it is worth considering a larger first phase of treatment to include the pelvic nodes to a dose of 50Gy in 25 fractions, followed by a second phase of treatment to the prostate itself of 18–24Gy in 9–12 fractions, although any survival benefit from this approach remains to be demonstrated.

Acute side effects of radiotherapy include dysuria, frequency, diarrhoea, lethargy, and erythema. Late effects include proctitis (diarrhoea, rectal bleeding, tenesmus: 30% mild, 5% severe), impotence (30–40%), and urinary incontinence (1–5%). If radiation is given to large pelvic fields, there is a risk of small bowel damage.

Brachytherapy
Low-dose rate (LDR) brachytherapy
Permanent radioactive seeds are implanted directly into the prostate via transperineal needles that are inserted with ultrasound guidance under general or spinal anaesthetic. Approximately 50–100 iodine-125 or palladium-103 seeds are implanted to achieve a prescribed dose of 145Gy. Patients are not suitable for LDR brachytherapy if the prostate is large (>50cc), if they have had a previous TURP or if they are at high risk of extracapsular extension or lymph node involvement. Generally, this technique is restricted to Gleason 6, PSA15, T2 or less disease—a similar group to those suitable for active surveillance. Patients should have a TRUS volume study to assess suitability for brachytherapy.

Although there is good evidence to confirm the efficacy of brachytherapy in terms of PSA control and biopsy findings, there are as yet no long-term survival data. The procedure has not been directly compared with external beam radiotherapy or radical surgery in randomized studies, but comparative and cohort studies show similar five-year biochemical recurrence-free survival and OS. The incidence of adverse events also appears to be similar to radiotherapy and prostatectomy.

High-dose rate (HDR) brachytherapy
HDR brachytherapy is suitable for intermediate–high-risk patients—a similar group to those suitable for large-field pelvic radiotherapy with prostate second phase. It is typically given as a boost followed by a shortened course of EBRT but can also be used as monotherapy. Treatment is delivered via catheters implanted with ultrasound guidance into the prostate under general anaesthetic. The catheter positions are confirmed on CT scanning and target volumes are contoured, along with the urethra and rectum as organs at risk. Dwell positions for the radioactive source are defined and an individual treatment plan is produced. HDR boost patients are typically treated in two or three fractions, six to 12 hours apart, often necessitating overnight stay with the catheters and template in situ. Typical doses are 17Gy in two fractions of HDR followed by 46Gy in 23 fractions of EBRT to the pelvis, but there is considerable regional variation.

Cryotherapy
Cryotherapy is a minimally invasive technique in which the prostate is frozen to temperatures of −140°C with

argon gas. Needles are inserted into the prostate through the perineum in a similar fashion to brachytherapy. A warming catheter is used throughout the procedure to protect the urethra, and particular attention should be paid to temperatures around the wall of the rectum. There is no long-term evidence of the success of cryotherapy as primary treatment of prostate cancer, with the literature restricted to short follow-up case series. However, reported biochemical control rates are good. Impotence rates are high at around 80% and there is a small (1–2%) risk of rectal perforation. Cryotherapy is not widely used as an initial treatment for localized prostate cancer, its use being mainly restricted to salvage therapy after previous radiotherapy.

High intensity frequency ultrasound (HIFU)
HIFU is administered via a transrectal probe, causing the prostate to heat to very high temperatures leading to cell death. As with cryotherapy, long-term outcome data is poor and reports are limited to relatively small case series. The most commonly reported side effects are urinary tract infection, impotence, and incontinence. Within the UK its use is mainly restricted to post-radiotherapy salvage treatment.

Role of endocrine therapy in localized disease

Neoadjuvant hormones
Patients undergoing radical radiotherapy are commonly treated with three months of neoadjuvant luteinizing hormone releasing hormone (LHRH) analogues. This approach may enable a reduction in the volume of tissue irradiated due to shrinkage of the prostate gland.

An RTOG study by Pilepich et al. (2001) looked at the role of androgen deprivation for two months before and during radiotherapy. Interestingly, the improvements in biochemical DFS and OS were confined to the better prognosis patients with low-grade disease (Gleason 6). Nevertheless, most institutions treat all radical radiotherapy patients with a period of neoadjuvant LHRH analogues.

The role of neoadjuvant endocrine therapy prior to radical prostatectomy is more controversial. A Cochrane review showed no overall or DFS advantage, but there were improvements in pathological variables such as organ-confined and clear margin rates.

Adjuvant hormones
There is good evidence of a benefit with prolonged endocrine manipulation in patients with locally advanced prostate cancer. An EORTC study (Bolla et al. 1997) compared radiotherapy alone versus radiotherapy with immediate androgen suppression started on the first day of radiotherapy and continued for three years. Five-year clinical DFS was 40% vs. 74% and OS was 62% vs. 78% in favour of the adjuvant endocrine group.

Prolonged adjuvant treatment for two to three years should be offered to all patients with high-risk disease (Gleason 8–10, clinical T3/4 tumours, or lymph node risk >30%). It may be that 18 months is sufficient, particularly if patients are struggling with the side effects of testosterone suppression. The role in low- and intermediate-risk patients is being assessed in randomized studies, but these patients are frequently treated with three to six months of LHRH analogues before and during radiotherapy.

It should be noted that LHRH analogues are not without side effects and can add considerably to the morbidity of patients undergoing radiotherapy.

There is no established role for adjuvant hormonal manipulation in patients undergoing radical prostatectomy, although the Cochrane review does suggest a benefit in DFS.

Postoperative adjuvant radiotherapy
There is increasing interest in the role of adjuvant radiotherapy to the prostatic bed following radical prostatectomy for patients with high-risk disease, particularly if there are positive surgical margins or if the PSA fails to suppress completely after surgery. Results from a randomized clinical trial have shown that adjuvant radiotherapy given after radical surgery for pathological T3N0M0 significantly reduces risk of metastasis by 29%, improves survival by 28%, and median survival by 1.9 years. We await the results of a UK study looking at immediate adjuvant radiotherapy versus deferred treatment on PSA relapse.

Further reading

Bolla M, Gonzalez D, Warde P, Dubois JB, Mirimanoff RO, et al. Improved survival in patients with locally advanced prostate cancer treated with radiotherapy and goserelin. *N Engl J Med* 1997 Jul 31; 337(5):295–300—available at: https://www.ncbi.nlm.nih.gov/pubmed/9233866

Choo R, DeBoer G, Klotz L, et al. PSA doubling time of prostate carcinoma managed with watchful observation alone. *Int J Radiat Oncol Biol Phys* 2001; 50:615–20.

Dearnley DP, Sydes MR, Langley, et al. Escalated-dose versus standard-dose conformal radiotherapy in prostate cancer: first results from the MRC RT01 randomised controlled trial. *Lancet Oncol* 2007; 8(6):475–87.

Pilepich MV, Winter K, John MJ, Mesic JB, Sause W, et al. From Clinical Guidelines Wiki. Citation. Phase III radiation therapy oncology group (RTOG) trial 86-10 of androgen deprivation adjuvant to definitive radiotherapy. *Intl J Radiat Oncol Biol Phys* 2001 Aug 1; 50(5):1243–52—available at: http://www.ncbi.nlm.nih.gov/pubmed/11483335

Zelefsky MJ, Leibel SA, Graham JD, et al. Dose escalation with three-dimensional conformal radiation therapy affects the outcome in prostate cancer. *Int J Radiat Oncol Biol Phys* 1998; 41(3):491–500.

8.11 Treatment of advanced disease for prostate cancer

Principles of management
- For patients with locally advanced disease and a high risk of micrometastases it is appropriate to offer primary endocrine therapy.
- Radical radiotherapy or surgery may add little or no additional benefit over hormone therapy alone in patients with T3b disease, a baseline PSA>50ng/ml, or those who are elderly or have significant comorbidities.
- Treatment in the advanced or metastatic setting is aimed at controlling the disease, symptoms, and PSA levels. It is sensible therefore to work through the treatment options systematically with the aim of maximizing the benefit obtained from each step

First-line treatment
- Treatment can be with surgical castration, LHRH analogues, or anti-androgens. Typically, LHRH analogues such as goserelin, leuprolide, or triptorelin are used in the first instance.
- LHRH analogues effectively reduce testosterone levels by eliminating the hormonal signals for its production. There are various formulations available, given by subcutaneous implants or injections.
- When commencing LHRH analogues, there is an initial release of testosterone ('flare') and patients should therefore be given anti-androgens for seven to ten days before the first LHRH analogue injection and continued for two weeks afterwards.
- Prolonged treatment with LHRH analogues results in significant toxicity due to reduction of testosterone levels. Side effects include hot flushes, weakness/loss of muscle bulk, weight gain, fatigue, osteoporosis/fracture risk, loss of libido and erectile function, lipid abnormalities, mood changes, poor concentration/memory, and disordered glucose metabolism.
- Management of hot flushes is often difficult but the following approaches have been tried with varying degrees of success: cyproterone acetate, diethylstilboestrol, megestrol acetate, clonidine, homeopathic remedies, sage, and selective serotonin reuptake inhibitors (SSRIs).
- Androgen receptor inhibitors, such as bicalutamide, effectively reduce the delivery of testosterone to the prostate without reducing serum testosterone levels and therefore tend to have a better side effect profile, although they can cause significant gynaecomastia and mastalgia. Erectile function is often maintained. However, evidence suggests they are less effective than LHRH analogues in terms of OS in metastatic disease, and so bicalutamide monotherapy is currently only licensed for use in locally advanced prostate cancer.
- Prophylactic radiotherapy to the breast buds or prophylactic tamoxifen 10–20mg/day can reduce and sometimes prevent the painful gynaecomastia. Typical radiotherapy doses are 8–8Gy in a single fraction or 15Gy in three fractions given on alternate days, using electron radiotherapy delivered to an 8–10cm circle around each nipple.
- First-line hormonal therapy is generally continued until there is evidence of intolerance or progression of disease, either with the development of new symptoms or PSA progression. There is no consensus on

the extent of rise in PSA which should trigger a change in treatment, but a doubling time of less than six months is a cause for concern.
- The typical duration of response to first-line endocrine therapy with LHRH analogues is 18–24 months.

Intermittent therapy
There is interest in intermittent endocrine therapy in patients established on treatment with good disease control. This has three possible benefits: patients are spared the side effects of treatment for a period of time, there is a cost saving, and also the potential of extending the period of efficacy of first-line therapy. Trials are ongoing but a systematic review of five small randomized studies showed no difference in survival but an improved quality of life when compared with continuous therapy. Patients spent a median of one year off endocrine treatment. A typical approach is to discontinue the LHRH analogue once the PSA has stabilized at a nadir (<4ng/ml) and restart when it rises above 10ng/ml.

Early chemotherapy
Traditionally reserved for castration-resistant prostate cancer, there is now good evidence from two large studies (STAMPEDE and CHAARTED) which suggests a significant survival benefit in favour of upfront docetaxel chemotherapy alongside the LHRH analogue. The STAMPEDE study showed a 22-month survival benefit in metastatic patients treated with early chemotherapy. This should be considered, particularly in younger men presenting with metastatic disease, although in the studies even those with no overt metastases but high presenting PSA levels or other adverse features were seen to benefit.

Second- and third-line treatments
- After failure of first-line LHRH analogue endocrine treatment (clinical or biochemical progression), the next step is combined or complete androgen blockade (CAB) or maximal androgen blockade (MAB) with the addition of anti-androgen therapy (e.g. 50mg of bicalutamide daily).
- Synthetic oestrogens such as diethylstilboestrol can result in a PSA response in patients failing CAB. There is a risk of thrombosis with oestrogen therapy—it is best avoided in men with a significant cardiovascular history, and in any case should be given with aspirin.

Hormone refractory disease
- There is no universally agreed definition of hormone refractory prostate cancer (HRPC), which usually is designated when combined androgen blockade is failing to control the PSA or symptoms.
- Even when disease is classed as hormone refractory, the LHRH analogue is continued. There is often still some activity of the androgen receptor on the cancer cells and stopping the androgen deprivation is likely to speed up the progression of the disease.
- Docetaxel is now well-established in this setting, with studies showing quality of life and OS benefits (in the region of 10–12 weeks) when compared with the previous standard regimen of mitoxantrone and prednisolone. It is unclear how the recent STAMPEDE trial

results will impact on the positioning of chemotherapy in future treatment pathways.

- Updated survival analysis of the TAX327 study, which randomized between three-weekly docetaxel, weekly docetaxel, and mitoxantrone (all given with prednisolone) showed OS figures of 19.2, 17.8, and 16.3 months respectively (Berthold et al. 2008).
- Doses of 75mg/m^2 of docetaxel are administered on a three-weekly basis for up to ten cycles.
- Low-dose oral steroids are typically given with the chemotherapy (prednisolone 5mg twice daily).
- Although low-grade neutropenia is fairly common, the rate of febrile neutropenic sepsis is surprisingly low (<3%) without need for granulocyte colony-stimulating factor support.
- There is also interest in second-line chemotherapy after failure of docetaxel. There is evidence of benefit from cabazitaxel in this setting. It does have a risk of neutropaenia and sepsis but is often well-tolerated and responses have been observed in patients who fail to respond to docetaxel.
- Abiraterone, an orally active inhibitor of 17alpha-monooxygenase (a member of the cytochrome p450 family), effectively suppresses testosterone production by both the testes and the adrenals to castrate levels. Abiraterone is administered with prednisolone to prevent symptoms of mineralocorticioid excess due to diversion of the steroid synthesis pathways. It is effective and licensed for use in metastatic castration-resistant prostate cancer both in chemotherapy-naïve and in post-docetaxel patients. In the post-chemotherapy COU-AA-301 study, OS was improved from 11.2 to 15.8 months when compared with steroids plus placebo. There were also significant improvements in PSA response, progression-free survival, and time to PSA progression. In a chemotherapy naïve study there was a 4.4-month survival benefit despite a high rate of crossover and subsequent therapies on progression. Side effects include hypertension, hypokalaemia, liver test abnormalities, and fluid retention, but it is generally well-tolerated. As with docetaxel chemotherapy, there is interest in bringing this forward in the treatment pathway to the hormone-sensitive metastatic setting rather than waiting for castration-resistance. The STAMPEDE trial showed similar survival benefits, although economically the cost of upfront abiraterone is much more significant due to its continuous nature and drug costs compared with six cycles of chemotherapy.

- Enzalutamide is a novel androgen-receptor signalling inhibitor with similar indications and benefits to abiraterone in the CRPC setting. In the post-chemotherapy setting, the AFFIRM trial revealed a 4.8 month OS benefit. It has the advantage that it can be given without concurrent steroids. The main side effect encountered in clinical practice is fatigue and a detrimental effect on concentration.
- Radium-223 is a radioisotope which localizes to bone. It is administered intravenously, usually monthly for six months, and can be effective in patients with multiple bone metastases, both in controlling or preventing bone symptoms and in improving OS. Side effects include gastrointestinal disturbance, fatigue, and bone marrow suppression.
- In patients not suitable for chemotherapy or who have been heavily pretreated, low-dose corticosteroids may be used. These can cause a fall in PSA levels (due to reduction in adrenal androgen production) and also have symptomatic benefits due to their anti-inflammatory effect and appetite stimulation.

Further reading

Berthold DR, Pond GR, Soban F, de Wit R, et al. Docetaxel plus prednisone or mitoxantrone plus prednisone for advanced prostate cancer: updated survival in the TAX 327 study. *J Clin Oncol* 2008 Jan 10; 26(2):242–5.

8.12 Detection and treatment of recurrence of prostate cancer

Significance of early detection of recurrence

- Following radical treatment with surgery, radiotherapy, or brachytherapy, disease will recur in a proportion of patients. This is often first detected with a rise in PSA levels following a post-treatment nadir.
- If the disease recurrence is localized to the prostate or prostate bed, there is potential for further curative interventions.
- Early detection of recurrence is therefore important to enable prompt salvage therapy in appropriate patients.

Postoperative recurrence

- A substantial proportion of patients who have undergone a radical prostatectomy (RP) for localized prostate cancer will have either persistently detectable PSA levels or a delayed rise in PSA. Approximately 25–40% of patients will experience recurrence after RP, manifested by a rising PSA, often without clinical or radiological evidence of disease.

- The optimum treatment for these situations is not known. The key question is whether the PSA is reflective of local or distant progression.
- For salvage radiotherapy to be most effective, treatment should be considered before the PSA is allowed to rise too high, when disease is more likely to be confined to the prostate bed. However, at low PSA levels, current imaging techniques are poor at detecting disease, making it difficult to differentiate local or distant recurrence and to target the radiotherapy appropriately.
- Theoretically any detectable level and/or rising PSA after RP should be considered as persistent or recurrent disease. The precise definition of biochemical failure varies from study to study. Though previous studies have suggested a threshold of 0.4ng/ml for biochemical failure, more recent work suggests that a PSA of >0.2ng/ml is an appropriate threshold to define PSA recurrence since these patients had a three-year PSA progression of 100%.

- A European Consensus statement on the management of PSA relapse in patients with prostate cancer defined PSA relapse after RP as a value of 0.2ng/ml with one subsequent rise.
- Ultrasensitive PSA assays that detect serum PSA levels of <0.01ng/ml may detect relapse several months or even years earlier than conventional assays, but the clinical utility is limited by higher rates of false positive results.
- Although biochemical recurrence is accepted as a surrogate endpoint for defining treatment outcome and as an indication for salvage treatment, the clinical significance in terms of OS and clinical DFS remains unclear. Even in men who develop biochemical recurrence, clinical progression may take many years to manifest and hence the benefit of local treatment in terms of prostate cancer-specific mortality is questionable. In one series of 1,132 patients, those with rising serum PSA after RP had a ten-year survival rate of 88% compared to 93% of those without biochemical recurrence.
- Current practice is to treat with salvage radiotherapy for a rising PSA, without the need for imaging or biopsy evidence of local recurrence, accepting that current techniques may not be sensitive enough to detect small volume local disease. Imaging is primarily aimed at excluding metastatic disease and hence patients who would not benefit from salvage radiotherapy. Current evidence suggests that bone scan and pelvic nodal assessment with CT or MRI should not be performed prior to commencing radiotherapy unless the PSA velocity is rapid, although there is no well-defined cut-off value. Functional imaging techniques such as PET or antibody scintigraphy may prove useful in identifying patients with early metastatic disease not evident on current standard techniques and these warrant further investigation.

Treatment of persistent PSA elevation

- It is not clear whether selective adjuvant radiotherapy for high-risk patients after RP is better than salvage radiotherapy for patients who develop biochemical relapse at a later date.
- This issue was addressed by a comparative study of postprostatectomy radiotherapy from two institutions, one adopting a prospective policy of adjuvant radiotherapy and the other salvage radiotherapy. The salvage group underwent radiotherapy after longer postoperative intervals (median, 40.3 months vs. 2.9 months; P<0.0001) and had higher PSA values before starting radiotherapy (4.5 vs. 0.86ng/ml; P=0.003), but radiotherapy was equally effective in either salvage or adjuvant setting when the pre-radiotherapy PSA level was <1ng/ml.
- The UK RADICALS study addresses this issue further. It is open to patients following radical prostatectomy where there is uncertainty about the need for postoperative radiotherapy. Patients are randomized between immediate radiotherapy to the prostate bed and delayed radiotherapy on PSA relapse. A second randomization amongst patients receiving radiotherapy is between no androgen deprivation therapy versus short-term (four months) and long-term (two years)

endocrine treatment. Given the uncertainty around adjuvant and salvage treatment following prostatectomy, eligible patients should be encouraged to take part in this study.

Salvage radiotherapy technique

- A CT scan of the pelvis is obtained for treatment planning and a three-dimensional conformal radiotherapy technique is used. The preoperative CT scan and the location of surgical clips in the fossa of the prostate and seminal vesicles are used to help define the CTV.
- CTV includes the prostatic bed, periprostatic tissue, and any residual seminal vesicle. In the majority of series, pelvic lymph nodes are not included in the CTV.
- The PTV for salvage radiotherapy includes a 1–1.5cm margin on the CTV. A lesser margin may be acceptable posteriorly for optimal sparing of rectum.
- After prostatectomy the bladder neck is pulled down into the prostatic fossa. Periprostatic bed surgical clips are typically located in the central lower aspect of the prostatic bed (from level with the top of pubic symphysis inferiorly) and in the upper region of the surgical bed (superior to the pubic symphysis and posterior to the bladder where the seminal vesicles are located).
- Radiotherapy dose is often limited by rectal tolerance, but the aim should be to treat to over 60Gy equivalent in 2Gy fractions. Studies have shown better biochemical control if doses of 66Gy and above are obtained and this would be considered standard in the UK.

Post-irradiation recurrence

- The rate of biochemical failure following radiotherapy reported in the literature varies widely (from 20% to 66%). By their very nature these figures are historical and it is difficult to know how they apply to new and improved radiotherapy techniques.
- Local recurrence following radical radiotherapy is more problematic to salvage. Surgery is more difficult due to post-radiation scarring, and many patients who underwent radiotherapy as the primary treatment may have been deemed unsuitable or unwilling for surgery in the first instance.
- There are various definitions of what constitutes a PSA relapse after radical radiotherapy, and for many years failure was defined as three consecutive rises in PSA. The 2005 ASTRO consensus group agreed the standard definition of biochemical failure after RT should be a rise in PSA by 2ng/ml or more above the post-treatment nadir.
- Patients are often offered a prostate biopsy following PSA relapse. It is important that the pathologist is aware the gland has been previously irradiated.
- Prior to considering local salvage therapy, clinically apparent metastases should be excluded using bone scans and pelvic MRI.
- Current salvage options include cryotherapy and HIFU. There are several published series with varying results.
- It is reasonable to consider a period of androgen deprivation prior to salvage therapy (three to six months),

to reduce the size of the gland and potentially decrease procedure-associated morbidity.

Distant recurrence

- In cases of patients with distant recurrence or the patient is not suitable for local salvage therapy, the mainstay of treatment is with endocrine therapy similar to advanced and metastatic disease.
- There is no clearly defined point at which endocrine treatment should be started. Although in practice many patients start endocrine therapy when they are diagnosed with metastatic recurrence, there is probably no detriment in waiting until the absolute PSA level climbs above 10ng/ml, the PSA velocity increases, or the patient becomes symptomatic.
- For patients with recurrence that is well-controlled on endocrine treatment, it is reasonable to consider a long-term policy of intermittent therapy.

8.13 Palliative care and symptom control for prostate cancer

Introduction

The natural history of prostate cancer is such that palliative care may be needed for a long period of time, often overlapping with active interventions as the disease progresses. It is important to involve palliative care services at an appropriate time and not to wait for the end-of-life setting.

Bone metastases

Radiotherapy

- EBRT is effective in controlling pain from bone metastases in approximately 80% of instances.
- Typical doses are 20Gy in five fractions or a single fraction of 8Gy. A trial comparing single and multiple fraction regimens found no difference in the speed of onset or duration of pain relief achieved.
- Re-irradiation to the same site at a later date is worth considering, particularly if the first treatment gave significant benefit.
- Prophylactic antiemetics should be given when large-field radiotherapy is used.

Bisphosphonates

- A systematic review of ten randomized trials reveals that the benefit of bisphosphonates in metastatic prostate cancer is unclear. Many of the trials were small and the outcomes measured were different.
- Only one trial (using zoledronic acid) confirmed a modest reduction in skeletal events (an absolute reduction in events of 8% compared with placebo) (Saad et al. 2002). Pamidronate did not reduce the frequency of skeletal events in two trials.
- Of the nine trials which evaluated pain, only one found a significant reduction, although the zoledronic acid trial did not specifically report on pain outcomes.
- It is reasonable to consider bisphosphonates for pain relief when other methods have failed.
- Denosumab, a monoclonal antibody that binds to and inhibits RANK-ligand, is effective in controlling bone pain and preventing skeletal events in a variety of solid tumours including prostate cancer.

Spinal cord compression

Spinal cord compression is a relatively common occurrence in late stage metastatic prostate cancer, and can occasionally be the presenting feature in previously undiagnosed individuals. Urgent MRI scan of the whole spine is indicated if patients present with neurological symptoms consistent with cord compression. Prompt treatment is essential to prevent permanent paralysis.

Decompressive surgery

For patients with previously good PS and relatively few metastases, consider decompressive spinal neurosurgery. If patients are correctly chosen, outcome in terms of function tends to be better following surgery and radiotherapy than following radiotherapy alone. In a randomized trial, significantly more patients were able to walk after the combined treatment (84% vs. 57%) (Patchell et al. 2005).

Radiotherapy

Aim to treat the involved vertebrae plus two vertebrae above and below if possible. Usual doses are 20Gy in five daily fractions. Patients should be started on high-dose steroids (e.g. dexamethasone 8mg twice daily) before commencing radiotherapy, and these can usually be tailed-off gradually on completion of treatment.

Obstructive uropathy

Patients may develop lower urinary tract symptoms due to prostatic enlargement or direct invasion into the base of the bladder or urethra. Flow studies and cystoscopy are appropriate, with a view to proceeding possibly to transurethral resection of the prostate for symptom relief. For men with significant prostatic enlargement and inadequately suppressed testosterone levels, 5-alpha reductase inhibitors may be beneficial. Some patients will require urinary catheters.

In severe cases, there may be significant back pressure, resulting in ureteric dilatation and hydronephrosis, necessitating ureteric stenting or nephrostomies.

Other symptoms

- Haematuria might be due to local invasion by the cancer and can be controlled with palliative doses of radiotherapy to the prostate/bladder. Patients should be examined cystoscopically to exclude other causes of haematuria such as radiation damage or unrelated bladder pathology. Sometimes bleeding points can be cauterized endoscopically.
- Bowel obstruction due to invasion of the prostate cancer is a rare but serious development. In the early stages it might be managed by diet, laxatives, and palliative radiotherapy. If the obstruction becomes more established, then defunctioning colostomy may be required.

Further reading

Parker C, Gillessen S, Heidenreich A, et al. Cancer of the prostate: ESMO clinical practice guidelines for diagnosis, treatment
and follow-up. *Ann Oncol* 2015; 26 (Suppl. 5):v69–77.

Patchell RA, Tibbs PA, Regine WF, et al. Direct decompressive
surgical resection in the treatment of spinal cord compression
caused by metastatic cancer: a randomised trial. *Lancet* 2005;
366(9486):643–8.

Saad F, Gleason DM, Murray R, et al. A randomized, placebo-
controlled trial of zoledronic acid in patients with hormone-refractory metastatic prostate carcinoma. *J Natl Cancer Inst* 2002;
94:1458–68.

Internet resources

European Association of Urology: http://uroweb.org
European Randomized Study of Screening for Prostate Cancer:
http://www.erspc.org
Memorial Sloan–Kettering Cancer Centre Prostate. Cancer
Prediction Nomograms: http://www.mskcc.org/applications/
nomograms/prostate/index.aspx
Partin Tables: http://www.http://urology.jhu.edu/prostate/
partintables.php
STAMPEDE (trial website): http://www.stampedetrial.org/

8.14 Testicular cancer overview

Epidemiology

In Western Europe, the incidence of malignant germ cell
tumours (MGCTs) has been rising by an annual rate of
3% during the last fifty 50 years, corresponding to a
two- to four-fold increased incidence rate.

Incidence of MGCT reveals large geographical variations. In general, the incidence is low in Asia and Africa
and high in Caucasians, especially in the northern part
of Europe, and among North Americans of European
origin. Denmark, Norway, and Sweden are among the
countries with the highest rates of testicular cancer (TC).
Danish or Norwegian males have a three to four times
higher risk to develop a MGCT compared to Finnish
males. TC is now the most frequent malignancy among
Caucasian males at ages 15–40 years.

> **Key points**
> • Most frequent cancer in 15–40-year-old males
> • Caucasians most affected
> • Rising incidence
> • Remarkable geographical variations

Aetiology

Causes for development of MGCT and its rising incidence remain obscure. However, most authorities
consider both genetic and environmental factors as
important.

Genetic factors

Approximately 2% of TC patients have a first-degree
family member who also is affected with this cancer.
The relative risk (RR) is eight to ten between brothers
and four to six between fathers and sons (Rapley 2007).
These RRs exceed those commonly observed in other
cancers (RR: 2–3) and indicate a genetic basis or an
extremely potent, yet unidentified, environmental risk
factor.

However, a large international consortium could not
reveal distinct genes as risk factors for TC. The authors
concluded that no single gene could account for the
substantial familial risk, since probably many genes contribute to the risk of MGCT.

Environmental factors

Despite numerous studies a consensus on the importance of environmental factors for the risk of MGCT
could not be reached yet.

However, substances with oestrogenic and anti-andro-
genic properties, so-called endocrine disrupters, are considered the most relevant substance classes.

Maternal oestrogens and industrial chemicals like pesticides, modified by polymorphic enzymes, might increase
the risk of MGCT development.

> **Key points of this simplified process**
> • Endocrine disrupters and genetic susceptibility
> • Decreased Leydig cell function → androgen
>   insufficiency
> • Disturbed Sertoli cell function → impaired germ cell
>   differentiation
> • Testicular dysgenesis syndrome

The testicular dysgenesis syndrome comprises the fol-
lowing features:
• Poor semen quality
• Cryptorchidism
• Hypospadia
• Testicular cancer

The first three findings are clinically more subtle, probably more prevalent, and not as reliably registered as
testicular cancer. Some authors consider the rising TC incidence as a 'whistle blower' for an increased prevalence
of sub-infertility and genital malformations.

Individuals at high risk

Presence of one or more of the components of the testicular dysgenesis syndrome indicates an increased risk
for TC development.

Cryptorchidism, i.e. the incomplete descent of one or
both testicles at birth, is associated with a seven- to eight-
fold risk to develop TC. Furthermore, sons and brothers
of men with TC are at increased risk to develop MGCT.
The more pronounced increased risk among brothers of
TC patients compared to their sons, might be related to
shared environmental risks.

> **Key points for individuals at risk**
> • Cryptorchidism
> • First-degree relative with TC
> • Poor semen quality/subinfertility

Pathology

Histological examinations should be performed of the
completely laminated testicle and spermatic cord.

In addition to staining with hematoxylin-eosin (HE) immunohistochemistry should be used:
- Mandatory:
  - Alpha fetoprotein (AFP)
  - Human chorionic gonadotropin (HCG)
- Recommended for detection of testicular intraepithelial neoplasia:
  - Placental alkaline phosphatase (PLAP)
  - Oct 3/4

Histology differentiates mainly between:
- Seminoma
- Non-seminoma

Seminoma

Seminoma is composed of homogenous cells and is found in approximately 50% of unselected TC patients (Horwich et al. 2006). Syncytiotrophoblastic cells may be encountered without impact on treatment or prognosis.

Non-seminoma

Non-seminoma can be heterogeneous and may be comprised of one or several components. These components are usually classified according to WHO and the British Tumour Panel which refers to most components as malignant teratoma (MT) (see Table 8.14.1).

The presence of both seminomatous and non-seminomatous components is found in 10–20% of unselected patients. Such combined tumours are treated as non-seminoma.

Teratoma

Teratoma is composed of slow growing somatic cell types of at least two germ layers (ectoderm, endoderm, mesoderm). The daunting variety of encountered structures,

Table 8.14.1 Summary of the classification of non-seminomatous testicular tumour

WHO	British Tumour Panel
Teratoma	Malignant teratoma (MT) differentiated
Embryonal carcinoma	MT undifferentiated
Choriocarcinoma	MT trophoblastic
Teratomacarcinoma	MT intermediate
Yolk sac tumour	Yolk sac tumour

e.g. hair, teeth, cartilage, etc., probably explains its Greek name meaning 'monster tumour'. In pre-pubertal children this testicular tumour is benign and enucleation is sufficient. In adults, however, this non-metastasing tumour is considered malignant due to its potential to grow and undergo malignant transformation into non-germ cell tumours, e.g. rhabdomyosarcoma, adenocarcinoma. Teratoma is resistant to radio- and chemotherapy and is therefore treated surgically. Prognosis does not differ between mature (adult-type differentiation) and immature teratoma (foetal differentiation).

> **Key points**
> - Somatic cell types of at least two germ layers
> - Slow growing
> - May transform into non-germ cell tumours
> - Resistant to radio- and chemotherapy

Embryonal carcinoma

Embryonal carcinoma consists of undifferentiated somatic cells with high metastatic potential. These cells resemble counterparts of human embryonic stem cells with the potential to differentiate into teratoma, choriocarcinoma, or yolk sac tumours. Syncytiotrophoblastic cells may be present but do not impact on treatment or prognosis.

Yolk sac tumours

Yolk sac tumours (synonym: endodermal sinus tumour) usually produce AFP. Pure yolk sac tumours are rarely seen in adults but may be found in mediastinal extragonadal germ cell tumours (EGGCT).

Choriocarcinoma

Choriocarcinoma is composed of syncytiotrophoblasts and cytotrophoblasts which may invade blood vessels, leading to primary extralymphatic metastases, e.g. liver, brain. Hemorrhage may occur with severe complications.

Testicular intraepithelial neoplasia (TIN)

TIN is considered the non-invasive precursor of all testicular MGCTs and is often found in the vicinity of these tumours. Spermatocytic seminoma is an exception to this rule.

Further reading

Horwich A, Shipley J, Huddart R. Testicular germ-cell cancer. Review. *Lancet* 2006; 367(9512):754–65.

Rapley E. Susceptibility alleles for testicular germ cell tumour: a review. *Intl J Androl* 2007; 30(4):242–50—available at: https://doi.org/10.1111/j.1365-2605.2007.00778.x

8.15 Clinical features, diagnosis, TIN, staging, and prognosis for testicular cancer

Clinical features

TC is the most common malignancy in 15–40-year-old males. The cure rate is approximately 90% and treatment of TC is considered a success story of evidence-based medicine.

Most TCs are comprised of malignant germ cell tumour (MGCT).

Typically, the diagnosis of MGCT is made in young men with a large and indolent testicle or a lump in an otherwise normal testicle. Pain may be caused by retroperitoneal lymph-node metastases, and persistent newly developed back pain in younger males should raise suspicion of TC prompting palpation of the testes and CT examination. More rarely, dyspnoea, haemoptysis, or seizures, caused by metastases in lungs and brain, respectively, indicate this disease. Tumours of unknown primary in younger males should always raise the suspicion of MGCT since these tumours are the most frequent solid malignancies in these patients.

> **Key points of clinical presentation of TC**
> - Enlarged painless testicle
> - A lump in an otherwise normal testicle
> - Persistent back pain
> - Gynecomastia or tender breasts
> - Rarely: haemoptysis, supraclavicular mass, or seizures
> - MGCT has to be ruled out in younger males with tumours of unknown primary

MGCT arising outside the testes, i.e. EGGCTs, account for about 2–5% of male MGCT. These tumours are located in the midline of the body in the retroperitoneal space, the anterior mediastinum, or in the brain in the pineal or suprasellar region. Differentiation between metastases from burnt-out testicular MGCT and EGGCT is difficult. In particular retroperitoneal tumours may represent metastatic TC rather than primary malignancies as one-third of patients harbour TIN and another third have testicular scar tissue, indicative of a 'burnt out' TC. Primary mediastinal EGGCTs have a poor prognosis and these tumours are over-represented among men with Klinefelter's syndrome (47 XXY) and Down's syndrome. Hematological malignancies such as megakaryoblastic leukaemia may be associated with these tumours as well.

Treatment initiation should not be delayed in critically ill patients in case of unequivocal elevation of AFP or HCG. If the histological diagnosis is not straightforward, immunohistochemistry and examination of isochromosome 12p should be performed.

> **Key points of EGGCTs**
> - Located in the body's midline (retroperitoneum, mediastinum, or brain)
> - Difficult: TC metastases or EGCCT?
> - Associated with chromosomal alterations
> - If histology not available: AFP↑/HCG↑ strongly supports diagnosis

Diagnosis

Demonstration of a solid testicular mass by ultrasound has to be followed by exploration by biopsies from the tumour, by retraction of the affected testicle through an inguinal incision, and examination of a frozen section.

The histological diagnosis distinguishes primarily between seminoma and non-seminoma which are treated differently.

The following tumour markers may be released by MGCT:
- HCG
- AFP
- Lactate dehydrogenase (LDH)

AFP production only occurs with non-seminoma and a histologically pure seminoma must be considered and treated as non-seminoma if there is no other explanation for the AFP elevation, such as liver disease or chemotherapy toxicity.

> **Key points serum AFP**
> - Normal level: <10μg/l or <14kU/l or <10ng/ml
> - ↑ defines non-seminoma
> - ↑ in 40–60% of non-seminoma patients
> - ↑↑ levels → yolk sac tumour
> - (↑) levels → possibly unrelated to TC, e.g. liver disease
> - Half-life: 5–7 days

HCG may be elevated in both seminoma and non-seminoma. Moderately elevated levels may stem from cross-reaction of the test assay with the α-chain of other glycoprotein hormones, e.g. luteinizing hormone (LH) or follicle-stimulation hormone (FSH). High levels are found in choriocarcinoma, which may metastasize haematologically to visceral organs such as lungs, liver, or brain.

> **Key points serum HCG**
> - Normal level: <5IU/l or <5mUI/ml
> - ↑ in 25–60% of men with disseminated TC
> - ↑↑ levels → choriocarcinoma → MR brain
> - (↑) levels → possible cross-reaction with LH, FSH in sub-gonadal patients
> - Half-life: 1–2 days

LDH is an enzyme which is elevated in most situations where there is high cellular turnover, such as infections or myocardial infarction, and is therefore the least specific marker for MGCT. However, LDH level predicts prognosis and helps to identify relapses at follow-up.

AFP, HCG, and LDH may be released by treatment-induced tumour lysis and elevation, a 'marker surge', during the first ten days after starting treatment should not be interpreted as tumour progression. However, persistent elevation, rise or slower decrease than calculated by respective serum half-lives may indicate insufficient treatment.

Table 8.15.1 Summary of the staging of testicular cancer

Stage	
I	Testicular tumour only
IM	Elevated levels of AFP and/or HCG without visible metastases
II	Infra-diaphragmatic lymphadenopathy
A: <2cm	
B: 2–5cm	
C: >5cm	
III	Supra-diaphragmatic lymphadenopathy
A: <2cm	
B: 2–5cm	
C: >5cm	
IV	Extralymphatic metastases (lung, liver, bone, etc.)

Pattern of metastases

TC spreads primarily through lymph vessels to the retroperitoneal lymph nodes. These are best assessed by CT of abdomen and pelvis. Metastases to visceral organs like lung, liver, or brain if the abdominal CT is normal is exceedingly rare. Choriocarcinoma is the exception from this rule as it spreads primarily through blood vessels, leading to visceral metastases. These tumours usually produce high serum levels of HCG and need magnetic resonance (MR) examination of the brain for complete staging (Table 8.15.1).

Mandatory diagnostic work-up
- Palpation of both testicles
- Ultrasound of both testicles
- Serum tumour markers (HCG, AFP, LDH)
- CT abdomen/pelvis
- CXR
- Histological diagnosis

TIN

Up to 9% of TC patients have TIN in their remaining 'unaffected' testicle. This proportion increases to approximately one-third in case of testicular atrophy (<12ml volume) and age <40 years. The majority of patients with TIN will develop a TC within ten years.

Prevalence of TIN
- <1% general population
- 2–3% among sub-/infertile males
- 4–9% in the remaining testicle of TC patients

Table 8.15.2 International prognostic classification of testicular tumour

Prognosis	Non-seminomatous MGCT	Seminomatous MGCT
Good	**56%** of patients fulfil all of the following: • No non-pulmonary visceral metastases • No mediastinal EGGCT • AFP <1,000 • HCG <5,000 • LDH <1.5 x UNL (upper limit of normal)	**90%** of patients are free from: • Non-pulmonary visceral metastases
5-y Progression-free survival (%)	89	82
5-y OS (%)	92	86
Intermediate	**28%** of patients fulfil the following: • No non-pulmonary visceral metastases • No mediastinal EGGCT And any of these: • AFP 1,000–10,000 • HCG 5,000–50,000 • LDH 1.5–10 x UNL	**10%** of patients do have: • Non-pulmonary visceral metastases
5-y Progression-free survival (%)	75	67
5-y OS (%)	80	72
Poor	**16%** of patients fulfil any of the following: • Non-pulmonary visceral metastases • Primary mediastinal MGCT • AFP >10,000 • HCG >50,000 • LDH >10 x UNL	No patients with seminoma have poor risk
5-y Progression-free survival (%)	41	
5-y OS (%)	48	

Source: data from International Germ Cell Cancer Collaborative Group. International Germ Cell Consensus Classification: A prognostic factor-based staging system for metastatic germ cell cancers. *J Clin Oncol* 1997 Feb; 15(2):594–603. 1997, American Society of Clinical Oncology.

- Up to 33% of TC patients <40 years with atrophic testicle
- Up to 33% in patients with EGGCT

Therefore, the possibility of a contralateral TC should be discussed with each patient. Self-examination after treatment is particularly important for these patients.

In high-risk patients, TIN is diagnosed by a testicular biopsy, which may be performed during orchiectomy of the affected testicle.

Important: use Bouin's or Stieve's solution NOT formalin.

Treatment of TIN in the contralateral testicle
- Orchiectomy
- Radiotherapy
- Surveillance strategy

Orchiectomy and radiotherapy are effective treatments but both will render the patients infertile. Surveillance by annually testicular ultrasound examination in combination with instruction about self-examination is a valid management option.

Staging
The Royal Marsden staging system is commonly applied in Western Europe, see Table 8.15.2.

Sensitivity to chemotherapy
The high curability of metastatic TC by cisplatin-based chemotherapy serves as a model for a curable neoplasm and is a remarkable clinical feature. The reasons behind

a two to four times higher sensitivity to cisplatin-based chemotherapy by TC compared to most other tumours are not yet fully understood, but the following findings are considered important.

MGCT cells lack or have only low activity of: drug export pumps, cisplatin-inactivation enzymes, efficient DNA repair system, especially the nucleotide-excision-repair system. High intrinsic levels of pro-apoptotic proteins, e.g. wild-type p53 or BAX, prompt cell death after chemotherapy. Furthermore, anti-apoptotic proteins such as BCL2 are either absent or present in only very low levels. However, all the above-mentioned features change under the selective pressure of sub-curative chemotherapy doses to more resistant ones until undifferentiated completely chemotherapy refractory clones emerge.

> **Key points**
> - Lack of drug-efficient export pumps
> - Inability to efficiently detoxify cisplatin
> - Inability to repair the respective DNA damage
> - Limited anti-apoptotic factors
> - Intact apoptotic cascade

Some of these features might as well explain the high radiosensitivity of seminoma.

Teratoma is slow-growing and resistant to radio- and chemotherapy. These non-seminoma components are common findings in residual masses and complicate the management of residual post-chemotherapy masses.

8.16 Management of low stage seminoma testicular cancer

Orchiectomy
Orchiectomy is usually the first step of treatment of TC and should be performed within one week of clinical diagnosis. However, in patients with advanced life-threatening TC, orchiectomy should not delay cisplatin-based chemotherapy (European Germ Cell Cancer Consensus Group 2008).

Organ-sparing surgery
Organ-sparing surgery many be considered in cases of:
- Bilateral testicular cancer
- Small (<2cm) solitary tumour
- Sufficient endocrine function
- Benign tumour
- Treatment at experienced centre

Clinical stage I
80% of seminoma patients present apparently without metastases, i.e. clinical stage I disease. Approximately 20% of those harbour micrometastases in the retroperitoneal lymph nodes. RPLND is the only approach providing both staging and cure for the majority of patients. In the hands of an experienced surgeon, a urologist performing at least ten RPLNDs per year, this operation is connected with low morbidity. Originally, all the retroperitoneal soft tissue within the diaphragm, ureters, and large iliac vessels was removed but characterization of typical landing zones, or areas of primary lymph drainage,

have allowed for removal of distinct templates for left- and right-sided testicular cancers.

After nerve-sparing (NS) RPLND, which aims at identification and preservation of sympathetic nerves, only a few patients (<10%) will experience retrograde ejaculation, the most common complication.

Approach
- Laparotomy
- Preparation of the retroperitoneal space
- Identification and preservation of sympathetic nerves and ganglions
- Removal of all tissue of the respective template (which includes numerous lymph nodes)

Advantages
- Curative for the vast majority of patients
- Accurate staging
- Low acute morbidity
- Only way to remove teratoma thereby preventing subsequent complications such as growing teratoma or malignant differentiation
- Only way to obtain 'control of the retroperitoneum', the most frequent site of late relapses
- Abdominal CT scans during follow-up become unnecessary
- Long observation data

Disadvantages
- Unnecessary treatment of approximately 50% of unselected patients (those without retroperitoneal micro-metastases)
- Outcome depends largely on the surgeon's experience.
- Disease outside the template is left untreated
- Risk of surgery-related complications such as infections, bowel perforation

Laparoscopic RPLND may reduce surgery-related complications such as lymphocele, bowel complications, infections, chylous ascites, and blood loss. However, lymph nodes between or behind the large vessels cannot be removed by this approach. This technique should only be used in a study setting since its efficacy both in terms of diagnostic and curative intent remains doubtful. Disease-specific survival rate approaches 100%, independent of which of the following three management strategies are applied:
- Radiotherapy
- Surveillance and treatment in case of relapse
- Carboplatin

Radiotherapy
Radiotherapy to para-aortic and ipsilateral pelvic lymph nodes represents adjuvant treatment. This approach exploits two features of seminoma:
- Extreme radiosensitivity
- Spread through the lymphatic vessels

During the last 50–60 years it has been the standard treatment of stage I seminoma.

Approach
- 20Gy, at 2.0Gy/fraction, five days/week
- Target: para-aortic lymph nodes
- Field size borders:
  - Upper border: upper edge T11
  - Lower border: lower edge of L 5
  - Ipsilateral (to primary tumour) border: renal hilum
  - Contralateral (to primary tumour): processes transversus included

Before 1999, prophylactic radiation included ipsilateral iliac lymph nodes as a 'dog-leg field'. Due to similar relapse rates and less acute toxicity para-aortic lymph node radiation became standard treatment (Fossa et al. 1999). Reduction of the radiation dose from 30 to 20Gy has further contributed to reduce toxicities (Jones et al. 2005).

Chemotherapy or extension of the radiation field to ipsilateral iliac, inguinal, or scrotal region may be considered for:
- Inguinal violation, e.g. by prior hernia operation
- Scrotal violation, e.g. trans-scrotal biopsy
- Advanced primary tumour, i.e. pT3–4

The advantages and disadvantages of adjuvant radiotherapy may be presented as follows:

Advantages
- Highly effective
- Mostly well tolerated
- Low relapse rate <5% (almost exclusively outside radiation field, obviating abdominal CT scans during follow-up)
- Long observation data

Disadvantages
- Unnecessary treatment to approximately 80% of unselected patients (those without retroperitoneal micro-metastases)
- Disease outside the radiation field is left untreated.
- Risk of long-term toxicity, e.g. radiotherapy-induced malignancies
- Risk of acute toxicity, e.g. nausea, fatigue, diarrhoea, peptic ulceration

Surveillance
Surveillance also called 'watchful waiting' or 'wait and see' is increasingly employed, since development of metastases, mostly to retroperitoneal lymph nodes, can be cured by subsequent radio- or chemotherapy.

Approach
- Frequent follow-up visits the first two to three years with decreasing frequency later on
- Salvage treatment by radio- or chemotherapy if metastatic disease found by radiological or clinical examination or by tumour marker elevation
- Unfortunately, surveillance has not been investigated in randomized trials and the long-term risk/benefit ratio remains uncertain

Advantages
- Avoidance of treatment and its toxicities to the majority of patients
- Salvage treatment highly effective

Disadvantages
- Late relapses may occur after two, five, and even ten years
- Long follow-up, including CT examinations, necessary
- Requires high degree of compliance
- May be psychologically demanding

Carboplatin
Carboplatin as adjuvant treatment of clinical stage I seminoma is considered equally effective as adjuvant radiotherapy.

Approach
- One course of carboplatin as single agent intravenously
- Dose: 7 x AUC (area under the curve), i.e. 7x (glomerular filtration rate (GFR) +25)

Advantages
- Highly effective
- Tolerated well, e.g. patients resume work earlier compared to radiotherapy, essentially due to less fatigue
- Convenient to administer
- Salvage treatment highly effective

Disadvantages
- Unnecessary and possibly harmful treatment to approximately 80% of unselected patients (those without retroperitoneal micro-metastases)
- Insufficient long-term observations

The most appropriate treatment may be chosen according to the two risk factors most predictive for micrometastases:
- Rete testis invasion
- Size of the primary tumour (>4cm)

International consensus

Following the Spanish Germ Cell Cancer Group, we recommend surveillance with treatment for relapse for patients with expected high compliance and without presence of risk.

Patients with expected low compliance and/or presence of one or both risk factors are advised to undergo adjuvant chemotherapy:

- Carboplatin x 1–2

Clinical stage II

Clinical stage II disease, i.e. presence of RPLN metastases, may be considered as advanced disease and treated by cisplatin-based chemotherapy.

However, non-bulky (<5cm) retroperitoneal lymph nodes metastases may be effectively treated by:

Radiotherapy

- Stage IIA, i.e. masses <2cm: 30Gy
- Stage IIB, i.e. masses 2–5cm: 36Gy

Approach

- 2Gy/day for five fractions/week
- Target: para-aortic lymph nodes

- Shielding of contralateral testicle
- Field size borders
  - Upper border: upper edge T11
  - Lower border: upper border of ipsilateral acetabulum
  - In CS IIA, same lateral boders as in CSI
  - In CS IIB, lateral boders modified to lymph nodes with 1.5cm safety margin

Relapse-free survival at six years is 95% for CS IIA and 89% for CS IIB and most patients with relapse are cured by cisplatin-based chemotherapy.

However, the risk of metastatic disease outside the radiation field increases by stage. We treat our CS II patients preferentially with cisplatin-based chemotherapy.

Further reading

Fossa SD, Horwich A, Russell JM, Roberts JT, et al. Optimal planning target volume for stage I testicular seminoma: a Medical Research Council randomized trial. *J Clin Oncol* 1999; 17:1146–54.

Jones WG, Fossa SD, Mead GM, et al. Randomized trial of 30 versus 20 Gy in the adjuvant treatment of stage I testicular seminoma: a report on Medical Research Council Trial TE18, European Organisation for the Research and Treatment of Cancer Trial 30942. *J Clin Oncol* 2005; 23:1200–8.

8.17 Management of low stage non-seminoma testicular cancer

Orchiectomy

Orchiectomy is usually the first step of treatment of TC and should be performed within one week after diagnosis. However, in patients with advanced life-threatening TC, orchiectomy should not delay cisplatin-based chemotherapy.

Organ-sparing surgery may be considered in case of:

- Bilateral testicular cancer
- Small (<2cm) solitary tumour
- Sufficient endocrine function
- Benign tumour
- Treatment at experienced centre

Clinical stage I

Approximately 80% of non-seminoma patients present without detectable metastases, i.e. CS I disease. Approximately 20–50% of these harbour micrometastases in the retroperitoneal lymph nodes. Disease-specific survival rate approaches 100%, independent of which of the following three management strategies are applied:

- Surveillance and treatment in case of relapse
- Adjuvant cisplatin-based chemotherapy

It is controversial whether all patients should be managed by active surveillance. Adjuvant chemotherapy, however, has several advantages and the patient himself should probably decide which of both strategies suits him best.

Surveillance

Surveillance aims at avoiding unnecessary and potentially harmful treatment in about 50% of patients. Compliance to a strict follow-up protocol is a prerequisite for this approach. MGCT metastases are then detected at an early stage, amenable to chemotherapy, surgery, or the combination of both.

Approach:

- Frequent follow-up visits the first two to three years with decreasing frequency later
- Finding of metastases by radiological or clinical examination or after tumour marker elevation
- Salvage treatment by cisplatin-based chemotherapy and/or surgery
- Unfortunately, surveillance has not been investigated in randomized trials and the long-term risk/benefit ratio remains uncertain

Advantages:

- Avoidance of treatment and its toxicities in approximately 50% of unselected patients
- Salvage treatment highly effective

Disadvantages:

- Long follow-up, including CT abdominal examinations
- Requires high degree of compliance and experience by patients and physicians, respectively
- Psychologically demanding

Cisplatin-based chemotherapy

Cisplatin-based chemotherapy as adjuvant treatment of CSI non-seminoma consists of one course of bleomycin, etoposide, cisplatin (BEP) (see 'Cisplatin-based chemotherapy', p. 228).

Approach:

- One course of BEP

Advantages:
- Abolishes small non-teratomatous MGCT systemically
- Lower dose of cytotoxic drugs than required for stage 2 or higher
- Convenient to administer
- Usually well tolerated

Disadvantages:
- Unnecessary and harmful treatment to approximately 50% of patients (those without retroperitoneal micro-metastases)
- Insufficient long-term observation means the risk of late relapses, treatment-induced malignancies, cardiovascular disease, etc. remains unknown
- Teratoma is left in place
- Possible selection of chemotherapy-resistant MGCT cells may complicate treatment at relapse

Management
Optimal management of clinical stage I non-seminoma remains controversial. However, most experts agree that identification of risk factors and tailoring of treatment accordingly should be pursued. Until now only one risk factor for micrometastases has been broadly accepted:
- Vascular invasion (VI) in the primary tumour

Roughly, every second patient with VI harbours micrometastases and adjuvant (prophylactic) treatment is recommended in patients with VI:
- One cycle of BEP
- NS-RPLND

Also, if compliance is expected to be low or if the prospect of watchful waiting appears too distressing for the patient adjuvant treatment is indicated. Absence of VI is associated with a relapse rate of 14–22% and surveillance is the recommended treatment strategy.

Clinical stage II
Small (<2cm) retroperitoneal lymph nodes metastases represent stage IIA and such patients may be cured by primary RPLND alone.

Larger retroperitoneal lymph-nodes, i.e. stage IIB/C, are treated as for advanced non-seminoma by cisplatin-based chemotherapy.

8.18 Prognosis and management of advanced testicular cancer disease

Prognostic grouping
Several algorithms had been developed for prognosis prediction and treatment adjustments for patients with advanced MGCT. By far the most important one has been established by the International Germ Cell Consensus Classification Group (IGCCCG). International experts retrospectively analyzed the outcome of a large number of patients with metastatic or extragonadal MGCT (non-seminoma n=5202, seminoma n=660).

Feasibility in the clinical setting was a priority and three features were the basis for prognostication:
- Serum level of tumour markers (AFP, HCG, LDH)
- Localization of the primary tumour (i.e. mediastinal EGGCT vs. the remainder)
- Presence of visceral metastases outside the lungs

Three prognostic groups were established according to five-year survival rate:
- Good (90%)
- Intermediate (80%)
- Poor (50%)

For seminoma only the presence of non-pulmonary visceral metastases confers an intermediate prognosis (approximately 10%). The remaining 90% have a good prognosis. Due to good treatment results, no poor prognosis group could be established for patients with seminoma (see Table 8.15.2).

Cisplatin-based chemotherapy
Introduction of cisplatin in the treatment of metastatic TC during the late 1970s by Einhorn et al. (1977) transformed this disease into a model for a curable neoplasm.

The three-drug regimen of BEP is today's gold standard.

Dosage
- Bleomycin 30,000IU day 1+8+15
- Etoposide 100mg/m^2 day 1–5
- Cisplatin 20mg/m^2 day 1–5
- Three-week interval between cycles

Treatment intensity is important and dose reduction and prolonged intervals should be avoided. However infections may delay the next cycle. Neutropenia without fever does not represent an indication for treatment delay. Granulocyte colony-stimulating factor (GCS-F) should not be used routinely, but may shorten prolonged periods of neutropenia and should be used in case of previous chemotherapy-induced serious infections with febrile neutropenia.

Carboplatin plays no role in conventional dose chemotherapy of patients with metastatic disease as it has been shown to be consistently inferior to cisplatin-based chemotherapy.

Good risk
Conventional chemotherapy followed by adjunctive surgery cures approximately 90% of patients with a good risk according to IGCCCG.

Patients with a good prognosis are primarily treated by three cycles of BEP.

If use of bleomycin is contraindicated, e.g. by compromised lung or kidney function, four cycles of etoposide, cisplatin (EP) may be given.

Alternative regimens have not been shown to be more effective (equal or higher cure rates and equal or less toxicities). Other chemotherapy regimens should therefore only be used in clinical trials.

Intermediate or poor risk

Only 16% of all patients with MGCT have a poor prognosis according to IGCCCG and survival of these patients is best if treated in centres which have high experience in the management of such patients. We recommend that patients with intermediate or poor prognosis are referred to hospitals specialized in the treatment of MGCT.

The standard treatment is four cycles of BEP.

Most experts agree that improvement of the survival rate of patients with intermediate or poor risk MGCT is a priority. Consequently, many randomized trials have been undertaken with more intensified treatment approaches, e.g. high-dose chemotherapy with stem cell rescue. However, no alternative regimen proved to be more effective; and most regimens caused higher toxicities.

Management of residual tumour

Seminoma

Residual tumours, especially those <3cm, consist usually of necrotic/fibrotic tissue. Surgical removal of such masses is more complicated than in non-seminoma because of desmoplastic reactions of seminoma and complete resection is sometimes impossible. Extensive biopsies should be taken and the presence of viable seminoma should prompt salvage chemotherapy. Positron emission tomography (PET) may identify residual seminoma, particularly in masses >3cm and salvage chemotherapy is the treatment of choice.

> **Key points residual seminoma**
>
> - <3cm → usually fibrosis/necrosis, follow with CT, PET optional
> - >3cm PET positive → salvage treatment (surgery, chemotherapy, or radiotherapy)
> - >3cm PET negative → follow with CT

Non-seminoma

As a rule, residual tumour should always be removed. Since the retroperitoneal lymph nodes represent the most frequent site of metastases most residual tumours are located in the retroperitoneal space. Post-chemotherapy (PC) RPLND is more challenging than primary RPLND and only experienced surgeons should perform this operation. The histological findings of PC-RPLND are:

- Necrosis (50%)
- Teratoma (35%)
- Vital non-teratomatous MGCT (15%)

It appears that only patients with either teratoma or vital MGCT benefit from this operation, whereas 50% of patients with necrosis alone will not.

This dilemma led to a need for an algorithm to reliably predict PC histology, but unfortunately no approach has been broadly accepted yet.

Small lesions are less likely to contain vital MGCT than larger ones. This relationship led to the recommendation to remove residual masses only if they exceed 1cm or 2cm in size. However, in lesions <2cm, teratoma and MGCT was present in 26% and 7% respectively of retroperitoneal lymph nodes. Five out of six patients with vital MGCT had residual lesions of <1cm.

Management of recurrence

More than 90% of patients who achieve a complete response to initial therapy are cured. A single lesion without tumour marker elevation may be cured surgically without chemotherapy. In patients with recurrent seminoma PET may help to differentiate vital MGCT from necrosis. In non-seminoma patients, however, PET is of limited value since teratoma, a common histology of recurrent masses, is PET negative.

In patients with systemic relapse, i.e. tumour marker elevation and/or multiple metastases, second-line or even third-line chemotherapy may lead to cure.

Whether second-line chemotherapy should consist of standard dose three-drug regimens or high-dose chemotherapy with autologous stem cell is controversial. Up till now, no randomized controlled trial has shown any survival benefit by intensifying treatment compared with the former approach.

Probably the most important TC clinical trial 'TIGER' aims to assess the efficacy of conventional dose versus high-dose chemotherapy. Inclusion of eligible patients to this trial is highly encouraged.

Four cycles of taxol, iphosphamide, cisplatin (TIP) have achieved >60% cure rate in patients relapsing after initial chemotherapy.

Four cycles of the following regimens are usually given:

- TIP
- VIP (etoposide (Vp-16), ifosfamide, cisplatin)
- VeIP (vinblastine, ifosfamide, cisplatin)

High-dose chemotherapy with two to three cycles of etoposide and carboplatin (iphosphamide or paclitaxel may be added) may alternatively be used. This intensive chemotherapy has been better tolerated more recently with the use of growth factor support (GCS-F) and mobilization of peripheral blood stem cells. Einhorn et al. (2007) achieved a four-year complete remission in 110 of 184 (63%) patients with relapsing or initially cisplatin-resistant TC by high-dose chemotherapy.

A retrospective analysis of 1,984 TC patients who relapsed after first-line cisplatin-based chemotherapy showed significantly better outcomes after high-dose chemotherapy compared with conventional dose chemotherapy. However, this retrospective trial does not preclude selection bias and does therefore not provide definitive answers.

Late relapses occur by definition at least two years—but may be encountered decades later—after successful primary treatment. Such recurrences are, if initially treated by chemotherapy, usually resistant to cisplatin. However, a seminoma patient with a single retroperitoneal mass after surveillance will respond well to either radio- or chemotherapy.

In non-seminoma patients, surgery is an extremely important treatment strategy which cures many patients with single lesions.

Achievement of a representative biopsy is important as almost all patients with teratoma alone will survive whereas 50% or more of patients with active MGCT will succumb to their relapse. Teratoma may differentiate by malignant transformation into, for example, rhabdomyosarcoma or adenocarcinoma, and demonstration of isochromosome 12 proves MGCT clonality. Complete removal is the treatment of choice, but if not feasible, chemotherapy relevant for the histology should be used.

Treatment of late recurrences is complex and requires individual treatment which should be restricted to specialized centres only.

Brain metastases occur in approximately 10% of patients with advanced MGCT. In patients with brain metastases at initial diagnosis survival is 30–40%, whereas those with systemic relapse or development of brain metastases during treatment have a dismal survival of 2–5%.

Treatment should comprise systemic chemotherapy and radiotherapy may be added. Neither the optimal sequence nor the role of surgery is defined yet.

Further reading

Einhorn LH, Donohue J. Cis-diamminedichloroplatinum, vinblastine, and bleomycin combination chemotherapy in disseminated testicular cancer. *Ann Intern Med* 1977 Sep; 87(3):293–8.

Einhorn LH, Williams SD, Chamness A, et al. High-dose chemotherapy and stem-cell rescue for metastatic germ-cell tumors. *N Engl J Med* 2007; 357:340–8.

8.19 Testicular cancer follow-up

Introduction

Today more than 90% of patients with testicular cancer are being cured, even after relapse. The follow-up programme must be designed to discover relapses as early as possible. The different biology of seminomas and non-seminomas should be reflected in the frequency and timing of the follow-up visits. Since approximately 2–3% of patients develop a new primary cancer in the contralateral testis, careful clinical examination of the remaining testis is important at every visit. Many of the patients have gone through heavy treatment comprising radiotherapy or chemotherapy and surgery. The follow-up visit should therefore also address late effects such as hypogonadism, sexual dysfunction, dyslipemias, cardiovascular disease, neurological symptoms, and fatigue.

The follow-up visits should look for:

- Recurrent disease
- New primary disease
- Late treatment effects

Follow-up

Early detection and treatment of relapse represents the primary objective of follow-up visits during the first five to ten years. Recommendations for the follow-up schedule need to be adapted according to national and institutional requirements. Many follow-up recommendations that have been published most likely expose testicular germ cell tumour (TGTC) survivors to unnecessary radiation, increasing the risk of a radiation-induced second cancer. Replacing CT by MRI scan would reduce this risk, but is not feasible for many European countries. However, effort should be made to reduce the frequency of CT scans and limit their overall number. PET-CT scanning has no role in the routine follow-up of TGCT patients.

Wait-and-see surveillance

Stage I disease confined to the testis may be cured by orchiectomy alone. Based on histopathological features however, stage I disease is stratified into high-risk and low-risk groups based on the probability of micrometastatic disease and risk of relapse. In seminomas, tumour diameter and invasion of rete testis accounts for up to 35% risk of relapse. In non-seminomas tumour invasion into blood and lymph vessels is associated with a 50% risk of relapse. Patients who carry one or two risk factors should be offered adjuvant treatment with a single course of carboplatin or radiotherapy to retroperitoneal lymph nodes in the case of seminomas, or one course of combination chemotherapy with BEP in the case of non-seminomas.

High-risk factors in seminomas

- Rete testis invasion
- Size of the primary tumor (>4cm)

High-risk factor in non-seminomas

- Vascular invasion

The follow-up schedules vary considerably between different institutions (see NCCN.org or SWENOTECA.org).

Further reading

Honecker F, Aparicio J, Berney D, et al. ESMO consensus conference on testicular germ cell cancer: diagnosis, treatment and follow-up. *Ann Oncol* 2018 Aug 1; 29(8):1658–86.

Internet resources

National Comprehensive Cancer Network: http://www.nccn.org

Swedish and Norwegian Testicular Cancer Group: https://www.swenoteca.org/

8.20 Penile cancer overview

Epidemiology
- Penile cancers account for <1% of all cancers in men, with an annual incidence of 1.5/100,000 in Western Europe. Incidence is higher in Africa, Asia, and South America, particularly in areas of low socioeconomic status.
- Peak age of occurrence is 60–80 years. Penile cancer is extremely rare in men <40 years.
- Incidence of penile cancer is generally falling, perhaps due to improved socioeconomic conditions.

Aetiology
- Risk factors for penile cancer include human papilloma virus (HPV) infection (types 16 and 18), smoking, multiple sexual partners, early age of first intercourse, and previous CIS.
- Circumcision is protective, although adequate hygiene with prepuce retraction confers similar benefit.
- Some reports suggest high rates of cervical cancer in female partners of men with penile cancer, lending support to the link with HPV infection.
- There is no recommendation for the use of HPV vaccine in boys.

Pathology
- Premalignant conditions include condylomata acuminata, leukoplakia (chronic irritation), and balanitis xerotica obliterans.
- Epithelial lesions with cytological changes of malignancy confined to the epithelium with no evidence of local invasion or metastases are known as CIS. Three distinct lesions have been described, but these may be variants of the same condition.
  - Bowen disease (CIS): solitary, grey plaque with shallow ulceration on the skin of shaft/scrotum. Approximately 10% progress to invasion.
  - Erythroplasia of Queryat: single/multiple shiny red plaques on glans/prepuce, with a velvety appearance. As many as a third progress to invasion.
  - Bowenoid papulosis: multiple pigmented plaques (very similar in appearance to Bowen disease) but tends to be in a younger age group and associated with HPV 16. Rarely becomes malignant.
- Invasive carcinoma: the majority (>90%) are SCCs. They range from well-differentiated exophytic papillomas to poorly differentiated ulcerative lesions.
- Verrucous carcinoma is an indolent variant which can present with bulky cauliflower-like lesions, accounting for approximately 5% of penile cancers. It is well differentiated and does not spread to lymph nodes.
- Other rare malignancies of the penis include melanoma, sarcomas (particularly Kaposi's sarcoma), BCCs, and metastases from bladder, prostate, or bowel primary tumours.

Clinical features
- Penile cancers present as erythematous patches, exophytic growths, nodules, or ulcers. There may be associated discharge from the prepuce.
- The differential diagnosis includes sexually transmitted diseases, CIS, balanitis, or condylomata.
- In patients with phimosis, the presentation may be with distal swelling of the penis. A dorsal slit or circumcision may be required for adequate examination and assessment.

Diagnosis
- Diagnosis is made by clinical appearance, biopsy of the lesion, and histological assessment. Investigations should include a full blood count, urea and electrolytes, and liver function tests.
- The inguinal, pelvic, and abdominal lymph nodes should be imaged with a CT or MRI scan. Clinically enlarged inguinal nodes can be assessed with FNA or biopsy. An MRI scan of the pelvis with an artificial erection may be useful in assessing cavernosal invasion, if penis preservation is intended.
- Ultrasonography may be useful in measuring the thickness of the lesion, and assessing the infiltration of the corpora and groin lymph nodes.
- PET/CT is reliable for identification of pelvic and distant metastases in patients with positive inguinal nodes. If PET/CT is not available, abdomino-pelvic CT and plain chest radiography are advisable.
- It is sensible to photograph the lesion before treatment for future reference.

Staging
Summary of penile cancer staging:
- Stage 1
  - T1N0: Invasion of subepithelial tissue
- Stage 2
  - T2N0: Invasion of corpora cavernosa
  - T1/2N1: Single superficial inguinal lymph node involvement
- Stage 3
  - T3N0/1: Invasion of urethra/prostate
  - T1–3N2: Multiple or bilateral superficial inguinal nodes
- Stage 4
  - T4N0–2: Invasion of adjacent structures
  - T1–4N3: Deep inguinal or pelvic nodes involved
  - M1: Distant metastases

8.21 Management of penile cancer

Management of non-invasive disease
- CIS can be treated with topical 5-FU or imiquimod, local excision, laser surgery, electro-dissection, or superficial radiotherapy.
- Topical 5-FU is applied twice a day. Patients should be warned to avoid contact with their hands and to abstain from sexual intercourse during the treatment.

Management of invasive disease
- The management of invasive disease is primarily surgical. The traditional approach of amputation has been superseded by more conservative techniques when possible.
- The aim of treatment is complete removal of the tumour with adequate margins and control of regional lymph nodes whilst retaining a functional penis.
- Radiotherapy is an alternative and potentially organ-sparing technique.

Role of surgery
For very small foreskin lesions, circumcision, and laser surgery can be curative.

For other T1/2 lesions of the glans, a glansectomy or partial amputation may suffice. Tumours are usually excised to 1.5–2cm of normal tissue proximal to the invasive margin. Recent reports suggest margins of 1cm are sufficient.

For larger tumours, particularly if the urethra is involved, total amputation is required. A perineal urethrostomy is formed. In cases where there is involvement of the scrotum or perineum, total emasculation is required, sometimes also involving a cystoprostatectomy and urinary diversion.

For T4 tumours, neoadjuvant chemotherapy followed by surgery, if adequate response, is advisable.

Radiotherapy
Both EBRT and brachytherapy techniques are used. There are no randomized trials comparing outcomes of surgery and radiotherapy, but amputation with good margins has the best long-term outcome with five-year survival approaching 90% while radiotherapy has a 30% long-term failure rate. For this reason, primary radiotherapy tends to be reserved for patients unfit for surgery, with locally advanced disease, and fixed inguinal lymphadenopathy or those who refuse total amputation. Circumcision should be performed in all patients, even if treated with radiotherapy.

If disease is limited to the glans, electron-beam radiotherapy gives a good dose distribution. A lead cut-out is fashioned with a 2cm margin around the tumour and Perspex® or bolus is placed over the cut-out section to ensure that the skin surface dose is 100%.

For more extensive disease, photon irradiation is appropriate. A common technique uses two lateral opposing fields with the penis held between two halves of a wax block. The block acts as an immobilization device and also as bolus to achieve adequate dose at the penis. The testes and groin are shielded with lead. The CTV for radiotherapy should include tumour with a 2cm margin and the entire circumference of the penile skin. The conventional dose is 60–4Gy in 30–32 daily fractions using 4–6MV photons.

Alternatively, a CT planned volume using two lateral oblique beams can be employed.

If there is residual disease following radiotherapy, surgical excision should be considered as a salvage treatment.

Side effects of radiotherapy to the penis
Early
- Mucositis
- Oedema of the prepuce
- Local infections
- Dysuria
- Difficulty with micturition

Late
- Telangiectasia/superficial necrosis
- Stenosis of the urethral meatus
- Deep fibrosis
- Loss of sexual function

Brachytherapy
As with EBRT, the local recurrence rates with brachytherapy are greater than with surgery, although there is the option of salvage surgery at recurrence. Patients are circumcised and catheterized before treatment. Brachytherapy is generally only suitable for T1/2N0 tumours of <4cm in size.

Two techniques are in use:
- The mould technique employs two Perspex® cylinders, the outer of which is loaded with iridium-192 wires. The device is worn for eight to ten hours per day for one week, giving a typical dose of 60Gy. Although reproducibility is poor with this technique, it is useful for superficial lesions and a relatively low dose to the urethra results in a low incidence of urethral stenosis. High-dose rate brachytherapy can also be delivered with this method.
- The interstitial technique involves insertion of radioactive implants under general anaesthetic. The implants are inserted at right angles to the penis, which is supported by foam blocks. One or two planes (at 20–30mm separation) with two to three sources each (at 12–15mm separation) are usually required. The target volume for treatment is the tumour with a 1–2cm margin and this is treated with 65Gy to the 85% isodose over one week using the Paris system. A 2mm lead shield is applied to the testes. Use of stilboestrol should be considered to prevent erections during the week of treatment. Local control rates of up to 90% have been reported for T1 tumours.

Management of lymph nodes
- Fifty per cent of patients with clinically enlarged nodes are found to have only reactive changes with no evidence of tumour involvement. Since nodal recurrence significantly reduces survival, the management of regional nodes is very important in penile cancer. Nodal staging is recommended for all patients with pT1G1 tumour and above.
- FNA and cross-sectional imaging may be of help in identifying truly positive nodes. Invasive staging methods include modified inguinal lymphadenectomy or dynamic sentinel node biopsy (DSNB).

- Radical inguinal lymphadenectomy should be considered for patients with clinically enlarged nodes (cN1/N2) or with pathological nodes on DSNB. There is controversy over the need for bilateral dissection, but prophylactic contralateral dissection is appropriate if the one side is heavily involved (some clinicians suggest contralateral dissection if more than two nodes are involved).
- Patients with cN3 disease are considered for neoadjuvant chemotherapy followed by radical inguinal lymphadenectomy in patients who respond to chemotherapy. Patients who are not unfit for chemotherapy, preoperative inguinal radiotherapy (45–50Gy in 2Gy daily fractions) may be considered.
- Patients with involvement of ≥2 inguinal nodes (pN2) and with extracapsular extension should be considered for ipsilateral pelvic lymphadenopathy.
- Although superficial lymphadenectomy is associated with a low morbidity rate, block dissection of the deep inguinal nodes has high morbidity (up to 80% will experience problems including lymphoedema, wound infection, necrosis, seroma, and vessel damage).
- In patients with inoperable nodal disease, palliative radiotherapy may prevent ulceration and leg oedema.

Chemotherapy
SCC of the penis is relatively responsive to chemotherapy, although responses tend to be short-lived. Small studies/case series suggest that adjuvant chemotherapy can improve the long-term survival of patients with radically resected pN2/N3 disease and therefore should be considered. There may also be a role for primary neoadjuvant chemotherapy in patients with fixed inguinal metastases. There are reports that up to 50% of these can be made resectable.

Taxol combined with cisplatin and 5-FU (TPF) has shown impressive response rates and therefore, is considered as the regimen of choice for adjuvant (three to four cycles) and neoadjuvant (four cycles) settings and recurrent disease. Alternative, chemotherapy regimens include cisplatin and 5-FU or cisplatin, methotrexate, and bleomycin.

There have been reports of combination chemoradiotherapy in early stage penile cancer, for example, with bleomycin. Given the success of chemoradiotherapy in head and neck, anal, and cervical SCCs one might expect benefit in penile cancer, but experience is limited and primary surgery remains the treatment of choice.

Prognosis
Overall five-year survival rates for cancer of the penis are 70%. Nodal status is the major determinant of prognosis. The five-year DFS rates of patients with N0 and N+ disease are approximately 80% and 30% respectively. The vast majority of recurrences occur in the first five years. Regular follow-up is needed for early detection of recurrences, especially local recurrence, which can be successfully salvaged.

Palliative treatment
For unfit patients or those with locally advanced disease, palliative treatment with EBRT is an option. A typical dose schedule is 21Gy in three fractions administered over one week.

Further reading
Hakenberg OW, Comperat EM, Minhas S, et al. EAU guidelines on penile cancer: 2014 update. *Eur Urol* 2015; 67:142–50.

Internet resources
The European Association of Urology: http://uroweb.org/

Chapter 9

Cancers of the female genital system

Chapter contents

9.1 Cervical cancer overview

Epidemiology
Cervical cancer is a significant health burden, being the fourth most common cancer worldwide in females, and seventh most common overall with a total of 527,000 cases diagnosed globally in 2012.

In the UK, in 2013, there were 3,207 cases of cervical cancer overall with incidence rates being higher in Scotland than in England. In 2011–13, over 50% of cases were diagnosed in females under the age of 45.

Almost all women who develop cervical cancer are infected with an oncogenic human papilloma virus (HPV) type, most frequently with types 16 or 18, and these two commonest subtypes account for around two-thirds of cases.

Eight HPV types—16, 18, 45, 31, 33, 52, 58, and 35 (in descending frequency)—account for almost 95% of cervical cancers.

Risk of cervical cancer is increased in the following situations:

- Women with multiple sexual partners (>6)
- Age of first sexual intercourse less than 14 years compared with age over 25 years
- Women with an uncircumsized partner
- Women with human immunodeficiency virus (HIV) or immunosuppression from other causes
- Women with concurrent sexually transmitted infections (STIs), e.g. chlamydia
- Smokers (risk 1.5 x higher in current vs. never smokers)
- Users of the combined oral contraceptive pill (risk doubled in current vs. never used)
- Young age at first pregnancy (<17 years vs. > 25 years)

Cervical cancer screening
Screening has been shown to be effective in the early identification of a pre-neoplastic stage, known as CIN (cervical intraepithelial neoplasia). Detection enables early treatment hence reducing the incidence of invasive malignancy. Cervical cancer is preventable and it should be a high priority in national screening programmes. The UK invites women aged 25–64 for screening on a three-yearly basis for those under 50, and five-yearly thereafter.

There are different methods of screening for cervical cancer. Historically, cervical cytology (Papanicolaou (Pap) smear) screening programmes were found to be successful in reducing cervical cancer incidence, but it is relatively resource-intensive. Pap smear screening involves a speculum examination of the cervix and vagina. A small brush is used to collect cells from the cervix which are then sent for further analysis in the laboratory. Squamous cell carcinomas (SCCs) are often easier to detect than adenocarcinomas, and there may be interobserver variability in interpreting the results.

HPV DNA testing can also be performed as a screening test, and co-testing where both Pap testing and HPV testing are done in conjunction, may increase diagnosis of earlier cervical abnormalities but is not known to impact on mortality.

Natural history and pathology
Most cervical carcinomas arise at the squamo-columnar junction between the ectocervix and endocervix. The greatest risk of neoplastic transformation coincides with periods of greatest metaplastic activity. Virally induced atypical squamous metaplasia developing in this region may progress to higher-grade squamous intraepithelial lesions (SILs). These dysplasias undergo spontaneous regression in 25–38% cases, persist in 50–60%, and progress to invasive cancers in 2–14%. Once tumour breaks through the basement membrane, it may penetrate the cervical stroma directly or through vascular channels. Invasive tumours may develop as exophytic growths protruding from the cervix into the vagina or as endocervical lesions that can cause massive expansion of the cervix. From the cervix, tumour may extend superiorly to the lower uterine segment, inferiorly to the vagina, or laterally into the paracervical spaces by way of the broad or uterosacral ligaments. Tumour may become fixed to the pelvic wall by direct extension or by coalescence of central tumour with regional adenopathy.

Cervical cancer usually follows a relatively orderly pattern of metastatic progression, initially to primary echelon nodes in the pelvis and then to para-aortic nodes, and subsequently distant sites. Even patients with loco-regionally advanced disease rarely have detectable haematogenous metastases at initial diagnosis. The most frequent sites of distant recurrence are lung, extrapelvic nodes, liver, and bone.

Histopathological types
Non-invasive disease:

- Cervical intraepithelial neoplasia
- SCC in situ
- Adenocarcinoma in situ
- Adenocarcinoma in situ, endocervical type
  Invasive disease:
- Squamous carcinoma: keratinizing, non-keratinizing, and verrucous
- Endometrioid adenocarcinoma
- Clear cell adenocarcinoma
- Adenosquamous carcinoma
- Adenoid cystic carcinoma
- Small cell carcinoma
- Undifferentiated carcinoma

SCCs and adenocarcinomas account for 90–95% of cervical cancers. Those with early stage disease are usually treated with surgery with or without adjuvant treatments if required, and those with more advanced disease are offered chemoradiation plus intracavitary brachytherapy as the primary modality. This will be discussed in more detail later in the chapter.

9.2 Clinical features, investigations, staging, and prognosis of cervical cancer

Clinical features

Early invasive disease may or may not be associated with any symptoms and may be an incidental finding during examination for vaginal bleeding for example.

The earliest symptom of invasive cervical cancer is usually abnormal vaginal bleeding, often post-coital. This may be associated with a clear or foul-smelling vaginal discharge. Pelvic pain may result from coexistent pelvic inflammatory disease or from loco-regionally invasive disease. Flank pain

may be a symptom of hydronephrosis, often complicated by pyelonephritis. The triad of sciatic pain, leg oedema, and hydronephrosis is almost always associated with extensive pelvic wall involvement from tumour.

Patients with very advanced tumours may have haematuria or urinary incontinence from a vesicovaginal fistula caused by direct extension of tumour into the bladder. Lower limb deep vein thrombosis (DVT), severe lower back ache, and bone pain typically in the lumbar region

---

Box 9.2.1 FIGO staging of carcinoma of the cervix uteri 2018

Stage I:
The carcinoma is strictly confined to the cervix uteri (extension to the corpus should be disregarded).
- **IA** Invasive carcinoma that can be diagnosed only by microscopy, with maximum depth of invasion <5mm[a]
  - **IA1** Measured stromal invasion <3mm in depth
  - **IA2** Measured stromal invasion ≥3mm and <5mm in depth
- **IB** Invasive carcinoma with measured deepest invasion ≥5mm (greater than stage IA), lesion limited to the cervix uteri[b]
  - **IB1** Invasive carcinoma ≥5mm depth of stromal invasion and <2cm in greatest dimension
  - **IB2** Invasive carcinoma ≥2cm and <4cm in greatest dimension
  - **IB3** Invasive carcinoma ≥4cm in greatest dimension

Stage II:
The carcinoma invades beyond the uterus, but has not extended onto the lower third of the vagina or to the pelvic wall.
- **IIA** Involvement limited to the upper two-thirds of the vagina without parametrial involvement
  - **IIA1** Invasive carcinoma <4cm in greatest dimension
  - **IIA2** Invasive carcinoma ≥4cm in greatest dimension
- **IIB** With parametrial involvement but not up to the pelvic wall

Stage III:
The carcinoma involves the lower third of the vagina and/or extends to the pelvic wall and/or causes hydronephrosis or non-functioning kidney and/or involves pelvic and/or paraaortic lymph nodes[c].
- **IIIA** Carcinoma involves the lower third of the vagina, with no extension to the pelvic wall
- **IIIB** Extension to the pelvic wall and/or hydronephrosis or non-functioning kidney (unless known to be due to another cause)
- **IIIC** Involvement of pelvic and/or paraaortic lymph nodes, irrespective of tumor size and extent (with r and p notations)[c]
  - **IIIC1** Pelvic lymph node metastasis only
  - **IIIC2** Paraaortic lymph node metastasis

Stage IV:
The carcinoma has extended beyond the true pelvis or has involved (biopsy proven) the mucosa of the bladder or rectum. A bullous oedema, as such, does not permit a case to be allotted to stage IV.
- **IVA** Spread of the growth to adjacent organs
- **IVB** Spread to distant organs

a Imaging and pathology can be used, when available, to supplement clinical findings with respect to tumour size and extent, in all stages.

b The involvement of vascular/lymphatic spaces does not change the staging. The lateral extent of the lesion is no longer considered.

c Adding notation of r (imaging) and p (pathology) to indicate the findings that are used to allocate the case to stage IIIC. For example, if imaging indicates pelvic lymph node metastasis, the stage allocation would be stage IIIC1r and, if confirmed by pathological findings, it would be Stage IIIc1p. The type of imaging modality or pathology technique used should always be documented. When in doubt, the lower staging should be assigned.

Reproduced with permission from Bhatla N, et al. Revised FIGO staging for carcinoma of the cervix uteri. *Int J Gynecol Obstet* 2019; 145(1). Copyright © 2019 John Wiley & Sons may all be presenting symptoms due to lymph nodal masses in the pelvis or para-aortic regions. Cachexia, cough, jaundice, and a left supraclavicular nodal mass may result from distant metastases.

Pretreatment evaluation and staging

Pretreatment evaluation

Complete physical and gynaecological examination is vital for clinical staging and usually includes examination under anaesthesia (EUA) to enable an accurate and complete examination.

Other tests are also required:

- Full blood count and biochemistry: to look for anaemia and renal impairment.
- Biopsy—punch, knife, colposcopy-guided, or conization: for histopathological diagnosis.
- Computed tomography scan (CT scan) of chest, abdomen, and pelvis: to look for regional lymphadenopathy, distant metastases, and evaluate presence of hydronephrosis.
- Magnetic resonance imaging (MRI) pelvis (preferred modality to assess and stage primary tumour accurately).
- Whole body positron emission tomography (PET) scan (optional).
- Cystoscopy/sigmoidoscopy: if clinical suspicion of bladder or rectal involvement. May be done during the EUA.

Staging

Staging is done at EUA jointly by gynaecological surgeons and radiation/clinical oncologists. The 2009 and most recent International Federation of Gynecology and Obstetrics (FIGO) staging of cervical cancer updates (2018) is given below in Box 9.2.1 and Table 9.2.1. Note: Staging in this chapter refers to the 2009 staging version unless specified.

The 2018 criteria have been updated to reflect the importance of size in the IB group of tumours and prognostic significance of lymph node status in stage III disease.

Salient features of FIGO staging

- Historically the staging of cervical cancer was based on clinical evaluation alone, and the clinical staging would not have been changed because of subsequent findings on imaging or histology reports. However, the new 2018 FIGO staging system does allow for imaging or histologically detected nodal disease to be classified within the IIIC subgroup and can be amended all stages. If staged as thus, a p (denoting pathology) or an r (denoting radiological) should be used to document how this decision was reached.
- When there is doubt as to the stage to which a particular cancer should be allocated, choice of the earlier stage is mandatory,
- Suspected bladder or rectal involvement should be confirmed by biopsy and requires histological evidence before upstaging is confirmed.
- Conization or amputation of the cervix is regarded as a clinical examination. Invasive cancers so identified are to be included in the reports.
- FNA of scan-detected suspicious lymph nodes may be helpful in treatment planning.

Table 9.2.1 FIGO staging of carcinoma of cervix (2018) notable updates

FIGO stage	Categories
IA	Invasive carcinoma diagnosed only by microscopy <5mm
IA1	Measured stromal invasion <3mm
IA2	Measured stromal invasion ≥3mm and <5mm
IB	Invasive carcinoma confined to the cervix or microscopic lesion greater than IA2
IB1	Invasive carcinoma ≥5mm depth stromal invasion and <2cm in greatest dimension
IB2	Invasive carcinoma ≥2cm in greatest size and <4cm
IB3	Invasive carcinoma ≥4cm in greatest size
IIIC	Involvement of pelvic and/or para-aortic lymph nodes irrespective of tumour size and extent (with r and p notations)
IIIC1	Pelvic lymph node metastasis only
IIIC2	Para-aortic lymph node metastasis

Adapted with permission from Bhatla N, et al. Cancer of the cervix uteri. *Int J Gynaecol Obstet* 2018; 143(S2):22–36. Copyright © 2018, John Wiley & Sons.

Prognosis

FIGO stage is the single most important prognostic factor for both survival and pelvic disease control rates in cervical cancer. Clinical tumour diameter is also strongly correlated with prognosis for patients treated with radiation or surgery. For patients with more advanced disease, other estimates of tumour bulk—such as the presence of medial versus lateral parametrial involvement (in FIGO stage IIB tumours) or the presence of unilateral versus bilateral parametrial or pelvic wall involvement—have also been correlated with outcome.

The Vienna data show high levels of both local control (LC) and cancer-specific survival (CSS) with their MRI-guided brachytherapy techniques. Tumours of 2–5cm had three-year LC rates up to 95%, and tumours >5cm 90%. Three-year CSS were 83% and 70% respectively for patients with tumours 2–5cm and >5cm in diameter.

Lymph node metastasis is also an important predictor of prognosis. For patients treated with radical hysterectomy for stage IB–IIA disease, five-year overall survival (OS) rates are much higher at 88–96% for patients with negative nodes and 50–74% for those with lymph node metastases and equivalent stage. The number of nodes dissected and positivity rates also have a bearing on the outcome after surgery. Survival rates for patients with positive para-aortic nodes treated with extended-field radiotherapy vary from 10% to 50% depending on the extent of pelvic disease and para-aortic lymph node involvement. For patients treated with radical hysterectomy, other histological parameters that have been associated with a poor prognosis are lymphovascular space invasion (LVSI), deep stromal invasion (10mm or more, or >70% invasion), and parametrial extension.

9.3   Management of cervical cancer

A thorough evaluation of the loco-regional disease extent and correct staging of the disease is essential before deciding on the appropriate treatment. The factors which influence the choice of local treatment include tumour size, stage, histological features, evidence of lymph node involvement, risk factors for complications of surgery or radiotherapy (RT), and patient choice.

Non-invasive disease (carcinoma in situ)

Extent of the disease is the most important factor in the treatment decision. The other factors that also influence the treatment decision include age of the patient, requirement for fertility preservation, and other medical conditions.

Ectocervical lesions only:
• Loop electrosurgical excision procedure (LEEP)
• Laser therapy
• Conization
• Cryotherapy

If the endocervical canal is involved:
• Laser or cold-knife conization: to preserve the uterus and avoid radiation
• Total abdominal or vaginal hysterectomy for the post-reproductive age group. This is particularly indicated when the tumour extends to the inner cone margin

Invasive disease

A surgical approach is usually recommended for those with early stage disease, with the definition of early stage from FIGO being stages IA1, IA2, or IB1. Essentially that means surgical options are considered in lesions confined to the cervix which are <4cm in size.

Radical RT is usually recommended therefore for lesions greater than IB1, and comprises a combination of chemoradiation usually with cisplatin, followed by subsequent internal brachytherapy insertions to deliver tumouricidal radiation doses.

There are a number of considerations in deciding on type of surgery. Women of child-bearing age may desire to preserve fertility if possible and the ability to carry a foetus by uterus-preserving surgery. High-risk histological types (e.g. small cell carcinoma) may influence surgical options, as may other high-risk features such as the presence of LVSI, or lymph node involvement.

Surgery for early cervix cancer
• Conization
• Radical trachelectomy
• Total abdominal hysterectomy

Conization
In patients with IA1 disease if no vascular or lymphatic channel invasion is present, and the margins of the cone are negative, conization alone may be appropriate in patients wishing to preserve fertility.

Recent data may also support the use of conization in stage IA2 disease in combination with laparoscopic lymph node dissection, but only where the cone margins are negative. This still needs further evaluation and is not standard therapy.

Radical trachelectomy
The trachelectomy can be done either via a vaginal or an abdominal approach, with the vaginal approach used for smaller lesions. It entails 'en bloc' resection of the cervix with 1–2cm of vaginal tissue and the proximal parametrial tissue. A permanent cerclage is placed just superior to the margin and the now 'neo-cervix' is stitched to the vaginal mucosal tissue. Fertility-sparing surgery such as this is not recommended for those with positive lymph node involvement, and lymph-node dissection should be done initially to ensure node-negative disease.

Total hysterectomy (abdominal or vaginal)
In patients with a IA1 lesion with no vascular or lymphatic involvement, the frequency of lymph node disease is very low and hence lymph node dissection is not required. The ovaries can be preserved in young women if required.

A modified radical hysterectomy is standard for stage IA2 disease (type II hysterectomy). This technique involves removal of the uterus, cervix, upper 1/4 of the vagina, and the parametria. Pelvic lymphadenectomy is done as part of the operation. Those with a higher stage disease, e.g. IB1 with tumours >2cm, tend to be offered a radical hysterectomy (type III) which involves removal of a greater amount of vaginal parametrial tissue.

Similar cure rates are obtained with either a surgical or radiotherapeutic treatment approach for stage IB squamous carcinoma of the cervix. The choice between initial surgical or radiotherapeutic management depends upon the age of the patient, desire to preserve ovarian function, comorbid conditions, and patient choice.

Adjuvant therapy after radical surgery

Adjuvant chemoradiation with external pelvic radiation therapy and concurrent weekly cisplatin chemotherapy is recommended if any one of the following high-risk factors is seen on final histopathology:
• Lymph node metastases
• Positive surgical margins
• Parametrial extension

The risk of recurrence after radical surgery is increased with the presence of positive nodes, positive parametria, or positive surgical margins (Peter's criteria). Adjuvant concurrent chemoradiation (using fluorouracil (5-FU) + cisplatin or cisplatin alone) improves survival compared with pelvic irradiation alone in such patients.

Transposition of the ovaries out of the pelvis can be done at surgery if the patient needs postoperative RT. Radiation dose to the ovaries can therefore be measured and limited to minimize toxicity to the ovaries. This may be done to minimize infertility risk and also reduce the chance of ovarian failure and premature menopause.

For patients who inadvertently had a hysterectomy for invasive cervical cancer, completion surgery is advocated. However, immediate second surgery is not practical so these patients should be considered as high risk and treated with adjuvant chemoradiation, although radical RT alone may be acceptable if combined chemoradiation is not possible.

Intermediate risk factors
- Deep invasion of cervical stroma
- LVSI
- Tumour size >4cm

Adjuvant RT is recommended if at least two of the listed factors are seen on final histopathology. The risk of recurrence is also increased in patients with uninvolved nodes but with large tumour volume, capillary-like space (CLS) involvement, and outer one-third invasion of the cervical stroma. Some also feel that adenocarcinomas are more likely to relapse locally (but not only locally) than SCCs of the cervix and warrant RT for local control.

Adjuvant whole pelvic irradiation reduces the local failure rate and improves progression-free survival (PFS) compared with patients treated with surgery alone.

Low risk factors
- All other patients with none of the previously mentioned risk factors (high or intermediate).
- No adjuvant therapy recommended in this group.

Radical radiotherapy
A combination of external beam pelvic irradiation, covering the cervix, uterus, parametria, and pelvic nodes, followed by intracavitary irradiation, primarily for the central disease is used. The aim is to deliver a dose equivalent of 80Gy to point A. The planned radical radiation/concomitant chemoradiation should be completed within eight weeks without significant treatment breaks as prolonged overall treatment time is associated with poor outcome. Compensation for treatment gaps (i.e. two treatments in one day) should be considered if they occur.

External beam radiation
Using 1.8–2Gy per fraction, a dose of 40–50Gy has traditionally been recommended. Fraction sizes of 1.8Gy are often used to reduce long-term small bowel toxicity, and typical UK practice is to deliver 45Gy in 25 fractions over five weeks.

Three-dimensional radiotherapy technique
Three-dimensional (3D) and intensity-modulated radiotherapy (IMRT) are increasingly being used in cervical cancer. These techniques allow for increased sparing of normal tissues and IMRT can also be used to differentially escalate the dose of radiation to high-risk disease. The target volumes are defined on the CT planning scan as follows:
- Gross tumour volume (GTV)—is defined by EUA and imaging. MRI is superior to CT scan in defining GTV. Stromal and parametrial invasion is best demonstrated on T2 weighted MRI images.
- Clinical target volume (CTV)—consists of the uterine body, upper vagina, parametria, and proximal uterosacral ligament in all patients. Further inclusion of vagina and pelvic ligaments in the CTV is based on the findings from the EUA. The CTV also includes the nodal regions at risk of metastasis—the parametrial, external iliac, internal iliac, obturator, and possibly the distal common iliac nodes. Inguinal nodes are included in the CTV if disease extends to the lower third of the vagina, and presacral nodes are included if there is posterior tumour extension. Since it is typically difficult to identify normal lymph nodes on the planning CT scan, the lymph nodes may be defined using major pelvic blood vessels as a surrogate target. In practice, in node-negative patients, the nodal CTV is marked as a 7–10mm margin around contrast

enhancing blood vessels. In cases of radiologically visible nodal disease, a margin of about 10mm is added to the macroscopic nodal disease.
- Planning target volume (PTV)—is usually delineated by adding a margin, to account for set-up errors and internal organ movement, e.g. of 15mm around the uterus and cervix (as these structures can move significantly) and 7–10mm around the nodal CTV depending upon local audit data. The PTV should be covered by 95–107% of the prescribed dose.
- The EMBRACE II group requires the concept of the internal tumour volume (ITV) to be contoured individually from the CTV, to develop a more personalized approach in cervix cancer. With the use of IMRT techniques and the steeper dose gradients which may spare non-target tissue, it is critical to ensure that if the target moves within the field, it should be covered suitably by the required dose. The ITV takes into account the tumour movement on a daily basis due to bladder and rectal filling for example.

Field-based technique
Use of either a two- or four-beam arrangement is typical, with a better dose distribution seen with the four-field brick, and AP-PA fields often reserved for those in whom the para-aortic nodes need to be included.

A guide to the radiation target volume is given below:

AP–PA target volume
- Superior border: L4–L5 interspace
- Inferior border: bottom of obturator foramina (or lower for vaginal involvement—3cm beneath palpable disease)
- Lateral border: 1cm lateral to pelvic brim

Lateral target volume
- Superior/inferior borders: same as AP–PA portals
- Anterior border: mid symphysis pubis
- Posterior border: 2cm anterior to sacral hollow. The width of the lateral volume should be approximately 10cm wide

Para-aortic nodes
Extended field RT, usually defined as up to the superior border of L1, has been reported to produce long-term disease control in women with involved common iliac or para-aortic nodes. Ideally these patients require combined chemoradiation rather than radiation alone as the nature of this level of nodal involvement clearly puts them at high risk.

Intracavitary brachytherapy
Brachytherapy plays a crucial role in achieving high cure rates with low toxicity. A good intracavitary insertion delivers a very high radiation dose to the cervix, upper vagina, and medial parametria without exceeding the tolerance doses for rectum, sigmoid colon, and bladder. The randomized trials comparing low dose rate (LDR) with high dose rate (HDR) brachytherapy in carcinoma of the cervix have shown that the two modalities are comparable in terms of local control and survival. Thus, either LDR or HDR brachytherapy may be used, taking into account the availability of equipment and other logistics of treatment delivery. HDR brachytherapy can be done as a day procedure in contrast to approximately 20 hours of continuous LDR treatment requiring an overnight inpatient stay. When intracavitary RT is used after external

beam radiotherapy (EBRT), a single application of LDR (27–30Gy to point A) after completion of EBRT or 2–4 applications of HDR (7–9Gy to point A) are often used.

Brachytherapy planning

Recently it has been recognized that brachytherapy planning techniques using 3D imaging yield better dose optimization. Based on 3D planning, using CT scan and/or MRI compatible applicators, the gynaecological GEC/ESTRO working group has put forward some recommendations for volume definition and dose–volume parameters. Cumulative dose–volume histograms (DVH) are essential for the evaluation of complex dose distribution.

Definitions of volumes of cervical cancer brachytherapy

The target volumes are delineated after the insertion of applicators and using CT scan and/or MRI the following treatment volumes are defined:

- High-risk CTV (HR-CTV): indicates the residual macroscopic disease with highest risk of local recurrence. The intent is to deliver the highest possible dose of RT to eradicate all residual macroscopic disease.
- Intermediate-risk CTV (IR-CTV): indicates an area with previous macroscopic disease but at the time of brachytherapy only residual microscopic disease at worst. The aim is to deliver at least 60Gy to this volume.
- Low-risk CTV (LR-CTV): denotes area with potential microscopic disease.

The organs at risk contoured should include bladder, rectum, and sigmoid.

Dose prescription

The prescription dose is planned to cover the target as completely as possible. The doses at point A (right, left, and mean), D100 for GTV, and D90 for HR-CTV and IR-CTV should be calculated. Doses to organs at risk should be calculated, for example—the D2cc (dose to 2cm^2) and correlated with toxicity. For details of 3D brachytherapy for cervical cancer, refer to Haie-Meder et al. 2005 in 'Further reading' (p. 243).

Concurrent chemoradiation with cisplatin chemotherapy

Five randomized phase 3 trials of radical RT alone versus concurrent cisplatin-based chemotherapy and RT, and a meta-analysis have shown an absolute benefit in OS and PFS with chemoradiotherapy in patients with stage IB2 to IVA disease as well as in high-risk patients after hysterectomy.

While these trials are somewhat heterogeneous in data, stage of disease, suboptimal doses of radiation, non-uniform usage for chemotherapeutic drugs, and different schedules and doses of cisplatin, a significant survival benefit for this combined approach is still shown. The risk of death from cervical cancer was decreased by 30–50% by use of concurrent chemoradiation. Based on these results, the National Cancer Institute (NCI) has recommended that 'strong consideration should be given to the incorporation of concurrent cisplatin-based chemotherapy with radiation therapy in women who require radiation therapy for treatment of cervical cancer especially in early stage disease'. However, one randomized clinical trial did not find any additional survival benefit of concurrent weekly cisplatin. A major criticism of this study was that nearly two-thirds of the patients with chemotherapy (CT) + RT had low haemoglobin, which was not corrected during RT as is generally recommended.

Concurrent chemoradiation as the new standard of care is reinforced by the results of a population-based study from Ontario which showed that there was a significant improvement in OS at the population level concordant with the widespread adoption of CT-RT. Collated data from 24 trials and 2,491 patients strongly suggested a benefit of adding chemotherapy for both disease-free survival (DFS) and OS with absolute benefits of 10% and 13% respectively. Due to statistical heterogeneity there was some suggestion that the benefit is greatest in stages I and II.

While chemoradiotherapy has been accepted as the new standard of care in many areas, it is worth remembering that these results were obtained from women in affluent countries who had better nutrition, performance status (PS), and renal parameters than the majority of patients in poorer countries and with more advanced disease. Therefore, in women with medical or social reasons which may preclude combined modality treatment, radical RT alone without compromising the doses and duration can still be considered as a standard treatment approach.

Locally advanced disease

The management of patients with stage IVA disease (invasion of bladder and/or rectum) has to be individualized, taking into account the extent of bladder/rectal involvement, parametrial infiltration, renal function, and the patient's PS. The treatment options include:

- Chemoradiotherapy +/− brachytherapy
- Neoadjuvant chemotherapy followed by concurrent chemoradiotherapy
- Radical RT alone
- Palliative RT/chemotherapy
- Pelvic exenteration
- Best supportive care (BSC)/palliative care

Neoadjuvant chemotherapy followed by concurrent chemoradiotherapy, concurrent chemoRT, or radical RT alone

Selected fit patients with good general and renal status can be treated with this approach with radical intent. High pelvic radiation doses are often used to prevent the patient dying with poorly controlled painful pelvic disease. Those with poor renal function can still receive radiation alone if PS allows.

Even those patients with borderline renal function or PS (e.g. glomerular filtration rate (GFR) 30–50ml/min) might benefit from reduced cisplatin doses capped at 40mg, rather than omitting it completely.

Palliative radiotherapy/chemotherapy

Patients who have a poor PS and extensive local disease may be best treated with palliative RT/chemotherapy. The major symptoms which may be palliated are vaginal bleeding, profuse discharge, and low back or pelvic pain due to local disease. A short palliative radiation regimen of 30Gy in ten fractions over two weeks could be appropriate and in a few patients who respond very well could be followed by an intracavitary application to prevent recurrent painful pelvic symptoms. Palliative chemotherapy is discussed on p. 249.

Surgical exenteration

Selected patients with stage IV disease who have no or minimal parametrial invasion may be treated with primary exenterative surgery, the extent of which (anterior, posterior, or total) depends on the extent of the lesion.

Best supportive care

Patients with poor general condition and/or extensive local disease may be offered BSC alone. In the presence of fistulae, consideration of a urostomy or colostomy might be of use in the palliation of troublesome symptoms.

Stage IVB

Radiotherapy may be used for palliation of central disease or symptomatic distant metastasis, and should be strongly considered as symptoms from uncontrolled pelvic disease may be difficult to manage later. The role of systemic therapy is discussed later (see section 9.5, 'Systemic CT in stage IVB or recurrent disease').

9.4 Recurrent cervical cancer

Management of patients who relapse after primary treatment

Treatment decisions should be based on the fitness of the patient, the site of recurrence and/or metastases, the extent of metastatic disease, and any previous treatments received.

Therapeutic options for local relapse after primary surgery

Relapse in the pelvis following primary surgery may be treated by either radical radiation or by pelvic exenteration. Radical irradiation (with concurrent cisplatin-based chemotherapy) may offer long-term control for a substantial proportion of those with isolated pelvic failure. Radiation dose and volume should be tailored to the extent of disease. 45–50Gy should be delivered to cover microscopic disease within the pelvis (CTV) and a boost to at least 64–66Gy should be delivered to gross macroscopic tumour (GTV). Pelvic exenteration may be an alternative (particularly if a fistula is present) to radical RT and concurrent chemotherapy in selected patients without pelvic sidewall involvement.

Where disease is metastatic or recurrent in the pelvis after failure of primary therapy and not curable, a trial of chemotherapy with palliative intent may be indicated.

Cisplatin is the single most active agent in cervical cancer and can be used as a single agent or in combination with another agent, e.g. a taxane. The median time to progression is measured in a number of months.

Local recurrence after primary radiotherapy

Selected patients with resectable recurrences should be considered for pelvic exenteration. Alternatively, in carefully selected patients with a small recurrence <2cm, a radical hysterectomy may be performed.

Patients being considered for exenterative surgery should be selected extremely carefully. Those with resectable central recurrences without evidence of intraperitoneal or extra pelvic spread and who have a dissectable tumour-free space along the pelvic sidewall are potentially suitable. The five-year survival for patients selected for treatment with pelvic exenteration is in the order of 30–60% and the operative mortality should be <10%.

Exenterative surgery should be undertaken only in centres with suitable facilities and expertise and only by teams who have the experience and commitment to look after the long-term rehabilitation of these patients. The prognosis is better for patients with a disease-free interval greater than six months, a recurrence 3cm or less in diameter, and no pelvic sidewall fixation.

9.5 Role of chemotherapy

Systemic CT in stage IVB or recurrent disease

Chemotherapy has a palliative role in patients with metastatic or recurrent cervical cancer after failure of surgery or RT. There are a number of chemo-therapeutic agents with activity in metastatic or recurrent cervical cancer. At present cisplatin is considered the most active cytotoxic agent, producing a response rate of 20–30% and a median survival of seven months.

Carboplatin is thought to have a similar efficacy in cervical cancer and can be substituted instead of cisplatin which can be quite toxic. A 2014 meta analysis reviewed 1,181 patients and showed no significant OS difference between the carboplatin and the cisplatin arms.

Although the older combination regimens failed to show an improvement in survival compared with cisplatin alone, the use of newer combinations has shown promise. In a phase 3 Gynecologic Oncology Group (GOG) study, paclitaxel + cisplatin were superior to cisplatin alone in terms of response, PFS and sustained quality of life (QoL) but not for OS. In another GOG study the combination of topotecan + cisplatin was superior to cisplatin alone for response, PFS, and OS. Therefore, selected patients with recurrent or metastatic disease of good PS could be offered one of these combination regimens.

Bevacizumab (an anti-VEGF (vascular endothelial growth factor) monoclonal antibody) in combination with cisplatin plus either paclitaxel or topotecan also showed an improved median OS of 3.7 months from 13.3–17 months in first-line metastatic disease.

In patients with poor PS, single-agent cisplatin or BSC continue to be appropriate choices.

Patients with distant metastases should be treated with palliative intent with chemotherapy or RT or symptomatic and supportive care only. Symptoms of recurrent/metastatic cervical cancer may include pain, leg swelling, anorexia, vaginal bleeding, cachexia, and psychological problems among others. The coordinated efforts of a team of professionals are required; this may include gynaecological oncologists, radiation and medical oncologists, palliative care physicians, specialized nursing staff, psychologists, and possibly stoma therapists. Relief of pain and other symptoms, with comprehensive support for the patient and her family, are paramount. Local treatment with radiation therapy is indicated to sites of symptomatic involvement in patients with metastatic disease for alleviation of symptoms, including pain arising from skeletal metastases, enlarged para-aortic or supraclavicular nodes, and symptoms associated with cerebral metastases. In view of the shortened life expectancy of patients with metastatic cervical cancer, palliative RT should be hypofractionated to allow adequate doses to be delivered over a short timeframe.

9.6 Treatment-related morbidity for cervical cancer

Introduction

Complications can be broadly divided into acute, subacute, and late. Acute complications manifest during treatment, subacute occur between three to six months following treatment, and late appear more than six months after treatment.

Surgery

The acute intraoperative and immediately postoperative complications include blood loss, ureterovaginal fistula (<2%), vesicovaginal fistula (<1%), paralytic ileus (1–2%), and postoperative fever (20–30%) secondary to DVT, pulmonary infection, pelvic cellulitis, urinary tract infection, or wound infection. The subacute complications include lymphocoele formation and lower extremity oedema. Risks of complications are increased if patients receive preoperative or postoperative irradiation. The late sequelae are due to extensive pelvic fibrosis which may result in ureteric obstruction, hydronephrosis, small bowel obstruction, or perforation.

Radiation therapy

During pelvic RT, most patients experience mild fatigue and mild to moderate diarrhoea which tend to respond to dietary modification and antidiarrhoeal medications. Some experience bladder irritation. These acute symptoms are increased when RT is combined with concurrent chemotherapy or includes extended fields. Patients receiving concurrent chemotherapy may additionally have haematological, neurological, or renal toxicity (cisplatin).

The late sequelae following radiation therapy which have been seen most frequently affect the rectum, bladder, and small bowel. These depend on the duration of follow-up, type of treatment modalities used, and estimated radiation doses to these organs. Reported grade III/IV late sequelae (toxicities requiring hospital admission or intervention) range from 5% to 15%.

Late rectal sequelae include chronic tenesmus, telangiectasia and profuse bleeding, rectal ulceration, and strictures. These are usually seen during the 18–36 months follow-up period. Treatment options are sucralfate or steroid enemas, argon plasma coagulation (APC), laser therapy, formalin applied to affected mucosa, or diversion colostomy.

Late bladder complications of haematuria, necrosis, or rarely vesico-vaginal or urethra-vaginal fistulae may occur. Hyperbaric oxygen therapy within six months of onset of haematuria may produce a good therapeutic response.

Late small bowel sequelae are chronic enteritis, subacute intestinal obstruction, perforation, or strictures. These sequelae are greater in patients undergoing radical surgery, especially transperitoneal pelvic lymphadenectomy, and adjuvant radiation ± chemotherapy.

Most patients treated with radical RT have telangiectasia and fibrosis of the vagina, resulting in significant vaginal shortening especially in the elderly, postmenopausal women, and those with extensive tumours treated with a high dose of radiation. These can be overcome to some extent by counselling for regular sexual activity and vaginal dilatation exercises.

9.7 Newer approaches to cervical cancer

Introduction

Over recent years, there has been rapid progress in radiation delivery techniques in parallel with advances in technology and imaging.

Newer external beam radiation techniques such IMRT, image guided radiation therapy (IGRT), and PET-CT guided radiation have also been explored in cervical cancers. However, these need further validation in clinical practice to understand their long-term benefit. Use of IMRT has already significantly reduced the incidence of bowel morbidity—a major issue in treating this disease.

In cervical cancer brachytherapy, the imaging modalities most commonly used are ultrasound, MRI, CT scan, and PET depending on their availability at various institutions. The GEC-ESTRO recommendations have recently been adopted in the USA and in Europe as a standard method of communication between centres using 3D imaging at the time of brachytherapy. These recommendations describe a GTV, which encompasses bright areas in the cervix on T2 weighted MRI; the HR-CTV, which encompasses the entire cervix and all visible or palpable disease at the time of brachytherapy; and the IR-CTV, which is a 1cm margin around this high-risk CTV plus the initial sites of involvement. The IR-CTV includes vaginal extension at the time of diagnosis that may have significantly decreased over time. The group also recommends starting with the standard method of dose prescription, either to point A or to the 60Gy reference volume, and then adjusting the loading pattern and dwell times to ensure comprehensive target coverage. All patients should have the D90, D100, and V100 recorded for the high-risk CTV. At this time, treatment of the full length of the tandem is recommended with modification if necessary of only the top dwell position based on dose to the sigmoid colon.

The European EMBRACE II study group is exploring the treatment of cervical cancer combining routine use of IMRT and daily IGRT with the aim of introducing a risk adaptive dose prescription protocol in locally advanced cervical cancer. It aims to stratify individual risk of nodal and systemic recurrence and enable adaptation of elective nodal volumes to occur, without decreasing local control rates in low-risk groups and improving systemic and para-aortic control in high-risk patients.

Data from the RetroEMBRACE and EMBRACE studies have shown evidence of dose and effect relationships for both target and organs at risk (OARs) confirming the need to deliver adequate target doses and minimize long-term toxicity in a highly curable disease.

There are ongoing studies looking at the timing and role of chemotherapy in cervix cancer. The RTOG trial is evaluating the role of adjuvant chemotherapy in the OUTBACK trial, delivering four cycles of carboplatin/ paclitaxel after completion of chemoradiation.

Furthermore, the INTERLACE trial is randomizing patients to chemoRT alone or neoadjuvant weekly chemotherapy with carboplatin/paclitaxel for six cycles before chemoRT. Until these trials show otherwise, the standard of care will remain concurrent chemoradiation.

Further reading

Haie-Meder C, Van Limbergen E, Barillot I, et al. Recommendations from Gynaecological (GYN) GEC-ESTRO Working Group (I): concepts and terms in 3D image based 3D treatment planning in cervix cancer brachytherapy with emphasis on MRI assessment of GTV and CTV. *Radiother Oncol* 2005; 74:235–45.

Marth C, Landoni F, Mahner S, et al. Cervical cancer: ESMO Clinical Practice Guidelines for diagnosis, treatment and follow-up. *Ann Oncol* 2018; 29(Suppl. 4):iv262.

Potter R, Haie-Meder C, Van Limbergen E, et al. Recommendations from Gynaecological (GYN) GEC-ESTRO Working Group (II): concepts and terms in 3D image based 3D treatment planning in cervix cancer brachytherapy—3D volume parameters and aspects of 3D image-based anatomy, radiation physics, radiobiology. *Radiother Oncol* 2006; 78:67–77.

9.8 Endometrial cancer

Introduction

In the UK, endometrial cancer is the fifth most common female cancer. Primary endometrial cancer arises from the glandular epithelium of the endometrium. The lifetime risk of endometrial cancer in the UK is one in 41. The incidence of endometrial cancer is highest in postmenopausal women, with a median age at presentation of 61 years. Approximately 5% of women with endometrial cancer are <40 years of age. Although the incidence of endometrial cancer has been increasing, mortality rates have generally declined.

Aetiology/risk factors

The majority of endometrial cancers are endometrioid in type (approximately 75%). These tumours often arise from a precursor lesion, severe atypical hyperplasia, and are associated with excessive endogenous or exogenous unopposed oestrogen stimulation. Up to 50% of women diagnosed with severe atypical hyperplasia are found to have invasive endometrial carcinoma in the hysterectomy specimen.

Risk factors for the development of endometrial cancer are:

- Obesity
- Early menarche
- Late menopause
- Prolonged anovulation
- Polycystic ovarian syndrome
- Nulliparity
- Infertility
- Diabetes mellitus
- Hypertension
- Unopposed oestrogen therapy
- Tamoxifen use in postmenopausal women
- Oestrogen-secreting ovarian granulosa cell tumour

- Hereditary predisposition—hereditary non-polyposis coli
- Tamoxifen use is associated with an increased risk of endometrial abnormalities, e.g. benign polyps, non-atypical hyperplasia, atypical hyperplasia, and malignancy. Any histological type of endometrial carcinoma may arise on a background of tamoxifen use. The effect is dose and duration dependent. There is much less evidence of its role in carcinogenesis in premenopausal women

Hereditary non-polyposis coli (Lynch syndrome)

Of endometrial cancer cases 2–5% are hereditary. Most hereditary endometrial cancers arise in women with hereditary non-polyposis colorectal cancer (HNPCC), which is an inherited autosomal dominant disorder arising from germline mutations in one or more mismatch repair genes (hMSH2; hMLH1; hMSH6; PMS1; and PMS2) leading to microsatellite instability (MSI). Women with HNPCC have a 40–60% lifetime risk of developing endometrial cancer.

Clinical features

History/presentation

- Postmenopausal bleeding (PMB) is the commonest presentation. Up to 10% women with PMB will be diagnosed with endometrial cancer.
- Premenopausal women may describe a significant change in menstrual pattern, e.g. increasingly heavy or irregular bleeding.
- Ninety per cent will have abnormal uterine bleeding.
- Persistent postmenopausal vaginal discharge may indicate pyometra associated with intrauterine pathology.
- Identification of endometrial thickening may be noted incidentally on imaging undertaken for other reasons.
- Abnormal endometrial cells may be noted incidentally on cervical cytology.

- Pain is not a significant feature.
- Presentation with the effects of metastatic disease is uncommon.

Examination

- Examination with a bivalve speculum may identify a cervical lesion or cervical extension of an endometrial lesion.
- Bimanual pelvic examination may reveal an enlarged uterus but is often normal.
- Rectal examination should be performed to assess operability if parametrial extension of tumour is suspected on vaginal examination.

Diagnosis

Ultrasound scan

The initial investigation of women with PMB is a transvaginal ultrasound scan.

Data from meta-analyses of trials indicate that endometrial thickness of >5mm on transvaginal ultrasound scan has a 96% sensitivity and 62% specificity for endometrial cancer. Of postmenopausal women 7–8% with an endometrial thickness of >5mm have endometrial cancer. The negative predictive value of an endometrial thickness of <5mm is 98%. The incidence of endometrial cancer where the endometrial thickness is <5mm is <0.5–1.7%. Women with endometrial thickness of 5mm require endometrial biopsy.

Women on tamoxifen commonly have benign subendometrial changes that mimic endometrial thickening on ultrasound scan. Ultrasound is therefore not discriminatory in the investigation of abnormal bleeding in these patients. Women with bleeding on tamoxifen treatment should undergo urgent hysteroscopy and endometrial sampling.

Endometrial sampling/hysteroscopy

Ultrasound scan is not helpful in diagnosing endometrial cancer in premenopausal women as specific cut-off levels for endometrial thickness do not accurately predict or exclude endometrial cancer. Premenopausal women with significant menstrual abnormalities should be investigated by endometrial biopsy ± hysteroscopy.

'Blind' endometrial sampling is accurate in diagnosing endometrial cancer where at least 50% of the uterine cavity is involved. Small or focal lesions may be missed by blind endometrial biopsy and hysteroscopy is recommended where focal thickening is seen on ultrasound scan.

Most women (approximately 80%) have outpatient endometrial sampling and/or hysteroscopy. A minority of women require investigation under general anaesthesia (dilatation, hysteroscopy, and curettage).

Screening

There is no population screening programme for endometrial cancer. Women with HNPCC may be offered annual screening with transvaginal ultrasound scan and endometrial sampling although the efficacy of screening in these women is unproven.

Pathology

Tumour classification

Primary endometrial cancers arise from the glandular epithelial elements within the endometrium. Different histological subtypes are recognized and classified

---

Box 9.8.1 WHO classification of epithelial tumours of the uterine corpus

Primary tumours
- Endometrioid adenocarcinoma
  - Secretory variant
  - Villoglandular variant
  - Ciliated cell variant
  - With squamous differentiation (this is distinct from squamous carcinoma)
- Mucinous adenocarcinoma
- Serous adenocarcinoma
- Clear cell adenocarcinoma
- Squamous cell carcinoma
- Transitional cell carcinoma
- Small cell carcinoma
- Undifferentiated carcinoma
- Mixed cell carcinoma

Note: the WHO classification does not currently include carcinosarcoma as an epithelial tumour although molecular evidence indicates that this is an epithelial tumour rather than a mesenchymal tumour.

Source: data from Kurman RJ, Carcangiu ML, Herrington S, Young, RH. *Tumours of the Female Reproductive Organs. WHO Classification of Tumours*. Lyon: IARC Press, 2014.

---

according to the World Health Organization (WHO) classification, based on cell type and pattern (see Box 9.8.1). Endometrioid carcinoma is the most common type (>75%). Less common types include serous, clear cell, and carcinosarcoma (previously called malignant mixed Müllerian tumour— see 'Uterine sarcomas', p. 251). Elements of different histological types may coexist in a single tumour. These cancers are classified as mixed tumours.

Tumour grade

Tumour grade is assessed for all endometrioid endometrial cancers. There are several grading systems. In the UK the FIGO grading system is used. It is based upon architectural abnormalities and is determined by the extent to which recognizable glands comprise the tumour compared to solid areas. Tumours are graded 1–3 with grade 1 tumours being low grade. Serous and clear cell tumours and carcino-sarcomas are considered high-grade tumours, as are undifferentiated tumours. Tumour grade is correlated with the risk of lymph node metastasis.

Pattern of spread

- See also 'Staging' (p. 245).
- Direct extension into myometrium and cervix.
- Transtubal metastasis to ovaries and peritoneal cavity.
- Lymphatic metastasis to pelvic lymph nodes.
- Para-aortic nodal involvement can arise directly via the lymphatic channels draining the upper uterus.
- Para-aortic involvement is less common in the absence of pelvic node metastasis.
- Lymphatic and haematogenous spread to vagina.
- Haematogenous spread to lungs.

- Serous and clear cell carcinomas have a tendency to early intraperitoneal spread.

Molecular features

Different histological subtypes of endometrial cancer exhibit different molecular characteristics suggesting different developmental pathways. Based on molecular differences, endometrial cancers can be broadly classified into two main groups: type I and type II tumours.

Type I tumours have the following characteristics:

- Grade 1 and 2 endometrioid tumours.
- Often arise in association with atypical hyperplasia, a precursor lesion.
- Associated with the risk factors shown listed earlier in this chapter under 'Aetiology/risk factors' (p. 243).
- Frequently exhibit mutations in the PTEN tumour suppressor gene, K-ras oncogene, and mismatch repair genes, or show evidence of microsatellite instability.
- Frequently exhibit oestrogen receptor (ER) and progesterone receptor (PgR).
- Associated with a better prognosis overall than type II tumours.

Type II tumours generally have the following characteristics:

- Non-endometrioid tumours, e.g. serous, clear cell, or grade 3 endometrioid tumours.
- Not associated with excess or unopposed oestrogens or other typical risk factors for type I tumours.
- Frequently arise in older postmenopausal women, on a background of atrophic endometrium.
- Recent evidence suggests the possible existence of a precursor lesion for serous tumours, endometrial intraepithelial carcinoma (EIC).
- Mutations of the p53 tumour suppressor are common in type II tumours (with the exception of clear cell tumours).
- Overexpression of epidermal growth factor receptor 2 (EGFR2) is commonly seen.
- Have a tendency to early extrauterine spread despite minimal invasion of the myometrium.
- Spread often occurs intraperitoneally with omental involvement.
- Associated with a worse prognosis than type I tumours.

Biomarkers and prognostic markers

Positive prognostic markers:

- Persistence of expression of ER and PgR

Negative prognostic markers are not currently clinically utilized as stage is a stronger predictor of outcome overall but include the following:

- P53 overexpression
- EGFR over expression
- Evidence of high proliferation rates such as Ki67

Investigations

Magnetic resonance imaging

MRI is commonly used to evaluate depth of tumour invasion into the myometrium as this is related to the risk of lymph node metastasis. Pelvic lymphadenopathy may be assessed although nodal metastasis cannot be definitively excluded on MRI.

Despite the common use of MRI, there is little evidence of benefit for routine pelvic MRI in women where the disease appears clinically confined to the uterine corpus. MRI may be used to evaluate the cervix where there is clinical suspicion of cervical involvement with tumour. Published series suggest that MRI findings accurately predict cervical extension and depth of myometrial invasion in 92% of cases.

In the UK, MRI is usually performed in order to identify women at high risk of extrauterine disease who need to have surgery performed by a specialist gynaecological oncologist.

MRI is used in the evaluation of suspected central pelvic recurrence.

Computed tomography

CT scan is inferior to MRI in the evaluation of myometrial invasion but is used in the evaluation of the upper abdomen and/or thorax where there is a higher risk of extrapelvic metastases, e.g. serous carcinoma, carcinosarcoma, or locally advanced disease.

CT scan is required for RT treatment planning (see 'Role of radiotherapy', p. 247), and is used in the evaluation of possible abdominal and extra-abdominal recurrence.

Examination under anaesthesia

EUA is indicated to determine operability where locally advanced tumour is suspected on outpatient examination or on imaging. Cystoscopy is indicated where bladder invasion is suspected.

Staging

FIGO staging (2009) of endometrial cancers which is based on both surgical findings and histopathology is shown in Box 9.8.2 (and is analogous to the T staging component of the 2017 tumour node metastasis (TNM)).

Box 9.8.2 FIGO staging of endometrial cancers 2009

Stage 0: carcinoma in situ
Stage I: limited to the body of the uterus
Ia: no or less than half (≤50%) myometrial invasion
Ib: invasion equal to or more than half (≥50%) of the myometrium
Stage II: cervical stromal involvement (endocervical glandular involvement only is stage I)
Stage III: local or regional spread of the tumour
IIIa: tumour invades the serosa of the body of the uterus and/or adnexa
IIIb: vaginal or parametrial involvement
IIIc: pelvic or para-aortic lymphadenopathy
IIIc1: positive pelvic nodes
IIIc2: positive para-aortic nodes with or without pelvic nodes
Stage IV: involvement of rectum and/or bladder mucosa and or distant metastasis
IVa: bladder or rectal mucosal involvement
IVb: distant metastases, malignant ascites, peritoneal involvement

Source: data from Creasman W. Revised FIGO staging for carcinoma of the endometrium. *Int J Gynaecol Obstet* 2009; 105(2):109. 2009, John Wiley & Sons.

Prognosis

Endometrial cancer has a better overall prognosis than other cancers of the female genital tract. The five-year survival rate across all stages is approximately 80%. This is due to early presentation with most women having stage I disease. Long-term outcomes for women with stage III/IV disease are significantly poorer.

Prognosis varies considerably depending on:
• Depth of myometrial invasion
• Stage
• Presence of LVSI
• Grade
• Histological subtype

Age >60 years was an adverse prognostic factor in a large randomized trial of adjuvant RT versus RT alone.

9.9 Management of endometrial cancer

Introduction

Surgery is the cornerstone of treatment for endometrial cancer and may be supplemented by adjuvant therapies. The majority of women have stage I disease at diagnosis (75%). Up to 10% of women have stage II cancer, and a further 15% stage III or IV disease. The extent of surgery varies according to stage of disease.

Surgery for stage I disease

Total laparoscopic hysterectomy and bilateral salpingo-oophorectomy

A standard surgical approach where disease is confined to the uterine corpus on examination is laparoscopically assisted vaginal hysterectomy and bilateral salpingo-oophorectomy (LAVH/BSO) or total laparoscopic hysterectomy and bilateral salpingo-oophorectomy (TLH/BSO). Peritoneal washings for cytology may be taken but as positive cytology does not affect staging they are not mandatory.

Laparoscopic surgery for endometrial cancer

The GOG-LAP2 study randomized >2,600 women with clinical stage I–IIa disease to laparoscopic staging and surgery for endometrial cancer versus laparotomy. Results demonstrate similar relapse rates (11.4% in the laparascopic group and 10.2% in the laparotomy group), with equivalent five-year OS (89.8%) but with significantly shorter hospital stay, fewer postoperative complications, and improved QoL scores in the laparoscopic arm. Consequently, laparoscopic surgery would be considered as standard of care. The use of robot assisted laparoscopy is increasing, particularly in the bariatric population.

Vaginal hysterectomy

In the case of severe comorbidity that prevents safe general anaesthesia for abdominal surgery, vaginal hysterectomy alone may be performed under regional anaesthesia. Vaginal hysterectomy (with or without adjuvant RT) can achieve five-year survival rates of 80–90% in very obese and/or medically compromised women.

Surgery for stage II disease

Radical hysterectomy, bilateral salpingo-oophorectomy +/– lymphadenectomy

Women with clinical stage II endometrial cancer may be treated with radical hysterectomy, BSO, +/– lymphadenectomy. Data from the SEER database show improved five-year survival (93%) following radical hysterectomy alone compared with standard hysterectomy (83%) alone for women with stage II endometrial cancer.

However, morbidity is significantly higher after radical hysterectomy than after standard hysterectomy and a significant proportion of women will not be considered fit enough for radical surgery. In practice many surgeons perform a standard hysterectomy and adjuvant RT is offered postoperatively.

Surgery for advanced endometrial cancer (stages III/IV)

Women with advanced disease are a heterogeneous group. Prognosis varies considerably within this group according to substage, i.e. women with stage IIIa disease have a better prognosis than those with stage IIIb or IIIc disease. In patients of good PS, maximal debulking should be undertaken where possible. If locally advanced disease is suspected, EUA should be performed to determine operability. If the patient is considered inoperable initially, primary RT or chemotherapy can be given and surgery considered secondarily following a clinical response.

In patients of good PS with metastatic disease, consideration should be given to palliative surgery. Good control of pelvic disease with palliation of vaginal bleeding and pelvic pain can be achieved by hysterectomy even when distant metastases are present. The role of more aggressive debulking surgery in advanced disease is uncertain.

Lymphadenectomy

The role of lymphadenectomy in endometrial cancer surgery is a controversial issue. Full pelvic and para-aortic lymphadenectomy is required for FIGO staging although the therapeutic role of lymphadenectomy continues to be debated. The UK Medical Research Council (MRC) trial, A Study in the Treatment of Endometrial Cancer (ASTEC) is the only large, adequately powered randomized study to address the role of lymphadenectomy in clinical stage I endometrial cancer. Women with clinical stage I disease were randomized to lymphadenectomy versus no lymphadenectomy. Most tumours had endometrioid histology. This study concluded that lymphadenectomy does not improve survival in women with clinical stage I endometrial cancer (89% survival with lymphadenectomy compared to 88% for women who did not have lymphadenectomy). Lymphadenectomy is associated with higher morbidity and mortality. This study has been criticized for having inadequate lymph node dissection, inadequate control of adjuvant therapies, and excessive numbers of low-risk patients. Indeed, retrospective data from the SEER and NCI databases and from Japan suggest that there may be an improvement in disease-specific survival in intermediate- and high-risk patients when compared with no lymph node dissection. It is generally accepted that in low-risk patients there is no value in lymphadenectomy but there may be a role in higher risk more advanced disease.

There have been no large randomized trials evaluating the role of lymphadenectomy in non-endometrioid endometrial cancers. A large series of 148 cases of fully staged serous endometrial cancers indicated that survival in true stage Ia and Ib disease was approximately 80% at five years. Similar results were seen for clear cell cancers. This may reflect understaging in other studies. Currently lymphadenectomy is advised in these tumours.

Omentectomy/omental biopsy

Omental biopsy/infracolic omentectomy may be performed in cases of serous endometrial cancer. Although omentectomy is not specifically featured in the FIGO staging system, serous tumours have a tendency to upper abdominal metastasis even when there is minimal myometrial invasion. Omental biopsy/omentectomy is associated with relatively little morbidity and many surgeons consider this to be a standard part of surgery for serous tumours.

Complications of surgery

Complications may be those that are seen with any surgical procedure, or specific to pelvic surgery.

General

- Haemorrhage
- Pulmonary complications—pneumonia, atelectasis

- Urinary retention
- Wound infection
- Thromboembolism—DVT, pulmonary embolism (PE)
- Haematoma

Specific to abdominopelvic surgery

- Bladder injury
- Ureteric injury
- Bowel injury
- Damage to major pelvic and abdominal blood vessels with major haemorrhage, e.g. at lymphadenectomy
- Neurological damage—genitofemoral and obturator nerves are at risk during pelvic lymphadenectomy
- Postoperative ileus
- Bladder dysfunction: more common with radical hysterectomy due to disruption of autonomic nerves in uterosacral ligaments
- Pelvic lymphocysts and lymphoedema following pelvic lymphadenectomy
- Hernia formation, e.g. through abdominal wound or vagina
- Ureteric fistula—secondary to ischaemia. Usually occurs as a late complication and is more common after radical hysterectomy followed by pelvic irradiation

Most complications are more common following radical surgery. Prophylactic antibiotics should be administered at the time of surgery and thromboprophylaxis used perioperatively and until the patient is fully mobile.

9.10 Role of radiotherapy

Introduction

RT may be used in the following situations:
- Adjuvant treatment after surgery
- Primary radical treatment
- Radical treatment of pelvic recurrence
- Palliation of advanced/metastatic disease

Adjuvant radiotherapy

RT is most commonly employed in the adjuvant setting following curative surgery. Data to support its use comes from the PORTEC and GOG-99 studies. It should be remembered that these studies used the FIGO 1998 staging rather than the currently used 2009 system. PORTEC 1 randomized high-risk stage 1 patients (IC G1, IB or IC G2, IB G3) to either observation or pelvic RT. The rate of local recurrence was significantly lower in the RT arm (4% vs. 14%) The majority of recurrences in the observation arm were in the upper vagina. There was no survival advantage and the reported toxicity was significantly higher in the RT arm (25% vs. 6%) The GOG study reported similar results. PORTEC 2 randomized between vaginal vault brachytherapy or pelvic RT and included intermediate/high-risk patients (age over 60 IC G1 or G2, or G3 +IB, or any age IIA G1–G3 with less than 50% myometrial invasion). The rates of vaginal recurrence were equivalent in the two arms and the pelvic recurrence rate in the brachytherapy arm was

below 5%. The rates of gastrointestinal toxicity were significantly greater in the pelvic RT arm. ESMO-ESGO-ESTRO guidelines for considering adjuvant RT based on these studies are shown in Table 9.10.1. However, the decision to proceed with pelvic RT, vaginal vault RT, or observation must be determined on an individual basis following a thorough assessment and frank discussion of the pros and cons.

External beam RT to the pelvis is typically delivered using either a 4-field box technique or IMRT to encompass the upper third of the vagina, residual parametrial tissues, paravaginal tissues, and internal, external, and common iliac lymph nodes. The presacral nodes may also be included. Schedules include 45Gy in 25 fractions, and 50.4Gy in 28 fractions. A single fraction of brachytherapy to the vaginal vault may also be delivered.

If brachytherapy is the sole mode of treatment it is typically delivered to the upper third of the vagina using a vaginal applicator and remote after loading devices. A typical high-dose rate schedule is 21Gy in three fractions prescribed at 0.5cm depth.

Radical radiotherapy

RT may occasionally be used as primary treatment in early endometrial cancer where comorbid conditions prevent surgery. This would usually be a combination of external beam RT and intracavity brachytherapy. For

Table 9.10.1 Adjuvant therapy for vaginal cancer

Risk group	Histology	Adjuvant treatment—if lymph node dissection	Adjuvant treatment—if no lymph node dissection
Low	Ia, G1–2, LVSI –ve	None	None
Intermediate	Ib, G1–2, LVSI –ve	Brachytherapy or none if age less than 60	Brachytherapy or none if age less than 60
High-intermediate	Ib, G1–2, LVSI +ve	Brachytherapy or none	Brachytherapy if G3 and LVSI–
	Ia, G3		Pelvic RT if LVSI+
High	Ib, G3	Pelvic RT or brachytherapy	Pelvic RT
	II, G1–2, LVSI –ve	Brachytherapy	Pelvic RT
	II, G3 or LVSI +ve	Pelvic RT	Pelvic RT
	III	Pelvic RT	

Source: data from Colombo N, et al. ESMO-ESGO-ESTRO consensus conference on endometrial cancer: Diagnosis, treatment and follow-up. *Radiother Oncol* 2015; 117(3):559–81. 2015, Elsevier Ltd.

very early tumours intracavity brachytherapy may be used as the sole modality. Typical RT schedules would include either 36Gy in six fractions using HDR brachytherapy alone or 45Gy in 25 fractions of external beam RT to the whole pelvis followed by HDR brachytherapy of 21Gy in three fractions. Cure rates of >65% can be achieved although the risk of recurrence is high (20%). Primary surgery is therefore advocated wherever possible.

Primary RT may also be indicated in cases of locally advanced cancer where the tumour is inoperable at presentation. Neoadjuvant chemotherapy may also be considered with a view to downstage the disease sufficiently to permit resection.

Treatment of pelvic recurrence

RT is a curative option for women with pelvic recurrence providing they have not received adjuvant pelvic RT. The cure rate is greater for women with isolated central pelvic recurrence than for women with pelvic side-wall disease. A dose of at least 60Gy is required and this is most likely to be achieved within the organ at risk constraints with IMRT.

Palliative radiotherapy

RT is an effective palliative treatment and may be used for:
- Problematic vaginal bleeding
- Vaginal metastases
- Symptomatic para-aortic metastases
- Bone pain secondary to bone metastases
- Cerebral metastases

Radiotherapy toxicity

RT toxicity may manifest as acute effects or late effects, some months or even years after treatment. Side effects range from mild to severe. Moderate late side effects occur in approximately 25% of women who receive adjuvant treatment. Severe toxicity affects up to 7% of women in clinical trials of adjuvant RT.

The risk of severe toxicity is dependent on total dose of radiation given as well as the fractionation schedule.

The following factors also increase the risk of severe side effects:
- Large treatment volume
- Previous pelvic or abdominal surgery including lymphadenectomy
- Inflammatory conditions affecting the pelvis, e.g. ulcerative colitis
- Conditions that impair the vascular supply to pelvic/abdominal organs, e.g. severe arteriopathy

Early effects

Early or acute effects are seen during treatment and affect approximately 60% of women. These usually resolve within four to six weeks following completion of treatment. These include:
- Abdominal cramps
- Diarrhoea
- Urinary frequency
- Urinary urgency
- Skin irritation
- Fatigue

Late effects

Late effects include:
- Radiation proctitis or radiation colitis
- Radiation cystitis
- Bowel/ureteric stricture or fistulae
- Vaginal bleeding or stenosis
- Lower limb lymphoedema
- Insufficiency fractures of the sacrum
- (Rarely) development of malignancy within the irradiated field (usually sarcomas)

Some late effects may respond to conservative or simple measures, e.g. dietary modification for bowel disturbances, steroid enemas for radiation proctitis, and argon laser photo coagulation for rectal bleeding. Where these are unsuccessful or where the complication is very severe or life-threatening, surgery may be required, e.g. bowel resection. There is a higher risk of anastomotic breakdown as irradiated bowel and ureter are poorly vascularized. Colostomy or urinary diversion may therefore be required.

9.11 Role of chemotherapy and hormonal agents

Chemotherapy

Chemotherapy may be considered in the following situations:

- Adjuvant treatment following surgery
- Neoadjuvant treatment of inoperable disease or recurrent disease
- Palliation of metastatic disease
- Palliation of recurrent disease

Adjuvant chemotherapy

The role of adjuvant chemotherapy is controversial due to limited high-quality data on which to base decisions. In individuals with high-risk disease (stage III or IV disease or clear cell or serous papillary histologies), many would advocate postoperative chemotherapy. A Cochrane analysis demonstrated an OS and a PFS advantage with the use of platinum containing regimens. In these studies, the regimens used included cisplatin + doxorubicin or cisplatin + doxorubicin + paclitaxel. Subsequently the GOG 209 study in advanced stage, chemotherapy-naive endometrial cancer patients has demonstrated equivalence between carboplatin and paclitaxel versus cisplatin, paclitaxel, and doxorubicin but with significantly less toxicity with the doublet as compared to the triplet regimen. Carboplatin and paclitaxel would be considered a standard option for adjuvant therapy.

An intermediate/high-risk disease group of patients can be defined on the basis of a combination of risk factors (see 'Adjuvant radiotherapy', p. 247). The value of adjuvant chemotherapy is also controversial in this group. A subgroup analysis of intermediate/high-risk patients in a Japanese study of pelvic RT versus a combination of cyclophosphamide, doxorubicin, and cisplatin demonstrated an improvement in both OS and PFS with adjuvant chemotherapy. A Cochrane review from 2011 also included some intermediate/high-risk patients and demonstrated a trend towards improved survival.

More recently PORTEC 3 has reported an OS advantage of approximately 5% across the trial cohort of intermediate and high risk with subgroup analysis demonstrating greater benefit in stage III cancers and high-grade serous histological subtypes. The ESMO guidelines suggest that chemotherapy be considered in all patients with either stage III disease or high-risk disease/serous histologies in the absence of lymphadenectomy/sentinel lymph nodes sampling.

Palliative chemotherapy

There is evidence from a further Cochrane review that combination regimens are active in advanced endometrial cancer and improve both QoL and OS. In light of the data from GOG 209 discussed earlier, it is considered reasonable to offer carboplatin and paclitaxel as first-line treatment as it is well tolerated and has similar activity to other more toxic regimens.

Hormonal agents

Systemic hormonal therapy is used to palliate symptoms in advanced and recurrent endometrial cancer. Hormonal treatments are associated with a favourable side effect profile compared with many cytotoxic drugs and they are therefore useful in medically unfit women where the goal of treatment is palliation.

Local progestin therapy delivered via an intrauterine device may be used as a palliative measure in low-grade tumours or as a holding measure in medically inoperable patients to allow time to improve fitness for surgery as, for example, to allow weight loss measures.

Progestogens

- Progestogen treatment has no benefit in the adjuvant treatment of endometrial cancer.
- Response rates with oral progestogens are approximately 10–25% in published studies of women with advanced and recurrent disease.
- Recommended regimens are medroxyprogesterone acetate 200–400mg daily or megestrol acetate 40–320mg daily in divided doses.
- Low-grade, slow-growing tumours are most likely to respond.
- The median progression-free duration is approximately four months. Median OS of approximately ten months is reported. Downregulation of PgRs shortens the duration of response.
- High-grade tumours often lack PgRs and therefore the beneficial effect may be limited.
- Tamoxifen and other selective ER modulators have been used in some studies with the aim of recruiting receptors and increasing the duration of response to progestogens. Median duration of response is similar to that seen with progestogens alone.

Aromatase inhibitors

- These drugs decrease oestrogen levels by blocking the aromatase enzyme.
- Response rates in phase 2 studies are low (approximately 9%) and duration of response limited.

9.12 Recurrence and metastasis

Introduction

The rate of recurrence of endometrial cancer is related to stage of disease. The overall rate of recurrence is 7–18%. Recurrence may occur locally, in the pelvis or at distant sites. The pattern of recurrence is influenced by the histological subtype and previous treatment modalities used.

A higher proportion of patients with disease relapse following adjuvant pelvic RT have recurrence at distant sites. Conversely, pelvic recurrence affects a higher proportion of women who receive adjuvant chemotherapy alone for high-risk disease.

Serous carcinomas have a tendency to spread intraperitoneally and more aggressive histologies predispose to distant disease.

Symptoms that may indicate recurrence

- Vaginal bleeding/persistent abnormal vaginal discharge
- Pelvic pressure symptoms
- Unilateral leg swelling or neuropathic pain
- New-onset central abdominal pain or back pain
- Symptoms from distant metastases are dependent on the affected organ(s)

Treatment options for recurrent and metastatic endometrial cancer

Treatment depends on the site(s) of recurrence, previous treatments used, and PS of the patient.

Surgery

Surgery is a curative option for previously irradiated women with a single recurrence at the vaginal vault. It is vital that other sites of disease are excluded by appropriate imaging, e.g. CT/MRI before embarking on surgery. PET-CT may also be undertaken to confirm isolated recurrence. Pelvic exenteration may be required to obtain tumour-free resection margins and if the bladder or bowel are involved with the tumour. Significant morbidity is 60–80% in some series and published perioperative mortality rates are as high as 16%. Careful patient selection is therefore very important.

Radiotherapy

Generally, women with pelvic recurrence who have not previously been exposed to pelvic radiation are treated with RT. Those who have received vault brachytherapy alone as adjuvant therapy can be safely retreated with radical doses of external beam RT. Isolated pelvic recurrence is curable and approximately 65% of women survive for at least five years after treatment with RT. In some cases it may be possible to deliver a curative dose using a combination of external beam and vaginal brachytherapy in the event of an excellent response to external beam but in most cases a dose of 60–65Gy will be delivered using external beam RT. The cure rate is lower for women with pelvic side wall disease reflecting the difficulty in delivering tumouricidal doses within the constraints of safe doses to the other pelvic viscera.

RT may be used with palliative intent in cases of extrapelvic disease, e.g. for pain from bony metastasis.

Chemotherapy

Chemotherapy is used in the palliative setting for metastatic or recurrent disease. In the case of large volume isolated pelvic recurrence it may be used before definitive RT to reduce the high-dose target volume.

Hormonal treatment

Hormonal treatment can provide good palliation with acceptable side effects in recurrent and widely metastatic disease although the duration of effect is limited. Oral progestogens are used most commonly.

Symptomatic measures

Treatment of symptoms associated with incurable recurrence is important, including the appropriate use of effective analgesia. Vaginal bleeding from advanced inoperable tumour or recurrent disease may respond to oral tranexamic acid, 3–4g daily in divided doses. Uterine artery embolization has also been used with good effect to treat acute haemorrhage from inoperable uterine tumours. Rarely a palliative surgical procedure may be considered in the case of advanced disease with an intact uterus causing intractable bleeding.

Further reading

Colombo N, Preti E, Landoni F, et al. Endometrial cancer: ESMO Clinical Practice Guidelines for diagnosis, treatment and follow-up. *Ann Oncol* 2013 Oct;24(Suppl. 6):vi33–8.

Talhouk A, McConechy MK, Leung S, et al. A clinically applicable molecular-based classification for endometrial cancers. *Br J Cancer* 2015; 113(2):299–310.

9.13 Uterine sarcomas

Introduction

- Uterine sarcomas represent a rare group of malignancies, the most common of which are leiomyosarcoma (LMS), low-grade or high-grade endometrial stromal sarcoma (ESS), and undifferentiated uterine sarcoma (UUS).
- Mixed epithelial and mesenchymal tumours of the uterus include adenosarcoma (AS) and carcinosarcoma (CS). CS (previously known as malignant mixed Müllerian tumours) were historically included within uterine sarcoma trials but have now been reclassified as aggressive carcinomas. They are included here as much of the early literature does not separate them from other uterine sarcomas.

Incidence/epidemiology

- Uterine sarcomas comprise about 3–7% of all uterine malignancies.
- Uterine sarcoma is two to three times more common in black women than Caucasians.
- Mean age of diagnosis is 60 years, with CS diagnosed more frequently in older women.
- Relative frequencies of different histological subtypes from SEER were reported as CS 53%, LMS 24%, ESS 14%, AS 5%, and sarcoma, not otherwise specified (NOS) 4%.

Aetiology

- Previous pelvic RT. The estimated absolute risk ranges from 0.003% to 0.8% after a latency period of 3–30 (median 17) years.
- Tamoxifen exposure (0.17 per 1,000 women-years but higher in CS) has been identified as a causative agent in a minority of patients
- Survivors of childhood retinoblastoma, and those with hereditary leiomyomatosis and renal cell carcinoma (a rare autosomal dominant condition caused by mutations in the fumarate hydratase gene), have been found to be at increased risk of developing uterine sarcoma.
- Black women and those over 50 years of age are at increased risk.
- Obesity, history of diabetes, and younger age of menarche have been suggested as additional risk factors.

Clinical features

- These depend on the stage at presentation, histological subtype, and grade of the tumour.
- In localized disease, patients may present with increased vaginal and PMB.
- Many uterine sarcomas are found unexpectedly at the time of routine hysterectomy.
- On vaginal examination a polypoidal lesion or mass protruding through the cervical os may be evident.
- Patients with advanced disease may present with an abdominal mass, abdominal pain, or symptoms of systemic disease such as lethargy, anorexia, and weight loss.
- Nodal disease is rare in uterine sarcomas but inguinal nodes should be excluded on examination.

Diagnosis

- Ultrasound or MRI is often performed with increased vaginal bleeding and a mass may be visible. MRI is the local imaging of choice.
- CT scan and fluorodeoxyglucose-PET (FDG-PET) are also used for diagnostic and staging purposes.
- Multiple benign leiomyomata may be visible and it may not be possible to distinguish LMS from the benign lesions.
- No imaging modality has yet been able to distinguish benign leiomyomata from LMS. Similarly, rapid growth rate has not been found to correlate with risk of malignancy.
- ESS are seen as infiltrative lesions.
- CS often present as large heterogenous polypoid structures which bulge through the cervical os.
- Pelvic and para-aortic nodes can be seen in CS but are rare in other uterine sarcomas.
- CA-125 is often elevated in CS.
- Biopsy may be performed prior to surgery but only examination of the entire uterus postoperatively gives an accurate diagnosis. In particular LMS are rarely diagnosed on preoperative biopsy.
- Biopsy of CS often only reveals the epithelial component.

Pathology

- LMS originate from the myometrium but are often large and protrude into the endometrium. They are predominantly high-grade lesions with a high mitotic rate. They usually express smooth muscle markers such as desmin, smooth muscle actin, and h-caldesmon, and are usually positive for CD10 (marker of endometrial stromal differentiation).
- The nomenclature for endometrial stromal tumours has been a cause of confusion over the years. Specifically, ESS was originally divided into low-grade and high-grade based on mitotic count, but subsequent studies showed that mitotic activity is prognostically irrelevant. Subsequently the 2003 WHO classification categorized endometrial stromal tumours into: endometrial stromal nodule (ESN) (a benign tumour), ESS (low-grade tumours resembling proliferative endometrial stroma that grow outwards into the myometrium and are usually CD10-positive), and undifferentiated endometrial sarcoma (UES) (pleomorphic tumours with no resemblance to endometrial stroma).
- However, it is increasing evident that the category of UES is too broad, and the latest 2014 WHO system has since reclassified these tumours:
  - ESN
  - Low-grade ESS (LGESS)
  - High-grade ESS (HGESS)
  - UUS
- LGESS is a slow-growing tumour with an indolent clinical course. The addition of a separate category of HGESS to the 2014 WHO classification was due

to the recent identification of an ESS with YWHAE-NUTM2A/B gene rearrangement, which has distinct morphological features and prognosis intermediate between LGESS and UUS.

- UUS is a high-grade, aggressive malignancy that lacks specific types of cellular differentiation and gene rearrangements.
- AS is a rare neoplasm that comprises benign epithelial and malignant stromal elements. AS with sarcomatous overgrowth (SO) (defined as the presence of pure sarcoma comprising at least 25% of the tumour) are highly malignant and tend to be larger and invade the myometrium compared to conventional AS.
- CS are dedifferentiated (metaplastic) carcinomas which have both malignant epithelial and sarcomatous components. The epithelial component is most commonly serous papillary or endometrioid carcinoma. The sarcomatous components can be homologous if it is native to the uterine tissue (e.g. LMS), or heterologous (e.g. chondrosarcoma). CS have been found to be monoclonal entities in which the epithelial component is frequently seen in metastatic lesions. For this reason they have been reclassified as a high-risk variant of endometrial adenocarcinomas. However, their poor prognosis more accurately reflects that of sarcomas.

Hormone receptors

- A significant proportion of uterine sarcomas express ER or PgR, although the degree of expression varies according to histology. The degree of ER and PgR expression is less than that seen in breast cancer.
- LGESS usually express ER and PgR and oestrogen-lowering therapy has been used as a treatment option. About 80% of LGESS are positive for ER-alpha, none for ER-beta, and 90% for PgR. ER and PgR are often negative in HGESS and UUS.
- ER and PgR are expressed in 40–87% and 38–80% of uterine LMS, respectively, and may be associated with a better outcome compared to receptor-negative disease.
- Most cases of AS showed ER and PgR positivity in the epithelial and stromal components, but this is significantly reduced or absent in AS with SO.

> Author tip: check ER and PgR status of uterine sarcomas. If strongly positive, oestrogen replacement therapy (HRT) would be inadvisable.

Molecular features

- About half of LGESS harbour the t(7;17)(p15;q21) translocation, producing the JAZF1-SUZ12 (formerly JAZF1-JJAZ1) fusion gene. The abnormality is also found in the benign ESN.
- HGESS are characterized by the t(10;17)(q22;p13) translocation, resulting in the YWHAE-NUTM2A/B (also known as YWHAE-FAM22A/B) fusion gene. These tumours tend to be positive for cyclin D1.
- AS with SO are more likely to have MYBL1 amplification or ATRX mutation. Their significance in AS is currently unknown.

Staging

Staging is according to the 2009 FIGO staging system and is based on surgical findings, although it does not reflect prognosis as well as for endometrial carcinoma. The staging for LMS and ESS are shown here.

- Stage I: tumour limited to uterus
  - IA: <5cm*
  - IB: >5cm*
- Stage II: tumour extends to the pelvis
  - IIA: adnexal involvement
  - IIB: involvement of other pelvic tissues
- Stage III: tumour invades abdominal tissues (not just protruding into the abdomen)
  - IIIA: one site
  - IIIB: >one site
  - IIIC: metastasis to pelvic and/or para-aortic lymph nodes
- Stage IV
  - IVA: tumour invades bladder and/or rectum.
  - IVB: distant metastasis

* Staging for AS is as above, except for stage I tumours: IA (tumour limited to endometrium/endocervix with no myometrial invasion); IB (≤half myometrial invasion); IC (>half myometrial invasion).

CS is staged using the endometrial carcinoma staging system. About 30% of patients have lymph node involvement at presentation.

Data from SEER showed that patients with AS were more likely to present with stage I disease (74.2%), compared to LGESS (54.7%), LMS (49.4%), CS (37.7%), and sarcoma, NOS (23.6%).

Prognosis

- Prognosis in uterine sarcomas is significantly worse than epithelial endometrial cancer of comparable stage.
- SEER analysis showed five-year OS rates of 78.7% for AS, 71.8% for LGESS, 41.9% for LMS, 39.1% for CS, and 20.5% for sarcoma, NOS. The survival patterns reflect those of disease stage at presentation.
- In a SEER study of 1,396 LMS patients, five-year disease-specific survivals of 75.8% for stage I, 60.1% for stage II, 44.9% for stage III, and 28.7% for stage IV were described.
- A SEER study of 831 women with LGESS showed five-year survivals of 91.7% for stage I, 52.8% for stage II, 61.5% for stage III, and 41.0% for stage IV. Late recurrences are common, even 20 years after initial surgery.
- YWHAE-NUTM2A/B-associated HGESS have intermediate prognosis between LGESS and UUS.
- Outcome of UUS is poor regardless of disease stage. In a series of 21 patients, the median PFS and OS were 7.3 months and 11.8 months, respectively. The respective one-year survivals were 35.7% and 80% for those with and without measurable disease respectively at time of treatment.
- Most patients with AS present with localized disease and therefore have a more favourable outcome. A SEER study demonstrated five-year survivals of up to 84% for stage I, 69% for stage II, 48% for stage III, and 15% for stage IV disease. However, this does not include AS with SO, which are more likely to present with advanced disease, recurrence, and have a much poorer outcome. For example, the recurrence rates among stage I patients were 77% versus 22% for those with and without SO, respectively.
- Five-year survivals for CS have been reported as 59% (stage I/II), 22% (stage III), and 9% (stage IV).

Prognostic factors

- Stage has consistently been identified as the most important prognostic factor for all uterine sarcomas. Other factors associated with a poor prognosis include old age, black race, local extension of tumour (myometrial invasion or lymphovascular invasion), and lack of primary surgery.
- In AS, the presence of SO is also a poor prognostic feature.
- In CS, elevation of serum CA-125 has been associated with a worse outcome.
- In LMS, factors associated with a poor prognosis were found to be old age, black race, big tumour, high grade, high mitotic index, advanced stage, and no primary surgical treatment. A Memorial Sloan–Kettering Cancer Center nomogram has been developed to predict five-year survival rates following surgery.

Patterns of relapse

- In LMS, pelvic and extrapelvic recurrences can occur. Extrapelvic metastases in LMS can occur in the liver, lung, lymph nodes, and bone.
- In LGESS, pelvic recurrence is more common although distant relapses to the lungs can occur.
- CS recur locally in the pelvis, throughout the peritoneum (as in epithelial ovarian cancer (EOC)), in the lymph nodes, lung, and bone.
- Brain metastases are rare in all subgroups. The patterns of relapse can be affected by treatment.
- Extrapelvic relapse has been shown to be more frequent in those who have had adjuvant RT.

Principles of management

Surgery remains the mainstay of uterine sarcoma treatment. The role of adjuvant therapy remains unclear and controversial but is often considered in patients at high risk of recurrence.

Surgical

- Standard surgical approach is a total abdominal hysterectomy and bilateral salpingo-oophorectomy. In young premenopausal women, oophorectomy may be individualized by taking into consideration the disease type/stage and hormonal receptor status.
- Removal of lesions by morcellation is contraindicated as this spreads disease within the pelvis and peritoneum. Any tumour found incidentally after morcellation should have a laparotomy to review for signs of spread within two months of primary surgery. Patients with unknown uterine lesions should be warned about the risks of morcellation in the event of unexpected finding of cancer.
- A single study has shown no improvement in survival for LMS with or without oophorectomy, but it is clear from the strong ER positivity of most of the remaining uterine sarcomas that oophorectomy remains an essential part of their surgery.
- Routine lymphadenectomy is advocated in CS as 20% with clinical stage I/II disease were found to have lymph node metastasis, and lymphadenectomy may be associated with improved survival.
- Routine lymphadenectomy in LGESS remains controversial. 5–10% of patients with LGESS have positive nodes, and nodal metastases are associated with poorer prognosis. However, routine lymphadenectomy has not been shown to improve survival, although it could provide prognostic information and help guide adjuvant treatment.
- Lymphadenectomy is not routinely performed for LMS, HGESS, and USS.
- Surgery also has a role in the management of isolated relapse or in resection of limited metastases as other soft tissue sarcomas.
- For resection of metastases there should be no evidence of disease elsewhere, a significant disease-free period with evidence of stable or slowly progressive disease.
- Resection of metastases in rapidly progressive disease is not advocated.

Radiotherapy

- External beam palliative RT is used extensively for symptomatic metastases in all uterine sarcomas.
- Treatment in the adjuvant setting, particularly for stage I/II, is more controversial and is usually not recommended although it could be considered for selected high-risk cases.
- Most evidence of adjuvant RT was derived from retrospective studies, which showed benefit in local control with adjuvant pelvic irradiation with doses of 40–50Gy.
- The phase 3 EORTC 55874 trial randomized patients with stage I/II uterine sarcomas to adjuvant pelvic RT (51Gy in 28 fractions) or observation. The trial took 13 years to accrue 103 LMS, 91 CS, and 28 ESS patients. The results demonstrated no benefit in local control or survival benefit of adjuvant RT in LMS and ESS. Some argue that the trial was underpowered to detect benefit in individual pathological groups.
- Results from large case series and the EORTC 55874 trial showed that adjuvant RT in CS appeared to decrease the rate of local recurrence but with no effect on OS.
- The peritoneal spread of CS led to the use of whole abdominal irradiation (WAI) in some studies. The GOG-0150 randomized phase 3 trial compared WAI with cisplatin and ifosfamide chemotherapy as post-surgical treatment in stage I–IV CS. This showed non-statistically significant lower rates of recurrence and death with chemotherapy than WAI, although there was no control treatment-free arm. As a result chemotherapy is preferred over WAI.

Chemotherapy (adjuvant)

- The evidence for adjuvant chemotherapy in uterine sarcomas comes from: (i) extrapolation from other soft tissue sarcoma studies; (ii) retrospective studies of all uterine sarcomas including all subgroups and CS; and (iii) smaller studies within specific subgroups.
- The evidence for adjuvant chemotherapy in soft tissue sarcoma is controversial as it is compounded by different histological subtypes with varied chemosensitivities being included as a group in the majority of studies, and the rarity of the disease means that most studies lacked statistical power to detect small changes in survival.
- In the first major meta-analysis published on adjuvant chemotherapy in soft tissue sarcomas, an overall benefit in PFS and time-to-distant metastases was seen

with doxorubicin-containing chemotherapy. There was also a trend towards improved survival although this did not reach statistical significance. Only one randomized trial included patients with uterine sarcomas and this did not show a survival benefit.

- With the increasing use of ifosfamide chemotherapy, four more trials were added to the original meta-analysis, and this demonstrated an absolute risk reduction of death of 6% with adjuvant chemotherapy, or a five-year survival of 46% (40% without chemotherapy).

- However, the subsequent phase 3 randomized EORTC 62931 trial failed to demonstrate a survival benefit with adjuvant doxorubicin and ifosfamide chemotherapy compared to observation in soft tissue sarcoma.

- There is no general consensus regarding the use of adjuvant chemotherapy in early stage uterine sarcomas. Consideration could be made for patients with completely resected high-grade and advanced stage disease (e.g. stage II and above) and subtypes with increased risk of recurrence (e.g. LMS, HGESS, UUS, AS, with SO, and CS). The dismal outcome and relative chemoresistant nature of UUS is also an argument against adjuvant treatment.

- Adjuvant gemcitabine and docetaxel chemotherapy has been shown in a small prospective study to improve PFS in stage I–IV high-grade uterine LMS patients compared with historical controls.

- A subsequent SARC 005 phase 2 trial of adjuvant gemcitabine and docetaxel, followed by doxorubicin, in uterus-limited LMS also suggested better PFS compared with historical controls. The GOG-0277 is a randomized phase 3 trial designed to compare this regimen with observation but had to be closed due to poor accrual.

- Studies of adjuvant chemotherapy in CS demonstrated improved recurrence rates and PFS, but not OS. It is often considered in stage IB disease or above.

- Adjuvant ifosfamide combined with cisplatin or paclitaxel have been shown to be beneficial in CS although they have not been compared with no treatment. Carboplatin combined with paclitaxel is also an active regimen in CS. Ifosfamide-paclitaxel and carboplatin-paclitaxel are preferred over ifosfamide-cisplatin for reasons of toxicity.

Hormonal treatment (adjuvant)

Oestrogen replacement and tamoxifen are contraindicated due to its agonistic effects on the uterus. They are associated with a poorer outcome in patients with LGESS.

- There is no evidence for hormonal treatment in the adjuvant setting for AS, LMS, HGESS, and USS, but it can be considered as an option in high-risk and receptor-positive disease.

- Data from retrospective studies supported the use of hormonal treatment for stage II–IV LGESS, including megestrol acetate, medroxyprogesterone acetate, aromatase inhibitors, and gonadotropin-releasing hormone analogues. The optimal treatment duration is unknown.

Chemotherapy (advanced/metastatic)

In advanced disease chemotherapy has an established role in the treatment of most uterine sarcomas.

- Originally the agents used were those which had the highest objective response rates (ORR) in soft tissue

sarcomas (doxorubicin +/− ifosfamide). The EORTC 62012 randomized phase 3 trial of advanced or metastatic soft tissue sarcomas showed that combination doxorubicin and ifosfamide resulted in better ORR (26% vs. 14%) and median PFS (7.4 vs. 4.6 months) compared with doxorubicin alone, although there was no difference in OS. As such single-agent doxorubicin is often recommended over combination treatment unless the specific goal is palliative tumour shrinkage.

- Recently the combination of doxorubicin and olaratumab (a human IgG1 monoclonal antibody against platelet-derived growth factor receptor alpha) was compared with doxorubicin alone in patients with advanced soft tissue sarcoma in a randomized phase 2 trial. Although there was no difference in ORR (18.2% vs. 11.9%) and median PFS (6.6 months vs. 4.1 months) between the treatment arms, median OS was significantly improved in the combination group (26.5 months vs. 14.7 months). However, when the results of the phase 3 Announce trail were revealed they showed that there was no survival benefit over a longer time period. Further work is being undertaken to understand the differences between phase 2 and phase 3 trials but olaratumab is no longer licensed for this use.

- Studies have suggested that different chemotherapeutic agents have specific roles in certain histological subtypes.

- Gemcitabine and docetaxel has an ORR of 16–18% in soft tissue sarcomas (higher in LMS, especially uterine LMS) and are often used as a second- or subsequent-line treatment. Results from the GeDDis trial in which this regimen was compared with doxorubicin in the first-line setting for all sarcoma subtypes showed it to be non-inferior but more toxic so that doxorubicin remains first-line treatment.

- Trabectedin works by a number of mechanisms including DNA binding, transcription regulation, and effects on the tumour microenvironment. It is used in soft tissue sarcomas and is particularly effective in myxoid/round cell liposarcoma and LMS. In a phase 3 randomized study comparing trabectedin with dacarbazine in metastatic liposarcoma and LMS after failure of conventional chemotherapy, ORR was found to be only 10% but clinical benefit rate (stable disease + ORR) was much higher at 34%, with a reported median PFS of 4.2 months. It is common that a period of disease stabilization may often occur for some time before a response is seen.

- Pazopanib is a multitargeted, orally active tyrosine kinase inhibitor. It was licensed for the treatment of metastatic, non-lipomatous soft tissue sarcoma (particularly synovial sarcoma and LMS) after the phase 3 PALETTE trial which demonstrated improvement in median PFS compared to placebo (4.6 months vs. 1.6 months) for patients who had progressed on chemotherapy. Improvement in OS was not statistically significant (12.5 months vs. 10.7 months). Pazopanib is no longer funded in the National Health Service (NHS).

- Other chemotherapeutic agents that have activity in sarcomas include ifosfamide, liposomal doxorubicin (particularly in elderly patients, or patients with cardiac impairment requiring an anthracycline in the first- or subsequent-line setting), dacarbazine, and oral cyclophosphamide.

- Eribulin, a microtubule inhibitor, was shown to be superior to dacarbazine in prolonging OS for patients with previously treated advanced liposarcoma in a randomized phase 3 trial, although this benefit was not seen with LMS.
- In uterine LMS, besides doxorubicin-based treatment, gemcitabine and docetaxel are also a recommended first- (ORR 36%) or second-line (ORR 27%) option. Single-agent gemcitabine also has activity (ORR 20.5%), as well as agents mentioned earlier. Ifosfamide generally has a low ORR in LMS.
- In LGESS, chemotherapy is rarely effective with response rates of less than 10%. Many of these respond to hormonal manipulation.
- HGESS and UUS are treated with drugs as with other soft tissue sarcomas, including doxorubicin-based regimens, gemcitabine-docetaxel, and ifosfamide. In a recent case series of metastatic HGESS (with confirmed YWHAE rearrangement), prolonged disease control was achieved particularly with anthracycline-based chemotherapy. In metastatic UUS, progression is rapid even in those who responded to chemotherapy.
- A current EORTC trial evaluating cabozantininb in high-grade uterine sarcomas which have responded to anthracycline-based chemotherapy is currently underway.
- AS without SO can be treated with hormonal therapy. AS with SO is highly aggressive and is treated in the same fashion as advanced soft tissue sarcoma, including doxorubicin, gemcitabine-docetaxel, and trabectedin.
- In CS, the most active single agents and their respective ORR are ifosfamide (29–36%), cisplatin (19%), paclitaxel (18%), doxorubicin (10–25%), and topotecan (10%). Combination regimens are more effective, and the following have been found to be superior to ifosfamide alone in phase 3 trials: cisplatin with ifosfamide (54%) and ifosfamide with paclitaxel (45%). Combination of carboplatin and paclitaxel has an ORR of 54% in a phase 2 trial. The latter two combinations are preferred over cisplatin-ifosfamide due to their better toxicity profile. The GOG-0261 randomized phase 3 trial aims to compare ifosfamide-paclitaxel with carboplatin-paclitaxel.

Hormonal treatment (advanced/metastatic)

- In advanced LMS, aromatase inhibitors have been associated with low ORR (~10%) but have a clinical benefit rate of up to 62.5%. It could be considered for patients with low-grade, strongly receptor-positive, and low-burden disease.
- Hormonal therapy is the primary treatment for recurrent or metastatic LGESS. Drugs include megestrol acetate, medroxyprogesterone acetate, aromatase inhibitors, and gonadotropin-releasing hormone analogues. A combined series and literature review suggested an ORR of 67% with aromatase inhibitors.

Support group

Sarcoma UK offers information and access to a growing support network for sarcoma patients and their carers.

Further reading

Benson C, Miah AB. Uterine sarcoma—current perspectives. *Int J Womens Health* 2017; 31(9):597–606.

Casali PG, Abecassis N, Bauer S, et al. ESMO Guidelines Committee and EURACAN: Soft tissue and visceral sarcomas: ESMO–EURACAN Clinical Practice Guidelines for diagnosis, treatment and follow-up, *Ann Oncol* 2018 Oct 1; 29(Suppl. 4):iv51–67.

El-Khalfaoui K, du Bois A, Heitz F, Kurzeder C, Sehouli J, Harter P. Current and future options in the management and treatment of uterine sarcoma. *Ther Adv Med Oncol* 2014 Jan; 6(1):21–8.

Internet resources

Sarcoma UK: http://www.sarcoma.org.uk

9.14 Epithelial ovarian cancer

Introduction, pathology, and clinical features

EOC is the seventh most common cancer in women worldwide, and sixth most common in the UK, with almost 300,000 (World Cancer Research Fund, American Institute for Cancer Research) new cases diagnosed worldwide in 2018 and about 7,500 women diagnosed with the disease each year in the UK. The signs and symptoms and signs of this disease are often non-specific and as a result the majority of cases are diagnosed at an advanced stage (stage 3/4 disease), when the prognosis is generally poor. Overall five-year survival rates for all stages are around 45% but less than 30% for women with stage 3 or 4 disease at diagnosis.

Risk factors

Hormonal and environmental factors

The median age of diagnosis of EOC is 63 years. Risk factors include nulliparity and late menopause (age >52), possibly due to an increased total of lifetime ovulations predisposing to malignant transformation. Early menarche (age <12) has been associated with increased risk in some studies, but not others. Whilst infertility is associated with increased risk of EOC, there is conflicting evidence on whether ovarian stimulation therapy increases the risk. However, a Cochrane review published in 2013 found no convincing evidence of increased risk with ovarian stimulation therapy. Use of hormone therapy in postmenopausal women appears to result in a small but statistically significant increased risk of developing EOC, with no significant difference between oestrogen only and oestrogen-progesterone preparations. Endometriosis and polycystic ovaries have been linked with an increased risk of EOC, but, perineal talc, and smoking have been discounted as causative factors.

Hereditary predisposition

BRCA 1 and BRCA 2

About 15% of all epithelial ovarian cancers have a hereditary predisposition, with the majority being linked to mutations in the Breast Cancer Susceptibility Gene (BRCA) 1 and BRCA 2. Features that may indicate a BRCA associated hereditary syndrome include early onset breast cancer (age <50 years), presence of ovarian cancer, male breast cancer, and an Ashkenazi Jewish ancestry. The life-time risk of ovarian cancer in women with the BRCA 1 mutation is about 40% and in those with the BRCA 2 mutation 10–20%.

Hereditary non-polyposis colon cancer
The HNPCC (or Lynch II) syndrome, which develops from inherited mutations in DNA mismatch repair genes, occurs less frequently and is more often associated with non-serous EOC. At-risk individuals have an increased lifetime risk of ovarian cancer (12%), colon cancer (70%), endometrial cancer (40–60%), and gastric cancer.

As over 15% of women who are diagnosed with high-grade serous ovarian carcinoma will have a germline BRCA mutation present, the National Comprehensive Cancer Network (NCCN) guidelines now recommend genetic testing for familial ovarian cancer syndromes in all women with high-grade ovarian cancer.

Risk reduction/prevention
It is important to identify women at high risk of ovarian cancer in order to discuss risk-reducing strategies. These may take the form of increased surveillance with regular examination, CA125 measurements, and transvaginal ultrasound scans and ultimately risk-reducing surgery.

There is evidence from the UKCTOCS trial that increased surveillance with multimodal screening (MMS) using CA125 and transvaginal ultrasound can detect ovarian cancer at an earlier stage. There was a stage shift with 40% of women diagnosed with stage I–IIIa disease in the MMS group compared to 26% in the no screening group (P<0.0001).

Bilateral salpingo-oophorectomy (BSO) is generally recommended in women known to have germline mutations in BRCA 1 or 2 at the age of around 35–40 years, depending on the affected gene and the age of onset of ovarian cancer in the family. Prophylactic BSO reduces the risk of ovarian cancer by >90% in these patients, although there remains an approximately 5% risk of primary peritoneal cancer two decades after BSO.

Screening
Two large trials have recently evaluated the role of screening with transvaginal ultrasound and/or CA125 measurements in reduction of mortality from ovarian cancer. The PLCO Cancer Screening Trial reported no difference in ovarian cancer deaths between screening and control groups. However, the UKCTOCS study, which randomized women to multimodal screening with longitudinal CA125 measurements and ultrasound scan (USS), USS alone, or no screening demonstrated that there was no significant reduction in mortality with screening over the 14 years of follow-up. However, a post-hoc analysis of the data showed a 28% reduction in mortality in years 7–14 in the MMS group compared to the no screening group, which had a median time to death of eight years. This illustrates the lag time of mortality benefit in long-term screening programmes. Further follow-up is required to establish if there is sufficient evidence to introduce a national UK screening programme.

Pathology
There are three major types of ovarian cancers:
- Epithelial (90%)
- Germ cell (5%) (see page 264)
- Sex cord-stromal tumours (5%)

Epithelial ovarian tumours are derived from the surface epithelium and the vast majority are sporadic (90–95%); 15% of epithelial tumours are of borderline malignant potential and the remainder are invasive cancers. There are at least five main types of epithelial ovarian cancer:
- High-grade serous adenocarcinoma (70%)
- Endometrioid adenocarcinoma (10%)
- Clear cell adenocarcinoma (10%)
- Mucinous adenocarcinoma (3%)
- Low-grade serous carcinoma (<5%)

High-grade serous carcinomas often originate from the epithelium of the distal fallopian tube and are the most common type of epithelial ovarian cancer. High-grade serous epithelial cancer of the ovary, fallopian tube, and peritoneum are considered as one disease due to shared clinical behaviour and treatment. They are particularly associated with BRCA mutations, carry TP53 mutations, and behave aggressively. Endometrioid cancers are similar to cells of the uterine lining and may occur as a result of endometriosis. Clear cell carcinomas are relatively uncommon, but occur most frequently in women in the fourth decade and in 50% of cases there is associated endometriosis. Clear cell carcinomas are relatively chemo-insensitive and have a worse prognosis than tumours of different subtypes diagnosed at the same stage. Mucinous tumours resemble cervical or intestinal cells and are more common in younger women. These tumours are usually unilateral (75–80%), benign, and often do not secrete CA125. Low-grade serous carcinomas are fundamentally different to their high-grade counterparts, usually contain a serous borderline component, and carry KRAS or BRAF mutations.

Clinical features
Key features of the history and examination of ovarian cancer are shown here. If symptoms persist for >2–3 weeks further investigations are warranted, especially in women aged 50 or over and where symptoms occur more than 12 times per month.

Key points: History
Clinical symptoms of ovarian cancer are often non-specific but may include the following:
- Pelvic or abdominal pain, bloating, early satiety
- Nausea, indigestion, constipation, or diarrhoea
- Vaginal bleeding, menstrual disorders, or dyspareunia
- Urinary frequency/urgency
- Fatigue, back pain
- Symptoms of bowel obstruction
- Unexplained weight loss

Key points: Examination
- Recto-vaginal examination: irregular solid pelvic mass may be palpable
- General physical examination: for evidence of metastatic spread, e.g. ascites, abdominal masses (omental thickening), lymphadenopathy, and pleural effusions

---

Further reading
Alsop K, Fereday S, Meldrum C, deFazio A, Emmanuel C, George J, et al. BRCA mutation frequency and patterns of treatment response in BRCA mutation-positive women with ovarian cancer:

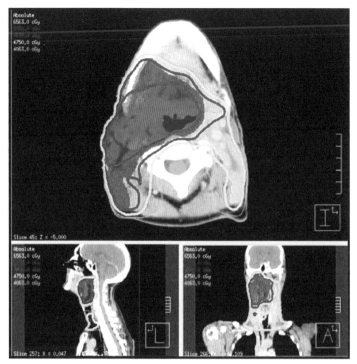

Fig. 3.1.1 IMRT dose plan for patient with oropharyngeal tumour

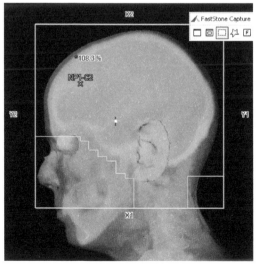

Fig. 5.8.1 Standard radiotherapy portals fields used for delivery of prophylactic cranial radiotherapy. The lens and oral cavity are shielded to reduce toxicity.

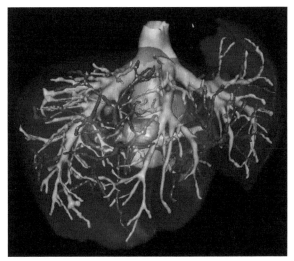

Fig. 7.7.5 A 3D model of the liver is reconstructed using preoperative CT data. On the model liver vasculature, bile ducts and the position of tumour nodules can be appreciated which aids in deciding on the optimal resection strategy.
(Visualization was performed with the Visual Patient™ planning software.)

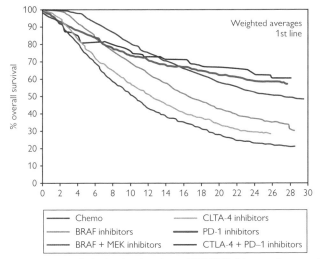

Fig. 10.3.1 Summary of outcomes reported in landmark trials evaluating BRAF/MEK inhibitors and immune checkpoint inhibitors in previously untreated advanced melanoma patients.
Reproduced with permission from Ugural S, et al. Survival of patients with advanced metastatic melanoma: the impact of novel therapies—update 2017. *Eur J Cancer* 2017; 87:247–57. Copyright © 2017, Elsevier Ltd.

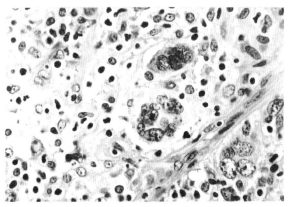

Fig. 12.1.1 Histological staining of an affected lymph node reveals the typical giant Hodgkin and Reed–Sternberg (H-RS) cells.

a report from the Australian Ovarian Cancer Study Group. *J Clin Oncol* 2012; 30(21):2654–63.

Banerjee S, Kaye SB. New strategies in the treatment of ovarian cancer: current clinical perspectives and future potential. *Clin Cancer Res* 2013; 19:961–8.

Ketabi Z, Bartuma K, Bernstein I, Malander S, Grönberg H, Björck E, Holck S, Nilbert M. Ovarian cancer linked to Lynch syndrome typically presents as early-onset, non-serous epithelial tumors. *Gynecol Oncol* 2011; 121(3):462.

Risch HA, McLaughlin JR, Cole DE, Rosen B, Bradley L, Kwan E, et al. Prevalence and penetrance of germline BRCA1 and BRCA2 mutations in a population series of 649 women with ovarian cancer. *Am J Hum Genet* 2001; 68(3):700–10.

Internet resources

PLCO: Prostate, Lung, Colorectal, and Ovarian Cancer Screening Trial: http://www.prevention.cancer.gov/major-programs/prostate-lung-colorectal

UK Collaborative Trial of Ovarian Cancer Screening: http://www.instituteforwomenshealth.ucl.ac.uk/women-cancer/gcrc/ukctocs

9.15 Investigations, staging, and prognosis for epithelial ovarian cancer

Special investigations

- Serum CA125: is raised in 80% of epithelial ovarian malignancies. Beware of false-positive results often due to endometriosis, benign ovarian cysts, pelvic inflammatory disease, first trimester pregnancy, liver cirrhosis, and other malignancies.
- Ultrasound scan of abdomen and pelvis (arrange if serum CA125 ≥35IU/ml).
- Transvaginal ultrasound: shows a complex ovarian mass with solid and cystic components.
- CT scan: chest, abdomen, and pelvis to assess extent of metastatic spread.
- MRI scan: pelvis.
- Staging/diagnostic laparoscopy.

Differential diagnosis

The diagnosis can be more difficult in patients with metastatic disease, and malignancies of the upper and lower gastrointestinal (GI) tract can also present with similar symptoms and signs. A serum CA125 : CEA ratio >25 is strongly indicative of an ovarian rather than a GI primary. The immunohistochemical cytokeratin profile of biopsy samples is often very helpful in confirming the diagnosis; a typical profile would include CK 7 positivity and CK 20 negativity. In women under 40 years old with suspected

Table 9.15.1 FIGO staging and prognosis for ovarian/fallopian tube tumours

FIGO stage	Description	Proportion of cases (%)	Five-year survival (%)
1	Tumour confined to ovaries or fallopian tubes(s)	–	–
1a	Tumour confined to one ovary (capsule intact) or fallopian tube; no tumour on ovarian or fallopian tube surface; no malignant cells in ascites/peritoneal washings	19.3	89.6
1b	Tumour involves both ovaries (capsules intact) or fallopian tubes; no tumour on ovarian or fallopian tube surface; no malignant cells in ascites/peritoneal washings	2.7	86.1
2	Tumour involves one or both ovaries or fallopian tubes with pelvic extension (below pelvic brim) or primary peritoneal cancer	–	–
2a	Extension and/or implants in uterus and/or tubes and/or ovaries	2.7	70.7
2b	Extension to other pelvic intraperitoneal tissues	4.2	65.5
3	Tumour involves one or both the ovaries/fallopian tubes or primary peritoneal cancer with microscopically confirmed peritoneal metastases outside the pelvis and/or regional lymph node metastasis	–	–
3a	Positive retroperitoneal lymph nodes only or microscopic extrapelvic (above the pelvic brim) peritoneal involvement (with or without positive retroperitoneal lymph nodes)	6.9	46.7
3b	Macroscopic peritoneal metastasis beyond the pelvis up to 2cm in greatest dimension (with or without retroperitoneal lymph node involvement). Includes extension to capsule of liver/spleen	6.6	41.5
3c	Peritoneal metastasis beyond the pelvis more than 2cm in greatest dimension (with or without retroperitoneal lymph node involvement). Includes extension to capsule of liver/spleen	18.0	32.5
4	Distant metastasis beyond peritoneal cavity	28.3	18.6
4a	Pleural effusion with positive cytology	–	–
4b	Hepatic and/or splenic parenchymal metastasis, metastasis to extra-abdominal organs (including inguinal lymph nodes and lymph nodes outside of the abdominal cavity	–	–

Source: data from Prat, J. Staging classification for cancer of the ovary, fallopian tube, and peritoneum. *Int J Gynecol Obstet* 2014; 124(1):1–5. Copyright © 2014, John Wiley & Sons; Heintz, APM, et al. Carcinoma of the Ovary. *Int J Gynecol Obstet* 2006; 95(S1):S161–92. 2006, John Wiley & Sons.

ovarian cancer, serum alpha fetoprotein (AFP), and beta human chorionic gonadotrophin (β-hCG) should also be measured, to identify possible germ cell tumours (dysgerminomas).

Staging

The most commonly employed staging system is the FIGO system (see Table 9.15.1), which is based on surgical findings taken at laparotomy Comprehensive staging (total abdominal hysterectomy (TAH), BSO, omentectomy, tumour debulking, peritoneal washings and biopsies, lymph node resection/sampling) is essential as this determines the need for further therapy, which strongly impacts on survival. It is evident that patients presenting with early stage (stage 1) disease have an excellent five-year survival in excess of 80%. Unfortunately, the majority of patients present with stage 3 and 4 disease and the five-year survival for stage 4 disease is <20%.

9.16 Early stage disease of epithelial ovarian cancer

Principles of treatment

- Optimal surgical cytoreduction
- Adjuvant chemotherapy in high-risk patients

Surgery

Surgery should include bilateral salpingo-oophorectomy, total hysterectomy, tumour debulking, and omentectomy. Optimal surgical cytoreduction (defined as residual disease ≤1cm in maximum tumour diameter) is associated with improved survival. Surgery also allows more accurate staging of disease, with evidence that complete surgical staging, including lymphadenectomy, can identify occult (stage 3 disease) in about 30% of cases originally thought to have stage 1 disease. This is important in deciding whether to recommend adjuvant chemotherapy, with results of a systematic review suggesting patients who have optimal surgical staging of their disease and low-risk (stage 1A or 1B) disease are unlikely to benefit from adjuvant chemotherapy, whereas those who have suboptimal debulking or high-risk disease benefit.

Chemotherapy

For patients with stage 1A or 1B disease, surgery alone is generally sufficient, with five-year survival >90%. However, specific pathological features place women at higher risk of recurrence, even with early stage disease. These include:

- Stage 1C or higher
- Clear cell histology
- High-grade disease (recurrence rates can be as high as 30%)

Two large randomized trials, ICON1 and ACTION (Adjuvant Chemotherapy in Ovarian Neoplasm), compared chemotherapy with observation only in patients with early stage disease. Combined analysis demonstrated that patients with high-risk early stage disease and those who had had suboptimally debulking surgery benefited from adjuvant chemotherapy, with five-year survival rates of 79% vs. 70% with observation in the ICON1. Furthermore, those patients with high-risk stage 1 disease who relapsed had survival rates comparable to patients with stage 3 disease (ICON 2003). Thus the current recommendations are that high-risk patients with early stage disease should receive adjuvant chemotherapy. Systemic treatment is generally either single agent carboplatin or carboplatin plus paclitaxel in combination. There have been no prospective randomized clinical trials comparing the two regimens in early stage ovarian cancer, but subgroup analysis from the ICON3 trial, and data extrapolated from trials in patients with advanced EOC (discussed in the next section), support using either carboplatin alone, or carboplatin plus paclitaxel, with a small increased benefit from the combination, which needs to be balanced against the increased risk of toxicity.

The optimal duration of adjuvant chemotherapy has also been investigated. A study by the Gynecologic Oncology Group (GOG157) compared three cycles of paclitaxel (175mg/m^2) and carboplatin (AUC 7.5) versus six in high-risk patients with stage 1 and 2 ovarian cancer. Five-year survival rates were similar in both arms (81% vs. 83%); hence patients with resected high-risk disease appear to derive the majority of benefit from adjuvant chemotherapy from the first three cycles of treatment. With subsequent cycles there is only a modest increase in survival but a significant increase in toxicity.

In summary, adjuvant chemotherapy is not recommended in the majority of patients with well-differentiated stage 1A (or 1B) ovarian cancer. In patients with early stage disease with poor prognostic features, carboplatin/paclitaxel chemotherapy is desirable (usually three to six cycles).

9.17 Advanced stage disease of epithelial ovarian cancer

Principles of treatment
- Optimal surgical debulking
- Carboplatin-based chemotherapy

Surgery
As with early stage disease, the extent of residual disease after primary surgery has been shown to be the most important predictive factor for survival in patients with advanced ovarian malignancy. There is now consensus that 'optimal debulking' should refer to surgical resection without any macroscopic residual disease, rather than <1cm residual disease as previously accepted. Studies have consistently indicated that specialist gynaecological-oncology surgeons are more likely than general surgeons to perform optimal surgery for ovarian cancer.

The standard of care is to offer debulking surgery followed by chemotherapy. In certain cases, where primary surgery is not considered suitable due to location or volume of disease or there are significant comorbidities at the time of diagnosis, neoadjuvant chemotherapy may be given first, followed by 'interval debulking surgery' (IDS), usually after three cycles of chemotherapy. The EORTC-NCIC randomized trial of primary (neoadjuvant) chemotherapy versus primary surgery in a group of women considered eligible for resection at diagnosis showed no detriment from delayed surgery; the hazard ratio (HR) for death was 0.98 (90% CI 0.84–1.13). The amount of residual disease after surgery in these patients was the strongest independent variable predicting OS. Postoperative mortality and adverse events including postoperative infections, haemorrhage, fistulae, and venous complications were higher in the primary debulking group compared with the interval debulking group. The CHORUS study also demonstrated the non-inferiority of primary chemotherapy followed by IDS, compared with primary surgery, in patients with stage 3 or 4 disease.

Chemotherapy
Despite advances in therapy, the majority of patients with stage 3 and 4 disease will not be cured. The primary goal of treatment in this group of patients is to prolong survival by the addition of chemotherapy following (or before) optimal surgical debulking. The two main chemotherapeutic agents are platinums and taxanes. Until the early 1990s cyclophosphamide/cisplatin represented the standard of care. The GOG111 study demonstrated that cisplatin plus paclitaxel was superior to cisplatin plus cyclophosphamide in patients with stage 3 and 4 disease (median PFS 18 vs. 13 months and median OS 38 vs. 24 months). The international OV-10 study also confirmed the superiority of paclitaxel/cisplatin over cyclophosphamide/cisplatin, and so in the mid-1990s paclitaxel/cisplatin became the accepted standard. Subsequently, a number of studies have demonstrated that cisplatin and carboplatin have similar efficacy in combination with paclitaxel. In the GOG158 study patients were randomized to six cycles of either paclitaxel 135mg/m^2 for 24 hours plus cisplatin 75mg/m^2 or paclitaxel 175mg/m^2 over three hours plus carboplatin AUC 7.5. In the OVAR-3 study patients received paclitaxel 185mg/m^2 over three hours plus either cisplatin 75mg/m^2 or carboplatin AUC 6. In both studies there was no significant difference in PFS or OS between treatment arms. Paclitaxel plus carboplatin causes more myelosuppression, whereas paclitaxel plus cisplatin causes more peripheral neuropathy and GI toxicity. Overall the carboplatin containing regime is better tolerated and easier to administer, and so has become the accepted standard of care. The GOG182-ICON5 study demonstrated that the addition of a third agent, such as gemcitabine, liposomal doxorubicin, or topotecan to paclitaxel/carboplatin does not improve PFS.

Two studies in advanced disease, ICON3 and GOG32, unexpectedly showed no difference in outcome after treatment with single-agent carboplatin (or cisplatin) compared to paclitaxel plus carboplatin (or cisplatin). These results have not been fully explained. However, a meta-analysis of the four first-line trials (GOG111, OVO-10, GOG32, and ICON3) does demonstrate an advantage, albeit relatively modest, of the two-drug combination. It is generally agreed that of the two drugs, platinum exerts the major effect, and in many patients single agent carboplatin represents an appropriate first-line treatment. However, a Japanese phase 3 trial of 637 patients, JGOG3016, demonstrated the superiority of weekly dose-dense paclitaxel in combination with standard three-weekly doses of carboplatin compared with three-weekly scheduling. The median PFS was 17.2 months in the standard three-weekly arm compared with 28 months in the dose-dense arm (HR 0.71; 95% CI 0.58–0.88). The three-year OS (median follow-up 42 months) was also substantially higher in the dose-dense arm (65.1% vs. 72.1%; HR 0.75; 95% CI 0.57–0.98). Both the ICON8 trial and MITO7 trial in Western populations demonstrated no difference in PFS for three weekly versus dose-dense chemotherapy. However, the MITO7 trial indicated reduced toxicity and improved QoL scores for the dose-dense weekly treatment.

There is also evidence that docetaxel may be as efficacious as paclitaxel in combination with carboplatin in the initial treatment of patients with all stages of ovarian cancer. Data from a randomized study comparing docetaxel/carboplatin with paclitaxel/carboplatin as first-line therapy demonstrated that the two regimens were similar in terms of PFS (15 months vs. 14.8 months respectively, P=0.707) and objective tumour response rates (58.7% vs. 59.5% respectively). The docetaxel/carboplatin arm was associated with less grade 2 or higher neurotoxicity than the paclitaxel-containing arm (11% vs. 30% respectively, P<0.001), but more grade 3–4 neutropenia (94% vs. 84% respectively, P<0.001). Global QoL scores were similar in both treatment groups, although a number of symptom scores favoured docetaxel.

Anti-angiogenic agents
Angiogenesis in ovarian cancer cells is mainly driven by vascular endothelial growth factor (VEGF). The most studied anti-angiogenic agent in EOC is bevacizumab, an intravenously administered recombinant humanized monoclonal antibody that blocks angiogenesis by inhibiting VEGF. Adding bevacizumab to chemotherapy has been evaluated in two major trials. In GOG218, patients with stage 3 or 4 disease who had undergone surgical cytoreduction were randomized to one of three arms: six cycles of standard (carboplatin and taxane) chemotherapy versus standard chemotherapy plus

concurrent bevacizumab 15mg/kg three-weekly versus standard chemotherapy plus concurrent bevacizumab followed by maintenance bevacizumab for 15 months. In the cohort that received maintenance bevacizumab there was a significant increase in median PFS compared with the chemotherapy only arm (14 months vs. 10 months).

The ICON7 trial evaluated patients with high-risk early stage disease or advanced disease. Patients were randomized after cytoreductive surgery to standard chemotherapy (carboplatin and paclitaxel) with or without 18 cycles of bevacizumab 7.5mg/kg (three weekly). The addition of bevacizumab improved ORR (67% vs. 48%) and, in patients at high risk of progression, a post-hoc subgroup analysis demonstrated an improvement in PFS (18 months vs. 14.5 months) and OS (37 months vs. 29 months). On this basis, adding bevacizumab to standard chemotherapy should be considered in patients with high-risk disease. The main toxicities associated with bevacizumab include hypertension, increased bleeding tendency, delayed wound healing, and bowel perforation, which may be of particular concern in patients with extensive intra-abdominal cancer. The ICON8b trial is currently evaluating the role of three weekly chemotherapy versus dose-dense chemotherapy both with concurrent bevacizumab followed by maintenance bevacizumab.

A number of other anti-angiogenic agents have been tested within phase 3 trials in the front-line treatment of advanced EOC. Pazopanib is an oral multikinase inhibitor that blocks angiogenesis by inhibiting VEGF receptors, platelet-derived growth factor receptors (PDGFRs), and the tyrosine kinase receptor C-KIT. In the AGO-OVAR16 study, maintenance treatment with pazopanib 800mg once daily (following primary treatment with surgery and chemotherapy) significantly improved median PFS compared with placebo in patients with advanced EOC (17.9 months vs. 12.3 months). However, this has not been adopted as a standard of care due to significant toxicity, with a third of patients discontinuing treatment due to adverse events. Nintedanib is an oral inhibitor of multiple kinases, including VEGFR, PDGFR, and fibroblast growth factor receptor (FGFR). In the AGO-OVAR12 study maintenance nintedanib after first-line chemotherapy significantly improved median PFS compared with placebo (27.1 months vs. 20.8 months) only in a subgroup of patients with <1cm residual disease post-debulking surgery.

Intraperitoneal chemotherapy

Advanced ovarian cancer is often confined to the peritoneal cavity and there is therefore a rationale for administering cytotoxic agents directly into the abdomen. The GOG172 study randomized 415 patients with residual disease ≤1cm to receive intravenous (IV) paclitaxel and cisplatin or IV paclitaxel followed by intraperitoneal (IP) cisplatin (day 1) and paclitaxel (day 8). A significant improvement in OS was demonstrated: 65.6 months in the IP arm compared with 49.7 months in the IV arm (P=0.03), despite only 42% of patients completing six cycles of IP chemotherapy. Grade 3/4 toxicity was significantly higher and QoL scores significantly worse in the IP arm. These results led to the National Cancer Institute (NCI) issuing a clinical alert in 2006 stating that patients with optimally debulked ovarian cancer should be considered for IP treatment.

A Cochrane review in 2016 of nine randomized control trials showed that IP chemotherapy increased PFS and OS but with increased complication rates compared to IV chemotherapy alone. However, due to continuing issues with excess toxicity and a lack of familiarity with the approach, and the view amongst many clinicians that no intraperitoneal regimen has been compared to the current standard of intravenous carboplatin and paclitaxel, there has not been widespread uptake of intraperitoneal treatment.

The PETROC/OV21 trial compared IV carboplatin and paclitaxel with IP carboplatin and IV/IP paclitaxel. The primary outcome was a nine-month progressive disease and rates were lower in the IP containing arm 24.5% vs. 38.6% with no increase in toxicity. However, there was no difference in PFS or OS. Analysis of two further trials are ongoing and will aim to resolve these issues further (JGOG3109 and GOG0252).

PARP inhibitors

Poly-ADP ribose polymerase (PARP) inhibitors initially demonstrated significant benefit for patients with a known germline BRCA mutation in a recurrent EOC setting. The SOLO 1 trial demonstrated that in women with BRCA1/2 mutations, maintenance olaparib following response to first-line platinum-based chemotherapy, the HR for PFS or death was 0.3 with the median PFS not reached by 54 months compared to 13 months in the placebo arm. The remarkable benefit of olaparib in this setting has led to use of olaparib in women with BRCA mutations as a maintenance treatment in the first-line treatment.

However, there is evidence from trials in the recurrent EOC setting that it is not only women with BRCA mutations who benefit from PARP inhibitors. The concept of 'BRCAness' refers to a clinical phenotype of platinum sensitivity and PARP inhibitor sensitivity in women without germline or somatic BRCA mutations. PARP inhibitors exploit the failure of homologous recombination (HR) in women with BRCA mutations. Homologous recombination deficiency (HRD) can be present due to other mutations beyond BRCA1/2. Several assays analyzing the HRD status of tumours are being employed in trial settings to identify the subgroups of women who may be PARP inhibitor sensitive due to a non-BRCA mediated HRD status.

In the first-line setting the PRIMA study has recently demonstrated that maintenance niraparib in all women, regardless of BRCA mutation status, improves PFS with a HR for PFS or death of 0.62 versus placebo. Subgroup analysis shows that the benefit is most marked in those with HRD with HR for PFS or death of 0.43 versus placebo. Further validation of HRD assays is required before their routine use in non-trial settings can be supported.

Combination treatment

There is a pre-clinical rationale that anti-angiogenic agents may sensitize HR proficient cells to PARP inhibition by promoting tumour hypoxia-induced DNA damage. This was the underlying hypothesis of the phase 3 PAOLA1 trial, which randomized women with platinum-sensitive ovarian cancer to receive either maintenance bevacizumab plus olaparib or a placebo. Whilst there was no PFS benefit overall in the combination arm, when women were stratified by tumour BRCA mutational status and HRD status, there were significant improvements in PFS with a HR of 0.43 in HRD positive patients without a BRCA mutation and a HR of 0.33 in HRD patients, including BRCA mutant tumours.

Further reading

Clamp AR, McNeish A, Dean D, Gallardo J, et al. ICON8: A GCIG Phase III randomised trial evaluating weekly dose- dense chemotherapy integration in first-line Epithelial Ovarian/ Fallopian Tube/ Primary Peritoneal Carcinoma (EOC) treatment: Results of Primary Progression- Free Survival (PFS) analysis. *Ann Oncol* 2017 Sep; 28(Suppl. 5):v605–49.

González-Martín A, Pothuri B, Vergote I, DePont Christensen R, et al. Niraparib in patients with newly diagnosed advanced ovarian cancer. *N Engl J Med* 2019 Dec 19; 381(25):2391–402.

Pignata S, Scambia G, Katsaros D, Gallo D, et al. Carboplatin plus paclitaxel once a week versus every 3 weeks in patients with advanced ovarian cancer (mito-7): a randomised, multicentre, open-label, phase 3 trial. *Lancet Oncol* 2014 Feb 28; 15(4):396–405.

Provencher DM, Gallagher CJ, Parulekar WR, Ledermann JA, et al. OV21/PETROC: a randomized gynecologic cancer intergroup phase II study of intraperitoneal versus intravenous chemotherapy following neoadjuvant chemotherapy and optimal debulking surgery in epithelial ovarian cancer. *Ann Oncol* 2018 Feb 1; 29(2):431–8.

9.18 Epithelial ovarian cancer: Recurrent disease

Principles of management

Of women with advanced stage 3c or 4 EOC 80–85% relapse after initial therapy. It is now well-established that the time to relapse after platinum-based therapy is a powerful predictor of future response to chemotherapy (both platinum and non-platinum regimens) and OS. Patients with a platinum-free interval of <6 months (platinum-resistant disease) generally have lower response rates to subsequent chemotherapy and a poorer prognosis compared to patients with a platinum free interval >6 months (platinum sensitive disease). Patients who progress on first-line chemotherapy are described as having platinum-refractory disease and further anticancer systemic treatment is rarely effective or in their best interests.

Chemotherapy

Although the majority of patients with advanced stage disease achieve a complete clinical remission with first-line therapy, disease will recur and the five-year survival rate for this group is around 30%.

The twin aims of therapy in this group of patients are prolongation of survival and symptom control. A number of factors, such as the platinumfree interval, the number of prior treatments, the potential cumulative toxicities of therapy, the patient's overall fitness (PS), disease volume, and symptoms impact on the decision to treat patients with recurrent disease.

At recurrence immediate treatment is not required in women who are asymptomatic as there is no evidence that early administration of chemotherapy impacts positively on survival. The MRC OV05/EORTC 55955 randomized trial reported no significant OS difference in patients who had second-line chemotherapy based on an increase in CA125 compared with patients who had chemotherapy started only after development of physical symptoms of relapse, which occurred on average about five months after CA125 rise (median OS from randomization was 25.7 months vs. 27.1 months respectively, median OS from end of first-line chemotherapy was 70.8 months).

Treatment of women with a platinum-free interval >6 months

Platinum-based therapy continues to be the principal regimen used to treat patients who recur at least six months after prior platinum therapy. Carboplatin monotherapy is easy to administer and well tolerated. Patients with a treatment-free interval of >24 months had response rates of around 60% following re-treatment with platinum.

Two randomized studies have demonstrated the benefit of combination chemotherapy in patients with platinum-sensitive recurrent disease. The ICON4/OVAR2.2 study compared single-agent carboplatin with paclitaxel and carboplatin and demonstrated a two-year survival rate of 50% vs. 57%, favouring combination chemotherapy. The Arbeitsgemeinschaft Gynaekologische Onkologie (AGO) group compared carboplatin alone with carboplatin plus gemcitabine and showed response rates of 30.9% vs. 47.2% and median survival of 5.8 vs. 8.6 months. In both studies combination therapy was associated with a modest overall increase in toxicity. Other combinations that are considered in this context include carboplatin with liposomal doxorubicin. The CALYPSO trial, designed as a non-inferiority study, compared carboplatin and paclitaxel with carboplatin and pegylated liposomal doxorubicin (PLD). The toxicity profile was shown to be better with carboplatin and PLD and there was an increase in the PFS. However, on further follow-up there was no improvement in OS.

Treatment of women with a platinum-free interval of <6 months

In patients with a platinum-free interval of <6 months, various platinum-sparing agents including liposomal doxorubicin, taxanes, gemcitabine, and oral etoposide are considered. These agents have similar response rates but different side effect profiles.

In the relapsed setting paclitaxel is generally used weekly at a dose of $80mg/m^2$. The SaPPrOC and OCTOPUS phase 2 trials have demonstrated weekly taxol response rates of 29–56% even in those patients who have developed resistance to prior platinum and paclitaxel (three-weekly schedule).

Liposomal doxorubicin at a dose of $50mg/m^2$ (four-weekly) has shown response rates of 26% in patients with platinum and taxane resistant disease. In a randomized phase 3 study of liposomal doxorubicin $50mg/m^2$ (four-weekly) versus topotecan overall response rates (20% vs. 17%) were statistically similar. OS was significantly better with liposomal doxorubicin in patients with platinum sensitive disease and comparable in patients with platinum resistant disease. Many clinicians favour liposomal doxorubicin because of ease of administration. However, at this dose toxicity, particularly palmar plantar erythrodysaesthesia is often a limiting factor. Several studies have demonstrated that doses of 40mg/m^2 (four-weekly) achieve response rates of 10–15% with a substantially improved adverse effect profile, which is essential in the palliative setting.

Hormones

Hormonal therapies have also been investigated in patients with recurrent ovarian cancer. A trial of high-dose megestrol acetate in a small group of patients with advanced disease has shown response rates of 10%. A trial of tamoxifen in recurrent disease demonstrated a complete response rate of 3.2% and partial response rate of 6.4%, with no correlation with receptor status. A retrospective analysis demonstrated that 40% of women receiving endocrine therapy with letrozole derived a clinical benefit, with either disease stabilization or shrinkage. Interestingly, patients who were most likely to benefit had a treatment-free interval >180 days and high levels of oestrogen receptor expression.

Surgery

The role of surgery followed by chemotherapy for women with disease recurrence has been evaluated in the DESKTOP III (Descriptive Evaluation of preoperative Selection KriTeria for Operability in recurrent OVARian cancer) and the GOG-0213 trials. DESKTOP III randomized 407 women with platinum-sensitive relapsed EOC to either secondary cytoreductive surgery followed by adjuvant chemotherapy or chemotherapy alone. There was an improvement in PFS from 14 to 19.6 months in the surgery plus chemotherapy arm and the OS data is not yet mature. However the GOG-0213 trial of 485 women demonstrated that there was no improvement in OS in the surgery arm compared to chemotherapy alone and there was significant surgical morbidity in the postoperative period. However, for selected patients, who have had long diseasefree intervals and limited sites of disease recurrence there may be a role for surgery for relapsed disease.

Novel therapeutic approaches

Anti-angiogenics

Bevacizumab is the most studied anti-angiogenic agent in EOC, as a single agent and in combination with chemotherapy. In the GOG170D trial bevacizumab 15mg/kg (three weekly) was given as a single agent to women with relapsed disease; 21% responded and 40% had a PFS of six months or more. In women with platinum-sensitive recurrent disease, the OCEANS trial of carboplatin and gemcitabine in combination with bevacizumab 15mg/kg (three weekly) demonstrated an improved PFS (8 months vs. 12 months) and an overall response rate (57% vs. 79%) with the addition of bevacizumab, but no significant increase in OS.

The AURELIA study evaluated the role of bevacizumab in patients with platinum-resistant disease. Bevacizumab (15mg/kg every three weeks or 10mg/kg every two weeks) in combination with chemotherapy significantly improved overall response rates (12% vs. 27%) and PFS (3.4 months vs. 6.7 months). Crossover at progression from the chemotherapy alone arm to single agent

bevacizumab was allowed, and may explain the lack of OS benefit.

Cediranib is an oral anti-angiogenic agent that targets VEGF receptors, as well as PDGFR and C-KIT. The ICON6 phase 3 trial evaluated platinum-based chemotherapy in combination with cediranib in women with platinum-sensitive relapsed EOC. The primary analysis demonstrated a significant 2.3-month extension (P<0.0001) in PFS with cediranib in combination with chemotherapy and as maintenance therapy compared to placebo. The mature survival analysis (85%) demonstrated an improvement in median OS of 7.4 months suggesting the potential value of cediranib in platinum-sensitive recurrent ovarian cancer. However, cediranib is not currently licensed for the treatment of relapsed EOC and is being further evaluated in women with relapsed EOC in the ICON9 trial.

PARP inhibitors

For patients with a known germline BRCA mutation PARP inhibitors have shown significant benefit in women with relapsed disease. These agents are generally well tolerated with predominantly haematological side effects. Olaparib, niraparib, and rucaparib have been licensed by the European Medicines Agency as maintenance treatment in patients with relapsed EOC regardless of BRCA mutational status.

Olaparib

SOLO2, a phase 3 trial of maintenance olaparib tablets at 300mg twice daily in women with a BRCA1/2 mutation with recurrent disease demonstrated a significantly improved PFS compared to placebo (19.1 months vs. 5.5 months). The benefit of olaparib maintenance was also demonstrated in Study 19, a large phase 2 trial of olaparib maintenance therapy in women with relapsed EOC. Study 19 demonstrated significantly improved PFS compared with placebo regardless of BRCA status. In those women with a BRCA mutation the PFS was 11 months versus four months in the olaparib and placebo arms respectively. The mature survival data of Study 19 also suggests an improved OS with olaparib maintenance treatment compared to placebo regardless of BRCA status (HR 0.73).

In women with a platinum-free interval of <6 months and a known BRCA mutation a phase 2 trial of patients with platinum-resistant ovarian cancer treated with olaparib capsules, 400mg twice daily, demonstrated an overall response rate of 31%. This led to the FDA approval of olaparib in the USA, but olaparib is not licensed in this setting in Europe.

Niraparib

The NOVA trial assessed maintenance niraparib versus placebo in women with relapsed platinum-sensitive disease and demonstrated a significant improvement in PFS in the niraparib arm in all women, regardless of BRCA or HRD status. Patients in the niraparib group had a significantly longer median duration of PFS than the placebo group of 21.0 months versus 5.5 months in the BRCA mutated cohort, compared with 12.9 months versus 3.8 months in the non-BRCA cohort for patients who had HRD tumours (hazard ratio 0.38; 95% CI 0.24–0.59) and 9.3 months vs. 3.9 months in the overall non-BRCA cohort (hazard ratio 0.45; 95% CI 0.34–0.61; P<0.001 for all three comparisons).

Rucaparib
Similarly, the ARIEL3 study assessed the use of rucaparib in women with relapsed platinum-sensitive disease regardless of BRCA mutation status. Maintenance rucaparib showed a significant benefit in PFS for all women compared to placebo (10.8 months vs. 5.4 months). This effect was most marked in the BRCA-mutant population at 16.6 months but in those with HRD, there was also a significant benefit of 13.6 months.

Combination treatment
A recent phase 2 trial in patients with relapsed platinum-sensitive ovarian cancer has demonstrated that the combination of olaparib and cediranib may be more active than olaparib alone, with a median PFS of 17.7 months versus 9 months respectively. A post-hoc exploratory analysis suggests greater activity for the combination in patients with wild type or unknown BRCA status (HR 0.32) compared with mutant BRCA patients (HR 0.55). The ICON 9 trial is currently evaluating the role of combined olaparib and cediranib maintenance treatment in women with recurrent ovarian cancer.

The AVANOVA/ENGOT-OV24, a chemotherapy sparing phase 2 trial randomized 97 women with relapsed platinum-sensitive disease to treatment with niraparib alone or niraparib in combination with bevacizumab. Patients receiving niraparib and bevacizumab had a median PFS of 11.9 months versus 5.5 months for niraparib alone, and this benefit was independent of their HRD status.

Immunotherapy
To date the single agent activity of immune checkpoint inhibitors has been disappointing in EOC. The PD1 inhibitor, avelumab was evaluated in both the frontline and relapsed treatment in the Javelin 100 and 200 trials respectively. The Javelin 200 trial demonstrated that there was no improvement in PFS or OS in combination with pegylated liposomal doxorubicin in the relapsed setting. In the front-line setting in women with advanced EOC the Javelin 100 trial was terminated early as interim futility analysis indicated that there was no benefit seen with the addition of avelumab to chemotherapy followed by maintenance treatment.

However, there are a number of trials assessing the activity of immune checkpoint inhibitors in combination with PARP inhibitors and anti-angiogenic therapies in an attempt to increase the immunogenicity of tumours and potentially sensitize tumour cells to PD-1/PD-L1 inhibitors. Trials such as ATHENA and FIRST in the front-line setting and CENTURION in relapsed disease, will hopefully demonstrate a benefit of combination therapy.

Future directions
There is often hyperactivation/mutation of TGFB in poor prognosis ovarian cancer. TGFB hyperactivation is thought to play a key role in the development of advanced ovarian cancer and renders an intrinsically more malignant phenotype, by promoting epithelial to mesenchymal transformation (EMT). The EMT phenotype is associated with poorer prognostic tumours, due to the promotion of dissemination, invasion, and migration of ovarian cancer cells and also immune evasion. Agents inhibiting TGFB could have significant potential in the treatment of EOC, either in combination with chemotherapy or immunotherapy. There is early preclinical evidence of TGFB inhibitors such as galunisertib inhibiting migration of ovarian cancer cell lines and this may be a potential area of future development.

9.19 Epithelial ovarian cancer: Palliative care issues and conclusion

Palliative care issues
The overall five-year survival rate of women with ovarian cancer is around 50%; however, many will experience multiple disease relapses during this period and contend with significant morbidity. Response rates to chemotherapy decline with subsequent treatments and there comes a point where toxicity will outweigh therapeutic benefit. At this time, supportive or palliative care only will be most appropriate for patients.

Due to the extensive spread of ovarian cancer within the abdomino-peritoneal cavity, bowel obstruction is a major end–of-life complication, with studies suggesting this complication develops in about 25–50% of patients. Once a provisional diagnosis of bowel obstruction has been made, a CT scan may be useful to determine the site of obstruction. Initial conservative measures to rest the bowel such as withholding oral intake and nasogastric tube suction should be instituted. A multidisciplinary approach is often required and a surgical opinion should be sought early on. However, obstruction at multiple levels is common and surgery may not be feasible. Other factors that also need to be taken into consideration when deciding on operability are the patient's overall condition, the aggressiveness of disease, the extent of disease, and the likely response to further chemotherapy. There are some data to suggest that there are no survival differences in chemotherapy-refractory patients treated surgically or conservatively. If surgery is not possible or is considered to be inappropriate, other palliative measures such as stent placement to expand the bowel may be considered in selected patients.

The majority of patients with advanced ovarian cancer and bowel obstruction are managed medically with a combination of octreotide, corticosteroids, analgesia, and antiemetics. Octreotide is a subcutaneously administered somatostatin analogue that blocks certain gut hormones that increase intestinal secretions such as vasointestinal peptide (VIP) and has been shown to provide symptom palliation by bowel decompression. Dexamethasone (8mg/day IV or SC) can improve pain, nausea, and vomiting in patients with bowel obstruction, an effect most likely to be due to its well-described antiemetic and anti-inflammatory effects. Adequate analgesia (often with a subcutaneous morphine infusion) and antiemetics is also recommended, although metoclopramide should be avoided because of its effects on bowel motility.

Often the most distressing feature of inoperable bowel obstruction for patients and their families will be the inability to maintain oral intake. A recent Cochrane review has concluded that the evidence base is too poor to recommend the use of total parenteral nutrition (TPN) in malignant bowel obstruction and based on the available evidence, parental nutrition does not appear to improve QoL or survival and can increase the risk of infection. Therefore, its use is not standardly advocated in patients with advanced ovarian cancer who have inoperable bowel obstruction. However, prospective trials should be considered in this setting to establish the role of TPN as some women may benefit significantly in terms of QoL and possibly survival from the judicious use of parenteral nutrition.

Conclusion

Ovarian cancer often presents non-specifically and early diagnosis is associated with improved OS. A multidisciplinary approach is required at all stages in the diagnosis and management of patients with early and advanced stages of disease. The mainstay of treatment is usually a combination of surgery and chemotherapy. Improvements in the treatment of relapsed disease have led to increases in life expectancy. However, recurrent disease is ultimately fatal and expert palliative care is essential. Novel therapeutic approaches, including anti-angiogenic agents and PARP inhibition have already shown considerable benefits and improved outcomes in the management of advanced ovarian cancer. Future studies are focusing on identifying combinations of these agents, biomarkers for treatment stratification and further novel agents that may further improve the QoL and survival of women with advanced ovarian cancer.

Further reading

Ledermann JA, Raja FA, Fotopoulou C, et al. Newly diagnosed and relapsed epithelial ovarian carcinoma: ESMO Clinical Practice Guidelines for diagnosis, treatment and follow-up. *Ann Oncol* 2018; 29(Suppl. 4):iv259.

9.20 Malignant ovarian germ cell tumours

Ovarian germ cell tumours (OGCT) are derived from embryonic germ cells and may undergo germinomatous or embryonic differentiation. They account for 20–25% of all ovarian tumours, the vast majority of which are benign teratoma. Malignant ovarian germ cell tumours (MOGCT) account for <5% of all ovarian cancers. OGCTs occur at one-tenth the frequency of testicular germ cell tumours.

Dysgerminoma, immature teratoma, yolk sac tumours, and mixed germ cell tumours make up >90% of all malignant germ cell tumours. Embryonal carcinoma, choriocarcinoma, and polyembryoma make up the remaining 5–10% and have the worst outcome.

Epidemiology

The incidence of MOGCT is 0.41 per 100,000 in the USA and 0.2 per 100,000 in the UK. MOGCT occur more frequently in Asian and black women than Caucasians (3:1). Although rare, MOGCT occur in children and young women, with a peak incidence in young women or adolescent girls and a median age at presentation of 18.

Aetiology

The exact aetiology is unknown. Five per cent of dysgerminomas are associated with phenotypic females who have a constitutional cytogenetic abnormality of all or part of the Y chromosome. These include pure gonadal dysgenesis (46XY), mixed gonadal dysgenesis (45X, 46XY), or complete androgen insensitivity (testicular feminization, 46XY). In these patients, dysgerminomas may develop within a gonadoblastoma (a benign ovarian tumour composed of germ cell and sex cord stroma).

Pathology

Germ cell tumour histologies mimic the developing embryo and are classified according to degree and character of cellular differentiation. The most recent version of the WHO classification (2014) of germ cell tumours is in the further reading list (p. 265).

Immature teratoma (36%) consists of variable amounts of tissue resembling early neural elements, cartilage, bone, muscle, etc. It is graded according to the proportion of tissue containing immature neural elements: I, II, and III if there are respectively 0–1, 2–3, and 4 low-power fields (x40) containing immature neuroepithelium.

Approximately 1% of mature cystic teratomas will undergo malignant degeneration. The most common secondary tumour is SCC. However, melanoma, sarcoma, adenocarcinoma, and others have been reported. Treatment is as for that of the secondary tumour histiotype.

Mixed germ cell sex cord-stromal tumours have a mainly benign clinical behaviour except in cases with a malignant germ cell component. Treatment for those with a malignant germ cell component is as for pure germ cell tumours.

Immunohistochemical and molecular features

Placental alkaline phosphatase (PLAP) is expressed in >95% of cases of dysgerminoma. OCT 3/4 is a marker for pluripotency and is expressed in all dysgerminomas and embryonal carcinomas. C-kit (CD117) is expressed in 87% of dysgerminomas.

Eighty-one per cent of dysgerminoma and other primitive germ cell tumours show gains in chromosome 12p.

Clinical features

- Abdominal pain (>85%). Particularly associated with rapidly growing tumours, i.e. dysgerminoma and yolk sac tumours (50% have symptoms of <1 week's duration)
- Abdominal distension (35%)
- Acute abdominal pain due to rupture, torsion, or haemorrhage (10%)

- Precocious puberty in premenarchal patients associated with increased β-hCG and/or oestrogen secretion, particularly with choriocarcinoma
- Abnormal vaginal bleeding (10%) in postmenopausal patients with increased β-hCG and/or oestrogen production
- Hirsutism if there is androgen secretion (some embryonal tumours)
- Primary amenorrhoea, undeveloped or absent secondary sexual characteristics, ambiguous genitalia secondary to gonadal dysgenesis

Examination

- Abdominal and/or adnexal mass (85% of patients)
- Ascites (20%)
- Lymphadenopathy—common route of dissemination of dysgerminoma
- Signs of distant spread—hepatomegaly, decreased air entry on chest examination, bony tenderness, particularly from choriocarcinoma, or yolk sac tumour

Investigations

The initial investigations include an abdominal ultrasound and/or transvaginal ultrasound. In suspected cases of germ cell tumours, serum tumour markers (AFP, β-hCG, and lactate dehydrogenase (LDH)) should be estimated in addition to CA125 for an undiagnosed pelvic mass.

Other investigations

- Full blood count (FBC), urea and electrolytes, liver function tests, calcium
- Chest X-ray (CXR)
- CT abdomen/pelvis if ultrasound does not show characteristics of dermoid cyst
- MRI if CT contraindicated or for further imaging if indicated
- Karyotyping for premenarchal patient with an ovarian mass

Diagnosis

Tumour markers

AFP and β-hCG can be used for diagnosis, to monitor response to treatment, and in post-treatment surveillance. LDH is raised in 88% of MOGCT and is associated with a high tumour burden.

Table 9.20.1 summarizes serum tumour markers associated with MOGCT.

Up to 5% of patients with dysgerminoma have elevated β-hCG due to the presence of multinucleated syncytiotrophoblastic giant cells. However, a β-hCG level of >100IU/l or an elevated AFP suggests the presence of non-dysgerminomatous elements in the tumour. All

Table 9.20.1 Serum ovarian germ cell tumour markers

	AFP	hCG	LDH
Dysgerminoma	–	–*	+
Yolk sac tumour	+	–	+/–
Embryonal carcinoma	+/–	+	+/–
Choriocarcinoma	–	+	+/–
Immature teratoma	+/–	–	+/–
Mixed germ cell tumour	+/–	+/–	+/–

AFP = alpha-fetoprotein

hCG = human chorionic gonadotrophin

LDH = lactate dehydrogenase

+ = always

+/– = sometimes present

* Rarely, if infiltrated with syncytiotrophoblastic giant cell

yolk sac tumours secrete AFP. Embryonal carcinoma may secrete both AFP and β-hCG. Immature teratomas may secrete AFP (30%) and choriocarcinomas always produce β-hCG.

Imaging

Most MOGCT are unilateral except dysgerminomas, which are bilateral in 10–15% of cases. Dysgerminoma appears as a multiloculated solid mass divided by fibrovascular septa on CT and MRI. There may be areas of high or low signal intensity due to fresh blood. Calcification is rare in dysgerminoma. Non-dysgerminoma appears as a large irregular heterogeneous mass lesion with solid and cystic components which may contain calcifications (40%), foci of fat, and areas of haemorrhage. All types of MOGCT may be associated with abdominal lymphadenopathy, peritoneal or omental disease, and liver metastasis.

There are no studies on the use of PET in OGCT; however, PET scanning as indicated in testicular germ cell tumours may be applicable to MOGCT.

Staging

MOGCT are staged according the FIGO staging for ovarian cancer (see 'Epithelial ovarian cancer', p. 255 and 'Investigations, staging, and prognosis for epithelial ovarian cancer', p. 257). Unlike EOC, most malignant germ tumours present at an early stage: 60–70% stage I, 25–30% stage II and III, and rarely stage IV.

Further reading

Kurman RJ, Carcangiu ML, Herrington CS, Young RH. WHO *Classification of Tumours of Female Reproductive Organs*. Vol. 6. 4th edition. Lyon: IARC, 2014.

9.21 Management of malignant ovarian germ cell tumours

General principles of surgery

Staging laparotomy follows the same principles as for EOC. Fertility preservation can be achieved even in extensive and metastatic disease without compromising the chances of cure. Patients with dysgerminoma have an increased risk of bilateral disease and should have a biopsy of the contralateral ovary. Patients with dysgenetic gonads and Y chromosome should have both ovaries removed, but the uterus may be left in situ for future assisted reproduction. The contralateral ovary should be carefully examined and biopsied if necessary.

Primary surgery

Surgery as the initial management is aimed at establishing the diagnosis, staging, and complete removal or optimal debulking of the tumour. Fertility-sparing surgery with unilateral salpingo-oophorectomy is the standard in young women with tumours confined to the ovary. For patients with advanced disease wishing to preserve fertility, optimal debulking is attempted with preservation of the contralateral ovary, fallopian tube, and uterus. Total hysterectomy and unilateral oophorectomy is appropriate for most women who have completed their family.

The role of routine lymphadenectomy as part of comprehensive surgical staging in adults is not defined.

Role of optimal cytoreduction

Although optimal cytoreduction is recommended whenever feasible, the role of such surgery is less well defined than for EOC. Considerations about likely morbidity may be more pertinent in determining optimal debulking of germ cell tumours compared with epithelial ovarian tumours. Though there are no randomized studies, retrospective series show a survival benefit for women with less bulky or completely resected disease. The largest series have shown DFS of 65–68% for patients who have had completely resected disease compared with 28–34% who have not. However, patients with dysgerminomas do uniformly well regardless of residual disease with long-term survival and in them optimal debulking may be less important.

Second-look laparotomy

In those with complete primary debulking and normal radiology and serum markers following chemotherapy, second-look laparotomy is not recommended due to the low incidence of viable residual tumour. Laparotomy is negative in >95% of patients with non-dysgerminomas and approaches 100% for dysgerminoma.

A second-look procedure would be recommended for a subset of patients with a teratoma (pure or mixed) and persistent radiological abnormalities and normal serum tumour markers to avoid growing teratoma syndrome. This syndrome results from continued growth of mature teratoma, which may cause local compressive symptoms or rarely undergo malignant transformation. Immature teratoma may undergo a transformation to benign mature teratoma following chemotherapy—a process known as chemotherapeutic retroconversion which is almost exclusive to this histotype.

For residual or progressive malignant disease following primary chemotherapy, the role of salvage surgery has not been established and chemotherapy remains the standard of care except for immature teratoma for which surgery and chemotherapy may be the treatment of choice.

Neoadjuvant chemotherapy

Patients presenting with bulky disease have been managed traditionally with primary surgery where possible. However neoadjuvant chemotherapy has increasingly been used to increase the chances of fertility-sparing surgery, to avoid morbidity at surgery and rapid tumour regrowth post operatively. Published data about neoadjuvant chemotherapy are sparse and further studies are needed but small series suggest comparable outcomes.

Postoperative management strategies

Stage IA dysgerminoma and stage IA, grade 1 immature teratoma are treated adequately with surgery alone followed by surveillance. The recurrence rate is relatively low at 15–25%, and recurrences can be effectively salvaged with chemotherapy. The overall cure rate for stage IA dysgerminoma with surveillance is 97%.

All other patients are treated with postoperative chemotherapy. RT has a limited, if any, role now but may still be an option for women with contraindications to chemotherapy, or in those who decline chemotherapy.

Surveillance

The role of surveillance rather than chemotherapy for stage IA/B of other histotypes is controversial. Results of small studies have supported this approach. It is likely that stage IB dysgerminomas can be managed with surveillance alone, given their chemosensitivity and high salvage rates, and many centres have adopted this policy.

It has also been proposed that surveillance be extended to patients with stage IA germ cell tumours of all histologies. In the UK, surveillance is an option for all patients with well-staged stage IA and B patients. An international trial of surveillance for stage IA non-dysgerminoma including children, adolescents, and adults is under development and should clarify the role of surveillance.

Adjuvant chemotherapy

The platinum-based regimen bleomycin, etoposide, and cisplatin (BEP) is the gold standard postoperative treatment. In a GOG study 93 patients with stages I–III completely resected non-dysgerminomatous MOGCT received three cycles of adjuvant five-day BEP (bleomycin 30,000IU IV weekly, etoposide 100mg/m^2 days 1–5, cisplatin 20mg/m^2 days 1–5 q21). Of these, 89 (96%) remained continuously disease-free at a median follow-up of 38.6 months. Two patients developed secondary haematological malignancies. This compares with the results of a previous series showing a DFS of 78% (n=54) in patients treated with VAC. This five-day BEP regimen remains the standard of care adjuvant chemotherapy.

Attempts to omit bleomycin from chemotherapy for metastatic testicular germ cell regimens, or replace cisplatin with carboplatin resulted in inferior outcomes. These results have been extrapolated to chemotherapy regimens for MOGCT though it is not known if the same applies to female germ cell tumours. Patients are considered to have received an optimal regimen if they have received one containing cisplatin and bleomycin.

Bleomycin terminology
30mg=30,000 international units (IU). In addition, some use IU/m^2 or mg/m^2. Note that mg refers to potency determined by bioassay rather than dry weight.

Tests at baseline pre-chemotherapy and during treatment
Pretreatment
- Bloods: FBC, U&Es, liver function tests (LFTs), Mg, LDH, hCG, and AFP
- Radiology: CXR, pulmonary function tests (PFTs), measured GFR, audiometry
- Clinical: full history and examination

During treatment
- Bloods: FBC, U&Es, liver function tests LFTs, Mg, LDH, hCG, and AFP before each cycle, and FBC weekly
- Radiology: CXR before each cycle (some centres also carry out PFTs)
- Clinical: recording of any toxicity, respiratory history, and chest auscultation before each cycle to monitor for pneumonitis

Three-day BEP
A three-day modified bleomycin, etoposide, and cisplatin (mBEP) regimen appears feasible and effective based on a study in 48 patients with stages I–IV MOGCT (bleomycin 15mg IV days 1–3, etoposide $120mg/m^2$ IV days 1–3, and cisplatin $40mg/m^2$ IV days 1–3 + G-CSF q21). Patients received either three courses of mBEP (completely resected stages I–III) or four courses (incompletely resected or stage IV). DFS at five years was 96%, with the two recurrences occurring in incompletely resected non-dysgerminoma. In testicular cancer, late ototoxicity was significantly more frequent in patients treated with three-day compared with five-day BEP.

Other small studies have substituted a lower dose of etoposide ($120mg/m^2$ days 1–3) and/or of bleomycin (10–15IU) to reduce toxicity with similar outcomes. However, there is no randomized trial to guide such a practice and five-day BEP remains the standard of care.

Alternative adjuvant regimens
Carboplatin and etoposide have been investigated as a less toxic regimen for those with completely resected stage IB–III dysgerminoma. The GOG study evaluated adjuvant chemotherapy with three courses of carboplatin ($400mg/m^2$ on day 1) and etoposide ($120mg/m^2$ on days 1–3 every four weeks) in 42 patients. None of the 39 evaluable patients developed recurrence at a median follow-up of 7.8 years. The regimen was well tolerated and has the advantage of minimal neurotoxicity compared with BEP.

Although this regimen is promising, the combination of carboplatin and etoposide awaits validation and has not replaced adjuvant BEP as standard treatment for dysgerminoma. However, it may be considered

as an alternative to BEP for patients with stage IB–III dysgerminoma for whom minimizing toxicity is critical or where reducing the number of treatment days is important.

POMB-ACE/POMB-ACE-PAV
Similar results to those obtained with adjuvant BEP have been reported for patients with OGCT receiving cisplatin, vincristine, methotrexate, bleomycin–actinomycin D, cyclophosphamide, and etoposide (POMB-ACE), though there are no direct comparisons. This regimen allows early exposure to the cytotoxic drugs in order to minimize the development of drug resistance. A study of 113 patients showed a ten-year DFS of 82%. These survival figures are lower than published results using BEP and other regimens (87–97%); however, a higher proportion of patients in this study had stage II–IV disease (80% vs. 31–69%). POMB-ACE is used instead of BEP as adjuvant treatment for poor prognosis tumours in some UK centres.

The POMB-ACE-PAV regimen additionally includes cisplatin, dactinomycin, and vinblastine. In a retrospective study of 20 patients (14 of whom had stage II–IV disease) who received this adjuvant regimen, 95% were disease-free at a median of 66 months. There were no treatment related deaths in either study.

Other treatments developed for intermediate and poor prognosis testicular germ cell tumours using dose intensified regimens have also been used to treat MOGCT, though patient numbers remain small.

Practical considerations for BEP chemotherapy
- Treatment should start within seven to ten days of surgery.
- Dose reductions or delays are not indicated unless serious complications arise.
- Lower threshold for delay if at the start of any treatment cycle neutrophils $<0.3–0.5 \times 10^9/L$, or platelets $<50 \times 10^9/L$. Delay therapy by three days and treat at full doses when recovered.
- Febrile neutropenia rate with five- and three-day BEP is approximately 10%. No dose reduction should be made provided haematological recovery has occurred by day 21.
- Bleomycin causes fever within 48 hours in 50% of patients. Hydrocortisone prevents this reaction. Paracetamol can be used as treatment.
- Bleomycin is not significantly myelosuppressive and should not be omitted based on FBC alone.
- Haematopoietic support is given in the first instance, as reductions in dose intensity may compromise cure.
- Patients should have a CXR before each cycle, and should be asked about respiratory symptoms and have a chest examination before each dose of bleomycin to monitor for pneumonitis.

Number of courses
Unlike in testicular tumours where validated risk stratification determines the type and number of cycles of chemotherapy, the optimal number of courses of chemotherapy for malignant OGCT is unclear.

Patients with completely resected stage IB–III non-dysgerminomatous tumours should receive three to four cycles of adjuvant BEP. Results from a GOG study suggest that three cycles are probably sufficient. In the absence of randomized controlled trials, many oncologists would administer three cycles for completely resected disease and four cycles for patients with macroscopic residual disease. For patients receiving four cycles, bleomycin is omitted after cycle 3 (total cumulative dose 270,000IU) to avoid lung toxicity. Total doses of >300,000IU are associated with increased risk of lung toxicity in patients receiving BEP for testicular germ cell tumours.

Cisplatin should only be replaced by carboplatin in women with significant neuropathy, nephropathy, or ototoxicity.

Adopting the principles of treatment from other chemosensitive tumours, common practice is to continue chemotherapy for two cycles after tumour markers return to normal. Up to six cycles may be needed depending on serum tumour marker status, bulkiness of residual disease, and histology. In those with initially raised tumour markers, failure to achieve a negative tumour marker status at four cycles is generally considered a failure of response. This should be treated as chemorefractory disease and salvage chemotherapy given (see 'Management of relapsed and refractory tumours', p. 268).

9.22 Prognosis, surveillance, and management of recurrence in malignant ovarian germ cell tumours

Prognostic factors

The most important prognostic factors are:
- Histiotype: dysgerminoma has the best prognosis among all histological types in all studies with cure rates of >95% even in advanced disease. There is a poor prognosis for yolk sac tumour and choriocarcinomas with <30% cure for advanced stages.
- Stage: see Table 9.22.1.

Other reported prognostic factors include:
- Amount of residual tumour (2cm) following primary surgery.
- Raised tumour markers at diagnosis: one-year survival of 90% for patients with raised β-hCG and AFP compared with 50% for those with normal markers.
- Grade of immature teratoma in addition to stage has been reported to be important. Five-year survival is 91% for grades I and II compared with 25% for those with grade III.
- For yolk sac tumours, stage and size of residual tumour are important prognostic factors.

Post-treatment surveillance

Approximately 75% of MOGCT recurrences occur within the first year and 90% within two years. Dysgerminomas may recur late, up to ten or more years after primary treatment. Patients are advised not to get pregnant within two years for this reason. The optimal post-treatment surveillance strategy has yet to be established. One reasonable strategy for patients treated with adjuvant chemotherapy might be:
- Clinical review every three months for the first two years, six monthly to three years, and annually to five years for non-dysgerminoma, and to ten years or more for dysgerminoma.

Table 9.22.1 Five-year survival for all MOGCT

FIGO stage	Five-year overall survival
I	100%
II	85
III	79
IV	71

- Tumour markers monthly for two years then with each clinical review thereafter.
- Radiographic imaging every three months for the first two years in patients whose initial tumour marker levels were not raised.
- Pelvic ultrasound every six months to three years for patient who had fertility-sparing surgery.
- CT imaging of the pelvis, abdomen, and chest (if abnormal at presentation) three months after completion of chemotherapy then as clinically indicated.

Management of relapsed and refractory tumours

Approximately 20% of advanced germ cell tumours will be resistant to treatment or will relapse at a later stage.

For patients relapsing >4 weeks after completion of chemotherapy (platinum sensitive), salvage chemotherapy regimens have been based on those used for testicular germ cell tumours, and incorporate ifosfamide and platinum. Active regimens include paclitaxel, ifosfamide, and cisplatin (TIP); etoposide, ifosfamide, and cisplatin (VIP); and vinblastine, ifosfamide, and cisplatin (VeIP), or BEP for those who have not previously received this regimen.

Disease which shows an incomplete response to first-line chemotherapy or relapses within four weeks of completing cisplatin chemotherapy has been described as either platinum-resistant or platinum-refractory. This group of patients rarely show long-term survival with conventional dose chemotherapy. These patients should be referred to a tertiary centre for consideration of alternative regimens. Although there are no positive randomized controlled trials, case series of testicular germ cell tumours favour high-dose chemotherapy (HDCT) with peripheral stem cell support. A retrospective series showed a DFS of 55% in patients with incomplete response to primary treatment (n=100). All patients also had surgery for residual disease after chemotherapy. Response rates compared favourably with VIP in the platinum sensitive group.

Patients failing second-line conventional dose chemotherapy should also be considered for trials or HDCT.

For patients with recurrent or resistant disease after multiple lines of chemotherapy or HDCT, response rates of 10–20% are seen with single agents such as oral etoposide, paclitaxel, gemcitabine, and oxaliplatin.

Salvage surgery

The value of salvage surgery in OGCT remains unclear. Although there are no randomized controlled trials to address this question, survival rates compare favourably with those seen in patients treated for relapse with chemotherapy alone and evidence suggests that salvage surgery is an important component of the management of relapse.

Issues of survivorship

Secondary malignancies

A dose-related risk of leukaemia is associated with administration of etoposide. Those treated with three to four cycles of BEP will receive 1,500–2,000mg/m^2, with a <0.5% risk of leukaemia. Patients requiring extended treatment or salvage chemotherapy will often receive >2,000mg/m^2, with an increase in the associated risk of malignancy of up to 5%.

Fertility and teratogenesis

Most studies do not suggest an adverse effect on fertility or increased risk of teratogenesis following fertility-preserving surgery and chemotherapy for MOGCT. Studies report success rates of 68–100% in those trying to conceive. From the available evidence, fertility may be unaffected or marginally affected by treatment for MOGCT. The risk of premature menopause is estimated at 3%.

The rates of malformation were slightly higher than the general population (3%). However, there was no difference among women who were and were not treated with chemotherapy (7.1% and 7.3% respectively). Miscarriages were in the expected range for the general population.

There is no evidence to suggest treatment predisposes to early pregnancy loss or congenital malformation of the foetus. Where fertility preservation is not possible or if the patient wishes no potential compromise to fertility, even if small, then embryo cryopreservation (or oocyte cryopreservation) is an option. The decision regarding assisted reproductive techniques must be weighed against the delay in starting therapy.

9.23 Sex cord-stromal tumours

Introduction and classification

Sex cord-stromal tumours (SCST) account for approximately 7% of all primary malignant ovarian neoplasms, and generally present early, have an indolent course, and a favourable prognosis.

Granulosa cell tumours

Granulosa cell tumours are the most common malignant SCST accounting for 70% of cases. They are considered to be low-grade malignancies.

Adult granulosa cell tumours

These account for 95% of all granulosa cell tumours. They commonly present at 40–60 years of age (median 50 years). There are no clearly identifiable risk factors. Macroscopically adult tumours are large (median size 12cm), unilateral tumours (92–98%), and often multicystic. These tumours are characterized by slow growth, early stage at presentation, and a late relapse. The overall prognosis is excellent, with long-term survival of 75–90%, attributable mainly to early stage at presentation.

Clinical presentation

- Abnormal vaginal bleeding due to hormonal secretion. Up to 70% secrete oestriol and up to 40% of patients will have oestrogenic symptoms.
- Abdominal pain and distension. Acute abdominal pain due to haemorrhagic rupture of the tumour into the abdominal cavity or torsion.
- Isosexual precocious pseudopuberty in premenarchal girls as a result of hormonal secretion, and infertility as a result of inhibin secretion. Rarely patients present with virilization or hirsutism if androgen secretion is present.

Investigations and diagnosis

Ultrasound

Most are large multilocular solid masses with a large number of locules, or solid masses of heterogeneous echogenicity. Haemorrhagic components are common.

All women with abnormal bleeding should have a transvaginal ultrasound.

Tumour markers

- Inhibin is the most useful clinical tumour marker and is raised in 95–100% of patients. However, it is not specific for granulosa cell tumours and may be raised in EOC.
- Oestriol is raised in 70% of patients.
- Müllerian-inhibiting substance (MIS) is highly specific and sensitive, but testing is not routinely available.

Endometrial biopsy

If this tumour is suspected preoperatively, endometrial biopsy should be carried out since endometrial hyperplasia is present in 25–50% of patients, and endometrial adenocarcinoma in 5–10% as a result of hyperoestrogenism. Granulosa cell tumour associated endometrial cancers are generally early stage, low-grade tumours.

Treatment

Surgery is the cornerstone of SCST management, both for primary treatment and relapsed disease, because of their characteristic localized presentation and slow growth.

Surgical treatment for early stage tumours is total abdominal hysterectomy and bilateral salpingo-oophorectomy (TAH-BSO). Pelvic and para-aortic lymphadenectomy is not required as part of routine staging, since the risk of involvement is low. Complete surgical staging is recommended, and the FIGO staging system is used, as for epithelial ovarian tumours. An endometrial curettage must be carried out to rule out concomitant endometrial carcinoma if an endometrial biopsy was not performed preoperatively. For advanced disease, complete cytoreduction is the goal, as for EOC.

Fertility-sparing surgery is an option for women of childbearing age with stage IA–C disease wishing to preserve fertility or avoid oestrogen therapy.

Adjuvant therapy

The selection of early stage patients for chemotherapy is controversial. Factors related to a relatively poor prognosis include tumour rupture, stage IC, size >10–15cm, and high mitotic index (4–10 mitoses per 10 high power field (HPF)). European guidelines suggest consideration of adjuvant therapy for patients aged over 40 years at the time of diagnosis, large tumour size (>5cm), bilaterality, high mitotic index, and atypia.

For most patients with stage I disease and no high-risk features (tumour rupture, stage IC, size >10–15cm, and 4–10 mitoses per 10 HPF), the long-term survival is >90%, and surgery alone may be sufficient. The NCCN guidelines recommend consideration of adjuvant platinum-based chemotherapy for women with high-risk stage I disease. Ruptured stage IC is the most clearly validated of the proposed high-risk factors, and some would advocate adjuvant chemotherapy for ruptured stage IC tumours, or stage 1C with high mitotic index. Some authors suggest treatment with less toxic carboplatin and paclitaxel, or carboplatin alone rather than BEP for stage I (see section 9.21, 'Management of malignant ovarian germ cell tumours').

Many studies recommend adjuvant chemotherapy for patients with completely resected stage II–IV disease. NCCN guidelines recommend platinum-based chemotherapy; three to four cycles of BEP or six cycles of carboplatin/paclitaxel are the preferred regimens.

RT may be an option for limited disease, if chemotherapy is undesirable or contraindicated, though the exact benefit is not quantified.

Recurrent disease or metastatic disease

Patients with recurrent disease should be considered for secondary tumour-reductive surgery if the disease-free interval has been prolonged, and particularly if disease is localized to the intraperitoneal space of the pelvis. Though survival benefit is unproven, postoperative platinum-based chemotherapy is usually given following surgery for relapse. BEP has been the most commonly used regimen for those who have not previously received this regimen. Carboplatin and paclitaxel are used in those who have received BEP previously or as an alternative to BEP. In patients with completely resected disease treated with chemotherapy, PFS is measured in years, and although most will eventually relapse, long-term DFS may be seen in around 15–20%.

Diffuse/unresectable disease is generally treated with chemotherapy. BEP (if not previously used) and carboplatin and paclitaxel may be the most appropriate regimens with similar response rates of 60–70%. For patients with measurable relapsed disease treated with BEP, complete pathological response at second-look laparotomy is seen in 37–46% of patients. Other platinum-based chemotherapy options include etoposide/cisplatin (EP), cyclophosphamide/adriamycin, cisplatin (CAP), and single-agent platinum.

RT is occasionally used to treat localized or symptomatic disease, since clinical responses and even long-term DFS have been seen in women with recurrent disease, particularly after surgery.

Overexpression of follicle stimulating hormone (FSH) receptors in some tumours, and secretion of oestrogen suggests a rationale for treatment of these tumours with hormonal agents. The gonadotrophin releasing hormone (GnRH) analogue leuprolide has perhaps been the most widely used, given at 7.5mg IM every four weeks or 22.5mg IM every three months. A response rate of 40% has been reported in one small series; however, others have failed to find a benefit. Other hormonal treatments with reported activity include oral megestrol acetate 160mg daily, tamoxifen, alternating biweekly cycles of megestrol 40mg twice daily for two weeks with tamoxifen 10mg twice daily for two weeks, and aromatase inhibitors.

Follow-up

Because of their tendency for late recurrence, long-term surveillance is required. The median time to relapse is four to six years. Common sites of recurrence are the upper abdomen (55–70%) and pelvis (30–45%). Approximately 15% of relapses occur at >10 years with the longest interval to relapse recorded being 40 years after diagnosis.

There is no consensus about a surveillance policy. Follow-up must include history, physical examination with pelvic examination, and tumour markers including inhibin and oestriol (if raised initially).

In patients who have had fertility-sparing surgery, additional imaging is often carried out, including pelvic ultrasound every six months with an annual CT scan of the abdomen and pelvis.

Prognosis

The prognosis depends upon the stage of disease at diagnosis and the presence of residual disease after surgery. Survival according to stage is shown in Table 9.23.1.

Juvenile granulosa cell tumours

Juvenile granulosa cell tumours are a variant that tend to occur in younger women, and have a different histopathology and natural history from adult tumours.

Approximately 90% of juvenile tumours occur in pre-pubertal girls. Juvenile tumours almost always secrete hormones and the majority of patients present with symptoms of isosexual puberty due to hyperoestrogenism. Occasionally, patients present with virilization as a result of androgen-secreting tumours.

The same guidelines for surgical staging and preservation of fertility apply to the juvenile form as for the adult counterpart. Surgical staging is particularly important since, although the overall cure rate is 95%, this is because almost all tumours present as stage I. Advanced-stage juvenile tumours are aggressive and less responsive to CT and RT, with short times to relapse. Combined small series show 25% survival for stage II–IV with relapse and death occurring within three years.

There is no consensus for adjuvant chemotherapy treatment of stage I disease. Some recommend platinum-based chemotherapy for all tumours of stage IB or greater, others for any 'natural' stage IC (i.e.

Table 9.23.1 Survival of granulosa cell tumours according to stage

FIGO stage	Five-year survival	Ten-year survival
I	90–100%	84–95%
II	55–75%	50–65%
III and IV	22–50%	17–33%

preoperative rupture or ascites), or alternatively for stage IC and a high mitotic index (20 per 10 HPF). For children with advanced stage juvenile granulosa cell tumours, adjuvant chemotherapy appears to contribute to long lasting complete remission and is usually recommended for those with stage IC disease, a high mitotic index (≥20 per 10 HPF), and advanced stage disease.

In advanced disease, adjuvant chemotherapy appears to contribute to long-term DFS, and should be given for stages II–IV. BEP is the most frequently used regimen, though carboplatin with paclitaxel has also been used, mainly for stage I disease.

For patients who relapse, surgery, RT, and CT have all been used. Responses have been seen with a number of different platinum and non-platinum containing regimens, notably BEP, paclitaxel, and carboplatin. However, few durable responses are seen. Hormone treatment with leuprolide has demonstrated stable disease in a number of cases.

Fibrosarcoma
Fibrosarcomas are rare, aggressive tumours with marked cellularity, moderate to marked nuclear atypia, and 4 mitotic figures per 10 HPF. They are treated as for other sarcomas with surgery ± CT ± RT.

Sertoli–Leydig cell tumours
These occur in women in their teens and 20s, with a mean age at diagnosis of 25 years. They can behave in a benign or malignant fashion depending on the degree of differentiation.

Sertoli–Leydig cell tumours are classified into five subtypes: well differentiated, intermediate, poorly differentiated, retiform, and mixed. Most tumours are low grade. Some Sertoli–Leydig cell tumours contain heterologous elements, which are associated with a poorer prognosis. Overall, 20% behave in a malignant fashion (metastasize or recur).

The majority present as stage I (97–98%) and are large (mean 16cm), and unilateral (95%). They commonly secrete androgens, and patients present with symptoms of androgen excess, abdominal swelling, or pain. A small number of Sertoli–Leydig cell tumours produce inhibin or AFP.

Since most patients present with unilateral stage I disease, fertility-sparing surgery may be carried out in those of childbearing age with a normal appearing contralateral ovary and uterus. Full surgical staging should be carried out as for EOC. Stage is the most important predictor of outcome. In patients with stage I poorly differentiated tumours, or heterologous elements of any stage, or stage

II or greater, adjuvant platinum chemotherapy seems reasonable in view of the higher risk of recurrence, though there are no randomized controlled trials to demonstrate a benefit. BEP or carboplatin and paclitaxel are the most commonly used regimens.

Case series have shown recurrence rates of 0%, 10%, and 60% for well differentiated, intermediate, and poorly differentiated tumours respectively. Tumours with heterologous elements have a 20% risk of recurrence. Two-thirds of recurrences will occur within the first year, and only 5% will occur after five years. Follow-up is with physical examination, including pelvic examination and measurement of serum testosterone, AFP, and inhibin. For patients who relapse, platinum-based chemotherapy is the mainstay of treatment.

Sex cord tumour with annular tubules (SCTAT) without Peutz–Jeghers syndrome
They are seen most frequently in women in their 20s, and present most commonly with abnormal uterine bleeding, and less frequently with abdominal pain, or isosexual puberty in the younger age group. Approximately 20% of patients will have metastatic disease at the time of diagnosis. Surgical staging and treatment follow the same principles as for other malignant SCTAT. Granulosa or Sertoli–Leydig cell tumour markers may be used for follow-up. In relapsed patients, responses to platinum-based chemotherapy have been seen, though optimal treatment has not been determined.

SCTAT associated with Peutz–Jeghers syndrome
These usually present in women in their 30s. Tumours are typically small (<3cm), multifocal, bilateral, calcified, and are always benign.

Gynandroblastoma
Gynandroblastoma is a very rare tumour accounting for <1% of SCST, consisting of a combination of granulosa and Sertoli or Sertoli–Leydig cell elements (with at least 10% of the minor component). They are usually large and benign (one malignant case reported).

Steroid or lipid cell tumours
There are three types of steroid or lipid cell tumours; stromal luteomas, Leydig cell tumours, and steroid cell tumours not otherwise specified (NOS). Together they account for <0.1% of all ovarian tumours. Stromal luteomas and Leydig cell tumours are benign tumours. Steroid cell tumours can be malignant and aggressive and for this reason intraoperatively discovered steroid cell tumours should be staged and aggressively cytoreduced.

9.24 Borderline ovarian tumours

Introduction

Borderline ovarian tumours (carcinomas of low malignant potential, or atypical proliferative tumours) account for 15% of ovarian tumours, with OS of 80–90%. They generally occur at a younger age (15 years earlier) than EOC (average at diagnosis of 40–60 years).

Clinicopathological features

Pathological criteria for a borderline tumour include a lack of obvious stromal invasion, and the presence of mitotic activity and nuclear abnormalities intermediate between benign and malignant tumours of a similar cell.

Histological subtypes of borderline tumours are:
- Serous (50%)
- Mucinous (46%)
- Endometrioid, clear cell, and transitional cell (4%)

The most common presentations are abdominal pain or pressure and abdominal distension. Approximately 25% will present asymptomatically as an incidental finding on clinical or radiological examination.

Serous borderline tumours: approximately 70% will present at stage I, 10% stage II, 20% stage III, and <1% stage IV. Survival for stage I tumours is virtually 100%. Survival for advanced stage tumours with non-invasive implants is 95%, whereas survival for tumours with invasive implants is 66%.

Mucinous borderline tumours: almost all present as stage I (95–100%) and are unilateral (>90%). Implants are generally not seen, and their presence should suggest the possibility of a misclassified mucinous carcinoma.

Endometrioid, clear cell and Brenner borderline tumours are almost always unilateral. Extra ovarian implants have not been well characterized due to their rarity.

Diagnosis

Accurate preoperative diagnosis is difficult. CA125 is raised in 40% of stage I and 90% of advanced stage borderline ovarian tumours, but lacks specificity. Appearances on ultrasound range from unilocular cysts to masses with solid and cystic components.

Staging

Staging is according to the FIGO system for ovarian carcinomas.

Treatment

Surgery

Surgery is the primary treatment of choice. When intraoperative frozen sections of an undiagnosed pelvic mass reveal a borderline tumour, surgical staging, as for epithelial carcinomas, is generally recommended, and results in an upstaging of approximately 25%. Lymphadenectomy does not improve survival and is not routinely required. A wedge biopsy of a clinically uninvolved contralateral ovary is unnecessary. Role of routine node sampling is debatable.

For women with borderline tumours who wish to preserve their fertility, unilateral salpingo-oophorectomy (USO) with staging is the first choice of conservative treatment as the recurrence rates are lower than for cystectomy. USO is considered appropriate and safe for clinical stage IA disease, and may be carried out even in advanced disease in the presence of a normal contralateral ovary, though this is more controversial.

One retrospective study carried out in early stage disease showed recurrence rates of 7% for USO and 23% for cystectomy. Comparative recurrence rates for radical surgery with TAH/BSO are 0–5%. Involvement of the resection margin following cystectomy is almost always associated with persistence or recurrence of tumours. Unlike most other tumours, almost all recurrences of borderline tumours can be salvaged surgically, often with further conservative surgery. Fatality rates following recurrence are 0–5%. Patients having any form of conservative surgery should be prepared for increased surveillance, with physical examination, ultrasound scan, and CA125.

Patients with advanced disease should have complete cytoreduction, and studies have demonstrated that patients with gross residual disease are at increased risk of recurrence and death.

Adjuvant treatment

Role of adjuvant chemotherapy is unclear. For patients with invasive implants, options include observation or treatment as for G1 epithelial carcinoma (NCCN guidelines). Most experts would recommend adjuvant chemotherapy after aggressive surgical debulking of advanced disease only if invasive implants are identified, since these represent small foci of invasive carcinoma, and their prognosis is poorer. Regimens used are as for EOC, with six courses of carboplatin ± paclitaxel.

Unexpected postoperative diagnosis of border-line tumours

Optimal management in this situation is not known. Most experts would try to avoid a second operation, except perhaps in cases of micropapillary borderline tumours, where the risk of invasive implants is higher. Careful follow-up is suggested for patients who have not been fully staged with clinical examination, CA125, and CT.

Residual or recurrent disease

Surgery should be considered whenever possible for recurrent disease, since in most cases disease is slow growing, and is thought to be comparatively resistant to other modalities.

Studies have shown that patients with optimally reduced disease at secondary cytoreduction have significantly better survival. Borderline tumours are thought to be relatively resistant to chemotherapy, hormonal treatment, and RT because of the low percentage of actively dividing cells.

Response rates appear highest for platinum-based chemotherapy and are of the order of 25–40%. Chemotherapy is usually considered for unresectable disease, or for tumours with a rapid growth rate which are symptomatic. Median survival from the time of first relapse is seven to eight years.

Follow-up

There is no consensus on follow-up schedules. Patients with surgically staged stage IA borderline tumours do not require any further follow-up. The suggested follow-up for other patients includes monitoring every three to six months for five years, followed by annual review. Patients

Table 9.24.1 Survival for borderline ovarian tumours according to stage

Stage	Five-year	Ten-year
I	99%	97%
II	98%	90%
III	96%	88%
IV	77%	69%

should have a physical examination including pelvic examination and CA125 estimation.

Patients who have undergone fertility-sparing surgery are at increased risk of relapse and should be monitored by transvaginal ultrasound in addition.

Prognosis

Stage and subclassification of extra-ovarian disease into invasive and non-invasive implants are the most important prognostic factors for serous borderline tumours (Table 9.24.1).

9.25 Uncommon ovarian tumours

Carcinosarcoma or malignant mixed Müllerian tumours

These are discussed in section 9.13 ('Uterine sarcomas').

Small cell carcinoma of the ovary

Small cell carcinoma is a rare form of ovarian cancer with a poor prognosis. It is divided into two types: hypercalcaemic (OSCCHT) and pulmonary (OSCCPT) of which the latter is extremely rare (less than 30 cases reported). OSCCHT occurs mainly in young women and is accompanied by hypercalcaemia in two-thirds of cases. OSCCPT typically occurs in postmenopausal women and histologically resembles pulmonary small cell carcinoma (PSCC). Approximately 50% of patients with OSCCHT will have localized disease at presentation. OSCCHT is characterized by mutation of the SMARCA4 gene (less commonly SMARCB1), and loss of expression on IHC can be used to distinguish these tumours from other similar tumours. Patients should have TAH/BSO staging and tumour reduction. The role of adjuvant CT and RT

is unclear; however, in view of their aggressive nature, chemotherapy is recommended and RT may be considered to improve local control. Cisplatin and etoposide (EP), or vincristine, adriamycin, and cyclophosphamide (VAC) are the most commonly used regimens. Case series show DFS of 33% for stage IA, 10% survival for stage IC, and 6.5% survival for stages II–IV.

Further reading

Ray-Coquard I, Morice P, Lorusso D, Prat J, Oaknin A, Pautier P, Colombo N. ESMO Guidelines Committee. Non-epithelial ovarian cancer: ESMO Clinical Practice Guidelines for diagnosis, treatment and follow-up. *Ann Oncol* 2018; 29(Suppl. 4):iv1–18.

Seong SJ, Kim DH, Kim MK, Song T. Controversies in borderline ovarian tumors. *J Gynecol Oncol* 2015; 26(4):343–49.

Internet resources

• National Comprehensive Cancer network: http://www.nccn.org

• Society of Obstetricians and Gynaecologists of Canada—Clinical Practice Guidelines: http://www.sogc.org/guidelines/

9.26 Gestational trophoblastic disease overview

Introduction

Gestational trophoblastic disease (GTD) is a rare complication of pregnancy. It includes a spectrum of inter-related tumours arising from tissues of placental origin. These include: hydatidiform mole (complete and partial), invasive mole, choriocarcinoma, placental site and epithelioid trophoblastic tumours (PSTT/ETT).

Gestational trophoblastic neoplasia (GTN) is a term used to describe persistent GTD and gestational trophoblastic tumours (GTT). GTN encompasses persistent and invasive mole, choriocarcinoma, and PSTT/ETT. GTN is almost always curable with preservation of fertility.

In the UK, patients diagnosed with GTD are registered at one of three reference centres: Ninewells Hospital in Dundee, Weston Park Hospital in Sheffield, and Charing Cross Hospital in London, for serial estimation of hCG concentration. Most molar pregnancies resolve spontaneously after evacuation of the uterus; however, 15% of complete moles and 0.5% of partial moles develop into GTN requiring chemotherapy.

Epidemiology

• Hydatidiform mole is the commonest variant of GTD and in the UK, it is around 1.5 per 1,000 live births.

• The incidence of choriocarcinoma is highly variable. For example, its incidence following term delivery is 1 per 50,000, while 3% of complete moles may develop into choriocarcinomas.

• PSTT and ETT are uncommon but important variants of GTD, constituting <1% of all trophoblastic tumours.

Aetiology

• Maternal age: complete moles are more common in women who become pregnant at <16 years or >40 years. Partial moles are less age-related.

• Previous pregnancies: history of previous molar gestation increases the risk of a subsequent occurrence by a factor of 10.

• Ethnicity: women of Asian origin have at least a two-fold increase in risk.

Table 9.26.1 Some features of complete mole and partial mole

	Complete	Partial
Foetal or embryonic tissues	Absent	Present
Hydatidiform swelling of chorionic villi	Diffuse	Focal
Trophoblastic hyperplasia	Diffuse	Focal
Scalloping of chorionic villi	Absent	Present
Karyotype	46XX; 46XY	69XXY; 69XYY

Pathology

Hydatidiform mole

Hydatidiform moles can be categorized as either complete (Figure 9.26.1) or partial on the basis of gross morphology, histopathology, and karyotyping (Tables 9.26.1 and 9.26.2).

Choriocarcinoma

Choriocarcinomas are characterized by:
- Absence of chorionic villi.
- Sheets of anaplastic cytotrophoblast and syncytiotrophoblast.
- Macroscopically they are soft, purple, and largely haemorrhagic.

Placental site and epithelioid trophoblastic tumour (PSTT/ETT)

PSTTs/ETTs consist mainly of intermediate trophoblasts and few syncytial elements; hence they secrete less hCG hormone. Macroscopically, they appear largely necrotic.

Clinical features

Complete hydatidiform mole (CHM)

Abnormal bleeding in early pregnancy is the most common presenting symptom occurring in up to 97% of cases. Uterine enlargement greater than expected for gestational age is still seen in over a quarter of the patients. Most cases are diagnosed in the first trimester of pregnancy by ultrasound scanning (see Figure 9.26.2).

Partial hydatidiform mole (PHM)

- Patients present with symptoms and signs of incomplete or missed miscarriage.
- Diagnosis is often made after histological review of curettings.

Gestational trophoblastic neoplasia

Up to 20% of trophoblastic diseases persist and patients usually present with irregular vaginal bleeding and/or elevated serum hCG. Excessive uterine enlargement, theca lutein ovarian cysts, and markedly elevated hCG are the main predictors of persistent trophoblastic disease.

Table 9.26.2 Summary of pathological features

Abnormality	Embryo	Hydrops	Trophoblast
Partial mole	Yes	Focal	Some excess
Complete mole	No	Extensive	Marked excess
Invasive mole	No	Extensive	Marked excess
Choriocarcinoma	No	No villi	Neoplastic
PSTT/ETT	No	No villi	Neoplastic

Metastatic disease occurs in 4% of patients after evacuation of complete molar pregnancy and rarely after other pregnancies (Table 9.26.3). Choriocarcinoma metastases can often bleed. Choriocarcinoma should be considered in any premenopausal woman presenting with metastatic disease with unknown primary.

Initial management

- Women with suspected molar pregnancy should undergo pelvic ultrasound scan, serum hCG measurement, and CXR.
- In complete moles, ultrasound scan may show a classical snowstorm appearance. The ultrasound scan picture of partial moles is more complex.
- Suction curettage is the method of choice for evacuation of complete mole. Medical termination of a complete mole, including cervical preparation, should be avoided where possible and oxytocic agents should only be commenced after the uterine cavity is evacuated because of the risk of embolization of trophoblastic tissue.
- In partial moles, suction curettage may be limited by the presence of foetal parts and therefore medical termination may be necessary.
- Sometimes it is difficult to diagnose molar pregnancy before uterine evacuation; therefore, it is recommended that all products of conception obtained after medical or surgical evacuation of the uterus and from therapeutic terminations with no foetal tissue should undergo histological examination.
- Women with persistent vaginal bleeding after nonmolar pregnancy should undergo a pregnancy test to exclude GTN. GTN should also be considered in women developing acute respiratory or neurological symptoms after any pregnancy.
- Follow-up: if the hCG level is normal, follow-up is then concluded in the case of PHM and continued for six months for CHM. Follow-up involves periodic assays of urine and/or serum hCG, initially weekly and then reduced to monthly depending on the rate of hCG fall.
- Patients with GTN are treated in specialist centres (e.g. in the UK in Sheffield or London).

Gestational trophoblastic neoplasia

Treatment is needed for persistent disease activity, which is unlikely to resolve spontaneously. In the UK only 5–8% of patients require chemotherapy whilst in Europe this figure is 12–15% and in North America 20–30%. These differences are explained by the different criteria for treatment in different centres.

Second uterine evacuation may be performed provided that:
- hCG elevation is low.
- There is a significant amount of intrauterine abnormal tissue on repeat ultrasound scan.

Further evacuations are contraindicated as they are associated with an increased rate of uterine perforation, haemorrhage, and infection without reducing the need for subsequent chemotherapy.

About 15–20% of complete moles and 0.5% of partial moles ultimately require chemotherapy. The indications for chemotherapy in the UK are shown in Box 9.26.1.

Patients who fulfil the treatment criteria are admitted and require the following assessment before starting treatment:

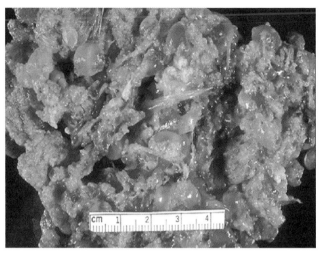

Fig. 9.26.1 Macroscopic appearance of complete mole.

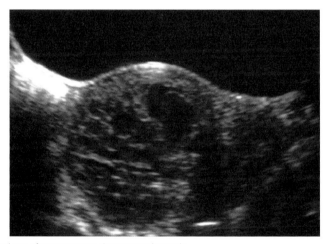

Fig. 9.26.2 Ultrasound scan of pregnant uterus showing complete mole.

Box 9.26.1 Indications for chemotherapy

- Serum hCG >20,000IU/l after one or two uterine evacuations.
- Static or rising hCG levels after one or two uterine evacuations.
- Persistent hCG elevation six months post-uterine evacuation.*
- Persistent vaginal bleeding with raised hCG levels.
- Pulmonary metastasis with static or rising hCG levels.
- Metastasis in liver, brain, or GI tract.
- Histological diagnosis of choriocarcinoma.*

* No longer considered as absolute indications.

Table 9.26.3 Incidence of common metastatic sites (%)

Lungs	78–93%
Vagina	5–16%
Pelvis	4–7%
CNS	8–15%
Liver	10%
Bowel, kidney, spleen	<5%
Other	<5%

Table 9.26.4 FIGO-adapted WHO prognostic scoring system

Score	0	1	2	4
Age (years)	<40	>40	NA	NA
Antecedent pregnancy	Mole	Abortion	Term	NA
Interval months from index pregnancy	<4	4–<7	7 –<13	≥13
Pretreatment serum hCG concentration (IU/l)	<10^3	10^3–<10^4	10^4–<10^5	≥10^5
Largest tumour size (including uterus) (cm)	<3	3–<5	≥5	NA
Site of metastasis	Lung	Spleen, kidney	Gastrointestinal	Liver, brain
Number of metastases	NA	1–4	5–8	>8
Previous failed chemotherapy	NA	NA	Single drug	2 drugs

NA = not applicable

Reproduced with permission from FIGO Committee on Gynecologic Oncology. Gestational trophoblastic neoplasia, FIGO 2000 staging and classification. *Int J Gynecol Obstet* 2004; 83(S1):175–7. Copyright © 2004, John Wiley & Sons.

- Complete history and physical examination.
- Blood tests:
  - Endocrine: hCG (broad spectrum assay), thyroid function
  - Haematology: full blood count
  - Biochemistry: liver and renal function
- Imaging:
  - CXR
  - Pelvic ultrasonography
- Other assessments should be performed as clinically indicated (see below).
- Central review of the histopathological specimen.

Before starting treatment, a prognostic risk score is calculated for each new patient using the FIGO-adapted WHO prognostic scoring system (Table 9.26.4). Patients then are categorized either low (score ≤6) or high (score 7) risk for treatment purposes.

Patients also should be staged according to FIGO criteria because this will encourage objective comparisons of data among centres in the UK and internationally (Table 9.26.5).

Central nervous system assessment
The risk of brain metastasis is greater in patients with:
- High-risk score
- Multiple pulmonary metastases
- hCG levels >50,000IU/l

It is therefore recommended that patients with any of these criteria should undergo MRI scan of the head, and, if clinically indicated, a lumbar puncture. Provided there is no clinical evidence of raised intracranial pressure, lumbar puncture allows estimation of hCG levels in cerebrospinal fluid (CSF). An abnormal value is interpreted when ratio of CSF to serum hCG level is >1 in 60.

Management of low-risk GTN
Low-risk GTN patients are those who have a risk score of six or less according to the WHO/FIGO classification (this includes the old WHO low risk 0–4 and intermediate risk 5–6). The majority of low-risk patients have disease that is limited to the pelvis; however, occasional patients have metastases (invariably to the lungs).

Patients with low-risk GTD (Figure 9.26.3) are often successfully treated with single-agent chemotherapy.

The most widely used single agents worldwide for low-risk GTD are methotrexate and dactinomycin. In the UK, patients with low-risk GTN are treated with intramuscular low-dose methotrexate with oral folinic acid rescue (see Box 9.26.2). This regimen is well tolerated provided the patient has normal renal function and maintains adequate hydration during treatment, since methotrexate

Table 9.26.5 FIGO staging system for GTD

Stage I	Disease confined to uterus
Stage II	GTD extends beyond uterus but is limited to genital structures
Stage III	GTD extends to lungs, with or without known genital tract involvement
Stage IV	All other metastatic sites

Reproduced with permission from FIGO Committee on Gynecologic Oncology. Gestational trophoblastic neoplasia, FIGO 2000 staging and classification. *Int J Gynecol Obstet* 2004; 83(S1):175–7. Copyright © 2004, John Wiley & Sons.

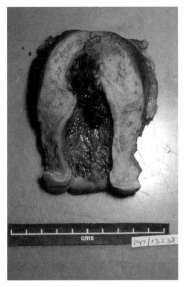

Fig. 9.26.3 Uterus showing penetrative invasive mole.

Box 9.26.2 UK low-dose methotrexate regimen

- Intramuscular methotrexate on alternate days for four doses.
- Oral folinic acid on alternate days.
- Seven days' rest between treatment cycles.

---

is excreted through the urine. 60–70% of the patients experience mild and <10% develop significant side effects. Occasionally patients develop methotrexate-induced liver damage which requires a change of treatment (Table 9.26.6). Methotrexate has two major advantages in that it does not cause alopecia and its long-term safety profile is excellent. There have been no recorded second malignancies.

An alternative is 'pulsed' dactinomycin regimen that employs a bolus dose repeated every two weeks. Dactinomycin may provide slightly higher cure rates than methotrexate. Therefore, many centres use it as a second-line treatment when methotrexate is inappropriate either due to resistance or toxicity.

Low-risk metastatic GTN

Patients with low-risk metastatic GTN have been treated successfully with single-agent chemotherapy, using methotrexate or dactinomycin. In the UK all patients with low-risk GTN receive single-agent methotrexate, whether they have metastases or not. However, in the USA, the approach is often more aggressive and some patients with low-risk metastatic GTN might be treated with combination chemotherapy.

Relapsed or resistant low-risk disease

Approximately 30% of patients with low-risk disease will develop single agent resistance and need salvage chemotherapy with or without surgery to achieve remission. In the UK, patients who develop resistance to methotrexate but with a low hCG level are changed to single-agent dactinomycin. Those with high hCG are changed to alternative chemotherapy: carboplatin or etopside, and dactinomycin (EA) or etoposide, methotrexate, dactinomycin/cyclophosphamide, and vincristine (EMA/CO).

Role of hysterectomy

The indications for hysterectomy are:

- To control excessive vaginal bleeding before or following the start of chemotherapy.
- The management of GTN which is resistant to chemotherapy.

Where the disease is limited to the uterus and the patient desires sterilization, hysterectomy can be integrated into the management plan. This approach was found to reduce the amount of chemotherapy needed to achieve remission and salvage those who developed resistance to chemotherapy.

Follow-up
During treatment
Before each cycle of treatment, hCG, full blood count, renal and liver function tests are checked.

Following completion of treatment
Once the treatment is concluded serum hCG is measured:

- Weekly for the first six weeks
- Monthly for the subsequent six months
- If remains normal; follow-up, with periodic urine hCG, for ten years.

Contraception
Provided there are no contraindications, oral contraceptives can be started once treatment has finished. Intrauterine contraceptive devices (IUCD and coil) are not recommended until the normal menstrual cycle resumes.

Management of high-risk GTN

Patients with high-risk GTN (with a prognostic score 7 or more) are more likely to have tumour resistant to single-agent chemotherapy. Therefore, they should be treated with combination chemotherapy from the start with or without adjuvant surgery.

The survival for patients treated in the UK with EMA/CO or MEA (methotrexate, etoposide, and dactinomycin) is 94%. In the USA patients with high-risk GTN are treated either with EMA/CO or MAC (methotrexate, dactinomycin, and cyclophosphamide or chlorambucil) chemotherapy, sometimes with RT or surgery.

Patients with high-risk GTN with widespread pulmonary metastases are at a higher risk of developing respiratory failure following the start of chemotherapy.

Treatment toxicity
EMA/CO is associated with higher levels of grade III/IV anaemia, neutropenia, and thrombocytopenia compared with MEA. Both regimens can result in grade II/III nausea (EMA/CO 23%, MEA 15%). The incidences of stomatitis and skin rash are similar in both regimens. MAC chemotherapy is associated with significant myelotoxicity which can be life threatening in about 6% of patients.

Table 9.26.6 Side effects from methotrexate treatment

Side effect	Mild (%)	Severe (%)	Comments
Mucositis/stomatitis	25%	<1%	Analgesic mouth wash (Difflam®) and low-dose corticosteroids
Conjunctivitis	25%		Hypromellose eye drops
Pleuritic chest pain	9–24%	1.2%	Simple analgesia. Avoid NSAIDs*
Skin rash	3%	1%	
Vaginal bleeding	15–20%	2%	
Haematological	<1%	<1%	

* Non-steroidal anti-inflammatory drugs

Source: data from Khan, F, et al. Low-risk persistent gestational trophoblastic disease treated with low-dose methotrexate: efficacy, acute and long-term effects. *Br J Cancer* 2003; 89(12):2197–201. 2003, Springer Nature Ltd.

Relapsed or resistant high-risk disease

About 20–30% of high-risk patients will develop resistance to first-line chemotherapy or relapse after treatment and need salvage treatment.

UK high-risk GTD regimen

Arm A:
- Etoposide infusion
- Methotrexate infusion
- Dactinomycin bolus
- Folinic acid commencing 24 hours after the start of methotrexate. Eight doses administered

Arm B:
- Cyclophosphamide infusion
- Vincristine infusion

Arms A and B are alternated weekly.

In general, salvage treatment with alternative agents (especially cisplatin) is needed for failed initial combination chemotherapy. Patients who develop resistance to EMA/CO are commonly treated with EP/EMA (P is cisplatin). The EP/EMA regimen is difficult to administer owing to both myelosuppression and the fact that even minor impairment of renal function caused by cisplatin can increase toxicities associated with methotrexate. An alternative effective and less toxic regimen is TE/TP.

In ultra-high-risk GTN (score ≥12 or patients with liver, brain, or extensive metastases), more intensive chemotherapy with regimens such as these should be considered from the start, often starting with low dose EP to reduce risk of treatment induced complications such as tumour lysis, haemorrhage, infection, and early death.

Salvage protocols for high-risk patients

EP/EMA
Arm A:
- Etoposide infusion
- Cisplatin infusion

Arm B:
- Etoposide infusion
- Methotrexate infusion
- Dactinomycin bolus

Arms A and B are repeated sequentially with seven days of rest interval between them.

TE/TP
Arm A:
- Paclitaxel infusion
- Etoposide infusion

Arm B:
- Paclitaxel infusion
- Cisplatin infusion

Arms A and B are alternated every 14 days.

Salvage surgery to remove the resistant disease, for example, by hysterectomy, thoracotomy, or craniotomy, may occasionally be required. High-dose chemotherapy with autologous stem cell rescue (ASCT) is considered, mainly as a consolidation strategy, in relapsed or rare GTNs where previous chemo-sensitivity has been demonstrated. In multiresistant disease there may also be role for novel agents such as the immune system checkpoint inhibitor pembrolizumab.

Role of surgery

Surgery during the treatment of high-risk GTN is used in selected patients with drug-resistant disease. Thoracotomy with pulmonary wedge resection is the commonly performed procedure. Hysterectomy after careful exclusion of other sites of metastatic disease may benefit selected patients. Women with high-risk GTN may undergo surgery for removal of primary tumour or metastases, or for the management of metastatic complications, such as haemorrhage or infection. A careful evaluation of the extent of disease should be carried out before proceeding with surgery. Prompt regression of hCG within one or two weeks of the surgical procedure predicts a favourable outcome.

Long-term complications of treatment

Patients treated with combination chemotherapy may be at a slightly higher risk of developing secondary tumours, such as myeloid leukaemia and colon and breast cancer. Multiple-agent chemotherapy may also result in premature menopause.

Follow-up

Patients are followed up as for low-risk GTN.

9.27 Special situations

Pulmonary metastases

CT scan of the thorax should be performed at presentation if the patient has respiratory symptoms, CXR shows disease, or for high-risk disease. If the patient is breathless at rest before treatment her respiratory function is likely to deteriorate further following initiation of chemotherapy. Other risk factors for developing respiratory failure include cyanosis, pulmonary hypertension, anaemia, and >50% lung opacification. Mortality rates approaching 100% have been reported in such patients although initiating chemotherapy with low dose EP significantly reduces risk of pulmonary haemorrhage, respiratory failure, and early death (Figure 9.27.1.). Due to the increased risk of haemorrhage, extracorporeal perfusion techniques and avoidance of mechanical ventilation are recommended.

Brain/central nervous system disease

Persistent GTD can readily metastasize to the brain, with an incidence as high as 8–15% and conferring a worse prognosis. The risk of central nervous system (CNS) metastases is increased with increased risk score, multiple pulmonary metastases, and when hCG level is >50,000IU/l (Figure 9.27.2).

Treatment of CNS metastases differs between centres. In the UK, chemotherapy with or without surgery or stereotactic RT are standard management while in the USA RT is often used simultaneously with systemic chemotherapy. Brain irradiation has a dual advantage of both being tumouorcidal and haemostatic.

As an alternative to brain irradiation, systemic chemotherapy regimens may be modified by increasing the

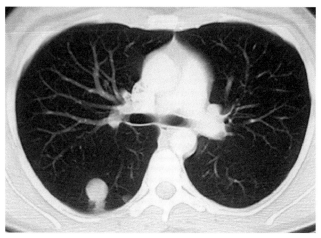

Fig. 9.27.1 CT scan of lung showing metastatic choriocarcinoma.

dose of systemic methotrexate and including intrathecal methotrexate to ensure maximum penetration of the drug to the CNS.

Surgery is reserved for patients with resectable cerebral metastases before chemotherapy or to evacuate intracranial haematoma or in cases where a patient develops resistance to chemotherapy, provided that there is no active disease elsewhere. Irrespective of differing treatment approaches on both sides of the Atlantic, cure rates are similar and range from 60% to 80%.

Some centres advise administering intrathecal methotrexate for patients considered to be at high risk of CNS metastases. However, in a study from Sheffield this was found to be unnecessary.

Other sites of metastasis

Liver metastasis has a poor prognosis. There is also a substantial risk of hepatic bleeding especially during the first course of chemotherapy. Irradiation of the whole liver in conjunction with chemotherapy has been advocated to reduce the risk of serious haemorrhage, but there is no conclusive evidence of benefit. Selective hepatic artery occlusion has been shown to be effective in controlling liver haemorrhage from choriocarcinoma. Hepatic resection might be necessary to control bleeding or to excise resistant foci. Nowadays, judicious but intensive chemotherapy cures many patients with liver metastases.

Metastatic trophoblastic tumours to the vagina are highly vascular and friable and can cause acute spontaneous haemorrhage. If the patient develops acute

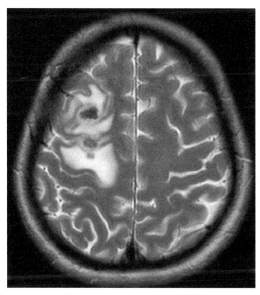

Fig. 9.27.2 CT scan showing brain haemorrhagic metastases of choriocarcinoma.

bleeding, surgical intervention might be necessary to control haemorrhage.

Placental site and epithelioid trophoblastic tumours (PSTT/ETT)

- These are rare forms of GTN arising from intermediate cytotrophoblast at the implantation site following any type of pregnancy.
- They have a variable clinical presentation, most commonly vaginal bleeding and their clinical course is unpredictable.
- Unlike other forms of GTN, PSTTs/ETTs have little syncytiotrophoblast and therefore secrete less hCG. hCG levels correlate neither with the volume nor with the malignant behaviour of the tumour.
- Thirty per cent of patients have metastases at the time of diagnosis. Unlike other forms of GTD, the WHO risk score is of limited value.
- After investigations, hysterectomy is the treatment of choice for patients with disease limited to the uterus. Patients with metastatic PSTT cannot be cured with surgery alone and treatment with multiagent chemotherapy is required. Data from the UK suggest EP/EMA as the best regimen. Other centres use EMA/CO. Additional intensified therapies such as high-dose chemotherapy and ASCT or immunotherapy could be considered in patients with poor prognostic features, e.g. metastatic disease or an antecedent pregnancy interval of >48 months.
- PSTTs/ETTs have a better prognosis when:
  - Tumour is limited to uterus.
  - Antecedent pregnancy is <4 years.
  - Distant metastases are absent at the time of diagnosis.

Twin molar pregnancy

The coexistence of normal intrauterine pregnancy and GTD (usually CHM) is rare and it occurs in <1 in 200 molar pregnancies (Figure 9.27.3). This situation poses both diagnostic and therapeutic dilemmas. It is often diagnosed late, associated with reduced live birth rates, and an increased risk of complications such as pre-eclampsia and bleeding. Despite these challenges once the 'normal' pregnancy is established, a successful outcome is likely. If the mole persists conventional chemotherapy is invariably successful.

The guidance in the UK is that 'if twin pregnancy is associated with a partial mole it would be allowed to proceed; in the case of association with complete mole the pregnancy may proceed after appropriate counselling'.

Fertility issues

After successful treatment of molar pregnancy (with preservation of the reproductive organs) patients should expect normal reproduction. One to two per cent of these patients will subsequently develop another molar pregnancy (a 60-fold increased risk). Patients with a history of molar pregnancy should have a first trimester ultrasound scan to confirm normal gestation. In the UK repeat hCG monitoring post pregnancy is now only recommended in women previously treated for GTN, with no requirement in patients who have had one previous mole that has not required chemotherapy.

It appears that the obstetric outcomes for patients with history of molar pregnancy are no different from those who have no such history. Neither low- nor high-risk treatments affect fertility or congenital abnormality rates in subsequent pregnancies.

Contraception

Following chemotherapy, women are advised not to conceive for at least 12 months after the conclusion of their treatment. Oral contraception can be safely given after evacuation. However, should pregnancy occur in this period a normal baby usually results. Intrauterine contraceptive devices should be avoided until hCG levels become normal because of the risk of uterine perforation and bleeding.

Internet resources

International Society for the Study of Trophoblastic Diseases: http://www.isstd.org

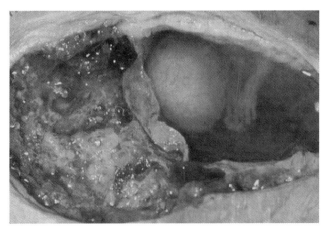

Fig. 9.27.3 Twin pregnancy showing coexisting normal foetus and complete mole.

9.28 Cancers of the vulva and vagina

Cancers of the vulva

Epidemiology
The incidence of vulval cancer appears to be increasing. Despite this, cancer of the vulva is rare, with approximately 1,313 new cases being diagnosed in the UK in 2013.

Aetiology
Age
It tends to be seen in older women, with 80% of cases occurring in the >60 years age group.

Human papilloma virus
HPV has been found to be responsible for approximately 30–50% of vulval cancers and up to 80% of vulval intraepithelial neoplasias (VINs). The development of vulval cancer is linked with the persistence of high-risk subtypes of HPV, mainly, 16, 18, and 31. HPV has also been found to be associated with multicentric disease of the lower genital tract, and concurrent lesions can be found in the vulva, cervix, vagina, and anus in patients infected with HPV.

Immunosuppression
Women with coexisting medical conditions that result in suppression of the immune system (e.g. HIV infection, on immunosuppressants) also appear to be at increased risk of developing vulval cancer.

Smoking
Studies have shown an association between smoking and the development of vulval tumours. The pathogenesis is thought to be due to the increased likelihood of persistent HPV infection, the direct damage of cells by the toxins found in tobacco, or alterations in local or cell-mediated immunity.

Chronic skin conditions and inflammation
Several chronic skin conditions predispose women to developing vulval cancer, and include lichen sclerosus, lichen planus, and Paget's disease. Of these, lichen sclerosus is the most common, with a 4–7% risk of malignancy. Studies suggest that the majority of vulval cancers will have lichen sclerosus, squamous cell hyperplasia, or differentiated VIN in the adjacent epidermis. Lichen planus is thought to coexist and possibly crossover with lichen sclerosus, and may have a similar risk of malignancy.

Vulvar intraepithelial neoplasia
The pathology and natural history of VIN is different from that of cervical intraepithelial neoplasia (CIN) and certainly more complicated. The evidence to show that VIN is linked with vulval cancer is based on clinical cancer developing with adjacent VIN, occult cancers found within areas of VIN, and reports of VIN progressing to cancer. The risk of developing vulval cancer in women is approximately 5–8%, and is more likely in women with high-grade VIN or VIN with high-grade multicentric disease.

Lifestyle and social background
It has been suggested that obesity may increase the risk of vulval cancer, while women who eat foods rich in vitamin A are reportedly less likely to develop it. SCCs are also said to be associated with poverty, nulliparity, early menopause, condylomata, and granulomatous inflammation.

Pathology
The majority of vulval cancers are squamous cell in origin; however, melanomas, basal cell carcinomas, adenocarcinomas, undifferentiated carcinomas, sarcomas, and metastatic tumours from a variety of primary sites have also been reported in the literature.

Squamous cell carcinoma
This is the most common type and is responsible for approximately 90% of all cases. It tends to be less aggressive, in the sense that it tends to develop slowly over years. Furthermore, adequate treatment and follow-up of VIN can reduce the risk of cancer development. Verrucous carcinomas are a slow growing type of SCC, and as the name suggests have the appearance of a large wart.

Vulval melanoma
After SCC this is the second commonest type of vulval cancer. Vulval melanomas cause 4% of all vulval cancers.

Adenocarcinoma
Paget's disease of the vulva can predispose to vulval adenocarcinoma and is found in 1–2% of women with vulval cancer.

Sarcomas
Sarcomas are responsible for <2% of all cancers of the vulva. They tend to be aggressive and therefore grow quickly. The types include leiomyosarcomas, rhabdomyosarcomas, angiosarcomas, neurofibrosarcomas, and epithelioid sarcomas.

Screening
- Currently there is no screening programme. Women should be educated about self-examination, and healthcare professionals are advised to examine the vulva during routine cervical smear taking.
- Vulval cytology obtained either using liquid-based cytology or the traditional Papanicolaou method may provide a clinically useful non-invasive method of screening for vulval cancer, although at present this remains a research tool. Biopsy and histology continue to remain the gold standard for diagnosis.

Clinical features
The most common symptoms that women with vulval cancer present with include itch or irritation, pain and soreness, a thickened, raised area of discoloration, an open sore or ulcer, vaginal discharge or bleeding, or a lump or swelling. However, these symptoms can be common, and the majority of these women will not have vulval cancer.

Diagnosis and staging
The size and location of the lesion should be documented, and any involvement of adjacent structures such as vagina, urethra, base of bladder, or anus, should be duly noted. Diagnosis of vulval cancer is made on clinical suspicion and confirmed by biopsy and histology. Vulval cancer is staged surgico-pathologically using the FIGO classification, and not clinically.

Vulval cancer spreads by direct extension to involve adjacent structures such as the vagina, urethra, and anus; by lymphatic channels to the inguinal and femoral nodes; and haematogenously to distant sites including the lungs, liver, and bone. Lymphatic metastases tend to occur earlier than haematogenous spread, with the overall incidence of lymph node metastases reported to be approximately 30%. Haematogenous spread tends to occur late, and is rare in the absence of nodal metastases.

Management of vulval cancer

Management should be individualized, as there is no 'standard' form of management for every woman.

Surgery

The aim of surgery in the management of vulval cancer is to remove sufficient tissue to prevent local recurrence. This is achieved with an adequate resection margin of at least 1cm. The choice of surgery as the primary form of treatment depends on whether it is felt that an adequate margin can be achieved (i.e. the stage and site of disease) and the woman's clinical condition. Groin lymphadenectomy allows the disease to be staged, identifies both microscopic and macroscopic metastases, and removes all nodal disease, thereby reducing the risk of groin recurrence. How radical the surgery depends on the size and location of the primary lesion, with radical vulvectomy being reserved for large tumours, and wide local excision for smaller ones.

The radical vulvectomy employs a triple incision technique, in which the groin node dissections are performed through separate incisions from that used for excision of the primary lesion. On the other hand, a butterfly (en bloc) incision is indicated in circumstances where, due to tumour site and size, a triple incision procedure would not allow complete removal of disease. However, skin bridge recurrences between the tumour and the groins in early stage disease appear to be uncommon.

Radical vulvectomies involving triple incisions are associated with a shorter operating time, less blood loss, a shorter hospital stay, and less wound morbidity compared with en bloc dissection, although, stage for stage and site for site, there is no significant difference in the recurrence rate, OS, or DFS between the two procedures. To date, there have been no randomized trials comparing the triple incision technique with the butterfly incision.

Early stage disease

Lesions <2cm in diameter that are confined to the vulva or perineum with stromal invasion of 1mm (FIGO stage 1A), can be managed by wide local excision without groin node dissection. This is because the risk of lymph node metastases is negligible (<1%). If the lesion is central, and the resection margin comes to within 1cm of the mid-line, bilateral groin node dissection should be carried out. To reduce the risk of recurrence, groin node dissection should involve removal of both the superficial inguinal as well as the deep femoral nodes. To date, there is no evidence to favour the use of prophylactic groin irradiation rather than primary surgery in early stage disease.

Advanced disease

Although the main form of treatment in women with advanced disease tends to be RT a small group of carefully selected patients may still benefit from surgical intervention. In those women with extensive disease where it is felt that adequate resection margins can be achieved, surgery in the form of radical vulvectomy, bilateral groin node dissection, and pelvic exenteration, or anovulvectomy with formation of end colostomy can be carried out with good results. The overall five-year survival rate in women with locally advanced disease treated by radical anovulvectomy has been reported to be 62%, and is comparable with that reported in other series of similar patients treated with other modalities.

Lateral lesions

Tumours are considered lateral if the lesion with a 1cm margin does not impinge upon any midline structure such as the clitoris, urethra, vagina, perineal body, and anus. In these tumours, ipsilateral groin node dissection alone may be performed. However, if the ipsilateral nodes are positive, contralateral lymphadenectomy should then be recommended.

Other lesions

Excision of other skin lesions such as VIN or lichen sclerosus should be considered as they may contain foci of invasion. The depth of tissue that needs to be removed is much more superficial than if malignancy is suspected.

Sentinel lymph node biopsy

The concept of sentinel node biopsy is based on the assumption that the first node to receive lymphatic drainage from the malignant tumour should be the first site of metastatic spread. In vulval cancer, there are numerous studies showing that if the sentinel node is free of metastatic disease then the other non-sentinel lymph nodes in the groin will also be negative. The benefit of sentinel node biopsy is the reduction in the need for a complete groin node dissection in women who do not have metastatic disease, with a resulting reduction in associated morbidity. Sentinel node excision in women with unifocal lesions of less than 4cm without clinically suspicious nodes on examination and with no radiological evidence of groin lymphadenopathy have resulted in recurrence rates of less than 3%, compared with those who underwent groin node dissection.

The current standard for sentinel node identification is with a combination of methylene blue dye, radioactive technetium, a preoperative radio-isotope scan, and the intraoperative use of a hand-held gamma probe. The preoperative assessment and surgical procedure has to be performed using a strict protocol. In addition, histological assessment of the sentinel node requires the use of ultra-staging techniques and immune-histochemistry.

Radiotherapy

RT may be given as a primary treatment in those women with larger, more advanced lesions involving the bladder or rectum, or who are considered unsuitable for surgery. It may also be used as an adjunct to surgery in patients who have inadequate surgical resection margins, or lymph node involvement. There appears to be improved survival in women with tumours with positive margins who receive adjuvant RT compared with those who do not.

Several studies suggest that adjuvant RT should be recommended in women with two or more nodal micrometastases in either groin, one macrometastasis (>5mm), or extracapsular spread in any node. In these situations, external beam RT should be administered to the pelvis and groins. It is uncertain, however, whether unilateral or bilateral adjuvant RT should be given to the groins in women with unilateral positive groin nodes.

In the radical setting, small fraction sizes are required to avoid unacceptable toxicity. 1.7Gy may be considered optimal but some centres will use 1.8Gy with a reduced total dose. Radical treatment usually requires an initial dose of 45–50Gy to the primary and nodal sites followed by either a second phase limited to the primary lesion, or brachytherapy to this area. Adjuvant therapy to the inguinal and lower pelvic nodes can be given using larger fraction sizes of up to 2Gy daily to avoid prolonged treatment times.

The possibility of managing the inguinal and pelvic lymph nodes by RT alone has been investigated in the past. While morbidity was reduced, the relapse rate was unacceptably higher. There are now further studies ongoing to assess the possibility of treating patients with positive sentinel nodes using more modern RT techniques ensuring adequate dose to the lymphatic drainage areas. Some centres will opt to combine chemotherapy with radiation.

Chemotherapy
The role of chemotherapy in the management of vulval cancer remains unclear. It has been used in combination with RT as a form of adjuvant treatment in women with node-positive disease, those with inoperable or unresectable tumours, or in women presenting with recurrence.

Although platinum and 5-FU have also been used in the management of recurrent vulval disease, there appears to be little consensus as to how best to integrate chemotherapy into the management of vulvar cancer. The role of postoperative adjuvant chemotherapy is unproven.

Chemoradiotherapy
Chemoradiation is a more recent advance in both the neoadjuvant and adjuvant treatment of vulvar cancer. This has involved the use of single-agent cisplatin or cisplatin and 5-FU, in combination with RT. There continues to be some discrepancy regarding the efficacy of chemoradiotherapy in treating vulval cancer, as some studies have shown a reduction in the local relapse rate, improved PFS and OS, while others have not.

Prognosis
Prognosis depends on both nodal status and the size of the primary lesion. In the absence of lymph node involvement, the five-year survival for vulval cancer exceeds 80% (all stages), whereas it is 50% with inguinal node and 10–15% with pelvic node metastases. The rate of nodal positivity appears to rise with increasing tumour depth. Furthermore, the incidence of vulval recurrence has also been shown to be related to the measured disease-free surgical margin on the histological specimen.

Post-treatment issues
Postoperative morbidities include wound breakdown, wound infection, lymphocyst formation, and lymphoedema. After a butterfly incision groin wound infection, necrosis, and breakdown has been reported in up to 85% of patients. These morbities are reduced to 44% if a triple incision is carried out, with major wound breakdown occurring only in 14% of women and are significantly lower in women who have undergone sentinel node biopsy.

Forty per cent of patients develop lymphocysts following groin lymphadenectomy, which, if large and problematic, can be managed by incision and drainage. The incidence of lymphocyst formation appears to increase with early and greater mobilization. Lymphoedema is a later complication, with an incidence of 62–69% following groin node dissection. The onset of lymphoedema occurs within three months in 50% of women, and in up to 85% of women by 12 months.

The development of complications following treatment with RT depends on several factors such as total dose, dose per fraction, the size of the radiation field, the radiation dose rate, the woman's general health, and associated treatments such as surgery and chemotherapy. These complications include vulval soreness, skin blistering, diarrhoea, urinary frequency, and the formation of fistulae (rectovaginal, vesicovaginal, and enterovaginal). The incidence of lower limb lymphoedema is also greater in those women who have been treated by surgery including lymphadenectomy, and adjuvant RT (groin and pelvis). In this group of patients, the prevalence of lymphoedema has been shown to be approximately 47%.

Many women who have been diagnosed with cancer, even when successfully treated, have a fear of recurrence. Follow-up clinics (at least up to five years initially), nurse specialists, and self-help groups can be very supportive and reassuring. However, as contact with the medical and nursing team becomes less common as the woman continues to recover, this can also be a source of anxiety for some. Sexual dysfunction is a consequence for many women diagnosed with and treated for any gynaecological cancer, and vulvar cancer is certainly no exception.

Recurrence and management
Recurrent vulval cancer appears to correlate most closely with the number of positive groin nodes. The recurrence rate for invasive SCC of the vulva appears to range from 15% to 33%. The most common sites of recurrence include the vulva (69.5%), groin nodes (24.3%), pelvis (15.6%), and distant metastases (18.5%).

Local vulval recurrences carry a better prognosis compared with groin or distant metastases, as these lesions tend to be more amenable to surgical excision. Groin recurrences are difficult to manage, and although RT would be the preferred first option, surgical excision should be considered in patients who have already received groin irradiation.

Recent advances
Newer surgical techniques include minimally invasive inguinal lymph node dissection (MILND). Initially carried out in patients with melanoma, MILND has been shown to provide an equivalent lymphadenectomy to the open procedure, while minimizing the severity of postoperative complications. However, the numbers have been small and, to date, this approach has not been subjected to any randomized controlled trials.

Cancers of the vagina
Epidemiology
Primary vaginal cancer constitutes 2% of female genital tract cancers, and Cancer Research UK estimates that approximately 240 new cases are diagnosed annually. It causes approximately 100 deaths in the UK each year and is responsible for one out of every 1,000 cancers diagnosed in women. Advances in diagnosis and treatment have made cure rates comparable with those of cervical cancer.

Aetiology

Age

Vaginal cancer tends to be most commonly seen in older women between the ages of 60–70 years, with >70% of cases occurring in this group. Vaginal cancer (clear cell carcinoma) in younger women is more common in those whose mothers were administered diethylstilboestrol during pregnancy.

Human papilloma virus

It is well established that the development of both pre-invasive and invasive vaginal cancer is associated with persistent infection with high risk oncogenic subtypes of HPV, especially 16.

Cervical intraepithelial neoplasia or cervical cancer

Up to 30% of women with primary vaginal cancer have a history of in situ or invasive cervical cancer treated in the preceding five years.

Vaginal intraepithelial neoplasia (VAIN)

VAIN is less common than CIN, and the relationship between VAIN and the development of invasive vaginal cancer remains unclear, but appears to be multifactorial.

Chronic conditions

A previous history of chronic vaginal irritation, the use of ring pessaries, and previous treatment with RT have been shown to be associated with the development of vaginal cancer.

Social background

Women with invasive disease have been found to be less well educated, have lower income, are more likely to have five or more lifetime sexual partners, have an early age at first intercourse, and be current smokers at diagnosis.

Pathology

Squamous cell carcinoma

80% of vaginal cancers are due to direct extension of adjacent tumours (e.g. cervical) or metastases (e.g. endometrial). Of the 20% that originate in the vagina (primary vaginal cancer), the most common histological type is squamous cell in origin, and accounts for >90% of cases. The association between the development of squamous cell vaginal carcinoma following either cervical or vulvar carcinoma reinforces the correlation between HPV and the development of multicentric disease.

Adenocarcinoma

Most vaginal adenocarcinomas tend to occur in women >50 years, with the exception of clear cell carcinoma. Clear cell adenocarcinoma is very uncommon, and is almost always associated with an exposure to diethylstilboestrol in utero. It is unusual before the age of 13, and most commonly presents between the ages of 17 and 22. Early stage disease is often curable but more advanced disease can result in both haematogenous and lymphatic metastases.

Papillary adenocarcinoma tends to arise from the connective tissue surrounding the vagina, and is less likely to spread via the lymphatics.

Adenosquamous carcinomas are also known as mixed epithelial tumours, and tend to be more aggressive. They are extremely rare and are found in up to 2% of women diagnosed with vaginal carcinoma.

Malignant melanoma

Malignant melanomas of the vagina are found in about 2% of women with vaginal cancer. They are more likely to develop in women in the fifth decade of life, and in the lower third of the vagina. Vaginal melanomas are harder to treat compared with malignant melanomas of the vulva.

Sarcoma botyroides

This vaginal tumour is extremely uncommon and is almost exclusively found in children under the age of five years. It arises from the lamina propria of the vagina and is of mesenchymal origin.

Screening

There is no national screening programme. Detecting and treating women with a history of CIN, VIN, and those undergoing cervical screening can prevent vaginal cancer developing.

Clinical features

Patients generally remain asymptomatic in both the preinvasive and early stages of vaginal cancer, and tumours are most commonly detected during routine cervical screening. Up to 20% of women with vaginal cancer remain asymptomatic at presentation.

In general, 80–90% of women will present with one or more of the following symptoms: intermenstrual, postcoital or postmenopausal bleeding, offensive or blood-stained discharge, dyspareunia, vaginal irritation, or a vaginal mass. With more advanced disease, women may also complain of pelvic pain, constipation, difficulty in micturition, and lower limb oedema.

Women with a history of HPV infection, CIN, or VAIN are at an increased risk of developing vaginal cancer and adequate follow-up of these women should be arranged.

Diagnosis and staging

The diagnosis is by clinical examination and histology. FIGO classifies vaginal tumours according to their site of involvement. Tumours extending to the external cervical os should be deemed cervical cancers, while tumours involving the vulva should be classified as vulval cancers. This emphasizes the necessity for, and vigilance during, the staging process, which incorporates an examination under anaesthesia, cystoscopy, proctoscopy, and sigmoidoscopy, depending on the site of the lesion.

Although the staging of vaginal cancer is made clinically, the concurrent use of radiological imaging allows an assessment of the tumour size and extent to be made. A combination of these influence the type of treatment the woman is offered, i.e. surgery versus RT. MRI provides a greater degree of resolution enabling the boundaries of the tumour to be assessed with greater accuracy.

The use of integrated PET/CT in gynaecological malignancies has increased in recent years, evolving into a potential method of assessing treatment response and disease progression.

Management of vaginal cancer

Vaginal cancer can be effectively treated, and when found in early stages can be curable. Factors to be considered when planning treatment for vaginal cancer are the stage, size, and location of the lesion; the presence or absence of the uterus; whether there has been previous pelvic irradiation; and the fitness of the woman. The management of each woman must therefore be individualized accordingly.

In women who have had a previous hysterectomy, 62% developed cancer in the upper third of the vagina, compared with 34% of women who had not had a hysterectomy.

Surgery

Surgical treatment of vaginal carcinoma can be curative in carefully selected women with early stage (I, small stage II) disease, and in women with stage IV disease in whom exenterative surgery is planned. Surgery is the treatment of choice if clear excision margins are achievable. However, the proximity of the bladder and the rectum can make vaginectomy potentially problematic.

In stage I disease, lesions at the apex, particularly on the posterior vaginal wall, may be treated with a partial vaginectomy or extension of a radical hysterectomy. More superficial lesions may be treated by wide local excision. Lesions that lie in the upper part of the vagina can be treated by radical hysterovaginectomy with removal of the parametria and paracolpos. In women who have had a previous hysterectomy, an upper vaginectomy and parametrectomy can be performed, although care must be taken to ensure adequate resection margins. Both procedures should also include bilateral pelvic node dissection.

In stage II disease, surgery should be reserved for those women with minimal extension outside the vaginal wall, and those with lesions in sites that would allow a procedure less aggressive than a radical vaginectomy.

Pelvic exenteration is rarely performed as a primary procedure, except in stage IVa disease. In these instances, the type of exenterative procedure performed will depend on the affected organs (bladder, rectum, or both). In these women, extension of the lesion to the pelvic side walls, or distant sites of metastases must be excluded before surgery if long-term cure is to be achieved.

Sentinel node detection

Sentinel node detection using technetium-labelled nanocolloid has been demonstrated in patients with primary and recurrent vaginal carcinoma. There appears to be a strong correlation between sentinel node status and histological findings at lymphadenectomy. Determining sentinel node status in women with vaginal cancer may have a role in planning treatment, when decisions between the benefits of radical surgery versus chemoradiotherapy/RT must be made.

Radiotherapy

RT continues to remain the treatment modality of choice unless clear resection margins can be obtained. The proximity of the vagina to the bladder and rectum can potentially limit treatment options and increase the risk of complications to these organs. IMRT is increasingly used to reduce normal tissue damage. However, movement of the target volume either between or even during treatment raises the risk of geographic miss. The position of the vagina in the pelvis can vary considerably with bowel and bladder filling. In order to ensure the target is not missed it is essential that the treatments are monitored by imaging. IGRT is thus an essential component of IMRT.

In early stage disease, intracavitary radiation may be used, while both intracavitary and external irradiation are required for larger and more advanced lesions. The use of both external irradiation and brachytherapy in treating vaginal cancer has been shown to achieve excellent results. Furthermore, it also allows vaginal preservation, albeit with a reduced functional capacity.

Women with advanced disease tend to be treated with chemoradiation rather than by RT alone. Prognosis in these women tends to be poorer compared to those with early stage disease, and although surgical salvage

may be required, primary RT does not appear to have any advantage over surgery.

Chemoradiotherapy

Most current evidence in the use of chemoradiotherapy in vaginal cancer stems from studies in cervical cancer. The use of platinum-containing regimens, namely, cisplatin and 5-FU-cisplatin, have been shown to improve OS and PFS in women with advanced disease (stage IIb, III, and IVa cervical carcinoma), bulky stage Ib disease, and high-risk early stage cervical carcinoma. Other studies have also shown an initial response rate as high as 60–85% with the concurrent use of 5-FU, mitomycin, and cisplatin with RT. The longer-term benefits, however, have been more variable. Chemotherapy alone appears to offer little benefit in the management of advanced (stage III and IV) disease.

HPV vaccine

Women who have had a previous anogenital cancer, especially cervical cancer, have a higher risk of developing vaginal cancer. However, evidence supporting HPV vaccination in vaginal cancer is limited and extends from studies in cervical cancer.

Prognosis

The reported overall five-year survival rate for vaginal cancer is 44%, which is poorer than that for both cervical and vulval cancer. Prognosis depends not only on the stage and location of the disease, but age, symptomatology, and differentiation. Women who present over 60 years of age, who are symptomatic at the time of diagnosis, have lesions in the middle and lower third of the vagina, and have poorly differentiated tumours, appear to have a poorer prognosis. The extent of involvement of the vaginal wall is also significantly correlated with survival, as is the stage of disease.

Post-treatment issues

Following surgical resection of the tumour, vaginal scarring and stenosis can be particularly problematic in sexually active women. Feelings of depression, grief, stress, and sexual dysfunction are frequently experienced by women following treatment which highlights the role of nurse specialists and psychosexual counsellors in the continuing care of these women.

Problems with urinary retention may occur in those who have undergone radical total vaginectomy. In patients who have received neoadjuvant RT, surgery may also result in the development of bladder and bowel fistulae.

Premenopausal women who require adjuvant RT often undergo a 'radiation menopause' which may also result in 'thinning' of the vaginal mucosa. HRT may have a role for some women.

Recurrence and management

The factors that affect the risk of recurrence are increased tumour bulk (specified by size in centimetres or FIGO stage), tumour site (upper lesions faring better), and tumour circumferential location (lesions involving the posterior wall faring worse). The major pattern of relapse appears to be pelvic. Increased tumour bulk increases the likelihood of metastatic relapse, as does failure to achieve local control of the tumour.

Recurrent vaginal cancer, with most cases presenting within two years of primary treatment, carries a grave prognosis. The five-year survival rate following recurrence is approximately 12%. In centrally recurrent vaginal cancers, there may be a role for pelvic exenteration or further RT. Studies have not shown any benefit to using either cisplatin or mitoxantrone in recurrent or advanced disease, and chemotherapy does not appear to play a role in the management of these tumours.

Recent advances

Laterally extended endopelvic resection (LEER) is a relatively new surgical technique based on developmentally derived surgical anatomy. It aims to increase the curative resection rate of tumours extending to and fixed to the pelvic side wall. In cases of lateral pelvic wall tumour fixation, the inclusion of pelvic side wall and pelvic floor muscles and the internal iliac vessel system allows a complete resection margin, described as an R0 excision. At a median follow-up period of 30 months, the five-year recurrence-free and disease-specific OS statistics have been shown to be 62% and 55% respectively. LEER has the potential to salvage selected patients with locally advanced and recurrent gynaecological malignancies, that extend to the pelvic side wall, that otherwise would not have been possible by a standard exenterative procedure.

Internet resources

Royal College of Obstetricians and Gynaecologists. RCOG Guideline—available at: https://www.rcog.org.uk/globalassets/documents/guidelines/vulvalcancerguideline.pdf

Cancers of the skin

Chapter contents

10.1 Introduction, clinical features, and staging of cutaneous melanoma

Epidemiology

Melanoma is the fifth most common cancer in the UK, accounting for 4% of all new cancer cases. It accounts for over 80% of skin cancer deaths. The incidence rate of melanoma is increasing worldwide, faster than any other cancer, due largely to environmental factors. In Europe, incidence has increased five-fold in the last 40 years. The lifetime risk of melanoma in the UK is around one in 55. In Australia, the risks are significantly higher, with lifetime risks of one in 25 for men and one in 35 for women. Melanoma incidence is highest in women under 35 years and older men. It is the third most common cancer among 15–35 year olds.

Survival rates have improved in the last ten years due to better detection of thinner melanomas which can be cured by surgery, while the last five years have recorded unprecedented improvements in the survival of patients with more advanced disease due to the introduction of new systemic therapies.

Aetiology

A number of factors are associated with increased risk of melanoma:

- Ultraviolet (UV) sun radiation (especially UVB) is the main risk factor for the development of cutaneous melanoma. Skin colour has a strong association with melanoma risk, with around a 20-fold increase in incidence in white compared with black skinned individuals. People with a history of blistering sunburn have a 2.5 times higher risk of melanoma.
- People with a strong family history and multiple atypical moles are at the greatest risk of melanoma and account for 10–15% of all patients diagnosed with this condition.
- Mutation in chromosome 9p21 tumour suppressor gene, cyclin dependent kinase inhibitor 2A (CDKN2A) accounts for 40% of hereditary melanomas, and CDK4 gene mutations confer a 60–90% lifetime risk of melanoma. CDKN2A mutation families also have a higher risk of pancreatic cancer (15% lifetime risk).
- Mutation of the melanocortin 1 receptor (MC1R) gene may contribute to the red hair/fair skin melanoma. MC1R mutation increases the risk of melanoma by two to four-fold and there is also an increased risk of non-melanoma skin cancer.
- Xeroderma pigmentosa is associated with a 600–1,000-fold increase in skin cancers including melanoma.
- BRCA2 mutation increases risk of melanoma 2.5–8-fold.
- Multiple benign naevi (>100) as well as multiple atypical naevi increase the risk of melanoma (RR 11).
- Immunosuppression: transplant recipients (RR 3) and patients with human immunodeficiency virus (HIV) or acquired immune deficiency syndrome (AIDS) (RR 1.5) have increased risk of melanoma.
- A previous melanoma incurs a 2–10% risk of a second melanoma and risk increases further with two previous melanomas.
- BRAF is a serine/threonine kinase which is a major player in the Ras-Raf-Mek-Erk mitogen activated protein kinase signalling transduction pathway that regulates cell growth, proliferation, and differentiation in response to various growth factors, cytokines, and hormones. BRAF gene mutations occur in approximately 45% of cutaneous melanomas; the most commonly occurring is the V600E mutation. There is an inverse relationship between BRAF mutation prevalence and age. Around 25% of melanomas have an NRAS mutation and in general, BRAF and NRAS mutations are mutually exclusive. Acral melanomas share a genetic aberration associated with mucosal melanomas, with around 10% having a mutation in the C-KIT gene.

Pathology

There are four histological variants of cutaneous melanoma:

- Superficial spreading melanoma is the most common type (70%). This often arises within a pre-existing naevus. It is common on the intermittent sun-exposed areas such as lower extremities of women and back in men.
- Nodular melanoma (10–15%) presents as a symmetrical, uniform, dark blue-black lesion. Most common site is the trunk and these tumours show rapid evolution. Amelanotic nodular melanomas occur and are often misdiagnosed.
- Lentigo maligna melanoma (10–15%) usually occurs on the chronic sun-exposed areas of the head and neck and hands of older people. Clinically, these are large (often >3cm) flat lesions with areas of dark brown or black discoloration. These lesions arise from the premalignant lesion called Hutchinson's freckle.
- Acral lentigenous melanomas, as the name suggests (acral = distal), occur on the palms, soles, and subungual regions. These tumours occur with the same frequency in white and non-white populations. While they account for only 2–8% of all melanoma in white-skinned people, they account for 40–60% melanoma occurring in non-white people. These tumours can be easily misdiagnosed as subungual haematoma.
- Desmoplastic melanoma is a locally aggressive variant occurring most often in the sixth to seventh decade of life and men are more commonly affected. It is common on the sun-exposed head and neck region.

Histological reporting of melanomas should include the type of melanoma, greatest (Breslow) thickness, radial or vertical growth phase, excision margins, and immunohistochemical staining pattern to confirm the diagnosis. Immunohistochemical stains used in melanoma include S100 (the most frequently used but it also stains benign melanocytes), HMB-45, MART-1, and tyrosinase. It is also possible to stain for the presence of the BRAF V600E mutant protein.

Clinical presentation

Patients usually present in primary care concerned about a new pigmented skin lesion or change in an existing skin lesion.

Initial evaluation includes a history of duration of the lesion, change of appearance over time, previous history of sun exposure, sun burn, previous skin cancers, any immunosuppressive treatment, and family history of melanoma and other cancers.

Clinical assessment includes detailed examination and a clinical photograph of the lesion, full skin examination, and examination for lymphadenopathy and hepatomegaly. Clinical risk factors for melanoma include itching, bleeding, ulceration, or changes in a pre-existing mole. The 'seven point checklist' is a useful tool recommended by the National Institute for Health and Clinical Excellence (NICE) (2005) for routine use in UK general practice to identify clinically significant skin lesions which require urgent referral. Weighting the features as major (2 points) and minor (1 point) provides better accuracy in referral (those lesions scoring >3).

Major features
- Change in size of a lesion
- Irregular pigmentation
- Irregular border

Minor features
- Inflammation
- Itch or altered sensation
- Larger than other lesions (diameter >7mm)
- Oozing/crusting of lesion

However, up to 50% of melanomas arise de novo, while others are non-pigmented, so identification of these tumour groups remains challenging.

There is no agreed screening protocol, although melanoma screening has been successfully implemented in Germany.

Diagnosis and management

Tissue diagnosis
The standard procedure is excision biopsy to include 2–5mm of clinical margin of normal skin with a cuff of subdermal fat. This helps to confirm diagnosis and provide guidance for subsequent management based on pathological Breslow thickness (mm). Full-thickness incisional biopsy from the thickest part of the lesion is acceptable as a mode of diagnosis in certain anatomical areas (e.g. face, ear, palm/sole) and for large lesions. Shave and punch biopsies are not recommended.

The pathology report should include Breslow thickness, Clark level, and mitotic index (for lesions <1mm), presence of ulceration, lateral and deep margin (mm)

size, presence of satellite lesions, evidence of vascular, and perineural invasion.

Staging
Breslow thickness and ulceration are the two most important prognostic factors of resected primary melanoma. Clark level was previously considered as a useful prognostic factor for melanoma of <1mm thickness, but mitotic index has now been confirmed as a more important prognostic marker in these thin melanomas (see Table 10.3.1).

Staging and follow-up
After resection of a primary melanoma, patients may be offered sentinel lymph node (SLN) biopsy as the most accurate method of staging loco-regional disease. Melanoma spreads locally, via the lymphatics initially to the regional lymph nodes, or to distant sites via the bloodstream. Monitoring of patients after resection of lower risk primary melanomas is focused around clinical assessment to identify loco-regional recurrence which might be amenable to surgical resection. For stage I–IIA (up to pT3a) melanomas, whose five and ten-year survival rates are greater than 94% and 88% respectively, whole body imaging is not recommended, but patients are followed clinically, usually for up to five years. In patients with thicker primary tumours (>4mm or >2mm ulcerated) or regional lymph node involvement, five-year survival rate varies widely from 93% for stage IIIA, to 32% for stage IIID. It is noteworthy in the new American Joint Committee on Cancer (AJCC) staging system that five-year survival for resected stage IIB and IIC disease is worse than stage IIIA and equivalent to stage IIIB. This has implications for communicating risk to patients, planning surveillance programmes, and offering adjuvant therapy. The most recent NICE guidance on melanoma management recommends surveillance imaging as part of follow-up for people who have had stage IIC melanoma with no sentinel lymph node biopsy (SLNB) or stage III melanoma and who would be candidates for systemic therapy as a result of early detection of metastatic disease. These guidelines predate introduction of adjuvant therapy.

10.2 Management of loco-regional disease for cutaneous melanoma

Primary surgery
Surgical excision with an adequate clinical margin is the standard treatment for primary melanoma. The excision margin refers to the clinically measured margin during surgery rather than the histopathological margin, since the tissue shrinks when fixed in formalin. A wider excision is usually undertaken as a second surgical procedure depending on the Breslow depth of the excised melanoma, but may need to be adjusted for cosmetic or functional reasons. In general, the recommended margins are: 1cm for melanomas <1mm in depth, 1–2cm for melanomas 1–2mm in depth, and 2–3cm for melanomas >2mm in depth. Depth of excision needs to be at least up to the muscle fascia to achieve local control.

Though there are no conclusive clinical trials, a margin of 5mm is recommended for melanoma in situ and a wider margin is recommended for desmoplastic

melanoma because of the increased risk of local recurrence due to contiguous subclinical spread.

The long axis of excision should be in the direction of the lymphatic drainage and parallel to the long axis of the limb to reduce the risk of lymphoedema.

Mohs micrographic surgery, a technique which aims for very narrow surgical margins, is not advisable for the treatment of melanoma. It may have a role in managing in situ melanoma.

Management of regional lymph nodes
Elective lymph node excision in the absence of palpable regional lymph node involvement has been shown conclusively not to confer any survival advantage for patients and is not recommended because of significant associated comorbidities. The role of elective node dissection in the case of a positive SLN has been hotly debated

(see the following section, 'Sentinel lymph node biopsy'), but results of the MSLT-2 trial suggest this should not be offered routinely.

Sentinel lymph node biopsy
The SLN is the node to which the lymph initially drains from a tumour before passing to the other regional nodes. In theory, the SLN is most likely to contain tumour cells and if none are present in this node, it is unlikely that other lymph nodes are involved.

The risk of SLN metastasis in melanoma depends on the thickness of the primary lesion. A tumour of <0.75mm thick has 1% SLN positivity rate; 0.75–1mm has 5%; and 1mm thickness has 8% risk, which steadily increases with increasing depth reaching 30% risk with 4mm thickness. A lesion >4mm thick has a 40% risk.

While SLN involvement has prognostic significance, the therapeutic benefit of removing it is uncertain. The MSLT-1 trial randomly assigned 2,001 melanoma patients with resected primary melanoma to undergo either wide excision and nodal observation with lymphadenectomy for nodal relapse, or wide excision and SLNB with immediate lymphadenectomy for nodal metastases detected on biopsy. The MSLT-1 investigators claimed that biopsy-driven lymphadenectomy prolonged disease-free survival (DFS), as well as distant DFS and melanoma-specific survival for patients with nodal metastases from intermediate-thickness melanomas. However, interpretation of this trial data is complex and currently the value of undertaking SLNB at the same time as performing wide local excision should be considered to be in providing optimal staging information.

The MSLT-2 trial showed that completion dissection was not associated with improved melanoma-specific overall survival (OS) versus observation in patients with sentinel-node metastasis, although a benefit was observed in regional disease control. Given that completion lymph node dissection (CLND) is associated with significant cost, complexity, and patient morbidity, this is now no longer recommended.

Management of microscopic lymph node involvement
Patients with clinically palpable regional lymph node disease are treated with surgical clearance of the lymph node basin. For some 30% of patients, surgery may be curative. After operation, support should be offered to manage lymphoedema (especially problematic with groin dissections), which may be contained with active physiotherapy and compression stockings.

CLND should include levels I–III in the axilla and clearance of the femoral triangle nodes in the groin. A therapeutic neck node dissection may include a superficial parotidectomy if clinically indicated. Despite radical surgery, risk of recurrence for many of these patients remains high and adjuvant therapy should be considered.

Adjuvant treatment
Adjuvant radiotherapy
Clinical trials to date suggest that adjuvant radiotherapy may assist in controlling disease within an irradiated field, but does not improve relapse-free survival or OS of treated patients. There is no proven role for radiotherapy (RT) after complete excision of primary cutaneous melanoma.

After regional lymph node dissection, several factors such as the number of lymph nodes involved (>3), size of lymph nodes (>3cm), location (neck), and extracapsular extension (ECE) predict for an increased risk of regional relapse. ECE is the single most important risk factor. Therefore, adjuvant RT would seem a sensible option for these patients. However, the evidence is limited to a single Australasian randomized study in which 250 high-risk patients received either RT, 48Gy in 20 fractions, or observation. In this trial, high risk was defined as: ≥1 parotid, ≥2 cervical or axillary, or ≥3 groin positive nodes; or extranodal spread of tumour; or minimum metastatic node diameter of 3cm (neck or axilla) or 4cm (groin). With median follow-up of 73 months, adjuvant RT was shown to reduce recurrence within the irradiated field (HR 0.52, P=0.023). Loco-regional symptoms and limb volumes were increased with adjuvant RT, particularly when irradiating inguinal regions, while long-term RT toxicity was relatively common. Therefore, adjuvant RT can probably only be justified as an option to treat high-risk resected melanoma involving the neck. Recent evidence that adjuvant systemic therapy significantly reduces risk of recurrence and improves OS, means that there will be far fewer indications for adjuvant RT.

Adjuvant systemic therapy
Following the introduction of new targeted agents and immune checkpoint inhibitors which can significantly improve survival of patients with metastatic melanoma (see Chapter 11, 'Cancers of the musculoskeletal system', p. 308), these agents have now been tested in the adjuvant setting. The first of these, ipilimumab, an anti-CTLA4 monoclonal antibody, reported an improvement in relapse-free survival (HR 0.75, P=0.0013). However, there were several treatment-related deaths. Two trials evaluating the anti-PD-1 monoclonal antibodies, nivolumab (CHECKMATE 238) and pembrolizumab (EORTC 1325/Keynote 054), have both shown significant gains in relapse-free survival with good patient tolerance. Furthermore, the most mature adjuvant therapy trial, Combi-AD has shown a 50% reduction in rate of relapse and a significant OS benefit following treatment with dabrafenib+trametinib in resected stage III BRAF mutant melanoma patients. All three treatments have been approved for routine use in National Health Service (NHS) patients. Trials are currently exploring the role of adjuvant therapy in resected stage IIB/C melanoma, as well as neoadjuvant approaches.

Further reading
Eggermont AMM, Blank CU, Mandala M, et al. Adjuvant pembrolizumab versus placebo in resected stage III melanoma. *N Engl J Med* 2018;378 (19):1789–801.

Eggermont AMM, Chiarion-Seleni V, Grob J, et al. Adjuvant ipilimumab versus placebo after complete resection of high-risk stage III melanoma (EORTC 18071): a randomised, double-blind, phase 3 trial. *Lancet Oncol* 2015; 16:522–30.

Faries MB, Thompson JF, Cochran AJ, Andtbacka RH, Mozzillo N, Zager JS, Jahkola T, et al. Completion dissection or observation for sentinel-node metastasis in melanoma. *New Engl J Med* 2017; 376:2211–22.

Gershenwald JE, Scolyer RA, Hess KR, Sondak VK, Long GV, Ross MI, et al. Melanoma staging: evidence-based changes in the American Joint Committee on Cancer Eighth Edition Cancer Staging Manual' *CA Cancer J Clin* 2017; 67:472–92.

Long GV, Atkinson V, Lo S, Sandhu S, Guminski AD, Brown MP, Wilmott JS, et al. Combination nivolumab and ipilimumab or nivolumab alone in melanoma brain metastases: a multicentre randomised phase 2 study. *Lancet Oncol* 2018; 19:672–81.

Morton DL, Thompson JF, Cochran AJ, et al. Final trial report of sentinel node biopsy versus nodal observation in melanoma. *New Engl J Med* 2014; 370:599–609.

Weber J, Mandala M, Del Vecchio M, et al. Adjuvant Nivolumab versus Ipilimumab in Resected Stage III or IV Melanoma. *N Engl J Med* 2017; 377(19):1824–35.

Internet resources

AJCC. Melanoma prediction tools: http://www.melanomaprognosis.net

NICE guideline 2015 [NG14]. Melanoma: assessment and management—available at: http://www.nice.org.uk/guidance/ng14#

10.3 Management of metastatic disease for cutaneous melanoma

Introduction

Untreated, metastatic melanoma has a poor prognosis, with median life expectancy of eight to ten months. Some patients with non-visceral metastases tend to live longer, while elevated serum lactate dehydrogenase (LDH) and brain metastases are poor prognostic factors, with median life expectancy as little as three to six months in these subgroups. Lymph node and skin metastases without other major organ involvement have the best prognosis (up to 18 months). Those with lung metastases in the absence of other visceral disease have an intermediate prognosis (up to 12 months median survival). Patients with other sites of visceral disease have a median survival of <6 months. These different patterns of metastases and associated outcomes are reflected in the AJCC staging criteria for metastatic melanoma (Table 10.3.1).

Treatment of metastatic melanoma depends on the site of disease spread, disease burden, overall fitness of the patient, and, more recently, molecular genotype. Until 2011, surgery was the only modality likely to offer

Table 10.3.1 AJCC Staging of malignant melanoma (2018)

Stage	Clinical staging	Pathological staging	Tumour node metastasis (TNM) description
IA	pT1aN0M0	pT1aN0M0 pT1bN0M0	pT1a: tumour of ≤0.8mm thickness without ulceration pT1b: tumour of ≤0.8mm thickness with ulceration or tumour of >0.8 mm but <1 mm
IB	pT1bN0M0 pT2aN0M0	pT2aN0M0	pT2a: tumour of >1 mm but ≤2mm thickness without ulceration
IIA	pT2bN0M0 pT3aN0M0	pT2bN0M0 pT3aN0M0	pT2b: tumour of >1 mm but ≤2mm thickness without ulceration pT3a: tumour of >2 mm but ≤4mm thickness without ulceration
IIB	pT3bN0M0 pT4aN0M0	pT3bN0M0 pT4aN0M0	pT3b: tumour of >2 mm but ≤4mm thickness without ulceration pT4a: tumour of >4mm thickness without ulceration
IIC	pT4bN0M0	pT4bN0M0	pT4b: tumour of >4mm thickness without ulceration
III	Any pT N1–3M0	Any pT N1–3M0	N1: metastasis in one regional lymph node N2: metastasis in 2–3 regional lymph nodes N3: Metastasis in ≥4 regional lymph nodes
IIIA		pT1–2a N1a/N2a	N1a: one clinically occult microscopic nodal metastasis N2a: microscopic disease in 2–3 nodes
IIIB		pT1–2a N1b–c/N2b pT2b–3a N1/ N2a/ N2b	N1b: clinically apparent macroscopic metastases N1c: satellite or in-transit metastases without regional nodal disease N2b: macroscopic disease in 2–3 nodes
IIIC		pT1–3a N2c/N3 pT3b, T4a, pT4b N1–N3	N2c: satellite or in-transit metastases with one regional nodal metastases
IIID		pT4bN3	
IV	Any pT any N M1	Any T any N M1	M1: distant metastasis M1a: skin, subcutaneous or lymph node metastases beyond regional nodes M1b: lung metastasis M1c: other non-central nervous system metastasis M1d: central nervous system metastasis

Source: data from Amin MB, Edge S, Greene F, et al. (eds). *AJCC Cancer Staging Manual.* 8th edn. Springer International Publishing. 2017, American College of Surgeons, pp. 563–85.

a chance of cure or life extension from melanoma, and dacarbazine was the only standard chemotherapy agent offered despite lack of survival benefit. However, unprecedented changes in melanoma developmental therapeutics have radically altered how inoperable melanoma is now managed.

Systemic therapy for metastatic melanoma

Up until 2011, no systemic therapy had convincingly been shown to improve survival of patients with metastatic melanoma. Dacarbazine was the international standard cytotoxic chemotherapy, offering at best a 15% objective response rate, while treatment within a clinical trial was an accepted first-line option. In 2011, two new agents—vemurafenib and ipilimumab—were licensed, with survival benefit for advanced melanoma patients confirmed in international randomized trials. They represent two very distinctive classes of agents: small molecule inhibitors of the MUTYH associated polyposis (MAP) kinase signalling pathway and monoclonal antibodies against immune checkpoint molecules.

MAP kinase pathway inhibitors

Vemurafenib was the first oral biological serine/threonine kinase inhibitor targeting BRAF which was licensed by the US Food and Drug Administration (FDA) in August 2011 (European Medicines Agency (EMA) licence in February 2012) for use in patients with advanced melanoma with a BRAFV600 gene mutation. Around 45% of all melanomas harbour a BRAFV600 mutation, providing a biomarker to identify those patients who will benefit from treatment. Randomized trials of vemurafenib and another BRAF inhibitor, dabrafenib, report consistent objective response rates around 50%, but virtually all patients treated will experience some tumour shrinkage. However, median progression-free survival is around six months, because of secondary resistance which develops on treatment. A key cause of resistance appears to be reactivation of the signalling pathway downstream of BRAF. Four international randomized trials (Combi-D, Combi-V, Co-BRIM, and Columbus (Dummer et al. 2018)) have confirmed that dual therapy with a BRAF and MEK inhibitor increases both progression-free survival and OS compared with BRAF inhibitor alone. Median survival of patients receiving combination BRAF/MEK inhibitors now extends beyond two years.

Use of these oral agents is associated with a number of chronic toxicities. Although frequency is high, most are manageable, not life-threatening, and compatible with normal daily living: hospitalization is rarely needed. The problematic skin toxicities associated with vemurafenib monotherapy—photosensitivity, rash, and occurrence of other skin lesions, ranging from benign (e.g. warts) to premalignant (e.g. keratoacanthomas) to malignant (squamous cell cancers)—are less prevalent with dabrafenib and combinations of BRAF/MEK inhibitors. Other common class toxicities include myalgia, arthralgia, and fatigue, while dabrafenib-containing regimens may generate fever and chills in the absence of infection and neutropaenia, which is an important education requirement for acute oncology teams. The most recently licensed combination regimen, encorafenib+binimetinib, appears to have a cleaner side effect profile. These agents can be given to patients with extensive disease burden including brain metastases and poor performance status such that patients who would normally be considered

beyond treatment with chemotherapy can be returned to good health for some months.

The combination regimens, dabrafenib+trametinib and encorafenib+binimetinig have been approved for use in the NHS.

BRAF is by far the most frequently mutated gene in melanoma. Other commonly mutated genes include NRAS (25% of melanomas), C-KIT (10% of acral and mucosal melanoma), and, in uveal melanoma only, GNAQ and GNA11. BRAF and NRAS mutations are generally mutually exclusive. New targeted therapeutics are being developed and tested in clinical trials for these patient subgroups with identified mutations: evidence of personalized (or 'precision') medicine in evolution.

Immunotherapy

Ipilimumab is a humanized monoclonal antibody blocking CTLA4, which, in effect, removes the brake from normal immunological controls. A series of international studies have confirmed that ipilimumab generates durable disease control in a minority of treated patients: around 20% of patients treated with ipilimumab remain alive beyond three years after completing treatment. A phase 2 trial of ipilimumab in patients with brain metastases reported disease control in the brain in 24% of asymptomatic and 10% of symptomatic patients, suggesting that these patients should not be excluded from receiving this drug.

Ipilimumab is straightforward to deliver to patients, being administered as four infusions three weeks apart, but has a range of complex immune-related side effects, such that around one in ten patients may experience severe life-threatening immune-related toxicities requiring hospitalization. The most common serious immune-related toxicities are colitis, skin reactions, hepatitis, and endocrinopathies, in particular, hypopituitarism. Currently, there is no predictive biomarker to select which patients will benefit from ipilimumab. Even so, this treatment is NICE approved for untreated and previously treated metastatic melanoma, irrespective of BRAF mutation status.

There are now increasing numbers of immune checkpoint molecules being identified as potential therapeutic targets. The most promising of these is programmed death-1, PD-1. Two monoclonal antibodies inhibiting PD-1—nivolumab and pembrolizuamb—have recently reported superior activity compared with ipilimumab. The KEYNOTE 006 trial reported improvements in response rate, progression-free survival and OS compared with ipilimumab, while immune-related adverse events were less frequent and less severe. The combination of nivolumab+ipilimumab has been compared to nivolumab and ipilimumab in the CHECKMATE 067 trial. The results are now mature, with four-year follow-up. Objective response rates of 58% versus 45% and 19% for nivolumb+ipilimumab, nivolumab, and ipilimumab, respectively, favour the combination arm. Four-year progression-free survival was 37%, 31%, and 9%; four-year OS was 53%, 46%, and 30%. These relatively modest survival gains with combination ipilimumab+nivolumab were associated with very high rates of grade 3 and 4 adverse events, occurring in 59% of treated patients, compared with 22% in the nivolumab and 27% in the ipilimumab arm (see Figure 10.3.1) (Hodi et al. 2018).

Both anti PD-1 monoclonal antibodies and ipilimumab+nivolumab are available for routine use in

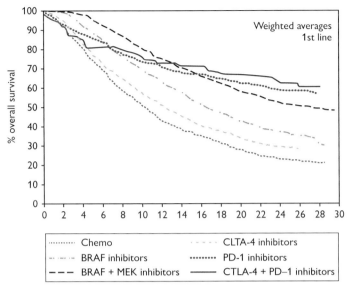

Fig. 10.3.1 Summary of outcomes reported in landmark trials evaluating BRAF/MEK inhibitors and immune checkpoint inhibitors in previously untreated advanced melanoma patients (see also colour plate).
Reproduced with permission from Ugural S, et al. Survival of patients with advanced metastatic melanoma: the impact of novel therapies—update 2017. *Eur J Cancer* 2017; 87:247–57. Copyright © 2017, Elsevier Ltd.

the UK. Decisions about which regimen to choose, and in BRAF mutant melanoma patients, whether to choose immunotherapy or BRAF targeted therapy first, are complex, unresolved, and largely clinically based currently. A huge amount of research aims to discover relevant biomarkers that might predict for both efficacy and toxicity, particularly associated with immunotherapy, including PDL1 expression, neoantigen load, molecular signatures, and the microbiome. None have yet proved so reliable to be used in the clinic.

Introduction of these new melanoma systemic therapies have clearly improved outcomes. Even so, the majority of treated patients will still die of their disease and many new targets are still being explored for their therapeutic potential.

Role of surgery
For an isolated metastasis, especially if the patient has had a long disease-free interval, surgery continues to be offered to patients. Accessible sites for surgical resection are soft tissue (skin, lymph nodes), but other sites where melanoma commonly metastasises may be amenable to surgery, including liver, brain, lung, bowel, and adrenal gland. Patients with up to three visceral metastases may be the best candidates for surgical resection and the five-year survival can be >20% after complete resection.

Surgery may also be used as an adjunct to maintaining patients on modern systemic therapies. Differential responses to both BRAF and immune checkpoint inhibitors are well recognized and surgical resection of a solitary site of disease growing in an otherwise stable patient may enable the patient to remain on systemic therapy for many more months. Furthermore, the potential to use systemic therapies to downstage large volume loco-regional melanoma and enable surgical clearance is now being evaluated.

Radiotherapy
RT is not a primary modality treatment except in elderly patients with extensive or unresectable lentigo maligna. However, it may be a useful option to palliate symptomatic metastatic disease. A new role to potentiate the benefits of immune activation (the 'abscopal' effect) is being explored in clinical trials (Hanna et al. 2015).

Brain metastasis
The brain is a frequent site for melanoma spread, especially in the end stages of life. Surgery or stereotactic radiosurgery should be considered for solitary or oligometastatic brain involvement. Whole brain radiotherapy (WBRT) may be offered to palliate symptoms in those patients with extensive brain involvement. There is negligible evidence that WBRT extends life, but it may help to control intracranial disease in the short term: most melanoma patients with brain involvement die of extracranial disease. There is no evidence that WBRT should be used as an adjuvant after surgery or radiosurgery for treating brain metastases.

Patients presenting with multiple brain metastases whose tumours carry a BRAF mutation are more likely to gain symptomatic benefit from targeted therapy and WBRT should be withheld in the first instance. For BRAF wild type patients with low volume, asymptomatic disease, ipilimumab+nivolumab generates remarkably high response rates (Long et al. 2018). Whether RT adds benefit over and above anti-PD-1 monotherapy is not certain.

Symptom management
Palliative RT is useful in controlling pain associated with brain metastases and remains a standard option for spinal cord compression not amenable to surgical decompression. Superficial metastases which are unresectable, rapidly enlarging, and about to ulcerate can also be treated with palliative RT.

Cytotoxic chemotherapy

In a very short time, cytotoxic chemotherapy has been replaced by modern systemic targeted and immunotherapies. However, since significant patients either do not respond or relapse after these treatments, traditional cytotoxic agents still remain options.

Dacarbazine is the standard intravenous chemotherapy drug for metastatic melanoma with a response rate of 15%. The median duration of response is three to six months and there is no evidence that dacarbazine extends patient survival. It is however easy to deliver to patients: it is administered three weekly at a standard dose of 1,000mg/m². It is usually well tolerated with modern prophylactic antibiotics.

Temozolamide is an oral analogue of dacarbazine which, unlike dacarbazine, crosses the blood–brain barrier. However, clinical trials have not shown any greater activity compared with dacarbazine, neither does it appear to have greater efficacy against brain metastases.

Combination chemotherapy regimens, e.g. carboplatin+paclitaxel, have higher response rates than dacarbazine and may be justified in an attempt to debulk high volume BRAF wild type melanoma.

Other immunotherapy strategies

Immunotherapies used in the past include interferon and interleukin-2 (IL-2). Interferon is a pleiotropic cytokine with a potential antitumour effect. IL-2 is a cytokine produced by CD4+ T lymphocytes. Its exact antitumour action is not known, but is thought to be due to stimulation and recruitment of natural killer cells and induction of other cytokines.

High-dose IL-2 is associated with response rates of 10–21% with rare cases of complete remission and this was the reason for the FDA licensing. However, toxicities are challenging and include hypotension, capillary leak syndrome, sepsis, and renal failure.

Multiple new immunotherapy approaches are being explored as more is being discovered about both the innate and adaptive immune system.

Vaccine approaches continue to be explored for melanoma. A randomized trial of a modified herpes virus, T-VEC, reported durable responses in distant sites when injected into accessible metastases. Adoptive T cell transfer is labour intensive, but has generated impressive outcomes in selected patients. Previously considered to be prohibitive due to cost, a single cell-based intervention may prove to be cost-effective compared to chronic administration of immune checkpoint inhibitor drugs and these approaches are now being tested in large-scale trials.

Isolated limb perfusion and isolated limb infusion

A small cohort of melanoma patients experience limited disease spread within the soft tissues of a single limb. In these patients, regional interventions may be an option. Isolated limb perfusion (ILP) with tumour necrosis factor A(TNF-A) and melphalan or melphalan alone under hypothermic conditions can establish good local control. This is only performed in a limited number of specialist centres, but can provide good clinical benefit.

Isolated limb infusion (ILI) is a simpler method of regional drug delivery, which may help to control disease within a distal limb (e.g. below knee or elbow). Response rates as high as 90% with complete response in 60–70% patients have been reported.

In approximately 50% of responders to regional limb interventions, the benefit may be sustained for more than a year, which may obviate or delay the need for systemic therapies. Thankfully, nowadays, limb amputation is rarely an appropriate intervention.

Other local interventions

Local disease may be controlled by a variety of other means, including cryotherapy, laser therapy, radiofrequency ablation, and electrochemotherapy. There is no high-quality evidence to directly compare these modalities.

Further reading

Ajithkumar T, Parkinson C, Fife K, Corrie P, Jefferies S. Evolving treatment options for melanoma brain metastases. *Lancet Oncol* 2015 Oct; 16(3):e486–97.

Dummer R, Ascierto PA, Gogas HJ, et al. Overall survival in patients with BRAF-mutant melanoma receiving encorafenib plus binimetinib versus vemurafenib or encorafenib (COLUMBUS): a multicentre, open-label, randomised, phase 3 trial. *Lancet Oncol* 2018; 19:1315–27.

Hanna GG, Coyle VM, Prise KM. Immune modulation in advanced radiotherapies: targeting out-of-field effects. *Cancer Letts* 2015; 368:246–51.

Hodi FS, Chiarion-Sileni V, Gonzalez R, et al. Nivolumab plus ipilimumab or nivolumab alone versus ipilimumab alone in advanced melanoma (CheckMate 067): 4-year outcomes of a multicentre, randomised, phase 3 trial. *Lancet* 2018; 19:1480–92.

Larkin J, Ascierto PA, Dreno B, et al. Combined vemurafenib and cobimetinib in BRAF-mutated melanoma. *N Engl J Med* 2014; 371:1867–76.

Larkin J, Chiarion-Sileni V, Gonzalez R, et al. Combined nivolumab and Ipilimumab or monotherapy in untreated melanoma. *N Engl J Med* 2015; 373:23–34.

Larkin J, Yan Y, McArthur GA, et al. Update of progression-free survival (PFS) and correlative biomarker analysis from coBRIM: Phase III study of cobimetinib plus vemurafenib in advanced BRAF-mutated melanoma. *J Clin Oncol* 2015; 33(suppl.): abstr 9006.

Long GV, Atkinson V, Lo S, et al. Combination nivolumab and ipilimumab or nivolumab alone in melanoma brain metastases: a multicentre randomised phase 2 study. *Lancet Oncol* 2018; 19:672–81.

Long GV, Stroyakovsky D, Gogas H, et al. Dabrafenib and trametinib versus dabrafenib and placebo for VAL600-mutant melanoma: a multicentre, double-blind, phase 3 randomized controlled trial. *Lancet Oncol* 2015; 386:444–51.

Robert C, Karaszewska B, Schachter J, et al. Improved overall survival in melanoma with combined dabrafenib and trametinib. *N Engl J Med* 2015; 372:30–9.

Robert C, Long GV, Brady B, et al. Nivolumab in previously untreated melanoma without BRAF mutation. *N Engl J Med* 2015; 372:320–30.

Robert C, Schachter J, Long GV, et al. Pembrolizumab versus ipilimumab in advanced melanoma. *N Engl J Med* 2015; 372:2521–32.

10.4 Non-cutaneous melanoma

Ocular melanoma

Ocular melanoma is a rare subtype of melanoma (incidence 2–8 per million per year in Caucasians), which can originate from any part of the uveal tract (choroid, iris, or ciliary body) or, even more rarely, the conjunctiva. More than 90% uveal melanomas arise in the choroid. The aetiology is uncertain but there are some studies which suggest a link with UV radiation and familial cases are very rare. The risks are higher in those who have had a cutaneous melanoma or have pale iris colour. The staging system differs from that of cutaneous melanoma and follows the AJCC staging system for eye cancer.

Outcomes for patients with uveal melanoma vary widely, but for patients with early tumours they are excellent: small uveal melanomas up to 3mm thickness have a 12% rate of metastases at ten years, while the rate rises to 50% for large melanomas >8mm thickness. An online tool, developed in Liverpool (the Liverpool Uveal Melanoma Prognosticator Online (LUMPO)) is available and generates an all-cause mortality curve based on age, sex, tumour size, ciliary body involvement, melanoma cytomorphology, closed loops, mitotic count, chromosome 3 loss, and presence of extraocular spread.

Certain cytogenetic features, e.g. chromosome 3 loss, chromosome 8 gain, and chromosome 1 loss correlate with reduced survival. Gains in chromosome 6p correlate with good prognosis. Long-term OS is <35% even with successful treatment of the primary.

Surgical enucleation used to be the standard treatment for primary uveal melanoma, but RT has replaced this for smaller tumours. RT can be administered by external beam, as a radioactive plaque (e.g. iridium-192) or with protons or other charged particles. Local control rates are similar with each technique. Vision is often lost in the irradiated eye with other complications occurring over time, including cataracts, glaucoma, retinopathy, and vitreous haemorrhage.

Metastatic disease when it occurs almost always involves the liver and is associated with a particularly poor survival, usually limited to <3 months. Although in most cases, liver metastases are multiple, in some cases, solitary, asymptomatic lesions are identified by surveillance imaging and should be considered for surgical resection, or other loco-regional intervention.

Metastatic uveal melanoma is even less responsive to cytotoxic chemotherapy than cutaneous melanoma. However, recent studies have identified a high prevalence (up to 80%) of activating mutations in either GNAQ or GNA11 genes and, at least in pre-clinical models, tumours with these mutations appear to respond to treatment with small molecule MEK inhibitors. Prospective clinical trials evaluating the role of MEK inhibitors have however proved disappointing. Uveal melanomas are almost exclusively BRAF wild type. Virtually all immune checkpoint inhibitor registration trials have excluded metastatic uveal melanoma patients, but real world studies have shown that the response rate to anti-PD-1 antibody therapy is around 5%. Therefore, these patients should be enrolled in clinical trials, where possible.

In 2015, national guidelines were published and endorsed by National Institute for Health and Clinical Excellence (NICE), recommending that uveal melanoma patients should have regular surveillance organized by regional specialist melanoma oncology teams including six-monthly imaging of the liver. Duration of surveillance is uncertain, but is recommended to be life-long for high-risk patients because recurrence can be late—in some cases, decades after treatment of the primary tumour.

Mucosal melanoma

Mucosal melanomas arise from melanocytes located in mucosal membranes lining the respiratory, gastrointestinal, and urogenital tract. They constitute <2% of all melanomas, with an incidence around two per million per year. The most common sites of presentation are the head and neck (up to 50%), female genital tract (25%), and anorectal region (20%), but they can arise from any mucosal membrane. Conjunctival melanoma is the only mucosal melanoma arising in a sun-exposed site.

They generally occur later in life (50–70s) than cutaneous melanoma, are more common in non-Caucasians, and slightly more common in women than in men. They tend to present late and have a very poor prognosis. Compared with cutaneous (80%) and uveal (75%) melanoma, five-year survival is only 25%. Over the years, the incidence of mucosal melanoma has remained relatively stable, unlike cutaneous melanoma. There is no specific staging system for mucosal melanomas. Their aetiology is not well understood, but they appear to be cytogenetically distinct from other melanomas: BRAF mutations are rare, while around 10% carry mutations and/or increased copy number of C-Kit.

Diagnosis is by full-thickness biopsy of the suspicious lesion and it is important to exclude the possibility of a metastasis from primary cutaneous or uveal melanoma. The treatment of choice is surgical resection with clear margins, but this is often difficult due to location and advanced stage of the tumour at presentation. RT has been used to try to improve local control, but has not been shown to improve survival. A study using carbon ions to minimize local morbidity showed good local control but five-year survival was still <30%. Cytotoxic chemotherapy is no more active than for cutaneous melanoma.

Head and neck mucosal melanoma

Mucosal melanomas of the head and neck region account for about 4% of head and neck malignancies, <1% of all head and neck melanomas, and most often arise in the nasal cavity and paranasal sinuses. Presenting symptoms include nasal obstruction, a mass, bleeding, or pain.

Complete surgical excision is the treatment of choice. Head and neck melanoma has a tendency to recur loco-regionally before developing distant metastasis and hence many clinicians consider RT as an adjuvant after surgery, though there is virtually no evidence that this improves either local control or survival.

In patients with localized tumours where surgery is not feasible, primary RT may be used to manage what can be quite unpleasant symptoms. Five-year survival is <30%, which reduces to <20% if lymph nodes are involved.

Female genital tract melanoma

Vulval melanoma

The most common site of melanoma arising in the female genital tract is the vulva; most arise from squamous epithelium and behave just like cutaneous melanoma. The most common histological types are lentiginous melanoma and nodular melanoma. A small proportion are true mucosal melanomas. Vulval melanoma accounts for <1% of gynaecological malignancies and occurs in older Caucasian women (median age 68 years).

Most patients present complaining of a perineal mass, bleeding, pruritus, pain, and/or discharge. One-third of patients have regional metastasis and one-quarter have distant metastasis at presentation. Prognostic factors include tumour thickness, ulceration, and nodal status.

As for any primary melanoma, surgery is the treatment of choice. Superficial lesions can be treated with wide excision. Central and thick lesions require aggressive surgery with bilateral vulvectomy and inguinal lymphadenectomy. SLNB can be undertaken by trained gynaecology surgeons, supported by melanoma plastic surgery teams.

Overall two-year survival is 50% with >70% for patients with a lesion <1mm thick, but <20% with nodal involvement.

Vaginal melanoma

Vaginal melanomas are extremely rare and mainly arise in the lower third of the vault. Patients frequently present with advanced disease, limiting the chance of complete surgical removal. Even if aggressive local intervention is possible, the recurrence rate is extremely high. Five-year survival rates range from 0–21%.

Anorectal melanoma

Primary mucosal melanomas can arise anywhere along the gastrointestinal tract, but well over 50% occur in the anorectal region. The majority occur in Caucasians over the age of 70 years. Anorectal melanoma comprises <1% of anorectal tumours. The usual presenting symptoms are bleeding per rectum, discomfort, and prolapse of a tumour mass. Most melanomas occurring in the gastrointestinal tract will be metastases from cutaneous melanoma, so careful pathological evaluation is key.

Around 30% of anorectal melanomas are amelanotic, so the pathological diagnosis is frequently unexpected after surgical resection. Around one-third of patients have regional or distant metastases at diagnosis. Primary tumour thickness and nodal involvement are less reliable prognostic factors.

The primary tumour needs to be assessed for resectability. If an adequate margin can be achieved, wide local excision with sphincter preservation is the best treatment option. One-third of patients may require abdominoperineal resection to accomplish a complete resection. In the absence of lymph node involvement, SLNB is not recommended, since this does not appear to have prognostic value in these patients.

If there is evidence of lymph node involvement, lymphadenectomy at the time of primary tumour surgery is advised.

Despite all treatment modalities, overall five-year survival for anorectal melanoma remains poor at about 20% and median survival is 14–20 months.

Systemic therapy for advanced mucosal melanoma

As for cutaneous melanoma, it is now important to genotype mucosal melanomas to identify BRAF and C-KIT mutations. Around 10% mucosal melanomas have a mutation in C-KIT. In contrast to BRAF, multiple types of mutations have been identified, only some of which appear to confer sensitivity to treatment with a kinase inhibitor selective for C-KIT mutant protein. These agents—including sunitinib and nilotinib and newer agents such as PLX3397—are being tested in clinical trials and are not established standard of care.

Currently, there is not standard adjuvant therapy after resection of mucosal melanoma.

Further reading

Carvajal RD, Schwartz GK, Tezel T, Marr B, Francis JH, Nathan PD. Metastatic disease from uveal melanoma: treatment options and future prospects. *Br J Ophthalmol* 2017; 101:38–44.

Lim L, Madigan MC, Conway RM. Conjunctival melanoma: a review of conceptual and treatment advances. *Clin Ophthal* 2013; 7:521–31.

Mahajlovic M, Vlajkovic S, Jovanovic P, Stefanovic V. Primary mucosal melanomas: a comprehensive review. *Int J Clin Exp Pathol* 2012; 5:739–53.

Internet resources

Liverpool Uveal Melanoma Prognosticator Online (LUMPO): https://mpcetoolsforhealth.liverpool.ac.uk/matsoap/lumpo3cr.htm

Melanoma Focus Uveal Melanoma Guidelines, January 2015: http://melanomafocus.com/wp-content/uploads/2015/01/Uveal-Melanoma-National-Guidelines-Full-v5.3.pdf

Ocula Melanoma Foundation: http://www.ocularmelanoma.org/other-online-resources.htm

10.5 Basal cell carcinoma

Introduction

Basal cell carcinoma (BCC) is a slow growing, locally invasive (hence called rodent ulcer), malignant epidermal skin tumour. The exact incidence is difficult to obtain although there is a worldwide trend towards increasing incidence. Approximately one million new cases are diagnosed per year in the USA.

Aetiology

The most important aetiological factors appear to be UV exposure and genetic predisposition.

Environmental factors

BCC is common in the sun-exposed area of the head and neck. Other risk factors include increasing age, male gender, fair skin, immunosuppression, vaccination scars, and arsenic exposure. Sunscreen use and a low-fat diet are thought to be protective.

Genetic factors

Aberrant activation of the hedgehog signalling pathway is a key driver in the pathogenesis of BCC. In sporadic BCC, loss of function mutations in the patched homologue 1 (PTCH1) gene are seen in 90% and activating mutations in smoothened homologue (SMO) in 10% of tumours.

BCC is a feature of a number of genetic conditions such as Gorlin's syndrome (basal cell naevus syndrome), Basex syndrome, and Rombo syndrome.

Basal cell naevus syndrome (Gorlin's syndrome) is an autosomal dominantly inherited condition due to mutations in PTCH1 on chromosome 9q22. It is associated with multiple (often hundreds) of BCCs, increased risk of other neoplasms (e.g. meningioma, ovarian fibroma, rhabdomyosarcoma), and bony developmental abnormalities.

Pathology

The common histological subtypes are superficial, nodular, and morpheoic (sclerosing). Other variants include micronodular, infiltrative, and basosquamous BCC which are aggressive with high risk of local recurrence. Perivascular and perineural invasion are also associated with aggressive tumours. BCC infiltrate tissues in a three-dimensional fashion. Lymph node metastasis is extremely rare except in those with multiple recurrences or uncontrolled primary tumour.

Clinical features

Clinical suspicion arises when there is any friable non-healing lesion on the skin. Some lesions manifest with brief bleeding and complete healing followed by recurrence of the lesion. BCCs can be locally invasive causing local tissue destruction but metastatic BCC is rare (<0.1%).

The common growth patterns are nodular, superficial, multifocal, and morpheoic. The sites affected are head and neck (52%), trunk (27%), upper limb (13%), and lower limb (8%).

- Nodular BCC, the commonest clinical subtype, occurs on the skin of the head and neck region of elderly patients. It presents as a shiny, pearly, telangiectatic papule or nodule. The pearly appearance becomes more prominent during skin stretching. Radially arranged dilated capillaries are often seen across the surface of lesion. With ongoing growth, tumour ulceration may occur which leads to central umbilication of the lesion with a raised rolled border. Islands of pigments may also be seen.
- Superficial BCC occurs on the trunk or limbs of young people. It presents as a well-defined, erythematous, scaling, or slightly shiny macular lesion. Stretching the lesion causes an increase in the degree of erythema, highlights the shiny surface, and reveals a peripheral thread-like pearly rim or islands of pearliness distributed throughout the lesion. These lesions will progressively enlarge and may reach 5–10cm in diameter. Biopsy is needed before definitive treatment.
- Morphoeic SCC typically presents as a pale scar and palpation reveals firm induration which extends more widely and deeply than is evident on inspection. It slowly enlarges to reach a large size. Biopsy is necessary.
- Pigmented BCCs are nodular BCCs with increased melanization leading to an appearance of a hyperpigmented translucent papule.

Examination

Clinical examination should be done in a well-lit area with the aid of a magnifier. Whole skin and regional nodal examination are necessary.

Diagnosis

Diagnosis is often clinical. Biopsy is indicated when there is clinical suspicion of an alternative diagnosis or if histological subtype may influence treatment decision. Punch or shave biopsy may be appropriate. Imaging of the local area, e.g. by computed tomography (CT), may be indicated when there is any suspicion of bone involvement and deep infiltration (particularly for a lesion close to the embryonic fusion lines such as the nasal vestibular region, or pre- and postauricular regions).

Treatment

Treatment is aimed at eradication of tumour with acceptable cosmetic and functional outcome. A number of treatment options are available for BCCs (see later in this section 'Treatment modalities in BCC', p. 299) and the choice of treatment in small BCCs depends on various factors (see later in this section 'Treatment of choice in BCC', p. 299). RT is indicated when cosmetic and/or functional outcome is better with RT compared with surgery and when there is a need to avoid complex plastic surgery.

Surgery

Wide excision (WE)

WE of simple lesions needs a 2–3mm margin whereas complex lesions, clinically poorly defined lesions, and recurrent disease need a margin of 3–5mm. An adequate microscopic margin is 0.5mm. Excision of the primary BCC should extend to fat to ensure adequate tumour control.

The most appropriate management after incomplete excision is debatable. The treatment options include re-excision, Mohs micrographic surgery (MMS), or RT. Adjuvant RT improves five-year recurrence-free survival from 61% to 91%. Observation is an option for frail elderly patients where further surgery and RT may not be appropriate.

Mohs micrographic surgery (MMS)

During this procedure, the tumour is excised and the entire peripheral and deep margins are examined by frozen section for residual tumour. Mapping and staining of excised tissue and a specialized tissue sectioning procedure enable precise localization of residual tumour and the process of excision continues until the margin is tumour free. It offers better histological analysis of tumour margin with maximal conservation of tissue compared with surgical excision. MMS is the treatment of choice for tumours with poorly defined borders (morphoeic), recurrent tumours, extensive disease, aggressive histological subtype, incompletely excised tumours, and BCCs at high-risk anatomical sites (mask area of face, scalp, embryonic fusion planes, periorbital area, and eyelid). In these situations, MMS offers better chances of cure than excision.

Curettage and desiccation

This is suitable for small lesions (<2cm) where >95% cure can be achieved. However, it is highly operator dependent. It is not recommended for morphoeic BCC, tumours >2cm, and recurrent BCC. It should also be avoided on areas of hair growth.

Cryosurgery

During cryotherapy BCC is destroyed with a clinically normal margin. However, it lacks the benefit of histological confirmation of a complete tumour removal. The best reported results are around 99% at five years. An important adverse outcome of cryotherapy is the obscuring of tumour recurrence by fibrous scar tissue.

Superficial treatments

Where surgery or RT are not an option, superficial treatments may be appropriate for low-risk superficial BCC, accepting that cure rates may be lower.

Topical imiquimod (5% cream)

Imiquimod is believed to act by boosting T helper 1 type immunity by inducing various cytokines. In superficial

BCC, it is reported to result in 79–82% histological clearance in randomized trials. In a meta-analysis of randomized and non-randomized studies, the pooled estimate of one-year tumour-free survival was 87%.

Photodynamic therapy (PDT)
PDT involves activation of a photosensitizing drug by visible light to produce activated oxygen species that destroy the cancer cells. Though there is good initial clearance (88%) with one or multiple treatments, the recurrence rates are higher than for other superficial treatments (27% at one year). Hence it is recommended only for situations in which established treatments are not feasible.

Radiotherapy
Primary RT results in 93–95% ten-year control rate for BCC of 2cm. RT details are given in the Box 10.5.1.

Adjuvant RT may be offered after incomplete excision where re-excision is not recommended and improves five-year survival from 61% to 91%.

Systemic therapy
The oral selective hedgehog pathway inhibitors vismodegib and sonidegib, have reported response rates of approximately 43–60% for locally advanced and 15–48.5% for metastatic BCC. However, these agents are associated with significant side effects, most frequently muscle spasm, alopecia, fatigue, weight loss, and dysgeusia. Toxicity leads to discontinuation of treatment in approximately 30–50% of patients. As with other targeted agents, acquired resistance typically develops, limiting the duration of response (7.6 months for metastatic BCC and 9.5 months in locally advanced BCC treated with vismodegib). Alternative regimens such as intermittent dosing (e.g. MIKIE trial) have been found to be equally effective as continuous treatment.

Box 10.5.1 Radiotherapy for BCC and SCC

Consent
- Acute reactions involve dermatitis and mucositis which resolve by six weeks following treatment.
- Late effects involve thinning of skin, alopecia, loss of sweating, change in colour, telangiectasia, and fibrosis.

Position and immobilization
- Depends on the site.

Type of radiation
Depends on depth of penetration needed and type of underlying tissue:

Depth of penetration
- 5mm deep lesion—superficial X-ray.
- >5mm–2cm deep lesion—orthovoltage X-ray or low energy electrons (4–6MeV).
- >2cm tumour—high energy electrons or photons.

Underlying tissue
- Bone—electrons are preferable to avoid increased absorbed dose from orthovoltage X-rays.
- Air cavities (e.g. near sinuses)—X-rays or photons preferred as dosimetry is difficult with electrons.

Treatment volume
- Well-defined BCC: 5mm margin around macroscopic tumour.
- Ill-defined BCC and SCC: 10mm margin.

Beam shaping
Custom-made lead cut out for X-rays and end frame cut-out for electrons. Crenellation of the margin of a round cut out gives a better cosmesis by blurring the edge of the radiation reaction.

Radiotherapy dose
The choice of fractionations depends on a number of factors such as size of tumour, importance of cosmetic outcome, travel logistics of patients, etc. Common RT fractionations are given in Table 10.5.1.

Special considerations

Electron planning
- Electron beam field is defined by 50% isodose and the 90% is 3–5mm inside the field. The planning target volume (PTV) needs to be enclosed within 90% isodose which needs a 5mm larger electron applicator than defined by PTV.
- At higher energies, isodoses close to the surface bow inwards which necessitates 1cm larger applicator diameter than the defined PTV to ensure homogenous dose to the tumour.
- Surface dose increases with electron energy, such that there is a need for bolus for lower energies.
- Bolus is also used to bring up high dose to surface to avoid radiation to underlying critical structures.
- Stand-off effect: fill the area with bolus/calculate correction.

Normal tissue shielding
- Lower eyelid and canthi tumours need corneal shielding.
- Lip tumours need buccal shields.
- Shields used with electrons should be coated with wax to absorb scattered radiation.
- When treated with electrons, tumours in the pinna and nasal regions need wax coated lead plugs in the external auditory canal and nose respectively to minimize normal tissue damage.

Table 10.5.1 Common radiotherapy fractionations

Indication	Dose fractionation
Basal cell carcinoma	
Lesion <3cm	36Gy in 8 fractions/3 fractions per week
	30–32Gy in 4 fractions/1–2 fractions per week
	18Gy single fraction
Lesion 3–5cm or nose/pinna/poorly vascular area	45Gy in 9 fractions/3 fractions per week
Lesion >5cm	50–55Gy in 15–20 fractions/3–4 weeks
	60Gy in 30 fractions/6 weeks
Squamous cell carcinoma	
Lesion <5cm	45Gy in 9 fractions on alternate days over 3 weeks
	45Gy in 10 fractions over 2–3 weeks
	55Gy in 20 fractions over 4 weeks
Lesion >5cm	55Gy in 20 fractions over 4 weeks
	60Gy in 30 fractions
Brachytherapy (HDR)	45Gy in 10 fractions
Postoperative nodal radiotherapy	50–60Gy in 25–30 fractions (boost up to a total of 66Gy in 33 fractions in the head and neck region if high-risk features)
Palliative RT	20Gy in 5 fractions
	8Gy single

Recurrence

Risk factors for recurrence include tumours >2cm, tumours occurring in high-risk sites ('mask area' of face, pre-auricular area, genitalia, hands, and feet), poorly defined borders, aggressive histologies (morphoeic, fibrosing, sclerosing, infiltrative), and presence of perineural spread. Recurrent tumours, those occurring in sites of previous RT and tumours occurring in the context of immune-suppression are also considered high risk.

Two-thirds of recurrences occur within two years of primary treatment and 20% occur in two to five years. Recurrences after non-surgical treatment are generally treated with surgical resection followed by plastic surgical repair. Recurrence after surgical treatment can be treated with surgery or RT.

The rate of recurrence depends on the mode of primary treatment. MMS has the lowest recurrence rate (1%). The reported recurrence rates with other treatments are: standard excision 10%, curettage and dessication 7.7%, RT 8.7%, and cryotherapy 7.5%.

Prognosis

Overall ten-year control rate is >90%. A number of factors influence prognosis. The important prognostic factors are size, depth of invasion, histological subtype (morphoeic, infiltrative, and basosquamous have higher recurrence rates), completeness of excision (incomplete excisions have a 30% recurrence rate), site of disease (lesions around nose, eyes, and ears have higher recurrence rates), and presence of perineural spread.

Treatment modalities in BCC

Surgical excision
- WE
- MMS

Surgical destruction
- Curettage and desiccation
- Cryosurgery
- Carbon dioxide laser

Non-surgical destruction
- Topical immunotherapy with imiquimod
- PDT
- RT

Treatment of choice in BCC

Surgery and RT are effective treatments for small and less invasive tumours. Large and deeply invasive lesions are treated with surgery with or without postoperative RT.

RT favoured in:
- Mid-face, nasal, inner canthus, lower eye lid, lip commissures (better function)
- Multiple superficial lesions difficult to excise (better cosmesis)
- Patients >70 years (long-term toxicity less of an issue)
- Patients who wish to avoid surgery.
- Patients prone to keloid formation.

Surgery is the choice in:
- Readily excisable lesions in those <70 years
- Lesions in hair-bearing areas or overlying lacrimal gland
- Recurrence after RT
- Multifocal disease especially with dysplastic skin
- Upper eye lid tumours (better function)
- Dorsum of the hand (better function)
- Below knee and other sites of poor vascularity (problem with healing and function)
- Invasion to bones and joints. (Cartilage invasion is not an absolute contraindication to RT. RT is, however, avoided in large pinna lesions with extensive, inflamed, or painful cartilage invasion.)
- Where RT is contraindicated, e.g. basal naevus syndrome, xeroderma

Further reading

Clark C, Furniss M, Mackay-Wiggan M. Basal cell carcinoma: an evidence-based treatment update. *Br J Dermatol* 2014; 15:197–216.

Conforti C, Corneli P, Harwood C, Zalaudek I. Evolving role of systemic therapies in non-melanoma skin cancer. *Clin Oncol (R Coll Radiol)* 2019; 31(11):759–68.

Veness MJ, Delishaj D, Barnes EA, Bezugly A, Rembielak A. Current role of radiotherapy in non-melanoma skin cancer. *Clin Oncol (R Coll Radiol)* 2019; 31(11):749–58.

Internet resources

British Association of Dermatologists: http://www.bad.org.uk
National Comprehensive Cancer Network: http://www.nccn.org
Skin Cancer Foundation: http://www.skincancer.org

10.6 Squamous cell carcinoma

Introduction

SCC is the second most common skin cancer constituting 20% of skin malignancies. Risk factors include exposure to ionizing or UV radiation, immunosuppression, scars, chronic wounds, smoking, and arsenic exposure. Congenital conditions such as oculocutaneous albinism and xeroderma pigmentosum are also associated with increased risk of SCC. It is common in sun-exposed areas and hence sunscreen is protective.

Pathology

In situ SCC (Bowen's disease) is limited to the epidermis and presents as a flat scaling pink lesion with irregular borders. There is no risk of metastasis, although progression to invasive SCC occurs in 3–11% of cases.

In situ SCC of the glans penis (erythroplasia of Queyrat) has 20% risk of metastasis and 30% can progress to invasive disease.

Invasive SCC is composed of a collection of atypical keratocytes which invade the dermis and deeper structures. Other histological variants are:

- Adenoid SCC: can metastasize in 3–19% and is associated with rapid local growth.
- Adenosquamous SCC: shows squamous appearance superficially and glandular appearance deeply. These are aggressive tumours.
- Spindle cell SCC: appears as ulcerated nodules or exophytic tumours and may be difficult to distinguish from sarcoma histologically. These tumours are aggressive with a tendency to perineural invasion and metastasis (25%).
- Verrucous SCC: appears like a large wart. These are slow growing, locally invasive, and do not metastasize.
- Keratoacanthoma: appears as a rapidly growing nodule with a central keratin plug. True lesions can undergo spontaneous regression but most are now viewed as SCC.

Clinical presentation

Typical presentation is a raised pink papule or plaque with erosion or ulceration. In advanced cases SCC present as large ulcerated masses with bleeding. Metastasis is primarily to the regional nodes (2–6%). The head and neck region is the commonest site in men whereas the upper limb followed by head and neck are the commonest sites in females. Only 8% of SCC arise on the trunk.

Examination should include the whole skin and regional lymph nodes.

Diagnosis

Tissue biopsy is essential for diagnosis. If there is suspicion of involvement of underlying structures (such as soft tissue or bone) CT or magnetic resonance imaging (MRI) can help determine tumour extent. Ultrasound or CT scan help to detect regional lymph nodes. Fine needle aspiration of the enlarged lymph node under radiological guidance is advised. Open surgical biopsy should be avoided. The role of sentinel node biopsy is evolving.

Treatment

Three factors that influence treatment of SCC are: the need for removal of tumour locally, the possibility of 'in-transit' metastasis, and regional nodal metastasis. Treatment options include:

- Surgical excision
- RT—used a primary treatment and adjuvantly after surgery
- MMS

Ablative techniques such as cryotherapy and curettage and electrodessication are generally not recommended for invasive SCC as these do not allow histological confirmation of adequate excision margins.

Surgery

Surgery is aimed at complete removal of the tumour and of any metastasis. Low-risk tumours of <2cm are excised with a minimal margin of 4mm whereas tumours of >2cm size, high-risk tumours (grade 2–4, in high-risk locations such as ear, lip, scalp, eyelids, and nose), and those extending into subcutaneous tissue need a minimum margin of 6–10mm. Depth of excision should be through normal underlying fat. The accepted minimal microscopic margin is >1mm.

Mohs micrographic surgery

MMS is indicated in high-risk tumours and recurrences. MMS allows a high cure rate with minimal tissue destruction. High-risk SCC include lesions of >2cm, depth of invasion >4mm, and Clark level IV or V, tumour involvement of muscle, nerve, or bone, scar carcinomas, high-grade (3–4) tumours, and tumours on ear and lip.

Tumours involving periocular and periauricular regions, recurrent tumours, tumours with poorly defined margins, and recurrences after RT are best treated with MMS.

Management of lymph nodes

The treatment of metastatic lymph nodes is primary surgery. Elective lymph node dissection is not routinely advised. There is some evidence that it may have a role in tumours of >8mm in depth. Patients with recurrent thick (>4mm) lesions in the vicinity of the parotid (temple, forehead, and preauricular area) are also considered for elective nodal treatment.

Radiotherapy

Principles of primary RT and treatment guidelines are the same as those for BCC (see section 10.5, 'Basal cell carcinoma', p. 296). Five-year control rate with RT is comparable with surgery with >93% for T1 lesions, 65–85% with T2, and 50–60% with T3–4 lesions. RT is indicated after incomplete excision when further surgery is not contemplated, as incomplete excision leads to 50% local recurrence.

After complete surgical excision postoperative RT to the primary tumour site is considered for patients with high-risk disease. High-risk disease includes: tumour invasion beyond subcutaneous tissue, recurrent disease, margin <5mm, perineural invasion (major or minor nerve), lymphovascular invasion, in-transit metastases, and nodal metastasis. Indications for postoperative nodal RT after primary surgical management of metastatic lymph nodes are:

- 3cm node
- Two positive nodes in neck and three nodes in axilla and groin
- Extranodal tumour extension
- Close or positive margin
- Skin involvement
- Major nerve involvement
- Parotid node metastases
- After salvage surgery for recurrent nodal metastases

The role of postoperative chemoradiotherapy for high-risk SCC is being evaluated. Palliative RT is used in metastatic disease to obtain symptom relief.

Systemic therapy

Distant metastases from cutaneous SCC are rare (3.7%). In patients with distant metastasis from SCC, cisplatin-based chemotherapy is the most effective. A commonly used combination is cisplatin with adriamycin, which has an overall response rate of >80% with complete response rate of 30%. However, responses are short-lived and survival is generally <2 years. Responses to the EGFR inhibitors gefitinib, erlotinib, and cextuximab have been reported in phase 2 trials.

Immunotherapy is being evaluated in SCC. A phase 1/2 study of cemiplimab, an anti-PDL-1 antibody, for patients with locally advanced and metastatic SCC, reported a 50% overall response rate including a 7% complete response rate. Cemiplimab is an approved treatment for patients with SCC when surgery and RT are not appropriate.

Recurrence

Most recurrences occur within two to three years. Treatment is individualized based on the extent of recurrence and previous treatment.

The reported recurrence rate with various treatments are as follows: MMS 3.1%, surgical excision 8.1%, and RT 10%.

Prognostic factors

- Grade of differentiation: grade 3–4 lesions are twice as likely to recur and three times more likely to metastasize than grade 1–2 lesions.
- Histological type: spindle cell carcinoma and adenosquamous carcinoma and desmoplastic subtypes have a high risk of recurrence and metastasis.
- Location of tumour: scalp, lips, pinna, nose, and genital lesions have a high risk of metastasis.
- Tumour size: risk of recurrence and metastasis increases with size of the tumour. Risk of recurrence is twice (15% vs. 7%) and risk of metastasis is three-fold (30% vs. 9%) in tumours >2cm compared with tumours of <2cm.
- Depth of invasion: tumours with depth <2mm seldom metastasize whereas those with >4mm have a high risk of recurrence and metastasis.
- Perineural invasion: occurs in 2.5% of tumours and its presence indicates a high risk of local recurrence (up to 50%) and distant metastasis (up to 35%).
- After lymphadenectomy, prognosis depends on number of positive nodes and presence of extranodal spread.
- Recurrence: local recurrence increases rate for further recurrence (25%) and lymph node metastasis (30%).
- Tumours in immunosuppressed patients and those arising from scars have a poor prognosis.

Outcome

Local control rate for SCC is 10–15% lower than for a similarly sized BCC.

Bowen's disease (in situ SCC)

Bowen's disease presents as a slow-growing erythematous plaque. Surgery, topical treatment, and RT are the options for treatment. RT dose is 40–50Gy in 10–20 fractions using 100–150KV superficial X-rays and results in 95–100% local control.

Keratoacanthoma

Keratoacanthoma presents as a rapidly enlarging lesion with a central keratin plug. Histologically, it is difficult to distinguish from SCC. In up to 20% of patients spontaneous regression may occur over six to 12 weeks. Treatment options include early excision and RT (similar to SCC).

Further reading

Conforti C, Corneli P, Harwood C, Zalaudek I. Evolving role of systemic therapies in non-melanoma skin cancer. *Clin Oncol (R Coll Radiol)* 2019; 31(11):759–68.
Veness MJ, Delishaj D, Barnes EA, Bezugly A, Rembielak A. Current role of radiotherapy in non-melanoma skin cancer. *Clin Oncol (R Coll Radiol)* 2019; 31(11):749–58.

Internet resources

British Association of Dermatologists: http://www.bad.org.uk
National Comprehensive Cancer Network: http://www.nccn.org
Skin Cancer Foundation: http://www.skincancer.org

10.7 Merkel cell carcinoma

Introduction

Merkel cell carcinoma (MCC) is a rare aggressive neuro-endocrine tumour of the skin. The estimated incidence is 0.44 per 100,000 people. The incidence is lower in the black population. The average age at presentation is 69 years. Males are more commonly affected (2:1 ratio). MCC commonly affects sun-exposed areas of the body with 50% occurring in the head and neck region (especially the periorbital region), 35% occurring in the extremities, and the rest in the trunk.

Aetiology

The exact aetiology is largely unclear but a number of risk factors have been reported. UV exposure increases the risk of MCC which tends to occur on sun-exposed sites. A higher incidence is also seen in patients receiving UVA treatment for psoriasis. Immunosuppression is a reported with risk factor with a higher incidence seen in patients with HIV infection, haematological malignancies, and post-transplant. With renal transplantation the estimated risk is 24 times that of the normal population and transplant-associated MCC tends to be aggressive. The relative risk of developing MCC in individuals with acquired immunodeficiency is approximately 13. Recently the MCC polyomavirus (MCPyV) has been found to be associated with MCC. MCPyV DNA has been detected in up to 80% of tumours and has been suggested to be involved in the pathogenesis of MCC.

Pathology

Histologically these tumours consist of small blue cells which are usually ovoid with scanty cytoplasm and fine granular nuclei. There will be numerous mitoses and apoptotic figures. The triad of vesicular nuclei with small nucleoli, abundant mitoses, and apoptosis is highly suggestive of MCC. There are three histological patterns: intermediate type which is the most common, followed by small cell, and the classic trabecular type.

MCC express neuroendocrine markers (NSE, synaptophysin, and chromogranin) and cytokeratin markers (cytokeratin 20 and CAM 5.2). CK-20 staining showing a 'perinuclear dot' pattern of cytokeratin is pathognomonic for MCC. S100 and LCA are negative; 95% of MCC express CD117. TTF-1 is negative in MCC and positive in small cell lung cancer (SCLC).

The minimal immunohistochemical panel for the primary tumour should preferably include CK-20 and TTF-1 whereas that for node biopsy should include CK-20 and pancytokeratins (AE 1/AE3).

Differential diagnosis includes poorly differentiated small cell neoplasms such as small cell carcinoma, lymphoma, and melanoma.

Clinical features

MCC present as red or violaceous nodules with a shiny surface, often with overlying telangiectasia. Spread through dermal lymphatics can result in the development of satellite lesions. The majority (73%) of patients present with localized disease, up to a third present with regional nodal metastases, and up to 5% present with distant metastases. MCC has a high rate of distant spread and 50% of patients go on to develop distant metastases. Liver, lung, bone, and brain are the common sites of distant metastasis.

Diagnosis and staging

Initial evaluation includes clinical examination of the whole skin surface and regional nodes. Imaging includes CT scan of the relevant nodal region as well as chest and liver, especially in node positive patients. Blood tests include full blood count and biochemistry.

Fluorodeoxyglucose-positron emission tomography (FEG-PET) although not used routinely, may be useful in staging and has both a high sensitivity (90%) and specificity (98%).

European (Lebbe et al. 2015) and National Comprehensive Cancer Network (NCCN) guidelines recommend SLNB to assess regional nodes for occult micrometastatic disease in clinically node negative disease. However, false negative rates of 13–30% have been reported and are particularly high in the head and neck region.

Staging is shown in Table 10.3.1.

- Stage I: tumours of <2cm with no nodal involvement
- Stage II: tumour or >2cm with no nodal involvement or tumours with deep tissue involvement without nodes
- Stage III: tumours with nodal or in-transit metastasis
- Stage IV: metastatic disease beyond nodal basin
  Note: 70–80% patients present with stage I–II, 10–30% with stage III, and 1–4% with stage IV disease.

Treatment

Stage I–III disease

Patients with loco-regional stage I–III disease are treated with WE of the primary tumour with adjuvant RT recommended to the primary site and if there is a high risk of loco-regional recurrence, additionally to the nodal basin.

Due to the risk of dermal lymphatic spread, a surgical margin of 1–2cm is used for WE of the primary tumour (some recommend 3cm). An excision margin of <2cm leads to 29% risk of local recurrence. MMS is also an option for the treatment of the primary tumour.

Clinically node negative disease (stage I/II) should be confirmed pathologically with SLNB or routine lymph node dissection. SNB should be carried out at the same time as that of WE to avoid disturbance of the lymphatic drainage. Approximately 30% patients have nodal disease on SLNB. If SLNB shows microscopic nodal involvement (stage IIIA disease) and in clinically node positive (stage IIIB) disease, lymph node dissection should be performed.

The role of adjuvant RT for stage I–III disease is unclear and although a number of studies have shown an improvement in local control with adjuvant RT, an OS benefit has not been clearly demonstrated. Most recommendations advocate postoperative RT to the primary site alone in most stage I and II disease with the exception of small (<1cm) tumours excised with wide margins and no adverse features (such as high lymphatic and vascular invasion (LVI) or immunosuppression) where close follow-up without RT is an option.

RT to the nodal bed may be avoided in immunohisto-chemically proven-negative SLNB; however, adjuvant RT is recommended if there is any risk of false negative SLNB such as after previous surgery, for primary tumours in the head and neck region, and failure to perform immunohistochemistry on SLNB.

In stage III disease adjuvant RT to the primary and nodal sites is recommended following lymph node dissection, particularly where there is multiple node involvement and/or presence of more than focal extracapsular extension.

In view of the risk of rapid repopulation after surgery, radiation should be started as soon as the wound is healed.

Based on retrospective reviews, adjuvant RT reduces local failure from 39–26% and the regional failure from 46–22%.

Primary RT is an option in those with comorbidities precluding surgery or where better cosmesis can be achieved with RT. Local control rates of 73–82% for stage I–III have been reported at two years.

RT dose to the primary tumour area ranges from 45 to 60Gy using 1.8–2Gy per fraction depending on the extent of the resection margin and residual disease. Nodal bed RT is given to a dose of 45–60Gy depending on the extent of the nodal involvement.

MCC is a radioresponsive tumour. RT doses range from 60–66Gy for macroscopic disease (primary RT, positive margins post surgery), 50–60Gy for microscopic disease (microscopic margin involvement, extracapsular nodal spread), to 45–50Gy in the adjuvant setting where there is no residual disease.

There is no proven role for adjuvant chemotherapy in stage I–III disease. In a small study, concomitant chemoradiotherapy and adjuvant chemotherapy has resulted in a three-year OS of 76%. The chemotherapy regimen is similar to that used for SCLC.

Stage IV disease

Stage IV disease is associated with a median survival of nine months. The common sites of metastases are liver, bone, lung, brain, and skin. Chemotherapy regimens have been derived from those used for SCLC. Etoposide and platinum combinations are the most commonly used in MCC with response rates of 60%. The combination of cyclophosphamide, doxorubicin (or epirubicin), and vincristine has an overall response of 76% with 35% complete response in non-randomized studies.

RT may be used to palliate symptoms such as pain, bleeding, and ulceration.

A number of newer agents are being studied in the management of MCC. These include anti-vascular endothelial growth factor receptor (anti-VEGFR) inhibitors (e.g. UKMCC1 study of pazopanib), immunotherapeutic agent such as ipilimumab and anti-PD-1 and anti-PD-L1 inhibitors (e.g. pembrolizumab and avelumab), and tyrosine kinase inhibitors (e.g. cabozantinib).

Follow-up

Most recurrences (90%) in MCC occur within two years of diagnosis and the median time of recurrence is about eight months. In one study most recurrences occurred at nodal (40%) or distant (39%) sites, but local (10%) and in-transit (11%) recurrences were also seen. This necessitates frequent follow-up to detect recurrences early. NCCN recommends follow-up every three to six months for the first two years, then every six to 12 months thereafter. The follow-up programme should include history and physical examination with a complete skin and regional lymph node examination.

Prognosis

Stage is the most important prognostic factor. The five-year DFS of stage I disease is 81%, stage II 67%, stage III 52%, and stage IV 11%. The median survival with node-negative disease is 40 months whereas that of node positive disease is 11 months. The median survival of patients with distant metastases is nine months.

Other poor prognostic factors include tumour >2cm, age >60 years, male gender, and lack of adjuvant RT.

Further reading

Lebbe C, Becker JC, Grob JJ, et al. Diagnosis and treatment of Merkel cell carcinoma. European consensus-based interdisciplinary guideline. *Eur J Cancer* 2015; 51(16):2396–403.

Prewett SL, Ajithkumar T. Merkel cell carcinoma: current management and controversies. *Clin Oncol* 2015; 27:436–44.

Steven N, Lawton P, Poulsen M. Merkel cell carcinoma—current controversies and future directions. *Clin Oncol (R Coll Radiol)* 2019; 31(11):789–96.

Internet resources

Merkel cell carcinoma information: http://www.merkelcell.org/

National Comprehensive Cancer Network (NCCN): http://www.nccn.org

10.8 Kaposi's sarcoma

Introduction

Kaposi's sarcoma (KS) is a low-grade multifocal vascular tumour associated with human herpesvirus 8 (HHV8)/Kaposi's sarcoma herpes virus (KSHV) infection.

KS lesions of all epidemiological forms are similarly comprised of HHV8-positive (LNA-1 immunoreactive) spindle-shaped tumour cells, vessels, and chronic inflammatory cells. Lesions evolve from an early patch, to plaque, and later tumour nodules.

KS affects patients of all ages, with a predilection for men. Epidemiological forms include:

- Classic KS affecting mainly elderly men of Mediterranean or Jewish origin. This has an indolent course with a median survival of years to decades.
- African KS endemic in central Africa, affecting both young patients and adults and has an aggressive course.

- AIDS-associated KS arising in HIV-infected persons (considered an AIDS-defining illness). AIDS-KS without highly active antiretroviral therapy (HAART) is 20,000 times more common than in the general population. In the post-HAART era (after 1996) this has diminished markedly to 3,500 times compared to the general population. It has an aggressive course.
- Iatrogenic KS associated with immunosuppression from drugs or following solid organ transplantation.

Clinical variants

KS regression can occur spontaneously (rare), following appropriate therapy, or after removal of immunosuppressive therapy.

KS flare (exacerbation) can occur with immune reconstitution inflammatory syndrome (IRIS) following HAART, after corticosteroids, and with rituximab therapy.

Clinical approach

- Patients may be asymptomatic, as the skin lesions are usually painless and non-pruritic. Skin lesions are multifocal, asymmetrically distributed, vary in size, and colour (pink, red, purple, brown to blue), and may be papular, plaque-like, bullous-like, indurated (woody) with a verrucous appearance, or fungating with ulceration and secondary infection.
- Intraoral KS lesions may cause pain, bleeding, ulceration, and affect mastication, speech, and swallowing.
- Conjunctival KS can cause red eyes, discharge, or visual disturbance.
- Gastrointestinal (GI) tract KS can cause weight loss, abdominal pain, nausea and vomiting, ileus, upper or lower GI bleeding, malabsorption, intestinal obstruction, or diarrhoea.
- Pulmonary KS can present with shortness of breath, fever, cough, haemoptysis, chest pain, and effusions.
- There may be associated psychosocial stress due to HIV stigma or cosmetic concerns.

Staging

Unique staging systems available for classic (stage I: maculonodular stage, stage II: infiltative stage, stage III: florid stage, and stage IV: disseminated stage) and AIDS-associated KS (AIDS Clinical Trials Group staging classification divided patients into good risk and poor risk based on extent of tumour, immune status, and severity of systemic illness) are used mainly for patients on trials.

Specific investigations

- HIV test (and if positive a CD4 cell count and HIV viral load).
- Chest imaging may show nodular, interstitial and/or alveolar infiltrates, pleural effusion, hilar and/or mediastinal lymphadenopathy, and only rarely a solitary nodule. Concomitant pulmonary infection must be excluded.
- Bronchoscopy can be used to identify pulmonary KS lesions.
- Faecal occult blood test (FOBT) is useful to screen for GI tract KS disease.
- GI endoscopy in symptomatic individuals may be helpful.
- CT scan, MRI, and PET may be helpful for evaluating deep nodal and visceral KS.
- Bone lesions which frequently go undetected on plain X-ray or bone scans are better detected by CT scan and MRI.
- Biopsy of a suspected KS lesion is encouraged to confirm the diagnosis. Laryngeal and pulmonary KS lesions may bleed significantly.
- Evaluate patients requiring systemic chemotherapy for hepatic, renal, and bone marrow function.

Treatment

- Treatment is aimed at symptom palliation, preventing progression, cosmetic improvement, and abatement of oedema, organ compromise, and psychological stress.
- Local therapy to manage bulky lesions and for cosmetic reasons.
- Surgical excision should be restricted for cosmetically disturbing lesions, to alleviate discomfort, or control local tumour growth such as for conjunctival KS obscuring vision.
- Indications for systemic chemotherapy include widespread skin involvement (>25 lesions), extensive oral KS, marked symptomatic oedema, rapidly progressive disease, symptomatic visceral KS, and KS flare.

Local therapy

- External beam radiation (8–20Gy)
- Laser therapy
- Cryotherapy
- PDT
- Topical panretinin gel (alitretinoin 0.1%)
- Intralesional vinblastine (0.2–0.3mg/ml solution with a volume of 0.1ml per 0.5cm^2 of lesion)

Systemic therapy

Liposomal anthracyclines including:
- Pegylated liposomal doxorubicin 20mg/m^2 every three weeks (response rate about 50%).
- Liposomal daunorubicin 40 mg/m^2 every two weeks.
- Taxanes including:
  - Paclitaxel 100 mg/m^2 every two to three weeks. Reduced steroid premedication should be used and in HIV-infected persons toxicity related to possible antiretroviral drug interaction must be monitored.
  - AIDS-associated KS patients should receive HAART. KS flare alone following HAART should not be considered as treatment failure or warrant change in antiretroviral regimen.

Alternative therapy

- Vinorelbine may be effective for AIDS-related KS in patients who have failed other therapies.
- Interferon-alpha, for patients with a robust immune system, has limited use due to toxicity.
- Thalidomide, COL-3, antiherpes therapy, and imatinib have shown therapeutic efficacy.
- For iatrogenic KS consider adjusting immunosuppressive therapy and use of sirolimus (rapamycin) in post-transplant KS.
- Current trials in advanced/recurrent KS are evaluating biological agents such as selumetinib, pomalidomide, bevacizumab, and pembrolizumab.

Further reading

Curtiss P, Strazzulla LC, Friedman-Kien AE. An update on Kaposi's sarcoma: epidemiology, pathogenesis and treatment. *Dermatol Ther (Heidelb)* 2016; 6(4):465–70.

10.9 Malignant skin adnexal tumours

Introduction
Malignant skin adnexal tumours represent 0.2% of skin cancers. These tumours generally exhibit a high risk of local recurrence and may be aggressive. The 2018 WHO classification is in the further reading list (p. 306).

Clinical presentation
Many of the malignant skin appendage tumours arise from their benign counterpart. These tumours present as longstanding single or multiple lesions which start to grow rapidly. Multiple tumours can often be due to inherited (autosomal dominant) conditions and are usually associated with various cutaneous and non-cutaneous pathologies. The anatomical distribution of various subtypes depends on the normal distribution of the adnexal structures from which the tumours arise. Specific features of commonly occurring skin appendage tumours are as follows:

- Extramammary Paget's disease: is an in situ adenocarcinoma arising in the anogenital region. It usually present as ill-defined erythema. Progression to invasive cancer is uncommon.
- Porocarcinoma: is the malignant counterpart of poroadenoma occurring in the elderly. It usually presents as a partially ulcerated, verrucous plaque, or polypoid tumour on the lower extremities, head and neck, and trunk. Up to 20% develop local recurrence and regional recurrence can also occur. Surgery is the treatment of choice. Even though metastatic porocarcinoma is thought to be resistant to RT and chemotherapy, there are reports of response to paclitaxel, cetuximab, and RT.
- Hidranocarcinoma: occurs as a solitary ulcerated nodule on the head and neck, trunk, or extremities of middle-aged or elderly people. Local recurrence is common even after optimal local treatment.
- Spiradenocarcinoma: presents in the middle-aged and elderly as a single large nodule on the extremities, trunk, and abdomen. Since it arises usually from a benign counterpart, patients often give a history of a long-standing nodule with recent increase in size and other associated symptoms. Loco-regional recurrences are common and 20% develop distant metastasis.
- Cylindrocarcinoma: occurs in the middle-aged and elderly and is common in women. These tumours present as a rapidly growing ulcerated or bleeding nodule on the scalp. Tumour spread is by local destructive invasion and nodal and distant metastases.
- Apocrine carcinoma: an aggressive tumour presenting as solitary or multiple lesions in the axilla or anogenital area. Nodal metastasis and visceral metastasis can occur.
- Malignant mixed tumour: often arises in the trunk or extremities of middle-aged women. It often presents as a solitary non-ulcerated or subcutaneous lesion. Lymph node metastasis is common.
- Trichilemmal carcinoma: usually present in older individuals as a solitary, exophytic, or polypoidal nodule over sun-exposed areas. It usually presents as a long-standing nodule with a rapid growth phase. It has a

non-aggressive course with local damage only and is therefore treated with WE alone.
- Pilomatrical carcinoma: usually arise on the skin in the head and neck region (60%) in the elderly. These tumours are locally aggressive (>60% recurrence with surgery alone) but can also metastasize to lungs, bones, and lymph nodes. Lower limb tumours have more aggressive behaviour. WE is the treatment of choice. The role of RT and chemotherapy is not known.
- Mucinous carcinoma: is a rare low-grade tumour presenting as a solitary slow-growing lesion in elderly men in the head and neck region. Metastases are rare.
- Adenocarcinoma: occurs usually in middle-aged adults in acral locations and have a high risk of local recurrence (50%). Adenocarcinoma also has a tendency for distant metastasis (up to 40%) which occurs mainly in the lungs (>70%). These tumours present as a firm tan-grey to white-pink rubbery nodule usually over the volar surface of the space between the nail bed and the distal interphalangeal joint.
- Microcystic adnexal carcinoma: is a locally destructive carcinoma often present as a sclerotic or indurated plaque with an intact dermis. The usual sites of involvement are mid face and lip. Wide local excision and Mohs surgery are the treatments of choice. Surgery is associated with a local recurrence rate of 50–60%. These are thought to be radioresistant tumours.

Principle of management
Non-invasive neoplasms (extramammary Paget's disease)
Wide local exision and MMS are the recommended treatments, which achieve a five-year DFS of >90%. Extensive inoperable neoplasms are treated with primary RT.

Invasive neoplasms
Complete surgical excision is the treatment of choice. MMS is being increasingly used. Patients with clinically enlarged nodes need regional lymphadenectomy whilst the role of elective lymphadenectomy is controversial. Role of sentinel node biopsy is evolving. The role of elective lymph node dissection is still controversial; some authors recommend it for patients with undifferentiated and recurrent tumours.

Adjuvant RT is individualized based on the surgical margins, type of tumour, and risk of loco-regional recurrence. It is generally recommended for tumour of >5cm, deep infiltration, close (<1mm) or positive margin, high-grade tumours, perineural infiltration, dermal lymphatic invasion, for positive nodes, and extranodal invasion. Patients with inoperable locally advanced tumours or who are medically unfit for surgery may be treated with primary RT delivering >55Gy in 1.8–2Gy per fraction. RT management is the same as for SCC of the skin (see section 10.6, 'Squamous cell carcinoma'). RT is also useful in a palliative setting.

A small number of patients present with metastatic disease and treatment is based on the fitness of patient, the site of disease, and symptoms. There is no accepted chemotherapy regimen. Cisplatin/fluorouracil (5-FU) based chemotherapy regimens are commonly used.

Other reported treatments include: methotrexate; bleomycin; a combination of doxorubicin, cyclophosphamide, vincristine, and bleomycin; and paclitaxel and cetuximab.

Prognosis and survival

Prognostic factors include size, histological type, and presence of metastasis. Reported ten-year DFS is 56% in node-negative patients and 9% in node-positive patients.

Further reading

Craig PJ. An Overview of Uncommon Cutaneous Malignancies, Including Skin Appendageal (Adnexal) Tumours and Sarcomas. *Clin Oncol (R Coll Radiol)* 2019; 31(11):769–78.

Elder DE, Massi D, Scolyer R, Willemze R. *WHO classification of skin tumours.* 4th edn. Vol II. No. 11. Lyon: IARC, 2018.

Perna AG, Smith MJ, Krishnan B, et al. Primary cutaneous adnexal neoplasms and their metastatic look-alikes. *Pathol Case Rev* 2007; 12:61–9.

10.10 Skin cancer in organ transplant recipients

Introduction

Recipients of solid organ transplants require lifelong immunosuppression to prevent rejection of the graft. An unfortunate consequence of chronic immunosuppression is an increased incidence of malignancy, of which skin cancer is the commonest. Whilst BCC is the commonest skin cancer in the general population, there is a particularly high incidence of SCC in organ transplant recipients (OTRs). The risk of SCC in OTRs is increased 65 times to that of the general population, and the risk of BCC is increased 6.1–10-fold. MCC is also seen more commonly in OTRs who have up to 24 times the risk of immuno-competent individuals.

Pathogenesis

The increased incidence of skin cancers is thought to be a result of both impaired immune surveillance resulting from chronic immunosuppression with immunosuppressant drugs and a direct carcinogenic effect of these drugs. Both cyclosporine and azathioprine increase the sensitivity of keratinocytes to UV radiation promoting photocarcinogenesis. Oncogenic viruses (e.g. human papilloma virus (HPV) and Merkel cell polymomavirus) have also been suggested to provide a link between immunosuppression and development of skin malignancies.

Risk factors

As in the general population, previous UV exposure is an important risk factor for the development of skin cancers, with lesions occurring most frequently in sun-exposed sites. Other risk factors include fair skin, previous history of skin cancer, and older age at the time of transplant. The risk of skin cancers in OTRs increases with increasing time since transplant (and hence duration of immunosuppression) and increasing degree of immunosuppression. A higher incidence of skin cancers is reported in heart transplant recipients compared with renal transplant, and the lowest risk is seen following liver transplant. This has been attributed to the differences in average age at the time of transplant and the degree of immunosuppression required post transplantation.

The type of immunosuppressive agent also appears to be important in determining the likelihood of developing skin cancer. A higher incidence of SCC is seen in patients receiving cyclosporine or azathioprine compared with those receiving tacrolimus or mycophenolate mofetil. The mTOR inhibitors sirolimus and everolimus are associated with a reduced risk of SCC, although not of Merkel cell carcinoma.

Voriconazole, an anti-fungal which is used to treat invasive aspergillosis in OTRs is also associated with an increased risk of skin cancer.

Clinical features

Skin cancers in transplant recipients occur at a younger age and behave more aggressively than in immunocompetent individuals. SCCs have higher rates of local and regional recurrence, a higher risk of distant metastases (8%), and higher rates of mortality. MCCs also behave more aggressively with higher rates of progression and reduced OS. Skin cancers after organ transplant can be multiple necessitating repeated treatments and leading to greater morbidity.

Management

Prevention

Patient education regarding increased skin cancer risk, need for self-examination, and UV protection is imperative. Use of regular high factor (SPF 50) sunscreen has been shown to reduce the incidence of both SCC and BCC in transplant recipients receiving immunosuppression.

In patients who develop multiple SCCs (five to ten per year), or SCCs with other high-risk features in addition to immunosuppression, systemic retinoids can be considered as chemoprevention to reduce the incidence of further SCCs. If adverse effects develop (e.g. hyperlipidaemia) the dose should be reduced gradually as abrupt cessation can result in a rebound effect with the development of multiple aggressive SCCs.

Pre-cancerous lesions such as actinic keratosis should be managed aggressively with topical imiquinod, topical 5-FU or PDT.

Treatment

Non-melanoma skin cancers arising in OTRs should be managed aggressively according to the same principles as 'high-risk' lesions in immunocompetent individuals. MMS is the preferred surgical approach and adjuvant RT is indicated if other risk factors for recurrence are present (see Box 10.5.1, p. 298).

Revision of immunosuppression should be considered, particularly in the case of multiple lesions or where there is a high risk of metastasis. Reduction of immunosuppression may reduce the incidence of further skin cancers and result in regression of existing tumours. The degree to which immunosuppression is reduced is determined by both the risk of morbidity and mortality from skin cancer and potential risk to allograft function from rejection. The recommended thresholds at which a reduction in immunosuppression and the anticipated risk of graft compromise has been published by the Task Force of the International Transplant Skin Cancer Collaboration.

The mTOR inhibitors everolimus or sirolimus have both immunosuppressive and antiproliferative properties. Conversion to an mTOR inhibitor reduces the risk of further non melanoma skin cancers, but side effects may limit their use.

Chemotherapy using cisplatin-based regimens has been used in the management of metastatic disease in OTRs; however, the potential for drug interactions, negative impact on graft function, and increased toxicity must be taken into consideration. EGFR inhibitors such as cetuximab and panitumumab are other treatment options. Cemiplimab, a PD-1 inhibitor, is an effective agent for metastatic and locally advanced SCC, but has not been studied in transplant patients. In post-transplant patients with advanced BCC, vismodegib is effective.

Further reading

Collins L, Asfour L, Stephany M, Lear JT, Stasko T. Management of non-melanoma skin cancer in transplant recipients. *Clin Oncol (R Coll Radiol)* 2019; 31(11):779–88.

Zwald F, Brown M. Skin cancer in solid organ transplant recipients: advances in therapy and management: part I. Epidemiology of skin cancer in solid organ transplant recipients. *J Amer Acad Dermatol* 2011; 65(2):253–61.

Zwald F, Brown M. Skin cancer in solid organ transplant recipients: advances in therapy and management: part II. Management of skin cancer in solid organ transplant recipients. *J Amer Acad Dermatol* 2011; 65(2):263–79.

Chapter 11

Cancers of the musculoskeletal system

Chapter contents

11.1 Bone tumours overview

Introduction

Primary malignant tumours of bone are rare and comprise a large number of histological subtypes.

- The most common are osteosarcoma, Ewing's family of tumours, and chondrosarcoma. Each of these has further subgroups which will be discussed in detail under their subheadings.
- The remaining subgroups are exceptionally rare and include the presentation of spindle cell sarcoma of bone, e.g. malignant fibrous histiocytoma (MFH), within the bone as a primary lesion. MFH of bone is treated as other primary bone tumours.

Epidemiology

- Osteosarcoma peaks in adolescence with a second peak in the >65-year age group.
- Ewing's sarcoma peaks at age 10–15 years but can occur at all ages.

- Chondrosarcoma increases in incidence with age >40 years.

Incidence

- There are 650 cases of bone sarcomas per year in the USA.
- There are 12 per million cases of childhood osteosarcoma per year in the UK.
- There are 5 per million cases of childhood Ewing's sarcoma per year in the UK.
- There are <2 per million cases of chondrosarcoma rising to seven per million in those >70 years in the UK.

Aetiology and risk factors

Most primary bone tumours arise spontaneously without a predisposing risk factor. However, for each subgroup there are recognized risk factors.

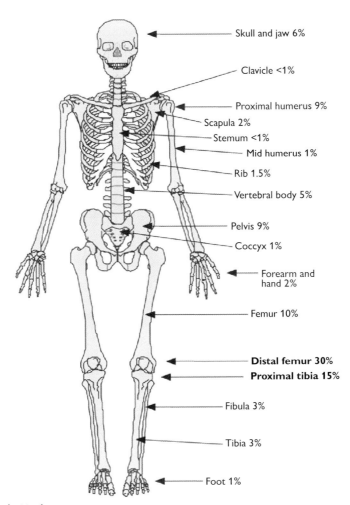

Skull and jaw 6%

Clavicle <1%

Proximal humerus 9%

Scapula 2%

Stemum <1%

Mid humerus 1%

Rib 1.5%

Vertebral body 5%

Pelvis 9%

Coccyx 1%

Forearm and hand 2%

Femur 10%

Distal femur 30%

Proximal tibia 15%

Fibula 3%

Tibia 3%

Foot 1%

Fig. 11.1.1 Sites of origin of osteosarcomas.

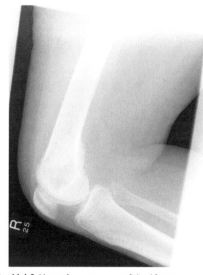

Fig. 11.1.2 X-ray of osteosarcoma of distal femur.

Osteosarcoma
- See Figures 11.1.1 and 11.1.2
- Prior radiotherapy (3% cases) with a time interval of 14 years (range 4–40 years)
- Chemotherapy with alkylating agents, especially if with anthracyclines and radiotherapy
- Paget's disease (1%)
- Chronic osteomyelitis (<1%)
- Genetic, e.g. Li–Fraumeni, hereditary retinoblastoma, Rothmund–Thomson syndrome

Ewing's sarcoma
- See Figure 11.1.3; also see Figures 11.3.1–11.3.3.
- Rarely after treatment for primary cancer in childhood

Chondrosarcoma
Increased risk in those with hereditary multiple exostosis or enchondromatosis syndromes (e.g. Maffucci syndrome). Presentation is at an earlier age in these groups (Figure 11.1.4).

Clinical features
There are some features which are common to many types of bone tumour:
- Localized bone pain usually presents for several months.

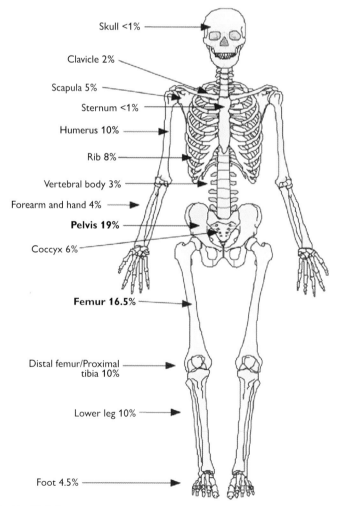

Skull <1%

Clavicle 2%

Scapula 5%

Sternum <1%

Humerus 10%

Rib 8%

Vertebral body 3%

Forearm and hand 4%

Pelvis 19%

Coccyx 6%

Femur 16.5%

Distal femur/Proximal tibia 10%

Lower leg 10%

Foot 4.5%

Fig. 11.1.3 Sites of origin of Ewing's sarcomas.

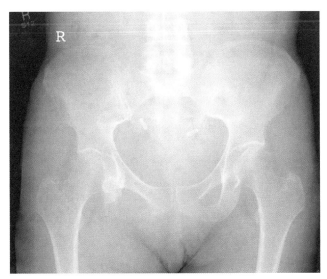

Fig. 11.1.4 X-ray of chrondrosarcoma eroding into pubis.

- Pain at night or at rest.
- Often a previous injury to the region has been noted and may result in delay in diagnosis.
- In advanced disease, systemic symptoms may be present. These include fever, weight loss, and lethargy. They occur more often in Ewing's sarcoma than any other bone sarcoma.

Diagnosis
- An X-ray of the affected area may be suggestive of a diagnosis but the majority of patients will require a diagnostic biopsy.
- Biopsy of localized disease should only be performed by a specialist sarcoma surgeon who will take into account possible future surgery and will minimize the risks of tumour spread to the skin or adjacent structures.
- Open incisional biopsy is usually performed but a core biopsy may be appropriate.
- Fine needle biopsies are not suitable for primary diagnosis but can be used to confirm metastatic disease.
- Biopsy is often performed under radiological guidance (fluoroscopy or ultrasound).
- Adequate drainage of the biopsy site is necessary as haematomas may also act to spread disease.
- The biopsy tract is often marked by clips to ensure it is removed at the time of definitive surgery.

Staging
Adequate staging includes:

- Optimal imaging of the primary site (magnetic resonance imaging (MRI)) and the entire bone to exclude intramedullary skip metastases.
- Computed tomography (CT) scan of the chest to exclude pulmonary metastases. For primitive neuroectodermal tumours (PNETs) arising in the lower half of the body, a CT of the pelvis and abdomen can be considered as there may be lymph node involvement.
- Bone scintigram to exclude bone metastases. If a CT-positron emission tomography (PET) scan is performed to exclude soft tissue metastases, a bone scintigram will not be required.
- Whole body MRI on short inversion time inversion recovery (STIR) sequence has been shown to be effective in detection of bone metastases which may not be visible with other forms of imaging.
- Bone marrow aspirate for the Ewing's family of tumours.
- Blood tests including lactate dehydrogenase (LDH) and alkaline phosphatase level (ALP) which have prognostic value in Ewing's tumours and osteosarcomas respectively.
- Staging is according to the American Joint Committee on Cancer (AJCC) staging for bone tumours.

Internet resources
Bone Cancer Research Trust: https://www.bcrt.org.uk
Sarcoma UK: http://www.sarcoma-uk.org

11.2 Osteosarcoma

Non-metastatic osteosarcoma

Introduction
Osteosarcoma is the most common type of bone cancer accounting for up to 35% of all primary bone tumours.

Incidence and age
There is a wide variation in incidence according to age.
- It has a peak incidence in those aged 15–19 at a rate of 1 per 100,000.
- Overall incidence is 0.2 per 100,000.
- Smaller second peak incidence occurs over the age of 65 associated with Paget's disease.

Presentation
Pain is the most common presenting symptom (especially at night or at rest). Pain is often associated with a recent injury. Systemic symptoms are rare, unlike Ewing's sarcoma.

Risk factors
- Previous radiotherapy. Most common secondary malignancy following treatment for childhood cancer.
- Chemotherapy, especially alkylating agents and anthracyclines. Increased risk is dose dependent. Chemotherapy plus radiotherapy.
- Paget's disease, although occurs in 1% patients with Paget's disease.
- Hereditary conditions (see below).

Genetics and biology
Several genetic syndromes predispose patients to the development of osteosarcoma. The most well-known are:
- Hereditary retinoblastoma due to a germline mutation in the retinoblastoma (Rb) gene on the long arm of chromosome 13. The relative risk of osteosarcoma is 500 times for limb osteosarcomas and 2,000 for skull osteosarcomas following irradiation for retinoblastoma.
- Li–Fraumeni syndrome in which there is a germline mutation in the p53 tumour suppressor gene. These patients have a relative risk of 15 for osteosarcoma at all sites.
- Several rarer syndromes which involve deficiencies of DNA repair mechanisms are also associated with a moderately increased risk of osteosarcoma, including Werner, Bloom, and Rothmund–Thomson syndromes.
- Unlike Ewing's sarcomas and many soft tissue sarcomas (STS) there are no characteristic chromosomal translocations, although loss of heterozygosity in the region of both Rb and p53 have been described.
- A significant number of osteosarcomas express insulin growth factor 1 receptor (IGF1-R) which is being explored as a therapeutic target.

Subtypes of osteosarcoma
Osteosarcomas are characterized as primary bone tumours in which there is a significant component of osteoid bone in addition to a malignant stromal environment. Several subtypes exist defined by the presence, absence, or relative amount of other components. Most (90%) are high-grade intramedullary tumours which fall into the following categories:
- Osteoblastic osteosarcoma (50%)
- Fibroblastic osteosarcoma (25%)
- Chondroblastic osteosarcoma (25%)

Further variants exist with distinct histologies:
- Telangiectatic osteosarcomas which are high grade and very vascular. They appear lytic on X-ray. They were previously thought to be more aggressive than intramedullary tumours but a recent study shows the same survival if given the same treatment.
- Small cell osteosarcoma which may resemble EFT (Ewing's family of tumours) but will not have the same genetic abnormalities or immunohistochemistry profile.
- Undifferentiated high-grade pleomorphic sarcoma of bone (previously known as malignant fibrous histiocytoma of bone) which lacks the osteoid component but responds to the same treatment as intramedullary osteosarcoma.
- Juxtacortical osteosarcomas which subdivide into low grade (paraosteal and periosteal) and high grade. Treatment differs from that for intramedullary tumours as surgery alone may be used in low-grade juxtacortical tumours.
- Extraosseous osteosarcomas which are extremely rare (<0.5% osteosarcomas in McCarter study). They are high-grade lesions which occur deep in the extremities of older patients with an overall survival (OS) of 50% at five years. They may occur as a secondary malignancy. They are generally treated as a STS with aggressive behaviour.

Principles of management of non-metastatic osteosarcoma

Surgery
- Complete surgical resection by specialist sarcoma orthopaedic surgeons is required for the best outcome.
- Limb-sparing surgery has evolved significantly in the past 30 years such that amputation is used less often.
- Extending endoprostheses have been developed to minimize the number of surgeries a growing child or young adult may require.

Chemotherapy
- Before the 1980s all patients with apparently localized disease had surgery but only 20–30% survived over five years. Most died of disseminated disease suggesting the presence of micrometastases in apparently early disease.
- A pivotal study showed that giving adjuvant chemotherapy improved survival from 17% to 66%.
- Neoadjuvant chemotherapy was subsequently developed to allow time to plan surgery. A study showed neoadjuvant therapy to be as efficacious as adjuvant chemotherapy.
- Methotrexate at doses up to $12g/m^2$ is used in addition to cisplatin and doxorubicin in younger patients and has been found to increase tumour necrosis.
- The bacterial cell wall mimic muramyl tripeptide (MTP) improved six-year survival to 78% in primary osteosarcomas when added to chemotherapy.
- The EURAMOS trial, a multicentre international study, stratified patients ≤40 years with resectable osteosarcoma according to response to two cycles of neoadjuvant MUTYH associated polyposis (MAP). The

good responders (<10% viable tumour) were randomized to four additional cycles of MAP with or without interferon 2b (IFN-2b). At the time of analysis, there was no difference in OS. The poor responders (>10% viable tumours) were randomized to MAP with or without ifosfamide and etoposide. There was no difference in survival.

- MAP chemotherapy remains the standard of care for young patients with resectable osteosarcoma.

Radiotherapy
Radiotherapy is markedly inferior to surgical resection of the primary tumour in terms of OS but has been used in patients who decline or who are unable to have surgery.

Prognosis/prognostic factors
Several factors have been associated with a poor prognosis which include:

- Age <14 years or >40 years
- Poor response (<90% necrosis) to neoadjuvant chemotherapy
- Pathological fracture
- Large tumour volume, which is also associated with lung metastases.
- Metastases at presentation with bone metastases having a worse prognosis than lung metastases.
- Primary tumours which are axial or extraosseous
- Secondary osteosarcoma
- Raised ALP or LDH
- Increased cadherin 11 expression

Other factors such as proliferative index are not associated with prognosis. The expression of c-erbB-2 has been shown to have no relation to prognosis in some studies but poor prognosis in others.

Metastatic osteosarcoma
Introduction
- 11.4% of osteosarcoma patients have metastases at the time of presentation.
- OS at five years ranges from 10% to 50%.
- Metastases may occur in the lungs (see Figure 11.2.1), bone, and bone marrow. Lymph node and brain metastases are exceptionally rare.
- Isolated pulmonary metastases have the best and bone metastases the worst prognosis.
- Up to 30% of patients with lung metastases survive >10 years with a combination of surgery, multiagent chemotherapy, and occasionally radiotherapy.

Principles of management
Although the chance of cure is small, patients particularly those with limited and potentially resectable lung metastases, should be treated aggressively with chemotherapy and surgery.

For those with large numbers of lung metastases or bone metastases, chemotherapy and radiotherapy can provide good palliation.

Chemotherapy
- The most effective agents are cisplatin, doxorubicin, methotrexate, and ifosfamide.
- Response rates are 20–40% although some tumours and metastases may not reduce in size. Calcification can occur in responding lung metastases.
- If metastases are present at diagnosis, combination chemotherapy should be used, as it is for localized

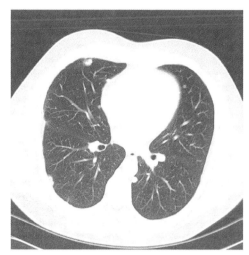

Fig. 11.2.1 Axial CT scan showing lung metastases from osteosarcoma. Typically these can be peripheral or pleural (causing bloody pleural effusions) or can be calcified. A calcified metastasis is seen at the top of the figure in the right lower lobe.

disease. In younger patients, cisplatin, doxorubicin, and methotrexate may be used. In older patients methotrexate is often omitted because of increased toxicity.

- If the patient has relapsed with metastases within one to two years of the original treatment, the same chemotherapy is unlikely to be useful. In these cases, ifosfamide with or without etoposide can be effective but is less so than chemotherapy given for metastases at presentation.
- High-dose methotrexate with folinic acid rescue can be effective if previously treatment was with cisplatin and doxorubicin alone.
- High-dose ifosfamide (12–15g/m^2) can be effective.
- High-dose treatment with stem cell rescue has shown no improvement in survival.
- Gemcitabine and docetaxel, a combination which has proved effective in some STSs, has shown activity in advanced osteosarcoma.
- Regorafenib and cabozantinib, two tyrosine kinase inhibitors have recently shown activity in metastatic osteosarcoma.
- Immunotherapy may have a role and the use of liposomal muramyl tripeptide-phosphatidyl-ethanolamine has been shown to produce a survival benefit in the adjuvant setting.

Surgery
Surgery in the metastatic setting should either be:
- Aimed at palliation of symptoms, e.g. resection of a large primary extremity tumour with low volume lung metastases.
- Performed with the intention of cure, e.g. resection of lung metastases.
- Lung metastases should be evaluated for resectability in conjunction with thoracic surgeons. Resection may follow chemotherapy.

Radiotherapy

Although osteosarcomas are relatively radioresistant tumours, radiotherapy has been successfully used:

- To control bone pain.
- In addition to chemotherapy and surgery, e.g. following resection of lung metastases some groups advocate whole lung radiotherapy as well as chemotherapy.
- To provide local control for some patients with advanced metastatic disease for whom resection of the primary tumour is inappropriate.
- In one review of 39 patients with high-risk, metastatic, or recurrent disease, 76% had clinical benefit from radiotherapy. The four-year survival of the group was 39% (Mahajan 2008). The median radiation dose was 30Gy in ten fractions with a range of 10–70Gy in 4–35 fractions.

Recurrent osteosarcoma

Introduction

Approximately 40% of patients treated for a primary osteosarcoma will have recurrence either locally or with metastatic disease. Those who recur locally only have a better prognosis than those with distant disease, but prognosis is worse than at initial presentation.

Management

Management of local recurrence may involve chemotherapy, surgery, or radiotherapy.

- Unless a significant time has passed (at least one year), repeating the same chemotherapy as given initially is unlikely to be beneficial due to the development of tumour resistance.
- Drugs are the same as those used for metastatic disease. Ifosfamide and etoposide can be effective, especially if not given previously. Cyclophosphamide and etoposide combination, gemcitabine and docetaxel combination, regorafenib and cabozantinib have shown activity.
- Surgery may be possible but limb-sparing surgery is less likely for local recurrence of extremity tumours.
- Radiotherapy may be useful for local control but is less effective than surgery.

Metastatic and recurrent osteosarcoma

Over 11% of recurrent osteosarcomas present with metastases and 40% with initially isolated disease relapse. Although the overall prognosis of these patients is poor, approximately 10–30% have a prolonged survival, predominantly those with resectable disease. Treatment should be aimed at cure for those with limited disease and effective palliation for those with more extensive disease. Chemotherapy has a primary role for these patients but surgery and radiotherapy also provide significant benefit.

Further reading

Bielack S, Smeland S, Whelan J, Marina N, Jovic G, Hook J, et al. Methotrexate, doxorubicin, and cisplatin (MAP) plus maintenance pegylated interferon alfa-2b versus MAP alone in patients with resectable high-grade osteosarcoma and good histologic response to preoperative MAP: first results of the EURAMOS-1 good response randomized controlled trial. *J Clin Oncol* 2015; 33(20):2279–87.

Mahajan A, Woo SY, Kornguth DG, Hughes D, Huh W, Chang EL, Herzog CE, Pelloski CE, Anderson P. Multimodality treatment of osteosarcoma: radiation in a high-risk cohort. *Pediatr Blood Cancer* 2008; 5(5):976–82.

11.3 Ewing's sarcoma

Introduction

- Described by James Ewing in 1921.
- Part of a spectrum of tumours called EFT. EFT includes PNET and Askin's tumour of the chest.

Incidence

- EFT comprise 3% of paediatric and adolescent malignancies in the USA and UK and are the second most common bone malignancy.
- Median age at diagnosis is 14 years although they can occur at any age.
- Highest in Caucasians with very low incidence in other racial groups.
- There is a male predominance with a 1.5:1 male to female ratio.

Presentation

- Most common site is long bone (53%) or axial skeleton (47%). Within presentations in the long bones, 52% occur distally and 48% proximally.
- Presenting symptoms in local disease are of pain, gradually increasing and worse at night (wakes from sleep).
- Median delay from symptoms to diagnosis is six to nine months.
- An associated soft tissue mass may be seen and is sometimes confused for a sign of infection; 25% have a soft tissue primary.
- Pelvic lesions are the most likely to present with metastatic disease (they are often large before being detected).
- Systemic symptoms may be present and are associated with advanced disease. Symptoms include fever, weight loss, and lethargy.
- Twenty-five per cent of patients have metastases at presentation.
- Subclinical metastases are present in 80–90% with apparently localized disease.

Prognostic factors

Poor prognosis is associated with metastases at presentation, especially non-pulmonary metastases, or pelvic or axial primary site, size >8cm, raised LDH, and age over 14 years.

Genetics

- EFT consistently have reciprocal translocations, usually between the EWS gene on chromosome 22 and FLI-1 on chromosome 11.
- t(11;22)(q24;q12) occurs in >85%.
- Other variants place EWS with other genes such as t(21;22)(q22;q12) EWS-ERG translocation which occurs in up to 10%.
- Due to consistency of the translocations these are used in diagnosis, either with cytogenetics, fluorescence in situ hybridization (FISH), or polymerase chain reaction (PCR).

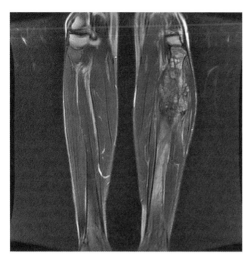

Fig. 11.3.1 Coronal section MRI (STIR sequence) of leg showing Ewing's sarcoma of left fibula with extensive soft tissue component.

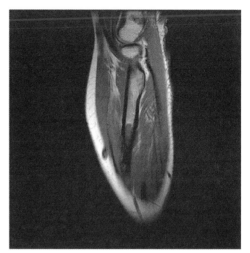

Fig. 11.3.2 MRI of left forearm showing Ewing's sarcoma of proximal radius with extensive intramedullary component but no soft tissue involvement.

Diagnosis and staging

- Initial X-ray may show:
  - A characteristic destructive lesion within the bone with periosteal reaction (onion skin appearance).
  - A soft tissue reaction (see Figure 11.3.1).
  - A pathological fracture (15%).
- Biopsy should be performed to confirm the diagnosis and exclude infection which in some cases may look similar radiologically. Biopsy should be:
  - Performed by a sarcoma specialist to allow for the tract to be removed during definitive surgery.
  - Of significant size such as a core or rarely an operative biopsy. Fine needle aspiration (FNA) cytology is not suitable for diagnosis but may be used to confirm relapse or metastases in a patient with confirmed EFT.
  - Sent for histology, microbiology, and cytogenetics or molecular pathology.
- Staging should be performed to help direct treatment.
  - MRI of primary lesion and remainder of that bone to exclude intramedullary skip lesions (Figure 11.3.2).
  - CT chest, bone scan (Figure 11.3.3), bone marrow biopsy.
  - PET scan is routinely used for the initial staging of patients with Ewing sarcoma (especially for primary bone tumours with a negative bone scan). It also plays a role to monitor response to chemotherapy/radiation therapy.
  - Blood tests including LDH.
  - Whole body MRI (STIR) may be considered to exclude occult bone metastases in otherwise localized disease.

Management of localized disease

- Without systemic treatment >80% with apparently localized disease will die of distant relapse.
- Multimodality treatment including chemotherapy, surgery, and/or radiotherapy is required.

Surgical management

- Should be undertaken by a sarcoma specialist.
- Aim for limb-sparing surgery if possible but need clear margins. Margins may be defined by compartment or joint. If a joint is involved joint replacement may be required. Pelvic tumours are the most difficult to resect especially if they involve the sacrum (sacral nerve involvement).
- Usually undertaken after induction chemotherapy to assess response and reduce risk of relapse.

Chemotherapy

- Combination chemotherapy pre- and postoperatively is usually given.
- Alkylating agents have highest response rate and have been combined with doxorubicin, vincristine, actinomycin D, and etoposide.

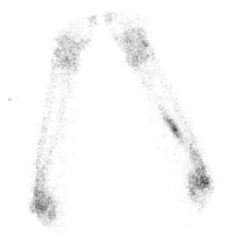

Fig. 11.3.3 Localized bone scan of Ewing's sarcoma of radius (same case as Fig. 11.3.2).

- International cooperation has allowed trials in this rare tumour with groups such as Intergroup Ewing's Sarcoma Study (IESS), the Children's Oncology Group, and the Euro-Ewing's Group which produced a series of trials.
- IESS-III showed that alternating ifosfamide and etoposide (IE) with vincristine, doxorubicin, and cyclophosphamide (VDC) improved survival from 54% to 69% in localized disease.
- The COG AEWS0031 showed that increasing dose-intensity by compressing the administration interval of VDC alternating with IE from three weeks to two weeks improved the event-free survival from 65% to 73% in localized disease. This regimen is considered by many the current standard of care for localized disease; however, its benefit in adults is unclear.
- High-dose treatment in localized low-risk disease has not been shown to improve survival.
- Response to chemotherapy at the time of surgery reflects prognosis.
- Stratifying treatment according to risk was investigated in the EURO-EWING 99 trial. In this non-inferiority trial, all patients received initially intensive induction chemotherapy consisting of vincristine, ifosfamide, doxorubicin, and etoposide (VIDE) followed by one course of vincristine, dactinomycin, and ifosfamide (VAI). Low-risk patients were randomized to standard treatment (VAI) and to less intense treatment (vincristine, dactinomycin, and cyclophosphamide (VAC)). Both groups had similar outcomes with disease-free survival around 75–78%. However, patients treated with the VAC regimen had a reduced incidence of renal tubular dysfunction. High-risk patients were randomized between standard treatment and high dose with stem cell rescue. This arm was prematurely closed because of lack of recruitment. Results are still awaited.
- The EURO-EWING 2012 trial randomized patients between the treatment strategy of two-week compressed interval VDC alternating with IE and the treatment strategy of VIDE induction followed by VAI/VAC consolidation. Results from this trial which completed early showed a survival benefit in the two-week compressed chemotherapy combination and has been adopted as the new standard of care.

Radiotherapy for localized disease
Unlike osteosarcomas, EFTs are radiosensitive and before chemotherapy was introduced, radiotherapy was a principal method of achieving disease control.
- Used as a primary method of local control in unresectable tumours, e.g. large pelvic tumours.
- Only used in addition to surgery with positive margins or significant soft tissue involvement.
- Studies have shown radiotherapy to have a worse outcome than surgery for local control but there may be some selection bias in that large pelvic tumours are more likely to be unresectable and be treated with radiotherapy alone compared with smaller limb tumours.
- Doses of 45–55Gy have been used. The lower dose has been found inadequate for local control and higher doses have been associated with second malignancy.
- Modern techniques of intensity modulated radiotherapy (IMRT), tomotherapy, and protons may reduce early and late side effects.

Prognosis in localized disease
Prognosis in localized disease has improved significantly since the introduction of chemotherapy.
- With combination chemotherapy and surgery or radiotherapy, five-year survival is 70%.

Management of advanced disease
Chemotherapy
- Some patients with limited pulmonary metastases may still be cured of their disease and many studies have examined the role of dose intensification to improve survival.
- The same combination chemotherapy agents are used in advanced disease as in localized disease.
- The benefit of high-dose treatment was examined within the EURO-EWING 99 trial. Patients were treated with standard induction therapy (VIDE plus VAI) followed by high-dose busulfan-melphalan and autologous stem-cell transplantation. OS was 34%. High-dose therapy remains experimental.

Surgery in advanced disease
- Surgery of the primary lesion may still be appropriate with limited pulmonary metastases if these respond to initial chemotherapy.
- Surgery may also be necessary for local control, especially if highly symptomatic.

Radiotherapy
- Radiotherapy can be used to treat either the primary tumour or metastatic lesions in advanced disease.
- The dose (radical or palliative) used for the primary will depend on the extent of other disease.
- Bilateral low-dose lung radiotherapy is often used as an adjunct to chemotherapy in responding patients with lung metastases.
- Unilateral lung irradiation is used for symptomatic bulky chest wall lesions.
- Palliative radiotherapy is used for painful bony metastases, including those causing spinal cord compression.

Prognosis of advanced disease
- With limited lung metastases and treatment with chemotherapy plus surgery or radiotherapy five-year survival of 20–40% can be expected.
- With more extensive disease five-year survival falls to <25%.
- All patients who are fit enough should be treated with combination chemotherapy initially as some will have prolonged responses.

Recurrence and management
- Recurrence usually occurs within the first two to five years and few of these patients survive.
- Relapse after five to ten years is associated with a survival similar to that of advanced disease at presentation.
- After ten years there are few relapses but it does occur. Late relapses have been reported in association with persistent infection and pregnancy.
- Treatment depends on the nature of relapse (local/systemic), nature of initial chemotherapy, and time from the end of primary treatment.
- Local recurrence in a limb previously treated with radiotherapy may be treated with surgery and chemotherapy.

- Isolated lung metastases after a long treatment interval may be suitable for surgical resection and further chemotherapy.
- To date, high-dose regimens remain experimental in this group.
- The type of chemotherapy depends on the initial regimen. The following regimens have shown activity in the relapsed or refractory setting: ifosfamide and etoposide, topotecan and cyclophosphamide (TC), irinotecan and temozolomide (IT) (Wagner, et al. 2007), carboplatin and etoposide combination, high-dose ifosfamide (IFOS) and regorafenib.
- The EORTC rEECur trial is randomizing patients with refractory or recurrent Ewing sarcoma to TC, IT, GD, and IFOS. Interim analyses have shown gemcitabine and docetaxel to be less active compared to other options.

- Trials of new agents such as IGF-IR antagonists are underway.

Further reading

Daldrup-Link HE, Franzius C, Link TM, et al. Whole body MR for detection of bone metastases in children and young adults. *Am J Roentgenol* 2001; 177(1):229–36.

Furth C, Amthauer H, Denecke T, et al. Impact of whole-body MRI and FDG-PET on staging and assessment of therapy response in a patient with Ewing sarcoma. *Pediatr Blood Cancer* 2006; 47(5):607–11.

Mahajan A, Woo SY, Kornguth DG, et al. Multimodality treatment of osteosarcoma: radiation in a high-risk cohort. *Pediatr Blood Cancer* 2008; 50(5):976–82.

Wagner LM, McAllister N, Goldsby RE, et al. Temozolomide and intravenous irinotecan for treatment of advanced Ewing sarcoma. *Pediatr Blood Cancer* 2007; 48:132–9.

11.4 Rare bone tumours

Chondrosarcoma

- Comprise <12% bone tumours.
- Third most common malignant bone tumour.
- More common over the age of 40.
- There are several subtypes including peripheral, central, dedifferentiated, mesenchymal, juxtacortical, and clear cell variants.
- The most common sites are pelvis (Figure 11.4.1), axial skeleton, and proximal limbs.
- As with other bone tumours, axial tumours have a worse prognosis than extremity tumours.
- Aetiology unknown. Some patients have a history of osteochondroma or enchondroma (Ollier's disease).

Rare genetic condition resulting in multiple exostoses (Maffucci syndrome) also confers increased risk.

- Presents with a mass which may be painful or painless or with symptoms due to local disease.
- Systemic symptoms are rare except with widely disseminated disease.
- Diagnosis may be suggested from plain X-rays but MRI should be undertaken for suspected sarcomas. Chondrosarcomas frequently exhibit calcification. MRI can also be used to assess soft tissue extension. The lesion often has a cauliflower-like appearance.
- As with other bone tumours an adequate biopsy should be performed at a specialist centre with sarcoma expertise.

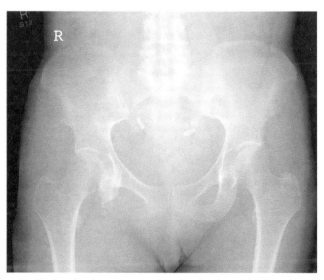

Fig. 11.4.1 X-ray of the pelvis showing a chondrosarcoma arising from the right pubis with local bone destruction. Note the presence of the tips of ureteric stents in the bladder.

- Local staging is determined by MRI with a CT scan of the chest to exclude lung metastases. PET is of no known benefit in staging these tumours.
- Staging system is as for other bone tumours.
- There are three grades of tumour from well to poorly differentiated. Five-year survival is >90% for a localized grade 1 tumour but reduces to 25% for a grade 3 tumour.
- The primary modality of treatment is surgery. Chemotherapy and radiotherapy have limited activity in chondrosarcoma but have been used for palliation in some cases. Proton therapy has shown some recent success. Dedifferentiated chondrosarcomas may respond to chemotherapy.

Giant cell tumour

- Less than 5% primary bone tumours.
- Most are benign but up to 10% can be malignant and 5% develop lung metastases.
- Malignant tumours are often secondary to radiotherapy.
- Peak age at presentation is 20–50 years.
- Most frequent sites are distal femur, proximal tibia, and distal radius.
- May also occur in fibula, distal tibia, pelvis, and spine.
- Presentation is usually due to pain as most occur near joint site. Pain increases with activity. Five to 10% are associated with a pathological fracture; 20% are associated with a joint effusion.
- Radiologically they can be distinguishable from other bone tumours on X-ray as they have an expansile lytic area ('soap bubble appearance') which is located close to the epiphysis. MRI is used to assess soft tissue and intramedullary extension.
- Staging should include chest CT scan as there is a possibility of lung metastases.
- A bone scintigram will show increased tracer uptake in the region of the tumour.
- Staging of giant cell tumours differs from other bone tumours (see Table 11.4.1).
- Surgery is the most effective treatment but often the whole tumour cannot be removed without leaving a residual deficit in the bone. This space is filled with bone graft material. Adding bone cement to the graft may reduce the risk of recurrence from 45% to <30%. Additional local treatments include cryotherapy and chemical adjuvants.

Table 11.4.1 Summary of staging for giant cell tumours of bone

Stage I	Benign latent giant cell tumours
	No aggressive activity
Stage II	Benign active giant cell tumours; imaging studies demonstrate alteration of cortical bone structure
Stage III	Locally aggressive tumours
	Imaging studies demonstrate a lytic lesion surrounding medullary and cortical bone
	There may be indication of tumour penetration through the cortex into the soft tissues

- Embolization is often used prior to surgery, especially for sacral tumours, to prevent excessive blood loss at the time of surgery.
- Radiotherapy can be used for these tumours but there is a risk up to 15% of secondary malignancy.
- Denosumab, a monoclonal antibody to RANK ligand, showed activity with an 86% response rate in patients with recurrent or unresectable giant cell tumour.
- Lung metastases may resolve after treatment of primary or can be resected.

Primary bone lymphoma

- Otherwise known as primary non-Hodgkin lymphoma (NHL) of bone.
- Mean age at presentation is 40–45 years.
- Males are affected almost twice as much as females.
- Presentation is with bone pain not relieved by rest and systemic ('B') symptoms (weight loss, fever, night sweats) are well described.
- Can present as a localized, solitary destructive lesion (stage IE), with associated local lymph node (stage IIE) or widespread bony disease (stage IV).
- X-rays show diffuse medullary mottling with lytic areas. MRI does not show a consistent picture as the appearance depends on the degree of fibrosis in the lesion.
- Bone biopsy should be performed with the same care and expertise as for other bone tumours. Immunohistochemistry should include lymphoid markers as this will affect treatment options.
- Staging should involve a CT scan of chest, abdomen, and pelvis to exclude distant nodal disease. PET is useful in excluding distant metastases but its role in assessment of primary lymphoma of bone in the absence of metastases has not been evaluated.
- Unlike most bone tumours, primary treatment is not surgery. Chemotherapy with CHOP-like (cyclophosphamide, hydroxydaunorubicin (doxorubicin), Oncovin® (vincristine), and prednisone) regimens has proved most effective, with or without rituximab.
- For localized disease in adults, external beam radiotherapy (EBRT) has been used with doses up to 40Gy with or without a boost of 10Gy to the tumour bed.
- In children excellent tumour control and survival rates are achieved in 90% with chemotherapy alone.
- There is a significant risk of secondary malignancy if anthracycline chemotherapy and radiotherapy are used as treatment.
- Pathological fracture and osteonecrosis may also occur if radiotherapy is combined with chemotherapy or doses >50Gy are used.
- Surgery is usually restricted to stabilization following impending or actual fracture.
- Prognosis is better in those aged <40, with localized disease and treated with combination therapy.
- Poor prognostic factors include pathological fracture and multifocal disease.

Langerhans cell histiocytosis of bone (eosinophilic granuloma)

- Incidence 0.5 per million per year.
- Predominantly in children five to ten years with a 2:1 male to female ratio.

- One manifestation of a rare syndrome that includes pituitary involvement, skin abnormalities, interstitial lung disease, and lytic bone tumours.
- Most common site is the skull followed by vertebra, femur, humerus, and ribs.
- Presents with painful swelling, spinal cord compression, or reduced joint movement.

- Can be isolated (>50%) or multiple lesions (<30%).
- Biopsy is necessary for diagnosis with immunohistochemical staining for CD1a and S100.
- Treatment may include corticosteroid injection, surgery, radiotherapy, and radiofrequency ablation.

11.5 Soft tissue sarcomas overview

Introduction
STSs represent a rare collection of heterogeneous tumours characterized by malignant growth of mesenchymal tissue.

Different subgroups can be divided by genetics, pathology, anatomical location, and clinical behaviour.

Incidence/epidemiology
- Less than 1% of malignant tumours with an incidence of 30 per million per annum.
- Median age at presentation depends on histological subtype. For example, rhabdomyosarcomas are most common in children and adolescents, whereas leiomyosarcomas predominate over the age of 40.

Aetiology
- Most cases arise de novo with no obvious predisposing factor.
- Known predisposing factors include familial cancer syndromes, prior radiotherapy and/or chemotherapy, chronic lymphoedema, or infection. Polyvinyl chloride is associated with angiosarcoma of the liver.
- Familial cancer syndromes include Li–Fraumeni, hereditary retinoblastoma, and familial gastrointestinal stromal tumour (GIST) tumours. Malignant peripheral nerve sheath tumours (MPNST) are more common in neurofibromatosis with inherited mutations in NF1 associated with a 10% lifetime risk of MPNST. Desmoid tumours and aggressive fibromatosis occur in those with APC gene mutations associated with familial adenomatosis polyposis (FAP).

Pathology
- There are >80 subtypes of STS. The most common are leiomyosarcoma, liposarcoma, synovial sarcoma, rhabdomyosarcoma, fibrosarcoma (several subtypes), MPNST, and alveolar soft part sarcoma.
- These are named after their supposed tissue of origin (e.g. leiomyosarcoma) or tissue which they most obviously resemble (e.g. liposarcoma).
- Many STSs are characterised and classified according to specific gene rearrangements.
- World Health Organization (WHO) guidelines classify them according to malignant potential in addition to morphology.

Clinical features
- Presentation depends on the stage of disease and histological subtype of sarcoma.
- Nine out of ten soft tissue masses will be benign.
- Risk factors for malignancy are:

- >5cm
- Deep to deep fascia
- Rapid growth
- Painful
- However, malignant tumours may be more superficial, painless, and <5cm.
- Systemic symptoms (fever, weight loss, anorexia, breathlessness) may be present in advanced disease, particularly if associated with extensive chest disease.

Diagnosis
- Because of their rarity and the need for complex management, sarcomas should be managed by specialist centres from diagnosis to treatment. Differential diagnoses may include infection, metastatic disease, and lymphoma.
- Correct diagnosis requires an adequate biopsy which, as for bone tumours, should not compromise later surgery.
- In some cases, when the mass is small and relatively superficial an excision biopsy can be undertaken.
- Biopsies are usually performed under image guidance (ultrasound or CT if deep).
- Samples should be sent to microbiology if infection is suspected.
- Pathology should be reviewed by an experienced sarcoma pathologist. Due to the difficulty of diagnosis even with immunohistochemistry, specialist techniques such as cytogenetics and PCR may also be used to identify translocation specific sarcomas.

Staging
Staging should include:
- MRI of primary to evaluate extension of tumour.
- CT scan of chest to exclude lung metastases.
- In certain rare subgroups (rhabdomyosarcoma, synovial sarcoma, clear cell, and epithelioid sarcomas), nodal disease may occur and therefore regional CT scanning may be appropriate (see Figure 11.5.1).
- The role of bone scintigraphy is less established in STSs than for bone sarcomas. PET has not been evaluated (except for GIST) in sufficient STSs.

Several staging systems exist, the most frequently used of which are the AJCC and Memorial–Sloan Kettering (MSK).
- AJCC staging can be used online (see 'Internet resources', p. 320).
- AJCC does not include histology or site which limits its use. It should not be used for non-extremity sarcomas.

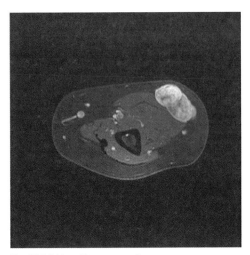

Fig. 11.5.1 Myxoid liposarcoma of arm.

For prognosis and management the key factors are whether it is localized or extensive/spread to other sites as this is what determines treatment. For many STSs a new app called 'Sarculator' can be found which has been validated for limb and retroperitoneal sarcomas.

Common subgroups of soft tissue sarcoma

Leiomyosarcoma
- Any site of body.
- Commonest subtype of uterine sarcoma.
- Most common sites of metastases are lung, except in uterine (liver). Soft tissue and bone metastases also occur.
- Chaotic karyotype.
- Variable grade and sensitivity to chemotherapy.

Liposarcoma
- Different subtypes with considerable differences in behaviour and management.
- Myxoid or round cell.
- Arise in limbs and spread to soft tissues (retroperitoneum, mediastinum).
- Propensity for bone metastases (especially spine) in up to 17% which may only be visualized on MRI. They are chemosensitive, e.g. to doxorubicin and trabectedin.

- Characteristic balanced translocation t (12;16) FUS-DDIT3.
- Well differentiated, often abdominal; tend to recur locally not systemically; and chemoresistant.
- Dedifferentiated tumours tend to occur in the retroperitoneum or abdomen. These are high-grade, chemoresistant tumours which have characteristic genetics with abnormalities in CDK4/MDM2.

Synovial sarcoma
- Predominantly in children and younger adults.
- Better prognosis in those aged one to ten years.
- Most common sites are limbs and trunk.
- Chemosensitive, especially to ifosfamide.
- Metastases predominantly in lungs.
- Balanced translocation t(X;18) between SX18 and SSX1 or SSX2.

Prognosis
Different prognostic factors predict for local and systemic recurrence.
- Size and grade best predict distant recurrence and OS.
- Other factors which predict survival include age, anatomical site, and histological subtype.
- Retroperitoneal and visceral tumours carry a worse prognosis than extremity tumours as, like EFT, they can grow to a very large size before they are detected.
- Specific tumour subtypes such as MPNST and leiomyosarcoma have a poorer OS.
- Increased proliferative activity as assessed by immunocytochemical stains has shown a correlation with poorer survival in at least three studies.
- In synovial sarcomas, a translocation-specific sarcoma, several studies have shown a poorer prognosis in SX18(SYT)-SSX1 gene fusion tumours than SS18(SYT)-SSX2. However other studies have not confirmed this finding.
- Involved resection margins and age >50 are worst for local recurrence.
- Specific histological tumour types with a higher rate of local recurrence include MPNST and fibrosarcomas.
- Nomograms have been developed, and validated, which help to predict survival based on these features. The best known is the MSK nomogram which can be found online (see 'Internet resources').

Internet resources
AJCC staging online: https://www.protocols.fccc.edu/fccc/pims/staging/sarcoma.html
MSK nomogram: http://www.mskcc.org/mskcc/html/443.cfm
Sarculator (app available for Iphone and Android devices)

11.6 Management of localized soft tissue sarcoma

Introduction
Surgical resection with wide margins remains the treatment of choice for STSs. Radiotherapy has a role in high-grade tumours and those with involved resection margins. Chemotherapy remains controversial in the adjuvant setting but may have a role in specific subgroups.

Surgery
Surgery from biopsy to definitive resection should be performed at a specialist sarcoma centre.

Resection must extend beyond the tumour to a wide margin.

An involved resection margin is the most important factor which predicts risk of recurrence. In two studies of patients who had surgery and radiotherapy, local recurrence was increased from 3–12% to 19–36% with uninvolved versus involved margins.

Margins must be defined in terms of compartments and fascial or skin borders as well as distance. For example, reporting a negative skin margin when the involved skin overlying the sarcoma has been removed represents a clear margin.

Although amputation and compartmentectomy reduce local recurrence rates compared with local resection, morbidity is significant. Surgery should be discussed within a sarcoma MDT to ensure morbidity is minimized with the use of radiotherapy if required.

Radical resection or combining radiotherapy with resection can reduce local recurrence to <10%. In specialist sarcoma centres amputation rates are <5% whilst maintaining good local control.

Amputation may be necessary in some cases because of involvement of vital structures, usually blood vessels, preventing radical resection.

Radiotherapy
Although surgery is the primary curative modality for STSs, radiotherapy has a significant role in the prevention and treatment of local recurrence. Many STSs are radiosensitive. The doses required (>60Gy) are higher than those used for many epithelial cancers due to the aggressive nature of many sarcomas. There is no evidence that radiotherapy improves OS.

The use of radiotherapy should be discussed in the context of an MDT but the following are appropriate reasons for postoperative radiotherapy:

- High-grade tumour
- Deep tumour
- Size >5cm
- Positive margins when re-resection is not possible
- Local recurrence which has been re-resected

For some patients who are unfit for surgery or in whom resection is technically not feasible, radiotherapy may be considered as a primary treatment modality. However, unless the tumour is very small and superficial, local control will not be as good as with surgery.

Proton therapy is increasingly being used in these patients to minimize late effects after treatment.

Limb sarcoma radiotherapy presents several challenges:

- Positioning and immobilizing the limb to ensure consistent placement and accurate dose to the tumour bed. Immobilization aids are used and the contralateral limb must be placed away from the treatment field.
- A wide 2cm margin is usually added to account for limb movement.
- Adequate dose must be delivered to the tumour bed but must not cross the fascial compartment to avoid lymphoedema. The risk of morbidity due to fibrosis, which significantly affects mobility, increases with treatment volume and dose.

Chest wall sarcoma presents other challenges:

- The tumour may be close to the heart or spinal cord making planning complex and potentially limiting doses delivered.
- Many sarcomas follow the pleural contour of the chest wall making it difficult to avoid significant lung volumes within the treatment field.

Other specific regions such as head and neck or retroperitoneal sarcomas pose their own problems which are discussed elsewhere (head and neck, STS special types, retroperitoneal).

Preoperative and postoperative radiotherapy
Postoperative radiotherapy is usually planned in two phases to take into account possible tumour spillage at the edge of the surgical procedure and then to focus on the central tumour bed. Planning must take into account preoperative scans to estimate tumour location, but should also encompass the surgical edges. Preoperative radiotherapy allows a single-phase approach. An ongoing trial, VORTEX, is examining the possibility of reducing the volume of the postoperative treatment comparing a single-phase treatment with a standard two-phase approach.

Radiotherapy has traditionally been given postoperatively but there are potential benefits to giving preoperative radiotherapy:

- Smaller treatment volume (and possibly dose).
- Tumour visible on planning scan.
- Reduction of tumour before surgery allowing a less morbid and complete operation.
- Reduction in significant late toxicity such as limb oedema, joint restriction, and fibrosis.

The concerns about preoperative radiotherapy are:

- It may affect interpretation of histology.
- It is associated with greater wound complications postoperatively. This study was stopped early due to a significant increase in acute wound complications (17–35%). Local control and OS was equivalent in the two groups, and further follow-up showed a reduction in late morbidity with preoperative radiotherapy.

Sarcomas represent one of the ideal tumour types for which IMRT, volumetric modulated arc therapy (VMAT), tomotherapy, and proton therapy can provide accurate planning, conformal dose delivery, and reduced long-term morbidity.

Adjuvant chemotherapy
The use of adjuvant chemotherapy in STSs remains controversial and is compounded by:

- Different histological subtypes of sarcoma with varied chemosensitivities being grouped together in the majority of studies.
- The development of new chemotherapy agents which may have greater efficacy in specific subgroups but

have not yet been studied in the adjuvant setting, e.g. gemcitabine/docetaxel in leiomyosarcomas.

• The rarity of the disease and need for international collaboration in trials which has only relatively recently been achieved.

There are some sarcomas, which tend to predominate in the paediatric setting, in which adjuvant treatment has been shown to be useful, e.g. rhabdomyosarcomas and the extra-skeletal Ewing's tumours such as PNETs. However, for the majority there is no consensus concerning the use of adjuvant chemotherapy.

There are two large meta-analyses that provide some guidance. The initial meta-analysis of 1,568 patients from 14 trials which used doxorubicin-containing chemotherapy showed a statistically significant improvement in local and distant recurrence if adjuvant chemotherapy was given. There was a trend towards an improved OS of 4% at ten years, but this was not statistically significant. The best evidence for adjuvant chemotherapy appeared to be for large (> 8cm), high-grade extremity sarcomas, but there was no absolute benefit for any specific subgroup.

Criticisms of this meta-analysis note the fact that many patients were included with tumours now known to be truly chemo-insensitive (e.g. GISTs) or which have been reclassified (e.g. carcinosarcomas). Recurrent tumours were also included. Some studies used only doxorubicin whereas others included additional drugs. The dose of doxorubicin was also variable from 50–90mg/m^2 although it is known that doses <60mg/m^2 are rarely effective in metastatic sarcoma.

A second updated meta-analysis conducted on 1,953 patients from 18 randomized trials using doxorubicin-containing therapy showed a statistically significant decrease in local and distant recurrence (similar to the previous meta-analysis). However, the combination of doxorubicin and ifosfamide therapy increased OS (absolute risk reduction of 11%). The main criticism of this meta-analysis is that it did not include the recent large EORTC trial (see below). Nevertheless, this analysis highlights the importance of combining ifosfamide with doxorubicin in the adjuvant treatment. This combination was studied in the following trials.

A study of 104 patients with large or recurrent sarcomas, many of whom were thought to have tumours of chemosensitive histologies (e.g. synovial sarcoma), were randomized to surgery alone versus intensive ifosfamide and epirubicin. Although initial results showed an improvement in OS this difference was not statistically significant on longer follow-up.

Another trial randomized 88 patients with high-risk extremity sarcomas to standard treatment or chemotherapy. The chemotherapy could be either epirubicin or epirubicin combined with ifosfamide. In this study the five-year survival was increased from 47% to 72%. The large number of treatment variables and the small number of studied patients makes interpretation of this result difficult but there is a move in some patients to consider neoadjuvant chemotherapy after this study.

An international multicentre EORTC study randomized 351 patients to standard treatment versus ifosfamide with doxorubicin. Over half had high-grade extremity tumours, 40% of which were >10cm. There was no significant difference in relapse-free survival or OS. This trial did include some low-grade tumours and many non-extremity tumours but they were balanced between the two arms of the trial.

Later, a pooled analysis of the two largest adjuvant trials of doxorubicin and ifosfamide-based chemotherapy (both EORTC) was negative. This negative result contrasts with the positive survival benefit seen in the updated meta-analysis. Finally, a trial comparing histology-tailored therapy to combination anthracycline and ifosfamide chemotherapy failed to show a difference in OS in high-risk STS subtypes of the extremities or trunk wall.

There have also been a number of retrospective reviews, some of which have shown a benefit, particularly for ifosfamide-containing chemotherapy, although others have not. A few studies have concentrated on tumours which are more chemosensitive in the metastatic setting such as synovial sarcoma.

The five-year metastasis-free survival was found to improve from 48% to 60% for the 61 patients of 215 with synovial sarcoma who received adjuvant chemotherapy in one study. However other studies have shown an initial benefit for chemotherapy in the first 12–24 months which is not sustained.

In many of these retrospective studies the outcome may have been affected by the fact that the majority of the patients who received chemotherapy had tumours of higher risk because of factors such as recurrence, size >10cm, and grade.

The use of adjuvant chemotherapy is not, therefore, routinely recommended outside a clinical trial, but the studies mentioned here should be discussed with patients in their particular situations and for some may offer a benefit that cannot yet be quantified.

Further studies alongside genomic data to evaluate patients most likely to respond are recommended.

Hyperthermia

Hyperthermia in conjunction with neoadjuvant chemotherapy with etoposide, ifosfamide, and doxorubicin has shown an improvement in local control from 16.2 to 31.7 months after a median follow-up of 24.9 months in a phase 3 trial. Its role in the management of STS needs to be further studied.

Treatment recommendations

Surgery remains the mainstay of treatment for STS. This should be performed by specialist sarcoma surgeons and clear margins should be the aim. Radiotherapy is recommended for the majority of cases except low-grade tumours which have been excised with a wide margin. The role of adjuvant chemotherapy for most subgroups remains controversial but could be considered within the context of a clinical trial.

Outcome

The prognosis for STSs depends on the histological subtype, size at presentation, grade of tumour, and age of the patient. This is highlighted in more detail for the most common subtypes of sarcoma.

More detailed information is available for each subtype using the Sarculator app.

Further reading

Davis AM, O'Sullivan B, Bell RS, et al. Preoperative versus postoperative radiotherapy in soft tissue sarcoma of the limbs. *Lancet* 2002; 359:2235–41.

Issels R, Abdel-Rahman S, Wendtner C-M, et al. Neoadjuvant chemotherapy combined with regional hyperthermia for locally advanced primary or recurrent high risk soft tissue sarcomas: long term results of a phase II study. *Eur J Cancer* 2001; 37:1599–608.

Petrioli R, Coratti A, Correale P, et al. Adjuvant epirubicin with or without ifosfamide for adult soft tissue sarcoma. *Am J Clin Oncol* 2002; 25:468–73.

11.7 Management of locally advanced and metastatic disease for soft tissue sarcomas

Introduction
The presentation of sarcoma may be with locally advanced or metastatic disease (see Figure 11.7.1). In the majority of cases this presentation carries a very poor prognosis. In other cases, patients present with limited metastatic disease a few years after their initial treatment for localized sarcoma and the prognosis is slightly better in this situation. In both cases treatment options depend on performance status, comorbidities, and histological subtype of sarcoma.

Median survival with metastatic disease is 12–18 months.

Chemotherapy
Systemic treatment with chemotherapy can be useful but its role is more complex than in other malignancies:

- There is little evidence that chemotherapy prolongs survival but it can provide significant benefits in symptom control.
- Tumours with a high response rate to chemotherapy (often high grade) do not necessarily have a better prognosis than those with a lower response rate.
- Response rates as determined by RECIST (Response Evaluation Criteria In Solid Tumors) criteria often do not reflect symptomatic benefit or disease control, especially in response to certain agents such as trabectedin.
- Different tumour types show different responses to chemotherapy in general and to specific drugs. The most chemosensitive tumours are synovial sarcoma, myxoid liposarcoma, and childhood rhabdomyosarcoma. Extraskeletal Ewing's tumours are also chemosensitive. The most chemoresistant tumours are dedifferentiated liposarcoma, alveolar soft part sarcoma, GIST, low-grade liposarcoma, and clear cell sarcoma.

- Trials of chemotherapy in advanced sarcoma, as in the adjuvant setting, have been hampered by inclusion of many resistant histological subtypes including GIST.

Single agent chemotherapy
Doxorubicin is a standard first-line agent with response rates of 20–25%. Doses <60mg/m^2 have been shown to be ineffective and >75mg/m^2 to have increased toxicity without clinical benefit.

Ifosfamide is often used as a second-line agent and has a response rate of 25% overall.

A review of an unselected group of patients with metastatic STS treated with doxorubicin-based chemotherapy showed a clinical benefit of 45% with a six-month progression-free survival (PFS).

Combination chemotherapy
In general, combination chemotherapy has been shown to improve response rates up to 46% but with no improvement in PFS or OS and with increased toxicity.

An EORTC trial compared single agent doxorubicin to doxorubicin-ifosfamide combination in patients with high-grade advanced STS. Despite achieving a higher response rate with the combination, there was no difference in OS.

The gemcitabine-docetaxel combination showed initial good activity in soft tissue. However, the UK GeDDiS trial comparing this combination to doxorubicin did not show any difference in OS.

High-dose treatment with stem cell rescue has shown no survival benefit.

There are a few special circumstances in which combined chemotherapy may be used first line:

- Life-threatening progressive disease.
- Preoperatively to downstage tumour and aim for resection.

Combination chemotherapy does have a role in tumours of childhood and adolescence such as rhabdomyosarcoma and extraskeletal Ewing's.

Specific therapies and histology
Recent studies have shown that some therapies are more effective in particular tumours:

- Ifosfamide-containing therapies are more active in certain subtypes (particularly synovial sarcoma) compared with others (including leiomyosarcoma).
- Taxanes and liposomal doxorubicin have been shown to be effective in angiosarcoma.
- Gemcitabine-docetaxel and gemcitabine-dacarbazine showed activity in leiomyosarcomas.
- Trabectedin has been shown to be effective in the treatment of liposarcomas, especially myxoid liposarcomas. It also has a >30% response rate in previously treated leiomyosarcomas and some activity in other sarcomas. Although complete and partial responses are rare, disease stabilization with a median duration of response of 16.5 months was reported in one study. A randomized trial compared trabectedin to dacarbazine in the third line in liposarcoma and for leiomyosarcoma showed a significant improvement in PFS.
- Eribulin, an antimitotic, improved OS in advanced leiomyosarcoma and liposarcoma compared to dacarbazine in the third line.

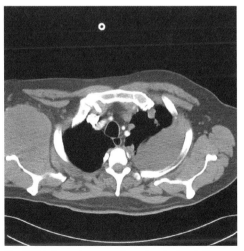

Fig. 11.7.1 Synovial sarcoma of scapula with pleural effusion and lung metastases.

- Aromatase inhibitors in endometrial stromal sarcoma and hormone positive leiomyosarcomas are active.

Targeted therapy

- Pazopanib, a multitargeted oral tyrosine kinase inhibitor, was shown to be effective in patients with STS progressing after a first-line therapy. The PALETTE trial randomized a variety of patients with STS (excluding liposarcomas and GISTs) to pazopanib versus placebo. There was three-month increase in PFS but no difference in OS.
- Imatinib had a response rate of 46% in dermatofibrosarcoma protuberans.
- The mTOR inhibitor everolimus had a response rate of 42% in angiomyolipomas. Sirolimus and temsirolimus were also active in perivascular epithelioid cell neoplasms.
- Other targeted therapies undergoing investigation are cediranib and sunitinib for alveolar soft part sarcoma, tivantinib and cabozantinib for clear cell sarcoma, axitinib for angiosarcomas, pazopanib, and sunitinib for solitary fibrous tumours, and nilotinib for pigmented villonodular synovitis and larotrectenib and entrectenib for *NTRK* fusion positive sarcomas.

Surgery

Despite the poor median OS with metastatic disease a small group of patients have a prolonged survival. The majority of these have disease which is amenable to surgery. Most of these patients will have isolated lung metastases or isolated intra-abdominal recurrence.

Pulmonary metastatectomy

Criteria for consideration of pulmonary metastatectomy are:

- No other sites of disease (including primary site).
- Complete resection appears possible.
- Long disease-free interval (preferably at least 18 months).
- Slowly progressive disease.
- Low number of metastases, preferably in one lung.

No randomized trial has evaluated the benefit of surgical resection of lung metastases but the five-year survival of patients selected using strict criteria is up to 40%.

The actual number of metastases which can be removed varies according to each institution but the prognosis decreases as the number of metastases increases.

In a single institutional study of 274 patients, having more than one lung metastasis, poor prognostic factors were shown to be metastases >2cm and a short disease-free interval of <18 months. Patients with all three factors had 0% chance of survival at five years compared with 60% survival if none of the factors were present.

Other surgery for locally advanced or metastatic sarcoma

Other situations in which surgery is considered in advanced sarcoma include isolated abdominal recurrence, as occurs with retroperitoneal sarcomas (see section 11.8, 'Retroperitoneal sarcoma') and soft tissue metastases elsewhere. As for lung metastases there are criteria which determine the appropriateness of further surgery:

- Isolated disease
- Resectable
- Long disease-free interval
- Slow growing
- Patient fit for surgery

In addition, consideration must be made for previous surgery and radiotherapy as this will affect the potential success and morbidity of the surgery. For this reason, multiple retroperitoneal surgeries are usually avoided.

Resection of liver metastases, other than for GIST, is performed rarely and there is little evidence that it is of benefit either in terms of survival or symptom control.

Chemotherapy after surgical resection

Since the development of metastases by definition confirms systemic disease, chemotherapy pre- or postoperatively may be considered. However, there are no trials to show that this is of benefit and the guidance is as that for adjuvant chemotherapy for sarcomas. It may be appropriate in paediatric type tumours such as rhabdomyosarcoma or synovial sarcoma, where young patients with advanced disease appear to have a better prognosis than adults with equivalent stage disease. It has also been suggested that giving chemotherapy before surgery allows evaluation of disease biology but this can also be assessed by a short interval chest X-ray or CT scan.

Radiotherapy

The majority of STSs are radiosensitive and radiotherapy can be an effective tool in disease and symptom control. Doses used, as with radical radiotherapy in sarcoma, range from 45 to 66Gy.

It may be used:

- To treat inoperable recurrence, particularly isolated recurrence and for chemoresistant tumours.
- Where there is skin infiltration.
- Over a chest drain site used to drain a malignant effusion.
- Following chemotherapy which may have reduced the tumour bulk (smaller field) but the symptoms are still present or likely to recur rapidly.
- If there is spinal cord compression or impending spinal cord compression.
- To relieve painful bone metastases.

Isolated limb perfusion

Some patients present with a massive limb sarcoma which may involve several compartments, neurovascular structures, or be inoperable due to other patient factors. This may occur as the initial presentation or as recurrence. These locally advanced tumours are often accompanied by significant symptoms and may be too large to be encompassed within a radiotherapy field. For some patients, systemic chemotherapy may not be appropriate due to comorbidities or histological subtype. For some there may be an option of isolated limb perfusion therapy (ILP).

- ILP involves isolating the circulation of the limb affected before perfusing it with recombinant tumour necrosis factor A (TNFA) and melphalan.
- Although this is a localized treatment it is associated with systemic symptoms such as fever and tachycardia.
- In some patients, surgery is then possible. In a small meta-analysis, limb salvage was obtained in 57–86% of patients. ILP was associated with the highest limb salvage rate and lowest complication rate.
- It is only available in a small number of specialist centres.

Treatment recommendations

- Metastatic STSs should be managed by a multidisciplinary team of sarcoma specialists who can discuss all available options.
- Where possible, and clinically indicated, surgery should be performed for isolated recurrence or metastasis as this appears to be associated with the best survival.
- Chemotherapy can give effective symptom control in many sarcomas but an understanding of the specific differences in histological subtypes is required. There is no evidence that combination chemotherapy improves survival but it is useful in special situations and in adolescent sarcomas.

- Radiotherapy should be used for specific indications.
- Isolated limb perfusion may be of benefit for a subgroup of patients.

Further reading

Hensley ML, Anderson S, Soslow R, et al. Activity of gemcitabine plus docetaxel in leiomyosarcoma (LMS) and other histologies: Report of an expanded phase II trial. *J Clin Oncol* 2004; 22(14s):9010.

Seddon B, Whelan J, Strauss S, Leahy M. GeDDiS: A prospective randomised controlled phase III trial of gemcitabine and docetaxel compared with doxorubicin as first-line treatment in previously untreated advanced unresectable or metastatic soft tissue sarcomas [abstract]. *J Clin Oncol* 2015; 33(suppl.):a10500.

11.8 Retroperitoneal sarcoma

Introduction

Retroperitoneal sarcomas (Figure 11.8.1) are a subgroup of STSs but are discussed separately here due to specialized management.

- Incidence is 3 per million per annum.
- Represent 13% of STSs.
- Most common histologies at this site are liposarcoma and leiomyosarcoma.
- Rarely present with symptoms until quite large. Many found incidentally when scanned for other reasons.
- Symptoms usually due to large mass such as abdominal swelling, leg swelling distal to the mass, pain if paraspinal or femoral nerve roots are involved.
- Median presenting size is 15cm.

Diagnosis

Diagnosis is often suggested by CT scan appearances, which may also indicate an alternative diagnosis such as lymphoma or germ cell tumour.

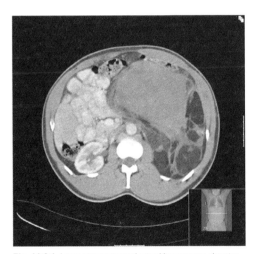

Fig. 11.8.1 Large retroperitoneal mixed liposarcoma showing elements of myxoid differentiation (posteriorly). In these tumours the kidney is often displaced across the midline.

- If operable a biopsy should be performed in collaboration with the surgeons who will perform the operation.
- If not operable a biopsy must be obtained to ensure correct management of an unsuspected alternative diagnosis.
- Sufficient material must be obtained to perform immunohistochemistry to exclude lymphoma, carcinoma, and germ cell tumours.
- Ideally samples should be sent for molecular analysis to characterize histology further, which may affect their future management.

Staging

Staging should include a CT scan of chest (to exclude pulmonary metastases), and abdomen and pelvis (to examine resectability). In retroperitoneal tumours, MRI often adds little information. Bone scintigrams and PET scans have not been demonstrated to be of value in these tumours.

The staging system used is often the AJCC system for limb sarcomas but this is of limited value given the usual size at presentation.

Surgery

Surgery is the treatment of choice and should be performed in a centre with sufficient experience in retroperitoneal surgery. Surgery is complex and may require resection of other structures such as kidney (20% cases), spleen, or bowel. Vascular involvement and metastatic disease are the two most common reasons for inoperability.

Clear resection margins should be the aim. If disease is found at the margins at histological review, re-resection should be attempted if technically feasible.

Chemotherapy

- Adjuvant chemotherapy is not standard treatment in these tumours and in one retrospective study was associated with worse outcome.
- In advanced disease chemotherapy has been used to aim for operability but there is no evidence it improves OS.
- In metastatic disease or inoperable recurrence, chemotherapy may have a role but is dependent upon

histology. Response according to histology is similar to that for other STSs. Leiomyosarcomas may respond to doxorubicin, gemcitabine with docetaxel, trabectedin, and pazopanib. Myxoid liposarcomas may also respond to doxorubicin, ifosfamide, and trabectedin. Dedifferentiated and low-grade liposarcomas are more chemoresistant, although a trial shows some response to trabectedin and to infusional ifosfamide.

Radiotherapy

Postoperative

Postoperative radiotherapy has not been shown to be of benefit in a randomized clinical trial. Several small retrospective or non-randomized studies have shown an improvement in local recurrence rates by up to 30% in completely resected tumours. However, there was no improvement in OS.

In those cases, where postoperative resection margins are involved, radiotherapy may be considered although the proximity of vital structures (kidney, small bowel) may limit the ability to deliver a sufficient dose. There are no randomized controlled trials examining the role of radiotherapy in this setting but a retrospective review including 17 patients with retroperitoneal tumours showed that local control appeared to be improved with radiotherapy. Doses of 64Gy are needed. This is technically challenging in this location but may be achievable with IMRT.

Preoperative

The presence of a large tumour provides some protection to the critical surrounding tissues (kidney, small bowel) if radiotherapy is given preoperatively. This allows higher doses to be administered to the tumour and it is technically easier to plan radiotherapy with the tumour in situ.

Two prospective pilot studies were combined and showed that in 54 patients given radiotherapy preoperatively for primary disease with a median dose of 45Gy (range of 18–50.4Gy), the five-year recurrence-free survival was 60% and OS was 61%. Survival was improved with doses >45Gy. Some patients were also treated concurrently with preoperative doxorubicin. One study used postoperative brachytherapy but this was associated with significant bowel toxicity and was not continued. The phase 3 EORTC STRASS trial failed to show a benefit of preoperative radiation therapy in retroperitoneal sarcoma.

A few pilot studies have also examined the possibility of intraoperative radiotherapy with postoperative radiotherapy. This has shown good local control rates but may be associated with additional toxicities such as damage to the ureters.

Prognosis

Prognostic factors associated with improved survival (in this order) are:

- Complete resection with uninvolved margins
- Grade of tumour
- No metastatic disease

In general, retroperitoneal tumours have a worse prognosis than other STSs of the same histology. This is taken into account in the MSK nomogram (see 'Internet resources') and Sarculator.

Further reading

Demetri GD, Schuetze S, Blay J, et al. Long-term results of a randomized phase II study of trabectedin by two different dose and schedule regimens in patients with advanced liposarcoma or leiomyosarcoma after failure of prior anthracyclines and ifosfamide. *J Clin Oncol* 2009; 27(15s):A10509.

Martin Liberal J, et al. Clinical activity and tolerability of a 14-day infusional Ifosfamide schedule in soft-tissue sarcoma. *Sarcoma* 2013; 2013: 868973.

Internet resources

MSK nomogram: http://www.mskcc.org/mskcc/html/443.cfm
Sarculator app available for iPhone and Android devices

11.9 Gastrointestinal stromal tumour

Introduction

GISTs are a rare subgroup of STSs which can occur anywhere in the gastrointestinal (GI) tract (Figure 11.9.1).

- Incidence is 15 per million per year for all GISTs and 3–4 million per year for high-grade GISTs.
- A small number are associated with a familial GIST syndrome in which there are germline mutations in the KIT gene. Rare paediatric cases are usually wild type with no KIT or PDGFRA (platelet-derived growth factor receptor A) mutation and tend to have a more indolent course. Mutations were identified in the succinate dehydrogenase (SDH) enzyme.
- Defined syndromes associated with GIST include Carney triad, Carney–Stratakis syndrome, and neurofibromatosis type 1.
- The most common sites are stomach (50%) and small bowel (25%). Rarely, they can occur in the colon and rectum (10%), omentum, peritoneum, and mesentery (7%), or oesophagus (5%).

- Presentation is most commonly with anaemia, abdominal mass, or as an incidental finding at endoscopy but abdominal pain may occur with larger tumours. Bowel obstruction is rare even with small bowel tumours.
- Patterns of spread include liver metastases (most common) and peritoneal metastases. Bone metastases occur rarely and late, often after years of treatment. Lung metastases (unlike other STSs) are exceptionally rare. Nodal metastases are also uncommon.

Diagnosis and staging

Diagnosis of GIST is often suspected at endoscopy or on CT scan due to the shape and location of the lesion. Biopsy preoperatively may not be necessary in certain circumstances unless preoperative therapy with imatinib is planned. The disease should be staged to determine operability. CT scan of the primary area and the liver is required. A PET scan is also useful as this may show small peritoneal or liver metastases undetectable by CT scan. Endoscopic ultrasound for upper GI GISTs may also be useful.

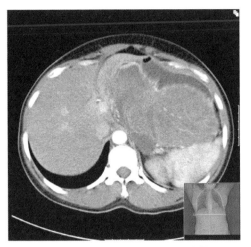

Fig. 11.9.1 Axial CT scan showing a large gastric GIST arising from the greater curvature of the stomach and compressing the stomach lumen.

Pathology and genetics

- The cell of origin is thought to be a precursor to the pacemaker cells of the GI tract, the interstitial cells of Cajal.
- The morphology can be spindle cell (70%), epithelioid (20%), or mixed type (10%).
- 95% of GISTs express c-KIT or the CD117 antigen.
- DOG-1 is as sensitive and specific as CD117 and often reacts in CD117-negative GISTs.
- Mutations in the KIT gene occur in >90% of cases. The exons most commonly affected are:
  - Exon 11 (66%)
  - Exon 9 (13%)
  - Exon 13 (1.2%)
  - Exon 17 (0.6%)
- In those cases with KIT mutations, constitutive activation of the KIT receptor occurs. Activation of KIT is thought to be pathogenetic in familial and sporadic cases.
- In an additional 7% of GISTs, mutations within the PDGFRA gene are found. These are more frequently associated with an epithelioid morphology and with primary site in the stomach. These tend to have a more indolent behaviour.
- The remaining cases, sometimes referred to as 'wild type' GIST, have mostly been found to have different mutations in NF or BRAF, or are SDH deficient. These have a different clinical course and often are not thought to respond to the same agents used in the majority of GIST subtypes.

Factors predicting malignant potential in GIST

The malignant potential of GISTs has been shown to be related to size of the tumour, mitotic rate, and location of the primary. Table 11.9.1 shows the National Institute of Health (NIH) consensus criteria for establishing risk based on size and mitotic count. All GISTs should be regarded as potentially malignant.

Table 11.9.1 Risk of aggressive behaviour in GISTs according to NIH consensus criteria

Risk	Size of tumour	Mitotic count
Very low risk	<2cm	<5 per 50 HPF (high power field)
Low risk	2–5cm	<5 per 50 HPF
	<5cm	6–10 per 50 HPF
Intermediate risk	5–10cm	<5 per 50 HPF
	>5cm	>5 per 50 HPF
High risk	>10cm	Any mitotic rate
	Any size	>10 per 50 HPF

Other features now shown to affect risk of aggressive behaviour are:
- Primary site: duodenal and small bowel GISTs are more aggressive than those arising in the stomach. This has been incorporated into a modified risk stratification.
- Tumour rupture spontaneously or at surgery.
- Location of the KIT mutation has been evaluated in several studies. Some have shown mutations in exon 9 to have a more aggressive course than exon 11.

More work is needed to clarify the prognostic role of mutational analysis.

Management
Localized disease
- Definitive curative treatment is only possible with resection of the primary tumour in the absence of metastases.
- High-risk (and intermediate-risk) tumours are, by definition, at risk of relapse after a clear resection.
- The definition of high risk remains unestablished, but the Miettinen classification is often used in practice.
- It is generally recommended to consider three years of adjuvant imatinib 400mg for resected high-risk GISTs.
- Imatinib is a tyrosine kinase inhibitor (TKI) which blocks signalling via KIT by binding to the adenosine triphosphate (ATP) binding pocket which is essential for phosphorylation and activation of the KIT receptor.
- The ACOSOG Z9001, EORTC 62024, and SSG XVIII phase 3 trials confirmed a significant decrease in relapse-free survival and an increase in OS in high-risk patients receiving adjuvant therapy. Further trials are establishing the optimal duration of adjuvant treatment.
- Mutational analysis also assists in making clinical decisions about adjuvant therapy (see later in this section, 'Location of mutations and response to TKIs', p. 328) Inoperable primary tumours may be rendered operable by the use of imatinib. Mutational analysis should be considered standard for all new cases and relapses of cases not previously tested.

Metastatic disease
Patients with metastatic disease should be treated initially with imatinib 400mg per day, unless mutations predicting resistance to imatinib therapy are found (see later in this section, 'Location of mutations and response to TKIs', p. 328).
- The median time to progression for metastatic disease on imatinib is 20–26 months.

- Imatinib should be continued without a break (except for toxicity) until progression. It has been shown that interrupting treatment is associated with progression, although many patients respond again after reintroduction of imatinib. The impact of interruption of imatinib on survival is uncertain.
- The introduction of imatinib therapy increased the median survival of advanced GIST from 18 to 57 months.

For patients with oligo-metastatic disease who have responded to imatinib, surgical resection, and/or radiofrequency ablation may be considered. At progression, dose escalation of imatinib to 800mg per day may enable temporary control of disease in 30–35% cases with a median time to progression of five months.

For patients progressing on imatinib therapy, sunitinib is the generally recommended second-line therapy. Sunitinib malate is a multitargeted TKI which has shown activity in GISTs which have progressed on imatinib. The median PFS in this clinical situation is six months; 68% patients achieved a partial response or stable disease on sunitinib.

Regorafenib, another multitargeted TKI, was active in patients refractory to imatinib and sunitinib. The median PFS was five months. Ripretinib has recently shown a significant improvement in PFS in the fourth-line.

In patients refractory to all TKI, imatinib rechallenge is a possibility, but duration of benefit is limited.

Other TKIs which have shown activity in GIST but are not in routine use are nilotinib, sorafenib, pazopanib, and cabozantinib.

Assessment of response

Assessment of response in GIST is performed by CT scanning but it has been shown that size criteria of response as defined by RECIST as suboptimal for measuring the activity of imatinib in these tumours.

FDG-PET (fluorodeoxyglucose-PET) can detect reduction in tumour activity within days of commencing imatinib or can visualize small liver metastases which may not be visible on CT scan. Similarly, it can detect increased activity should the tumour develop resistance (new mutations) once on imatinib.

Early response to treatment may not be associated with a significant size change. Choi (2004) described alternative criteria to evaluate GIST response. A 15% reduction in tumour density or 10% unidimensional reduction in tumour size was a better predictor of response than RECIST. Choi's criteria have been shown to correlate better with survival than RECIST.

Location of mutations and response to TKIs

There is a correlation between location of KIT or PDGFRA mutation and response to imatinib or sunitinib:

- Patients with an exon 11 KIT mutation have a greater chance of response to imatinib (67–84%) than those with an exon 9 (40–48%) or no (0–39%) mutation at a dose of 400mg per day.
- Exon 11 responses were also of a longer duration (576 days) than exon 9 (308 days) or those without a mutation (251 days).
- Higher-dose imatinib (800mg per day) has been shown to be of greater benefit in PFS in patients with exon 9 mutations.
- Of the 7% patients with PDGFRA mutations, tumour with the commonest mutation (D842V) is resistant to imatinib but others may respond.
- Sunitinib has been shown to be more effective against exon 9 mutant GIST than standard dose imatinib and also appears to be effective against wild-type disease.
- Secondary mutations that confer resistance to imatinib occur more commonly after prolonged exposure (hence in exon 11 mutant tumours) and may respond to sunitinib.

Further reading

Casali P, Le Cesne A, Velasco AP, et al. Imatinib failure-free survival (IFS) in patients with localized gastrointestinal stromal tumours (GIST) treated with adjuvant imatinib (IM): the EORTC/AGITG/FSG/GEIS/ISG randomized controlled phase III trial (abstract). J Clin Oncol 2013; 31(Suppl. abstr. 10500)—available at: http://meetinglibrary.asco.org/content/114179-132

Choi H, Charnsangavej C, de Castro Faria S, et al. CT evaluation of the response of gastrointestinal stromal tumors after imatinib mesylate treatment: a quantitative analysis correlated with FDG PET findings. AJR Am J Roentgenol 2004; 183(6):1619–28.

Dematteo RP, Ballman KV, Antonescu CR, et al. Adjuvant imatinib mesylate after resection of localised, primary gastrointestinal stromal tumour: a randomised, double-blind, placebo-controlled trial. Lancet 2009; 373:1097.

Joensuu H, Eriksson M, Sundby Hall K, et al. One vs three years of adjuvant imatinib for operable gastrointestinal stromal tumour: a randomized trial. JAMA 2012; 307:1265.

11.10 Future directions in soft tissue sarcoma

Overview

The development of molecularly targeted therapy for GIST in the form of imatinib and sunitinib has raised the hope that other sarcomas will prove similarly treatable. However, whereas the target in GIST is an activating mutation in KIT or PDGFRA resulting in an altered receptor tyrosine kinase, which can be inhibited by a small molecule, the majority of sarcomas with a defined molecular abnormality have a balanced translocation resulting in multiple alterations in gene expression. Most of these are not easily amenable to pharmaceutical intervention. A better understanding of oncogenic signalling pathways and the identification of predictive biomarkers is crucial in the development of targeted therapy. Nevertheless, work is ongoing to exploit this information for new drug development.

Other active areas of research include the development of insulin-like growth factor 1 receptor monoclonal antibodies in Ewing sarcoma and cyclin dependent kinase 4 inhibitors in liposarcoma. Breakthroughs in the field of immuno-oncology allowed the development of immune checkpoint inhibitors. The combination of programmed cell death-1 (PD-1) inhibitors with chemotherapy, targeted therapy, and radiation therapy may benefit certain subtypes of sarcoma and will be investigated thoroughly in the following years. International collaboration is key for research and development in this rare tumour group. With the advent of next generation diagnostic technology, there is genuine hope that major advances will be seen in the field of sarcoma in the next decade.

Tumours of the haemopoietic system

Chapter contents

12.1 Hodgkin lymphoma

Origin and history

Hodgkin lymphoma (HL) is one of the neoplastic diseases of the lymphatic tissue. In 1832, Thomas Hodgkin first described the disease in his historic paper entitled 'On Some Morbid Appearances of the Absorbant Glands and Spleen'. In 1898 and 1902 Carl Sternberg and Dorothy Reed contributed the first microscopic descriptions of the pathognomonic Hodgkin and Reed–Sternberg (H-RS) cells (Figure 12.1.1).

Hodgkin had already assumed that it was an autonomous lymphatic process rather than an inflammatory condition, autoimmune process, or infectious disease like tuberculosis. Despite fragments of evidence for the malignant nature of HL for a very long period of time, the malignant clonal origin of H-RS cells from germinal centre-derived B lymphocytes was shown only recently. However, the mechanisms that drive the proliferative activity and the causes that hinder the cells from undergoing apoptosis, programmed cell death in the germinal centre, are still not fully understood.

Early in the disease process, HL is typically restricted to the lymph nodes. Lymphatic structures are often breached with progression of disease, which then results in organ involvement, mainly of the bone marrow, liver, or lungs. Without effective treatment, the classic form of HL is fatal. However, since the first descriptions of HL, therapeutic strategies have developed from surgery, herbs, and arsenic acid to sophisticated stage- and risk-adapted treatment regimens including modern polychemotherapy and radiotherapy. Currently about 80% of patients achieve long-term disease-free survival (DFS), rendering this entity one of the most curable human cancers.

For patients with newly diagnosed HL, current treatment strategies aim at maintaining the high standard of cure reached for all stages and further improving outcome. At the same time, efforts are made to minimize or prevent therapy-induced complications, such as infertility, cardiopulmonary toxicity, and second malignancies. Ongoing trials for patients with early stage disease try to define the minimal treatment needed for cure with the least acute and long-term toxicity. Over the last few years, there has been a trend towards combining chemotherapy and radiotherapy. Recent studies have predominantly investigated lower doses and smaller fields of radiation and a possible reduction of chemotherapy in terms of number of drugs or cycles given. For patients with advanced stage disease, new schedules of established drug combinations with higher dose density and intensity have been developed. Furthermore, ongoing studies are trying to use new diagnostic tools, such as fluorodeoxyglucose-positron emission tomography (FDG-PET) to enable a response-adapted therapy. Detection of early response during chemotherapy or of a satisfactory response after chemotherapy might allow reduction of treatment cycles or render consolidation radiation unnecessary.

Depending on previous treatment given, approaches for relapsed HL consist of radiotherapy, chemotherapy, and high-dose chemotherapy followed by autologous stem cell transplantation. In recent years, the introduction of effective salvage protocols and a better understanding of prognostic factors have remarkably improved the management of relapsed HL. For patients who relapse after many previous treatments novel approaches using radioimmunoconjugates, monoclonal antibodies, and more recently small molecules targeting signal transcription pathways have demonstrated some clinical efficacy; most of these approaches, however, are still experimental.

Histology

The World Health Organization (WHO) classification defines two types of HL: 1) classical type of HL (cHL) with the subtypes of nodular sclerosis (NS), mixed cellularity (MC), lymphocyte depleted (LD), and lymphocyte-rich classical HL (LRCHL); and 2) nodular lymphocyte predominant HL (nLPHL). There is a substantial variation in the frequency of occurrence between the different subtypes.

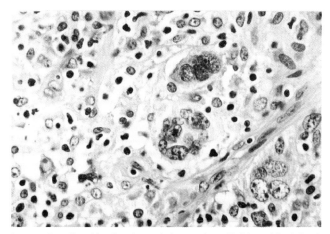

Fig. 12.1.1 Histological staining of an affected lymph node reveals the typical giant Hodgkin and Reed–Sternberg (H-RS) cells (see also colour plate).

Epidemiology

In the Western world, the annual incidence of HL is about two to three per 100,000 persons at risk, and has remained constant over the last decades. As a result of clinical progress in recent years, the mortality rate has dropped, particularly in the 1990s, from earlier rates >2 to a current mortality rate of about 0.5 per 100,000. In Asia, HL occurs only at a very low rate of about 0.6/ 100,000, but Asians who migrate to Western countries will develop HL as frequently as locally born natives. More men than women develop HL with a ratio of 1.4:1. Four out of five males and three out of four females develop HL before the age of 60, which is very early compared to most other malignancies. In industrialized countries, the age at onset has historically shown two peaks, one in the third decade and a second for patients >50 years. However, in more recent analyses, the second peak seems to have disappeared, because non-Hodgkin lymphomas (NHLs) were misclassified mainly as lymphocyte-depleted HL in the past (Table 12.1.1).

There is a noteworthy difference in the timing of onset of HL between developing and industrialized countries: in developing countries, the disorder usually appears during childhood and the incidence decreases with age, whereas in industrialized countries the first peak is seen in young adulthood. Furthermore, in economically developed countries, the early occurrence of HL is often related to better maternal education, early birth order, low number of siblings and playmates, and single-family dwellings. The incidence of HL by age also depends upon histological subtype. Among young adults, the most common subtype is NS HL occurring at a higher frequency than the MC subtype. The frequency of MC increases with age, while NS subtypes reach a plateau in the group >30 years of age.

Pathophysiology

For a long time HL was considered an infectious disease, as indicated by its former designation 'lymphogranulomatosis'. The giant mono- and multinucleated H-RS cells typically account for <1% of the affected tissue in cHL, which made systematic analyses difficult in the past. The detection of their malignant clonal origin in microdissected cells by polymerase chain reaction (PCR) was demonstrated only recently. H-RS cells are derived from germinal-centre B cells in >90% of cases. However, in a small group of patients the H-RS cells exhibit T cell characteristics.

HL can be distinguished from other types of malignant lymphoma by the presence of characteristic tumour cells, H-RS cells, in a background of non-neoplastic cells such as lymphocytes, histiocytes, neutrophils, eosinophils, and monocytes. The histological subclassification of HL considers both the morphology and immunophenotype of the H-RS cells and the composition of the cellular background. The WHO classification differentiates between cHL with CD30-positive H-RS cells and nLPHL with CD20-positive lymphocyte predominant (LP) cells. In cHL, immunophenotyping demonstrated that H-RS cells stain positive for CD15 in about 80% and for CD30 in about 90% of cases. The activation of B-cell antigens has only been reported in few cases. In contrast, the LP cells in nLPHL are scattered in the nodular structures and are usually CD45-positive. They express B-cell associated antigens such as CD20 in 98% of cases, but also express CD19, CD22, CD79a, and epithelial membrane antigen (EMA); however they lack CD15 and CD30 expression.

Despite enormous efforts and progress in basic research, many key questions concerning transforming events and pathways, oncogenic viruses, and the exact mechanism(s) by which H-RS cells proliferate and resist apoptosis in the germinal centre still remain unanswered. Some reports suggest that NF-κB is a central effector of malignant transformation in cHL by downregulation of an anti-apoptotic signalling network. LMP1 as an Epstein–Barr virus (EBV) encoded gene may also induce tumorigenesis by triggering NF-κB activation.

Viral infections (e.g. EBV) have been implicated in the pathogenesis of HL by several studies. Patients with a medical history of EBV-related mononucleosis have a two- to three-fold increased risk of developing HL. In about 50% of cases of cHL in Western countries, EBV DNA is present in the H-RS cells, predominantly in the MC subtype. In contrast, patients with low socioeconomic status and those from developing countries show EBV-positive H-RS cells in about 90% of cases.

However, since EBV is not present in the tumour cells of a substantial proportion of patients in the Western world, other viruses might be involved in the transformation process of HL in these cases. To date, the role of other viruses in the pathogenesis of HL is uncertain and other transforming mechanisms must also be taken into account.

Genetic components seem to contribute to the appearance of this malignancy. Family members of patients affected by HL are at a three- to nine-fold increased risk of developing the same disease. Furthermore, the analysis of monozygotic twin pairs and the remarkable proportion in which both twins are affected strongly supports the idea of HL as a genetically imbalanced disorder. However, no specific mechanisms of inheritance or evidence for a genetic translocation unique to cases of familial HL have been identified so far and familial HL only appears to play a role in a small subset of HL patients.

Table 12.1.1 WHO classification of Hodgkin lymphoma.

	Frequency (%)
Classical Hodgkin lymphoma:	
Nodular sclerosis Hodgkin lymphoma (grades 1 and 2)	60–70
Mixed cellularity Hodgkin lymphoma	20–30
Lymphocyte-rich classical Hodgkin lymphoma	3–5
Lymphocyte-depleted Hodgkin lymphoma	0.8–1
Nodular lymphocyte-predominant Hodgkin lymphoma	3–5

Source: data from Harris NL. Hodgkin's disease: classification and differential diagnosis. *Mod Pathol* 1999; 12:159–76. 1999, Springer Nature Ltd.

12.2 Clinical features, diagnosis, and staging for Hodgkin lymphoma

Clinical features

In most cases, swollen indolent lymph nodes localized in the cervical or supraclavicular region (60–70%) are noticed first, but lymph nodes at other sites can also be affected. Almost two-thirds of patients with newly diagnosed cHL have radiographic evidence of intrathoracic involvement. Symptoms caused by a large mediastinal mass include a feeling of pressure, cough, venous congestion, or even dyspnoea owing to tracheal compression or pericardial or pleural effusions. Hepato- or splenomegaly may indicate hepatic or splenic involvement, but affected organs can also be of normal size. In advanced stages, adjacent regions such as lung, pericardium, chest wall, or bone may also be affected and patients sometimes suffer from bone pain, neurological, or endocrinological symptoms. Compared with NHL, bulky infradiaphragmatic lesions with obstructive symptoms are rare in HL. Bone marrow involvement occurs in <10% of newly diagnosed patients.

About 40% of patients, especially those with initial abdominal involvement or advanced stage disease, report systemic 'B-symptoms' which are defined as fever >38°C, drenching night sweats, or weight loss >10% within the previous six months (with no other cause). Other symptoms include pain at the site of nodal involvement shortly after drinking alcohol, pruritus, or fatigue. Compared with cHL, nLPHL usually begins with localized disease that is rather slowly growing with involvement of only one peripheral nodal region, usually a cervical, axillary, or inguinal lymph node.

Diagnosis and staging

Physical examination should include a thorough inspection and palpation of possibly involved nodal regions, as well as thoracic auscultation and examination of the abdomen, liver, spleen, and spine. An excisional biopsy of a suspicious lymph node should be performed to confirm the initial diagnosis of HL. Adequate material should be obtained but 'debulking' to reduce tumour mass does not improve the prognosis. The assessment of bone marrow is important for disease staging. However, with the advent of PET imaging, bone marrow biopsies can be omitted if PET scanning was performed at initial staging.

Accurate staging procedures and assessment of risk factors are essential to allocate patients to appropriate treatment groups. Clinical staging (CS) methods have become less invasive in recent years. They usually include computed tomography (CT) scans of the neck, thorax, abdomen, and pelvis, PET, and bone marrow biopsy. In some cases, additional or alternative procedures including magnetic resonance imaging (MRI) or a liver biopsy may be indicated. Pathological staging procedures such as laparotomy or splenectomy to assess occult infradiaphragmatic disease are no longer used routinely. They are associated with possible acute or long-term side effects, such as an overwhelming postsplenectomy infection (OPSI) syndrome. Furthermore, better imaging techniques and the introduction of systemic chemotherapy for most patients with early stage disease have restricted invasive measures to a very few patients for whom the initial diagnostic findings give conflicting or unclear results.

The differential diagnosis of HL includes all types of benign or malignant lymph node swelling due to infectious or reactive disease or other types of lymphoma or solid tumours. Infectious lymphadenopathy can be of bacterial (e.g. purulent or tuberculous), viral (e.g. EBV, human immunodeficiency virus (HIV), cytomegalovirus (CMV)), fungal (e.g. coccidomycosis), or parasitic (e.g. toxoplasmosis) origin. Reactive lymphadenopathy can be associated with sarcoidosis as well as other diseases of the soft tissues or the skin or can be drug-induced (e.g. by diphenylhydantoin). Malignant causes include metastases from other solid tumours, leukaemias, or NHL. The differential diagnosis between certain types of HL and NHL can be very challenging and should be performed by an experienced haematopathologist. Occasionally, a composite lymphoma, comprising both HL and NHL, is diagnosed.

HL patients are usually treated according to stage and risk factors. The histological subtype—except for the nodular lymphocyte predominant type—does not influence the treatment decision. The stage of HL at diagnosis is determined according to the Ann Arbor classification depending on the number of nodal regions involved and their distribution on one (stage I+II) or both (stage III) sides of the diaphragm or on organ involvement (stage IV). The presence (B) or absence (A) of systemic symptoms further characterizes severity of disease. Clinical, biological, and serological risk factors further influence the choice of treatment. The Cotswolds modification (proposed in 1989 during a meeting held in the Cotswolds, England) of the Ann Arbor classification uses information from staging and treatment collected over 20 years. Information about prognostic factors such as mediastinal mass, other bulky nodal disease, extranodal extension of disease, and the extent of subdiaphragmatic disease is included in this classification (Figure 12.2.1).

Generally, patients with clinical stage I and II without risk factors are allocated to the early stage favourable group, and those with risk factors to the early stage unfavourable group. Patients with stage III and IV disease are assigned to the advanced stage risk group. Besides stage and B-symptoms, most groups have included larger tumour burden as a relevant prognostic factor (bulky disease >10cm or a large mediastinal mass >1/3 of thoracic diameter).

However, there are still small differences in the definition of risk factors used and the classification of certain subgroups of HL patients among the different study groups in Europe and the USA. In the USA, patients are usually either allocated to early or advanced stages. More patients, even those with low tumour burden, are included in the advanced stage group. These patients then receive more therapy than in most European countries, which must be considered when comparing the data.

Prognostic factors define the likely outcome of the disease for an individual patient at diagnosis. Such analysis may be used to inform a patient, or in the context of clinical trials, to describe the study population or guide data

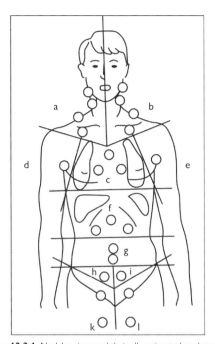

Fig. 12.2.1 Nodal regions and their allocation to lymph node areas; regions above the diaphragm: Waldeyer´s ring, upper cervical/nuchal/submental/cervical region, supraclavicular region, infraclavicular region (area a/b); upper/lower mediastinal region, lung hilum (area c); and axillary region (area d/e). Regions below the diaphragm: spleen and spleen hilum, liver hilum, coeliac region (area f); mesenteric and para-aortic region (area g); iliac region (area h/i); and inguinal region (area k/l).

analysis. For clinicians, the most important use of prognostic factors is to select appropriate treatment strategies. In an attempt to define the risk for patients with advanced HL more precisely, a variety of clinical and laboratory parameters have been analyzed to construct a prognostic index. The International Prognostic Score (IPS) consists of seven factors that have been shown to be significantly related to an unfavourable prognosis when present at initial diagnosis: serum albumin <4g/dl, haemoglobin <10.5g/dl, male sex, age <45 years, stage IV disease, leukocytosis >15.000/mm^3, lymphocytopenia <600/mm^3, and/or <8% of white cells. This score has maintained its validity in patients treated with current standard approaches.

Prognostic factors may be used to identify patients either for treatment intensification or treatment reduction. Reduction may be achieved by creating a modified protocol or by including these patients in the early stage group.

Intensification by early high-dose chemotherapy with haematological stem cell support has not shown a clinically relevant long-term survival benefit compared with conventional treatment. Since clinical and biological factors so far have not been able to select patients with advanced-stage disease who will progress during therapy or experience an early relapse, new molecular, genetic, or biological parameters that reliably predict response and outcome are awaited.

12.3 Treatment of early stage Hodgkin lymphoma

Definition and prognostic groups

According to current knowledge, risk-adapted therapy can be stratified into three groups: early favourable, early unfavourable, and advanced stage. Patients in the early stage favourable group are those with clinical stage I and II disease at diagnosis without risk factors. Those with certain risk factors are allocated to the early stage unfavourable group.

Early stage favourable HL

Radiotherapy

In the treatment of early stages, extended-field radiotherapy (EFRT) was considered standard treatment for a long time. The extended-field strategy delivers radiation to all initially involved and adjacent lymph node regions, leading to large irradiation fields compared with involved-field radiotherapy (IFRT), which is restricted to the initially involved lymph node regions only. With the successful introduction of MOPP and ABVD chemotherapy for advanced stages in the 1980s, the shift from radiation alone to additional chemotherapy in early stages was accelerated by the recognition of long-term toxicity and mortality related to large radiotherapy fields and doses. Longer follow-up of patients who underwent EFRT showed the development of

severe late effects as competing causes of death, including heart failure, pulmonary dysfunction, and secondary malignancies. Furthermore, though complete remission was generally achieved, there was a high risk of relapsing from first-line treatment when EFRT alone was given. Two different strategies were explored to prevent these relapses: either using even more intensive radiotherapy or adding chemotherapy for early favourable stages to control occult lesions. The latter strategy produced better outcomes and at the same time enabled reduction of radiotherapy to the involved field for this risk group.

Thus radiotherapy alone is almost obsolete, with one exception: patients with a first diagnosis of nLPHL clinical stage IA without risk factors are usually not included in ongoing trials for HL. On the basis of the very favourable prognosis of this subtype, European groups currently recommend treatment with 30Gy IFRT only. This less toxic strategy seems to produce similar responses for nLPHL IA patients to those obtained with combined modality treatment and better tumour control than with anti-CD20 antibody treatment. Compared with nLPHL stage IA patients, advanced nLPHL stages at initial diagnosis have less favourable outcomes and are therefore treated according to protocols used for cHL.

Chemoradiotherapy and chemotherapy

Most centres and groups in Europe and the USA have accepted combined modality treatment, consisting of two cycles of ABVD, followed by 20Gy IFRT as the standard of care for early favourable stage disease. Several randomized trials have confirmed the superiority of combined modality treatment over radiotherapy alone. Other trial results have led to reduced radiation fields and doses as well as decreased chemotherapy drug combinations and duration of treatment.

The Southwest Oncology Group (SWOG) demonstrated that patients treated with combined modality therapy consisting of three cycles of doxorubicin and vinblastine followed by subtotal lymphoid irradiation (STLI) had a markedly superior outcome in terms of freedom from treatment failure (FFTF) than those receiving STLI alone (94% vs. 81% at three years). Another study from Milan showed that STLI can be effectively replaced by IFRT after short duration ABVD (adriamycin, bleomycin, vinblastine, dacarbazine) chemotherapy, while maintaining the same progression-free survival (PFS) (97%) and overall survival (OS) (93%) at five years. The European Organization for Research and Treatment of Cancer (EORTC) and the Groupe d'Étude des Lymphomes de l'Adulte (GELA) demonstrated that combined modality with either six courses of EBVP (H7F trial) or three of MOPP (mustine, vincristine, procarbazine, prednisone)/ABV (adriamycin, bleomycin, vinblastine) (H8F trial) followed by IFRT yielded a significantly better event-free survival than that achieved by subtotal nodal irradiation alone. The aim of their H9F trial was to evaluate a possible dose reduction of radiotherapy (36Gy or 20Gy or no radiotherapy) after administering six cycles of EBVP. However, the arm without radiotherapy was closed prematurely due to a higher relapse rate than expected.

Although EBVP was used instead of ABVD in this setting, the use of chemotherapy alone in early favourable stages should currently still be regarded as experimental. A combined modality approach was also used in the HD7 trial by the German Hodgkin Study Group (GHSG). In this trial, two cycles of ABVD plus EFRT were shown to be superior to EFRT alone in terms of FFTF (88% vs. 67% at seven years). OS was equal in both arms due to effective salvage treatment. Further improvement in treatment seems difficult due to the already excellent long-term survival rates. Thus, strategies to reduce drug dose and toxicity while maintaining efficacy are being pursued. In the subsequent HD10 trial of the GHSG, a possible reduction in chemotherapy from four to two cycles of ABVD and/or IFRT from 30 to 20Gy was evaluated. The final analysis revealed no significant differences in FFTF and OS between patients receiving four or two cycles of ABVD or those receiving different doses of radiotherapy (30Gy or 20Gy). The GHSG follow-up HD13 trial then evaluated whether it is possible to omit the presumably less effective drugs, bleomycin or dacarbazine, from the ABVD regimen and patients were randomized between two cycles of ABVD, ABV, AVD, or AV (adriamycin, vinblastine) followed by 30Gy IFRT. However, the arms without dacarbazine (ABV and AV) were closed prematurely for safety reasons because there was more progressive disease in these arms. The recent final analysis also showed impaired tumour control among patients who had received AVD chemotherapy. Ongoing and recently completed trials incorporated PET as a tool to help evaluating early response and reduce chemotherapy or avoid radiation for some patients with very good prognosis. Results from larger randomized trials such as the UK RAPID trial and the EORTC/LYSA/FIL H10 study are available showing decreased tumour control in patients who do not receive radiation even with a negative PET after chemotherapy. However, OS is still excellent when a PET-based approach is applied. Generally, mature data from more prospective trials are needed for final conclusions regarding this issue.

Early stage unfavourable HL

Patients with early stage unfavourable (intermediate) HL are generally treated with combined modality treatment. However, the ideal chemotherapy and radiation regimens have not yet been clearly defined. Optimization of therapy in this risk group is being attempted by reducing radiation doses and field sizes in a similar manner to that for early favourable stages.

Several trials seem to indicate that the reduction of field size does not compromise the efficacy of treatment. A trial from Italy comparing STLI with IFRT after four cycles of ABVD in patients with early favourable and unfavourable stages reported a similar treatment outcome in both arms. In the H8U trial, the EORTC randomized patients between six cycles of MOPP/ABV + 36Gy IFRT, four cycles of MOPP/ABV + 36Gy IFRT, and four cycles MOPP/ABV + STLI. There was no difference between the groups in terms of response rates, failure-free survival, or OS. The largest trial investigating radiotherapy reduction was conducted by the GHSG: in the HD8 trial, patients were randomized to two alternating cycles of COPP/ABVD plus radiotherapy to either extended (arm A) or involved field (arm B). Final results at five years as well as a follow-up analysis at ten years did not show any significant differences between the two arms in terms of FFTF and OS, but more toxicity was reported in patients treated with EFRT.

In early unfavourable stages, efforts were made to improve the efficacy of chemotherapy by altering drugs and schedules as well as the number of cycles. In the past, alternation or hybridization of a MOPP-like regimen with ABVD did not produce better outcomes when compared with ABVD alone. Furthermore, studies in advanced stage HL indicated that ABVD alone is equally effective and less myelotoxic than alternating MOPP/ABVD, and both are superior to MOPP alone. Thus, a combined modality treatment consisting of four courses of ABVD followed by 30Gy IFRT is considered standard treatment for patients with early stage unfavourable HL. Despite the excellent initial remission rates obtained with ABVD and radiotherapy, approximately 15% of patients with early unfavourable stages relapse within five years and about another 5% suffer from primary progressive disease. These outcomes are similar to those in patients with advanced stage disease, treated with more intense regimens. Thus, study groups evaluated regimens for the early unfavourable group that had been previously tested for the treatment of advanced stages.

In the EORTC/GELA H9U trial, patients were randomly assigned to six cycles of ABVD, four cycles of ABVD, or four cycles of BEACOPP-baseline, followed by 30Gy IFRT in all arms. After a median follow-up of four years, no significant difference was observed between the three different treatment arms with respect to event-free survival (EFS) or OS. The final results of the GHSG trial HD11 did not show significantly better results with BEACOPP-baseline in comparison with ABVD either. However, these results led the GHSG to a further intensification of treatment. Thus for this patient group, the HD14 trial for early unfavourable stages introduced the BEACOPP escalated regimen, which had shown high efficacy in the treatment of advanced HL. Patients were randomized to 2x BEACOPP escalated + 2x ABVD or 4x ABVD followed by 30Gy IFRT. This '2+2'combination was associated with improved tumour control in comparison with ABVD alone and was therefore adopted as standard of care for the treatment of younger patients with early unfavourable HL within the GHSG. Results of the HD17 study published in 2020 reported that omission of radiotherapy in patients who achieved a complete metabolic response after 2+2 combination did not result in a loss of tumour control.

12.4 Treatment of advanced stage Hodgkin lymphoma

Definition

Patients in the advanced stage risk group are those with clinical stage III and IV disease at diagnosis or special risk factors, which slightly differ between the various European and US study groups.

Prognosis

Before the introduction of combination chemotherapy, >95% of patients with advanced HL succumbed to their disease within five years. The remission rates achieved with MOPP were a major breakthrough and MOPP was subsequently used successfully for many years in advanced stage disease, with long-term remission rates of nearly 50%. The regimen was then replaced by ABVD, after a series of large multicentre trials had proved the superiority of ABVD and alternating MOPP/ABVD over MOPP alone. Hybrid regimens such as MOPP/ABV were only as effective as alternating MOPP/ABVD and even rapidly alternating multidrug regimens such as COPP/ABV/IMEP did not result in better outcome. However, more acute toxicity and a higher incidence of leukaemia were reported after the MOPP/ABV combination as compared with ABVD.

Treatment options

Chemotherapy

Different study groups have tried to improve the cure rates achieved with ABVD by developing new regimens with additional drugs by increasing dose intensity using colony-stimulating factors and modern antibiotics. These new approaches include multidrug regimens such as Stanford V, MOPPEBVCAD, VAPEC-B, ChlVPP/EVA, and various BEACOPP variants.

Stanford V was developed as a short-duration, reduced-toxicity programme and was given weekly over 12 weeks. Consolidating radiotherapy to sites of initial disease was used. With an estimated five-year FFP (freedom from progression) of 89% and OS of 96%, it seemed to be a promising strategy when used at a single centre. However, a prospective randomized multicentre comparison with MOPPEBVCAD and ABVD showed that Stanford V was clearly inferior in terms of response rate and PFS so that the authors concluded that ABVD was still the best choice when it was combined with optional, limited irradiation. These conflicting results may be partly explained by the use of less radiotherapy in the randomized setting and better treatment quality in single-centre studies. The Manchester group developed VAPEC-B, an abbreviated 11-week chemotherapy programme and conducted a randomized comparison with the hybrid ChlVPP/EVA. After five years, EFS and OS were significantly better with ChlVPP/EVA than with VAPEC-B.

The GHSG HD9 trial compared COPP/ABVD, BEACOPP-baseline, and BEACOPP-escalated. Results from 1,195 randomized patients showed a superiority of escalated BEACOPP over BEACOPP-baseline and COPP/ABVD at five years. The follow-up data at ten years confirmed these results. The subsequent GHSG HD12 trial aimed at de-escalating chemotherapy and radiotherapy by comparing eight courses of BEACOPP-escalated with four courses of escalated and four courses of baseline BEACOPP, with or without consolidation radiation to initial bulky and residual disease. However, no significant difference regarding toxic events between the arms could be detected and a reduced efficacy of the reduced chemotherapy schema could not be excluded. In the GHSG follow-up HD15 trial, patients were randomized between eight courses of BEACOPP-escalated, six courses of BEACOPP-escalated, or eight courses of BEACOPP-14, which is a time-intensified variant of BEACOPP-baseline. Additional radiotherapy was only given to residual PET-positive lesions larger than 2.5cm. The final analysis of this study revealed the best outcome for patients treated with six cycles of BEACOPP-escalated. Six cycles of BEACOPP-escalated followed by PET-guided radiotherapy was therefore adopted as standard of care within the GHSG.

The question whether escalated BEACOPP is superior to ABVD alone was addressed in a number of randomized studies and a large network meta-analysis. While prospective trials have consistently shown an improved tumour control and a non-significant trend towards a better OS with escalated BEACOPP, the results of the meta-analysis also indicated a superior OS with escalated BEACOPP. The survival advantage was 10% at five years.

Further intensification of first-line therapy in high-risk patients by directly administering high-dose chemotherapy and autologous stem cell transplantation after four instead of eight cycles of ABVD did not improve outcome compared with conventional treatment. BEACOPP chemotherapy is generally associated with more haematological toxicity, sterility, and secondary leukaemia when compared with ABVD. Nevertheless, cardiotoxicity and pulmonary side effects are similar with both regimens, especially when combined with radiotherapy.

At present, several prospective clinical studies are evaluating the combination of ABVD and BEACOPP variants in combination with the antibody–drug conjugate brentuximab vedotin which has shown impressive single agent activity in heavily pretreated patient with cHL. In addition, these trials are investigating whether early PET-guided treatment stratification is possible in patients with

Table 12.4.1 The ABVD and the BEACOPP escalated protocol

Doxorubicin	25mg/m^2	i.v.	Days 1 + 15
Bleomycin	10mg/m^2	i.v.	Days 1 + 15
Vinblastine	6mg/m^2	i.v.	Days 1 + 15
Dacarbazine	375mg/m^2	i.v.	Days 1 + 15
Bleomycin	10mg/m^2	i.v.	Day 8
Recycle Day 29			
Etoposide	200mg/m^2	i.v.	Day 1–3
Doxorubicin	35mg/m^2	i.v.	Day 1
Cyclophosphamide	1,250mg/m^2	i.v.	Day 1
Vincristine	1.4mg/m^2	i.v.	Day 8
Procarbazine	100mg/m^2	p.o.	Day 1–7
Prednisone	40mg/m^2	p.o.	Day 1–14
G-CSF		s.c.	From Day 8
Recycle Day 22			

advanced HL. However, mature results of these trials are pending (Table 12.4.1).

Elderly patients with HL

Although the general health and performance status (PS) of elderly HL patients may vary considerably, age at diagnosis remains an unfavourable risk factor, particularly for patients with advanced stage disease. For most study groups, patients are considered 'elderly' if they are >60 years. Factors such as more aggressive disease, more frequent diagnosis of advanced stage, comorbidity, poor tolerance of treatment, failure to maintain dose intensity, shorter survival after relapse, and death due to other causes contribute to the poorer outcome of elderly patients. A retrospective analysis of GHSG trials showed that elderly patients have a poorer risk profile, more treatment-associated toxicity, a lower dose-intensity, and higher mortality as major factors for poorer outcome. Generally, elderly patients without major comorbidities

who are sufficiently fit to tolerate standard therapy have a treatment outcome comparable to that of younger patients. In the GHSG HD9$_{elderly}$ trial, patients aged 66–75 years with advanced stage HL were treated with either COPP/ABVD or BEACOPP baseline. Tumour control appeared to be better with the BEACOPP regimen, but toxicity was higher, resulting in no differences in FFTF or OS. Based on these results, the BEACOPP protocol should not be applied in HL patients aged over 60.

Whenever possible, elderly patients should be treated with a doxorubicin-containing regimen. Large radiotherapy fields should be avoided. At present, ABVD represents a reasonable choice for older HL patients in a good general condition. In case of lung comorbidities, bleomycin may be omitted from the protocol. Alternative protocols consist of the PVAG and the VEPEMB protocols that have shown good results and a tolerable toxicity profile in older HL patients.

12.5 Management of relapsed Hodgkin lymphoma

Treatment options

The majority of HL patients achieve complete remission with current first-line treatment. Patients who relapse still have a chance of being cured with adequate salvage treatment. Depending on first-line therapy, there are various treatment options. Conventional chemotherapy is usually the treatment of choice for patients who relapse after initial radiotherapy only. In contrast, those who relapse after prior chemotherapy should receive high-dose chemotherapy (HDCT) followed by autologous stem cell transplantation (SCT). Other experimental options, such as allogeneic SCT and monoclonal antibodies are being evaluated for multiply pretreated patients. Depending on the duration of remission after first-line treatment, most study groups categorize failures into three subgroups: early relapses, late relapses, and primary progressive HL.

Recurrence after radiotherapy

Conventional chemotherapy is the treatment of choice for patients who relapse after initial radiotherapy for early stage disease. The survival of these patients is similar to that of patients with advanced stage HL initially treated with chemotherapy.

Recurrence after chemotherapy

The best treatment for recurrent HL after primary chemotherapy is high-dose chemotherapy. A number of salvage protocols that can be given prior to high-dose chemotherapy and autologous stem cell transplantation have been developed during the last decade. Those include DHAP (dexamethasone, high-dose cytarabine, cisplatin), ICE (ifosfamide, carboplatin, etoposide), and IGEV (ifosfamide, gemcitabine, vinorelbine). So far, two randomized trials have demonstrated the superiority of HDCT followed by autologous SCT over conventional chemotherapy. The British National Lymphoma Investigation (BNLI) reported that patients with relapsed or refractory HL receiving high-dose BEAM (BCNU (carmustine), etoposide, cytarabine, melphalan) with autologous SCT fared significantly better than those treated with conventional dose mini-BEAM. The three-year EFS was 53% versus 10% for those treated with conventional chemotherapy. In the HDR1-trial of the GHSG, chemosensitive patients relapsing after initial chemotherapy were randomized between four cycles of Dexa-BEAM and two cycles of Dexa-BEAM followed by BEAM and autologous SCT. The final results at five years demonstrated a higher FFTF in the transplanted group when compared with the group receiving conventional salvage chemotherapy (55% vs. 34%).

The European HDR2 intergroup study evaluated whether treatment results can be improved by the introduction of a sequential high-dose chemotherapy programme prior to autologous stem cell transplantation. Unfortunately, the promising results of the pilot study could not be confirmed in the randomized setting and no superiority in comparison with the standard treatment could be demonstrated. Thus, two to four cycles of a salvage protocol followed by high-dose chemotherapy and autologous stem cell transplantation remained the standard of care in patients with relapsed HL who respond to chemotherapy.

For patients with primary progressive disease during first-line treatment or within 3 months after the end of first-line therapy, conventional salvage chemotherapy has given disappointing results in the vast majority of patients. Therefore, these patients should be treated with high-dose chemotherapy followed by autologous stem cell transplantation whenever possible. The effectiveness of HDCT and autologous SCT in patients with biopsy-proven primary refractory HL was shown by the Memorial Sloan–Kettering Cancer Center in a study of 75 consecutive patients. At a median follow-up of ten years for surviving patients, the EFS, PFS, and OS rates were 45%, 49%, and 48% respectively. Chemosensitivity to second-line chemotherapy was predictive for a better survival.

The success of HDCT followed by autologous SCT does not depend only on obvious factors such as tumour burden or chemosensitivity. A prognostic score based on treatment outcome of patients with relapsed HL also identified the time to relapse, the clinical stage at relapse, and the presence of anaemia as independent risk factors.

Recurrence after HDCT and autologous SCT

Depending on the patient's physical condition, there are several options. In some patients, allogeneic SCT can be discussed; however, it cannot yet be considered an alternative standard treatment in patients with relapsed HL. So far, the advantages of a potential graft-versus-lymphoma effect are offset by a high transplant-related mortality (TRM). As shown in a matched-pair analysis, TRM might be significantly reduced by employing a reduced-intensity conditioning regimen (RIC). A study by Peggs et al. (2005) using RIC in 49 HL patients showed the potential for durable responses in patients who have previously had substantial treatment for HL. Allogeneic SCT following RIC might thus become an appropriate strategy in selected subgroups of young poor-risk patients; however, the number of patients treated is still small, requiring further clinical studies to define clear indications.

Depending on age, number, and character of relapses, previous therapies and presence of concomitant diseases, it should be carefully evaluated whether a curative or a palliative approach is appropriate. A palliative regimen can achieve satisfactory pain control, improve general condition, and lead to partial, sometimes rather long-lasting remissions. Drugs such as gemcitabine, vinorelbine, vinblastine, idarubicin, or etoposide are mostly given as monotherapy which can be combined with corticosteroids. The most promising alternative is gemcitabine which proved to be an effective and well tolerated drug, even for patients with multiple relapses of HL.

Experimental strategies in the treatment of HL include passive immunotherapy based on monoclonal antibodies to specifically target malignant cells and drugs that modulate the tumour microenvironment and the immune system. Other more recent promising drugs include the antibody–drug conjugate brentuximab vedotin as well as the anti-PD1 antibodies nivolumab and pembrolizumab which have shown promising single agent activity in heavily pretreated patients with classical HL. Further antibody-based drugs and small molecules are currently undergoing investigation in phase 2 studies.

Further reading

Peggs KS, Hunter A, Chopra R, Parker A, Mahendra P, et al. Clinical evidence of a graft-versus lymphoma effect after reduced intensity allogeneic transplantation. *Lancet* 2005; 365:1906–8.

12.6 Long-term toxicities and fertility issues of Hodgkin lymphoma

Surveillance and long-term toxicities

During follow-up of HL patients, attention should be paid to two crucial areas. First, more than two-thirds of relapses occur within 2.5 years and >90% within five years after initial treatment. The patient should therefore be given a schedule for follow-up visits and examinations (Table 12.6.1). Second, a number of long-term toxic effects related to treatment of HL can occur. They include minor disorders such as endocrine dysfunction, long-term immunosuppression, and viral infections. Serious impairments include lung fibrosis from bleomycin and irradiation, myocardial damage from anthracyclines and irradiation, sterility, growth abnormalities in children, opportunistic infections, psychological and psychosocial problems, and fatigue. Potentially fatal effects include the overwhelming postsplenectomy infection (OPSI) syndrome after splenectomy or spleen irradiation, and secondary neoplasms. Acute myeloid leukaemia and myelodysplastic syndrome are mostly observed within the first three to five years and secondary NHL mainly at 5–15 years after initial treatment. Solid tumours, such as lung or breast cancer can also occur decades after initial treatment and sometimes multiple tumours develop.

Fertility issues

Due to the substantially improved long-term survival in young patients with HL undergoing chemotherapy, preservation of fertility becomes an increasingly important issue. Regimens such as COPP, MOPP, or BEACOPP containing alkylating agents such as procarbazine or cyclophosphamide often lead to therapy-induced infertility, whereas ABVD is less gonadotoxic. For men, cryopreservation of semen prior to therapy is possible; strategies for women include ovarian cryopreservation with auto- or xenotransplantation; in vitro maturation of thawed primordial follicles followed by fertilization and embryo transfer has successfully been established.

Data on co-treatment to preserve ovarian function is still scarce. A retrospective analysis from the GHSG demonstrated that the rate of therapy-induced amenorrhoea is higher in women receiving eight cycles of escalated BEACOPP than in women treated with ABVD alone, COPP/ABVD, or standard BEACOPP. Moreover, amenorrhoea after therapy was most pronounced in women with advanced stage HL, in those >30 years at treatment, and in women who did not take oral contraceptives during chemotherapy. Administration of oral contraceptives or gonadotropin-releasing hormone agonists during chemotherapy may possibly result in lower rates of ovarian failure, but larger studies are awaited.

Further reading

Behringer K, Goergen H, Hitz F, et al. Omission of dacarbazine or bleomycin, or both, from the ABVD regimen in treatment of early-stage favourable Hodgkin's lymphoma (GHSG HD13): an open-label, randomised, non-inferiority trial. *Lancet* 2015; 385(9976):1418–27.

Böll B, Görgen H, Fuchs M, et al. ABVD in older patients with early-stage Hodgkin lymphoma treated within the German Hodgkin Study Group HD10 and HD11 trials. *J Clin Oncol* 2013; 31(12):1522–9.

Eichenauer DA, Aleman BMP, André M, et al. ESMO Guidelines Committee. Hodgkin lymphoma: ESMO Clinical Practice Guidelines for diagnosis, treatment and follow-up. *Ann Oncol* 2018; 29(Suppl. 4):iv19–29.

Engert A, Plütschow A, Eich HT, et al. Reduced treatment intensity in patients with early-stage Hodgkin's lymphoma. *N Engl J Med* 2010; 363(7):640–52.

Hasenclever D, Diehl V. A prognostic score for advanced Hodgkin's disease. International Prognostic Factors Project on Advanced Hodgkin's Disease. *N Engl J Med* 1998; 339(21):1506–14.

Table 12.6.1 Follow-up assessment for Hodgkin lymphoma: information for HL patients concerning follow-up examinations

Examination time point	First year			Second to fourth year	Fifth year onwards
	Month 3	Month 6	Month 12	Every six months	Annually
Physical examination	X	X	X	X	X
Case history	X	X	X	X	X
Laboratory tests:					
Blood count and differential distribution	X	X	X	X	X
ESR, CRP	X	X	X	X	X
TSH	X	X	X	X	X
CT[a] (if partial response)	X[a]		X		
CXR (if no CT)	X		X	X[b]	X
Lung function		X			
Abdominal ultrasound	X		X	X[b]	X

a Further CT scans are recommended according to findings in final restaging and follow-up.

b Imaging examinations annually.

CRP: C-reactive protein; CT: computed tomography; CXR: chest X-ray; ESR: erythrocyte sedimentation rate; TSH: thyroid stimulating hormone.

Küppers R, Engert A, Hansmann ML. Hodgkin lymphoma. *J Clin Invest* 2012; 122(10):3439–47.

Moccia AA, Donaldson J, Chhanabhai M, et al. International Prognostic Score in advanced-stage Hodgkin's lymphoma: altered utility in the modern era. *J Clin Oncol* 2012; 30(27):3383–8.

Radford J, Illidge T, Counsell N, et al. Results of a trial of PET-directed therapy for early-stage Hodgkin's lymphoma. *N Engl J Med* 2015; 372(17):1598–607.

Raemaekers JM1, André MP, Federico M, et al. Omitting radiotherapy in early positron emission tomography-negative stage I/II Hodgkin lympho-ma is associated with an increased risk of

early relapse: Clinical results of the preplanned interim analysis of the randomized EORTC/LYSA/FIL H10 trial. *J Clin Oncol* 2014; 32(12):1188–94.

Skoetz N, Trelle S, Rancea M, et al. Effect of initial treatment strategy on survival of patients with advanced-stage Hodgkin's lymphoma: a systematic review and network meta-analysis. *Lancet Oncol* 2013; 14(10):943–52.

von Tresckow B, Plütschow A, Fuchs M, et al. Dose-intensification in early unfavorable Hodgkin's lymphoma: final analysis of the German Hodgkin Study Group HD14 trial. *J Clin Oncol.* 2012; 30(9):907–13.

12.7 Non-Hodgkin lymphoma

Introduction

Non-Hodgkin lymphomas (NHLs) are a group of lymphoid malignancies of varying subtypes arising from B cells, T cells, natural killer (NK) cells, or their precursors with a range of clinical behaviours requiring different treatment strategies. There is a high incidence in Europe, USA, and Australia and the lowest incidence in Asia. Around 14,000 new cases are diagnosed each year in the UK and 72,000 cases in the USA. The median age is 65 although aggressive B-cell lymphomas are the predominant NHL in younger adults. The male to female ratio is 1.5:1.

Aetiology

The aetiology of NHL is largely unknown. Autoimmune disease and immunodeficiency are known to predispose to NHL. Sjögren's disease (associated with marginal zone lymphomas of salivary gland) and rheumatoid arthritis are linked with NHL. Immunodeficiency (both acquired and inherited) and solid organ transplantations increase the risk of NHL. In patients with AIDS, NHL is the second most common malignancy, and its incidence is declining due to antiretroviral therapy. A number of infective agents are associated with various types of NHL. These include:

- EBV: associated with post-transplant immunoproliferative disorders, immunodeficiency associated lymphomas (e.g. HIV associated primary central nervous system (CNS) lymphoma), Burkitt lymphoma, etc.
- Human herpesvirus 8 (HHV-8): associated with primary effusion lymphoma, and plasmablastic lymphoma in Castleman disease.
- Human T-lymphotropic virus 1 (HTLV-1): associated with adult T-cell lymphoma/leukaemia.
- Hepatitis C virus (HCV): associated with extranodal and splenic marginal zone B-cell lymphoma.
- *Helicobacter pylori*: associated with gastric marginal zone B-cell lymphoma of mucosa-associated lymphoid tissue (MALT) type. Eradication of *H. pylori* can lead to regression of this type of lymphoma.

Prior radiotherapy and chemotherapy also increase the risk of NHL. Obesity is associated with an increased risk of diffuse large B-cell lymphoma (DLBCL) and genome-wide association studies (GWAS) have identified multiple susceptible loci that are associated with an increased risk of follicular lymphoma and marginal zone lymphomas.

Some studies suggest that sun exposure and alcohol may be protective against NHL.

Pathology

The cell of origin is different for each subtype of lymphoma. Classification is by the updated WHO modification of the REAL (revised European and American lymphoma) classification system which is broadly divided into B cell, T cell/natural killer cell, and Hodgkin disease. Immunophenotyping has a significant role in the classification of NHL. Table 12.7.1 gives a summarized classification showing common varieties of NHL, and their cytogenetic and molecular characteristics. B-cell lymphomas constitute >90% of NHL, and T-cell lymphomas approximately 10%. Immunohistochemistry based on the expression of cell surface antigens and immunoglobulin proteins, which in turn depends on the type of lymphocyte and its stage of differentiation, is important diagnostically and to determine causality. B-cell lineage is indicated by pan B-cell markers (CD22, CD19, and CD20) and T-cell lineage by T-cell markers (CD3, CD2, CD7, CD4, and CD8). Immunophenotyping using flow cytometry is used in the subclassification of NHL. The markers of mature B-cell NHL include surface Ig heavy and light chains, CD79a, CD19, CD20, and CD22. Antibodies such as CD5, CD10, CD23, and cyclin D1 are used to subtype NHL (see Table 12.7.1). In the majority of lymphomas there is good reproducibility (>85%) in the diagnoses except in Burkitt-like lymphoma, lympho-plasmacytic lymphoma, and marginal zone B-cell lymphoma of nodal type (<60%).

Chromosomal translocations and molecular rearrangement are used to confirm diagnosis. The most common chromosomal abnormality in NHL is t(14;18) (q31;q21), which is found in >80% of follicular lymphomas and >25% of diffuse large B-cell lymphoma. Follicular lymphoma and diffuse large B-cell lymphoma constitute >50% of adult NHL. Next-generation sequencing (NGS) studies have led to significant understanding of the pathogenesis, progression, and prognosis of different subtypes of NHL. Table 12.7.2 summarizes the recent advances in the molecular knowledge of NHL.

The REAL classification is important for management and prognostication. Based on biological behaviour there are three categories of NHL: indolent (low grade), aggressive, and highly aggressive.

- Indolent lymphomas (e.g. follicular, small lymphocytic, lymphoplasmacytic, etc.) usually occur in older adults and are characterized by a waxing and waning course. More than 80% of patients with indolent lymphomas present with advanced stage disease with a high risk of involvement of bone marrow. Some of the tumours

Table 12.7.1 A summary of WHO–REAL classification of NHL

Type of NHL	Biological behaviour	Immunohistochemistry
B-cell neoplasms (>90%)		
Precursor B-cell neoplasms	Highly aggressive	B-cell marker (CD19, PAX-5) positive
Precursor B lymphoblastic leukaemia/lymphoblastic lymphoma	Low grade	TdT+, CD99+, CD10+
Mature B-cell neoplasms (83%)	Low grade	Rearrangement of Ig heavy chain gene
CLL/small lymphocytic lymphoma (17%)	Low grade	CD20+, CD3−, CD10−, CD5+, CD23+
Lymphoplasmacytic lymphoma (0.9%)	Low grade	CD20+, CD3−, CD10−, CD5−, CD23−
Splenic marginal zone lymphoma (0.4%)	Low grade	CD20+, CD3−, CD10−, CD5−, CD23−
Extranodal marginal zone lymphoma of MALT type (3.8%)	Low grade	CD20+, CD3−, CD10+, CD5−
Nodal marginal zone B-cell lymphoma (1.5%)	Low grade	CD20+, CD3−, CD10−, CD5+, CD24−, PRAD1+
Follicular lymphoma (12%)	High grade	CD20+, CD3−
Mantle zone lymphoma (2.2%)	Favourable group, of DLBCL	
Diffuse large B-cell lymphoma (23%)		
Mediastinal large B-cell lymphoma (0.1%)		
Burkitt lymphoma (1.4%)	Highly aggressive	CD20+, CD3−, CD10−, CD5−, Tdt−
T-cell and NK-cell neoplasms (7%)		
Precursor T-cell and NK-cell neoplasms (0.9%)	Highly aggressive	CD20−, CD3+, CD30+, CD15−, EMA+, ALK+
Precursor T-lymphoblastic leukaemia/lymphoblastic lymphoma		
Peripheral T-cell and NK-cell neoplasms (3.8%)	Low grade	CD30+
T-cell prolymphocytic leukaemia (0.1%)	High grade	
Aggressive NK-cell leukaemia (0.2%)	Highly aggressive	
Adult T-cell lymphoma/leukaemia (0.1%)	Low grade(MF)	
Mycosis fungoides/Sézary syndrome (1.5%)	Low grade	
Primary cutaneous anaplastic large cell lymphoma (0.3%)	High grade	
Peripheral T-cell lymphoma (1.4%)		
Anaplastic large cell lymphoma (1%)	Different behaviour (e.g. nodal disease aggressive and skin disease indolent)	

Table 12.7.2 Cytogenetic characteristics of common varieties of NHL

Type of NHL	Cytogenetic abnormality	Genes involved
Mature B-cell neoplasms:		
CLL/small lymphocytic lymphoma	17p13 del	TP53
Lymphoplasmacytic lymphoma	t(9;14)(p13;q32)—50%	pax-5
Splenic marginal zone lymphoma	7q21–32 deletion	CDK6
Extranodal marginal zone lymphoma of MALT type	t(11;18)(q21;q21)—50%	api2/mlt
Nodal marginal zone B-cell lymphoma	t(1;14)(p22;q32)	bcl-10
Follicular lymphoma	t(14;18)(q32;q21)—90% t(2;18)(p11;q21) t(18;22)(q21;q11)	bcl-2
Mantle zone lymphoma	t(11;14)(q13;q32)—70%	bcl-1/cyclin D1
Diffuse large B-cell lymphoma	der (3)(q27)—35%, t(14;18) (q32;q21)	bcl-6 bcl-2
Mediastinal large B-cell lymphoma (0.1%)	9p gain	REL
Burkitt lymphoma (1.4%)	t(8;14)(q24;q32)—80% t(2;8)(p11;q24)—15% t(8;22)(q24;q11)	c-myc
T-cell and NK-cell neoplasms:		
Anaplastic large cell lymphoma	t(2;5)(p23;q35)—70–80%% t (1;2)(q25;p23)—10–20%	npm/alk tpm3/alk

can transform to high-grade, large-cell lymphoma. Indolent lymphomas are not curable.

- Aggressive lymphomas can occur in any age group. These tumours are fast growing and untreated are fatal within a year or two. Diffuse large B-cell lymphomas and some of the T/NK cell lymphomas fall into this category. Patients can present with all stages of disease and bone marrow involvement indicates a poor prognosis. Approximately 70–80% of patients achieve complete remission (CR) with combination chemotherapy, of whom two-thirds are cured.

- Burkitt and lymphoblastic lymphomas constitute the highly aggressive category of NHL. These subtypes are common in children and young adults and are very fast growing. These tumours present with advanced stage and a high incidence of bone marrow and CNS involvement. With combination chemotherapy some patients with these tumours can be cured, especially those who present with early stage disease.

12.8 Clinical features of non-Hodgkin lymphoma

Introduction
The clinical presentation of patients with NHL is extremely variable. Patients most commonly present with painless lymph node enlargement. In indolent lymphoma, lymphadenopathy may wax and wane. Other symptoms are due to specific organ involvement, e.g. abdominal pain due to obstruction by bulky disease, spinal cord compression, etc.

Constitutional symptoms, known as B symptoms (fever >38°C, night sweats, unintended weight loss of >10% of body weight during the last six months) occur in up to 50% of patients.

Diagnosis
The most important step in treating patients with NHL is an accurate histopathological diagnosis. Diagnosis of NHL and its subtypes is based on the histopathological, immunohistochemical, and genetic evaluation of an adequate sample of tissue. A fine needle aspiration or cytology is therefore not appropriate for the initial diagnosis of lymphoma. An excisional lymph node biopsy or a generous incisional biopsy of an involved organ is the preferred method of obtaining a sample. If these methods are not possible, a cutting core biopsy is the best option.

An image-guided core biopsy might be the only option in certain situations where there is no easily accessible lymph node, e.g. where there is retroperitoneal involvement.

Diagnostic standards for the classification of malignant lymphomas are laid down in the 2014 edition of the WHO classification of haematopoietic tumours. Conventional histological examination of paraffin-embedded sections, immunohistochemistry, and genetic tests (fluorescence in situ hybridization (FISH) analyses, cytogenetics, molecular genetics, e.g. PCR) are mandatory to provide an accurate diagnosis. Gene expression profiling and DNA sequencing are being increasingly used in clinical practice.

Staging
Once the diagnosis of NHL is established, detailed staging must be undertaken to determine sites of involvement by the lymphoma. This is the basis for the choice of the most appropriate therapy.

Initial evaluation of a patient with NHL should include a careful history and clinical examination. The presence or absence of constitutional symptoms should be noted. The PS of the patient should be assessed using the Karnofsky or ECOG (Eastern Cooperative Oncology Group) score.

A complete physical examination should be done with particular attention to location and size of enlarged lymph nodes including Waldeyer's ring and size of the liver and spleen.

Laboratory studies should include a complete blood count with careful examination of a peripheral blood smear to evaluate for the presence of circulating lymphoma cells. Serum biochemical tests should include an assessment of renal and hepatic function and the uric acid level. Lactate dehydrogenase (LDH) can identify patients with a high tumour mass and is a prognostic factor in indolent and aggressive lymphomas.

Serological testing for HIV and hepatitis should be performed before starting therapy.

A bone marrow biopsy (BMB) has been part of the standard staging evaluation. In patients with bone marrow involvement on PET-CT scan, a BMB is not required. In patients with DLBCL with no bone marrow disease on PET-CT scan, a BMB is only indicated if the presence of a discordant histology would affect management. In all other situations, a unilateral biopsy of at least 2.5cm in length is recommended with immunohistochemistry and flow cytometry.

Standard imaging studies include CT scans of the neck, chest, abdomen, and pelvis, as well as other apparently involved sites. The major criterion for recognition of nodal involvement is that of size. Detection of lymphoma in normal sized lymph nodes is not possible.

PET scan is being increasingly used for pretreatment assessment and is essential for response assessment. PET scan is the preferred method of staging for FDG-avid lymphomas and CT scan for non-avid lymphoma (e.g. small lymphocytic lymphoma, lymphoblastic lymphoma, marginal zone, etc.). A diagnostic lumbar puncture is recommended in patients with neurological symptoms or in patients presenting with sinus or testicular involvement.

Colonoscopy should be performed in mantle cell lymphoma, which often involves the bowel. Gastroduodenal endoscopy and endoscopic ultrasound are mandatory in gastric MALT lymphomas.

If anthracyclines are included in the treatment regimen, an echocardiogram should be performed.

Other diagnostic procedures may be useful in specific patients.

Based on the results of the diagnostic procedures, patients are assigned to an Ann Arbor stage I–IV. The suffix A or B reflects the absence or presence of constitutional symptoms. However, constitutional symptoms do not confer an unfavourable outcome for NHL and therefore these suffixes are not needed for NHL.

Assessing response to treatment in NHL

An end of treatment PET-CT scan is essential for response assessment. A five-point-scoring system (Deauville score) as below is recommended for reporting PET-CT:

- No uptake.
- The highest uptake in site(s) of lymphoma is less than or equal to the uptake in the mediastinum.
- The highest uptake in site(s) of lymphoma is more than the uptake in the mediastinum but less or equal or the uptake by the liver.
- Uptake is greater than the uptake by the liver.
- New sites of uptake or substantial increase in the standardized uptake value (SUV) in previous sites of lymphoma. X—new area of uptake unlikely to be related to lymphoma.

Complete metabolic response (CMR) in NHL is defined as score of 1–3 with or without a residual mass with no evidence of FDG-avid disease in marrow. Partial metabolic response (PMR) is defined as a score of 4 or 5 with reduced uptake compared with baseline scan. A score of 4 or 5 with no significant change in FDG uptake from baseline is defined as no metabolic response (stable disease), whereas a score of 4 or 5 with increased SUV from baseline and/or new FDG avid sites consistent with lymphoma is considered as progressive metabolic disease.

Prognosis

Clinical prognostic markers

The International Prognostic Index (IPI) has been developed based on data from patients with aggressive B-cell and T-cell lymphoma who were treated with an anthracyclin-containing regimen. Based on five risk factors that correlate with survival, all patients can be stratified into different prognostic groups as follows:

- Age >60 years
- Serum LDH concentration greater than normal
- ECOG PS ≥2
- Clinical stage III or IV
- Number of involved extranodal disease sites >2

The prognostic groups include low risk (IPI 0–1), low–intermediate risk (IPI 2), high–intermediate risk (IPI 3), and high risk (IPI 4).

While incorporation of treatment with rituximab has improved prognosis in all four risk groups, the IPI retains its clinical relevance. The age-adjusted IPI (aaIP1) defines four prognostic categories for patients ≤60 years based on risk factors of stage III–IV, PS 2–4, and serum LDH above normal.

- Low risk (no-risk factors)
- Low–intermediate risk (1 risk factor)
- High–intermediate risk (2 risk factors)
- High risk (3 risk factors)

The IPI can also be applied to indolent lymphomas, but the Follicular Lymphoma International Prognostic Index (FLIPI) score has been shown to be more discriminatory.

The FLIPI score comprises five adverse factors: age >60 years, advanced stage, haemoglobin level <12.0g/l, elevated serum LDH, and involvement of more than four extranodal sites. The FLIPI defines three risk groups: low risk (0–1 adverse factor), intermediate risk (2 adverse factors), and poor risk (3 adverse factors). The addition of rituximab has significantly improved OS of CD20+ indolent lymphomas. The FLIPI2 is the new scoring system which is useful for patients treated with immunochemotherapy. It comprises five adverse factors: age >60 years, bone marrow involvement, haemoglobin level <12.0g/dl, greatest diameter of the largest involved node >6cm, and serum beta-2 microglobulin level greater than the upper limit of normal. The FLIPI2 defines three risk groups: low risk (no risk factor), intermediate risk (1–2 risk factors), and high risk (3–5 risk factors).

Molecular prognostic markers

Most clinical risk factors are based on surrogate markers. Molecular genetic analysis adds important information for lymphoma biology and prognosis.

Gene expression profiling in DLBCL allows differentiation between a germinal centre B-cell (GCB) and an activated B-cell (ABC) type. These two subgroups can be considered distinct diseases. In the GCB type the cell of origin is a germinal centre B cell and in the ABC type it is a postgerminal centre B cell. When treated with rituximab-chemotherapy, the clinical outcome is much better in the GCB type with a three-year survival of 85% versus 69% in the ABC type (P=0.032).

Lymphomas with mutations of MYC gene and either BCL2 or BCL6 ('double-hit') have a poor prognosis with immunochemotherapy.

In follicular lymphomas, a new prognostic model (m7-FLIPI) incorporates ECOG PS and mutation of seven genes (EZH2, ARID1A, MEF2B, EP300, FOXO1, CREBBP, and CARD11). It is yet to be adopted into routine clinical practice.

12.9 Treatment of low-grade disease

Introduction

By far the most prevalent subtype of low-grade lymphoma is follicular lymphoma, the second most common B-cell lymphoma in the Western world. Follicular lymphoma accounts for approximately 20% of all lymphomas with an annual incidence of three per 100,000. The clinical course of follicular lymphoma is highly variable and characterized by a continuous pattern of relapse. Most patients present with advanced disease and with the availability of monoclonal antibodies, the median survival has improved from eight to ten years to 15 years or more. Spontaneous regression (up to 12%) occasionally occurs.

Transformation to an aggressive histological type occurs in up to 40% and is associated with a poor prognosis.

The WHO classification divides follicular lymphoma into three grades: grade I (0–5 centroblasts/high power field (HPF)), grade II (6–15 centroblasts/HPF), and grade III (>15 centroblasts/HPF). Grade III is subdivided into IIIA (most cells are centrocytes) and IIIB (with sheets of centroblasts). Grade IIIA is treated similarly to follicular lymphoma whereas IIIB behaves aggressively and should therefore be treated like a diffuse large B-cell lymphoma.

Early stage

Only about one-third of patients with follicular lymphoma present initially with limited stages I and II or stage III limited (with up to five involved lymph nodes). Patients with stage I and II disease are considered for involved-site radical radiotherapy to a dose of 24Gy in 12 fractions. A recent retrospective study of patients staged with PET-CT reported a five-year freedom from progression (FFP) of 74.3% for stage I and 48.1% with stage II disease. Almost 90% of patients achieved a CMR after radiotherapy and the five-year OS was 95.8%. 2.5% of patients developed in-field or marginal relapses whereas 25.8% developed distant relapses. Watchful waiting or rituximab monotherapy is an option if radiotherapy is not appropriate (e.g. patient choice to avoid side effects, or large radiotherapy portal).

Patients with early stage bulky disease should be treated like patients with advanced disease.

Advanced stage

In patients with advanced disease stage III and IV, no curative treatment is yet established. The treatment options include watch and wait, single agent rituximab with or without maintenance or a combination of chemotherapy with rituximab. Previous clinical trials using different chemotherapy regimens could not demonstrate a survival benefit for early initiation of chemotherapy compared with deferred treatment. A recent phase 3 trial compared watch and wait with rituximab (rituximab induction 375mg/m weekly ×4) or rituximab induction followed by maintenance treatment (375mg/m² once every two months ×12) in asymptomatic patients with advanced stage follicular lymphoma. While there was a significant difference in the time to start of new treatment, with 54% of patients in the watch and wait group needing treatment within three years compared with 12% of patients who received maintenance rituximab, three-year survival was similar in both groups (94% vs. 97%).

In the absence of a clear survival benefit with early treatment, the goal of treatment in these patients must be to improve quality of life and delay the impact of treatment-related toxicity. Based on these data, treatment in advanced follicular lymphoma should be initiated only when lymphoma-associated symptoms occur.

In practice, treatment is indicated most frequently due to potential or actual local compressive disease or impairment of organ function, bulky disease, constitutional symptoms, or rapid disease progression. Other indications are bone marrow infiltration with consequent haematopoietic impairment, massive hepatosplenomegaly, or transformation to an aggressive lymphoma.

The treatment options include rituximab monotherapy or rituximab in combination with CHOP, CVP (cyclophosphamide, vincristine, prednisolone), or bendamustine. There are four prospective trials and a meta-analysis showing the benefit of the addition of rituximab to chemotherapy in terms of PFS and OS. The Italian FOLL05 trial showed that the combination of R-CHOP (rituximab, cyclophosphamide, doxorubicin, vincristine, prednisone) and R-FM (fludarabine and mitoxantrone) is superior in terms of time to failure (TTF) and PFS compared with R-CVP. However, R-CHOP has a better toxicity profile compared with R-FM. The three-year PFS in this study was 95%. A German phase 3 trial compared six cycles of CHOP with six cycles of single agent bendamustine and both groups received rituximab on day 1 of each cycle of chemotherapy. At a median follow-up of 24 months, R-bendamustine resulted in a better median PFS (69.5 months vs. 31.3 months, P<0.0001) compared with R-CHOP. The toxicities were also fewer in the R-bendamustine group.

Because of the high relapse rate in follicular lymphoma, maintenance therapy with different agents has been investigated for improving outcome. Interferon-alpha has been shown to prolong OS when given as maintenance therapy but its toxicity profile precluded widespread use. The intergroup PRIMA phase 3 study evaluated the role of two years of rituximab maintenance in patients with follicular lymphoma responding to first-line immunochemotherapy. Six-year PFS was better with rituximab maintenance (59% vs. 43%, P <0.001), but there was no improvement in OS. A German phase 3 trial failed to show any improvement in OS with autologous stem cell transplantation (ASCT) after initial immunochemotherapy.

Relapsed disease

All patients should have a biopsy to rule out aggressive transformation. Treatment of relapse depends on the symptoms and treatment-free interval. Patients with low volume relapse may be observed. In patients with early relapse (<12–24 months) treatment with rituximab-containing chemotherapy combinations or radioimmunotherapy may be used.

Over the past few years it has been shown in two large randomized trials that rituximab maintenance has a clear clinical benefit in relapsed or refractory follicular lymphoma after induction with chemotherapy alone and rituximab plus chemotherapy. In the EORTC trial 20981, 465 patients were initially randomized to six cycles of CHOP or R-CHOP. Responders were randomized to maintenance with rituximab once every three months for a maximum of two years or observation. Rituximab maintenance yielded an impressive improvement of median PFS from second randomization of 51.5 months versus 14.9 months with observation. OS was improved with 85% at three years versus 77% and the hazard ratio was 0.52. In a second prospective randomized trial of the GLSG, patients with recurring or refractory follicular lymphoma and mantle cell lymphoma (MCL) were randomized to four courses of FCM (fludarabine, cyclophosphamide, mitoxantrone) alone or combined with rituximab. Responders were randomized to rituximab maintenance comprising two further courses of four-times-weekly doses of rituximab after three and nine months. Response duration was significantly prolonged by maintenance therapy after R-FCM and PFS was doubled. OS was improved with 82% versus 55% at three years.

In conclusion, both trials demonstrated that rituximab maintenance therapy significantly prolongs OS in relapsed follicular lymphoma with a low rate of clinically relevant side effects.

The role of consolidating autologous stem cell transplantation in first remission was evaluated in three randomized trials from the pre-rituximab era. In conclusion, none of these studies could show a relevant improvement in long-term outcome. In addition, the risk of secondary neoplasms after stem cell transplantation has to be considered.

Multiple studies have also shown the efficacy of radioimmunotherapy (RIT) both as a single agent and in combination with chemotherapy. By conjugating a radio-isotope to an anti-CD20 antibody, radiation is directly delivered to the tumour cell. Ibritumomab tiuxetan, an yttrium-90 labelled radioimmunoconjugate, is registered in Europe to treat relapsed follicular lymphoma. One recently presented trial has demonstrated a significant benefit for ibritumomab consolidation after initial chemotherapy without rituximab. Other studies are underway looking at personalized vaccines and oral targeted therapies that work by inhibiting the enzyme SKY kinase (e.g. biovax ID and fostamatinib).

Treatment recommendations

In patients presenting with stage I and II disease without bulky disease, involved-site radiotherapy (24Gy in 12 fractions) is the treatment of choice with curative potential.

To date there is no standard treatment in advanced follicular lymphoma. To achieve long PFS, rituximab in combination with chemotherapy such as CHOP FM, or bendamustine should be administered. Rituximab monotherapy or a brief course of immunochemotherapy with full course of rituximab is an alternative in elderly patients with comorbidities. Rituximab maintenance for two years significantly prolongs PFS in primary disease. Ibritumomab tiuxetan with or without prior reinduction is an effective and safe treatment in first and subsequent relapses. The role of autologous transplantation in relapse is being evaluated in clinical trials.

12.10 Diffuse large B-cell lymphoma

Introduction

Diffuse large B-cell lymphoma (DLBCL) constitutes 30–60% of NHL. Treatment approach depends on age, IPI, and feasibility of dose intensification.

Early stage disease (stage I–II)

Approximately 30–40% patients with DLBCL present with limited stage disease. Those with non-bulky disease are treated with three cycles of R-CHOP chemotherapy followed by involved-site radiotherapy (30–36Gy). However, six cycles of R-CHOP chemotherapy may be an alternative if radiotherapy is likely to result in significant morbidity (e.g. oropharyngeal, salivary gland, or pelvic region). Patients with bulky limited stage disease are treated with six cycles of R-CHOP with involved-site radiotherapy to bulky disease or intensified R-ACVBP (doxorubicin, vindesine, cyclophosphamide, bleomycin, and prednisolone).

Advanced stage disease

Approximately 60–70% patients present with advanced disease and they are considered for six to eight cycles of R-CHOP or clinical trials. Patients aged 60–80 years are considered for six to eight cycles of R-CHOP whereas patients aged >80 years or unfit for standard chemotherapy are considered for R-miniCHOP or replacement of doxorubicin with gemcitabine, etoposide, or liposomal doxorubicin.

Patient with ≥2 risk factors, especially those with more than one extranodal disease or increased LDH, are considered for CNS prophylaxis with intravenous high-dose methotrexate.

Primary mediastinal B-cell lymphoma

Primary mediastinal B-cell lymphomas present with bulky mediastinal disease associated with pleural or pericardial effusions. Staging and prognostication are similar to nodal DNBCL and PET/CT scan is essential for diagnosis and treatment response assessment.

Standard treatment is rituximab based immunochemotherapy (R-CHOP, dose-dense CHOP, or a dose intense regimen such as DA-EPOCH-R). While consolidation mediastinal radiotherapy is recommended (30–36Gy), its role in patients with CMR is not known. The IELSG-37 is a current randomised clinical trial evaluating the role of consolidation radiotherapy after CMR.

Patients who do not achieve CMR after first-line treatment are considered for high-dose chemotherapy and autologous stem cell transplantation, particularly if residual disease is confirmed on biopsy.

Patients who remain disease free after 18 months are considered to be cured and those who relapse are considered for salvage treatment similar to nodular DLBCL.

12.11 Mantle cell lymphoma

Introduction

Mantle cell lymphomas constitute 4–9% of all lymphomas and have an aggressive and variable clinical behaviour. The median age at presentation is 60 years with patients generally presenting with advanced stage disease. Conventional chemotherapy remains a non-curative approach with a median survival of three to six years. However, the addition of rituximab, dose-intensified chemotherapy, and autologous stem cell transplantation have improved the median survival to more than ten years.

Clinical presentation includes extensive lymphadenopathy, involvement of blood and bone marrow and marrow, and splenomegaly and involvement of extranodal sites such as the gastrointestinal (GI) tract and CNS.

Immunohistochemistry shows tumour cells are typically CD5+, CD20+, and CD23– with the majority expressing cyclin D1. The chromosomal translocation t(11:14) (q13; 32) is characteristic of MCL.

Staging is as for other lymphomas; on PET/CT imaging the sites of disease show low to intermediate SUVs.

Prognostic index

The Mantle Cell International Prognostic Index (MIPI) is based on prognostic factors of age, ECOG PS, LDH levels, and white blood cell (WBC) count (Hoster et al. 2008).

First-line therapy

As a result of the aggressive clinical course of mantle cell lymphoma, a watch and wait strategy is not generally recommended. However, a subset of patients characterised by splenomegaly and bone marrow involvement may have an indolent course and a period of watch and wait is justified in this group of patients.

Patients with non-bulky stage I–II disease may be treated with three to four course chemotherapy (R-CHOP) followed by involved site radiotherapy (30–36Gy). Radiotherapy alone for these patients may lead to an early relapse within one year.

Patients with stage I–II disease with large tumours or adverse prognostic factors are treated with primary systemic treatment followed by consideration for consolidation radiotherapy if appropriate.

Younger patients (≤65 years) with stage III–IV disease may be considered for dose-intensified immunochemotherapy (e.g. R-CHOP, high-dose cytarabine) followed by consideration of autologous stem cell transplantation and rituximab maintenance. Older patients and patients with comorbidities may be considered for conventional immunochemotherapy (R-CHOP) followed by rituximab maintenance.

An early dose-intensified phase 2 study of rituximab plus hyper-CVAD (cyclophosphamide, vincristine, doxorubicin, and dexamathasone) alternating with high-dose methotrexate/cytarabine in newly diagnosed mantle cell lymphoma reported a median TTF of 4.6 years and the median OS was not reached after ten years of follow-up. Among patients ≤65 years, the median TTF was 5.9 years and 64% of patients were projected to live beyond ten years. The Nordic MCL2 study reported a median OS and response duration of more than ten years and a median event-free survival of 7.4 years with intensive induction immunochemotherapy followed by ASCT. The European MCL network trial compared six courses of R-CHOP followed ASCT (Arm A) with alternating courses of R-CHOP (x3) and R-DHAP (x3) followed by ASCT (Arm B) in patients aged <65 years with stage II–IV MCL. At median follow-up of 51 months, the TTF (88 months vs. 46 months, P=0.0382) and OS were superior with arm B compared with arm A. The phase 3 LyMa trial evaluated the role of maintenance rituximab (consisting of one infusion of rituximab ($375mg/m^2$) every two months for three years) after ASCT in patients aged <66 years with stage II–IV disease. This study showed that maintenance rituximab leads to a 60% reduction in risk of progression and a 50% reduction of risk of death. The four-year PFS (82.2% vs. 64.6%, P=0.0005) and OS (88.7% vs. 81.4%, P=0.0413) were better with rituximab maintenance. Thus patients ≤65 years are treated with dose-intensive immunochemotherapy followed by ASCT and rituximab maintenance.

Immunochemotherapy (R-CHOP x6–8 or R-bendamustine x6) is the treatment of choice for the elderly (>65 years) and patients who are not suitable for the intensive chemotherapy. In frail patients, less intensive immunochemotherapy (e.g. VADC, PEP-C) may be considered for palliation.

Second-line therapy

Second-line treatment depends on the efficacy of previous treatment and duration of disease control. Relapses within 12 months of previous treatment should be treated with non-cross resistant regimens (e.g. bendamustine, R-BAC) or newer agents.

In a phase 2 study, patients with relapsed or refractory mantle cell lymphoma were treated with bendamustine, a nitrogen mustard compound, and rituximab (BR regimen). The CR rate was 60% and the median PFS was 30 months. The addition of cytarabine with BR regimen (R-BAC) improved the CR rate to 70% but was associated with significant cytopenias. In a phase 2 study with 155 patients with relapsed mantle cell lymphoma, bortezomib was administered for up to 17 cycles. Response rate in 141 assessable patients was 33% including 8% CR/Cru (Cru indicates CR unconfirmed). Median time to progression was 6.7 months with a median OS of 23.5 months. The most common adverse event of grade 3 or higher was peripheral neuropathy (13%). Temsirolimus, an inhibitor of the mammalian target of rapamycin kinase (mTOR), has shown activity in a phase 2 trial conducted by the North Central Cancer Treatment Group. Twenty-nine patients with relapsed or refractory MCL received temsirolimus 25mg intravenously every week as a single agent for at least six cycles. The overall response rate was 41% with one complete response and ten partial responses. The median time to progression was six months. Haematological toxicities were the most common toxicities observed (50% grade 3). In a phase 3 study, high-dose temsirolimus (175mg) led to an objective response rate (ORR) of 22% and PFS of 4.8 months.

A study of ibrutinin (a brutons tyrosine kinase inhibitor) led to an ORR of 68% with a CR of 21%.

In patients who previously have had conventional chemotherapy, high-dose chemotherapy and ASCT is an option.

Further reading

Hoster E, Dreyling M, Klapper W, Gisselbrecht C, van Hoof A, et al. A new prognostic index (MIPI) for patients with advanced-stage mantle cell lymphoma blood. German Low Grade Lymphoma Study Group (GLSG) and the European Mantle Cell Lymphoma Network. 2008 Jan 15; 111(2):558–65.

12.12 Cutaneous non-Hodgkin lymphomas

Epidemiology

Primary cutaneous lymphomas present in the skin without evidence of extracutaneous disease at the time of diagnosis. This group of lymphomas has to be differentiated from secondary involvement of the skin by primary systemic lymphomas.

The annual incidence is one per 100,000 with a much higher overall prevalence because most primary cutaneous lymphomas are indolent malignancies with a long survival.

Primary cutaneous lymphomas differ considerably in their clinical course and outcome from systemic lymphomas. They are classified according to the WHO–EORTC classification (2005) and primary cutaneous lymphomas are generally divided into lymphomas with an indolent or an aggressive clinical course.

Approximately 75–80% of primary cutaneous lymphomas are T-cell lymphomas and the remainder are B-cell lymphomas. Mycosis fungoides (MF) and primary cutaneous CD30+ lymphoproliferative disorders account for approximately 90% of cutaneous T-cell lymphomas.

Primary cutaneous CD30+ lymphoproliferative disorders include primary cutaneous anaplastic large cell lymphoma and lymphomatoid papulosis. Both entities can only be differentiated by their clinical course.

The remaining group of primary cutaneous T-cell lymphomas constitutes <10% of all cases and is very heterogeneous in terms of clinicopathological features. Prognosis of this group is poor.

Primary cutaneous B-cell lymphomas are subclassified as primary cutaneous marginal zone B-cell lymphoma, primary cutaneous follicle centre B-cell lymphoma, and primary cutaneous diffuse large B-cell lymphoma, leg-type.

Clinical features

MF typically presents with erythematous patches, plaques, and tumours usually in areas not often exposed to sunlight. Most patients have multiple lesions and ulceration can occur. The lesions can be atrophic and dyspigmented. The course of the disease is indolent.

The lesions of MF can be classified into four groups: T1 and T2 with patches and plaques affecting less or more than 10% of body surface, T3 with tumours >1cm, and T4 with erythroderma affecting >80% of body surface.

In T1 disease outcome is excellent and patients with T2 disease also have a median OS of more than ten years.

Patients with erythrodermic MF have a median survival of five years and those with visceral involvement have an even worse survival of only one or two years.

Sézary syndrome (SS) is defined as an erythrodermic cutaneous T-cell lymphoma with haematological evidence of leukaemic involvement and can be preceded by MF. Sézary cells are atypical cerebriform mononuclear cells circulating in the peripheral blood. However, morphological features alone are prone to interobserver variability. Therefore, the diagnosis of SS should be made primarily on the basis of objective molecular or flow cytometric evidence of a clonal abnormal T-cell population in the peripheral blood.

The clinical behaviour of the disease is aggressive.

MF and SS are classified according to the TNMB (tumour node, metastasis, blood) staging system.

Primary cutaneous marginal zone B-cell lymphoma and primary cutaneous follicle centre B-cell lymphoma usually show an indolent clinical behaviour. The former presents characteristically with violaceous solitary or multiple papules or nodules located mainly on the extremities. Spontaneous resolution may occur. In some cases, association with *Borrelia burgdorferi* has been reported.

Primary cutaneous follicle centre B-cell lymphoma preferentially involves the head and trunk with solitary or grouped plaques and tumours. The presence of multiple lesions is not of prognostic importance.

In both entities, transformation into a DLBCL is extremely rare.

Cutaneous relapses are common in both types. However, extracutaneous dissemination rarely occurs.

The five-year survival is excellent, >95% in both entities.

In contrast, primary cutaneous diffuse large B-cell lymphoma, leg-type, behaves aggressively, and affects predominantly elderly patients. This entity typically presents as red solitary or multiple nodules on the leg but can also rarely be found at other sites. Both cutaneous relapses and extracutaneous dissemination are frequent.

With a five-year survival of only 50%, prognosis is significantly worse than for the other two entities.

Investigations and staging

All patients should be fully staged to exclude extracutaneous disease and investigations include full clinical examination, full blood count (FBC), biochemistry, and imaging studies including PET/CT scan. Bone marrow examination is needed for aggressive or intermediate lymphomas. Flow cytometry of peripheral blood is indicated in patients with SS. MF/SS is staged according to the TNMB staging.

Management of cutaneous T-cell lymphoma

In patients with early stages of MF, topical therapy with mechlorethamine or bexarotene, superficial radiotherapy, and phototherapy (psolarens +UVA (PUVA)) are appropriate treatment options.

Patients with more advanced disease will require some form of systemic treatment. Total skin electron beam therapy (TSEBT) is appropriate in patients with generalized thickened plaques or tumorous disease due to its depth of penetration. The rate of complete response is >80% but the long-term outcome is not affected. TSEBT should be followed by an adjuvant therapy such as mechlorethamine or PUVA to prolong the duration of response.

Patients with erythroderma are difficult to manage. Electron beam therapy often leads to severe desquamation. Patients without evidence of circulating peripheral cells are suitable candidates for low-dose PUVA. Initial doses must be very low to avoid phototoxic reactions.

In patients with leukaemic or nodal involvement, systemic treatment usually in combination with topical therapy is required.

Extracorporal photophoresis (ECPP) can be used for patients with erythroderma and a low number of circulating cells. ECCP is usually administered every four weeks, but the frequency can be increased to twice monthly.

Systemic therapy can be with a single agent or a combination. Methotrexate, chlorambucil, and gemcitabine are active agents. Low-dose methotrexate leads to an overall response rate of 30–50%. A number of single agents are evaluated in progressive and relapsed MF/SS. The orally administered retinoid bexarotene can achieve response rates of 50%, and has been approved by the European Medicines Agency as a second-line treatment after at least one prior systemic therapy. Bexarotene is teratogenic. Liver function and serum lipids must be carefully monitored. Pegylated doxorubicin achieved an overall response rate of 80% in patients with relapsed and refractory MF in one trial. Vorinostat, an oral histone deacetylase inhibitor was evaluated in patients with progressive or relapsed MF/SS. An objective response was achieved in 30%. Remarkably, vorinostat seems not to be cross-resistant to other agents. Alemtuzumab, an anti-CD52 monoclonal antibody leads to an overall response of up to 55% in erythrodermic MF. Superiority of one agent has not been shown so far.

Most frequently used combination chemotherapy regimens include cyclophosphamide, vincristine, and prednisone with or without doxorubicin. There are no trials comparing single-agent chemotherapy with combination chemotherapy.

High-dose chemotherapy followed by autologous stem cell transplantation in patients with advanced disease has been shown to induce high response rates in most patients but the responses were predominantly of short duration (time to progression just over two months). In contrast, allogeneic transplantation seems to induce long-term durable remissions of >3 years.

Management of cutaneous B-cell lymphoma
Treatment options include local and systemic treatment modalities.

Due to their indolent course and the excellent outcome in primary cutaneous marginal zone and follicle centre B-cell lymphoma, a watch-and-wait strategy is adequate management in most cases with asymptomatic lesions.

In patients with limited symptomatic skin lesions, local excision or radiotherapy (20–36Gy) are the first choices of treatment. Both modalities result in nearly 100% CR. However, local recurrence or relapse at distant sites occurs in approximately one-half of the patients.

Cutaneous relapses can be treated in the same way as the initial lesion and do not worsen prognosis.

In patients with extensive skin lesions rituximab is the treatment of choice. Treatment schedules vary in different studies, but most patients have been treated with rituximab once weekly for four to eight weeks.

Oral chlorambucil is a treatment option often used in Europe.

Multiagent chemotherapy is rarely indicated in these types of cutaneous lymphomas except for patients who develop extracutaneous disease.

Primary cutaneous diffuse large B-cell lymphoma, leg-type, should be treated like systemic diffuse large B-cell lymphomas. Solitary or localized lesions are treated with R-CHOP with or without involved site radiotherapy whereas multifocal disease is treated with R-CHOP.

12.13 Extranodal involvement of non-Hodgkin lymphoma

Epidemiology
Primary extranodal NHLs are defined as those that clinically present with a predominantly extranodal tumour mass amenable to focal treatment, e.g. by radiotherapy. Regional or distant nodal involvement is common and does not exclude this diagnosis. However, in some cases, primary extranodal disease will be hard to distinguish from secondary spread of a disseminated primary nodal lymphoma.

Extranodal lymphomas occur frequently. The proportion of primary extranodal NHL is approximately 25–30%. Extranodal lymphomas can arise from almost any anatomical site of the body, even from those which normally do not contain lymphoid tissue.

The most commonly involved sites are the skin, stomach, brain, small intestine, and Waldeyer's ring.

Histologically, nearly 50% of all extranodal lymphomas are diffuse large B-cell lymphomas. It is the most common histological subtype in the testis, brain, bone, thyroid, and sinuses.

The majority of the remaining group arise from mucosa associated lymphoid tissue (MALT). This subtype is termed extranodal marginal-zone lymphoma of MALT-type and represents 5–10% of all NHLs. The most commonly involved sites are the stomach, small intestine, orbits, salivary glands, and the lung. Chronic antigenic stimulation from either infectious agents or autoimmune diseases plays a major role in the pathogenesis of MALT lymphoma. For gastric MALT lymphoma, chronic infection with *Helicobacter pylori* has been demonstrated as an aetiological factor. Furthermore, *Borrelia burgdorferi* and *Chlamydia psittaci* may be involved in the pathogenesis of at least a subset of cutaneous and ocular adnexal marginal-zone lymphoma. More recently, immunoproliferative small intestine disease (IPSID) was found to be associated with *Campylobacter jejuni*. Chronic inflammatory diseases such as Sjögren's syndrome in the salivary glands, myoepithelial sialadenitis (MESA), and Hashimoto's thyroiditis have also been associated with MALT lymphoma.

CNS lymphoma
Primary CNS lymphoma may involve the brain, cerebrospinal fluid, and eyes without systemic involvement. Approximately 10–20% patients have ocular involvement.

Risk factors for development of this tumour are congenital and acquired immunodeficiencies such as iatrogenic immunosuppression in organ allograft recipients and infection with HIV, implicating an important role of the immune system in the pathogenesis of this lymphoma. In immunocompromised patients, EBV genomic DNA can be detected in nearly all cases. In the era of highly active antiretroviral therapy the incidence of HIV-related primary CNS lymphoma has decreased again. However, most patients with CNS lymphoma are immunocompetent. EBV seems not to play a pathogenic role in these patients.

The median age at diagnosis is 60 years in immunocompetent patients and 30 years in HIV patients. Initial symptoms are related to size and site of the tumour lesion. Primary CNS lymphoma often has a rapidly progressive course. Systemic dissemination is rare. Early diagnosis and rapid initiation of therapy are crucial. The finding of characteristic features on CT scan and MRI should prompt a stereotactic biopsy. Corticosteroids should be avoided before biopsy whenever possible. Patients should have cytological examination and flow cytometry of the cerebrospinal fluid (CSF) and CT scan of the chest, abdomen, and pelvis.

Histologically, tumours are predominantly classified as diffuse large B-cell lymphomas. The growth fraction is usually high with >80% positivity for Ki67.

Resection of the tumour provides no relevant therapeutic benefit and does not prolong survival.

With a median OS of only 12 months, whole-brain radiation alone does not result in durable tumour control and is associated with a high risk of neurotoxicity in older patients.

High-dose methotrexate with or without whole brain radiation therapy (WBRT) prolongs survival in patients with primary CNS lymphoma (>24 months) compared with WBRT alone. However, the combination of chemotherapy and radiation has been associated with delayed neurotoxicity.

Recently methotrexate-based multiagent chemotherapy regimens have been evaluated. The IELSG32 randomized phase 2 study evaluated three different regimens namely methotrexate and cytorabine; methotrexate, cytorabine, and rituximab; methotrexate, cytorabine, thiotepa, and rituximab (MATRix). The MATRix regimen led to better a complete response rate of 49% compared with 23% with methotrexate-cytabine and 30% with methotrexate-cytarabine-rituximab. Grade 4 haematological toxicity was also highest with the MATRix regimen.

In the IELSG32 trial, patients who have had a response or stable disease, underwent a second randomization between WBRT and carmustinethiotepa conditioned ASCT. There was no difference in two-year PFS between WBRT (80%) and ASCT (69%, P=0.17). However, the risk of long-term neurocognitive impairment is not known.

For patients aged ≤70 years, the IELSG32 trial has established a new standard of care. This group of patients are treated with high-dose methotrexate-based chemoimmunotherapy followed by WBRT or ASCT. The choice between WBRT and ASCT is made based on feasibility for ASCT (e.g. adequate stem cell collection, good PS) and on consideration of potential neurocognitive impairment after WBRT. Patients aged >70 years with good performance status and without any significant comorbidities may be considered for methotrexate-based chemotherapy. Radiation therapy may be deferred until relapse to minimize the risk of treatment-related neurotoxicity. Salvage whole brain radiation therapy is an effective regimen for recurrent and refractory primary CNS lymphoma.

The prognosis of HIV-associated primary CNS lymphoma is generally worse and depends on the CD4+ cell count. Whereas patients with a CD4+ cell count >200/μL can achieve a long-term remission, those with a CD4+ cell count <200/μL do not respond to chemotherapy. These patients may respond to highly active antiretroviral therapy.

Bone lymphoma

In most cases, involvement of the bone is secondary in patients with advanced stage lymphoma whereas primary bone lymphoma is rare. The median age at diagnosis for primary bone lymphoma is 45–60 years and the most commonly involved sites are the femur, pelvic bone, and the spine. The presenting symptoms include localized bone pain (80–90%) and a tumour mass (30–40%). Depending on the involved site a pathological fracture (10–15%) or spinal cord compression (15%) can occur. To establish diagnosis an open biopsy is required. Diffuse large B-cell lymphoma is the most common histological diagnosis. Staging investigations are similar to other high-grade lymphomas. MRI scan is better in defining the local extent of disease and cortical bone changes.

Three different prognostic groups (patients <60 years, patients >60 years and IPI 0–3, and IPI 4–5) with significantly different OS at five years of 90%, 61%, and 25%, respectively, could be identified. Patients receiving rituximab plus CHOP had a significantly better three-year PFS than those who received CHOP only (88% vs. 52%).

The current standard of care is therefore six to eight cycles of R-CHOP. The role of radiotherapy is not defined. Patients with completely metabolic disease (CMR) may be observed without consolidation radiotherapy. However, patients without CMR are treated with involved field radiotherapy to a dose of 30–36Gy.

Radical surgery does not improve outcome.

Testicular lymphoma

Primary testicular lymphoma is a rare disease representing 1–2% of all NHLs.

The estimated annual incidence is 0.2 per 100,000. However, it is the most common malignancy of the testis in men >60 years. In most cases patients present with unilateral painless scrotal swelling.

The vast majority of these lymphomas are diffuse large B-cell lymphomas. Other histological subtypes including Burkitt's and lymphoblastic lymphoma are rare. Histological diagnosis is usually established by initial orchiectomy. In spite of providing local tumour control, orchiectomy alone is not curative.

The diagnostic work-up is the same as for other lymphomas. In approximately 80% of cases at initial presentation, stage I or II is diagnosed. Distant relapses are frequent and occur predominantly in other extranodal tissues like the CNS, the contralateral testicle, the skin, soft tissues, and lung and pleura.

In a retrospective survey by the International Extranodal Lymphoma Study Group (IELSG), prognostic factors and clinical outcome in 373 patients with primary lymphoma of the testis were analyzed. The median age of patients was 66 years. Prophylactic intrathecal chemotherapy was given to 18% of patients. Although 80% of all patients had stage I or II disease, clinical outcome was significantly worse than in diffuse large B-cell lymphomas at other sites. The five-year OS was only 48% and the survival curves did not reach a plateau. Fifty-two per cent of patients relapsed at a median follow-up of 7.6 years. The majority of relapses (72%) occurred at extranodal sites. Fifteen per cent relapsed in the CNS, mainly in the brain parenchyma up to ten years after presentation. Advanced disease at diagnosis was a risk factor for

CNS relapse. Patients receiving prophylactic intrathecal chemotherapy had better PFS than without. A low IPI, no B-symptoms, the use of anthracyclines, and prophylactic contralateral scrotal radiotherapy were significantly associated with longer survival in multivariate analysis. Recurrence in the contralateral testis was common in patients without prophylactic scrotal radiotherapy. Systemic chemotherapy alone does not seem to be effective in preventing relapses in the contralateral testis because the testis is an immunological sanctuary site.

Benefit from prophylactic cranial radiation has not been clearly shown so far.

The efficacy of CNS and contralateral testicular prophylaxis in addition to combination therapy with rituximab and CHOP was analyzed in a prospective single-arm trial conducted by the IELSG. In a preliminary analysis three-year OS was 86% and three-year PFS 77%. Recurrence in the contralateral testicle was not seen and the number of CNS relapses was slightly decreased.

Based on these data, patients with stage I–II primary testicular lymphoma should be treated with six to eight courses of R-CHOP followed by prophylactic irradiation of the contralateral testis (25–30Gy). Although data are not convincing, prophylactic intrathecal therapy should always be considered. The treatment of advanced testicular lymphoma is similar to advanced stage nodal DLBCL. However, all patients should be considered for CNS prophylaxis and prophylactic testicular radiotherapy.

Further reading

Cheson BD, Fisher RI, Barrington SF, et al. Recommendations for initial evaluation, staging, and response assessment of Hodgkin and Non-Hodgkin lymphoma: the Lugano Classification. *J Clin Oncol* 2014; 32 :3059–67.

Dreyling M, Geisler C, Hermine O, et al. Newly diagnosed and relapsed mantle cell lymphoma: ESMO Clinical Practice Guidelines for diagnosis, treatment and follow-up. *Ann Oncol* 2014; 25(Suppl. 3):iii83–92.

Dreyling M, Ghielmini M, Marcus R, et al. Newly diagnosed and relapsed follicular lymphoma: ESMO Clinical Practice Guidelines for diagnosis, treatment and follow-up. *Ann Oncol* 2014; 25(Suppl. 3):iii76–82.

Illidge T, Specht L, Yahalom J, et al. Modern radiation therapy for nodal non-Hodgkin lymphoma-target definition and dose guidelines from the International Lymphoma Radiation Oncology Group. *Int J Radiat Oncol Biol Phys* 2014; 89(1):49–58.

Martelli M, Ferreri A, Di Rocco A, Ansuinelli M, Johnson PWM. Primary mediastinal large B-cell lymphoma. *Crit Rev Oncol Hematol* 2017; 113:318–27.

Tilly H, Gomes da Silva M, Vitolo U, et al. Diffuse large B-cell lymphoma (DLBCL): ESMO Clinical Practice Guidelines for diagnosis, treatment and follow-up. *Ann Oncol* 2015; 26(Suppl. 5):v116–25.

Vitolo U, Seymour JF, Martelli M, et al. ESMO Guidelines Committee. Extranodal diffuse large B-cell lymphoma (DLBCL) and primary mediastinal B-cell lymphoma: ESMO Clinical Practice Guidelines for diagnosis, treatment and follow-up. *Ann Oncol* 2016; 27(Suppl. 5):v91–102.

Willemze R, Hodak E, Zinzani PL, et al. Primary cutaneous lymphomas: ESMO Clinical Practice Guidelines for diagnosis, treatment and follow-up. *Ann Oncol* 2013; 24(Suppl. 6):vi149–54.

12.14 Adult acute lymphoblastic leukaemia

Introduction

Acute lymphoblastic leukaemia (ALL) is a malignant neoplasm of the lymphocyte precursor, characterized by aberrations in proliferation and differentiation of leukaemic lymphoblasts leading to failure of the normal immune response and decreased normal haematopoiesis.

Epidemiology and aetiology

ALL represents <1% of adult cancers, but 25% of all childhood cancers. In adults, the incidence increases with age, being five per million in those aged 25–50 and 12 per million in those aged >60 years. ALL occurs slightly more frequently in males than in females.

Although a small percentage of cases are associated with inherited genetic syndromes, and many environmental factors (ionizing radiation, chemicals, electromagnetic fields, viruses) have been investigated as potential risk factors, the cause remains largely unknown.

Clinical features

Initial signs and symptoms reflect bone marrow infiltration and extramedullary disease. Signs of bone marrow failure include anaemia, neutropenia, and thrombocytopenia, clinically responsible for fatigue and pallor, fever, and petechiae, easy bruising, and bleeding. Other signs include weight loss, bone pain, and symptoms due to CNS or other extramedullary infiltration. A mediastinal mass is present in about half of T-cell ALL cases.

Laboratory studies

Peripheral blood

The WBC count may be abnormally low, within the normal range, or abnormally high. Haemoglobin level and platelet count are generally low and patients may require transfusions.

Bone marrow

A complete morphological and immunological examination of the bone marrow is required to establish the diagnosis of ALL. The French–American–British (FAB) classification, which recognized three subtypes of ALL—L1 (30%), L2 (60%), L3 (10%)—was strictly based on morphology and cytochemistry, whereas the current WHO classification also incorporates immunophenotyping and cytogenetics.

Immunophenotyping

The majority of ALL cases (75%) have phenotypes that correspond to those of B-cell progenitors (CD19, CD22, CD79). Additional subclassification within B-lineage into pro-B ALL, common ALL, pre-B, or mature B is made according to the expression of CD10, cytoplasmic immunoglobulin (Ig) μ heavy-chain proteins, surface, or cytoplasmic Ig+ or Ig–.

T-cell ALL (25%) is identified by the expression of T-associated surface antigens (CD3, CD7, CD5, or CD2). T-ALL subtypes comprise early T-ALL, thymic (cortical

T-ALL CD1a+) and mature T-ALL. ALL blasts coexpress myeloid markers in 15–50% of adults.

Flow cytometry allows the identification of an immunophenotype specific to the leukaemic blasts. This can be used in tandem with molecular techniques for monitoring the level of minimal residual disease (MRD) which correlates with outcome.

Cytogenetic and molecular biology

Genetic alterations are identified in >65% of cases. In addition to standard cytogenetic analysis, molecular techniques (reverse transcriptase PCR (RT-PCR), Southern blot) and FISH can identify translocations that are not detected by routine analysis of the karyotype.

Important genetic alterations in B-lineage ALL include t(9;22) and/or BCR-ABL (30–35%), t(1;19) and/or E2A-PBX1 (3–4%), t(12;21) and/or TEL-AML1 (1–3%), a variety of MLL gene rearrangements: t(4;11) and/or MLL-AF4 (3–4%), or 11q23 aberrations (<5%), and hyperdiploidy defined as >50 and <67 chromosomes or a DNA index of 1.16 or higher.

In T-ALL, elevated expression of HOX11, HOX11L2, SIL-TAL1, and CALM-AF10 is associated with different subtypes. HOX11L2 and SIL-TAL1-positive T-ALL have poorer outcomes than thymic T-ALL overexpressing HOX11. NOTCH1 activating mutations are identified in up to 50% of T-ALL and may be targeted by G-secretase inhibitors. NUP214–ABL1 aberration is detected in 4% of T-ALL cases and may be targeted by imatinib therapy.

Ph+ chromosome t(9;21) represents historically the strongest adverse cytogenetic prognostic features. Other high-risk cytogenetic features include del(7p), del(7p), +8, MLL translocations, t(1;19), t(17;19), and t(5;14). Very high-risk cytogenetics comprise t(4;11), t(8;14), complex karyotypes (≥ 5 abnormalities), hypodiploidy, and triploidy.

Nowadays, microarrays and next generation sequencing provide new approaches to profile ALL genomes. New subtypes of ALL harbouring submicroscopic genetic alterations have been identified, of which several have implications for risk stratification and targeted therapeutic intervention.

Genes involved encode proteins with key roles in lymphoid development (PAX5, IKZF1, EBF1), transcriptional regulation (ETV6, ERG), lymphoid signalling (BTLA, CD200, TOX, BLNK, VPREB1), cell-cycle regulation and tumour suppression (CDKN2A/B, RB1, PTEN), and drug responsiveness (NR3C1). IKZF1 encoding IKAROS has been identified as one of the most clinically relevant tumour suppressors in ALL. Deletions or mutations of IKZF1 are associated with a poor outcome in BCR-ABL+ adult ALL. A subset of BCR-ABL-negative B-ALL with IKZF1 alterations exhibit a gene-expression profile similar to BCR-ABL+, named BCR-ABL-like ALL. BCR-ABL-like ALL has a poor prognosis. In addition to IKZF1, other genetic alterations have a prognostic impact on ALL: CRLF2 rearrangements, activating mutations of JAK1/2, CDKN2A/B deletions, TP53 or CREBBP deletions/mutations have unfavourable outcomes in terms of response to chemotherapy, OS, and incidence of relapse. In T-lineage ALL, NOTCH1 and/or FBXW7 mutations have been associated with a favourable outcome, while N/K-RAS mutations or PTEN deletions/mutations demonstrated a worse outcome.

Prognostic significance of MRD

In the past, the classic prognostic factors were clinical features (age >50 years, WBC >30G/l in B-lineage), immunophenotyping (pro-B, early-T, mature-T), cytogenetics and molecular biology (t(9;22)/BCR-ABL, t(4;11)/MLL-AF4), and response to treatment (late achievement of response). MRD following induction and early consolidation therapy stands out as the most sensitive individual prognostic marker to define the risk of relapse following CR achievement, and ultimately that of treatment failure or success. A prospective monitoring for MRD should be considered in patients achieving CR after initial induction therapy to enable recognition of high-risk patients with suboptimal MRD response, to whom consolidation with allogeneic SCT may be offered. Patients showing complete MRD response, considered as standard-risk patients, can avoid allogeneic SCT. Molecular complete remission may be defined as a level of MRD (evaluated by molecular analysis of gene rearrangements or of gene fusion transcripts) below the detection limit of clone-specific PCR, which is generally 10^{-4}.

Treatment

In contrast to childhood ALL, which shows cure rates of approximately 90%, adults with ALL have a worse prognosis. Most of the therapeutic advances in adult ALL have arisen from successful adaptation of ALL treatment strategies in children. However, current treatments lead to only 30–40% long-term survivors in adult ALL. Comparisons demonstrate that adolescents with ALL significantly benefit from paediatric rather than adult chemotherapy regimens. Differences in drugs and dose intensity of many chemotherapeutic agents (such as asparaginase, vincristine, corticosteroids, and methotrexate, earlier CNS leukaemia prophylaxis) may explain the superior results with paediatric regimens. Although no major differences were demonstrated in terms of achievement of CR, CR is more rapidly obtained with paediatric regimens. These results have led to new paediatric-inspired therapeutic approaches that have improved the long-term EFS rate of newly diagnosed Ph-negative ALL to 60% or higher.

Induction chemotherapy

Induction chemotherapy should contain at least vincristine, daunorubicin, prednisone/dexamethasone, and asparaginase. Some groups also administer, to all patients or specific subgroups, cyclophosphamide, cytarabine, methotrexate, and/or mercaptopurine. Induction therapy can be preceded by a prephase with corticosteroids in order to detect poor responders and to avoid acute tumour lysis syndrome. Intensive combination therapy has resulted in CR proportions of 80–90%. Whereas a limit for intensification of myelotoxic drugs seems to have been reached, intensification with non-myelotoxic drugs (such as vincristine, steroids, or asparaginase) is still possible. Dexamethasone has replaced prednisone for better antileukaemic activity and achievement of higher levels in the CSF. In B-precursor ALL, higher doses of anthracyclines may be associated with improved results. Results of T-ALL have improved with the combination of cytarabine and cyclophosphamide added to the conventional drugs. Supportive care is of increasing importance during induction, including the concomitant application of haematopoietic growth factors throughout chemotherapy. CR is currently morphologically defined as a reduction of blast cells to <5% together with return of marrow cellularity and function to normal levels and the disappearance of all extramedullary manifestations.

Consolidation chemotherapy

Consolidation therapy is administered after CR is achieved. Cycles of consolidation chemotherapy in large studies are very variable. The type, duration, and intensity of consolidation may be adapted to the initial features, the response to prephase, the remission status, and/or level of MRD at the end of induction therapy. Several studies have demonstrated that late modified reinduction improves outcome. In general, it seems that intensive application of high-dose methotrexate is beneficial. There is also an important role for dose intensification of asparaginase. The role of high-dose anthracyclines, podophyllotoxins, and high-dose cytarabine is more questionable. Stricter adherence to protocols with fewer delays, dose reductions, or omission of drugs may be important factors for therapeutic improvement.

Central nervous system treatment

The diagnosis of CNS ALL requires the presence of more than five leukocytes per microlitre in the CSF and the identification of lymphoblasts in the CSF differential cell count. False-negative CSF results may occur in patients with predominantly cranial nerve involvement. Effective CNS prophylaxis not only reduces the risk of isolated CNS relapse but also improves general outcome. CNS prophylaxis includes intrathecal (IT) chemotherapy (methotrexate, cytarabine, steroids), high-dose systemic chemotherapy (methotrexate, cytarabine, asparaginase), and cranial or craniospinal irradiation, if there is CNS involvement initially. The use of IT liposomal cytarabine may reduce the number of IT injections and improve efficacy.

Maintenance chemotherapy

After consolidation, maintenance therapy given over 1.5–2 years is still standard in ALL. Omission of maintenance therapy has been associated with shorter DFS rates. Daily doses of mercaptopurine and weekly doses of methotrexate are the backbone of maintenance, and are eventually combined with monthly pulses of vincristine and corticosteroids. No clear advantage has been demonstrated with intensified versus conventional maintenance doses. Patients with mature B-ALL do not require maintenance. In T-ALL, the benefit of maintenance chemotherapy has been questioned.

Allogeneic stem cell transplantation

Allogeneic SCT is the most potent post-remission antileukaemic therapy in adult ALL. A myeloablative conditioning regimen followed by rescue with infusion of HLA-matched haematopoietic stem cells is generally used in Ph+ ALL and non-Ph+ high-risk ALL. A recent meta-analysis concluded that allogeneic SCT in first CR is recommended in high-risk but not in standard-risk ALL. Recent protocols tend to avoid SCT in standard-risk patients who are confirmed to be MRD-negative given the good results of paediatric-based chemotherapy. The survival rate with matched related allogeneic SCT in first CR is about 50% (range 20–80%). The increasing use of unrelated donors, umbilical cord blood, haploidentical donors, and reduced intensity SCT have expanded the opportunity for more patients to undergo SCT. In large prospective trials, results are similar between allogeneic related SCT and allogeneic matched unrelated donor (MUD) SCT, with however, higher relapse rates for sibling and higher mortality for MUD SCT. Although haploidentical SCT remains investigational, this approach has shown promising results in conjunction with high-dose post-transplant cyclophosphamide in very high-risk ALL. Reduced-intensity conditioning facilitates SCT in elderly patients and in those with comorbidities. In second CR, the outcome of SCT is superior to that of chemotherapy. Intensity of therapy before SCT, conditioning regimens, and immunosuppressive therapy after SCT may influence outcomes.

Autologous stem cell transplantation

Autologous SCT is inferior to allogeneic SCT. No significant difference has been detected in several randomized studies between autologous SCT and chemotherapy. Autologous SCT may be of interest in certain situations such as MRD negativity after consolidation.

New therapeutic agents

Advances in the understanding of molecular mechanisms of disease, and the successful model of imatinib in Ph+ disease, have led to the development of several new therapeutic approaches in ALL.

Therapy with monoclonal antibodies is an attractive treatment approach in ALL. Its use may be most promising in the setting of MRD. To date, the most promising data concern the anti-CD20 antibody (rituximab), which has been successfully integrated into therapy of mature B-ALL, B-precursor ALL, and Ph+ ALL. Other actively investigated monoclonal antibodies are the anti-CD22 epratuzumab (a naked humanized monoclonal antibody) and inotuzumab ozogamicin (an anti-CD22 monoclonal antibody bound to calicheamicin). Studies integrating anti-CD52 (alemtuzumab) are also ongoing. Bi-specific monoclonal antibodies constitute a new generation of compounds. Blinatumomab, a bi-specific monoclonal antibody with a CD3-binding site for the T cells and a CD19 site for the target B leukaemia cells, has been shown to be highly effective in treating adult B-precursor ALL in haematological CR but with MDR positivity and in adults with active refractory/relapsed B-lineage ALL.

T cells can be genetically modified to express chimeric antigen receptors (CARs) that recognize specific targets on leukaemia cells. Preclinical and first clinical data are encouraging, but CAR activity in B-cell lineage ALL remains to be established.

A number of other novel agents are being investigated. New types of asparaginase are emerging: the pegylated *Escherichia coli* derived L-asparaginase shows less immune response and a prolonged half-life; asparaginase *Erwinia chrydanthemi* is immunologically distinct from the *E. coli* L-asparaginase; L-asparaginase-loaded red blood cells are a new option that showed a reduction in the number and severity of allergic reactions and fewer coagulation disorders. Other potential new agents include liposomal agents (liposomal vincristine), mTOR inhibitors, JAK inhibitors, and the purine analogues. In T-lineage ALL, attention must be paid to the new nucleoside analogues (clofarabine, forodesine, and nelarabine).

Subset specific approaches

Philadelphia chromosome–positive ALL

New molecular therapeutic strategies with imatinib and other new TKIs (dasatinib, nilotinib, bosutinib) have led to considerable improvement in the treatment of this unfavourable subgroup. The efficacy of imatinib has been explored as front-line therapy combined with chemotherapy, given either simultaneously or as an alternating regimen. Efficacy analyses based on BCR-ABL transcript levels showed a clear advantage of the simultaneous over the alternating schedule. Adding imatinib to consolidation chemotherapy may increase the proportion of PCR negativity and decrease the relapse rate prior to SCT. A higher proportion of patients can proceed to SCT in first remission. The DFS after transplant at three years was 75–80%. Nevertheless, there are still challenges including the selection of pre-transplant therapy, the use of TKIs after transplant, and the development of therapeutic strategies to overcome disease resistance. TKIs combined with minimal chemotherapy are able to yield high CR rates, low toxicity, and three-year OS at about 45% in elderly patients. Reduced-intensity conditioning or non-myeloablative SCT could be considered as consolidation therapy in this patient population. MRD after SCT is predictive of relapse. Imatinib has been used as a treatment for MRD after transplantation in order to abort relapse. Most relapses are associated with the T315I mutation. Ponatinib is a pan-BCR-ABL inhibitor with activity against all mutants, including the T315I mutation. Combined with chemotherapy, it is a promising approach to overcome TKI resistance.

Burkitt's ALL

Outcome with conventional ALL therapy for mature B-ALL was poor, with long-term DFS of <10%. Mature B-ALL is now generally treated in separate studies with short intensive cycles. Hyperfractionation of cyclophosphamide, and use of different non-cross-resistant agents together formed the basis of many dose-intensive programmes. Intensive early prophylactic IT therapy, in addition to intensive systemic methotrexate and cytarabine, significantly reduced the rate of CNS recurrence. CR is now achieved in about 90% of patients and two-year DFS rates have increased to 60–80%. Disease recurrence is rare after the first year in remission. Recent integration of anti-CD20 before each chemotherapy cycle appears very promising with 70–80% OS.

ALL in the elderly

Increasing age is the most adverse factor for CR rate and is also associated with shorter remissions. The remission rate ranges from 30% to 70%. The OS at three years was estimated to be only 7–19% in patients aged 60 years and older. Older patients with ALL have often been excluded from clinical trials by eligibility criteria. Very few clinical trials have focused on therapies designed specifically for older patients, and fewer still have sufficient numbers to deal with the clinical and biological heterogeneity within this age group.

Salvage therapy

The outcome of salvage therapy remains unsatisfactory. CR rates range from 10% to 50% and long-term DFS is poor, although more intensive reinduction chemotherapy programmes followed by allogeneic SCT may achieve durable remissions. Although SCT is superior to chemotherapy with long-term DFS rates of 20–40% in salvage therapy, only 30–40% of patients who achieved a second CR were eligible for SCT and <50% had enough time before disease recurrence to undergo SCT. In this setting, the use of innovative drugs may open the door to effective rescue treatments which may significantly increase the effective role of SCT for this group of patients.

Further reading

Bassan R, Hoelzer D. Modern therapy of acute lymphoblastic leukemia. *J Clin Oncol* 2011; 29:532–43.
Faderl S, O'Brien S, Pui CH, et al. Adult acute lymphoblastic leukemia: concepts and strategies. *Cancer* 2010; 116:1165–76.
Ribera JM. Optimal approach to treatment of patients with Philadelphia chromosome-positive acute lymphoblastic leukemia: how to best use all the available tools. *Leuk Lymphoma* 2013; 54:21–7.

12.15 Adult acute myeloid leukaemia

Introduction

Acute myeloid leukaemia (AML) is a malignancy that is characterized by infiltration of bone marrow by abnormal haematopoietic progenitors that disrupt normal production of erythroid, myeloid, and/or megakaryocytic cell lines.

Epidemiology and aetiology

AML is diagnosed in people of all ages. The median age at diagnosis ranges from 66 to 71 years. The risk increases about ten-fold from age 30 (ten cases per million population) to age 70 (100 cases per million population). Sex distribution (male to female) is approximately 1:1 in patients <60 years, but 2:1 in those >60 years. Although the cause of AML in most patients is unknown, several factors are associated with its development: exposure to toxic chemicals (benzene, toluene), prior treatment with antineoplastic cytotoxic agents (alkylating agents, podophyllotoxin derivatives or other inhibitors of DNA topoisomerase II activity), exposure to radiation, and inherited disorders (Fanconi's anaemia) or genetic abnormalities, such as Down's syndrome. This suggests that these factors trigger a malignant transformation through the action of different oncogenes.

Clinical features

Clinical features comprise those caused by a deficiency of normal functioning cells and those due to the proliferation of the leukaemic cell population. Haematological symptoms include anaemia (fatigue), thrombocytopenia (haemorrhage), and neutropaenia (infection, fever). Infiltrative disease may include adenopathy, hepatomegaly, splenomegaly, skin, or CNS involvement. High WBC count (>100G/l) may be associated with hyperviscosity, intracerebral and/or pulmonary leukostasis, or haemorrhage. This is a poor prognostic factor for early death. Although there are no studies proving an advantage with leukapheresis, this procedure should be carefully considered in those patients.

Older patients may present with myelodysplasia (MDS), an indolent disorder characterized by progressive cytopenias, which may last for several months or even years before converting into AML.

Laboratory studies

Peripheral blood

The WBC count may be abnormally low, within the normal range, or abnormally high. Haemoglobin level and platelet count are generally low and patients may require transfusions.

Bone marrow

A complete morphological and immunological examination of the bone marrow is required to establish the diagnosis of AML. The FAB classification recognized eight subtypes of AML—M0 minimal myeloid differentiation (3%), M1 poorly differentiated myeloblasts (15–20%); M2 myeloblastic with differentiation (25–30%); M3 promyelocytic (5–10%); M4 myelo-monoblastic (20%); M5 monoblastic (2–9%); M6 erythroblastic (3–5%); M7 megakaryoblastic (3–12%)—strictly based on morphology and cytochemistry (most AML cells have positive reactions to myeloperoxydase and Sudan black stains; esterase stains can differentiate myeloid from monocytic leukaemia; periodic acid–Schiff positivity indicates acute biphenotypic leukaemia or undifferentiated leukaemia with lymphoblastic features). Currently AML is categorized on the basis of the WHO Classification of Tumours of Haematopoietic and Lymphoid Tissues in several distinct entities which are mostly defined by the underlying cyto- and molecular-genetic aberrations.

Trephine biopsy of bone marrow for histology analysis is not routinely performed, but may be useful in the presence of failure of marrow aspiration.

Immunophenotyping

Myeloid markers include CD13, CD14, CD15, and CD33, with >90% of leukaemia cells demonstrating positivity to some of these antigens. CD34 is also frequently found in AML blasts and is a marker of poor prognosis.

Cytogenetics and molecular biology

Cytogenetic abnormalities are found in >85% of patients by classical cytogenetic and/or molecular analyses. Cytogenetic abnormalities at presentation are the most important prognostic factor. In cases of normal or failed cytogenetic examination, FISH is recommended to detect abnormality such as an MLL fusion transcript. Three cytogenetic groups can be distinguished:

- A favourable group with core binding factor (CBF) leukaemias (inv(16), t(16;16), or t(8;21)) and t(15;17). This group represents at most 10% of patients and involves mainly patients <60 years of age.
- An unfavourable group with monosomies or partial deletions of chromosome 5 or 7, or with abnormalities involving three chromosomes complex abnormalities. This group constitutes about 30–40% of all patients, on average older (>50–60 years) often with an antecedent haematological disorder or AML related to therapy.
- The remaining 50–60% of patients fall into a group whose prognosis is intermediate.

Additional prognostic markers have become available through the identification of mutations in, or altered expression of, disease genes that predict response to treatment. The P-glycoprotein transmembrane transporter proteins are the product of the multidrug resistance gene (MDR-1). Most of the studies attempting to overcome MDR-1 have been negative. Unfavourable prognosis is associated with overexpression of specific genes including: the Wilms tumour gene, WT1; the genes for the apoptosis regulators B-cell lymphoma protein, BCL2, and BCL2-associated X protein, BAX; the brain and acute leukaemia cytoplasmic gene, BAALC; the ectropic viral integration site 1 gene, EVI1; the FMS-like tyrosine kinase type 3 gene, FLT3 (especially in the form of internal tandem duplication (ITD); and KIT, ERG, and the mixed-lineage leukaemia gene, MLL. Isocitrate dehydrogenase (IDH1 and IDH2), TET2, and DNMT3A encode enzymes that promote DNA methylation, resulting in gene silencing and maintenance of proliferative homeostasis. The impact of these gene mutations on survival remains controversial. Some mutations confer a more favourable prognosis; most notably, mutations in the gene for CCAAT enhancer binding protein-A (C/EBP-A), CEBPA, and nucleophosmin, NPM1. These prognostic determinants have been particularly important for patients with AML and a normal karyotype (CN-AML), identifying within this group two genotypes, NPM1+ FLT3-ITD− and CEBPA+ FLT3-ITD−, which are associated with a favourable risk profile, comparable with that of CBF AML. Within the group of patients with CBF leukaemia, a c-Kit mutation identifies a subgroup at high risk of relapse.

Prognostic factors

Outcome is influenced by patient features such as age, comorbidities and PS, as well as disease characteristics including type of AML (de novo, treatment-related, secondary after MDS or myeloproliferative disease), and the genetic profile. From a more practical clinical perspective, AML can be grouped into four risk groups according to the recommendations of the European LeukemiaNet (Figure 12.15.1). Approximately 50% of non-promyelocytic AML patients under the age of 60, and 90% over the age of 60, relapse after initial therapy. European LeukemiaNet favourable risk groups have the lowest risk of relapse (10–35%) and usually receive combination chemotherapy. Relapse is highest in the adverse risk group varying from 70–90% with chemotherapy to 30–50% with myeloablative transplantation.

Treatment

Induction chemotherapy

The combination of an anthracycline (daunorubicin, idarubicin) in conjunction with cytarabine (3+7) remains the standard of care of induction therapy in patients considered medically fit. Typically the anthracycline (daunorubicin at 45–60mg/m^2/day) is given for three days, whereas cytarabine is given at 100–200mg/m^2 daily for seven days by constant infusion. With this regimen, the CR rate for younger adults (<60 years) is 60–80% and the OS rate is approximately 30%. Among older adults (> 60 years), the CR rate is 40–55%, but there are only 10–15% long-term survivors. Numerous randomized trials have attempted to identify which anthracycline should be combined with cytarabine. The general consensus favours idarubicin, which is generally administered at a dose of 12mg/m^2 daily for three days. Additional drugs may include etoposide and mercaptopurine. The use of high-dose cytarabine in induction for younger adults has been debated. Higher doses of daunorubicin (60–90mg/m^2) have recently suggested superior response rates. Other strategies to improve the CR rate include combination of fludarabine with cytarabine, sequential therapy followed by high doses of cytarabine, timed sequential chemotherapy, or the addition of growth factors for either haematological support or priming to

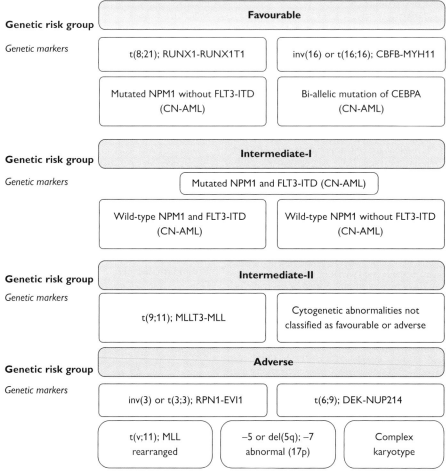

Fig. 12.15.1 European LeukemiaNet genetic prognostic risk groups.
Source: data from: Döhner H, et al. Diagnosis and management of acute myeloid leukemia in adults: recommendations from an international expert panel, on behalf of the European LeukemiaNet. *Blood* 2010; 115(3):453–74. 2010, American Society of Hematology.

recruit leukaemia cells into the cell cycle to render them more susceptible to cytotoxic chemotherapy.

Supportive care during remission induction treatment should routinely include red blood cell and platelet transfusions when appropriate, prophylactic oral antibiotics, and empirical broad-spectrum antimicrobial therapy for febrile neutropenic patients.

Rates of therapy-induced mortality increase with increasing age, abnormal organ function, and poor PS. An ambulatory (PS <3) adult aged <50 years would be expected to have an induction mortality rate of <5–10%. This rate might be 10–20% at age 60 years, 20% at age 70–79 years, and 30–40% at age 80 years and above.

Cytological CR is characterized by a percentage of bone marrow blast cells <5%, calculated on at least 200 nucleated cells in an aspirate sample with marrow spicules, absence of cells with Auer rods, and resolution of peripheral blood cytopenia.

It has been shown that failure to achieve an early response (clearance of blasts to a percentage lower than 10–15% in bone marrow at day 14–16) has an important prognostic value. A second course of induction therapy can be recommended in those patients with persistent leukaemia at early assessment.

In patients ineligible for intensive chemotherapy, treatment options are limited with low-dose cytarabine and the hypomethylating agents, decitabine or azacitidine, resulting in CR rates of between 10% and 30%.

Consolidation chemotherapy

After achieving CR, post-remission therapy is mandatory to prevent relapse. Consolidation chemotherapy may comprise the same drugs used for induction therapy or non-cross-resistant drugs. Increasing the intensity of post-remission therapy is beneficial in younger adults, but not in older adults. Usually consolidation chemotherapy combines cytarabine at different dosages with other drugs. The advantage associated with more intensive doses of cytarabine ($3g/m^2$ x 6 doses) was found to be significant for patients who have not previously received high-dose cytarabine. The beneficial effect of high-dose cytarabine was mainly restricted to CBF leukaemias as well as CN-AML, where at least two cycles should be given. In contrast to younger patients, high-dose cytarabine appears too toxic in patients >60 years of age. In these patients, a beneficial advantage has been noted with lower-dose out-patient combination chemotherapy compared to one course of intensive consolidation therapy. Patients eligible for transplant should receive a shorter consolidation.

Although not formally evaluated, chemotherapy-based maintenance treatment after completion of intensive consolidation therapy does not seem to influence survival and is nowadays not recommended.

Allogeneic stem cell transplantation

Allogeneic SCT is considered to be the treatment with the strongest anti-leukaemia effect. Considerable progress has occurred in the area of allogeneic SCT, making this option available to a greater number of patients with AML. However, the benefit of this procedure on OS may be compromised by treatment-related mortality (TRM). In first CR, an integrated risk-adapted approach has been proposed for younger patients taking into account: the risk of relapse, TRM of allogeneic SCT, and transplant-specific parameters as reflected by the haematopoietic cell transplantation comorbidity index (HCT-CI) and the European Group for Blood and Marrow Transplantation (EBMT) score.

Indications for standard allogeneic SCT

There is a marked diversity in the risk of relapse according to the (cyto)genetic profile. Allogeneic SCT represents the most appropriated post-remission therapy in patients with low HCT-CI and EBMT scores in the intermediate, poor, and very poor categories. No beneficial effect on survival could be demonstrated for an allogeneic SCT in CBF-AML. Similarly, no beneficial effect on survival could be shown in CN-AML with the genotype NPM1+/FLT3-ITD and those with double mutant CEBPA. In the intermediate-risk category, which comprises mainly AML with CN-AML, DNMT3A mutations and RUNX1 mutations were found to be associated with an unfavourable prognosis. In this risk group, allogeneic SCT is preferable in cases for which a matched donor is available and in the absence of comorbidities reflected by an EBMT and HCT-CI score <2. Most patients in the poor or very poor risk group should be offered an allogeneic SCT if a CR is achieved and even if a CR is not achieved. The low rate of relapse following allogeneic SCT has been confirmed in all donor/no donor comparisons but has not translated into a consistent survival advantage. Therefore allogeneic SCT from an HLA-matched family donor represents the best option for prevention of relapse in patients with unfavourable or intermediate AML (except NPM1+ or CEBPA+ and FLT3-ITD−). Age limits have also commonly been part of eligibility criteria for standard allogeneic SCT.

Outcome of allografts beyond first remission is inferior to that in first remission, owing to an increase in both TRM (25–35%) and relapse (40–45%).

Reduced-intensity conditioning

Despite its wide use, to date there have been no prospective comparative studies. The most important reason for reduced-intensity conditioning (RIC) is age or significant comorbidity. RIC regimen classically involved minimally toxic total body irradiation of 2Gy, most often with fludarabine before, and a combination of cyclosporine and mycophenolate mofetil after, allogeneic SCT. However, a fludarabine/busulfan/ATG (antithymocyte globulin) regimen demonstrated a lower relapse rate. A number of regimens with augmented antitumour activity have been designed, such as the FLAMSA regimen that incorporates both intensive pretransplantation cytoreduction and early administration of donor lymphocyte infusions (DLI). RIC regimens were used for both related- and unrelated-donor transplantations. The postgrafting immunosuppression both enhanced engraftment and mitigated serious graft-versus-host disease (GVHD). Serial analyses for chimerism were performed on days 28, 56, 84, 180, and 360 after SCT. The OS rate at two years was 48%, and patients receiving SCT during first CR had two-year OS rates of 44% (related SCT) and 63% (unrelated SCT). Cumulative incidences of acute GVHD (grades 2–4) were 35% at 180 days after related SCT and 42% after unrelated SCT. The probability of chronic GVHD was 36% at two years. Engraftment is generally prompt as indicated by the percentages of donor chimerism during the first 180 days after transplantation.

Alternative-donor transplantation

Few MUD transplantations take place during first CR in AML patients with unfavourable cytogenetics. Patients who did not have a sibling are assigned to MUD, if a donor is available. The risk of GVHD, graft failure, and mortality increases progressively with the number of HLA disparities, emphasizing the importance of high-resolution HLA typing and the selection of donors with preferably no more than one mismatched allele out of ten.

Allogeneic SCT from a haplotype mismatched relative emerges as a viable alternative option for AML patients without matched donors and/or those who urgently need transplantation, especially when the donor shows alloreactivity of natural killer cells towards the recipient.

Cord blood has now become established as a suitable source for haematopoietic transplantation. Even two HLA disparities between donor and recipient can be tolerated for a cord blood transplant. Promising results in terms of reduction of transplant-related mortality have been reported in adults given two different cord blood units. Compared to MUD transplants, several advantages exist: the immaturity of the immune system allowing a less restrictive HLA-compatibility requirement, a shorter time for transplant, and the absence of any risk for donors.

Disease relapse after allograft

The outcome for patients with recurrent disease after allograft remains extremely poor. In patients with no evidence of GVHD who relapse more than 12–18 months after SCT, a second allograft can be proposed, although there is no evidence that use of a different stem cell donor is beneficial. DLI also has the capacity to salvage a proportion of patients who have achieved CR after salvage therapy. Conventional myelosuppressive chemotherapy is associated with significant toxicity. Azacitidine in combination with DLIs is an active treatment in high-risk patients who have relapsed after allogeneic SCT.

Autologous stem cell transplantation

Data about superiority of autologous SCT in first CR over standard dose consolidation are controversial.

Autologous SCT has been shown to improve EFS without any effect on OS, compared with consolidation chemotherapy. Five-year OS rates of 45% in high-risk and 64% in favourable-risk patients have been observed. A significant reduction in relapse incidence has been reported in favourable- and intermediate-risk AML. Stem cell harvest is usually performed after the last consolidation chemotherapy cycle. The collection of stem cells is potentially contaminated by clonogenic leukaemia cells surviving previous cytotoxic therapies, so that the efficacy of the treatment is strongly dependent on good in vivo purging with chemotherapy. Autologous SCT should be done within a period not exceeding six months from first CR. Different non-randomized trials have provided evidence in favour of a reduced relapse rate when ex vivo purging with mafosfamide is employed. No evidence supports maintenance chemotherapy after autologous SCT performed in patients with a first CR. Vaccination with high-density dendritic cells generated from autologous leukaemic blasts in combination with interleukin-2 administration might elicit antileukaemia T cell responses and represents a promising approach in consolidation therapy of patients treated with autologous SCT.

Minimal residual disease

Measurement of the disease burden during treatment and follow-up allows post-remission strategy and pre-emptive salvage treatment to be adapted before overt haematological relapse occurs. MRD can be evaluated by polymerase chain reaction and multiparameter flow cytometry. Consistently, either negativity or marked reduction of MRD at different time points was associated with lower risk of relapse. Inversely, a marginal reduction in MRD levels was associated with relapse. Thus, intensification of post-remission with an allogeneic SCT in first CR can be envisaged if MRD levels stay either positive or above a distinct level whatever was the (cyto)genetic profile of AML. A steady increase in MRD levels during the follow-up period was closely associated with haematological relapse. Thus, the initiation of a pre-emptive salvage therapy intervention during molecular relapse may be advantageous.

New and targeted therapies

Several novel agents have emerged recently for therapy for AML. Among these are drugs that specifically bind to the surface of the AML blasts such as the anti-CD33 Mylotarg® (gemtuzumab ozogamicin). Great progress has been achieved in middle-aged and older patients by using gemtuzumab ozogamicin at the dose of 3mg/m^2 on days 1, 4, and 7 as adjunct to intensive induction therapy. Agents have been designed to inhibit the multidrug-resistant (MDR) protein FLT3 (PKC-412, CEP-701, MLN518, SU11248) and other tyrosine kinases, the processes of angiogenesis (antivascular endothelial growth factors), apoptosis (anti-BCL-2), and methylation (histone deacetylases: decitabine, azacitidine). New nucleoside analogues (clofarabine, troxacitabine) have shown activity in AML. The development of these agents, coupled with new insights into the molecular pathogenesis of the disease offers hope for significant progress in the treatment of AML.

Subset specific approaches

Acute promyelocytic leukaemia

Several developments over the past 30 years have made acute promyelocytic leukaemia (APL) the most curable of all types of AML. APL is more frequent in the Mediterranean countries. Chromosome aberrations other than t(15;17), CD56 expression, or short PML/RARA isoform are adverse prognostic factors. A stratification system has been developed that distinguishes low-risk patients with a WBC count <10G/l and platelets >40G/l, high-risk patients with WBC count >10G/l, whereas others are at intermediate risk.

A sizable fraction of patients develop fatal haemorrhages during the diagnostic evaluation. The disease should therefore be managed as a medical emergency, starting supportive measures (frozen plasma, fibrinogen, platelet support) and all-trans retinoic acid (ATRA) therapy to reverse the ongoing coagulopathy. Addition of ATRA to chemotherapy is of clear benefit and represents the current standard approach for newly diagnosed APL. ATRA should be used together with anthracyclines during induction and, probably, during post-remission therapy. Anthracyclines are so effective in APL that there is probably no reason to administer cytarabine. Idarubicin has shown a slight survival advantage when compared with daunorubicin. The ATRA syndrome (25% of patients) is the major toxicity of ATRA and is characterized by fever and leakage of fluid into the extravascular space producing fluid retention, dyspnoea, effusions, and hypotension. It is treated effectively with high doses of methylprednisolone or dexamethasone. Development of a PCR test to detect the characteristic t(15;17) provides a sensitive and highly specific means to detect relapse. The achievement of molecular remission rates of 90–99% in patients receiving at least two further cycles of anthracycline-based chemotherapy after induction has led to the adoption of this strategy as the standard for consolidation. Randomized studies have shown a benefit from administering ATRA maintenance intermittently or continuously.

Studies have also demonstrated the activity of arsenic trioxide (ATO) in APL by a slightly different mechanism. ATO is currently regarded as the best option in the context of relapsing APL. Arsenic trioxide produces CR rates of 80% in relapsed APL and may be more effective than ATRA. Its role in previous untreated disease and in postinduction therapy in newly diagnosed APL has also been explored. In second-line therapy, the choice of transplant modality is mainly based on PCR status achieved after reinduction.

Based on the activity of these agents and pre-clinical evidence of synergy, combination strategies have been tested in first-line therapy. A European consortium compared a regimen of ATRA and ATO with standard therapy with ATRA and idarubicin. This study established a new standard front-line treatment, without the use of cytotoxic chemotherapy, at least in patients with low-risk disease.

AML in the elderly

Older age is generally associated with increased comorbidities, more marginal PS, and the presence of more adverse disease features, including antecedents of haematological disorder and adverse risk cytogenetics. The intensive induction approach remains the best treatment option for carefully selected patients. This selection process should consider host-related (age, chronic organ dysfunctions, PS, infection at baseline) as well as AML-related (cytogenetics) selection criteria. There is no confirmed postremission strategy in elderly patients once CR has been achieved. High-dose consolidation courses, with or without high-dose cytarabine, are usually too toxic to benefit most patients. Beneficial effects associated with prolonged therapy with lower doses of chemotherapy have been reported. Allogeneic SCT after reduced-intensity conditioning is being used with increased frequency from either matched related or unrelated donors. With lower predicted rates of response and higher probability of toxicity, a significant proportion of older patients will not be considered good candidates for, and might not benefit from, intensive chemotherapy. Physicians might therefore decide to offer palliative or supportive care only. However, studies have shown that patients receiving even low-intensity therapy do better than those receiving only supportive care. In this setting, hypomethylating agents, such as azacitidine and decitabine, have shown significant activity and an OS benefit. With azacitidine, CR rates range from 15% to 20% and median OS ranges from 19 to 24.5 months in patients with 20–30% bone marrow blasts and less proliferative disease. Decitabine treatment produces

similar response rates and a survival benefit in responding patients (7.7–14.4 months). The former principle of achieving CR with intensive chemotherapy to convey a favourable outcome might not apply to these agents. Other lower-intensity combinations and prolonged consolidation/maintenance strategies are currently under investigation. Prolonged maintenance with new agents is also being investigated.

Further reading
Cornelissen JJ, Gratwohl A, Schlenk RF, et al. The European LeukemiaNet AML Working Party consensus statement on allogeneic HSCT for patients with AML in remission: an integrated-risk adapted approach. *Nat Rev Clin Oncol* 2012; 9:579–90.

Döhner H, Estey EH, Amadori S, et al. Diagnosis and management of acute myeloid leukemia in adults: recommendations from an international expert panel, on behalf of the European LeukemiaNet. *Blood* 2010; 115:453–74.

Schlenk RF. Post-remission therapy for acute myeloid leukemia. *Haematologica* 2014; 99:1663–70.

12.16 Chronic myeloid leukaemia

Introduction
Chronic myeloid leukaemia (CML) is a myeloproliferative disorder characterized by an acquired mutation affecting haematopoietic stem cells. The mutation results in a reciprocal translocation between the long arms of chromosomes 9 and 22, t(9;22)(q34;q11), producing a shortened chromosome 22, first identified in 1960, and termed the Philadelphia (Ph) chromosome (Nowell and Hungerford 1960).

Epidemiology
- CML is rare with an annual incidence of 1.6 per 100,000.
- Median age at diagnosis is 55 years. It is very rare in children and the incidence increases with age.
- There is a slight male preponderance with a male to female ratio of 1.4:1. Females have a survival advantage.

Aetiology
In most patients, there is no known aetiological factor. There are no ethnic, geographical, socioeconomic, or hereditary associations. Radiation exposure is the only known aetiological factor predisposing to CML.

Pathology and cytogenetics
The Philadelphia translocation relocates the 3′ segment of ABL, the human homologue of the Abelson murine leukaemia proto-oncogene, encoding a non-receptor tyrosine kinase (TK), from the long arm of chromosome 9 to the 5′ segment of the breakpoint cluster region (BCR) gene in the long arm of chromosome 22. BCR encodes a protein with serine-threonine kinase activity. The resulting fusion gene is translated to a chimeric protein, BCR-ABL, with constitutive leukaemogenic TK activity. Cytokine-independent cell growth and haematopoietic cell transformation are mediated by BCR-ABL through increased transcriptional activity via signal transducer and activator of transcription (STAT)-5 recruitment, enhanced proliferation from RAS activation, and reduced

apoptosis secondary to phosphatidylinositol 3-kinase (PI3K)/protein kinase B (Akt) activation.

- Ph chromosome is detected in 95% of patients with CML, 5% of children, and 15–30% of adults with ALL, and 2% of patients with AML.
- Variant Ph chromosome translocations, involving one or more additional chromosomes arise in 5–10% of patients with Ph chromosome-positive CML (Huret 1990). Variant Ph translocations are associated with a similar response to treatment when compared with patients with a classic Ph chromosome.
- 5–10% of patients with clinical features typical of CML are Ph chromosome-negative, of whom 30–50% demonstrate the BCR-ABL molecular rearrangement by RT-PCR. These patients have the same outcome as those expressing the Ph chromosome.
- Patients lacking the Ph chromosome and BCR-ABL molecular abnormality are classed as atypical CML, require different treatment, have a different prognosis and should be considered as a separate disease entity (Kurzrock et al. 1990).
- Breakpoints within ABL span a region of >300kb at its 5′ end, and within BCR localize to three main breakpoint cluster regions, resulting in three fusion transcripts, each encoding a BCR-ABL hybrid protein.
- p210$^{BCR-ABL}$, a 210kDa fusion protein occurs in most patients with CML and a third of patients with Ph chromosome-positive ALL. The breakpoint occurs within the major breakpoint cluster region (M-bcr), a 5.8kb area between BCR exons e12 and e16.
- p190$^{BCR-ABL}$ arises very rarely in CML and in two-thirds of patients with Ph chromosome-positive ALL. Breakpoints are identified in the minor breakpoint cluster region (m-bcr), spanning an area of 54.4kb between exons e2′ and e2. It is associated in CML with monocytosis at presentation and a worse prognosis than for patients with p210.

- p230$^{BCR-ABL}$ is associated with chronic neutrophilic leukaemia, and arises from a breakpoint cluster region (μ-bcr) downstream of BCR exon 19. Reduced TK activity relative to p190$^{BCR-ABL}$ is reflected in a less aggressive clinical course.

Evidence from studies utilizing highly sensitive (10^{-8}) RT-PCR demonstrates the presence of BCR-ABL in up to 30% of healthy individuals, suggesting that BCR-ABL is not the only genetic abnormality involved in the pathogenesis of CML (Bose et al. 1998).

Clinical features

Natural history

Three disease phases are recognized: chronic phase (CP), accelerated phase (AP), or blastic transformation.

- 90–95% of patients present in CP. Median survival is three to five years if they are not treated with a thymidine kinase inhibitor (TKI). There is a 3–4% annual risk of transformation to blast phase.
- AP is characterized by increasing maturation arrest, blast count, organomegaly, and clonal evolution. Most frequent secondary chromosomal abnormalities are trisomy 8, monosomy 17, duplicate Ph chromosome; trisomy 19, 21, 17, and deletion 7 are found in <10% of cases. Median survival without treatment is one to two years. In most patients, disease progresses to blast phase after four to six months.
- Blast phase (BP) resembles acute leukaemia with >20% blasts in peripheral blood or marrow. Lymphoid blast phase occurs in 20–30%, myeloid in 50%, and undifferentiated in 25%. Median survival without treatment is three to six months with lymphoid blast phase.

AP and blast phase may be combined as advanced phase disease. Different criteria have been proposed to define the three phases of disease and Table 12.16.1 details the WHO criteria. The classification systems provide prognostic information for patients and clinicians, and standardization for clinical trials.

Table 12.16.1 WHO criteria for CML AP and BP

CML AP diagnosed by presence of one or more:

10–19% peripheral blood or bone marrow blasts

>20% peripheral blood basophils

Platelets <100 x 10^9/L unrelated to therapy,
or >1000 x 10^9/L unresponsive to therapy

Persisting or increasing splenomegaly unresponsive to therapy

Persisting or increasing WBC (>10 x 10^9/L unresponsive to therapy

Any new clonal aberration during therapy

Additional clonal abnormalities in Ph cells at diagnosis that include major route abnormalities (second Ph, trisomy 8, isochromosome 17q, trisomy 19), complex karyotype, or abnormalities of 3q26.2

CML BP diagnosed by presence of one or more:

≥20% peripheral blood or bone marrow blasts

Extramedullary involvement excluding liver and spleen, including lymph nodes, skin, CNS, bone, and lung

Source: data from Arber DA, et al. The 2016 revision to the World Health Organization Classification Of Myeloid Neoplasms and Acute Leukemia. *Blood* 2016; 127(20):2391–405. 2016, American Society of Hematology.

Symptoms and signs

- Insidious onset. Diagnosis is often made following an incidental finding of leucocytosis on routine full blood count in an asymptomatic patient. Approximately 50% patients in Europe are asymptomatic at diagnosis.
- Non-specific constitutional symptoms of weight loss, night sweats, and low-grade fever characterize the hypermetabolic state.
- Splenomegaly is the most common physical finding (40–50%). Patients report abdominal discomfort, 'fullness' and early satiety related to splenomegaly and/or hepatomegaly. Splenic infarction is associated with left upper quadrant pain. The spleen extends 5cm below left costal margin in over 50% of patients at diagnosis.
- Hyperviscosity and leukostasis may occur in patients presenting with marked leukocytosis and WBC >300 × 10^9/L. Fundoscopy may demonstrate papilloedema, fundal haemorrhages, and venous obstruction. Priapism, confusion, visual disturbance, cerebrovascular accidents, and tinnitus are also reported secondary to leukostasis. Leukapheresis may transiently reduce WBC.
- Suspect transformation to blast phase if bleeding, petechiae, fever secondary to infection, and bone pain are prominent symptoms. Other features of transformation include headaches, arthralgia, and pain from splenic infarction.

Diagnosis

- *Full blood count, peripheral blood film, and preferably 1,000 cell differential count performed by microscopy* (Goldman 2007). High WBC. Left shifted leucocytosis, with all stages of granulopoiesis visible; predominant neutrophils and myelocytes. Mild basophilia and eosinophilia also seen. Platelet count may be elevated, normal, or low. Mild anaemia is common; usually normochromic normocytic.
- *Bone marrow aspirate and trephine biopsy.* Bone marrow markedly hypercellular with expansion of the myeloid cell line and progenitors; all stages of maturation present with myelocyte peak. <10% myeloblasts and promyelocytes in CP. Trephine biopsy allows assessment of fibrosis by reticulin stain.
- *Bone marrow or peripheral blood cytogenetics.* Confirms diagnosis by demonstrating presence of Ph chromosome. May reveal possible additional chromosomal abnormalities. Allows detection of clonal evolution in AP and blast phase.
- *FISH on bone marrow or peripheral blood cells.* Detects Ph chromosome and can be designed to also allow detection of prognostically important deletions of the derivative chromosome 9, der(9).
- *Real-time quantitative PCR (RT-PCR) for BCR-ABL transcripts.* Results expressed as ratio of BCR-ABL transcripts to number of copies of control gene (Hughes et al. 2006).
- *Upper abdominal ultrasound/CT scan.* Confirms presence of splenomegaly and/or hepatomegaly.
- *Serum urate level.* Hyperuricaemia associated with marked leucocytosis and high cell turnover.
- *Human leucocyte antigen (HLA) typing at diagnosis on patient and siblings if fit and aged <65 years.*

Differential diagnosis

- *Leukaemoid reactions secondary to inflammation, infection or malignancy.* Absent Ph chromosome, evidence of secondary disorder.

- *Myeloproliferative disease.* Essential thrombocythaemia characterized by absent Ph chromosome and possible presence of Jak2 mutation. Myelofibrosis excluded by Ph chromosome.
- *Myelodysplasia.* Absent Ph chromosome, dysplasia and maturation arrest on bone marrow aspirate and peripheral blood film.
- *Chronic neutrophilic leukaemia.*

Staging and prognosis

Accurate identification of disease phase at diagnosis is essential.

Patients in CP are further differentiated according to low, intermediate, and high risk determined by a prognostic score based on clinical and laboratory factors. The most extensively used system is the Sokal score (based on age, spleen size, percentage blasts, and platelet count); this was later modified to include basophil and eosinophil counts, as the Hasford score (Sokal et al. 1984; Hasford et al. 1998). These scoring systems were derived from OS figures for patients treated predominantly with busulfan or interferon-alpha (Sokal and Hasford systems respectively). The EUTOS (European Treatment and Outcome Study) score estimates the chances of achieving a complete cytogenetic response (CCyR) after 18 months of TKI therapy.

The timing and degree of haematological, cytogenetic, and molecular response also predicts outcome (Table 12.16.2).

Additional high-risk factors include deletion der(9), secondary chromosomal abnormalities in Ph-positive cells at diagnosis, clonal evolution, and less than MCyR after 12 months imatinib therapy.

General management

Patients who present with life- or organ-threatening features of leucostasis such as deterioration in the level of consciousness, bleeding, or priapism may need temporary cytoreduction with hydroxyurea (40mg/kg/day) while waiting for confirmation of the diagnosis. The dose should be tapered before its discontinuation.

Patients should be adequately hydrated (2.5–3l/day) and urine pH should be optimized at 6.4–6.8 (for uric acid clearance) with sodium bicarbonate to avoid tumour lysis syndrome. Patients with symptomatic hyperuricemia are treated with allopurinol.

Treatment of chronic phase

The treatment of CML has been revolutionized with the advent of molecularly targeted TKIs. With modern treatment, almost 90% patients are alive with normal blood counts and in molecular remission after five years. Imatinib mesylate is a TKI with activity against BCR-ABL, ABL, c-kit, stem cell factor receptor, and platelet-derived growth factor receptor (PDGFR). Imatinib binds to the inactive non-adenosine triphosphate (ATP)-binding conformation of BCR-ABL, stabilizing the kinase in its inactive form. ATP binding is competitively inhibited,

Table 12.16.2 Definitions of response to treatment

Complete haematological response (CHR)	
Platelets	$<450 \times 10^9$/L
White blood cells (WBC)	$<10 \times 10^9$/L
Differential	No immature granulocytes
	Basophils <5%
Spleen	Not palpable
Cytogenetic response (CyR)	
	% Ph+ metaphases by chromosome banding analysis (CBA)
Complete (CCyR)	0 or <1%
	BCR-ABL+ nuclei by iFISH out of ≥200 cells
Partial (CyR)	1–35%
Minor	36–65%
Minimal	66–95%
No	>95
Molecular response (MR)	
Major (MMR)	BCR-ABL transcript level ≤0.1% on the international scale
Deep MR MR⁴	BCR-ABL transcript level 0.01% on the international scale or BCR-ABL not detectable with at least 10,000 ABL or 24,000 GUS transcripts
MR⁴·⁵	BCR-ABL transcript level 0.0032% on the international scale or BCR-ABL not detectable with at least 32,000 ABL or 77,000 GUS transcripts

Source: data from Baccarani M, et al. European LeukemiaNet recommendations for the management of chronic myeloid leukemia: 2013. *Blood* 2013; 122(6):872–84. 2013, American Society of Hematology.

preventing substrate phosphorylation, resulting in inhibition of CML cell proliferation and induction of apoptosis.

The superiority of imatinib (400mg daily) was demonstrated by the International Randomized Study of Interferon and STI571 (IRIS) trial in 1,106 newly diagnosed patients with CP CML. Estimated CCyR rate at 18 months was 76% in the imatinib group and 14% in the interferon-cytarabine arm (O'Brien et al. 2003). Five-year estimated cumulative rate of CCyR was 87%, EFS 83%, and OS 89% in the imatinib group (Druker et al. 2006). At a median follow-up of 10.9 years, 65.6% of patients treated with first-line interferon alfa plus cytarabine crossed over to imatinib due to disease progression or lack of response (31.5%), unacceptable side effects (26.2%) or patient preference (8.0%) (Hochhaus et al. 2017a). Ten-year estimated OS was 83.3%, EFS 79.6%, and the rate of progression to the accelerated phase or blast crisis 92.1% in the imatinib group.

Toxicities include peripheral and periorbital oedema in 60%, diarrhoea or nausea in around 50%, musculoskeletal pain in 47%, rashes in 40%, and fatigue in 39% (Druker et al. 2006). Severe, grade 3/4, adverse effects are rare with imatinib. Myelosuppression occurs most frequently, followed by hepatotoxicity. Less severe side effects are more common. The drug is teratogenic requiring use of contraception in men and women. Serious adverse events are highest in the first year of treatment and decline subsequently (Hochhaus et al. 2017a).

Second generation TKIs
Dasatinib is a competitive Src- and ABL-kinase inhibitor, binding active and inactive forms, with 300-fold greater potency than imatinib. In a randomized controlled study of first-line dasatinib (100mg once daily) versus imatinib (DASISION) in chronic phase CML, dasatinib resulted in a higher CyCR (77% vs. 66%, P=0.007) and major molecular response (46% vs. 28%, P<0.0001) than imatinib (400mg once daily) at a minimum follow-up of 1 month (Hochhaus et al. 2010). The median time to CyCR was shorter with dasatinib compared with imatinib (3 months vs. 6 months) (Jabbour et al. 2014). However, five-year estimated OS (91% for dasatinib and 90% for imatinib) and PFS (85% for dasatinib and 86% for imatinib) were similar (Cortes et al. 2016).

Nilotinib, a derivative of imatinib, exhibits 30- to 50-fold greater in vitro potency. A randomized phase 3 trial (the ENEST study) reported higher rates of CyCR (80% vs. 65%, P<0.001) and major metabolic response (44% vs. 22%, P<0.001) at 12 months with nilotinib (300mg once daily) compared with imatinib (Saglio et al. 2010). At five years, more than 50% of patients in the nilotinib arms and 31% in the imatinib arm achieved molecular response (Hochhaus et al. 2016).

Choice of first-line treatment in chronic phase
The first-line treatment options for CP CML are imatinib (400–800mg daily), dasatinib (100mg daily), or nilotinib (300mg twice daily) (Hochhaus et al. 2017b). While dasatinib and nilotinib are associated with higher rates of major molecular response (MMR) compared with imatinib 400mg daily, the five-year OS is similar (85–95%). A recent meta-analysis estimates that imatinib 800mg daily is associated with 30% higher probability of MMR at 12 months compared with imatinib 400 mg daily (Hoffmann et al. 2017).

The choice of first-line TKI depends on treatment intent, age and comorbidities of the patient, and the side effect profile of the drug. For example, patients with high risk of developing pleural effusion (e.g. pre-existing lung disorders or hypertension) should avoid dasatinib.

Response assessment and treatment modifications
RT-PCR for BCR-ABL transcripts is the cornerstone for monitoring patients response to TKIs. All patients need RT-PCR at three months. All patients should have at least one bone marrow aspirate and cytogenetic assessment for documenting CCyR. After CCyR, monitoring peripheral blood BCR-ABL transcript levels every three months is recommended (Goldman 2007). The interval of monitoring may be increased to six months after achieving a repeated MMR (BCR-ABL transcript level 0.1%, 3 log reduction from standardized baseline). Table 12.16.2 shows measurement of various responses.

A patient with an 'optimal' response is continued on treatment with first-line TKI. Optimal response is defined as ≤35% Ph+ metaphases and BCR-ABL <10% at three months, 0% Ph+ metaphases and BCR-ABL <1% at six months, and BCR-ABL <0.1% at 12 months. Approximately 50% of patients on first-line TKI who achieve and maintain deep molecular response (DMR) could discontinue treatment for several years without disease relapse (Rea and Cayuela 2017). However, this may be considered on an individual basis and monitoring with RT-PCR is needed four to six weeks after discontinuation of treatment.

A patient with a 'warning' response (defined as 36–95% Ph+ metaphases and BCR-ABL >10% at three months, 1–65% Ph+ metaphases and BCR-ABL 1–10% at six months, and BCR-ABL 0.1–1% at 12 months) should be monitored closely and treatment changed if there are features of failure.

TKI failure is defined as no CHR (complete haematological response) and >95% Ph+ metaphases at three months, >35% Ph+ metaphases and BCR-ABL >10% after six months, ≥1% Ph+ metaphases and BCR-ABL >1% at 12 months, or relapse or loss of MMR anytime. All patients with treatment failure should have a bone marrow examination to assess the phase of CML and rule out clonal evolution.

Second and subsequent lines of treatment
Patients who remain in chronic phase without evidence of clonal evolution continue on TKI. While increasing the dose of imatinib to 600–800mg daily may be effective in mildly resistant mutations, studies suggest that early switch to an alternative TKI may be more effective, in terms of higher rates of CHR, CCyR, and MMR (Giles et al. 2013, Cortes et al. 2016, Shah et al. 2016). Second-line TKIs after previous imatinib include nilotinib, dasatinib, or bosutinib.

Dasatinib is licensed for the treatment of imatinib-resistant CML. At eight months, CHR is achieved in 90% and MCyR in 52% of imatinib-resistant or intolerant patients in CP treated with 70mg dasatinib twice daily (Hochhaus et al. 2007). It is superior to high-dose imatinib in patients failing imatinib 400mg daily, with MCyR in 52% on dasatinib and 33% for imatinib 800mg (Kantarjian et al. 2007). The higher discontinuation rate is due to toxicities, including pleural and pericardial effusions.

Bosutinib is a dual Src- and ABL-kinase inhibitor active against CML cell lines. In a phase 2 trial of 228 patients including more than two-thirds with imatinib resistant disease, bosutinib 500mg once daily resulted in MCyR at six months in 31% and CCyrR in 41% (Cortes et al. 2016).

The most common toxicities were diarrhoea (84%), nausea, vomiting, and rash.

Ponatinib is a third-generation TKI, which is 500-fold more potent than imatinib in inhibiting BCR-ABL and is the only TKI which is active against CML with a T315I mutation. Ponatinib 45mg daily achieved a MCyR of 56% at 12 months in patients who developed resistance or intolerance to second-generation TKIs or with a T315I mutation (Cortes et al. 2013). The serious toxicities include veno-occlusive disease, pancreatitis, hypertension, and severe skin rashes.

Allo-HSCT

Transplant rates have decreased significantly since the introduction of TKIs. Allo-HSCT (allo-haematopoietic stem cell transplantation) is a therapeutic option for CP CML after failure of at least two TKIs and CML with a T315I mutation after a trial of ponatinib. Patients should be considered for allo-HSCT early during the development of AP. It is also the only curative option for CML in BP.

High treatment-related mortality (TRM), lack of a suitable sibling donor, and poorer outcome from unrelated donor transplants limit eligibility for allo-HSCT. Response is monitored following allo-HSCT as for TKI therapy.

Accelerated and blastic phases

Newly diagnosed patients presenting in accelerated phase should receive initial TKI. In a study, imatinib resulted in a CHR of 82% and CCyR of 43% with an estimated four-year survival of 53% (Kantarjian et al. 2005). Responders who have an appropriate donor and are fit for transplant should proceed to allogenic stem cell transplantation, which is a standard approach.

In BP, TKIs (imatinib and dasatinib) result in a haematological response of 42–55% and a major CyR of 16–25% with a two-year estimated survival of less than 28%. Allogenic bone marrow transplantation remains the only potentially curative approach (with a durable remission in 10%) in this group of patients.

Relapsing CML

For patients with TKI resistant disease, omacetaxine mepesuccinate has shown a haematological response rate of 67% with a median PFS of seven months in a phase 2 study of 46 patients. Another palliative treatment option is hydroxyurea.

Relapses after allogenic transplants may be treated with infusions of buffy-coat leukocytes or isolated T cells obtained by pheresis from the bone marrow transplant donor, which leads to durable remission in 50% of patients.

Further reading

Baccarani M, Deininger MW, Rosti G, et al. European LeukemiaNet recommendations for the management of chronic myeloid leukemia: 2013 *Blood* 2013; 122(6):872–84.

Bose S, Deininger M, Gora-Tybor J, Goldman JM, Melo JV. The presence of typical and atypical BCR-ABL fusion genes in leukocytes of normal individuals: biologic significance and implications for the assessment of minimal residual disease. *Blood* 1998; 92:3362–7.

Cortes JE, Kim DW, Pinilla-Ibarz J, le Coutre P, et al. A phase 2 trial of ponatinib in Philadelphia chromosome-positive leukemias. *N Engl J Med* 2013 Nov 7; 369(19):1783–96.

Cortes JE, Saglio G, Kantarjian HM, Baccarani M, Mayer J, Boque C, et al. Final 5-year study results of DASISION: the dasatinib versus imatinib study in treatment-naive chronic myeloid leukemia patients trial. *J Clin Oncol* 2016; 34:2333–40.

Druker BJ, Guilhot F, O'Brien SG, et al. Five-year follow-up of patients receiving imatinib for chronic myeloid leukaemia. *N Engl J Med* 2006; 355:2404–17.

Giles FJ, Hong F, Mauro MJ, et al. Rates of peripheral arterial occlusive disease in patients with chronic myeloid leukemia in the chronic phase treated with imatinib, nilotinib, or non-tyrosine kinase therapy: a retrospective cohort analysis. *Leukemia* 2013; 27(6):1310–15.

Goldman JM. Recommendations for the management of BCR-ABL positive chronic myeloid leukaemia. BCSH approved document 2007—available at: https://b-s-h.org.uk/media/16262/cml_bcr-abl_270707.pdf

Hasford J, Pfirrmann M, Hehlmann R, Allan NC, Baccarani M, et al. A new prognostic score for survival of patients with chronic myeloid leukemia treated with interferon alfa. *J Natl Cancer Inst* 1998; 90:850–8.

Hochhaus A, Kantarjian HM, Baccarani L, et al. Dasatinib induces notable hematologic and cytogenetic responses in chronic phase chronic myeloid leukemia after failure of imatinib therapy. *Blood* 2007; 109:2303–9.

Hochhaus A, Kantarjian H, Shah NP, Cortes J, Shah S, et al. Dasatinib versus imatinib in newly diagnosed chronic-phase chronic myeloid leukemia. *N Engl J Med* 2010 Jun 17; 362(24):2260–70.

Hochhaus A, Larson RA, Guilhot F, Radich JP, et al. Long-term outcomes of imatinib treatment for chronic myeloid leukemia. *N Engl J Med* 2017b; 376(10):917–27.

Hochhaus A, Saglio G, Hughes TP, et al. Long-term benefits and risks of frontline nilotinib vs imatinib for chronic myeloid leukemia in chronic phase: 5-year update of the randomized ENESTnd trial. *Leukemia* 2016; 30(5):1044–54.

Hochhaus A, Saussele S, Rosti G, et al. Chronic myeloid leukaemia: ESMO Clinical Practice Guidelines for diagnosis, treatment and follow-up. *Ann Oncol* 2017a; 28 (Suppl. 4):iv41–51.

Hoffmann VS, Hasford J, Deininger M, Cortes J, Baccarani M, Hehlmann R. Systematic review and meta-analysis of standard-dose imatinib vs. high-dose imatinib and second generation tyrosine kinase inhibitors for chronic myeloid leukemia. *J Cancer Res Clin Oncol* 2017; 143(7):1311–18.

Hughes T, Branford S. Molecular monitoring of BCR-ABL as a guide to clinical management in chronic myeloid leukaemia. *Blood Rev* 2006; 20:29–41.

Huret JL. Complex translocations, simple variant translocations and Ph-negative cases in chronic myelogenous leukaemia. *Hum Genetics* 1990; 85:565–8.

Jabbour E, Kantarjian HM, Saglio G, Steegmann JL, Shah NP, et al. Early response with dasatinib or imatinib in chronic myeloid leukemia: 3-year follow-up from a randomized phase 3 trial (DASISION). *Blood* 2014 Jan 23; 123(4):494–500.

Kantarjian HM, Pasquini R, Hamerschlak N, et al. Dasatinib or high dose imatinib for chronic-phase chronic myeloid leukemia after failure of imatinib therapy. *Blood* 2007; 109:5143–50.

Kantarjian H, Talpaz M, O'Brien S, Giles F, Faderl S, et al. Survival benefit with imatinib mesylate therapy in patients with accelerated-phase chronic myelogenous leukemia—comparison with historic experience. *Cancer* 2005; 103(10):2099–108.

Kurzrock R, Kantarjian HM, Shtalrid M, Gutterman JU, Talpaz M. Philadelphia chromosome-negative chronic myelogenous leukemia without breakpoint cluster region rearrangement: a chronic myeloid leukemia with a distinct clinical course. *Blood* 1990; 75:445–52.

Nowell P, Hungerford D. A minute chromosome in human chronic granulocytic leukemia [abstract]. *Science* 1960; 132:1497.

O'Brien SG, Guilhot F, Larson R, et al. Imatinib compared with interferon and low-dose cytarabine for newly diagnosed chronic-phase chronic myeloid leukaemia. *N Engl J Med* 2003; 348:994–1004.

Rea D, Cayuela JM. Treatment-free remission in patients with chronic myeloid leukemia. *Int J Hematol* 2017 Oct; 108(4):355–64.

Saglio G, Kim DW, Issaragrisil S, le Coutre P, Etienne G, et al. Nilotinib versus imatinib for newly diagnosed chronic myeloid leukemia. *N Engl J Med* 2010 Jun 17; 362(24):2251–9.

Shah NP, Rousselot P, Schiffer C, Rea D, et al. Dasatinib in imatinib-resistant or -intolerant chronic-phase, chronic myeloid leukemia patients: 7-year follow-up of study CA180-034. *Am J Hematol* 2016 Sep; 91(9):869–74.

Sokal JE, Cox EB, Baccarani M, Tura S, Gomez GA, et al. Prognostic discrimination in 'good-risk' chronic granulocytic leukaemia. *Blood* 1984 Apr; 63(4):789–99.

12.17 Chronic lymphocytic leukaemia

Introduction, clinical features, and staging

Chronic lymphocytic leukaemia (CLL) is a malignant clonal expansion of B-lymphocytes. It is considered part of the 'Mature B-cell Neoplasms', as classified by the WHO. The malignant lymphocytes are commonly identified in the blood, bone marrow, and lymphoid organs, and may also be found in other organs in the body.

Epidemiology

CLL is the most common leukaemia in the Western world. It is seen more frequently with increasing age and has a median age at diagnosis of 72 years. It is twice as common in males as it is in females. CLL is uncommon in Asian populations. The incidence appears unaffected by migration. The age-adjusted incidence is 4.2 per 100,000 population per year.

Aetiology

Familial relative risk associated with CLL is one of the strongest for any cancer with a six-fold increased risk in first-degree relatives (FDRs) of cases. This translates to a lifetime cumulative risk of 2.3% in FDRs. Risks are highest for siblings of affected cases and for FDRs of patients diagnosed at a younger age. Genome-wide association studies (GWAS) have provided unambiguous evidence of genetic susceptibility to CLL, having identified >40 genetic loci associated with disease risk. No consistent environmental factors contributing to CLL risk have been identified thus far.

Pathogenesis

The cell of origin of CLL is controversial. The current model postulates that CLL with an unmutated immunoglobulin heavy-chain variable (IGHV) region (U-CLL) is derived from a pre-germinal centre B cell, whereas CLL with mutated IGHV (M-CLL) originates from a post-germinal centre B cell. The current biological model defines an event (e.g. abnormal response to antigenic stimulation) inducing the formation of a clonal B-cell population with a CLL phenotype. Further events—in combination with the development of a suitable microenvironment—support proliferation of this clone. Proliferation centres form focal aggregates located in the bone marrow and lymph nodes, and their presence is unique to CLL. Interactions between CLL and accessory cells are critical for providing growth and survival signals to CLL cells. CLL cells outside of these proliferation centres (e.g. cells circulating in the blood) are considered part of the non-proliferative compartment. The B-cell receptor (BCR) is important in the pathogenesis of CLL, controlling clonal expansion, differentiation, and interaction with the tumour microenvironment.

High throughput sequencing (HTS) has revealed recurrent somatic mutations in CLL. These occur in genes such as NOTCH1, SF3B1, and BIRC3 which, in addition to known mutations in genes such as TP53, provide insight into the pathophysiology of CLL. Furthermore, HTS has demonstrated the clonal heterogeneity in CLL, as well as the clonal evolution that occurs in patients receiving treatment.

Diagnosis

The diagnosis of CLL may be suspected in an individual with a lymphocytosis; however, the differential diagnosis of lymphocytosis includes non-malignant conditions such as infection (non-clonal proliferation) and other lymphoproliferative disorders (LPDs). The International Workshop on CLL (iwCLL) recommends that a full blood count, peripheral blood smear, and immunophenotyping be carried out to identify features consistent with a diagnosis of CLL:

- Clonal lymphocytosis $>5 \times 10^9$/L sustained for >3 months.
- Typical morphology—small lymphocytes with clumped chromatin, absent nucleoli, and scanty cytoplasm. Smear cells are frequently produced by the crushing of lymphocytes but this is not specific to CLL.
- Typical immunophenotype—clonality is also established by demonstrating restricted light chain expression (e.g. by flow cytometry).

Five markers encompassing the CLL score have been defined which differentiate CLL from other LPDs (Table 12.17.1).

Scores in CLL >3, in other B-cell malignancies <3.

Monoclonal B-cell lymphocytosis (MBL) is thought to precede almost all cases of CLL and is defined as a clonal lymphocyte count $<5 \times 10^9$/L with no lymphadenopathy or disease related symptoms and a typical CLL phenotype. When primarily confined to lymph nodes, with a peripheral lymphocyte count $<5 \times 10^9$/L and an absence of cytopenias caused by clonal marrow infiltrate, the disease is termed small lymphocytic lymphoma (SLL).

Symptoms

CLL is usually diagnosed in asymptomatic patients following detection of a lymphocytosis from a full blood count. Some patients consult a doctor because of lymphadenopathy, and 5–10% of patients at presentation have systemic symptoms such as weight loss, pyrexia, night sweats, and tiredness. Occasionally symptoms may be related to immunodeficiency, autoimmune complications such as haemolytic anaemia (AIHA) or immune thrombocytopenia, and bone marrow failure.

Signs

- Lymphadenopathy (generalized or local)—50–90% of cases, commonly cervical, supraclavicular, and axillary
- Splenomegaly—25–55% of cases
- Hepatomegaly—15–25% of cases
- Other organ involvement

Table 12.17.1 Flow cytometry scoring system for the diagnosis of CLL

| Marker | Score points | |
	1	0
SmIg	Weak	Moderate/strong
CD5	Positive	Negative
CD23	Positive	Negative
FMC7	Negative	Positive
CD22 or CD79b	Weak/negative	Moderate/strong

Reproduced with permission from Matutes E, et al. The immunological profile of B-cell disorders and proposal of a scoring system for the diagnosis of CLL. *Leukemia* 1994; 8(10):1640–5. Copyright © 1994, Springer Nature Ltd.

Table 12.17.2 Clinical staging systems in CLL

Risk	Binet[1]		Rai (original)[2]	
Low	A	<3 lymphoid areas involved	0	Lymphocytes >15 x 10^9/L
Intermediate	B	≥3 lymphoid areas involved	I	Lymphocytes >15 x 10^9/L + lymphadenopathy
			II	Lymphocytes >15 x 10^9/L + splenomegaly and/or hepatomegaly
High	C	Hb <10g/dl and/or platelets <100 x 10^9/L	III	Lymphocytes >15 x 10^9/L + Hb <11g/dl
			IV	Lymphocytes >15 x 10^9/L + Plt < 100 x 10^9/L

Lymphoid areas for Binet staging (each area counts as 1 area): head and neck (including Waldeyer ring), axillae, groins, palpable spleen, palpable liver.

[1] *Source:* data from Binet JL, et al. A new prognostic classification of chronic lymphocytic leukemia derived from a multivariate survival analysis. *Cancer* 1981 Jul 1; 48(1):198–206.

[2] *Source:* data from Rai KR, et al. Clinical staging of chronic lymphocytic leukemia. *Blood* 1975; 46 (2):219–34.

Investigations

Other tests performed at diagnosis may include:

- Serum chemistry.
- Direct antiglobulin test—to investigate autoimmune haemolysis.
- Serum immunoglobulins—hypogammaglobulinaemia can occur and may be clinically significant.
- Beta 2-microglobulin (B2M).
- Viral infectious disease status (HIV, hepatitis B and C) and CMV in patients treated with alemtuzumab, idelalisib, or allogenic stem cell transplant (risk of reactivation).
- Plain chest radiograph.
- Bone marrow aspirate and trephine are not necessary unless there is uncertainty about the diagnosis or pretreatment.
- Lymph node biopsy—if transformation is suspected or the diagnosis is unclear.
- Fluorescent in situ hybridization (FISH)—will aid diagnosis when the CLL flow cytometry score is low and will identify cytogenetic abnormalities (e.g. 17p deletion) with prognostic information (pretreatment).
- TP53 and IGHV mutation status (pretreatment).
- CT scan—to provide a baseline assessment of lymphadenopathy and splenomegaly.
- Organ function assessment—determined by medical history and toxicity profile of planned treatment.

Staging

The two most commonly used clinical staging systems were devised by Binet and Rai. Classification results in low, intermediate, and high-risk groups (see Table 12.17.2).

Since their initial description, the survival times associated with each clinical stage are likely to have changed due to improvements in CLL management. However, these staging systems are still useful in standardizing patient care as well as informing on prognosis.

In up to 10% of patients, the CLL can transform to lymphoma and in the majority of cases this is clonally related to the CLL clone. The most common transformation is that resembling DLBCL, termed Richter's Transformation. This is heralded by a sudden clinical deterioration with rapid enlargement of lymph node(s) associated with systemic symptoms. The clinical outcome is poor with median survival of approximately six months.

Prognostic factors

In addition to the Rai and Binet staging described earlier, many other prognostic factors have been investigated. Male gender and high B2M are associated with a worse outcome.

Standard cytogenetic analysis of CLL cells is limited by the inability to obtain reliable metaphase cells for analysis. FISH can detect abnormalities in approximately 80% of cases; the most common are:

- 13q deletion: approximately 55% of patients
- 11q deletion: 10–20% of patients
- 12q trisomy: 15–20% of patients
- 17p deletion: 5–10% of patients

These cytogenetic abnormalities have important prognostic implications. Del(17p) usually results in loss of TP53—a tumour suppressor gene. These patients respond poorly to current chemoimmunotherapy, are at greater risk of transformation, and exhibit shorter survival times. Del(11q) involves ATM, which encodes a protein which interacts with p53 in response to DNA damage. Del(11q) deletions are more commonly seen in younger patients and are associated with poorer outcome. When del(13q) deletion is the sole cytogenetic abnormality it confers a better prognosis. Studies have provided conflicting evidence regarding the implications of trisomy 12.

The median survival of patients with mutated IGVH is 25 years compared to eight years for patients with unmutated IGVH.

Increased levels of CD38, detectable by flow cytometry, are associated with poorer prognosis.

With the advent of HTS, a large number of genomic prognostic factors are being evaluated to better understand disease biology and the association between specific abnormalities and patient outcome.

A pooled analysis of international trial data has proposed a prognostic scoring system (the CLL International Prognostic Index, CLL-IPI) incorporating the above clinical, laboratory, and genetic information.

12.18 Treatment for chronic lymphocytic leukaemia

Overview

Indications for treatment are defined by the international workshop iwCLL. Not all patients with CLL will require treatment. In patients with low-risk, asymptomatic CLL (Binet A/Rai 0), observation rather than immediate treatment is the current standard of care. This includes patients with adverse prognostic factors such as 17p deletion in whom no other indication for treatment exists. Many of these patients do not need specialist follow-up and can be monitored by a general practitioner with regular blood tests every three to six months. Patients with intermediate-risk (Binet B/Rai I and II) and high-risk (Binet C/Rai III and IV) CLL usually benefit from the initiation of treatment. However, some patients can be monitored until they exhibit symptoms of 'active disease':

- Progressive marrow failure (Hb <10g/dl or platelet counts <100 × 10^9/L, although a stable platelet count of <100 × 10^9/L may not require therapeutic intervention).
- Massive (≥6cm below the costal margin), progressive or symptomatic splenomegaly.
- Massive (≥10cm longest diameter), progressive or symptomatic lymphadenopathy.
- Progressive lymphocytosis (increase of ≥50% over two months or a doubling time <6 months) in the absence of a secondary cause.
- Autoimmune complications not responsive to steroid therapy.
- Symptomatic extranodal involvement.
- Disease-related systemic symptoms:
  - Unintentional weight loss (≥10% in six months).
  - Fever ≥38°C for ≥2 weeks in the absence of infection.
  - Significant fatigue (i.e. ECOG PS ≥2).
  - Night sweats ≥1 month in the absence of infection.

First-line therapy

There are several treatment options available and these are likely to increase over the coming years. They include purine analogues (e.g. fludarabine, pentostatin), alkylating agents (e.g. cyclophosphamide, chlorambucil), monoclonal antibodies (e.g. rituximab, ofatumumab, obinutuzumab), and 'targeted' therapies such as Bruton's tyrosine kinase (BTK) inhibitors (e.g. ibrutinib), PI3K inhibitors (e.g. idelalisib), and B-cell lymphoma 2 (BCL2) inhibitors (e.g. venetoclax). Choice of therapy is based upon patient characteristics, tumour characteristics, and goals of therapy. Where possible, patients should be enrolled in a clinical trial.

Pretreatment assessment

Of significant importance is defining the 'unfit' patient with CLL, which is not always synonymous with older age. An individual aged 75 years may be 'fitter' than an individual aged 60 with multiple comorbidities. Various scores have been employed to give a more objective assessment of comorbidity. Generally clinicians will divide patients into three groups: those fit for more intensive regimens, those not suitable for intensive therapy, and those not fit for treatment at all. Clinical trials do not employ uniform entry criteria to capture these patient groups. Therefore, the treating clinician needs to evaluate and extrapolate trial data carefully.

Untreated fit patients with no TP53 abnormality

Fludarabine, cyclophosphamide, and rituximab (FCR) is the current recommended first-line treatment in younger, fit patients with no TP53 abnormality. Toxicity is related to myelotoxicity and infectious complications. FCR has been shown to be superior to FC in a randomized controlled trial, with higher overall response rates (ORR) (95% vs. 88%) and complete response rates (CRR) (44% vs. 22%), longer median PFS (52 months vs. 33 months), and OS at three years (87% vs. 83%), with similar rates of severe infections and treatment-related deaths. This regimen is particularly effective in patients with mutated IGHV where about 60% remain progression-free at ten years.

Fludarabine-based therapy has demonstrated superiority to chlorambucil; this is apparent in long-term data from phase 3 trials. FCR therapy appears to overcome the adverse prognosis of del(11q) but patients with del(17p) have a poor prognosis and an alternative approach should be taken. In fit patients, FCR continues to show superior results compared to bendamustine and rituximab (BR) in a randomized trial from the German study group (CLL10 study). FCR is however associated with greater toxicity.

Emerging evidence supports the use of 'targeted' therapies in untreated fit patients without a TP53 abnormality. A recent oral presentation of the phase 3 ECOG-ACRIN E1912 trial demonstrated in most younger adults with CLL that ibrutinib plus rituximab when compared to FCR improves PFS and OS with fewer serious adverse events. The benefit of ibrutinib and rituximab was less clear in patients with IGHV-mutated CLL.

Untreated patients with TP53 abnormality

Patients with del(17p) or a TP53 mutation are at significant risk of not responding to or relapsing soon after initial treatment with chemoimmunotherapy such as FCR. Ibrutinib has now replaced alemtuzumab and steroids as the standard of care in this patient cohort. Evidence supporting the use of ibrutinib in previously untreated CLL patients with a TP53 abnormality is extrapolated from its use in trials in relapsed/refractory CLL as well as smaller trials in the treatment-naïve population. Idelalisib and rituximab or venetoclax are also effective treatments for this patient group when ibrutinb is unsuitable.

Untreated unfit patients

Chlorambucil-based regimens remain the standard treatment in patients unfit for more intensive therapy. The addition of an anti-CD20 antibody (rituximab, ofatumumab, or obinutuzumab) improves RR, PFS, and OS compared to chlorambucil alone. The CLL11 trial randomized patients to chlorambucil, rituximab-chlorambucil, or obinutuzumab-chlorambucil. Treatment with obinutuzumab-chlorambucil or rituximab-chlorambucil increased the ORR and prolonged PFS when compared with chlorambucil (median PFS, 27 months with obinutuzumab-chlorambucil vs. 16 months with rituximab-chlorambucil vs. 11 months with chlorambucil). Treatment with obinutuzumab-chlorambucil, when compared with chlorambucil, prolonged OS (hazard ratio (HR) for death 0.41; 95% CI 0.23–0.74). Treatment with obinutuzumab-chlorambucil, when compared with rituximab-chlorambucil, resulted in prolongation of PFS (HR 0.39; 95% CI 0.31–0.49), higher CRR (21% vs. 7%), and improved OS. Although infusion-related reactions and neutropenia were more common with obinutuzumab-chlorambucil than with rituximab-chlorambucil, the risk of infection was not increased.

Bendamustine in combination with rituximab is an acceptable alternative to FCR for patients with comorbidities such as decreased renal function. Bendamustine monotherapy has demonstrated improved ORR when compared with chlorambucil alone, although survival benefits have not been demonstrated.

As with fit untreated patients, emerging evidence supports the use of ibrutinib in unfit, untreated patients. The Alliance A041202 trial demonstrated that single agent ibrutinib improved 24-month PFS (87% vs. 74%) when compared to BR. The RESONATE-2 trial found ibrutinib therapy resulted in higher PFS (89% vs. 34%) and OS (95% vs. 84%) rates at 24 months when compared to chlorambucil. Finally, in the iLLUMINATE trial, a higher PFS (79% vs. 31%) with similar OS at 30 months was observed with ibrutinib-obinutuzumab when compared to chlorambucil-obinutuzumab. The role of an anti-CD20 in combination with ibrutinib in unfit, treatment-naïve CLL patients is currently not clear.

Response criteria

The iwCLL has published the most recent response criteria (Hallek et al. 2018).

For therapies with a definitive duration (e.g. FCR), disease response assessment should be >2 months after the end of treatment. For continued therapies, disease response assessment should be performed >2 months after patients achieve their maximum response (or at a time predefined in the protocol).

The use of sensitive multicolor flow cytometry, polymerase chain reaction, or high-throughput sequencing can detect MRD to <1 CLL cell in 10,000 leukocytes. Prospective clinical trials have provided evidence that treatment which eradicates MRD can result in improved clinical outcomes. However, this goal must be balanced with minimizing treatment-related toxicity and ensuring a good quality of life.

Follow-up after treatment

Many patients undergoing chemotherapy for CLL/SLL will have an initial complete response or partial response. Except for those patients who undergo potentially curative HSCT, disease relapse invariably occurs. Following initial therapy, patients are reviewed at regular intervals, with a consultation, examination, and blood tests, with a focus on monitoring for therapy-related complications or relapse.

If relapse is suspected, this must be confirmed:
- Full blood count, peripheral blood film, FISH, and immunophenotyping—this can confirm disease relapse in most cases as well as identifying adverse prognostic factors (e.g. del(17p)).
- If histological transformation is suspected (rapid progression of lymphadenopathy, infiltration of uncommon extranodal sites, systemic symptoms, or an elevated lactate dehydrogenase), a lymph node biopsy is mandatory. FDG-PET scanning may assist in deciding an appropriate biopsy site.

- Bone marrow biopsy (particularly if cytopenias are present, but often used to assess disease burden).

Relapsed or refractory CLL

The choice of treatment should take into account the response to previous therapy, presence of adverse genetics (TP53), and patient fitness.

In patients with disease relapse occurring earlier than the median predicted PFS for prior therapy and for those with a TP53 abnormality, 'targeted' therapy is preferred. Options include ibrutinib, idelalisib-rituximab, and venetoclax with or without rituximab. The choice of treatment is dependent on side effect profile of each agent and prior exposure to 'targeted' treatment. The optimal length of treatment (years/life-long) for these agents is unknown. Current practice is to continue treatment until progressive disease or unacceptable toxicity. Many of the clinical trials have shown a benefit across the different CLL disease subgroups.

Ibrutinib is generally well tolerated and in patients who respond, a lymphocytosis is observed followed by a reduction in lymphadenopathy and improvement in symptoms and blood counts. The RESONATE trial, which compared ibrutinib to ofatumumab in relapsed/refractory CLL, found a favourable PFS (59% vs. 3%) and OS (74% vs. 65%) with ibrutnib at 36 months. The efficacy of ibrutinib in relapsed/refractory CLL with del(17p) has also been demonstrated in the phase 2 RESONATE-17 trial, with a 24-month OS of 75%. In a recent phase 2 study, the addition of rituximab to ibrutinib did not appear to improve PFS. Unwanted effects of ibrutinib include atrial fibrillation, hypertension, transient diarrhoea, infection, transaminitis, an increased risk of bleeding, skin rash, and cytopenia.

Idelalisib has shown therapeutic activity in relapsed/refractory CLL as a single agent or, as now used in clinical practice, in combination with rituximab. A phase 3 trial demonstrated idelalisib-rituximab had a superior ORR (84% vs. 16%) when compared to placebo plus rituximab. Another randomized phase 3 trial compared ofatumumab-idelalisib versus ofatumumab. With a median follow-up of 16 months, the addition of idelalisib improved the ORR (75% vs. 18%) although OS was similar. As with ibrutinib, idelalisib therapy results in a transient lymphocytosis. Significant unwanted effects include an increased risk of opportunistic infection such as *Pneumocystis jirovecii* pneumonia (PJP), hepatotoxicity, diarrhoea, colitis, intestinal perforation, and pneumonitis.

Venetoclax has demonstrated efficacy in CLL both with and without rituximab. In a phase 2 single-arm study of patients with del(17p) CLL, the majority of whom had relapsed/refractory disease, venetoclax demonstrated an 77% ORR with an estimated 24-month PFS of 54%. An interim analysis of a phase 2 trial of venetoclax in patients who have relapsed/refractory disease following ibrutinib or idelalisib found an ORR 65% and 67% and 12-month PFS of 75% and 79% respectively. Finally, the phase 3 MURANO trial randomized patients with relapsed/refractory CLL to venetoclax-rituximab or BR. Venetoclax-rituximab showed superior 24-month PFS (85% vs. 36%) and OS (92% vs. 87%). Tumour lysis syndrome (TLS) is an important unwanted effect on commencement of venetoclax. As well as a dose escalation regimen, TLS risk stratification with appropriate prophylaxis is necessary when commencing venetoclax.

In patients with disease relapse occurring later than the median predicted PFS (late relapse) the same therapy may be considered, particularly if minimal toxicity was associated with the initial treatment.

As the only definitive curative option HSCT may be considered in younger fit patients; however observational studies suggest patients in complete remission at the time of transplantation have an improved prognosis and therefore treatment should be given to achieve this before HSCT.

Management of complications and supportive care

Patients with CLL are at risk of infection due to disease burden, treatment, hyposplenism, and immune dysfunction. Patients should receive immunization against pneumococcus, haemophilus influenza B, and annual influenza, but should not receive any live vaccines. While on treatment, prophylactic anti-PJP and antiviral medications should be given for patients receiving immunosuppressive therapy. In addition, antifungals should be given to those receiving steroids. Hypogammaglobulinaemia is a common occurrence in patients with CLL, and infusion with regular intravenous immunoglobulin (IVIG) may be beneficial in patients with severe or recurrent infections. Hepatitis B reactivation has been observed in patients following monoclonal antibody therapy—serology should be sent prior to therapy and appropriate antiviral therapy given to those at risk of reactivation.

For autoimmune complications, steroids, IVIG, or rituximab may be useful. Staging of a patient with CLL should not take place when there are autoimmune complications; this may result in overstaging the patient, resulting in unnecessary chemotherapy administration.

The destruction of a large volume of CLL cells as a consequence of the initiation of certain therapies, results in large amounts of phosphate and other products which co-precipitate with calcium in the kidneys, leading to hypocalcaemia, and sometimes to renal failure. Hyperuricaemia further contributes to this problem. Rasburicase, (a recombinant version of urate oxidase) can be used for patients at high risk of developing TLS, or allopurinol for patients with moderate or low risk.

Symptom control

Rituximab and corticosteroids can result in short-term partial responses with minimal toxicity. Splenectomy may be useful in patients with splenomegaly and significant cytopenias unresponsive to chemotherapy or refractory AIHA. Radiation therapy to bulky lymphoid tissue is an option for patients with bulky disease compromising nearby structures.

Further reading

Hallek M. On the architecture of translational research designed to control chronic lymphocytic leukemia. *Hematology Am Soc Hematol Educ Program* 2018; 1:1–8.

Hallek M, Cheson BD, Catovsky D, Caligaris-Cappio F, Dighiero G, Dohner H, et al. iwCLL guidelines for diagnosis, indications for treatment, response assessment, and supportive management of CLL. *Blood* 2018; 131(25):2745–60.

Schuh AH, Parry-Jones N, Appleby N, et al. Guideline for the treatment of chronic lymphocytic leukaemia: A British Society for Haematology Guideline. *Br J Haematol* 2018; 182:344–59.

Internet resources

BCSH Guidelines: https://b-s-h.org.uk/guidelines/guidelines/treatment-of-chronic-lymphocytic-leukaemia/

Cancer Research UK: http://www.cancerresearchuk.org

Macmillan Cancer Support: Chronic Lymphotcytic Leukaemia: https://www.macmillan.org.uk/cancer-information-and-support/leukaemia/chronic-lymphocytic-leukaemia-cll

NICE: http://www.nice.org.uk/

UKCLL Forum: http://www.ukcllforum.org

12.19 Hairy cell leukaemia

Introduction

Hairy cell leukaemia (HCL) is a chronic B-cell lymphoproliferative disorder that tends to present in late middle age with an incidence of one to three per million. There are classical and variant subtypes which are characterized by the clonal proliferation of mature B cells that are typically found in the peripheral blood and bone marrow. These cells have a characteristic 'hairy' morphology owing to cytoplasmic projections and a typical immunophenotype that is distinct from other chronic B-cell lymphoproliferative disorders. Recent advances in our understanding of the genetic mutations that are almost universal in classical HCL have translated directly into patient benefit. Data are now supportive of using new targeted signalling pathway inhibitors for patients with disease refractory to standard therapies.

Clinical presentation

HCL has a male predominance (3:1) with a median age of 63 at diagnosis. Many patients are relatively well at initial presentation and the diagnosis may be made as part of investigations for unexplained cytopenias. Other patients may be unwell at presentation as a consequence of neutropenia or anaemia, and many have symptoms and signs of splenomegaly. Peripheral lymphadenopathy is generally not a feature of this disease. Systemic 'B' symptoms are not common at initial presentation, but may become more problematic with advanced disease. However, it is well recognized that HCL patients have a higher incidence of non-specific symptoms including arthralgia, weight loss, myalgia, and skin rashes. HCL typically responds very well to treatment with patients enjoying protracted periods in remission when symptoms are minimal and patients usually have a good quality of life.

Laboratory features

HCL can present with profound neutropenia (<0.5 x 10^9/L), monocytopenia (<0.1 x 10^9/L) and a variable low-level lymphocytosis which is typically less than 10 x 10^9/L in classical HCL (cHCL). This can occasionally be as high as 100 x 10^9/L in HCL variant (HCLv). There is commonly a normochromic normocytic anaemia at presentation which can occasionally be exacerbated by a direct antiglobulin test positive haemolytic anaemia. Examination of the blood film typically reveals lymphoid cells with characteristic cytoplasmic projections which give the hairy appearance recognized in the name of the condition. These cells are typically twice as large as normal lymphocytes and possess round to oval shaped nuclei with an open chromatin pattern. Some cHCL patients have very few hairy cells in the peripheral blood at presentation and the cells are easily missed without careful examination of the blood film. Bone marrow aspiration is generally unsuccessful providing only a 'dry tap'—this is due to an increase in reticulin fibres. However, bone marrow trephine biopsy examination reveals sheets of abnormal lymphoid cells with reduced normal haematopoiesis and fibrosis. Immunophenotyping of blood or bone marrow through flow cytometry is the mainstay for diagnosing HCL with classical hairy cells expressing the common B-cell antigens CD19, CD20, and CD22 but also co-expressing CD11c, CD25, CD103, and CD123. Additional immunohistochemistry of the bone marrow biopsy demonstrates CD20, tartrate-resistant acid phosphatase and DBA.44 positivity, the latter two of which, when combined, have near 100% sensitivity for cHCL. Rarely, histological analysis of splenic tissue from biopsy can also be used to make the diagnosis, demonstrating infiltration and expansion of the red pulp with hairy cells. In recent years, molecular analysis has identified the V600E mutation of the BRAF gene in almost all cases of cHCL. The BRAF V600E mutation is also very common amongst other cancers including melanoma, colorectal cancer, thyroid cancer, and non-small cell lung carcinoma. The BRAF gene encodes a member of the serine/threonine protein kinase family that is important in mediating cell division and differentiation. Downstream effectors of BRAF include MEK (mitogen-activated protein kinase) which phosphorylates ERK (extracellular signal-regulated kinase) and contributes to increased cell proliferation. In recent years, there has been considerable interest in the development of small molecule inhibitors to exploit these novel targets in cHCL with the advantage of bypassing conventional chemotherapy options that have less favourable side effect profiles.

Management

The majority of patients presenting with HCL tend to be well at diagnosis and do not require immediate intervention. The indications for treatment are primarily symptomatic; e.g. painful splenomegaly, significant fatigue interfering with activities of daily living and PS, or progressive cytopenias producing symptoms of infections, anaemia, or bleeding. The use of α-interferon in cHCL was first described in 1984, producing 30% CR and 56% partial remission rates. This was rapidly superseded by the introduction of the purine analogues pentostatin (2-deoxycoformicin), that functions through the inhibition of adenosine deaminase (an enzyme important for lymphocyte proliferation), and cladribine (2-chloro-2'deoxyadenosine) which induces cell death through directly preventing DNA repair. Biweekly pentostatin was shown to produce CR rates of >70% and proven to be significantly superior to α-IFN in randomized trials. Large retrospective studies have shown patients treated with either agent had an overall CR rate of 80% with median relapse-free survivals as long as 16 years. As a result, these two drugs have become standard first-line therapy for patients with cHCL. CR in cHCL is defined as complete clearance of hairy cells from the peripheral blood and bone marrow with resolution of cytopenias and organomegaly, whilst PR constitutes a normalization of cytopenias with at least 50% resolution in organomegaly and bone marrow infiltration. Patients who attain PR after first course cladribine, may be given a second course to achieve CR or may equally well be treated further at disease progression. Many patients require repeat courses of purine analogues, potentially over decades, and a progressive shortening of response tends to be the rule. Relapses that occur within two years of remission are usually treated next with the alternative purine analogue, whilst those occurring after two years may be retreated with the same agent. Patients receiving purine analogues for cHCL require prophylaxis against pneumocystis infections and herpesvirus reactivation due to long-term significant suppression of CD4 lymphocyte counts. Additionally, both drugs carry long-term risks of transfusion associated graft versus host disease (ta-GVHD) therefore patients will have a lifelong requirement for ir-radiated blood if ever transfused in the future. Adjuncts to purine analogues in the form of immunotherapies have been explored in recent years, particularly in the relapse setting, to augment treatment responses. The B-cell-specific differentiating antigen CD20 is expressed across all B-cell malignancies, and has been demonstrated to have the highest level of expression on hairy cells. Rituximab is an anti-CD20 monoclonal chimeric antibody that induces B-cell depletion through antibody-dependent cell-mediated and complement-dependent cytotoxicity and induction of apoptosis—and in retrospective studies has shown additional benefit when treating relapsed cHCL in combination with purine analogues, delivering CR rates as high as 89%. Whilst its current use is in combination with purine analogues at relapse, the use of rituximab with purine analogues versus single agent in de novo or relapsed cHCL is currently being addressed in clinical trials. Limited data suggest that HCLv may respond better to purine analogues when combined with rituximab, rather than purine analogues alone. The immunotoxin conjugates LMB-2 and moxetumomab pasudotox that target CD25 and CD22 respectively have been evaluated for their use in HCL in clinical trials, having shown promise in early trials, with the latter recently receiving approval for use in relapsed or refractory HCL. More recently, targeted kinase inhibition with the thymidine kinase inhibitor vemurafenib has shown considerable efficacy against BRAFV600E mutated melanoma and small numbers of heavily pretreated cHCL patients, having a limited sideeffect profile. Smaller clinical trials have recently demonstrated short oral courses of vemurafenib to be highly effective in relapsed or refractory hairy cell leukaemia. Interestingly, reactivation of the downstream MEK and ERK pathway was noted in a number of patients treated with BRAF inhibition, suggesting potential mechanisms of resistance, and there is currently interest in developing targeted inhibitors of these, potentially adding further options to the armamentarium of therapies for cHCL in the future. MEK inhibition has since been successfully used in a patient with relapsed HCL demonstrating resistance to prior therapy with vemurafenib, highlighting a novel therapeutic option that requires further testing in a formal trial setting. Finally, early data suggests ibrutinib, a targeted inhibitor of the Bruton tyrosine kinase that has licensed indications in other B lymphoproliferative disorders, may have efficacy in HCL. However, the rarity of the disease and particularly the rarity of patients with relapsed/refractory disease makes prospective trial design to explore these new agents challenging.

Further reading

Basheer F, Bloxham DM, Scott MA, Follows GA. Hairy cell leukemia—immunotargets and therapies. *Immunotargets Ther* 2014; 24(3):107–20.

Caeser R, Collord G, Yao W, et al. Targeting MEK in vemurafenib-resistant hairy cell leukemia. *Leukemia* 2019; 33:541–5.

Follows GA, Sims H, Bloxham DM, Zenz T, Hopper MA, Liu H, Bench A, Wright P, Van't Veer MB, Scott MA. Rapid response of biallelic BRAF V600E mutated hairy cell leukaemia to low dose vemurafenib. *Br J Haematol* 2013; 161(1):150–3.

Grever MR, Abdel-Wahab O, Andritsos LA, et al. Consensus guidelines for the diagnosis and management of patients with classic hairy cell leukaemia. *Blood* 2017; 129(5):553–60.

12.20 Myelodysplastic syndrome overview

Introduction

The myelodysplastic syndromes (MDSs) are a heterogeneous group of clonal haematopoietic stem cell diseases characterized by dysplasia and ineffective haematopoiesis in one or more of the major cell lineages. The dysplasia may be accompanied by an increase in the myeloblasts in the bone marrow but the number is <20%, which is the requisite threshold recommended for the diagnosis of acute myeloid leukaemia.

Epidemiology and aetiology

MDS occurs predominantly in older adults (median age 70 years), with a non-age incidence of three per 100,000 but rising to 20 per 100,000 over the age of 70 years.

MDS occurs as primary or de novo disorder and an increasing number of therapy-related disease or 'secondary MDS/AML' have been recognized as a result of chemotherapy/radiation therapy for other malignant disorders. In 'de novo' MDS, possible aetiologies include viruses and exposure to benzene/petrochemicals. Cigarette smoking increases the risk by two-fold. Some inherited haematological disorders, such as Fanconi's anaemia are also associated with an increased incidence of MDS.

Secondary MDS/AML may represent as many as 10–15% of all MDS and AML diagnosed each year. Two major types are recognized based on the causative agents:

- Alkylating agents/radiation related: usually occur five to six years (range of 10–192 months) following exposure to the mutagenic agents. The risk for occurrence is related to the total cumulative dose of the alkylating agent and the age of the patient.
- Topoisomerase II inhibitor related: usually has a shorter latency period and develops at a median interval of 33–34 months (range 12–130 months) from the time of institution of the implicated agents. Major agents are etoposide and teniposide but anthracyclines like doxorubicin are also implicated.

Classification

In 2008, WHO published a new classification scheme for MDS to improve its prognostic value (see 'Further reading' p. 369).

Diagnosis

The minimal initial evaluation for patients clinically suspected to have MDS includes a comprehensive history and physical examination, complete blood count with leukocyte differential which usually shows one or more cytopenias, bone marrow aspiration and biopsy with iron stain, and cytogenetic studies, erythropoietin levels, and iron studies.

Other investigations to exclude transient or reactive causes for macrocytic anaemia or isolated cytopenias such as vitamin B12 and folate levels, hepatic and renal functions, screen for viral infections/alcohol/toxins, and thyroid function should be done.

Morphological considerations

Assessment of the degree of dysplasia and hence the diagnosis of MDS requires high-quality smear preparation and staining.

The blood and marrow aspirate smears should be examined for dysplasia, the percentage of blasts and monocytes, and for ringed sideroblasts.

Cells counted as 'blasts' include myeloblasts, monoblasts, and megakaryoblasts. Small dysplastic megakaryocytes are not blasts and erythroid precursors are also not counted as blasts except in rare cases of 'erythroleukaemia' in which primitive erythroblasts account for the majority of the cells. In myelomonocytic proliferations, promonocytes are included as 'blast equivalents'. Substitution of the percent of CD34+ cells determined by flow cytometry for a visual blast count on morphology is misleading and is discouraged.

Dyserythropoiesis is manifested principally by alterations in the nucleus including budding, internuclear bridging, karyorrhexis, multinuclearity, and megaloblastoid changes; cytoplasmic features include ring sideroblasts, vacuolization, and periodic acid–Schiff positivity, either diffuse or granular.

Dysgranulopoiesis is characterized primarily by small size, nuclear hypolobulation (pseudo-Pelger–Huët), and hypersegmentation, hypogranularity, and pseudo-Chediak–Higashi granules.

Megakaryocyte dysplasia may be characterized by hypolobulated micromegakaryocytes, non-lobulated nuclei in megakaryocytes of all sizes, and multiple widely separated nuclei.

The marrow is usually hypercellular or normocellular and the cytopenias result from ineffective haematopoiesis.

A bone marrow biopsy, although not always necessary, can provide valuable diagnostic and prognostic information such as disruption of normal marrow architecture in the form of abnormal localization of immature precursors (ALIPs).

Immunophenotypic considerations

Enumeration of CD34+ cells by flow cytometry provides diagnostic and prognostic information.

No single abnormality is specific for MDS, but an abnormal light scatter of dysplastic cells, abnormal antigen density, loss of antigens, and dys-synchronous expression of antigens that are normally coexpressed during myeloid maturation have all been reported in MDS and may even correlate with the grade of the disease (Stetler-Stevenson et al. 2001)

Cytogenetics and molecular aspects
The importance of cytogenetic abnormalities in the prediction of survival and in assessing the risk of transformation to acute leukaemia is well known and cytogenetic studies have been included in most of the classification and predictive scoring systems developed for MDS (Greenberg et al. 1997). Clonality in MDS is demonstrated by deletional defects, i.e. monosomy 7 occurring in at least two of 30 cells, and additional defects, i.e. trisomy 8 occurring in one or more of 30 cells examined. Clonal chromosomal abnormalities are detected in 40–70% of cases of de novo MDS cases. Deletions of part or all of chromosome 5 and/or 7 and complex chromosomal abnormalities account for 90% of karyotypic changes in therapy related MDSs (t-MDS).

The de novo '5q- syndrome' is recognized as a specific type of MDS which occurs primarily in women, is characterized by normal or increased platelet counts, megakaryocytes with hypolobulated nuclei, refractory macrocytic anaemia, an isolated del(5q) chromosome abnormality, and a favourable clinical course.

Other cytogenetic abnormalities with prognostic significance are included in the International Prognostic Scoring System (IPSS).

Molecular abnormalities involved in the pathogenesis of MDS are multiple and incompletely understood. However, some of the mechanisms resulting in an imbalance between apoptosis and proliferation pathways are:
- Uncontrolled proliferation: RAS (NRAS), JAK2, PDGRFB mutations
- Loss of apoptotic mechanisms: p53 mutation
- Differentiation block: c-fms pathway, granulocyte colony stimulating factor (G-CSF) receptor mutations
- Constitutive activation of tyrosine kinases: flt 3 pathway
- Epigenetic mechanisms: methylation of genes like p15, e-cadherin
- Aberrant immune surveillance: increased T regulatory cells
- Aberrant gene 5q-: block of ribosomal protein RPS14 expression.

Specific diagnostic issues
Reactive or transient cytopenias
- Morphologic dysplasia is not specific to MDS.
- Reactive dysplasia is seen in conditions like megaloblastic anaemia, exposure to toxins like arsenic and alcohol, and after cytotoxic and growth factor therapy.
- Dyserythropoiesis is common in situations of 'stressed haemopoiesis' like haemolysis, recovery from cytotoxic therapy, or transplantation.
- Cytogenetic abnormalities or raised percentage of blasts are uncommon.

Unexplained cytopenias
- Unexplained persistent cytopenias with little or no morphologic dysplasia can be a challenging problem and can be seen commonly in older adults.
- If not associated with a clonal cytogenetic abnormality, they should be monitored at regular intervals.
- A small proportion will evolve into MDS—morphologically and cytogenetically.

Hypocellular MDS
- A minority of MDS patients have a hypocellular bone marrow (<30% cellularity in patients <60 years old; <20% cellularity in patients 60 years old).
- Differentiating between hypocellular MDS and aplastic anaemia (AA) can be very difficult. Features favouring MDS are neutrophils with pseudo-Pelger–Huët nuclei and/or hypogranular cytoplasm in blood smears and dysplastic granulopoiesis and megakaryocytopoiesis and normal or raised blasts in the bone marrow.
- Abnormal antigen expression of CD34+ cells measured by multiparameter flow cytometry, the number of HbF containing erythroblasts, and the percentage of Ki67+ cells, have also been reported to be helpful in separation of AA from MDS.
- Although the identification of a clonal chromosomal abnormality at the time of presentation is generally considered as indicative of MDS, patients with clonal chromosomal abnormalities have been included in some series of AA.
- It is necessary to exclude other diseases with hypocellular bone marrow specimens that may masquerade clinically as AA or MDS, particularly hypocellular AML, hairy cell leukaemia, and large granular lymphocytosis.

Myelodysplastic syndrome/myeloproliferative disorders (MDS/MPD)
The MDS/MPD category includes clonal myeloid disorders that have both dysplastic and proliferative features at presentation.

Disorders included in this category of WHO classification are:
- Chronic myelomonocytic leukaemia (CMML)
- Atypical chronic myeloid leukaemia
- Juvenile myelomonocytic leukaemia (JMML)
- Myelodysplastic/myeloproliferative disease, unclassifiable

Further reading
Greenberg P, Cox C, LeBeau MM, et al. International Scoring System for evaluating prognosis in myelodysplastic syndromes. *Blood* 1997; 89:2079–88.

Stetler-Stevenson M, Arthur DC, Jabbour N, et al. Diagnostic utility of flow cytometric immunophenotyping in myelodysplastic syndromes. *Blood* 2001; 98:979–87.

Swerdlow SH, et al. WHO Classification of Tumours of Haematopoietic and Lymphoid Tissues. *IARC WHO Classification of Tumours*, Vol. 2, 4th edn. IARC, 2008.

12.21 Clinical features, staging, and prognosis of myelodysplastic syndrome

Clinical features

- Signs and symptoms of the disease are those associated with cytopenias, i.e. symptoms of anaemia, bleeding/petechiae with thrombocytopenia, or infections because of neutropenia.
- Many patients can be asymptomatic and MDS is diagnosed on routine screening blood tests.
- Infection remains the principal cause of death in patients with MDS. Although fungal, viral, and mycobacterial infections can occur, they are rare in the absence of concurrent administration of immunosuppressive agents.
- Autoimmune manifestations can be seen in about 14% of MDS patients—the most common are cutaneous vasculitis and monoarticular arthritis.
- Acute febrile neutrophilic dermatosis (Sweet's syndrome) is the most common vasculitic condition in MDS.
- Although connective tissue disorders such as relapsing polychondritis, polymyalgia rheumatica, Raynaud's phenomenon, and Sjögren's syndrome, inflammatory bowel disease, pyoderma gangrenosum, and glomerulonephritis have been reported in association with MDS, a causal relationship has not been established.

Staging and prognosis

- The IPSS was revised in 2012. In this system, percentage of marrow blasts, specific cytogenetic abnormalities, and number of cytopenias were used in combination to define five risk groups for OS and AML evolution: very low, low, intermediate, high, and very high.
- The overall median survival was 8.8. 5.3, 3.0, 1.6, and 0.8 years for the five groups respectively.

- The time for disease in 25% of patients in each of the five risk groups to evolve into acute leukaemia was 'not reached' for very low risk, and was 10.8, 3.2, 1.4, and 0.73 years for the low-, intermediate-, high-, and very high-risk groups respectively.
- The impact of age is a major prognostic parameter for OS in MDS, but not for leukaemic transformation. Adverse impact of older age is more apparent on the lower-risk group than the high-risk group categories. Most patients with low- and intermediate-risk MDS, die because of the consequences of bone marrow failure rather than transformation to AML, while many patients with IPSS high-risk disease would be considered by some already to have AML.
- Other factors have been shown to add significant prognostic information to that provided by the IPSS. One of these is the mutation and/or loss of the heterozygosity of the tumour suppressor gene p53. This defect is commonly noted in MDS, especially in older patients and following exposure to alkylating agents and is associated with complex karyotypic changes, an increased tendency to evolve into AML, reduced responses to chemotherapy, and shorter OS. Other molecular mutations shown to have an impact on prognosis are ASXL1, IDH1, IDH2, RUNX1, TET2, EZH2, N-RAS, and K-RAS. Other prognostic factors which have been studied are:
  - Transfusion dependence
  - CD34 positivity of bone marrow nucleated cells
  - Increased expression of the Wilms' tumour gene
  - Increased serum beta-2 microglobulin concentration
  - Decreased platelet mass
  - Abnormal localization of immature precursors

12.22 Treatment for myelodysplastic syndrome

Introduction

The IPSS score at diagnosis, blood transfusion dependence, bone marrow cellularity, and comorbidities of the patient guide management of MDS. Supportive care has previously been the standard of care for patients with MDS and may still be the only care appropriate for some. However, the following key advances in MDS emphasize better outcomes with state-of-the-art treatment leading to supportive care being an important scaffold in the definitive treatment of MDS.

Key advances

- The FDA approval of three drugs, azacytidine, decitabine, and lenalidomide, for the treatment of MDS.
- Recognition of transfusion dependence and iron overload as independent adverse prognostic factors that affect overall and leukaemia-free survival.
- Evidence that the treatment of iron overload also significantly increases OS.

Supportive care

This consists of monitoring blood counts, blood product replacement, treatment of infections, and iron chelation.

Indications for supportive care

- Patients not suitable for definitive treatment.
- During and pending a response to definitive treatment.
- Failure to respond or loss of response to active drugs.

Monitoring blood counts

- In low-risk MDS, monitoring blood counts for disease progression may be the only requirement.

Platelet transfusions

- Bleeding may be due to thrombocytopenia or platelet dysfunction (even with normal counts).
- Treatment with platelet transfusions to maintain a threshold of 10×10^9/L if the patient is not septic or bleeding, 20×10^9/L if septic, and higher if surgery is contemplated.

Blood transfusions

- Eighty per cent of patients are anaemic at presentation.
- Correctable causes such as iron, vitamin B12, or folate deficiency, thyroid and liver dysfunction, autoimmune haemolytic anaemia, and PNH (paroxysmal nocturnal haemoglobinuria) should be excluded.
- Blood transfusions are usually introduced for symptomatic anaemia (Hb 8g/dL; higher if there is a history of cardiac impairment).

Iron chelation therapy

- In low-risk MDS, where long-term transfusion therapy is anticipated, iron chelation is recommended when ferritin >1000mcg/l or 25 units of blood have been transfused.
- Ophthalmological and audiometric review are prerequisites to commencing desferrioxamine or deferasirox as both can cause sensorineural hearing loss and lenticular opacities.
- Creatinine clearance of at least 60ml/min is necessary before commencing deferasirox
- Desferrioxamine 20–40mg/kg subcutaneously over 12 hours, five to seven days a week is commenced to achieve a target ferritin of <1000mcg/l. The dose of desferrioxamine is reduced to <25mg/kg once ferritin levels are <2000mcg/l.
- Deferasirox (Exjade®, Novartis) an oral iron chelator is commenced at 20–30mg/kg/day. Renal and liver function monitoring is recommended with the use of deferasirox.

Management of infections

- There is no evidence for a role for prophylactic antibiotics or antifungal drugs.
- G-CSF therapy in severe neutropenia may be used to maintain a neutrophil count >1 × 10⁹/L.
- Episodes of neutropenic sepsis are treated as emergencies according to local protocols.

Differentiation therapy

Erythropoietin stimulating agents

- Recombinant human erythropoietin (EPO) or darbepoietin alpha (Aranesp®, its hypersialyated derivative with a longer half-life) can be used to stimulate erythropoiesis in MDS.
- Factors predicting EPO responsiveness include <10% bone marrow blasts; low or Int-1 IPSS, serum EPO levels <200U/l, transfusion independence, and a short time between diagnosis and treatment.
- The presence of del 5q- with or without additional cytogenetic abnormalities reduces response duration from a mean of 24 months to 12 months but does not affect response rates.
- Treatment of anaemia with erythropoiesis stimulating agents (ESAs) reduces the risk of progression to AML, and responders to EPO/G-CSF combination have a longer OS of 53 months compared with 23 months in non-responders.
- Patients are selected on the basis of the ESA predictive score: see Table 12.22.1.
- EPO/darbepoietin may be commenced for symptomatic anaemia at Hb between 9–11g/dl.
- If the Hb is lower than this, initial transfusion support in addition to an ESA may be necessary.
- A front-loading schedule utilizes 30,000–60,000 units of erythropoietin SC per week initially for six to eight

Table 12.22.1 Predictive score for treatment of MDS with G-CSF and EPO

Parameter	Value	Score
Serum erythropoietin	<500U/L	0
	>500U/L	1
Blood transfusions	<2U/month	0
	>2U/month	1

Predicted response rate pre-treatment: score 0=74% score 1=23%, and score 2=7%.

weeks aiming for a target haemoglobin of 12g/dl. If the increment in Hb is <1g/dl in this time frame, GCSF 300mcg SC twice a week is added.
- Lower doses of GCSF 150mcg SC once or twice a week may be sufficient.
- If no response is obtained in a further eight weeks a de-escalation of EPO should ensue.
- On obtaining a response EPO should be continued at the same dose until the target Hb is reached before lowering the dose.
- Darbepoietin is administered less frequently (weekly to once every three weeks) with doses between 150 and 300mcg/week.
- It is effective in MDS even in patients who have failed EPO therapy. Dosing starts at 300mcg SC once every one to three weeks accompanied by G-CSF weekly. The median time to response is usually six to eight weeks.
- Ferritin levels in ESA treated patients need to be maintained above 100ng/l by parenteral rather than oral supplementation.
- Loss of response to ESAs may accompany disease progression. Variability in EPO manufacturing is a historic cause of loss of response with reticulocytopenia.

Cytokines

- The recombinant human GSF has been used in MDS in combination with erythropoietin or to support neutropenic patients with a neutrophil count <0.5 × 10⁹/L.
- It may be used in neutropenic sepsis.
- Though supportive data is lacking, it may be used to prevent infections in patients who have had previous severe or life-threatening infections.

Immunosuppressive treatment (IST)

Autoimmune suppression of haemopoiesis due to cytotoxic T lymphocytes occurs in approximately 50% of patients with MDS (Kochenderfer et al. 2002). This immune component is a potential therapeutic target particularly in hypoplastic MDS.

Antithymocyte globulin with cyclosporine

Antithymocyte globulin (ATG) with or without cyclosporine evokes haematological improvement in a third of patients.

- Clinical features predicting response to IST include:
  - Age <60 years
  - <6 months of red blood cell transfusion dependence
  - Hypocellular marrow
  - The presence of a PNH clone
  - HLA DR15 phenotype

- ATG is administered via a central line after a test dose (1mg of ATG in 100ml of normal saline over one hour).
- Severe anaphylaxis is a contraindication to treatment with ATG.
- Horse ATG (lymphoglobulin) 15mg/kg/day for five days or rabbit ATG (thymoglobulin) 3.75mg/kg/day for five days are equivalent treatment doses infused daily over 12–18 hours.
- Reverse barrier nursing, premedication with hydrocortisone and piriton, and daily platelet transfusion to maintain platelets at >30 × 10^9/L is necessary.
- Prednisolone 1mg/kg is given from day 5 of ATG until day 14 and is rapidly tapered over five days to prevent serum sickness.
- Serum sickness manifesting as urticarial rash and joint pains may occur seven to ten days later and responds to 100mg IV hydrocortisone six-hourly.
- Cyclosporin 5mg/kg is commenced on day 14 after starting ATG to achieve target trough levels of 150–250mc/ml. The median time to a response is three months.

Immunomodulatory drugs (IMIDs)

Thalidomide 100–400mg orally daily yields erythroid responses in 13% of patients, but not neutrophil or platelet responses. Neurotoxicity, fatigue, constipation, and sedation are dose limiting.

Lenalidomide (derivative of thalidomide CC5013, Celgene Revlimid®) is particularly effective in treating patients with an interstitial deletion of 5q. It is FDA approved for low or Int-1 transfusion dependent MDS with a del 5q.

- Dosing: 10mg daily or 10mg daily for 21 out of 28 days orally as a cycle of treatment. Recurrent cycles of treatment are necessary. Lower dose scheduling of 5mg daily is being studied.
- Teratogenicity is a potential problem and pregnancy tests/contraception are advised in patients with reproductive potential.
- Responses: three trials have established the efficacy of lenalidomide in transfusion dependent MDS who had failed or had a poor predictive score for EPO MDS.
- The best responses are in patients with a deletion 5q (some with additional cytogenetic abnormalities) who experienced 76% erythroid response and 67% transfusion independence. Accompanying cytogenetic responses occurred in 73%.
- The incidence of response is lower (43% erythroid response) in transfusion dependent low/Int-1 MDS without del 5q.
- The median duration of response is two years.
- Myelosuppression is the predominant toxicity with grade 3 or more neutropenia and thrombocytopenia seen in >50% of patients. G-CSF administration may ameliorate this.
- Predictors of response to lenalidomide:
  - Interstitial deletion of 5q
  - Myelosuppression in the first eight weeks of treatment
  - RBC transfusions <4 units in eight weeks
  - Low-risk IPSS
  - Age <70 years
  - Low ECOG score

- Cytogenetic response predicts prolonged survival and reduced risk of leukaemic transformation

Epigenetic therapies

Epigenetic changes such as methylation of promoters of genes or deacetylation of histones modulate gene expression reversibly. As these changes are frequent in all cancers including MDS, they offer a therapeutic target. Epigenetic therapies include the both the DNA methyltransferase inhibitors (DNMTI) and histone deacetylase (HDAC) inhibitors.

DNA methyltransferase inhibitors

5-azacytidine

- 5-azacytidine-Vidaza® (Pharmion) and its analogue 5-aza-2'deoxycytidine Decitabine® (Dacogen) are emerging as first-line therapies for Int-2 and higher MDS.
- FDA approval for 5-azacytidine includes the treatment of all subtypes of MDS whereas 5-aza-2'deoxycytidine has been approved for IPSS Int-1 or higher MDS.
- 5-azacytidine is a pyrimidine analogue that is chemically synthesized and incorporated into both DNA and RNA.
- It can be administered intravenously or subcutaneously.
- The recommended dose is 75mg/m^2 daily for seven days every 28 days (constitutes one cycle) for at least four to six cycles of treatment.
- Local skin reactions (treated with topical steroid cream) and nausea and vomiting (premedicate with granisetron/odansetron) are the commonest side effects.
- Almost all patients develop grade 3–4 neutropenia.
- The transfusion requirements particularly for platelets may increase in the first few cycles and then decrease once a response is obtained.
- Medians of four to six cycles of treatment are needed for a response. An increase in platelet counts may be the first sign of a response. Once a response is seen therapy is continued indefinitely.

In the CALGB 9221 phase 3 randomized controlled trial 5-azacytidine was compared with best supportive care. Cross over of patients into the 5-azacytidine arm was permitted. An overall response of 60% with 7% CR, 16% PR, and 37% haematological improvement (HI) was observed. The median duration of response was 18 months and a significant disease modifying activity was observed. The time to progression to AML was prolonged by six months.

A phase 3 randomized controlled trial comparing 5-azacytidine to physicians' choice treatment (best supportive care, or low-dose cytarabine 20mg/m^2 SC for 14 days every 28 days or AML induction chemotherapy) for high-risk MDS showed OS was significantly prolonged to 24.4 months for patients treated with 5-azacytidine whereas for the comparator arm this was 15 months. The time to progression to AML was prolonged to 26.1 months with 5-azacytidine and transfusion independence was observed in 45% of patients.

5-azacytidine should be considered as first-line treatment for patients with high-risk MDS, not fit for intensive chemotherapy and stem cell transplant.

Decitabine

Decitabine is an analogue of azacytidine that only incorporates into DNA. A low-dose schedule of 20 mg/m^2 IV for five days every four weeks yielded promising results with 32% CR, 1% PR, and 13% HI in phase 1/2 studies.

For both drugs altered doses, schedules of administration, and synergistic combinations are being studied.

Histone deacetylase inhibitors

Chromatin with acetylated (negatively charged) histones is in the open configuration and transcriptionally active. Deacetylation of histones leads to chromatin being tightly configured and inaccessible to the transcriptional machinery. HDACs prevent deacetylation of histones enabling transcription of genes. The exact mechanism by which this group of drugs is effective in MDS is unclear.

Sodium valproate, sodium phenyl butyrate, arsenic trioxide, and suberoylanilide hydroxamic acid (SAHA) are examples of HDAC inhibitors. They have been used as single agents and in combination therapy with DNMTI and AI transretinoic acids. Whilst responses have been achieved, their exact place in the treatment of MDS is to be determined.

Novel therapies

Imatinib

Imatinib mesylate (Glivec®, Novartis), a tyrosine kinase inhibitor, is useful in the treatment of chronic myelomonocytic leukaemia associated with eosinophilia, characterized by the presence of a t(5;12) (q33; p13) with an ETV6-PDGFR mutation.

Treatment with imatinib 400mg orally daily led to clinical responses in four weeks followed by molecular responses.

Chemotherapy

Conventional AML induction type chemotherapy is used for remission induction in good performance, high-risk MDS particularly when consolidation with an allogeneic stem cell transplant is possible.

- Daunorubicin combined with cytarabine (DA or fludarabine, high-dose cytarabine; G-CSF and idarubicin (FLAG/FLAG Ida) have been used.
- Prolonged time to neutrophil recovery has been a problem with FLAG/Ida and is often associated with morbidity such as invasive fungal infections.
- The role of these chemotherapies and various novel agents is being studied in the NCRN AML 18 trial open to patients at least 60 years old with high-risk MDS or AML.

Stem cell transplantation

- Despite more treatment options becoming available to patients with MDS, haemopoietic stem cell transplantation remains the only modality with a curative potential.
- Non-myeloablative stem cell transplants that are immunosuppressive rather than myeloablative have enabled transplants in this elderly group of patients.

- For low risk or Int-1 MDS, delaying transplantation until progression, and for Int-2 or higher MDS early transplant, are associated with the best life expectancy.
- The non-relapse mortality using fludarabine 125mg, busulphan 8mg, and campath 100mg is approximately 10% in the first 100 days and one-year OS 70%.
- OS at three years varies from 30% for high-risk to 60% for low-risk MDS. Increased risk of relapse, graft-versus-host disease, and infections contribute to morbidity and mortality.
- The AML 16 trial is studying the role of non-myeloablative transplants in elderly patients.

Treatment algorithm

- Risk stratify patient based on their IPSS-R, transfusion requirement, PS, and comorbidities. Institute supportive care as necessary.
- Low-risk patient if bone marrow hypocellular and <60 years, HLA DR15 or good PS, consider ATG/cyclosporin.
- Normocellular, becoming transfusion dependent, assess EPO/G-CSF predictive score to determine a trial of EPO.
- Del 5q with or without additional cytogenetic abnormalities, lenalidomide is the treatment of choice. Consider lenalidomide for low-risk MDS who have failed EPO therapy.
- High-risk MDS, treatment with 5-azacytidine should be considered (may be followed by consolidation with an allograft).
- In young and fit patients, AML induction chemotherapy consolidated by an allogeneic stem cell transplant should be considered.
- Eligible patients should be considered for trials of novel agents.

Further reading

Greenberg P, Cox C, LeBeau MM, et al. International Scoring System for evaluating prognosis in myelodysplastic syndromes. *Blood* 1997; 89:2079–88.

Kochenderfer JN, Kobayashi S, Wieder ED, Su C, Molldrem JJ. Loss of T-lymphocyte clonal dominance in patients with myelodysplastic syndrome responsive to immunosuppression. *Blood* 2002; 100:3639–45.

Montalban-Bravo G, Garcia-Manero G. Myelodysplastic syndromes: 2018 update on diagnosis, risk-stratification and management. *Am J Hematol* 2018; 93(1):129–47.

Stetler-Stevenson M, Arthur DC, Jabbour N, Xie XY, Molldrem J, et al. Diagnostic utility of flow cytometric immunophenotyping in myelodysplastic syndrome. *Blood* 2001; 98(4):979–87.

Internet resources

National Cancer Institute: http://www.cancer.gov/cancertopics/pdq/treatment/myelodysplastic/healthprofessional/allpages#Reference4.52

NCCN guidelines for treatment of MDS: http://www.nccn.org/professionals/physician_gls/PDF/mds.pdf

12.23 Multiple myeloma

Introduction

Multiple myeloma accounts for approximately 10% of haematological malignancies. In almost all patients disease evolves from an asymptomatic premalignant stage termed monoclonal gammopathy of undetermined significance (MGUS). In some patients, an intermediate asymptomatic premalignant stage referred to as smouldering multiple myeloma (SMM) can be recognized clinically. The diagnosis of active myeloma requires 10% or more clonal plasma cells on bone marrow examination (or biopsy proven plasmacytoma), and one or more myeloma defining events (MDE). MDE include evidence of end-organ damage (hypercalcaemia, renal insufficiency, anaemia, or bone lesions) secondary to the underlying plasma cell disorder, clonal bone marrow plasma cells ≥60%, serum free light chain (FLC) ratio ≥100 provided involved FLC level is ≥100 mg/l, and there is more than one focal lesion on MRI.

Epidemiology

The annual incidence is approximately four per 100,000. The disease is twice as common in African–Americans compared with Caucasians, and slightly more common in males than females. The median age at diagnosis is 66 years.

Aetiology

The aetiology of myeloma is not known; however, important advances have occurred that shed light on the pathogenesis of the disease. The first pathogenetic event is the establishment of the premalignant phase, MGUS. MGUS is thought to occur as a result of specific cytogenetic events triggered by infection or immuno-suppression. The cytogenetic changes associated with MGUS are immunoglobulin heavy chain (IgH) gene translocations (45% of MGUS) or trisomies (45%), or both (approximately 10%).

There are five recurrent IgH translocations seen in MGUS, and they involve fusion of the IgH locus on chromosome 14q32 with one of five partner chromosome loci. The partner chromosome loci and the corresponding genes dysregulated are: 11q13 (CCND1 [cyclin D1 gene]); 4p16.3 (FGFR-3 and MMSET); 6p21 (CCND3 [cyclin D3 gene]); 16q23 (c-maf); and 20q11 (mafB). Approximately 45% of MGUS are not associated with IgH translocations, but have evidence of trisomies, usually of the odd numbered chromosomes with the exception of 13; a small proportion of MGUS has both IgH translocations and trisomies.

Once MGUS is established it progresses to myeloma or related malignancy at a constant rate of 1% per year. The specific second-hit that initiates this progression is unknown, but several additional cytogenetic events are felt to be important including Ras mutations, p16 methylation, abnormalities involving the myc family of oncogenes, secondary translocations, and p53 mutations. In addition, the bone marrow microenvironment undergoes marked changes with progression, including induction of angiogenesis, suppression of cell-mediated immunity, and paracrine loops involving cytokines such as interleukin-6 and VEGF (vascular endothelial growth factor). Lytic bone lesions in myeloma are caused by an imbalance between the activity of osteoclasts and osteoblasts. There is an increase in RANKL (receptor activator of nuclear factor-kappa B ligand) expression by osteoblasts (and possibly plasma cells) accompanied by a reduction in the level of its decoy receptor, osteoprotegerin (OPG). This leads to an increase in RANKL/OPG ratio, which causes osteoclast activation and bone resorption. In addition, there is inhibition of osteoblast differentiation resulting in the type of osteolytic bone destruction without evidence of new bone formation that is characteristic of myeloma.

Clinical features

The most common presenting symptoms of myeloma are fatigue and bone pain. Osteolytic bone lesions and/or compression fractures, that can be detected on routine radiographs, MRI, or CT scans, are the hallmark of the disease, and cause significant morbidity (Figures 12.23.1–12.23.3). Bone pain may present as an area of persistent pain or migratory bone pain, often in the lower back and pelvis. Pain may be sudden in onset when associated with a pathological fracture, and is often precipitated by movement. Extramedullary expansion of bone lesions may cause nerve root or spinal cord compression. Anaemia occurs in 70% of patients at diagnosis and is the primary cause of fatigue. Hypercalcaemia is found in one-fourth of patients while the serum creatinine is elevated in almost one-half. Other symptoms may result from infections, hypercalcaemia, painful radiculopathy, or spinal cord com-pression.

On physical examination, pallor is the most frequent finding. The liver is palpable in about 5% of patients and the spleen in 1%. Tenderness may be noted at sites of bone involvement. Occasionally, extramedullary or bone plasmacytomas may be visible and/or palpable.

Diagnosis

A complete blood count, serum creatinine, and calcium are the essential tests in the diagnostic evaluation of suspected myeloma. A normocytic, normochromic anaemia is present initially in approximately 75% of patients but eventually occurs in almost all patients with multiple myeloma. The serum creatinine value is increased initially in almost half of patients. The major causes of renal insufficiency are light-chain cast nephropathy ('myeloma kidney') and hypercalcaemia. Myeloma kidney is characterized by the presence of large, waxy, laminated casts in the distal and collecting tubules. The casts are composed mainly of precipitated monoclonal light chains. Hypercalcaemia is present in 15–20% of patients initially.

Myeloma is characterized by the presence of monoclonal immunoglobulins in the serum and/or urine in almost 98% of patients but the presence of M proteins is not diagnostic of myeloma. Conditions such as MGUS, Waldenström macroglobulinaemia, and amyloidosis are also associated with M proteins and need to be differentiated from myeloma. M proteins can be detected by serum protein electrophoresis (SPEP) in 82% of patients with myeloma, and by serum immunofixation electrophoresis (IFE) in 93%. Up to 20% of patients with myeloma lack heavy-chain expression in the M protein, and are considered to have light-chain myeloma. The M protein in these patients is detected mainly in the urine, and

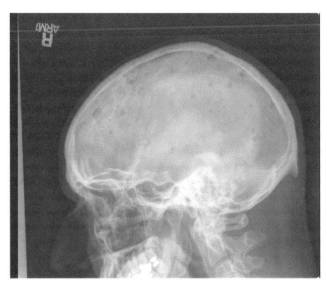

Fig. 12.23.1 Skull radiograph showing multiple lytic lesions in myeloma.

thus addition of urine protein electrophoresis (UPEP) increases the sensitivity of detecting M proteins in patients with myeloma to 98%. The serum free light chain (FLC) assay can be used instead of urine studies when screening for myeloma since it is as sensitive as urine studies in detecting light chain myeloma. Currently only 1–2% of patients with myeloma will have no detectable M on any of these tests; these patients have true non-secretory myeloma.

Low-dose whole body CT, or PET-CT, of all bones including long bones is needed to detect lytic bone lesions in myeloma. Conventional roentgenograms (referred to as skeletal surveys) are less sensitive and are recommended only if low-dose CT or PET-CT is not available. Bone lesions in myeloma have a characteristic punched-out appearance. Osteoporosis and/or fractures can also be present. MRI studies may be needed to further evaluate symptomatic areas, or to rule out focal lesions in patients who are suspected to have myeloma but have no bone lesions on CT or PET-CT.

A unilateral bone marrow aspiration and biopsy is indicated in all patients with myeloma. By definition, all patients with myeloma should have 10% or more clonal bone marrow plasma cells or a biopsy proven

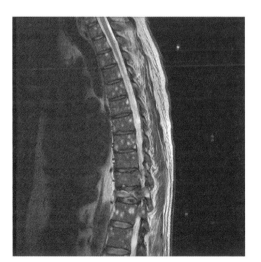

Fig. 12.23.2 MRI sagittal section showing myeloma involving T11 vertebral body with compression fracture.

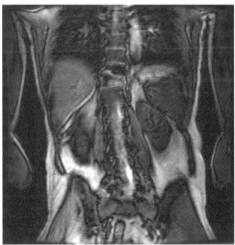

Fig. 12.23.3 MRI coronal section showing myeloma involving T11 vertebral body with compression fracture.

Table 12.23.1 International Myeloma Working Group diagnostic criteria for multiple myeloma and related plasma cell disorders

Disorder	Disease definition
Non-IgM monoclonal gammopathy of undetermined significance (MGUS)	All three criteria must be met: • Serum monoclonal protein (non-IgM type) <3g/dl • Clonal bone marrow plasma cells <10%* • Absence of end-organ damage such as hypercalcemia, renal insufficiency, anaemia, and bone lesions (CRAB) that can be attributed to the plasma cell proliferative disorder
Smouldering multiple myeloma	Both criteria must be met: • Serum monoclonal protein (IgG or IgA) ≥3g/dl, or urinary monoclonal protein ≥500mg per 24h and/or clonal bone marrow plasma cells 10–60% • Absence of myeloma defining events or amyloidosis
Multiple myeloma	Both criteria must be met: • Clonal bone marrow plasma cells ≥10% or biopsy-proven bony or extramedullary plasmacytoma Any one or more of the following myeloma defining events: • Evidence of end-organ damage that can be attributed to the underlying plasma cell proliferative disorder, specifically: • Hypercalcemia: serum calcium >0.25mmol/l (>1mg/dl) higher than the upper limit of normal or >2.75mmol/l (>11mg/dl) • Renal insufficiency: creatinine clearance <40ml per minute or serum creatinine >177micromol/l (>2mg/dl) • Anaemia: haemoglobin value of >2g/dl below the lower limit of normal, or a haemoglobin value <10g/dl • Bone lesions: one or more osteolytic lesions on skeletal radiography, CT, or PET-CT • Clonal bone marrow plasma cell percentage ≥60% • Involved: uninvolved serum free light chain (FLC) ratio ≥100 (involved free light chain level must be ≥100mg/l) • >1 focal lesions on MRI studies (at least 5mm in size)
IgM monoclonal gammopathy of undetermined significance (IgM MGUS)	All three criteria must be met: • Serum IgM monoclonal protein <3g/dl • Bone marrow lymphoplasmacytic infiltration <10% • No evidence of anaemia, constitutional symptoms, hyperviscosity, lymphadenopathy, or hepatosplenomegaly that can be attributed to the underlying lymphoproliferative disorder
Light chain MGUS	All criteria must be met: • Abnormal FLC ratio (<0.26 or >1.65) • Increased level of the appropriate involved light chain (increased kappa FLC in patients with ratio >1.65 and increased lambda FLC in patients with ratio <0.26) • No immunoglobulin heavy chain expression on immunofixation • Absence of end-organ damage that can be attributed to the plasma cell proliferative disorder • Clonal bone marrow plasma cells <10% • Urinary monoclonal protein <500mg/24h
Solitary plasmacytoma	All four criteria must be met: • Biopsy-proven solitary lesion of bone or soft tissue with evidence of clonal plasma cells • Normal bone marrow with no evidence of clonal plasma cells • Normal skeletal survey and MRI (or CT) of spine and pelvis (except for the primary solitary lesion) • Absence of end-organ damage such as CRAB that can be attributed to a lymphoplasma cell proliferative disorder
Solitary plasmacytoma with minimal marrow involvement**	All four criteria must be met: • Biopsy-proven solitary lesion of bone or soft tissue with evidence of clonal plasma cells • Clonal bone marrow plasma cells <10% • Normal skeletal survey and MRI (or CT) of spine and pelvis (except for the primary solitary lesion) • Absence of end-organ damage such as CRAB that can be attributed to a lymphoplasmacell proliferative disorder

* A bone marrow can be deferred in patients with low-risk MGUS (IgG type, M protein <15g/l, normal free light chain ratio) in whom there are no clinical features concerning for myeloma.

** Solitary plasmacytoma with 10% or more clonal plasma cells is considered as multiple myeloma.

plasmacytoma. If a lower extent of involvement is detected, one may be dealing with an erroneous diagnosis or there is a sampling error due to patchy marrow involvement. Clonal is defined as a kappa/lambda ratio on immunohistochemistry or flow cytometry that is >4:1 or <1:2. Based on these tests, myeloma is diagnosed by the following criteria:

- Clonal bone marrow plasma cells 10% or biopsy proven plasmacytoma; and
- Any one or more of the following myeloma defining events:
  - Evidence of end organ damage that can be attributed to the underlying plasma cell proliferative disorder, specifically lytic bone lesions, anaemia, hypercalcaemia or renal failure
  - Clonal bone marrow plasma cell percentage ≥60%
  - Involved: uninvolved serum FLC ratio ≥100 (involved FLC level must be ≥100mg/l)
  - >1 focal lesions on MRI studies (at least 5mm in size)

The main differential diagnosis is between myeloma, MGUS, smouldering myeloma, macroglobulinaemia, and primary amyloidosis. These disorders are distinguished from each other using the criteria listed in Table 12.23.1.

MGUS and SMM are precursor conditions to myeloma that are asymptomatic and need no therapy. They lack the end-organ damage that is required for the diagnosis of multiple myeloma. MGUS and smouldering myeloma are distinguished from each other because they have different rates of progression to myeloma or related malignancy, 1% per year in the case of MGUS, and approximately 10% per year in the case of smouldering myeloma. Not all patients with an M protein and evidence of possible end-organ damage have myeloma. It must be reasonably established that the end-organ damage is likely to be related to the underlying plasma cell disorder rather than an unrelated process. For example, bone lesions in a patient with MGUS due to an unrelated metastatic carcinoma may be mistaken for multiple myeloma. In this case, the presence of a small M protein and <10% plasma cells in the bone marrow makes metastatic carcinoma with an unrelated MGUS more likely. If there is any doubt, a biopsy of one of the lytic lesions is needed.

Myeloma is differentiated by flow cytometry from polyclonal reactive plasmacytosis that occurs in conditions such as autoimmune diseases, metastatic carcinoma, chronic liver disease, acquired immunedeficiency syndrome (AIDS), or chronic infection.

12.24 Staging, prognosis, and treatment response criteria for multiple myeloma

Staging

The median survival of myeloma is approximately five to seven years. However, some patients can live >10 years. Older staging systems such as the Durie–Salmon staging system and the International Staging System relied primarily on tumor burden and host characteristics. However, prognosis in myeloma is affected not only by these factors, but also the underlying cytogenetic abnormalities. In fact it is impossible to determine prognosis in a patient with myeloma without considering the presence or absence of adverse cytogenetic abnormalities.

Revised International Staging System

The Revised International Staging System (RISS) adopted by the International Myeloma Working Group (IMWG) takes into account host factors (serum albumin), tumor burden (beta-2 microglobulin) and determinants of disease biology (presence of high-risk cytogenetic abnormalities or elevated lactate dehydrogenase level. The three adverse cytogenetic abnormalities considered in the RISS are t(4;14), t(14;16), and del 17p (Table 12.24.1). In a study of 4,445 patients with newly diagnosed multiple myeloma from 11 international trials, the five-year survival rate of patients with stage I, II, and III RISS was 82%, 62%, and 40%, respectively. The RISS allows outcome in clinical trials to be compared with each other more readily. It is easy to assess and reproducible. The RISS has two important limitations. The first is that it is not useful unless the diagnosis of myeloma has already been made. The RISS for multiple myeloma has no role in MGUS or smouldering (asymptomatic) multiple myeloma,

and cannot distinguish these two premalignant disorders from myeloma. Secondly, the RISS classifies patients using a composite system, and thus cannot be used to determine therapeutic strategies.

Prognosis

Age, RISS stage, haemoglobin concentration, creatinine, calcium, albumin, and extent of bone marrow involvement are all significant predictors of survival in myeloma. Plasmablastic morphology, circulating plasma cells, and LDH are additional independent risk factors for survival. The most important independent predictors of survival are discussed in the following sections.

Performance status

PS is probably the single most powerful predictor of outcome in myeloma, but its value has not been highlighted in the literature. PS is also a key determinant of transplant eligibility. Patients with poor PS are not candidates for stem cell transplantation. PS is assessed usually by the ECOG scale, which grades patients from 0 to 4 based on activity level. Patients who are fully functional are classified as 0, while patients who are bedridden are classified as 4. Patients with slight limitations in activity are classified as 1, those with significant limitations but are up and about >50% of waking hours are classified as 2, and those who have some activity but are up and about <50% of time are classified as 3.

In one study, an ECOG PS of 3–4 had a greater adverse impact on outcome (hazard ratio 1.9, 95% CI 1.6–2.4) than any other single variable.

Table 12.24.1 Revised International Staging System for myeloma

Stage	Frequency (% of patients)	Five-year survival rate (%)
Stage I • ISS stage I (serum albumin >3.5, serum beta-2-microglobulin <3.5) and • No high-risk cytogenetics • Normal LDH	28	82
Stage II • Neither stage I or III	62	62
Stage III • ISS stage III (serum beta-2-microglobulin >5.5) and • High-risk cytogenetics [t(4;14), t(14;16), or del(17p)] or elevated LDH	10	40

Source: data from Palumbo A, et al. Revised International Staging System for Multiple Myeloma: A Report From International Myeloma Working Group. *J Clin Oncol* 2015; 33(26): 2863–9.

Conventional metaphase cytogenetics

Abnormalities detected by conventional metaphase karyotyping especially deletion of chromosome 13 and hypodiploidy have been associated with poor prognosis in myeloma. However, in many instances, it is unclear whether the adverse prognostic effect is secondary to the underlying cytogenetic abnormality or simply a reflection of the higher proliferative rate of plasma cells that is needed in order to get an informative result on this test.

Molecular cytogenetics

Cytogenetic abnormalities are present in most if not all patients with myeloma if sensitive interphase FISH techniques are used. The most common cytogenetic changes include deletion chromosome 13 (30–55% of patients), deletion 17p13.1 (10%), t(11;14)(q13;q32) (15–20%), t(4;14)(p16.3;q32) (15%), and t(14;16)(q32;q23) (5%).

The presence of t(4;14)(p16.3;q32), t(14;16)(q32q23), t(14;20)(q32;q11), del 17p, gain 1q, and del 1p which are detected by interphase FISH (or metaphase spectral karyotype imaging) are associated with adverse prognosis in myeloma. The t(4;14) (p16.3;q32) abnormality results in dysregulation of the fibroblast growth factor receptor 3 (FGFR3) and MMSET. The t14;16 translocation dysregulates the c-maf oncogene, while deletions involving 17p13 result in p53 inactivation. In contrast, presence of trisomies is associated with a favourable prognosis.

Risk stratification of myeloma

The specific prognostic factors used to stratify patients into high-risk and standard-risk myeloma to guide therapeutic strategy are del 17p or IgH translocations t(4;14) or t(14;16) on FISH studies. Presence of any one or more of these high-risk factors classifies a patient as having high-risk myeloma. Patients with none of the features are considered to have standard-risk disease. The median survival of high-risk myeloma is only two to three years even with tandem stem cell transplantation, compared to >7–10 years in patients with standard-risk myeloma. In an ECOG clinical trial of 351 patients, the presence of t4;14, t(14;16), or del 17p were associated with poor prognosis (median survival 25 months).

Treatment response criteria

Uniform response criteria are required to monitor effectiveness of therapy in patients and to evaluate new drugs and interventions in clinical trials. Several response criteria have been developed for myeloma over the years that define various categories of response and progression.

In 2016, the IMWG published updated uniform response criteria that are to be used in future clinical trials and in clinical practice (Table 12.24.2). The IMWG criteria are critical for purposes of calculating PFS and time to progression (TTP). With the development of new therapies, we are now beginning to achieve deep responses, deeper than CR as defined by the IMWG criteria. MRD detection can occur now at a sensitivity of one cell in $>10^{-5}$ using next generation flow cytometry and sequencing techniques. MRD negative is defined as no evidence of myeloma cells using one of these validated techniques with a sensitivity of at least 1 in 10^{-5} or greater.

12.25 Treatment for multiple myeloma

Untreated patients

The treatment of newly diagnosed multiple myeloma is rapidly evolving. The introduction of thalidomide, bortezomib, and lenalidomide, has prolonged the survival of multiple myeloma significantly. More recently, there have been several additional new drugs such as carfilzomib, pomalidomide, panobinostat, elotuzumab, ixazomib, and daratumumab that have shown significant clinical activity in myeloma and are entering into clinical practice.

The first step in the treatment of myeloma is to exclude MGUS and SMM which do not require therapy. The next step is to determine whether the patient is a potential candidate for stem cell transplantation because initial therapy differs accordingly. Transplant eligibility is determined by a variety of factors including age, PS, and comorbidities. In most countries, age 65 is considered as the upper limit for ASCT.

The third step is risk stratification into high- and standard-risk myeloma based on specific prognostic markers. Presence of del 17p or IgH translocations

Table 12.24.2 International Myeloma Working Group criteria for response and progression in myeloma

Response category	Response criteria
Minimal residual disease (MRD) negative	Absence of phenotypically aberrant clonal plasma cells by nerve growth factor (NGF) on bone marrow aspirates using the EuroFlow standard operation procedure for MRD detection in multiple myeloma (or validated equivalent method) with a minimum sensitivity of 1 in 10^5 nucleated cells or higher (Flow MRD negative); or
	Absence of clonal plasma cells by next generation sequencing on bone marrow aspirates in which presence of a clone is defined as less than two identical sequencing reads obtained after DNA sequencing of bone marrow aspirates using the LymphoSIGHT platform (or validated equivalent method) with a minimum sensitivity of 1 in 10^5 nucleated cells or higher (sequencing MRD negative)
Complete response (CR)	Negative immunofixation on the serum and urine; and
	Disappearance of any soft tissue plasmacytomas; and
	<5% plasma cells in bone marrow; and
	If the only measurable disease is FLC (free light chain), a normal FLC ratio
Partial response (PR)	50% reduction of serum M-protein; and
	Reduction in 24-hour urinary M-protein by 90% or to <200mg per 24 hours;
	If the only measurable disease is FLC, a ≥50% reduction in the difference between involved and uninvolved FLC levels;
	If the only measurable disease is bone marrow (BM), a ≥50% reduction in BM plasma cells (PCs) (provided the baseline PCs was ≥30%); and
	If present at baseline, ≥50% reduction in the size (SPD) of soft tissue plasmacytomas
Progressive disease (PD)	Increase of 25% from lowest response value in:
	Serum M-component (absolute increase must be 0.5g/dl); and/or
	Urine M-component (absolute increase must be 200mg/24 hour); and/or
	If the only measurable disease is FLC, the difference between involved and uninvolved FLC levels (absolute increase must be >10mg/dl); and/or
	Definite development of new bone lesions or soft tissue plasmacytomas or ≥50% increase from nadir in the size of existing bone lesions or soft tissue plasmacytoma or >50% increase in circulating plasma cells (minimum of 200 cells/l) if this is the only measure of disease

SPD, sum of the produce of the maximal perpendicular diameters of measured lesions. *Source:* data from Kumar, S et al. International Myeloma Working Group consensus criteria for response and minimal residual disease assessment in multiple myeloma. *Lancet Oncol* 2016; 17(8): e328–e346.

t(4;14) or t(14;16) on FISH classifies a patient as having high-risk myeloma.

The approach to treatment of symptomatic newly diagnosed multiple myeloma is outlined in Figure 12.25.1. Table 12.25.1 lists the most common regimens used in the treatment of newly diagnosed myeloma.

Initial treatment of patients eligible for transplantation

Patients who are determined to be candidates for ASCT are typically treated with three to four cycles of induction therapy followed by stem cell harvest (Figure 12.25.1).

The most common regimens used in the treatment of newly diagnosed MM in patients who are candidates for ASCT are bortezomib, lenalidomide, dexamethasone (VRd), daratumumab, lenalidomide, dexamethasone (DRd), bortezomib, thalidomide, and dexamethasone (VTD), and bortezomib, cyclophosphamide, dexamethasone (VCD). Induction therapy is usually given for three to four cycles and is then followed by stem cell harvest. In a randomized trial conducted by the Southwest Oncology Group (SWOG), PFS and OS were significantly superior with VRd compared with lenalidomide plus dexamethasone (Rd). A recent randomized trial also found that VTD is superior to VCD. Based on these data, VRd or VTD are the preferred regimens for initial therapy in transplant eligible patients.

The low-dose dexamethasone regimen (40mg once a week) is preferred in all regimens to minimize toxicity. In a randomized trial conducted by the Eastern Cooperative Oncology Group (ECOG), the low-dose dexamethasone approach was associated with superior OS and significantly lower toxicity. Similarly, the once-weekly subcutaneous schedule of bortezomib is preferred in all regimens. The neurotoxicity of bortezomib can be greatly diminished by administering bortezomib once a week instead of twice-weekly, and by subcutaneous administration instead of the intravenous route. Higher doses of dexamethasone, and twice-weekly bortezomib can be considered if a rapid response is desired as in the case of patients with acute renal failure due to cast nephropathy, extensive extramedullary disease, plasma cell leukaemia, or impending cord compression.

Initial treatment of patients not eligible for transplantation

Patients who are not transplant candidates are treated with nine months of VRd followed by lenalidomide maintenance. A recent randomized trial found that DRd is superior to Rd in terms of response rate and PFS. Based on these data, VRd or DRd are the preferred regimens for initial therapy in patients not eligible for transplantation.

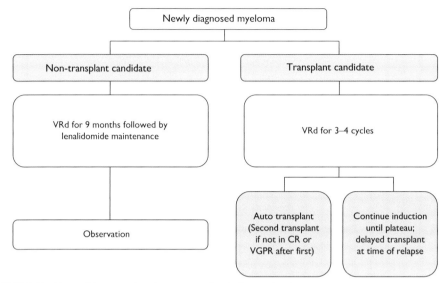

Fig. 12.25.1 Algorithm outlining approach to the treatment of newly diagnosed myeloma. CR complete response; VGPR very good partial response; VRd bortezomib, lenalidomide, dexamethasone.

In many countries or in patients with limited insurance or financial means, 12–18 months of a bortezomib-based triplet such as VCd or bortezomib, melphalan, prednisone (VMP) are reasonable alternatives.

Treatment of high-risk myeloma
Patients with high-risk myeloma tend to do poorly with median OS of approximately two to three years even with tandem ASCT. The quadruplet regimen of daratumumab, bortezomib, lenalidomide, dexamethasone (Dara-VRd) has shown high activity with high stringent complete response rates (sCR) and MRD negative rates. This may therefore be an option for indication in the future. Selected high-risk myeloma patients may also be candidates for tandem ASCT.

Acute renal failure due to cast nephropathy
The diagnosis of light chain cast nephropathy can be made presumptively if the circulating FLC levels are high in the presence of MM and acute renal failure. However, a renal biopsy is required if serum FLC levels are below 500mg/l. Patients presenting with acute renal failure due to light chain cast nephropathy need urgent treatment to lower circulating FLC levels with a triplet regimen that does not require major dose adjustment such as VCD or VTD. The role of plasmapheresis to remove circulating light chains is controversial, and randomized trials indicate a lack of benefit. However, the trials so far have had some limitations, and the risk of the intervention is minimal compared with the major impact on prognosis that occurs if renal dysfunction is not reversed. Therefore, plasmapheresis or dialysis using high cut-off filters to rapidly reduce FLCs is recommended. Close monitoring of serum FLC levels and creatinine are needed for the first few weeks.

DVT prophylaxis
Deep vein thrombosis (DVT) is a major complication of thalidomide and lenalidomide based therapy.

For most patients, aspirin alone can be used as DVT prophylaxis as long as patients are receiving low-dose corticosteroids (e.g. dexamethasone 40mg once a week or prednisone), and provided no concomitant erythropoietic agents are used. On the other hand, patients receiving thalidomide or lenalidomide in combination with high-dose steroids or doxorubicin need higher intensity thromboprophylaxis with coumadin (target INR 2–3) or low-molecular-weight heparin (equivalent of enoxaparin 40mg once daily).

Autologous stem cell transplantation
Although not curative, ASCT improves complete response rates and prolongs median OS in myeloma by approximately 12 months. The mortality rate is 1–2%. Melphalan 200mg/m^2 is the most widely used preparative (conditioning) regimen for ASCT.

There is little doubt that ASCT prolongs survival in myeloma, but its timing (early versus delayed) is controversial. Survival is similar whether ASCT is done early (immediately following three to four cycles of induction therapy) or delayed (at the time of relapse as salvage therapy). Overall, given the inconvenience and side-effects of prolonged chemotherapy, insurance, and other issues we still favour early ASCT, especially for patients <65 years of age with adequate renal function. However, given effective new agents to treat myeloma, some patients and physicians may choose to delay the procedure. The need for early ASCT is an important question for future clinical trials.

With tandem (double) ASCT, patients receive a second planned ASCT after recovery from the first procedure. Two randomized trials found better EFS and OS in recipients of double versus single ASCT. In both trials, the benefit of a second ASCT was restricted to patients failing to achieve a complete response or very good partial response (VGPR) with the first procedure. A tandem ASCT can be therefore considered in high-risk patients

Table 12.25.1 Common regimens used in the treatment of newly diagnosed myeloma

Regimen	Usual dosing schedule*
Lenalidomide-dexamethasone (Rd)	Lenalidomide 25mg oral days 1–21 every 28 days
	Dexamethasone 40mg oral days 1, 8, 15, 22 every 28 days
	Repeated every 4 weeks
Bortezomib-melphalan-prednisone (VMP)**	Bortezomib 1.3mg/m² intravenous days 1, 8, 15, 22
	Melphalan 9mg/m² oral days 1–4
	Prednisone 60mg/m² oral days 1–4
	Repeated every 35 days
Bortezomib-thalidomide-dexamethasone (VTD)**	Bortezomib 1.3mg/m² intravenous days 1, 8, 15, 22
	Thalidomide 100–200mg oral days 1–21
	Dexamethasone 20mg on day of and day after bortezomib (or 40mg days 1, 8, 15, 22)
	Repeated every 4 weeks x 4 cycles as pretransplant induction therapy
Bortezomib-cyclophosphamide-dexamethasone** (VCD)	Cyclophosphamide 300mg/m² orally on days 1, 8, 15, 22
	Bortezomib 1.3mg/m² intravenously on days 1, 8, 15, 22
	Dexamethasone 40mg oral days 1, 8, 15, 22
	Repeated every 4 weeks†
Bortezomib-lenalidomide-dexamethasone (VRd)**	Bortezomib 1.3mg/m² intravenous days 1, 8, 15
	Lenalidomide 25mg oral days 1–14
	Dexamethasone 20mg on day of and day after bortezomib (or 40mg days 1, 8, 15, 22)
	Repeated every 3 weeks†
Carfilzomib-lenalidomide-dexamethasone (KRd)	Carfilzomib 27mg/m² intravenously on days 1, 2, 8, 9, 15, 16 (Note: cycle 1, day 1 and 2 carfilzomib dose is 20mg/m²)
	Lenalidomide 25mg oral days 1–21
	Dexamethasone 20mg on day of and day after bortezomib (or 40mg days 1, 8, 15, 22)
	Repeated every 4 weeks
Daratumumab-lenalidomide-dexamethasone (DRd)	Daratumumab 16mg/kg intravenously weekly x 8 weeks, and then every 2 weeks for 4 months, and then once monthly
	Pomalidomide 4mg oral days 1–21
	Dexamethasone 40mg days 1, 8, 15, 22
	Pomalidomide-dexamethasone repeated in usual schedule every 4 weeks
Elotuzumab-lenalidomide-dexamethasone (ERd)	Elotuzumab 10mg/kg intravenously weekly x 8 weeks, and then every 2 weeks
	Lenalidomide 25mg oral days 1–21
	Dexamethasone 40mg days 1, 8, 15, 22
	Lenalidomide-dexamethasone repeated in usual schedule every 4 weeks
Ixazomib-lenalidomide-dexamethasone (IRd)	Ixazomib 4mg oral days 1, 8, 15
	Lenalidomide 25mg oral days 1–21
	Dexamethasone 40mg days 1, 8, 15, 22
	Repeated every 4 weeks

*All doses need to be adjusted for performance status, renal function, blood counts, and other toxicities.

**Doses of dexamethasone and/or bortezomib reduced based on subsequent data showing lower toxicity and similar efficacy with reduced doses.

† The day 22 dose of all three drugs is omitted if counts are low, or after initial response to improve tolerability, or when the regimen is used as maintenance therapy; when used as maintenance therapy for high-risk patients, further delays can be instituted between cycles.

Adapted with permission from Rajkumar SV, Multiple myeloma: 2016 update on diagnosis, risk-stratification, and management. *Am J Hematol* 2016; 91(7): 719–34.

who fail to achieve a complete response or very good partial response (>90% reduction in M protein level) with the first ASCT.

Allogeneic transplantation

Conventional allogeneic transplants are unacceptable for most patients due to high treatment-related mortality rates. Non-myeloablative conditioning regimens (mini-allogeneic transplantation) have reduced treatment related mortality rates. But results are conflicting, and the role of allogeneic strategies in myeloma remains unresolved. At this time, allogeneic transplantation for myeloma remains investigational for most patients.

Maintenance therapy

Three randomized trials have shown better PFS with lenalidomide as post ASCT maintenance therapy. A survival benefit has been seen in one trial. One concern is an increased risk of second cancers with lenalidomide maintenance. Lenalidomide maintenance is recommended following initial therapy in standard risk patients.

In patients with high-risk MM, bortezomib-based maintenance may be of value. In a randomized trial, patients receiving two years of bortezomib given every other week as post-transplant maintenance had superior outcomes compared with thalidomide maintenance. This benefit was particularly seen in patients with high risk myeloma.

Refractory and relapsing myeloma

Almost all patients with myeloma eventually relapse. If relapse occurs >6 months after stopping therapy, the initial chemotherapy regimen should be reinstituted. Patients who have cryopreserved stem cells early in the disease course can derive significant benefit from ASCT as salvage therapy. In general, patients who have indolent relapse can often be treated with single agents. In contrast, patients with more aggressive relapse often require therapy with a combination of active agents. Given the non-curable nature of myeloma, patients with relapsed disease typically continue on one drug/regimen until relapse or toxicity and then try the next option. The regiments discussed in untreated patients (Rd, VRd, VCD, VTD) can all be used in relapsed/refractory patients. Several additional treatment options are also available (Table 12.25.2).

Thalidomide and thalidomide-based regimens

The finding of increased angiogenesis in myeloma and the antiangiogenic properties of thalidomide led to the investigation of thalidomide in myeloma. As a single agent, thalidomide produces response rates in about 25–35%

of patients with relapsed/refractory MM. High response rates can be achieved by using thalidomide in three-drug combinations such as cyclophosphamide, thalidomide, dexamethasone (CTd), or VTd.

Thalidomide is a teratogenic agent. Its use in pregnancy is absolutely contraindicated. Most countries have programmes in place to prevent teratogenicity through strict restrictions for women of child-bearing potential.

Bortezomib and bortezomib-based regimens

Bortezomib is a proteasome inhibitor approved for the treatment of patients with relapsed and refractory multiple myeloma. Bortezomib is effective in relapsed myeloma in various triplet combinations such as VRd, VCD, and VTD.

Lenalidomide

Lenalidomide belongs to a class of thalidomide analogues termed immunomodulatory drugs (ImiDs). Two large phase 3 trials have shown significantly superior time to progression with Len/Dex compared to placebo plus dexamethasone in relapsed myeloma. Typical dosing of lenalidomide for myeloma is 25–30mg per day on days 1–21 of a 28-day cycle, with dose adjustments based on toxicity. The lenalidomide-low-dose dexamethasone combination Rd is the backbone of several myeloma treatment regimens.

Carfilzomib

Carfilzomib is a keto-epoxide tetrapeptide proteasome inhibitor approved for the treatment of relapsed

Table 12.25.2 New regimens used in the treatment of relapsed refractory myeloma

Regimen	Usual dosing schedule*
Pomalidomide-dexamethasone (Pom/Dex)	Pomalidomide 4mg days 1–21
	Dexamethasone 40mg oral days 1, 8, 15, 22
	Repeated every 4 weeks
Carfilzomib-pomalidomide-dexamethasone (KPd)	Carfilzomib 27mg/m^2 intravenously on days 1, 2, 8, 9, 15, 16 (Note: cycle 1, day 1 and 2 carfilzomib dose is 20mg/m^2)
	Pomalidomide 4mg oral days 1–21
	Dexamethasone 40mg days 1, 8, 15, 22
	Repeated every 4 weeks
Elotuzumab-lenalidomide-dexamethasone (ERd)	Elotuzumab 10mg/kg intravenously weekly x 8 weeks, and then every 2 weeks
	Lenalidomide 25mg oral days 1–21
	Dexamethasone 40mg days 1, 8, 15, 22
	Lenalidomide-dexamethasone repeated in usual schedule every 4 weeks
Ixazomib-lenalidomide-dexamethasone (IRd)	Ixazomib 4mg oral days 1, 8, 15
	Lenalidomide 25mg oral days 1–21
	Dexamethasone 40mg days 1, 8, 15, 22
	Repeated every 4 weeks
Daratumumab-bortezomib-dexamethasone (DVd)	Daratumumab 16mg/kg intravenously weekly x 8 weeks, and then every 2 weeks for 4 months, and then once monthly
	Bortezomib 1.3mg/m^2 subcutaneously on days 1, 8, 15, 22
	Dexamethasone 20mg on day of and day after bortezomib (or 40mg days 1, 8, 15, 22)
	Bortezomib-dexamethasone repeated in usual schedule every 4 weeks
Panobinostat-bortezomib**	Panobinostat 20mg orally twice weekly 3 weeks on, one week off
	Bortezomib 1.3mg/m^2 subcutaneously once weekly 3 weeks on, one week off

*All doses need to be adjusted for performance status, renal function, blood counts, and other toxicities.

**Dose of bortezomib reduced based on subsequent data showing lower toxicity and similar efficacy with reduced doses.

Adapted with permission from Rajkumar SV, Multiple myeloma: 2016 update on diagnosis, risk-stratification, and management. *Am J Hematol* 2016; 91(7): 719–34.

refractory myeloma. In a phase 3 trial of 792 patients, carfilzomib, lenalidomide, dexamethasone (KRd) was associated with better response rates, PFS, and OS compared with Rd, with two-year survival rates of 73.3% versus 65.0%, respectively (P=0.04) (Stewart et al. 2015). Carfilzomib has lower risk of neurotoxicity than bortezomib, but a small proportion (5%) of patients may experience serious cardiac side effects.

Pomalidomide

Pomalidomide is an analogue of lenalidomide and thalidomide approved for the treatment of relapsed refractory myeloma. As with Rd, the doublet regimen of pomalidomide plus dexamethasone (Pd) is a reasonable option for patients with indolent relapse. But more often, pomalidomide needs to be administered in combinations such as pomalidomide, bortezomib, dexamethasone (PVd), or carfilzomib, pomalidomide, dexamethasone (KPd).

Panobinostat

Panobinostat is a pan-deacetylase inhibitor active in the treatment of relapsed and refractory MM. It blocks the aggresome pathway, an alternative route for cells to bypass the lethal effects of proteasome inhibition. In a randomized trial of 768 patients, bortezomib/dexamethasone plus panobinostat was associated with superior PFS compared with bortezomib/dexamethasone plus placebo; median PFS 12 months versus 8.1 months, respectively (P<0.0001). The main side effect is severe diarrhoea in approximately 25% of patients, and care should be exercised when using this drug.

Elotuzumab

Elotuzumab is a monoclonal antibody targeting the signalling lymphocytic activation molecule F7 (SLAMF7). It has shown activity in relapsed MM when combined with Rd. In a phase 3 trial of 646 patients, elotuzumab plus Rd was superior to Rd in terms of PFS, with median PFS 19.4 months versus 14.9 months, respectively (P<0.001).

Daratumumab

Daratumumab is a monoclonal antibody targeting CD38, and is active in relapsed, refractory MM. In a phase 2 trial, daratumumab as a single agent produced a response rate of approximately 30% in heavily pretreated patients. In a phase 3 trial, DRd was superior to Rd.

Ixazomib

Ixazomib is an oral proteasome inhibitor that is active in relapsed refractory myeloma. It is analogous to bortezomib but has the advantage of once-weekly oral administration. Compared with bortezomib it has more GI adverse events, but lower risk of neurotoxicity.

Other options

Other promising agents that are under investigation for the treatment of myeloma include marizomib and oprozomib, two new proteasome inhibitors; filanesib, a kinesin spindle protein inhibitor; dinaciclib, a cyclin dependent kinase inhibitor; and venetoclax, a selective BCL-2 inhibitor.

Several other options exist for relapsed/refractory disease. Intravenous methylprednisolone is a reasonable option, particularly in patients with severe cytopenias and poor performance. Conventional combination chemotherapy regimens can be effective in relapsed/refractory disease. Intravenous melphalan at a dose of 25mg/m^2

is another active regimen, but usually requires transfusion and growth factor support. Liposomal doxorubicin in combination with bortezomib is also effective in relapsed/refractory disease.

Supportive care and treatment of complications

Hypercalcaemia

Hydration plus a single dose of pamidronate 60–90mg intravenously over two to four hours, or zoledronic acid 4mg intravenously over 15 minutes, will normalize the calcium levels within 24–72 hours in most patients.

Skeletal lesions

Surgical fixation of fractures or impending fractures of long bones may be needed. Local radiation should be limited to patients with disabling pain due to a myeloma lesion that has not responded to conventional therapy, and patients with spinal cord compression.

Bisphosphonates (pamidronate or zoledronic acid) are recommended as secondary prophylaxis in patients with multiple myeloma who have one or more lytic lesions on skeletal X-rays. Such therapy can reduce the incidence of osteolytic bone lesions. Avascular osteonecrosis of the jaw (ONJ) is a risk with bisphosphonate therapy. The standard recommendation is at least one to two years of monthly bisphosphonate therapy following diagnosis in patients with myeloma bone disease. Denosumab can be used in selected patients who are unable to tolerate bisphosphonates.

Vertebroplasty or kyphoplasty are helpful in patients with vertebral fractures to decrease pain and help restore height.

Renal insufficiency

Non-steroidal anti-inflammatory agents, dehydration, infection, and radiographic contrast may contribute to acute renal failure in myeloma. Patients with acute or subacute renal failure due to light-chain cast nephropathy should be treated with regimens such as VCd or VTd to reduce the tumour mass as quickly as possible. A trial of plasmapheresis should be considered in these patients in an attempt to prevent irreversible renal damage.

Anaemia

Iron, folate, or B12 deficiency must be recognized and treated. Treatment of the underlying disease and renal failure often leads to improvement in the haemoglobin level. Transfusions, erythropoietin (40,000U subcutaneously weekly) or darbepoietin (200mcg subcutaneously every two weeks) are useful in patients with persistent symptomatic anaemia despite antimyeloma therapy.

Infections

Newly diagnosed patients should receive prophylaxis with levofloxacin for the first two to three months. Trimethoprim-sulfamethoxazole should be used at prophylactic doses to prevent pneumocystis infection in patients who are receiving significant doses of dexamethasone.

Hyperviscosity syndrome

Infrequently patients with multiple myeloma develop hyperviscosity syndrome. Plasmapheresis promptly relieves the symptoms and should be done regardless of the viscosity level if the patient has signs or symptoms of hyperviscosity.

Further reading

Palumbo A, Avet-Loiseau H, Oliva S, et al. Revised International Staging System for multiple myeloma: a report from International Myeloma Working Group. *J Clin Oncol* 2015; 33:2863–69.

Rajkumar SV, Dimopoulos MA, Palumbo A, et al. International Myeloma Working Group updated criteria for the diagnosis of multiple myeloma. *Lancet Oncol* 2014; 15(12):e538–48.

Rajkumar SV, Kumar S. Multiple myeloma: diagnosis and treatment. *Mayo Clin Proc* 2016; 91(1):101–19.

Stewart AK, Rajkumar SV, Dimopoulos MA, et al. Carfilzomib, lenalidomide, and dexamethasone for relapsed multiple myeloma. *N Engl J Med* 2015; 372(2):142–52.

Internet resources

International Myeloma Foundation: http://www.myeloma.org

Mayo Stratification for Myeloma and Risk Adapted therapy. http://www.msmart.org

Multiple Myeloma Research Foundation: http://www.multiplemyeloma.org

12.26 Solitary plasmacytoma

Epidemiology and aetiology

Solitary plasmacytomas are uncommon relative to multiple myeloma, with an incidence that is approximately one-tenth of myeloma. The aetiology and epidemiology are similar to multiple myeloma. In over half of the cases, a solitary plasmacytoma is a precursor to myeloma.

Solitary plasmacytomas may be confined to bone (solitary bone plasmacytoma) or occur in extramedullary sites (extramedullary plasmacytoma). Patients with solitary plasmacytoma are at risk for progression to multiple myeloma. Increased microvessel density detected in the initial diagnostic tissue specimen has been associated with an increased risk of progression to multiple myeloma, suggesting that the evolution to systemic disease may be dependent on an angiogenic switch.

Solitary plasmacytoma of bone

Solitary bony plasmacytomas may occur anywhere in the axial or appendicular skeleton. Common sites of involvement include the spine, ribs, femur, humerus, and skull.

Solitary extramedullary plasmacytoma

Extramedullary plasmacytoma is localized to the upper respiratory tract (nasal cavity and sinuses, nasopharynx, and larynx) in >80% of cases, but can also occur in the GI tract, CNS, urinary bladder, thyroid, breast, testes, parotid gland, or lymph nodes.

Clinical features

Pain is the most common clinical symptom of solitary bone plasmacytoma. In general, clinical symptoms depend on the site of involvement. For example, a solitary bone plasmacytoma in the spine may manifest as back pain or can cause spinal cord compression and extremity weakness. Similarly, symptoms related to extramedullary plasmacytomas reflect the region of involvement.

In over half the patients, solitary plasmacytoma is a precursor to multiple myeloma, but in many the lesion is truly solitary and curable. Over 50% of patients with a solitary bone plasmacytoma are alive at ten years, and DFS at ten years ranges from 25% to 50%. Progression to myeloma, when it occurs, usually appears within three years, but patients must be followed indefinitely. Prognosis is better in patients with solitary extramedullary plasmacytoma, with ten-year DFS rates of approximately 70–80%.

Diagnosis

Diagnostic criteria are listed below. A whole body CT, or PET-CT, or MRI of the spine and pelvis is essential to ensure that the lesion is solitary. Serum and urine protein electrophoresis and immunofixation must be done, and may reveal a small monoclonal protein. By definition, bone marrow does not show evidence of a clonal plasma cell disorder. If the bone marrow shows evidence of clonal plasma cells (less than 10%), it is considered as solitary plasmacytoma with minimal marrow involvement.

Diagnostic criteria for solitary plasmacytoma

- Biopsy proven solitary lesion of bone or soft tissue with evidence of clonal plasma cells
- Normal bone marrow with no evidence of clonal plasma cells
- Normal skeletal survey and MRI of spine and pelvis
- Absence of myeloma defining events or end-organ damage such as anaemia, hypercalcaemia, renal failure or additional lytic bone lesions that can be attributed to a plasma cell proliferative disorder

Treatment

Treatment consists of radiation to a dose of 40–50Gy to the involved site. Patients with solitary plasmacytoma with minimal marrow involvement are treated identically.

Prognosis

The risk of progression to myeloma over three years is 10% in patients with solitary plasmacytoma. In patients with solitary plasmacytoma with minimal marrow involvement the risk of progression over three years is 60% in those with a solitary bone lesion and 20% in those with a solitary extramedullary lesion. Patients with a baseline serum M protein >1g/dl have a high risk of persistent M protein following radiation therapy to the involved site. Persistence of an M protein one year or more after radiation therapy has been associated with an increased probability of progression to multiple myeloma in patients with solitary bone plasmacytoma. The ten-year myeloma-free survival was 29% in patients with a persistent serum or urinary M protein compared to 91% in those in whom the M protein was not detectable following radiation therapy. An abnormal serum free light chain ratio at baseline is a risk factor for progression to multiple myeloma.

Further reading

Caers J, Paiva B, Zamagni E, et al. Diagnosis, treatment, and response assessment in solitary plasmacytoma: updated recommendations from a European Expert Panel. *J Hematol Oncol* 2018; 11(1):10.

Kyle RA, Therneau TM, Rajkumar SV, Offord JR, Larson DR, et al. A long-term study of prognosis in monoclonal gammopathy of undetermined significance. *N Engl J Med* 2002 Feb 21; 346(8):564–9.

Rajkumar SV, Dimopoulos MA, Palumbo A, et al. International Myeloma Working Group updated criteria for the diagnosis of multiple myeloma. *Lancet Oncol* 2014; 15(12):e538–48.

12.27 Monoclonal gammopathy of undetermined significance

Introduction
Almost all patients with multiple myeloma and Waldenström macroglobulinaemia evolve from a pre-malignant stage termed monoclonal gammopathy of undetermined significance (MGUS), although in most patients this is unrecognized clinically due to the asymptomatic nature of the condition.

Epidemiology and aetiology
MGUS is an asymptomatic premalignant disorder characterized by limited monoclonal plasma cell proliferation in the bone marrow and absence of end-organ damage (Kyle et al. 2010). It is the most common plasma cell dyscrasia, prevalent in approximately 3% of the general population 50 years of age and older. The prevalence increases with age: 1.7% in those 50–59 years of age, and >5% in those >70 years. Age-specific incidence is higher in males than females. MGUS is also twice as common in African-Americans compared with Caucasians.

MGUS is associated with a life-long risk of progression to multiple myeloma or a related disorder. The rate of progression of MGUS to multiple myeloma or related malignancy is 1% per year. However, the true lifetime probability of progression is substantially lower when competing causes of death are taken into account, approximately 11% at 25 years. The risk of progression with MGUS does not diminish with time.

The aetiology of MGUS is not known. MGUS is characterized by evidence of genomic instability on molecular genetic testing. The trigger for this genomic instability is not well understood, but current evidence suggests that in many cases antigenic stimulation or immunosuppression may be a key factor. Thus the current hypothesis for the pathogenesis of MGUS is that infection or immunosuppression triggers proliferation of plasma cells, and cytogenetic errors at this time (either immunoglobulin heavy chain translocations or hyperdiploidy) contribute to the development of MGUS.

Diagnosis
Since MGUS is asymptomatic, its identification is usually incidental, and occurs when serum and urine electrophoresis and immunofixation studies are performed during the investigation of patients with a wide variety of medical conditions, including suspected myeloma, hypercalcaemia, neuropathy, renal failure, etc.

MGUS is defined by a serum M-protein concentration <3g/dl, <10% plasma cells in the bone marrow, and absence of lytic bone lesions, anaemia, hypercalcaemia, and renal insufficiency that can be attributed to a monoclonal plasma cell disorder (see Multiple myeloma, Table 12.23.1).

Serum protein electrophoresis and immunofixation
Agarose gel serum protein electrophoresis (SPEP) and immunofixation are the preferred methods of detection of serum monoclonal (M) proteins. M proteins appear as a localized band on SPEP. After recognition of a localized band suggestive of an M protein on SPEP, immunofixation is necessary for confirmation, and to determine the heavy- and light-chain class of the M protein. In addition, immunofixation is more sensitive than SPEP, and allows detection of smaller amounts of M protein.

Quantitative immunoglobulin studies
Quantitation of serum immunoglobulins is performed by nephelometry and is a useful adjunct to protein electrophoresis in patients with MGUS, SMM, and other plasma cell disorders.

24-hour urine protein electrophoresis and immunofixation
Urine studies are needed when evaluating suspected monoclonal plasma cell disorders since a subset of patients with myeloma and amyloidosis may have an M protein restricted to the urine and absent on serum studies.

Serum free light chain assay
The serum FLC assay allows quantitation of free kappa (κ) and lambda chains. An abnormal kappa/lambda FLC ratio indicates an excess of one light chain type over the other, and is interpreted as a surrogate for presence of monoclonal light chains. The FLC assay can eliminate need for urine studies when evaluating a patient with a suspected monoclonal plasma cell disorder.

It is also useful in assessing prognosis in MGUS, SMM, myeloma, plasmacytoma, and light chain amyloidosis.

Risk stratification of MGUS
A risk stratification system can be used to predict the risk of progression of MGUS based on three risk factors: size of the serum M protein, the type of immunoglobulin, and the serum FLC ratio. Patients with three adverse risk factors, namely an abnormal serum FLC ratio, non-IgG MGUS, and a high serum M protein level (15g/l), had a risk of progression at 20 years of 58% (high-risk MGUS) compared to 37% in patients with any two of these risk factors present (high/intermediate-risk MGUS), 21% with one risk factor present (low/intermediate-risk MGUS) and 5% when none of the risk factors were present (low-risk MGUS). In fact, the low-risk MGUS subset (constituting almost 40% of the cohort) had a lifetime risk of only 2% when competing causes of death are taken into account.

Treatment
The current standard of care for MGUS is observation alone, without therapy (Kyle et al. 2010). For patients

with low-risk MGUS a baseline bone marrow and bone survey may be deferred if there are no worrisome features for myeloma or related disorder. Patients with MGUS may benefit from risk stratification as discussed earlier to guide follow-up. Patients with low-risk MGUS can be rechecked in six months, and then once every two to three years or when symptoms worrisome for myeloma or related disorder occur. All other subsets of patients need to be rechecked in six months and then yearly thereafter.

Further reading

Go RS, Rajkumar SV. How I manage monoclonal gammopathy of undetermined significance. *Blood* 2018; 131(2):163–73.

Kyle RA, Durie BG, Rajkumar SV, et al. Monoclonal gammopathy of undetermined significance (MGUS) and smoldering (asymptomatic) multiple myeloma: IMWG consensus perspectives risk factors for progression and guidelines for monitoring and management. *Leukemia* 2010; 24(6):1121–7.

Rajan AM, Rajkumar SV. Diagnostic evaluation of monoclonal gammopathy of undetermined significance. *Eur J Haematol* 2013; 91:561–62.

12.28 Smouldering myeloma

Introduction

In almost all patients, multiple myeloma evolves from the premalignant stage termed MGUS. In some patients, an intermediate asymptomatic but more advanced premalignant stage referred to as SMM is recognized clinically. Both MGUS and SMM represent asymptomatic plasma cell disorders, but the latter needs to be differentiated from MGUS in the clinical setting because progression to myeloma or related malignancy is markedly higher, approximately 10% per year in SMM compared with 1% per year in MGUS. However, a separate biological stage of SMM with a unique pathogenetic mechanism probably does not exist. The classification of MGUS and SMM is done only for clinical purposes. In fact, patients clinically diagnosed as SMM are most likely a mix of patients with biological premalignancy (MGUS) and early myeloma.

SMM accounts for approximately 15% of all cases with newly diagnosed multiple myeloma. The prevalence estimates for SMM are not reliable since some studies include asymptomatic patients with small lytic bone lesions on skeletal survey and/or abnormalities on MRI.

As for MGUS and active myeloma, almost all patients with SMM appear to have evidence of genomic instability manifested as IgH translocations or hyperdiploidy on molecular genetic testing.

Diagnosis

SMM is defined by the presence of an IgG or IgA M-protein level >3g/dl in the serum or 10–60% clonal plasma cells in the bone marrow in the absence of myeloma defining events or anaemia, renal insufficiency, hypercalcaemia, or skeletal lesions that can be attributed to the underlying plasma cell disorder. Often, a small amount of M protein is found in the urine, and the concentration of normal immunoglobulins in the serum is decreased.

Testing to differentiate SMM from multiple myeloma is as described for MGUS (see section 12.27, 'Monoclonal gammopathy of undetermined significance'; and Table 12.23.1, p. 376).

Note that patients with serum IgM monoclonal protein 3g/dl and/or bone marrow lymphoplasmacytic infiltration 10%, and no evidence of end-organ damage such as anaemia, constitutional symptoms, hyperviscosity, lymphadenopathy, or hepatosplenomegaly that that can be attributed to a plasma cell proliferative disorder are considered to have smouldering Waldenström's macroglobulinaemia (also referred to as indolent or asymptomatic Waldenström's macroglobulinaemia), an asymptomatic condition similar to SMM, but associated with a risk of progression to Waldenström's macroglobulinaemia rather than multiple myeloma.

Treatment

The standard of care thus far is observation alone until evidence of progression to myeloma. Patients with SMM need more frequent follow-up than those with MGUS, at least every three to four months.

Two randomized trials have now shown that lenalidomide may prolong time to end-organ damage, and a survival benefit has been noted in one of these trials. Based on these data, lenalidomide or lenalidomide plus dexamethasone can be considered in patients with high-risk SMM. Therapy with bisphosphonates can also be considered for high-risk patients. Several clinical trials are ongoing to determine the best strategies to delay progression and improve survival in SMM.

Prognosis

The risk of progression of SMM to multiple myeloma is approximately 10% per year for five years, 3% per year for the next five years, and 1.5% per year thereafter. Thus the risk decreases with time in contrast to MGUS where the risk of progression does not change with time.

The presence of occult bone lesions on MRI increases the risk of progression in patients otherwise defined as having SMM. The median time to progression is significantly shorter with an abnormal MRI compared with normal MRI, 1.5 years versus five years, respectively.

Risk stratification

A risk-stratification model is useful in assessing prognosis of SMM using three risk factors: bone marrow plasmacytosis >20%; serum M spike >2g/dl; and FLC ratio >20. Patients with two to three risk factors are considered to have high-risk SMM and these patients have a cumulative probability of progression at two years of 50%.

Further reading

Rajkumar SV, Landgren O, Mateos MV. Smoldering multiple myeloma. *Blood* 2015; 125:3069–75.

12.29 Waldenström's macroglobulinaemia

Epidemiology and aetiology

Waldenström's macroglobulinaemia is a clonal IgM monoclonal protein secreting lymphoid/plasma cell disorder, which currently also includes the entity referred to previously as lymphoplasmacytic lymphoma. A majority of patients with Waldenström's have a recurrent mutation of the MYD88 gene (MYD88 L265P).

Clinical features

The median age at diagnosis is approximately 65 years, with a slight male predisposition. The typical symptoms at presentation are weakness and fatigue due to anaemia. Other clinical manifestations include constitutional symptoms (fever, night sweats, and weight loss), hepatosplenomegaly, lymphadenopathy, hyperviscosity, cryoglobulinaemia, and sensorimotor peripheral neuropathy. Patients with hyperviscosity may present with headaches, epistaxis, blurred vision, somnolence, and seizures. Unlike multiple myeloma, osteolytic bone lesions and immunoglobulin heavy chain translocations are not seen in Waldenström's macroglobulinaemia.

Diagnosis

The diagnostic hallmark is the presence of an IgM monoclonal protein on serum immunofixation. The serum protein electrophoresis often reveals a fairly large spike, but in some patients the M spike may be small despite significant tumour burden. Anaemia is a major presenting symptom, and is normochromic, normocytic. The erythrocyte sedimentation rate is typically very high. Bone marrow biopsy reveals infiltration by clonal lymphoplasmacytoid cells. Serum viscosity may be elevated, usually in proportion to the size of the serum monoclonal protein.

Criteria for diagnosis of Waldenström's macroglobulinaemia

The diagnostic criteria for Waldenström's macroglobulinaemia require IgM monoclonal gammopathy (regardless of the size of the M protein), 10% or greater bone marrow infiltration (usually intertrabecular) by small lymphocytes that exhibit plasmacytoid or plasma cell differentiation, and typical immunophenotype (e.g. surface IgM+, CD5+/−, CD10−, CD19+, CD20+, CD23−) that satisfactorily excludes other lymphoproliferative disorders including chronic lymphocytic leukaemia and mantle cell lymphoma (Table 12.29.1).

Differentiation from IgM MGUS and smouldering Waldenström's macroglobulinaemia

The presence of <10% lymphoplasmacytic infiltration in the absence of end-organ damage represents IgM MGUS and not Waldenström's macroglobulinaemia; such patients have a risk of progression to symptomatic disease at a rate of 1.5% per year. On the other hand, patients with serum IgM monoclonal protein 3g/dl and/or bone marrow lymphoplasmacytic infiltration 10%, and no evidence of end-organ damage such as anaemia, constitutional symptoms, hyperviscosity, lymphadenopathy, or hepatosplenomegaly that can be attributed to a plasma cell proliferative disorder are considered to have smouldering Waldenström's macroglobulinaemia (also referred to as indolent or asymptomatic Waldenström's macroglobulinaemia), an asymptomatic condition similar to SMM, but which is associated with a risk of progression to Waldenström's macroglobulinathemia.

Waldenström's macroglobulinaemia and lymphoplasmacytic lymphoma

Historically, patients with an IgM M protein <3g/dl meeting criteria for Waldenström's macroglobulinaemia were once classified as 'lymphoplasmacytic lymphoma with an IgM M protein'. However, except for hyperviscosity, the clinical picture, therapy, and prognosis in these patients is no different from that of patients classified as having Waldenström's macroglobulinaemia who have an IgM protein level >3g/dl. By the current definition, such patients are considered to have Waldenström's macroglobulinaemia regardless of the size of the serum M protein.

Treatment

Patients with Waldenström's macroglobulinaemia who are asymptomatic do not need immediate therapy. The indications for therapy are anaemia or thrombocytopenia (platelet count <100,000) which are thought to be related to Waldenström's macroglobulinaemia; constitutional symptoms such as weakness, fatigue, night sweats, or weight loss; hyperviscosity; symptomatic cryoglobulinaemia; and significant hepatosplenomegaly or lymphadenopathy.

Initial therapy

The main options for initial therapy are: bendamustine plus rituximab (BR) and dexamethasone, rituximab, and cyclophosphamide (DRC). Recently, ibrutinib has been approved for the treatment of Waldenström's macroglobulinaemia, and represents an additional option. Ibrutinib is an irreversible and selective inhibitor of Bruton tyrosine kinase, a signalling molecule in the B-cell antigen receptor cascade which has been implicated in many B-cell malignancies. The choice of initial therapy varies according to cost and drug availability in various countries. Patients should where possible be treated in clinical trials.

Relapsed disease

Options listed for initial therapy can be tried at the time of relapse if there is an adequate interval between cessation of therapy and relapse. Ibrutinib is an orally administered drug that is very active in relapsed disease. In clinical studies, overall investigator response rate is >80%. The most common side effects with ibrutinib are low blood counts, GI symptoms, rash, muscle spasms, and fatigue.

Bortezomib, rituximab, and dexamethasone is an option for relapsed disease. Purine nucleoside analogues, fludarabine, or cladribine, are also effective. Response rates are approximately 50–80%. Cladribine at a dose of 5mg/m^2 intravenously over two hours for five days, repeated once after 28 days if needed, is an excellent choice particularly for patients with high tumour burden. The need for further cycles is determined by extent of response to the first two cycles as well as observed toxicity.

Alkylators such as chlorambucil may be still of value in older patients with refractory disease. Chlorambucil is administered orally in a dosage of 6–8mg/day with dose

Table 12.29.1 Diagnostic criteria

Disorder	Diagnostic criteria
IgM MGUS	Serum IgM monoclonal protein <3g/dl; and
	<10% clonal bone marrow lymphoplasmacytic infiltration; and
	No evidence of anaemia, constitutional symptoms, hyperviscosity, lymphadenopathy, or hepatosplenomegaly that can be attributed to a lymphoproliferative disorder
Smouldering (asymptomatic) Waldenström's macroglobulinaemia	Serum IgM monoclonal protein 3g/dl and/or bone marrow lymphoplasmacytic infiltration 10%; and
	No evidence of end-organ damage such as anaemia, constitutional symptoms, hyperviscosity, lymphadenopathy, or hepatosplenomegaly that can be attributed to a lymphoproliferative disorder
Waldenström's macroglobulinaemia	IgM monoclonal gammopathy (regardless of the size of the M protein); and
	>10% bone marrow lymphoplasmacytic infiltration (usually intertrabecular) by small lymphocytes that exhibit plasmacytoid or plasma cell differentiation and a typical immunophenotype (surface IgM+, CD10−, CD19+, CD20+, and CD23−); and
	Evidence of end-organ damage such as anaemia, constitutional symptoms, hyperviscosity, lymphadenopathy, or hepatosplenomegaly that that can be attributed to a lymphoproliferative disorder

adjustments based on blood counts. Other active regimens include fludarabine plus rituximab, fludarabine plus cyclophosphamide, R-CHOP (rituximab, cyclophosphamide, doxorubicin, vincristine, prednisone), lenalidomide, and carfilzomib. Selected patients may be candidates for autologous stem cell transplantation.

Supportive care
Patients with refractory anaemia or anaemia during chemotherapy will benefit from erythropoietin and/or red cell transfusions. Plasmapheresis is indicated for the treatment of hyperviscosity syndrome. Plasmapheresis may need to be continued on an intermittent basis until a therapeutic response is achieved with one of the treatment options discussed earlier.

Prognosis
The median survival is greater than five years. Adverse prognostic factors include age >70 years, haemoglobin <9g/dl, weight loss, and cryoglobulinaemia. The risk-stratification model proposed by Morel and colleagues is useful in determining prognosis. It is based on a set of three adverse prognostic factors: age 65 or higher, albumin <4.0g/dl, and cytopenias. Cytopenia restricted to one haematopoietic lineage is scored as one risk factor, while two or more cytopenias are scored as two risk factors. Patients with 0–1 risk factors (low risk), 2 risk factors (intermediate risk), and 3–4 risk factors (high risk) have five-year survival rates of 87%, 62%, and 25%, respectively.

Further reading
Oza A, Rajkumar SV. Waldenstrom macroglobulinemia: prognosis and management. *Blood Cancer J* 2015; 5:e394.

12.30 Amyloidosis

Epidemiology and aetiology
Amyloid is the term given to a fibrillar proteinaceous material deposited in various tissues that is detected with Congo-red staining showing a characteristic apple-green birefringence under polarized light. It consists of rigid, linear, non-branching fibrils, 7.5–10nm in width, aggregated in a B-pleated sheet conformation. There are several distinct types of amyloidosis which are classified based on the protein composition of the amyloid material (Table 12.30.1).

AL (immunoglobulin light chain) amyloidosis refers to the type of amyloidosis derived from the variable portion of a monoclonal light chain and occurs as a result of a clonal plasma cell proliferative disorder. AL amyloidosis may be localized (a benign disorder) or systemic. AL amyloidosis was previously referred to as primary systemic amyloidosis or primary amyloidosis. Occasionally AL amyloid fibrils may be detected in a localized area such as larynx, bladder, or carpal tunnel without any systemic disease, and this is termed localized AL amyloidosis. Localized AL amyloidosis is a benign disorder that does not require any systemic therapy and is distinct from AL amyloidosis which is by definition a systemic disease. The pathogenesis of AL amyloidosis is not well understood. It involves aberrant de novo synthesis and abnormal proteolytic processing of light chains.

Clinical features
The median age at diagnosis of AL amyloidosis is 65 years. The clinical manifestations vary greatly, and depend on the dominant organ involved. Nephrotic syndrome, restrictive cardiomyopathy, and peripheral/autonomic neuropathy are common presenting syndromes. Patients may also have associated macroglossia, carpal tunnel syndrome, and purpura involving the neck, face, and eyes. Immunofixation reveals an M protein in the serum or urine in almost 90% of patients at diagnosis. The serum free light chain assay is abnormal in most patients. Approximately 10% of patients with systemic AL amyloidosis have myeloma, and vice versa, but usually one of the two disorders dominates the clinical picture.

The clinical features of other forms of amyloidosis depend on the type of organ involvement.

Diagnosis
The diagnosis of systemic AL amyloidosis requires:
• Presence of an amyloid-related systemic syndrome.
• Positive amyloid staining by Congo red in any tissue.
• Evidence that amyloid is light-chain related established by direct examination of the amyloid using

Table 12.30.1 Classification and treatment of common forms of amyloidosis

Type of amyloidosis	Constituent amyloid protein	Treatment
AL (primary) amyloidosis	κ or λ immunoglobulin light chain	Bortezomib, cyclophosphamide, dexamethasone (VCd); autologous stem cell transplantation in selected patients
AA (secondary) amyloidosis	Protein A	Treat underlying infection or inflammation
Transthyretin (ATTR) amyloidosis	Mutant transthyretin	Liver transplantation for selected patients
Familial ATTR	Wild-type transthyretin	No specific therapy
Senile amyloidosis		

mass spectrometry (MS)-based proteomic analysis, or immuno-electron microscopy.

• Evidence of a monoclonal plasma cell proliferative disorder.

Approximately 2–3% of patients with AL amyloidosis will not meet the requirement for evidence of a monoclonal plasma cell disorder listed; the diagnosis of AL amyloidosis must be made with caution in these patients (see Table 12.31.1 in 'POEMS syndrome' section). AL amyloidosis should be suspected when patients with nephrotic syndrome, axonal neuropathy, or restrictive cardiomyopathy display evidence of a plasma cell proliferative disorder and/or a serum or urine monoclonal protein. It should be differentiated from localized amyloidosis which can be derived from immunoglobulin light chains in many patients. Localized amyloidosis, unlike systemic AL amyloidosis, is typically benign and is treated primarily for symptom relief as needed.

Treatment

AL amyloidosis

The standard treatment for AL amyloidosis is VCd. Selected patients may be treated with ASCT in specialized centres with significant experience with the procedure. Patients with AL amyloidosis with 10% or more clonal plasma cells in the bone marrow may require induction therapy prior to ASCT. A randomized trial found that stem cell transplantation was not superior to melphalan and high-dose dexamethasone. However, interpretation of this trial is confounded by the high treatment-related mortality observed in the transplant arm. The goal of therapy in AL amyloidosis is to achieve and maintain an involved serum FLC level of less than 40 mg/l. Second-line treatment options include daratumumab and carfilzomib. Patients with AL amyloidosis require significant supportive care based on the nature of organ involvement such as treatment of nephrotic syndrome, malabsorption, neuropathy, and heart failure.

Other forms of amyloidosis

Treatment for other forms of amyloidosis varies depending on the type of amyloidosis (Table 12.30.1).

Prognosis

Survival varies greatly depending on the type of amyloidosis. In systemic AL amyloidosis, survival is greatly dependent on the dominant organ involved. Cardiac amyloidosis has the worst outcome. The number of major organs involved is another major factor that influences outcome. Patients not eligible for stem cell transplantation have an estimated median survival of 18 months, compared with >40 months for those eligible for transplantation. Elevated levels of cardiac troponin T levels and N-terminal pro-brain natriuretic peptide (NT-proBNP) levels are associated with an adverse prognosis. Elevated uric acid levels, and failure to achieve a serum free light chain level less than 40mg/l is also associated with an adverse outcome.

Further reading

Dispenzieri A, Lacy MQ, Kyle RA, et al. Eligibility for hematopoietic stem-cell transplantation for primary systemic amyloidosis is a favorable prognostic factor for survival. *J Clin Oncol* 2001; 19:3350–6.

Gertz MA. Immunoglobulin light chain amyloidosis: 2014 update on diagnosis, prognosis, and treatment. *Am J Hematol* 2014 Dec; 89(12):1132–40.

Rajkumar SV, Dimopoulos MA, Palumbo A, et al. International multiple myeloma. *Lancet Oncol* 2014; 15(12):e538–48.

Rajkumar SV, Gertz MA. Advances in the treatment of amyloidosis. *N Engl J Med* 2007; 356:2413–15.

12.31 POEMS syndrome

Introduction

POEMS (polyneuropathy, organomegaly, endocrinopathy, monoclonal protein, skin changes) syndrome is defined by the criteria listed in Table 12.31.1. It is a rare, atypical, plasma cell proliferative disorder variously referred to in the literature as osteosclerotic myeloma, Crow–Fukase syndrome, PEP (plasma cell dyscrasia, endocrinopathy, polyneuropathy) syndrome, and Takatsuki syndrome.

Clinical features

The median age at presentation is approximately 50 years. Almost all patients have either osteosclerotic lesions or Castleman's disease. The major clinical features are a predominantly motor chronic inflammatory demyelinating polyneuropathy, sclerotic bone lesions, and a varying number of associated abnormalities such as hepatomegaly, hyperpigmentation, hypertrichosis, gynaecomastia, testicular atrophy, clubbing, polycythaemia, thrombocytosis, and Castleman's disease. Biopsy of an osteosclerotic lesion may be necessary for the diagnosis. In almost all cases the immunoglobulin light chain type is lambda. The diagnostic criteria are listed in Table 12.31.1.

Table 12.31.1 Diagnostic criteria for AL amyloidosis and POEMS syndrome

Disorder	Disease definition
AL amyloidosis	1. Presence of an amyloid-related systemic syndrome (such as renal, liver, heart, gastrointestinal tract, or peripheral nerve involvement).
	2. Positive amyloid staining by Congo red in any tissue (e.g. fat aspirate, bone marrow, or organ biopsy)
	3. Evidence that amyloid is light-chain related established by direct examination of the amyloid using mass spectrometry (MS)-based proteomic analysis, or immuno-electron microscopy
	4. Evidence of a monoclonal plasma cell proliferative disorder (serum or urine M protein, abnormal free light chain ratio, or clonal plasma cells in the bone marrow)
	Note: approximately 2–3% of patients with AL amyloidosis will not meet the requirement for evidence of a monoclonal plasma cell disorder listed above; the diagnosis of AL amyloidosis must be made with caution in these patients
POEMS syndrome	All four criteria must be met: • Polyneuropathy • Monoclonal plasma cell proliferative disorder (almost always *lambda*) • Any one of the following three other n major criteria: 　1. Sclerotic bone lesions 　2. Castleman's disease 　3. Elevated levels of vascular endothelial growth factor (VEGF)* • Any one of the following six minor criteria. 　1. Organomegaly (splenomegaly, hepatomegaly, or lymphadenopathy) 　2. Extravascular volume overload (oedema, pleural effusion, or ascites) 　3. Endocrinopathy (adrenal, thyroid, pituitary, gonadal, parathyroid, pancreatic)** 　4. Skin changes (hyperpigmentation, hypertrichosis, glomeruloid hemangiomata, plethora, acrocyanosis, flushing, white nails) 　5. Papilledema 　6. Thrombocytosis/polycythaemia
	Note: not every patient meeting the above criteria will have POEMS syndrome; the features should have a temporal relationship to each other and no other attributable cause. Anaemia and/or thrombocytopenia are distinctively unusual in this syndrome unless Castleman disease is present.
	*The source data do not define an optimal cut-off value for considering elevated VEGF level as a major criterion. We suggest that VEGF measured in the serum or plasma should be at least three- to four-fold higher than the normal reference range for the laboratory that is doing the testing to be considered a major criteria.
	** In order to consider endocrinopathy as a minor criterion, an endocrine disorder other than diabetes or hypothyroidism is required since these two disorders are common in the general population.

Treatment

If the lesions are in a limited area, radiation therapy (40–50Gy) is the treatment of choice. For patients with widespread osteosclerotic lesions, treatment is similar to myeloma.

Prognosis

POEMS syndrome may have an indolent or a fulminant course. In one study of 99 patients, median survival was 13.8 years. If unchecked, the clinical course is characterized by progressive disabling neuropathy, inanition, anasarca, and pulmonary demise.

Further reading

Dispenzieri A. POEMS syndrome: update on diagnosis, risk-stratification, and management. *Am J Hematol* 2015 Oct; 90(10):951–62.

Rajkumar SV, Dimopoulos MA, Palumbo A, et al. International Myeloma Working Group updated criteria for the diagnosis of multiple myeloma. *Lancet Oncol* 2014; 15(12):e538–48.

12.32 Heavy chain disease

Introduction

The heavy-chain diseases (HCDs) are characterized by the presence of an M protein consisting of a portion of the IgH chain in the serum or urine or both, and are classified based on the type of heavy chain that is involved.

Gamma heavy chain disease (γ-HCD)

Patients with γ-HCD often present with a lymphoma-like illness. The electrophoretic pattern often shows a broad-based band more suggestive of a polyclonal increase than an M protein. Treatment is indicated for symptomatic patients and consists of chemotherapy similar to myeloma or NHL.

Alpha heavy chain disease (α-HCD)

This is the most common form of HCD, and occurs in patients from the Mediterranean region or Middle East. Most commonly, the GI tract is involved, resulting in severe malabsorption with diarrhoea, steatorrhoea, and loss of weight. The usual treatment is with antibiotics. Patients who do not respond adequately to antibiotics are treated with chemotherapy similar to that used to treat NHL.

Mu heavy chain disease (σ-HCD)

This disease is characterized by the demonstration of a monoclonal μ-chain fragment in the serum. Treatment is with corticosteroids and alkylating agents.

12.33 Histiocyte disorders

Introduction

The primary histiocyte disorders are rare conditions that occur most often in children. They remain incompletely defined both in terms of phenotype and biological behaviour, and pose a significant challenge from the standpoint of nosology. The clinical presentation is variable and ranges from self-limiting to lethal disease. Recent studies suggest that many, but not all, of the histocyte disorders represent malignant rather than inflammatory conditions. Nevertheless, identification of the cell of origin within the context of normal histiocyte development (ontogeny) and correlation of biological behaviour with aspects of histiocyte morphology, immunophenotype, and clonality remain important. The primary focus of this review is Langerhans cell histiocytosis (LCH).

Epidemiology

Many patients with LCH are children, with a peak between one to three years of age, and a predilection for males (male to female ratio 3–4:1). The annual incidence in children <15 years has been estimated to range from 0.5 to 1 cases per 100,000 children. In adults, LCH is probably underdiagnosed given the heterogeneous clinical presentation, and the variety of specialists involved in patient care. The prevalence in adults is estimated at one to two cases per one million population. In one study of 274 adult patients, 52% were men, and the median age at diagnosis was 35 years. Although familial LCH has been reported, most cases are sporadic in nature.

Aetiology

The aetiology of primary histiocyte disorders remains unknown. Clonality studies indicate that in most LCH cases, the pathological cell (Langerhans cell (LC)) is clonally derived. However, the frequent spontaneous regression of LCH lesions, and the inability to propagate LC in ex vivo culture or in immune-deficient mice, support the view that LCH is not a conventional neoplasm. The most well accepted environmental risk factor is cigarette smoking which is virtually universally associated with the pulmonary form of adult LCH, which, in contrast to other forms of systemic LCH, represents a reactive proliferation of LC. LCH has also been postulated to result from an abnormal cytokine microenvironment, wherein immune cells such as macrophages and T-lymphocytes produce cytokines (tumour necrosis factor-alpha, various interleukins) that inhibit normal maturation of LC. This cytokine dysregulation may explain several features that are often associated with active disease, including presence of eosinophils within LCH lesions, elevated erythrocyte sedimentation rate (ESR), and thrombocytosis. Recent studies have shown that somatic mutations in genes involved in the mitogen-activated protein kinase (MAPK) pathway including BRAF V600E are present in half of the patients, supporting a neoplastic origin, even in pulmonary LCH.

Classification

On the basis of morphological, ultrastructural, and functional features, two major categories of histiocytes are recognized: 1) dendritic cells (DC) that play a key role in antigen presentation to lymphocytes, and include LC (skin, bronchial, and gut epithelium), interstitial DC/dermal dendrocytes (IDC) (counterpart of LC in parenchymal organs), and follicular DC (FDC) (germinal centre of lymph nodes); and 2) phagocytes, which may be freely mobile, such as circulating monocytes, or fixed within tissues, such as Kupffer cells of the liver or alveolar macrophages of the lung. There exists a close relationship between histiocytes that results in phenotypic and functional overlap, with specific cell characteristics being governed by the stage of development as well as the cytokine microenvironment. The 2016 WHO classification of haematopoietic and lymphoid tumours divides histiocyte disorders into three categories: myeloid-derived macrophage disorders (familial and secondary haemophagocytic syndromes, Rosai–Dorfman disease, histiocytic sarcoma), myeloid-derived dendritic cell disorders (LCH, Langerhans cell sarcoma, juvenile xanthogranuloma, Erdheim–Chester disease, interdigitating dendritic cell sarcoma, blastic plasmacytoid dendritic cell neoplasm), and stromal-derived dendritic cell disorders (FDC sarcoma). LC exhibit low levels of lysozyme and are CD14−, CD1a+, S-100+, Langerin+, and factor XIIIa−. In contrast IDC, which represent the putative precursor cell for most non-LCH myeloid-derived dendritic cell disorders, are typically CD14+, Factor XIIIa+, CD68+, Fascin+, CD1a−, and S-100−. Myeloid-derived macrophage disorders exhibit lesional cells that are CD14+, CD68+, CD163+, Fascin+, S-100+, and CD1a−.

Clinical features

LCH presents as several overlapping syndromes: unifocal disease, most often involving bone (lytic lesions involving skull, ribs, pelvis, or femur), which present as a painless isolated lesion, or cause pain, fracture, deformity, dental problems, or hearing loss; extension into adjacent soft tissue may compromise vital structures (e.g. spinal cord, optic nerve). Less common sites of unifocal involvement include skin (seborrhea-like or papular rash), lymph node, or lung—in adults, isolated pulmonary involvement is a distinct condition and is considered an LCH variant. Multifocal LCH can affect a single system (most often bone), or multiple systems—the latter is subclassified into two groups, based on whether there is 'risk organ' involvement (spleen, liver, lungs, and bone marrow). Risk organ compromise

(<15% of paediatric cases) may be accompanied by hypoalbuminaemia, oedema, ascites, jaundice, and/or coagulopathy (liver); tachypnoea, dyspnoea, and/or chest pain from pneumothorax (lung); and cytopenias (bone marrow involvement and/or hypersplenism). 15–50% of cases have pituitary/hypothalamic involvement, presenting as diabetes insipidus (DI) or growth retardation that may predate the LCH diagnosis—risk factors for DI include multisystem disease and involvement of craniofacial bones. CNS involvement (cerebellum, brainstem) may be seen late in the disease, with ataxia, dysarthria, or visual problems. Poor prognosis features include 'risk organ' involvement, multisystem disease, CNS involvement, and/or poor early (six weeks) response to therapy—a 30–50% mortality has been reported in the presence of such features, as compared to <10% in their absence. In addition, >50% of children with multisystem involvement suffer from late sequelae of the disease (DI, short stature, orthopaedic deformities, cognitive dysfunction, pulmonary fibrosis, etc.). Survival of adults with isolated pulmonary LCH has been reported to be significantly shorter than that of age- and sex-matched control subjects.

Diagnosis

The diagnosis of histiocyte disorders rests on pathological examination of the involved organ or tissue. Recognition of characteristic histiocyte cytomorphology, as displayed by haematoxylin and eosin (H&E) stain, may allow for a presumptive diagnosis of this condition. A definitive diagnosis however additionally requires demonstration of characteristic tennis racket-shaped Birbeck granules in lesional cells by electron microscopy (present in 1–75% of LC), and is considered the 'gold standard'. The CD1a antigen is a more convenient but less specific marker, and also allows for definitive diagnosis of LCH when detected in lesional cells by immunostaining. The frequency of positive tests varies according to the specific organ or tissue examined. For instance, it may be difficult to demonstrate Birbeck granules or positive staining for the CD1a antigen in CNS lesions. Staining for S-100 is also commonly employed in the evaluation of histiocyte disorders, but its presence is not specific for LC; other cell types (e.g. interstitial or indeterminate histiocytes), reactive activated macrophages, and naeval cells and chondrocytes are also S-100+. Langerin, a novel C-type lectin specific to LC cells, is an endocytic receptor that induces the formation of Birbeck granules. Langerin expression, as detected by immunohistochemistry, appears to be a highly sensitive and relatively specific marker for LCH. It is virtually uniformly coexpressed with CD1a in LCH lesions, and in contrast, is rarely expressed in proliferative disorders involving non-LC histiocytes. Determining the mutational profile is now becoming routine with implementation of next generation sequencing.

Treatment

Treatment of LCH is individualized and based upon patient age, risk group, number of lesions, and site(s) of involvement. Treatment options range from a 'wait-and-see' approach, to local approaches (curettage, intralesional steroids, radiation, topical steroids, or nitrogen mustard), to corticosteroids in combination with single- or multiagent chemotherapy (vinblastine and etoposide are mainstays; other active agents include 6-mercaptopurine, and 2-chlorodeoxyadenosine), to myeloablative therapy with allogeneic stem cell rescue. In the paediatric population, several randomized multicentre clinical trials have been conducted under the auspices of the Histiocyte Society, with the recent LCH III study regimen demonstrating improved survival of patients with 'risk organ' involvement with intensification and prolongation of treatment. For adults, expert recommendations from the Euro-Histo-Net offer invaluable guidance. BRAF inhibitors such as vemurafenib and MEK inhibitors such as cobimetinib have been shown to produce high remission rates in BRAF mutant and wild-type patients, respectively.

Further reading

Allen CE, Merad M, McClain KL. Langerhans-Cell Histiocytosis. *N Engl J Med* 2018 Aug 30; 379(9):856–68.

Abla O, Jacobsen E, Picarsic J, Krenova Z, Jaffe R, et al. Consensus recommendations for the diagnosis and clinical management of Rosai-Dorfman-Destombes disease. *Blood* 2018 Jun 28; 131(26):2877–90.

Diamond EL, Dagna L, Hyman DM, Cavalli G, Janku F, et al. Consensus guidelines for the diagnosis and clinical management of Erdheim-Chester disease. *Blood* 2014 Jul 24; 124(4):483–92.

Internet resources

Histiocytosis Association: https://www.histio.org/

Endocrine tumours

Chapter contents

13.1 Thyroid cancer overview

Epidemiology

Malignancies of the thyroid gland are the commonest endocrine malignancy but comprise <1% of cancer incidence overall in the UK. Over the last decade thyroid cancer has been increasing worldwide; incidence rates have increased by two-thirds (66%) in the UK (see 'Internet resources', p. 396). The highest incidence is seen in North and Central America, and Australasia, with the lowest incidence in Africa.

Histological types

Classification is according to the cell of origin. Of those of epithelial cell origin, the differentiated papillary and follicular carcinomas are the most common; anaplastic or undifferentiated thyroid carcinomas are less frequent. Medullary carcinomas originate from the parafollicular C cells. Finally, primary thyroid lymphomas can also occur. Reporting of histopathology should be performed by a histo/cytopathologist with a special interest in thyroid malignancy.

Several genetic alterations have been identified in the molecular pathogenesis of thyroid cancer, leading to activation of the mitogen-activated protein kinase (MAPK) and phosphatidylinositol 3-kinase (PI3K) pathways. RET-PTC translocations and BRAF point mutations are frequently seen in papillary thyroid cancer, and RAS point mutations in follicular and poorly differentiated thyroid cancer. Gain-of-function mutations in the transmembrane tyrosine kinase RET are seen in virtually all patients with hereditary medullary thyroid cancer (MTC) and in approximately 50% of sporadic cases.

Molecular-based markers have the potential to improve the diagnosis of thyroid nodules and the risk stratification of thyroid cancers.

Aetiology

Papillary

- The majority are idiopathic
- Radiation exposure particularly during childhood
- Inherited conditions:
  - Familial adenomatous polyposis (FAP)
  - Cowden's disease
  - Gardner's syndrome
- As an isolated inherited syndrome
- BRAF and RET mutations are frequently seen

Follicular

- Endemic goitre associated with iodine deficiency
- RAS mutations are common

Medullary carcinoma thyroid

- 80% are sporadic
- Inherited conditions:
  - MEN syndromes
  - Familial medullary thyroid cancer (FMTC) syndrome
- RET mutations are common

Anaplastic carcinoma thyroid

- History of other thyroid pathology:
  - Differentiated thyroid cancer (20%)
  - Multinodular goitre (50%)
- Multiple mutations have been reported in anaplastic thyroid cancer including p53, RAS, BRAF, β-catenin, PIK3CA, Axin, APC, and PTEN

Clinical features

Well-differentiated thyroid carcinoma

Most commonly presents with a slow growing or pre-existing enlarging solitary nodule. The female-to-male ratio ranges from 1.5:1 to 4:1. Lymphadenopathy is unusual with follicular tumours and is more common in papillary tumours. Papillary carcinomas are frequently multifocal. Symptomatic metastases at presentation are uncommon.

Approximately 80% of well differentiated thyroid cancers are papillary. There are many types of papillary thyroid cancer (PTC). Classic PTC is the most common (70–80%). The second most prevalent type is the follicular variant of PTC which has increased in incidence in recent decades. These tumours are frequently encapsulated and have a low malignant potential, with lymph node metastases being rare. Non-invasive encapsulated tumours (no vascular or capsular invasion), which behave very similarly to follicular adenomas, have recently been renamed as non-invasive follicular thyroid neoplasm with papillary-like nuclear features (NIFTP). NIFTP represent a pre-invasive stage of encapsulated follicular variant papillary carcinoma. The tall cell, columnar, and diffuse sclerosing variants of papillary thyroid cancer are more aggressive.

Oncocytic change can occur in any thyroid type, benign or malignant, but is most often associated with follicular neoplasms. Oncocytic (Hürthle cell) follicular carcinomas are associated with a decreased likelihood of iodine uptake. There is conflicting evidence as to whether Hürthle cell carcinoma has equivalent or worse prognosis compared with other types of differentiated thyroid cancer.

Medullary carcinoma thyroid

These patients are typically older than those with differentiated cancer with a mean age at presentation of 50–60 years. A solitary thyroid nodule is the commonest presenting feature. Cervical lymphadenopathy is common. There may be symptoms of local invasion such as hoarse voice or dysphagia. Diarrhoea and flushing may occur as a result of calcitonin secretion. Rarely Cushing's syndrome may be seen.

Anaplastic carcinoma thyroid

Patients are older than those with other forms of thyroid malignancy. Mean age is 65 years. Presentation is with a rapidly growing thyroid mass. Symptoms and signs of local invasion are common, including dysphagia, stridor, hoarse voice due to paralysis of the vocal cords, and evidence of superior vena cava (SVC) obstruction. There may be skin involvement with erythema or ulceration. Pain is a common feature. The mass may be fixed to underlying structures. Lymphadenopathy is often seen. There may be symptoms of metastatic disease and systemic symptoms such as fever, weight loss, and lethargy. The important differential diagnosis is that of thyroid lymphoma.

Diagnosis

Initial thyroid function tests should be performed. Elevated thyroid hormones make a malignant diagnosis extremely unlikely, as it is rare for any form of thyroid malignancy to be associated with oversecretion of thyroid hormones. Fine needle aspiration (FNA) with ultrasound guidance is the investigation of choice. Anaplastic thyroid cancer and lymphomas may require a core biopsy. The diagnosis of follicular thyroid cancer cannot be made on a biopsy since it requires evidence of capsular or vascular invasion. All follicular lesions diagnosed by FNA (Thy3f) require further evaluation with a hemithyroidectomy.

Additional investigations will depend on the clinical presentation and may include:

- Three-dimensional imaging with computed tomography (CT) or magnetic resonance imaging (MRI), particularly if there is clinical evidence of local invasion. MRI may be preferred as it avoids the use of iodine containing contrast. However, recent evidence suggests that iodine contrast is generally cleared from the body within four weeks, so this is unlikely to have a significant impact on postoperative radioactive iodine treatment.
- Thyroid autoantibodies if underlying Hashimoto's thyroiditis is suspected.
- Calcitonin and carcinoembryonic antigen (CEA) in suspected medullary carcinoma.
- Flow volume loop if there is evidence of airway obstruction.

Staging

The recommended pathological staging is by the tumour node metastasis (TNM) staging system. There are a number of other postoperative staging systems in use for differentiated thyroid cancers which are used for assessing prognosis. The TNM and MACIS (metastases, age, completeness of resection, invasion, size) have been shown to be the best predictors of outcome in validation studies. The American Joint Committee on Cancer (AJCC)/TNM staging system is optimized to predict survival in patients with cancer whilst the American Thyroid Association (ATA) and British Thyroid Association (BTA) risk stratification systems are designed to predict risk of disease recurrence. The AJCC/TNM staging system for differentiated and anaplastic thyroid cancer has recently been updated to the eighth edition. Most of these modifications mean that more patients will be classified as lower stage in the eighth edition compared to the seventh edition. This reflects the low risk of death from thyroid cancer for the majority of patients.

Staging of differentiated thyroid cancer

T1 and T2 tumours are defined as ≤2cm and ≤4cm in greatest dimension respectively. The T1 category may be further divided into T1a and T1b depending on whether they are ≤ or >1cm respectively. T3a tumours are larger than 4cm in maximum dimension. In the eighth edition the presence of microscopic extrathyroid extension does not influence T stage. The presence of gross radiological or clinical extrathyroid extension categorizes tumours as T3 if only the strap muscles are invaded, as T4a if the subcutaneous soft tissues, larynx, trachea, oesophagus, or recurrent laryngeal nerve are invaded, and T4b if the tumour invades the prevertebral fascia or encases the carotid artery or mediastinal vessels.

In the eighth edition of the TNM staging system, pathological confirmation of lymph node stasis is not required. The N0 category is therefore divided into N0a and N0b, the latter representing patients with no preoperative clinical or radiological evidence of disease but with histological involvement after surgery. N1a disease is defined by clinical or radiological evidence of unilateral or bilateral disease in level VI or VII (pretracheal, paratracheal,

prelaryngeal/Delphian, retropharygeal, or upper mediastinal lymph nodes). N1b disease includes metastases to unilateral, bilateral, or contralateral cervical nodes (levels I, II, III, IV, or V) or retropharyngeal lymph nodes.

The definitions of stage according to the eighth edition uses an age cut-off of 55 years. All patients younger than 55 years are classified as either stage I or II depending on the presence or absence of distant metastases (M1) respectively. Patients who are five years or older with metastatic disease are classified as stage IVB. Patients in the older age category without metastatic disease and T1 or T2 disease are classified as stage I or stage II depending on the absence or presence of clinical lymph node involvement respectively (N1a or N1b disease). Older patients with tumours >4cm or gross invasion of the strap muscles (T3a or T3b) are classified as stage II. Older patients with T4a or T4b disease are divided into stage III and IV respectively.

In addition to the factors included in the TNM staging system, other clinical factors are important in initial risk stratification of differentiated thyroid cancer. These include the presence of microscopic extrathyroidal extension, number, size, and location of involved lymph nodes, extranodal extension, presence and extent of vascular invasion, completeness of surgical resection (R status), and the histological subtype. Other staging and prognostication systems which incorporate these factors are in use.

Other staging/prognostication systems in use

- MACIS (see Table 13.1.1)
  - Composite scoring system for 20-year survival probability
  - Score = 3.1 (age <40 years) or age x 0.08 (age 40 years or more):
    - + 3 if metastasis
    - +1 if incomplete resection
    - +1 if invasion seen
    - + 0.3 x size in cm
- AMES: age metastasis extent size
- AGES: age grade extent size
- De Groot: thyroid limited disease, nodal disease, extrathyroidal extension, metastases
- European Organisation for Research and Treatment of Cancer (EORTC): age, sex, histology, invasion, distant metastases
- National Thyroid Cancer Treatment Cooperative Society (NTCTS): age, size, multicentricity, invasion, nodal metastases, distant metastases

Staging of anaplastic thyroid cancer

T stage is the same as for differentiated tumours. However, anaplastic tumours are categorized as stage IVA if they are confined to the thyroid, stage IVB if there is clinical evidence of lymph node involvement, and stage IVC in the presence of distant metastases.

Staging of medullary thyroid cancer

T1 and T2 tumours are defined as ≤2cm and ≤4cm in greatest dimension respectively. T3 tumours are

Table 13.1.1 MACIS score

MACIS score	<6	6–6.99	7–7.99	>8
20-year survival	99%	89%	56%	24%

larger than 4cm in maximum dimension or microscopic extrathyroid extension The presence of gross radiological or clinical extrathyroid extension categorizes tumours as T4a if the subcutaneous soft tissues, larynx, trachea, oesophagus, or recurrent laryngeal nerve are invaded, and T4b if the tumour invades the prevertebral fascia or encases the carotid artery or mediastinal vessels. Patients are classified as stage I if they have T1N0M0 disease and as stage II if they have T2–3N0M0 disease. Stage III disease involves level VI and VII lymph nodes (T1–3 N1a). Stage IVA comprises patients with T4a disease or N1b disease, stage IVB includes patients with T4b disease, and stage IVC includes patients with metastatic disease.

Internet resources

Cancer Research UK: Thyroid Cancer Statistics: https://www.cancerresearchuk.org/health-professional/cancer-statistics/statistics-by-cancer-type/thyroid-cancer

13.2 Treatment of differentiated thyroid cancer

Surgery

Thyroid

In recent years there has been a trend towards less aggressive surgery. Hemithyroidectomy without radioactive treatment in lower risk patients has been shown to be as effective as total thyroidectomy in retrospective studies.

Hemithyroidectomy is appropriate surgery for:

- Papillary thyroid cancer diameter <1cm and no evidence of nodal involvement.
- Follicular thyroid cancer diameter <1cm with minimal capsular invasion.
- Follicular thyroid cancer in patients <45 years old with tumour diameter <2cm.

In addition to these patients there is an intermediate group of patients for whom it may be appropriate to perform a lobectomy after multidisciplinary team (MDT) and patient discussion. This includes patients with unifocal tumours >1 to ≤4cm in diameter, age <45 years, with no extrathyroidal spread, no familial disease, no lymph node involvement, no angioinvasion, and no distant metastases.

Patients with tumours >4cm in diameter will require total or near total thyroidectomy with complete removal of virtually all thyroid tissue, preserving the recurrent laryngeal nerve. Total thyroidectomy is also recommended for tumours of any size with multifocal disease, bilateral disease, extrathyroidal spread, familial disease, and those with clinically or radiologically involved lymph nodes and/or distant metastases. Patients with widely invasive follicular tumours should be treated with total thyroidectomy. In addition patients with Hürthle cell carcinomas >1cm should undergo total thyroidectomy.

Parathyroid glands should be conserved where possible. It is recommended that where the vascular supply is compromised they may be reimplanted into muscle.

Lymph nodes

As for thyroidectomy, the extent of surgery depends on assessment of the risk of metastatic spread. Elective dissection of level VI (anterior compartment) nodes may be considered in higher risk patients with papillary thyroid cancer with one or more risk factors for nodal involvement:

- Age ≥45 years of age
- Multifocal or bilateral tumours
- Tumour diameter >4cm
- Evidence of extrathyroid disease
- Adverse histological subtype
- Male
- Evidence of involved lateral lymph nodes

Patients with palpable level VI nodes should have dissection of central compartment nodes. If there is evidence of lateral compartment (levels II–V) involvement this should be confirmed with FNA or frozen section and a selective lateral neck dissection of levels IIa–Vb should be performed, preserving the accessory nerve, sternocleidomastoid muscle, and internal jugular vein.

Postoperative management

All patients should have serum calcium measured postoperatively as profound transient hypocalcaemia may occur. Triiodothyronine (T3), 20mcg three times daily or thyroxine (T4), 150–200mcg should be commenced as thyroid hormone replacement. Thyroglobulin is a protein secreted both by normal thyroid tissue and by differentiated thyroid carcinomas. It is used as a tumour marker. Serum thyroglobulin (TG) should be measured at least six weeks postoperatively.

Radioiodine ablation

After thyroidectomy some residual normal thyroid tissue may remain, making thyroglobulin unreliable as a tumour marker. Radioiodine remnant ablation (RRA) eliminates residual thyroid tissue. In patients who have undergone total thyroidectomy, radioiodine ablation, and who are free of disease, thyroglobulin should be undetectable. It also allows identification and possible elimination of occult micrometastatic disease. In high-risk patients, i.e. patients with gross extrathyroidal extension, M1 disease and patients age >45 with T3 disease, RRA has been shown to decrease the risk of recurrence and death. The benefit of RRA in other patients is less clear and so potential benefit must be weighed up against toxicity and potential to cause second malignancies.

Decision-making for radioiodine administration should be within the MDT setting and the BTA guidelines aim to assist this process (see 'Internet resources', p. 401).

Indications for radioiodine ablation

Currently radioiodine ablation is definitely recommended for those with differentiated tumours >4cm in diameter, any tumour with gross extrathyroidal extension, or distant metastases.

There is no indication for RRA in patients with tumours with all three of the factors below:

- ≤1cm unifocal or multifocal
- Classical papillary or follicular variant of papillary or follicular carcinoma minimally invasive without angioinvasion
- No invasion of the thyroid capsule

In all other cases the indication for RRA is uncertain and one or more of the following risk factors may identify patients who are at high risk of recurrence who may benefit:

• Larger tumour size
• Extrathyroidal extension
• Unfavourable cell type (tall cell, columnar, or diffuse sclerosing papillary cancer, poorly differentiated elements)
• Widely invasive histology
• Multiple lymph nodes involved, large lymph nodes, high ratio of positive to negative lymph nodes, extracapsular nodal spread

Procedure for ablation

In order to maximize the efficiency of radioactive iodine, the patient is advised to commence a low iodine diet, and avoid other sources of iodine, e.g. contrast from CT imaging and amiodarone before radioiodine administration. The patient is rendered hypothyroid either by the use of recombinant human thyroid stimulating hormone (rhTSH) or thyroxine hormone withdrawal (THW). rhTSH has been shown to be as effective and better tolerated in patients with lower risk disease; and rhTSH is recommended for patients with pT1 to pT3, no metastases, and R0 disease (no residual microscopic disease). For higher risk patients or patients with recurrent or metastatic disease rhTSH is not licensed due to a lack of trial evidence, but observational studies suggest it may be as effective as THW. rhTSH should be used in higher risk patients when medically indicated, e.g. history of severe depression, cardiac disease, frailty and comorbidity, or high-volume metastatic disease.

0.9mg rhTSH is given by intramuscular injection once daily for 48 hours before administration of radioiodine. When THW is used, thyroxine (T4) is stopped four to six weeks before treatment and replaced with shorter-acting T3. Two weeks before therapy, T3 replacement is discontinued completely.

Patients are admitted to a specialist facility with appropriate lead shielding and sanitation. Consent is confirmed (Box 13.2.1) and pregnancy or lactation are excluded.

Box 13.2.1 Consent for radioiodine: information for patient

Early effects
• Sialoadenitis and taste changes
• Nausea
• Neck pain and swelling
• Radiation cystitis, gastritis
• Bleeding/oedema in metastases

Late effects
• Dry mouth and taste changes
• Dry eyes due to lacrimal gland dysfunction
• Epiphora due to nasolacrimal duct stenosis
• Risk of second malignancy <1%—leukaemia, bladder, breast, salivary glands
• Pulmonary fibrosis—miliary pulmonary disease and multiple doses of iodine-131
• Male infertility—rare with cumulative doses <5.5GBq
• Increase in miscarriage rate in first year after treatment

Patients are advised to avoid pregnancy for six months or fathering a child for four months after radioactive iodine. Stimulated TSH and thyroglobulin are measured. 1.1 or 3.7GBq of radioiodine is administered orally as a drink or capsule. Patients remain in isolation until safe levels are measured by medical physics staff. During isolation patients are advised to keep hydrated, empty the bladder frequently, and to take prescribed laxatives to avoid constipation. These measures minimize absorbed dose of radiation. An uptake scan using a gamma scintillation camera is performed two to ten days after radioiodine administration.

Activity of radioactive iodine

Meta-analysis of randomized trials has shown no difference in efficacy between 1.1GBq and 3.7GBq for low- and intermediate-risk patients. Patients with pT1–2, N0 disease who underwent R0 resection should receive 1.1GBq. The dose for patients with pT3 and/or N1 disease should be decided by the MDT, taking other risk factors into account.

Post ablation measurement of thyroglobulin and the uptake scan are useful in the diagnosis of residual disease. In these patients, with elevated thyroglobulin and positive uptake scans, management is according to the site of disease. If residual neck disease is found, consideration should be given to further surgery. If the residual disease is not amenable to surgery, a therapy dose of radioiodine (5.5MBq) is administered.

Dynamic risk stratification

Dynamic risk stratification should be performed six to nine months after radioiodine ablation for all patients with R0 disease. This allows potential modification of the post-surgical risk; so, for example, some patients who were deemed high risk after their surgery may be lower risk after a good response to RRA. This facilitates a more personalized approach to treatment, follow-up, and prognosis.

Stimulated thyroglobulin is measured and neck ultrasound is performed. Cross sectional or diagnostic uptake scans may be performed if indicated. The response to initial therapy may thus be divided into excellent, indeterminate, or incomplete (Table 13.2.1).

Follow-up and further management

Thyroid stimulating hormone (TSH) is thought to stimulate tumour growth. Retrospective data has shown improvements in relapse-free survival when TSH levels are undetectable. This is achieved by administration of T4 in supra-physiological dose which both replaces endogenous thyroid hormones and suppresses TSH release from the pituitary by negative feedback on the hypothalamus. However, adverse effects of long-term TSH suppression include an increased risk of osteoporosis, atrial fibrillation, cardiac disease, and death. In recent years there has been increasing concern that TSH suppression may be overtreatment in lower risk patients.

Patients with tumour ≤1cm and low risk of recurrence after hemithyroidectomy do not require TSH suppression or long-term follow-up and can be discharged to the care of the GP with annual TSH measurement and thyroxine only in the event of overt hypothyroidism.

Low-risk patients with tumours >1 to <4cm who have not received RRA do not require TSH suppression and their TSH levels should be maintained in the low normal range between 0.3mU/l and 2mU/l.

Table 13.2.1 Response criteria after radioiodine ablation

Excellent response: patients are low risk	All of the following:
	Suppressed and stimulated TG<1mcg/l
	No evidence of disease on neck ultrasound scan (USS)
	Other imaging (if performed) negative
Indeterminate response: intermediate risk	Any of:
	Suppressed TG<1mcg/l and stimulated ≥1 and <10mcg/l
	Neck USS: non-specific changes or stable sub-centimetre nodes
	Non-specific changes on other imaging
Incomplete response: high risk	Any of:
	Suppressed TG ≥1mcg/l or stimulated >10mcg/l
	Rising TG values
	Persistent or newly identified disease on cross-sectional and/or nuclear imaging

Following initial treatment with total thyroidectomy and RRA, all patients should be suppressed to <0.1mU/l before dynamic risk stratification at six to nine months. T4 dose is adjusted by 25mcg every six weeks until a TSH level of <0.1mU/l is achieved. Most patients require a T4 dose of 175–200mcg.

In patients with an excellent response to treatment, the serum TSH should be suppressed to between 0.3mU/l and 2mU/l.

In patients with an indeterminate response to treatment, the serum TSH should be suppressed to between 0.1mU/l and 0.5mU/l for five to ten years, at which time the need for continuing TSH suppression should be re-evaluated.

In patients with an incomplete response to treatment, the serum TSH should be suppressed to <0.1mU/l indefinitely. These high-risk patients need lifelong follow-up, both because of the risk of curable late relapses and to monitor and manage the toxicity of supra-physiological thyroid replacement.

Patients are initially reviewed to ensure satisfactory T4 dose. When levels are stable they are seen 6–12 monthly. At review, apart from clinical examination, thyroid function tests, TG, and serum calcium are estimated. Assessment of toxicity of T4 replacement is made and in some cases dose may be reduced despite unsuppressed TSH levels depending on the risk and toxicity. Baseline DEXA (dual-energy X-ray absorptiometry) scan for bone mineral density is performed and follow-up imaging and bisphosphonates are prescribed as necessary. Patients who have had calcium abnormality requiring long-term replacement should be assessed by an endocrinologist.

In patients with elevated stimulated TG but no evidence of residual disease, a repeat stimulated TG is performed after six months and often the TG level will have fallen. In these patients it is important to ensure that the uptake scan is not spuriously negative as a result of inadequate TSH stimulation or iodine contamination. If the TG level is rapidly rising, it is suggestive of occult metastatic disease and hence further assessment with other imaging modalities is required. Fluorodeoxyglucose-positron emission tomography (FDG-PET) may be helpful in those with elevated TG. If no disease is identified, management options lie between expectant or empirical use of therapy doses of radioiodine.

Management of recurrent disease

Recurrent disease usually manifests as elevated unstimulated TG (5% will relapse without elevation in TG and 25% of patients will have antithyroglobulin antibodies making serum TG levels unreliable). Ultrasound scan of the neck is performed to identify the site of recurrence, which may be thyroid bed or cervical lymph nodes. As for residual disease, local recurrence is managed by surgery where possible. In patients with inoperable or soft tissue metastatic disease, a therapy dose of radioiodine is administered in the same way as an ablation dose. A dose of 5.5MBq is usually given. (Lower doses are used in renal impairment.) Following treatment an uptake scan is performed as per ablation scan. In those with uptake, further doses of radioiodine are given every six months. Treatment is continued until uptake ceases or there are concerns regarding bone marrow suppression or lung fibrosis. In patients with skeletal metastases, radioiodine can be less effective and may require additional treatment with palliative external beam radiotherapy (EBRT). Patients with known bony metastases may benefit from bisphosphonates or denosumab. Before use of bisphosphonates a dental assessment is essential.

Patients with solitary brain metastases should be considered for surgical excision or stereotactic ablative radiotherapy (SABR) if good performance status (PS) and with otherwise controlled disease. Otherwise whole-brain radiotherapy is used. In some cases, stereotactic boosts may be employed.

Role of external beam radiotherapy

Radiotherapy is not commonly used in differentiated thyroid cancer because the majority take up radioiodine. The evidence for the use of EBRT is unclear. The majority of studies are retrospective and surgical procedures, use of radioiodine, and TSH suppression are variable. It is therefore difficult to draw conclusions. Many studies show no benefit. However, this may reflect the inclusion of many low-risk patients diluting the benefits to those at high risk of relapse. There does appear to be reduction in local recurrence in those with high-risk features such as older age, gross extrathyroidal extension, and extensive extranodal spread. EBRT should therefore be considered in patients with a high risk of recurrence/progression with gross evidence of local tumour invasion at surgery with significant macroscopic residual disease or residual or recurrent tumour that does not take up radioiodine.

The target volume includes the entire thyroid bed, and draining lymph nodes (levels III–VI); this may be adjusted depending on the operative findings and pathology results. Ideally 60Gy in 30 fractions is delivered using intensity-modulated radiotherapy (IMRT).

Targeted therapy

Sorafenib is an oral kinase inhibitor of vascular endothelial growth factor receptors (VEGFR) 1–3, RET, RAF (including BRAF V600E), and platelet-derived growth factor-β. Sorafenib (400mg orally twice daily) has been shown to significantly improve median progression-free survival (PFS) from 5.8 months to 10.8 months in a phase 3 randomized double-blind trial of patients with radioactive iodine-refractory locally advanced or metastatic differentiated thyroid cancer. Targeted therapy agents are associated with a significant incidence of adverse effects and a small risk of death. Common adverse effects of sorafenib include hand–foot skin reaction, diarrhoea, alopecia, rash, desquamation, arthralgia, hypertension, and fatigue.

Lenvatinib is an oral inhibitor of VEGFR 1–3, fibroblast growth factor receptors 1–4, RET, c-kit, and platelet-derived growth factor-α. Lenvatinib (24mg per day) has been shown to significantly improve median PFS from 3.6 to 18.3 months in a phase 3 randomized double-blind trial of patients with progressive radioactive iodine-refractory locally advanced or metastatic differentiated thyroid cancer. The benefit of lenvatinib was also seen in patients who had already received tyrosine kinase inhibitor (TKI) treatment. Common toxicity included hypertension, diarrhoea, fatigue/asthenia, anorexia, weight loss, and nausea; 97.3% of patients had treatment-related adverse effects, and 75.9% had grade 3 or higher toxicity.

Due to their significant toxicities which may impact on quality of life, and the lack of overall survival (OS) benefit, the use of TKIs is indicated when there is symptomatic disease that is resistant to radioactive iodine and/or clinically significant disease with radiographic progression.

Role of chemotherapy

There is no role for chemotherapy in the adjuvant setting. It may be used as palliative therapy in patients with symptomatic progressive disease for whom there are no further therapeutic options. Numerous agents have been used, none of which have shown dramatic activity or prolonged responses. Single agents include doxorubicin and cisplatin. Combination regimens include doxorubicin, cisplatin, and bleomycin.

Prognosis

Overall the prognosis of differentiated thyroid cancer is excellent with long-term survival >90%. Anticipated ten-year disease-specific survival rates with the use of the eighth edition of TNM are 98–100%, 85–95%, 60–70%, and <50% for stage I, II, III, and IV respectively.

13.3 Treatment of medullary carcinoma thyroid

Evaluation

The management of these patients is complex and should be undertaken within a team with experience of the management of MTC. The biology of MTC has unique implications for the development and structure of clinical services and management. Twenty-five per cent of MTC is familial, inherited in an autosomal dominant fashion, necessitating a comprehensive and integrated approach to both patient and their family. When MTC arises within a familial syndrome, assessment, and management of other endocrine tumours is required.

Up to 20% of patients will have metastatic disease at presentation. This does not preclude extensive neck surgery since retrospective series have demonstrated a survival advantage for surgery even in the face of advanced disease. Baseline serum calcitonin and carcinoembryonic antigen (CEA) should be measured. Calcitonin is almost invariably elevated. Neck disease should be evaluated with ultrasound and CT. Staging of the chest and abdomen is with CT. Even in the absence of obvious familial disease, MEN (multiple endocrine neoplasia) syndromes should be considered. Screening for phaeochromocytoma with 24-hour urinary catecholamines and metanephrines should be undertaken and serum calcium should be measured in order to exclude hyperparathyroidism.

Surgery

Thyroid

The optimum procedure is total thyroidectomy. In all inherited and one-third of sporadic MTCs the disease is multifocal. There is no role for more conservative surgery. Effective treatment of the primary tumour limits the risk of aerodigestive tract compromise, and may assist in the control of calcium levels.

Lymph nodes

There is a high risk of nodal involvement in all forms of MTC. Up to 50% of patients will have metastases to level VI nodes. Elective dissection of level VI and VII nodes is standard practice. This approach appears to reduce the risk of relapse and probably improves survival. The management of the rest of the neck is more controversial. The risk of metastasis to the ipsilateral and contralateral neck nodes ranges from 20% to 60%. Bilateral selective neck dissection of levels IIa–Vb is recommended if palpable nodes are identified. In the clinically normal neck either routine modified neck dissection or sampling followed by dissection for positive nodes is undertaken. If there is suspicion of upper mediastinal nodal involvement, sternotomy and dissection may be considered.

Postoperative management

There is high risk of hypocalcaemia secondary to hypoparathyroidism so serum calcium should be closely monitored and replaced intravenously or orally as necessary. T4 should be commenced with the intention of rendering the patient euthyroid.

Postoperative baseline levels of calcitonin should be measured. It is recommended that serum calcitonin measurement be delayed until four to six months postoperatively as this appears to be the most predictive level.

Role of external beam radiotherapy

The role of adjuvant radiotherapy is controversial. There are no randomized studies investigating the value of radiotherapy in medullary carcinoma of the thyroid. Most retrospective studies have shown a prolongation in time to relapse after radiotherapy. However, others have shown no benefit. In patients who are unable to undergo complete resection, postoperative radiotherapy may improve relapse-free survival. A dose of 50–60Gy in 25–30 fractions may be delivered to the thyroid bed, bilateral cervical, and upper mediastinal nodes using IMRT.

There is no role for radioiodine as parafollicular cells do not demonstrate iodine uptake.

Follow-up

Follow-up should be lifelong as late relapse can occur and those with inherited genetic mutations are at risk of new malignancies. Patients who undergo complete resection and who have undetectable calcitonin postoperatively are at low risk of relapse and persisting disease is unlikely. They are reviewed six-monthly with clinical examination, with particular reference to the thyroid bed. Serum calcitonin levels are measured at each visit and assessment of adequacy of T4 replacement is made.

Prognosis

Overall the ten-year survival is 50–69%. Patients may survive for many years even with a significant tumour burden. This makes the risk–benefit decisions for additional intervention for persistent or recurrent disease difficult. A number of factors affect prognosis.

- Stage at presentation: using the AJCC/UICC (International Union against Cancer) system, a study with median follow-up of four years showed risk of death is 0% for stage I disease and rises to 13%, 56%, and 100% for stage II, III, and IV respectively.
- Preoperative calcitonin levels: levels above 500pg predict for failure to achieve biochemical remission after surgery due to occult metastatic disease.
- Postoperative serum calcitonin: those with normalization of calcitonin levels postoperatively have a five-year recurrence rate of 5%.
- Age at diagnosis: age over 40 years confers a poorer disease-free survival (DFS) (95% vs. 60%). Risk of dying rises by 5% for each year of age.
- MEN3 (formerly MEN2B): the MEN3 genotype has a more aggressive pattern of disease and as such a worse prognosis than sporadic or other inherited forms of the disease.

Other factors which impact adversely on outcome include:

- Exon 16 mutations
- Elevated CEA levels
- Low levels of tumour calcitonin staining
- Male gender

Recurrence and management

Persistently elevated calcitonin or CEA postoperatively is highly suggestive of persistent disease. Calcitonin levels rise in proportion to disease extent. As outlined previously, complete surgical excision appears to predict for good outcome. Patients with elevated postoperative calcitonin should be carefully reassessed for evidence of metastatic disease and residual neck disease. This may require high-resolution ultrasound of the neck, conventional three-dimensional imaging, FDG-PET (although this is only shown to have adequate sensitivity when calcitonin levels are >500pg). In some cases, selective intravenous calcitonin measurements with or without pentagastrin stimulation can be helpful in identifying site of residual disease, particularly in the neck. In patients with isolated residual disease in the neck or mediastinum

or no evidence of disease, further neck dissection should be considered. This may result in biochemical cures of up to 35%.

In patients relapsing with elevated calcitonin at a later date a similar approach is employed. Where possible, further surgery is attempted. Surgical excision of metastatic disease is also appropriate in solitary or small volume metastatic disease as this can be helpful in the control of hypercalcaemia and symptoms from calcitonin secretion.

EBRT is used in patients with inoperable recurrence. There is some data to suggest it may delay progression. Radiotherapy is also utilized in the palliation of symptoms of pain, particularly in the case of bony metastatic disease.

The management of disseminated disease must be tailored to the individual. Often the pace of disease may be slow and in the absence of symptoms systemic therapy may be inappropriate. Systemic therapy should be reserved for patients with rapidly progressive disease or those with symptoms uncontrolled by other palliative measures.

Radiolabelled somatostatin analogues and or 131 I-MIBG therapy may be useful in a small subgroup of patients.

Diarrhoea may be managed with the use of loperamide or codeine. Patients with severe flushing or diarrhoea found to have large liver metastases may benefit from embolization procedures.

Patients with known bony metastases may benefit from bisphosphonates or denosumab.

Targeted therapy

Vandetanib, a RET, epidermal growth factor receptor (EGFR), and VEGFR inhibitor, and cabozantinib, a RET, VEGFR, and MET inhibitor have been approved for the treatment of metastatic or unresectable progressive MTC. Both vandetanib and cabozantinib have been shown to significantly prolong PFS in randomized double-blind placebo-controlled studies.

Common adverse events of vandetanib include diarrhoea, rash, nausea, hypertension, and headache. Common cabozantinib-associated adverse events include diarrhoea, hand–foot skin reaction, decreased weight and appetite, nausea, and fatigue. Cabozantinib increases the risk of gastrointestinal (GI) perforations and fistulas as well as haemorrhage.

Genetic counselling

The RET mutation is a proto-oncogene causing constitutive activation of the RET tyrosine kinase which results in uncontrolled downstream signalling. A number of cysteine mutations at 10q22 have been identified including those at exons 10, 11, 13, and 16.

An underlying familial RET mutation is identified in 25% of patients. In some there may be no obvious family history despite the presence of a germline mutation. The presence of an inherited RET mutation predicts for early development of C-cell hyperplasia and of MTC. This can occur before the age of five in MEN2A and before 18 months in MEN3.

The early identification of germline mutations allows the possibility of prophylactic thyroidectomy at a young age preventing the development of thyroid malignancy. It is therefore advocated that all patients with a diagnosis of MTC are referred for genetic screening. The counselling process should include discussion that in MEN2 families prophylactic thyroidectomy will not negate the risk of other associated malignancies although screening for these can be undertaken. Furthermore, rare kindreds of

MEN2 do not have any known RET mutation. Therefore, a negative result does not entirely exclude a heritable form of MTC. In these patients if there is a clear family history it may be possible to perform annual screening with stimulated calcitonin and neck ultrasound in relatives of the index case.

Prophylactic surgery should be in the form of thyroidectomy in disease-free relatives. This should be performed before one year in MEN3 (central lymphadenectomy should also be undertaken), between five and ten years in MEN2A, and after age ten in carriers of familial thyroid cancer. Lymph node dissection is not routinely recommended except in MEN3 unless there is risk of occult disease. As more information becomes available from individual mutation phenotypes this will help in management of unaffected carriers.

13.4 Treatment of anaplastic carcinoma thyroid

Role of surgery

The majority of patients present with locally advanced or metastatic disease. The disease is usually rapidly progressive and so surgery only has a role in a minority of patients. Those with small tumours not yet invading adjacent structures are best served by complete excision. Surgery also has a role in airway management in advanced disease; over half of patients have airway compromise.

Role of radiotherapy

Radiotherapy is the mainstay of treatment of this disease. It does not confer a survival advantage. The majority of patients will initially respond to treatment but local relapse typically occurs within weeks or months of completing treatment. Some patients will demonstrate rapid disease progression during radiotherapy. Attempts to accelerate treatment with hyperfractionated schedules of radiotherapy have not improved survival rates or had a dramatic impact on rates of local control. Although not expected to cure disease, radical doses are required in order to achieve the best rates of local control. Typically doses of between 50Gy and 60Gy are delivered in fractions of 2Gy daily over approximately six weeks.

Palliative dose regimens may be appropriate in patients who have metastatic disease at presentation. Anaplastic tumours do not concentrate radioiodine and there is no role for radioiodine therapy in these patients.

Role of chemoradiation

Attempts have been made to improve outcome by combining radiation with chemotherapy. Various combinations have been reported as individual cases or small series. The majority of other reports use hyperfractionated accelerated schedules. All of these regimens are associated with significant grade 3 and 4 toxicities. Another approach to improve outcomes has been to add full dose systemic therapy to radiotherapy. After surgery, patients received two cycles of doxorubicin $60mg/m^2$ with cisplatin $120mg/m^2$ followed by accelerated radiotherapy to a dose of 55Gy using 1.25Gy twice daily fractionation. This was followed with a further four cycles of full dose chemotherapy. This approach gave an OS of 27% at three years and a median survival of ten months. However, significant grade 3 or 4 toxicity was seen with haematological toxicity in >70%.

Follow-up

These patients are followed-up regularly in a multidisciplinary clinic. The rapidly progressive nature of this disease means they should have clinic access at short notice. Routine review includes assessment of neck and airway together with examination for evidence of metastatic disease.

Prognosis

The outcome in this patient group is very poor. Median survival is between 5 months and 12 months and one-year survival 20–40%. Factors predicting for poorer outcome include:

- Disease extending beyond the thyroid
- Tumour diameter >6cm
- Older age
- Male gender
- Dyspnoea at presentation
- Incomplete excision
- Distant metastases
- Leukocytosis

Progression and systemic management

Local progression is often inevitable despite aggressive initial local treatment. This often proves difficult to manage and early involvement of the palliative care team is vital. Systemic therapy does not seem to improve survival but may induce initial response. Single-agent or combination regimens may be considered for palliation. Targeted therapy has generally limited efficacy in anaplastic thyroid cancer and responses are very short-lived. However, recently a phase 2 study reported a benefit of dabrafenib (a BRAF inhibitor) and trametinib (a MEK inhibitor) in 16 patients with BRAF V600E–mutated anaplastic thyroid cancer. Although follow-up is currently limited, a confirmed overall response rate of 69% and prolonged survival represents a meaningful therapeutic advance in this disease.

Palliative radiotherapy may be used for treatment of symptomatic localized metastases. In the majority of cases, death results from airway obstruction and unless carefully managed can be especially distressing for patients and family. Tracheostomy and endotracheal stenting can have a role although do not always prevent this mode of death.

Heliox can be helpful and some advocate nebulized epinephrine.

Opiates and short-acting benzodiazepines are helpful in reducing the symptoms and anxiety associated with terminal airway obstruction.

Further reading

Amin MB, Edge S, Greene F, et al. (eds). *AJCC Cancer Staging Manual 8th edition*. Springer International Publishing, 2017.

Internet resources

British Thyroid Association Guidelines for the Management of Thyroid Cancer—available at: https://www.british-thyroid-association.org/current-bta-guidelines-and-statements

Cancer Research UK. Thyroid cancer statistics—available at: http://www.cancerresearchuk.org/health-professional/thyroid-cancer-statistics

13.5 Primary thyroid lymphoma

Introduction
Primary thyroid lymphomas (PTLs) constitute 1–5% of thyroid malignancies and <2% of extranodal lymphomas. The usual age of occurrence is 50–80 years and females are affected more than male (3–4:1). Hashimoto's thyroiditis appears to be the only known risk factor (60 times higher).

Pathology
PTLs are almost always non-Hogkin lymphoma (NHL). The two most common subtypes are diffuse large B-cell lymphoma (DLBCL) and mucosa-associated lymphoid tissue (MALT) lymphoma. DLBCL (50–70%) are positive for CD5, CD10, CD20, CD23, CD43, CD30, and bcl-2 oncogene whereas MALT lymphomas (30%) are positive for CD5, CD10, and CD23. Rarely Hodgkin lymphoma and Burkitt's lymphoma may occur.

Clinical features
A rapidly enlarging neck mass is the most common (70–90%) presentation followed by pressure symptoms (30%) such as dysphagia, stridor, and hoarseness. Ten per cent of patients have associated B symptoms and up to 10% may have hypothyroidism. Occasionally lymphoma may present as a solitary nodule.

Investigations
Ultrasound of the thyroid with needle biopsy or excision biopsy is needed to confirm diagnosis. Given the high frequency of Hashimoto's thyroiditis with lymphoma, the addition of flow cytometry, immunoperoxidase studies, and polymerase chain reaction may be necessary to establish monoclonality and subtype. CT and MRI scans are helpful in local staging. Other investigations include full blood count, biochemistry including serum lactate dehydrogenase (LDH) and B2 microglobulin, thyroid function tests, CT scan of the chest, abdomen, and pelvis, and bone marrow biopsy. PET should be interpreted cautiously as it can be falsely negative in MALT lymphoma and can show diffuse uptake (false positive) in Hashimoto's thyroiditis. However, SUV (standardized uptake value) in large cell lymphomas tends to be >6 whereas in inflammatory conditions it is usually <6. Some centres advise gastroscopy in MALT lymphoma to exclude gastric involvement.

Staging
- IE: disease localized within the thyroid (50% of patients)
- IIE: disease localized within the thyroid and regional nodes (45% patients)
- IIIE: lymph nodes involving both sides of diaphragm (<5%)
- IVE: disseminated disease (<5%)

Treatment
Treatment of PTL depends on the histological subtype and stage. These tumours are both radio- and chemosensitive. Combination treatment with rituximab, chemotherapy and EBRT provides the best OS rates. This approach is based on treatment of extranodal lymphoma, although there is some evidence from studies comparing treatment modalities for PTL.

Localized DLBCL is treated with combination chemotherapy (CHOP-rituximab for three courses) and radiotherapy. Some suggest six to eight courses of CHOP-R alone. However, a retrospective study showed that combined modality treatment results in fewer relapses than with single modality treatment (<10% vs. 37–43%). It should be noted that the role of rituximab is not fully evaluated in PTL.

Advanced stage DLBCL is treated mainly with chemotherapy. Some advocate local radiotherapy to all patients irrespective of stage.

Since MALT lymphomas are indolent, localized disease is treated with EBRT. However, bulky IE and stages IIE–IVE are treated with single agent rituximab alone or chemoimmunotherapy.

Surgery
There is no role for radical surgery as a single-modality treatment and it is likely to result in increased morbidity. It may have a role for palliation of obstructive symptoms developing while on chemotherapy and radiotherapy.

Prognostic factors and survival
Stage is the important prognostic factor. Stagewise five-year survivals are 80% for IE, 50% for stage IIE, and <36% for stages IIIE and IVE. Other reported poor prognostic factors include tumours of >10cm size, presence of pressure symptoms, mediastinal involvement, and rapid tumour growth. MALT lymphoma presents at an early stage, and has an indolent behaviour with a five-year DFS of 96%.

Relapse
Relapse is common with DLBCL and principles of management are similar to any recurrent DLBCL. If feasible, high-dose chemotherapy with autologous transplantation is considered.

Further reading
Hoskin PJ, Diez P. Recommendations for radiotherapy technique and dose in extra-nodal lymphoma. *Clin Oncol* 2016; 28(1):62–8.

Stein SA, Wartofsky L. Primary thyroid lymphoma: a clinical review. *J Clin Endocrinol Metab* 2013; 98(8):3131–8.

13.6 Parathyroid cancer

Epidemiology

These are extremely rare tumours, with an incidence of 0.015 per 100,000 in the USA. They may occur slightly more frequently in Japan than elsewhere. They affect males and females equally and are commonest in the fourth and fifth decades. Parathyroid cancer occurs in <1% of all patients with primary hyperparathyroidism.

Aetiology

Aetiology is largely unknown; the majority are probably sporadic. A minority occur as part of familial hyperparathyroidism, either within the MEN1 complex or as an autosomal dominant condition comprising benign and malignant parathyroid tumours. Mutation in the tumour suppressor gene CDC73 (previously known as HRPT2) which encodes parafibromin has been identified in these patients. Sporadic parathyroid malignancies also commonly show mutations of CDC73. Absence of expression of retinoblastoma protein and overexpression of cyclin D1 has also been identified. Other factors implicated included radiation exposure to the neck, and pre-existing parathyroid adenomas.

Pathology

The differential lies between carcinoma and adenoma. The distinction may not be easy to make. Macroscopically malignant tumours are typically hard lobulated structures often enclosed in a fibrous capsule while benign tumours are softer and reddish in colour without a capsule. Microscopically chief cells are seen, arranged in sheets in a uniform lobular pattern, separated by fibrous trabeculae. Occasionally transitional cells may be identified or a mixed picture is seen. The differentiation from adenoma relies on the presence of mitoses and evidence of capsular or vascular invasion although these may be seen in adenomas.

Clinical features

The vast majority of tumours are functioning and patients present with symptoms of hypercalcaemia, including fatigue, weakness, nausea, vomiting, dehydration, polyuria, polydipsia, and confusion. The hypercalcaemia, and its associated symptoms and signs, is generally more severe than in those patients with primary hyperparathyroidism due to benign adenomatous or hyperplastic disease. Neck masses are seen in 30–70%. Local invasion may cause voice changes due to involvement of the recurrent laryngeal nerve causing vocal cord palsy. Lymphadenopathy is rare. Renal disease, including renal colic, nephrolithiasis, and renal failure are common. Bone disease may manifest as pain or pathological fracture. Less commonly recurrent pancreatitis and peptic ulcer disease are seen.

Diagnosis

Diagnosis may be difficult as tumours are often small. The condition may be mistaken for primary hyperparathyroidism. A number of factors make malignancy more likely.

- Age <60 years
- Palpable neck mass (30–76%)
- Elevated parathyroid hormone—typically three to ten times the upper limit of normal compared to one to two times the upper limit of normal in primary hyperparathyroidism

- Elevated serum calcium, alkaline phosphatase (ALP), α- and β-subunits of human chorionic gonadotropin (hCG)
- Presence of vocal cord palsy in the absence of previous surgery
- Renal and skeletal disease

Neck ultrasound may be required to identify a parathyroid mass. CT may be required to investigate evidence of local invasion. Metastatic disease occurs in <1% at presentation so routine screening for metastatic disease is not required. Skeletal survey will demonstrate features of bone disease including osteopenia.

In patients with suspected recurrent disease, ultrasound scan, thallium-201 technetium scanning, or FDG-PET may be helpful in identifying sites of recurrence.

Staging

There is no universally accepted staging system. Commonly the distinction between localized disease and metastatic (lymphatic or distant) is the only system used.

Treatment

Surgical treatment

The mainstay of treatment in these patients is en bloc excision of parathyroid mass and any invaded tissues, with a wide margin, including the ipsilateral thyroid gland and isthmus. It is important to maintain the integrity of the tumour capsule to reduce the risk of tumour spillage. Often the diagnosis is made after surgery in which case further surgery may be indicated particularly if the calcium remains elevated. The role of lymph node dissection is unclear. Any clinically involved lymph nodes should be dissected and many advocate prophylactic ipsilateral neck dissection in view of the difficulties in managing recurrent disease. However, the risk of lymph node involvement at diagnosis is <5% and there may be considerable morbidity attached to neck dissection.

Postoperatively calcium levels may drop precipitously requiring large replacement doses for prolonged periods.

In cases of recurrent hypercalcaemia sometime after surgery, careful reassessment of the neck with ultrasound or MRI should be undertaken with a view to re-excision of locally recurrent disease which may be curative.

Surgery also has a role in metastatic disease. Persistently elevated calcium, uncontrolled by other means may justify metastatectomy even in the face of advanced disease.

Radiotherapy

The paucity of controlled trials in this rare condition means that the role of radiotherapy is uncertain. It has been shown in case series to reduce the risk of local recurrence in the adjuvant setting. The presence of vascular or capsular invasion may predict for local recurrence and these may be used as an indication for postoperative radiotherapy. There are case reports of its use as primary therapy in patients unfit for surgical intervention. It is also used palliatively in the control of symptomatic metastases.

Medical treatment

The main difficulty in patients with metastatic disease is control of hypercalcaemia and this is usually the cause of death rather than extensive metastatic disease. Measures to control serum calcium include hydration, diuretics, and bisphosphonates although care may be required in the face of renal impairment. Endocrinology input is invaluable.

Chemotherapy has been used for metastatic disease. Agents shown to have activity include dacarbazine, either as single agent or in combination with fluorouracil (5-FU) and cyclophosphamide. In a non-functioning parathyroid carcinoma, prolonged partial response was reported with a combination of methotrexate, cyclophosphamide, doxorubicin, and lomustine.

Genetic screening

Referral for genetic screening should be considered in all patients with parathyroid carcinoma. The presence of a mutation would make a second primary more likely in the setting of apparent disease recurrence which would underline the need to reassess the neck. Relatives found to be carriers of HRPT2 may be surveyed with serum calcium and parathyroid hormone levels. However, during the counselling process it should be noted that surveillance in this manner is not infallible since not all tumours are functioning.

Recurrence

Recurrent disease typically occurs between two and five years from initial resection, and usually presents as recurrent hypercalcaemia. Recurrence is most frequently local, but may be difficult to identify as they may be small and multifocal.

Prognosis

The prognosis is very variable, with ten-year survival rates of 40–86% reported. The rule of thirds applies; with one-third cured by aggressive surgical management. One-third has slowly progressive disease, relapsing many years after the original presentation. The final third develop aggressive, rapidly progressive disease and fail to receive significant benefit from medical interventions.

Further reading

McClenaghan F, Qureshi YA. Parathyroid cancer. *Gland Surg* 2015; 4(4):329–38.

13.7 Adrenocortical carcinoma

Introduction

Adrenocortical carcinoma (ACC) is a rare malignancy with heterogenous manifestations and poor prognosis. The estimated prevalence is 4–12 per million adults. The age distribution is bimodal with a first peak at 3.5 years and second peak at 57 years of age. There are no proven aetiological factors. ACC is rarely reported in MEN1, Li–Fraumeni syndrome, and Wiedemann–Beckwith syndrome.

Clinical features

Approximately 60% of patients present with features of adrenal steroid hypersecretion. Benign adrenocortical tumours secrete a single class of steroid whereas ACC can secrete various steroids. Rapidly progressing Cushing's syndrome with or without virilization is the most common presentation. Androgen secreting tumours in women may lead to features of virilization whereas oestrogen secreting tumours in males lead to gynaecomastia and testicular atrophy. Aldosterone producing tumours present with hypertension and hypokalaemia.

Non-secreting tumours present with abdominal discomfort or back pain due to mass effect. Rarely patients may present with fever, weight loss, and anorexia.

Diagnosis

Initial investigations include imaging (CT chest and abdomen) and hormonal work-up. Size of tumour on CT scan remains one of the best indicators of malignancy. Tumours >6cm are highly suspicious for malignancy. On CT scan, ACCs are irregularly enhancing non-homogenous masses. Apart from the size of the adrenal mass, imaging characteristics are also helpful in distinguishing benign from malignant lesions. Measurement of Hounsfield units (HU) in unenhanced CT may be useful in distinguishing benign from malignant lesions. A value of >10HU (indicating low fat content) has a sensitivity of 71% and specificity of 98% to diagnose ACC. On MRI scan, ACCs present as isointense to liver on T1-weighted and intermediate to increased intensity on T2-weighted images. MRI is also useful

in identifying invasion of adjacent organs and the inferior vena cava (IVC), and hence in planning surgery. Recent studies suggest ACC has a high uptake on FDG-PET.

All patients should have endocrine assessment prior to surgery. This helps to:
* Establish the steroid secretory profile.
* Plan surgery and postoperative management.
* Establish tumour markers for follow-up.
* Exclude a pheochromocytoma.

Biopsy of adrenal tumour is controversial because of the theoretical risk of needle tract metastases. However, it may be acceptable if primary surgical management is not feasible and the diagnosis cannot be established with non-invasive measures.

Pathological assessment

Differentiation between benign and malignant tumour is based on macroscopic and microscopic features. Nuclear atypia, atypical and frequent mitoses (>5 per 50 high power field (HPF)), vascular and capsular invasion, and necroses are suggestive of malignancy.

Staging

A summary of the World Health Organization (WHO) (2010) staging for ACC is as follows:
* Stage I: localized tumour of ≤5cm
* Stage II: localized tumour of >5cm
* Stage III: locally invasive or tumours with regional lymph node metastases
* Stage IV: tumour invading adjacent organs or distant metastases

Management

Multidisciplinary management involves surgeons, oncologist, and endocrinologist.

Surgery

Complete removal of tumour offers the best chance for cure in patients with stage I–III disease. Presence of tumour thrombus in the IVC or renal vein does not preclude a complete excision. While open surgery remains the standard of care, laparoscopic adrenalectomy has been increasingly performed. The main concern with laparoscopic adrenalectomy (LA) for ACC is the risk of recurrence and intraperitoneal dissemination. The risk of recurrence is associated with advanced stage (III and IV), tumour spillage during LA, or a positive margin. Therefore adequate staging needs to be obtained prior to opting for laparoscopic approach. Recently updated European Society of Endocrine Surgeons guidelines suggest LA for stages I and II diseases only. Postoperative hormone levels should be assessed to indicate the completeness of resection of functional tumours.

The role of tumour debulking in the presence of metastatic disease is not established. It may have a role in selected patients to control hormonal excess and to facilitate other therapies.

In selected patients with ACC and liver metastases, major liver metastactomy was shown to improve long-term survival (five-year survival 39%).

Radiofrequency thermal ablation is an alternative to surgery for lung and liver metastases.

Radiotherapy

Radiotherapy has an established role in the palliation of bone and brain metastases. The role of primary radiotherapy in inoperable adrenocortical tumour is not well established. Adjuvant tumour bed radiotherapy in completely resected stage III and high-risk (tumour >8cm with invasion of blood vessels and Ki67 index >10%) stage II adrenocortical cancer may reduce local recurrence, though not proven in a randomized trial setting. Radiotherapy should be started within three months of surgery.

Chemotherapy

Mitotane (o,p'-DDD) is a specific drug for the treatment of adrenocortical cancer. It is cytotoxic to adrenocortical cells and inhibits steroidogenesis. It was approved for clinical use by Food and Drug Administration (FDA) in 1970 and by the European Medicine Agency in 2004. It leads to an objective response in 25% of cases and control of hormonal hypersecretion in the majority. A mitotane blood level of at least 14mg/l seems to improve the tumour response rate. However, >80% patients experience some side effects. The main side effects are GI (nausea, vomiting, diarrhoea, anorexia, mucositis) or CNS (lethargy, somnolence, depression, dizziness, polyneuropathy). It also induces adrenal insufficiency and increased metabolic clearance of glucocorticoids. Hence all patients need high-dose gluococorticoid replacement (e.g. 50mg hydrocortisone daily) which helps to minimize mitotane induced side effects.

The starting dose of mitotane is 2g/daily in four divided doses. The daily dose is increased by 1g every one to two weeks until the maximum tolerated dose (usually 6g/daily in two to four divided doses) or a serum level of 14–20mcg/dl is reached. The dose limiting toxicities are anorexia and nausea.

The role of adjuvant mitotane has not been established. An international consensus panel recommended adjuvant mitotane for patients with incompletely resected tumours and/or tumours with a high proliferation rate (Ki67 index of >10%). The optimal duration of adjuvant mitotane is not known and many authors recommend a minimum of two years.

A randomized trial ADIUVO, looking at adjuvant mitotane versus observation in completely resected stage I–III disease with Ki67 index of <10%, is currently closed.

Combination chemotherapy

Several combinations have been tried with dismal results. Cisplatin with or without etoposide appears to have activity in ACC. A combination of mitotane with streptozotocin has yielded a response rate (partial and complete) of 36%.

The commonly used combination regimens are cisplatin, etoposide, and doxorubicin (EDP) with mitotane (Berruti regimen) and EDP with streptozocin (Khan regimen). The FIRM-ACT randomized controlled trial showed that response rates (23.2% vs. 9.2%) and PFS (5 months vs. 2.1 months) were significantly better with the Berruti regimen than the Khan regimen as the first-line treatment for inoperable stage III–IV disease. There was no difference in OS and toxicities between the two arms.

Patients with Cushing's syndrome need medical treatment to control symptoms and complications of Cushing's syndrome. Ketoconazole is commonly used and it can be combined with mitotane. Other agents include etomidate, metyrapone, and aminoglutethimide.

Survival and prognosis

Overall outcome depends on the tumour stage as well as completeness of resection. Tumours of >12cm in spite of complete resection have a poor prognosis. Other reported prognostic factors include high mitotic rate, atypical mitoses, tumour necrosis, and tp53 mutation. The reported five-year survival is 60% for stage I, 58% for stage II, 24% for stage III, and 0% for stage IV. Median survival of stage IV patients is <12 months. Cortisol secreting tumours are associated with worse prognosis, partially attributable to morbidity associated with Cushing's syndrome.

Follow-up

Patients with hormonal markers need three-monthly hormonal assays to detect a tumour recurrence. Since surgical salvage of a local or metastatic recurrence is feasible, all patients need imaging of the abdomen and chest for at least five years.

Further reading

Libé R. Adrenocortical carcinoma (ACC): diagnosis, prognosis, and treatment. *Front Cell Dev Biol* 2015 Jul 3; 3:45.

Internet resources

Adrenal Cancer Support: http://www.adrenalcancersupport.org
European Network for the study of adrenal tumours: http://www.ensat.org/
Orphanet. The portal for rare diseases and orphan drugs—available at: http://www.orpha.net

13.8 Neuroendocrine tumours

Introduction

Neuroendocrine cells are cells that receive neuronal input from nerve cells via neurotransmitters and as a consequence of this input, release hormones into the blood stream. As a result, these cells serve to integrate the nervous and endocrine systems. These cells are diffusely distributed in the body, and give rise to an uncommon group of tumours called neuroendocrine tumours (NETs). Although they may arise in any part of the body such as the adrenal glands (phaechromocytomas), thyroid (medullary thyroid cancer), nervous system (paraganglioma), skin (Merkel cell tumours), etc. the most common site of origin is the gastroenteropancreatic neuroendocrine tumour (GEP NET) system, which accounts for over half of all NETs.

Epidemiology

NETs comprise 2% of all malignant GI tumours with an incidence of approximately one per 100,000 in the UK, with approximately 600 people diagnosed each year. The Surveillance, Epidemiology, and End Results (SEER) database from the USA, however, shows that the incidence of these tumours has been increasing over the last 30 years rising now to 4.4 per 100,000. These tumours can occur at any age, with a mean age of 50–60 years.

Aetiology

The aetiology of these tumours remains largely unknown. Most tumours are sporadic, but they may be associated with hereditary endocrine syndromes such as
- MEN
- Familial paragangliomatosis
- Von Hippel–Lindau syndrome
- Tuberous sclerosis

Pathology and grading

NETs are defined as epithelial tumours with predominant neuroendocrine differentiation. Terminology and classification of NETs can be confusing as there are multiple competing systems for staging and grading (WHO, TNM) because of the variety of sites at which these tumours may occur. The grading of GEP NETs, however, has evolved to reflect two distinct categories of tumours, based on morphology and cell proliferation rates into:
- Well differentiated NETs: these show solid, trabecular, or glandular patterns, fairly uniform nuclei, salt and pepper chromatin, and granular cytoplasm. These are divided into grade 1 (G1) and grade 2 (G2) tumours based on Ki67 index values of ≤2% and 3–20% respectively.
- Poorly differentiated NETs: these are high-grade carcinomas with clinical and morphological characteristics similar to small or large cell tumours of the lungs. These have a high Ki67 proliferation index of >20%.

The grading of NETs has a significant prognostic implication. In the SEER registry the survival for well and moderately differentiated tumours (G1 and G2) ranges from 33 to 223 months whilst poorly differentiated (G3) tumours do worse with a prognosis of 5–34 months.

Terminology

Pancreatic neuroendocrine tumours (pNETS)

These can sometimes produce a range of bioactive products. Such tumours are called functioning tumours, and are associated with symptoms and syndromes related to the specific hormones they secrete: Zollinger–Ellison syndrome (gastrin overproduction), hypoglycaemic syndrome (caused by insulinomas), Verner–Morrison syndrome, or VIPoma (vasoactive intestinal peptide overproduction), etc.

Carcinoid tumours

Originally used in 1907, the term carcinoid (or carcinoma like) is generally used to refer to G1/G2 well differentiated GI NETs (functioning or non-functioning).

Clinical features

Clinical features are highly variable and patients may remain asymptomatic for years with the more indolent tumours. As a result of the indolent nature of well differentiated NETs, these often present late with metastatic disease.

More common features of GEP NETs include vague abdominal pain, acute appendicitis (if the primary site is the appendix), change in bowel habits, or bowel obstruction.

Patients with functioning hormone secretory tumours may present with symptoms specific to the hormone.

The secretion of serotonin and other vasoactive substances such as tachykinin and bradykinin cause the carcinoid syndrome in patients with carcinoid tumours with metastases in the liver. The liver inactivates the bioactive products of carcinoid tumours, explaining why patients who have GI carcinoid tumours have the carcinoid syndrome only if they have liver metastases. Symptoms of the carcinoid syndrome include:
- Flushing (35%)
- Abdominal pain (70%)
- Diarrhoea (60%)
- Bronchospasm
- Telangiectasia of the face
- Sweating

Carcinoid heart disease (CHD)

In post-mortem studies carcinoid heart disease is seen in up to 50% of patients. Carcinoid heart lesions are characterized by plaque-like, fibrous endocardial thickening that involves the right side of the heart, resulting in right-sided heart failure in the majority of cases.

Carcinoid crisis

This is a potentially life-threatening form of the carcinoid syndrome, which is triggered by tumour manipulation (e.g. at surgery), or due to anaesthesia, chemotherapy, or peptide receptor radionuclide therapy (PRRT) in patients with extensive tumour bulk. Symptoms include severe diarrhoea, flushing, arrhythmias, and altered blood pressure. It is treated with intravenous octreotide infusions at a rate of 50–100 mcg/h. Patients with functioning tumours undergoing surgery should receive intravenous octreotide prophylactically for 24 hours before and at least 24 hours after surgery to prevent the crisis from occurring.

Diagnosis

Many NETs are diagnosed incidentally, during radiographic, endoscopic, or surgical procedures. Once detected, clarification may be needed as to the site of the primary tumour and whether the tumour is functional. There are various blood tests, urine tests, and imaging tests that can aid in this diagnosis. Ultimately a biopsy should be performed and certain immunostains should be used to make a correct pathological diagnosis.

Specific blood tests that are useful include:

• Fasting gut hormones
• Serotonin (5-hydroxytryptamine) levels
• Chromogranin A
• Adrenocorticotropic hormone
• Cortisol
• Calcitonin
• Pituitary hormone screen

Perhaps the most useful initial test to perform is measurement of 24-hour urinary 5-hydroxyindoleacetic acid (5-HIAA, a breakdown product of serotonin). This has a specificity of almost 100% but a lower sensitivity (35%). Errors may occur due to the ingestion of certain drugs and foods. These include substances such as caffeine, bananas, ethanol, and certain nuts. Diet should always be checked before performing the test. Urinary catecholamine may also be measured.

If the tumour has been confirmed biochemically it must still be localized. The main imaging techniques used for this purpose are:

• CT (or MRI) of chest/abdomen/pelvis with contrast
• Somatostatin receptor scintigraphy (Octreoscan®)
• Gallium-68 DOTATE PET scan (where available)
• Barium studies/endoscopy/colonoscopy (if intestinal problems)
• Cardiac evaluation with ECHO cardiogram

GEP NETs often contain high concentrations of somatostatin receptors; these can be radiolabelled using a somastatin analogue, octreotide (indium-111 pentetreotide), which can then be imaged by an Octreoscan®. These receptor scans have also been shown to be predictive of clinical response to treatment with somatostatin analogues. Where available a 68Ga DOTATE PET scan should be performed as it has a higher sensitivity and specificity compared with an Octreoscan® and provides incremental information.

Once a site for biopsy has been established, tissue should be sent for specific immunostains including:

• CD56 (neuroendocrine marker, including small cell)
• Chromogranin
• Synaptophysin
• Gastrin/other gut hormones
• Ki67 (MIB1) marker of proliferation to establish grade of tumour

Management

Surgical management

Surgical resection of the primary, and where possible, of the metastatic disease, remains the gold standard first-line therapy for fit patients. Five-year survivals of up to 60–80% may be achieved with resectable metastatic disease. The minimum requirements for resection with curative intent are: resectable G1/G2 liver disease, absence of right heart insufficiency, absence of an unresectable lymph node, or extra-abdominal disease or peritoneal carcinomatosis. Surgery is not advocated for G3 tumours. In unresectable disease, subtotal resection may be considered as a palliative procedure in patients who suffer from severe hormonal disturbances refractory to medical therapy, or to debulk disease and reduce local symptoms. Orthotopic liver transplant may be considered in judiciously selected patients with diffuse liver metastases and intractable symptoms.

Loco-regional and ablative techniques

In patients with unresectable disease, loco-regional liver directed therapies can be effective in both relieving symptoms and achieving local control of liver metastases. Radiofrequency ablation is the most commonly used procedure, and there is good emerging data supporting its use. Seventy per cent of patients experience lasting resolution of symptoms for over a year. Radiofrequency ablation (RFA) may also be used as an adjunct to surgery to allow complete tumour removal. Other techniques employed include cryotherapy and laser induced thermotherapy (LITT), but these techniques do not have as good an evidence base as RFA and are not commonly used.

Liver metastases from NETs are highly vascular, and derive 80–90% of their blood supply from the hepatic artery. This combined with the fact that the normal liver derives most of its blood supply from the hepatic vein, provides an attractive rationale for the use of hepatic artery embolization to treat these metastases. Various strategies employed include bland embolization for vascular occlusion, chemoembolization with agents such as doxorubicin or mitomycin C, or the use of selective internal radiotherapy (SIRT) with yttrium-90 microspheres. Outcomes are similar for bland or chemoembolization, and currently SIRT is considered investigational in the management of liver metastases from NETs.

Medical management

Somatostatin analogues

Cell surface somatostatin receptors are expressed in over 70% of NETs, and therefore can be used as a target for imaging and therapeutic approaches. There are two long acting somatostatin analogues (SSAs) in use: octreotide LAR (Sandostatin®) and lanreotide (Somatuline Autogel®).

Somatostatin can inhibit the release of a number of GI peptide hormones, and therefore these agents are used as first-line therapy for control of hypersecretory symptoms from functional NETs. SSAs may also have antitumour, antiproliferative activity through triggering pro-apoptotic pathways.

Two recent randomized trials—PROMID (Sandostatin® LAR versus placebo in metastatic midgut NETs) and CLARINET (lanreotide autogel versus placebo in metastatic enteropancreatic NETs) have shown evidence of significant improvement in time to progression (TTP) and PFS. This effect was seen regardless of the functional status and tumour bulk, and based on these results SSAs have now been incorporated into the European and American guidelines as first-line therapy for progressive metastatic GEP NETs.

The preparations are given as four weekly injections. Sandostatin® LAR is administered intramuscularly, whilst lanreotide is administered as a deep subcutaneous injection. The drugs are usually well tolerated, but a third of patients may develop nausea, abdominal discomfort, and diarrhoea. These effects generally wear off after the first few weeks. Long-term use of SSAs is associated with an increased risk of developing cholesterol gallstones.

Interferon alpha

Interferon can have an antitumour effect through a variety of mechanisms. These include T-cell stimulation, cell cycle arrest, and the inhibition of angiogenesis. Early trials of interferon in NETs were conducted prior to the introduction of SSAs, and showed significant palliation of hormonal symptoms such as diarrhoea and flushing, with a 50% improvement in tumour markers. Subsequent to the development of SSAs, in vitro studies suggested a synergistic action between interferon and SSAs, resulting in various trials to assess the efficacy of this combination in the clinical setting. Results did show a trend towards better survival, although this did not reach statistical significance. The use of interferon is limited in clinical practice due to its side effects, which include flu-like symptoms with fevers, chills and myalgia, depression, and myelosuppression.

Systemic chemotherapy

The role of chemotherapy in NETs differs depending on whether the tumour is of GI or pancreatic origin. GI NETs are relatively insensitive to chemotherapy with response rates of around 10–20%, probably due to the slow proliferative rate of these tumours. Chemotherapy in GI NETs is therefore reserved for patients with progressive disease, when all other avenues of treatment have been exhausted, and the patient remains of good PS. The most commonly used chemotherapy regime is streptozotocin and 5-FU. Trials of chemotherapy have shown better results with combination rather than single agent chemotherapy, and with combinations that contain streptozotocin.

In contrast to GI NETs, pancreatic NETs show a much greater chemosensitivity and therefore chemotherapy is more frequently used in these cases, either at initial presentation or on progression after initial therapy. Combinations of streptozotocin-based chemotherapies remain the backbone of treatment. Combination of 5-FU and streptozotocin has been shown to be superior to streptozotcin alone, with response rates of 63% for the combination as opposed to 36% for single agent streptozotocin. Triplet combination chemotherapy with cisplatin, capecitabine, and streptozotocin has been investigated, and although response rates were better, there was no evidence of a survival advantage. The addition of cisplatin was associated with greater toxicity. In phase 2 trials another oral agent, temozolamide, has been shown to have response rates of up to 45%.

High grade (G3) neuroendocrine carcinomas (NECs) have a poor prognosis with median survival of approximately five months. These tumours share various pathological and cytological similarities with small cell lung cancers, and are treated according to similar principles. Chemotherapy is therefore considered the first-line option, and a combination of cisplatin and etoposide is the most commonly used regimen.

Peptide receptor radionuclide therapy (PRRT)

With the successful utilization of SSAs in nuclear imaging for the diagnosis and staging of NETs (octreoscans), the next natural step was to increase the administered activity of the radiopharmaceutical and use the SSAs as a vehicle for targeted radiotherapy. The radiolabels of choice are yttrium-90 and lutetium-177, and the most commonly used peptides for coupling are DOTATOC and DOTATATE. Yttrium and lutetium are both beta emitters and have shown similar efficacies. However, lutetium PRRT appears to have less toxicity and is more commonly used. There are no prospective trial data available on PRRT and data is limited to retrospective case series. In the largest series of 304 patients, 177Lu DOTATATE was associated with a radiological response rate of 30% and a median time to progression of 40 months.

Molecular targeted therapies

There are currently two novel targeted agents in use for the treatment of pancreatic NETs—everolimus (an mTOR inhibitor) and sunitinib (a TKI).

Phase 3 trials with everolimus (RADIANT-3 trial, everolimus versus placebo) showed an impressive difference in median PFS of 11 months versus 4.6 months. There was no observed OS difference but this could be because of the crossover design of the study. The effect of everolimus on PFS in non-functioning GI NETS has been the subject of trial in the RADIANT-4 study, the results of which are currently awaited. The main side effects of everolimus include stomatitis, rash, fatigue, and diarrhoea. Symptomatic interstitial pneumonitis is observed in approximately 2% of cases.

Whilst phase 2 studies have shown no activity with sunitinib in GI NETS, its efficacy is well established in phase 3 trials in patients with pancreatic NETS (pNET). The trial which randomized pNETs to sunitinib or placebo, showed a PFS of 11.4 versus 5.5 months in favour of sunitinib. Although no OS difference was observed, this again could be due to the crossover design of the study. The main side effects of sunitinib include diarrhoea and palmar plantar erythema.

Prognosis and conclusion

The prognosis for NETS is very variable due to the wide spectrum of disease, and varies greatly between well and poorly differentiated tumours. Patients with well differentiated (G1/G2) tumours have a 75–80% five-year survival, whilst poorly differentiated (G3) tumours have a five-year survival of approximately 7%. Prognosis also depends on the stage of the tumour (90% five-year survival for stage 1 versus 57% five-year survival for stage 4 disease). Patients presenting with the carcinoid syndrome have a worse prognosis than those that are non-secretory, and the development of carcinoid heart disease and right heart failure is a poor prognostic factor.

There have been many recent advances in the management of NETs as outlined, and a multidisciplinary approach is essential in the management of these patients. Early liver directed therapies and new novel agents have significantly improved OS. Although a number of therapies are now available to treat NETs, the exact sequence in which these should be deployed to achieve maximum benefit remains unclear and studies of sequential treatments are required to address this issue.

Internet resources

European Neuroendocrine Tumor Society https://www.enets.org/

UK and Ireland Neuroendocrine Tumour Society (UKI NETS): https://www.ukinets.org/

Chapter 14

Paediatric tumours

Chapter contents

14.1   Leukaemia

Introduction
Leukaemia is the commonest cancer (accounting for >40% of cases) in children. It is a clonal proliferation of stem cells which leads to bone marrow failure and tissue infiltration.

Epidemiology
Incidence per 100,000 under 16:
- Acute lymphoblastic leukaemia (ALL): 4 per 100,000
- Acute myeloid leukaemia (AML): 0.7 per 100,000
- Chronic myeloid leukaemia (CML): 0.2 per 100,000
- Myelodysplastic syndromes (MDS)/proliferative disorders: 0.3 per 100,000

Peak incidence of ALL is two to five years. Approximately 85% of paediatric ALL is of precursor-B-cell origin whereas T-cell ALL is more common in adolescence. AML, CML, and MDS occur at all ages.

Aetiology
Genetic predisposition
Chromosome fragility. Increased incidence in children with Fanconi's (10–15% will develop AML), Bloom's syndrome (ALL), and ataxia telangiectasia (ALL). DNA repair defects including Li–Fraumeni syndrome, BRCA, and MSH2 mutations are associated with increased familial risk of leukaemias and solid tumours.
Trisomy 21 (Down's syndrome) predisposes to ALL (15 times increased risk) and AML. Trisomy 21 results in disturbed foetal haemopoiesis in the liver and acquisition of GATA1 mutations which are present in blast cells of transient abnormal myelopoiesis (TAM) and in the blasts of myeloid leukaemia of Down's syndrome (ML-DS), which may develop in up to 20% of children, post TAM.

Recent genome-wide association studies have shown that single nucleotide polymorphisms of ARID5B, IKZF1, CEBPE, CDKN2A, and GATA3 are associated with an increased risk of ALL.

Therapy-related
Topoisomerase II inhibitors (particularly VP16 (etoposide) and VM26 (teniposide) cause secondary MDS and AML, characterized by an 11q23 rearrangement within two to five years of exposure. Alkylator exposure is associated with the development of MDS/AML with partial or whole deletions of chromosome 7 and has delayed presentation with preceding latent phase of myelodysplasia.

Sporadic
There is 100% concordance of clonally identical 11q23 infant ALL in monozygotic twins consistent with a prenatal origin and metastasis in the placental circulation. There is limited concordance in identical twins and the high incidence of t12:21 in non-leukaemic Guthrie cards suggest the need for a second hit (only 1% of children born with a preleukaemic clone will develop leukaemia).

Clinical features
History and symptoms
Acute leukaemia has a short (two to four weeks) history. CML often presents with hyperviscosity.
- Symptoms of marrow failure:
  - Poor feeding, lethargy, bleeding, infection

- Symptoms of organ infiltration:
  - Bone pain, limping, fracture
  - Headache and (rarely) meningism
  - Cough, stridor from mediastinal mass (T-ALL)
  - Confusion, dyspnoea, deafness, visual disturbance are signs of hyperviscosity
  - Central nervous system (CNS) manifestations occur in 2–3% of ALL cases, and present with features of raised intracranial pressure or cranial nerve involvement

Examination
- Pallor, bruising
- Lymphadenopathy and hepatosplenomegaly
- Gum infiltration, signs of superior vena cava (SVC) obstruction
- Papilloedema, cranial nerve palsy
- Chloroma is present in 10% of AML patients.

Diagnosis
- Full blood count and blood film
- Clotting screen with fibrinogen
- Renal profile and urate
- Chest X-ray (CXR) to exclude mediastinal mass
- Bone marrow aspirate and trephine
- Immunophenotyping and cytogenetics
- Save material for testing for minimal residual disease (MRD)
- Diagnostic lumbar puncture

Management
Supportive care
Treatment of infection
Neutropenic sepsis is the commonest cause of non-leukaemic death. Prompt intervention with broad-spectrum antibiotics and circulatory support is essential. Early empirical therapy of fungal infection is common practice. Non-neutropenic fever is often caused by central venous line infections.

Treatment of bleeding
Platelet transfusions may be required and clotting abnormalities should be corrected with fresh frozen plasma and cryoprecipitate.

Treatment of anaemia
Blood transfusion is usually necessary and is required in most children when Hb <7g/dl. Caution must be taken in children with a high white cell count (WCC) due to the risk of hyperviscosity.

Prevention of tumour lysis
Hyperhydration with $3L/m^2$ of fluid and reduction of urate with either allopurinol or for bulk disease, rasburicase, a potent urate oxidase that converts urate to allantoin (a readily excreted soluble metabolite), should be employed.

Treatment of hyperviscosity
Hyperhydration and aggressive chemotherapy will usually result in resolution of hyperviscosity. Coagulation support is often necessary. Leucopheresis is rarely indicated and if used must be accompanied by chemotherapy

(steroid in ALL, anthracycline in AML) to prevent rebound leucostasis.

Curative therapy: risk-directed protocols

Multiagent chemotherapy is very effective for acute leukaemia giving 88% five-year event-free survival (EFS) in ALL, and 62% five-year EFS in AML.

Prognostic factors (see Table 14.1.1) are widely used in risk-directed protocols in which the most intensive therapy is reserved for those at highest risk of relapse. It is now clear that for children receiving homogeneous therapy, cytogenetics and response to treatment as measured by MRD are the strongest prognostic indicators.

In acute leukaemia, bone marrow transplant (BMT) is reserved for very high-risk disease in CR1 (first complete remission) and treatment of relapse.

Treatment of acute lymphoblastic leukaemia

Treatment is divided into four phases:
* Induction: four weeks of corticosteroid, vincristine, asparaginase, and anthracycline achieves remission in 98% of cases.
* CNS prophylaxis through regular intrathecal methotrexate and/or high-dose systemic methotrexate.
* Intensification/re-induction: at present all risk groups benefit from intensive re-induction.
* Maintenance: oral 6MP/methotrexate for up to three years from diagnosis is required. The benefit of pulses of vincristine and steroid during maintenance is unclear.

Subgroup-specific therapy

Infant ALL

This has a unique biology with MLL rearrangement, and a pro-B immunophenotype. The relatively poor prognosis seen in the past has improved with a protocol based on post-induction intensification with high-dose cytarabine and methotrexate. The role of an ALL/AML hybrid regimen is also being studied. Very high-risk patients (age <6 months, MLL rearrangement and WCC >300 x 10^9/L) proceed to stem cell transplant (SCT) in CR1.

Philadelphia-positive ALL

This is associated with a poorer prognosis and these patients are treated with imatinib with intensive chemotherapy. In the UK most proceed to SCT in CR1. Dasatinib, a second-generation TKI, is being currently studied as the initial treatment.

Relapse

Prognosis depends on site and timing of relapse. Re-induction chemotherapy is followed by BMT in those with an early relapse (<6 months from end of treatment) or high levels of MRD at week 5 of re-treatment. It is not clear whether the addition of allogeneic transplantation after second CR in late-relapse improves the cure rate. Full systemic therapy is required for isolated extramedullary relapse. Up to 50% of relapses are cured.

Treatment of acute myeloid leukaemia

Involves up to five courses of anthracycline and cytarabine-based intensive chemotherapy. In the UK transplantation is no longer offered to children in CR1.

Table 14.1.1 Prognostic factors of childhood acute leukaemia

Acute lymphoblastic leukaemia

	% of patients	Five-year event-free survival (%)
Clinical features		
NCI standard risk (age 1–10, WCC <50 x 10^9/L)	62	>90
NCI high risk (age < 1 or >10, and/or WCC >50 x 10^9/L)	38	Up to 80
Cytogenetics	25	94
Tel/AML-1 fusion gene	25	85
High hyperdiploidy (>50 chromosomes)	2	40
Hypodiploidy (<44 chromosomes)	2	35
iAMP 21 Philadelphia positive	3	55
MLL gene arrangement (infant ALL)	80	50
Response to therapy		
Day 8/15 marrow >25% blasts	14	70
No CR day 35	2	40
MRD <0.01% day 28	35	95

Acute myeloid leukaemia

	% of patients	Five-year overall survival (%)
Cytogenetics (MRC classification)		
Favourable (t8:21, t15:17, inv 16)	31	76
Intermediate (11q23, normal)	61	52
Poor (–7, –5, del3q, complex)	7	40
Response to therapy		
Day 35 marrow >15% blasts	16	23

Note: outcomes for ALL are illustrative and are derived from composite outcomes of recent, UK, US, and European trials. AML outcomes are based on UKAML X.

ALL acute lymphoblastic leukaemia; AML acute myeloid leukaemia; CR complete remission; MLL mixed lineage leukaemia; MRC Medical Research Council; MRD minimal residual disease; NCI National Cancer Institute; WCC white cell count.

Subgroup-specific therapy

Down's syndrome

TAM spontaneously resolves in the majority of cases but low-dose cytarabine may be needed to treat symptomatic children. Twenty per cent of children with TAM will develop AML within three years. AML of DS is uniquely sensitive to cytarabine. Relapse is very rare but toxicity leads to an event-free survival (EFS) of 85%. Consequently, anthracycline is now reduced in induction and high-dose cytarabine is given during consolidation to reduce toxicity and infective complications.

AML M3

AML M3 (acute promyelocytic leukaemia (APML)) is treated with ATRA (all-transretinoic acid) and chemotherapy. ATRA causes selective proteolytic degradation of PML-RARA and allows normal differentiation of promyelocytes. Serial MRD monitoring allows identification of molecular relapse, which can be treated with arsenic trioxide. BMT is considered in those with persistent MRD.

Relapse

All relapsed patients undergo re-induction and those who remit are considered for bone marrow transplantation. Patients who relapse within one year of diagnosis have a very poor outcome (20% EFS).

Treatment of chronic myeloid leukaemia

Children with CML often present with symptoms of hyperviscosity and leucopheresis may be indicated. Children with CML are often treated with first-line imatinib, which leads to a complete haematological response of 98% with a CyCR of 61–91% and a MMR at 12 months ranging from 31% to 67%. Patients who relapse on imatinib or who have an inadequate response are considered for second-generation TKIs such as dasatinib or nilotinib. With the success of TKI, the role of allogenic transplant in childhood CML is still undefined.

Myelodysplasia/myeloproliferative disorders

MDS in children is rare and the diagnosis should be made with caution in those without a clonal cytogenetic abnormality. MDS is commonly seen in Down's syndrome, Fanconi anaemia, Diamond–Blackfan, neurofibromatosis, and Schwachmann–Diamond syndrome.

Juvenile myelomonocytic leukaemia is analogous to adult chronic myelomonocytic leukaema. It is characterized by a monocytosis $>1 \times 10^9/L$, $< 20\%$ blasts, high HbF, WCC $>10 \times 10^9/L$, hypersensitivity to granulocyte-macrophage colony stimulating factor (GM-CSF), and clonal abnormality including monosomy 7. Massive hepatosplenomegaly (in more than 95% children) and skin rashes are also a feature. There is an association with neurofibromatosis and Noonan's syndrome and two-thirds of patients will have defects in the RAS signalling pathways (inactivation of NF1, mutations in PTPN11). Treatment is with allogenic haematopoietic stem cell transplantation (HSCT), sometimes preceded by AML type chemotherapy for cytoreduction. Disease recurrences occur in 30–40% cases after HSCT and a second HSCT should be considered.

Refractory anaemia with ring sideroblasts is not seen in children. The presence of ring sideroblasts indicates either X linked ALA synthase deficiency or a mitochondrial cytopathy.

Further reading

Creutzig U, van den Heuvel-Eibrink MM, Gibson B, et al. Diagnosis and management of acute myeloid leukaemia in children and adolescents: recommendations from an international expert panel. *Blood* 2012 Oct 18; 120(16):3187–205.

Hasle H. Myelodysplastic and myeloproliferative disorders of childhood. *Hematol Am Soc Hematol Educ Program* 2016; 1:598–604.

Locatelli F, Niemeyer CM. How I treat juvenile myelomonocytic leukemia. *Blood* 2015; 125(7):1083–90.

Madhusoodhan PP, Carroll WL, Bhatla T. Progress and prospects in pediatric leukemia. *Curr Probl Pediatr Adolesc Health Care* 2016; 46(7):229–41.

Tanizawa A. Optimal management for pediatric chronic myeloid leukemia. *Pediatr Int* 2016; 58(3):171–9.

14.2   Lymphoma

Introduction

Lymphomas account for 8–10% of all childhood cancers. Non-Hodgkin lymphoma (NHL) in children is aggressive, often leading to symptoms from tissue infiltration or compression of vital structures.

Classification and incidence per 100,000 population:

- Hodgkin lymphoma (HL): 0.3 per 100,000
- NHL: 0.6 per 100,000

Non–Hodgkin lymphoma

NHLs are aggressive, high-grade malignancies of B and T lymphocytes, often pathologically indistinguishable from leukaemia but do not diffusely involve the bone marrow. In practice only three World Health Organization (WHO) NHL categories of NHL are seen: mature B-cell lymphoma (55%) including Burkitt's lymphoma (BL) and diffuse large B-cell lymphoma (DLBCL); lymphoblastic lymphoma (B and T cell) (25%); and anaplastic large cell lymphoma (5%).

Aetiology

Genetic predisposition

- Chromosome fragility: increased incidence in children with Bloom's syndrome and ataxia telangiectasia (T-NHL).
- Congenital immune deficiency/dysregulation: increased incidence in Wiskott–Aldrich syndrome and autoimmune lymphoproliferative syndrome.
- X-linked lymphoproliferative disease (XLP): defects in expression of SAP (SLAM associated protein) lead to failed T and NK cell control of Epstein–Barr virus (EBV) and the development of EBV positive lymphoma.
- Infection–endemic Burkitt lymphoma.
- Epstein–Barr virus: 100% of endemic African BL is EBV genome positive. Endemic BL is restricted to areas in which malaria is holoendemic, supporting a role for chronic immune stimulation by *Plasmodium falciparum*. The role of EBV in sporadic BL is much less clear.

- Immune suppression: advances in transplant technology have revealed the central role of T-cell immunity in the control of EBV. EBV post-transplant lymphoproliferative disorder (PTLD) is an increasing feature of alternative donor BMT and solid organ grafts.

Clinical features

History and symptoms
- Lymphadenopathy, especially cervical in HL
- Abdominal pain and distension secondary to an abdominal mass. Occasional jaundice due to cholestasis
- Cough, wheeze, shortness of breath, and signs of SVC obstruction secondary to a mediastinal mass
- Fever, weight loss, night sweats
- CNS symptoms and cranial nerve palsy

Examination
- Large 'rubbery' lymph nodes, especially cervical
- Hepatosplenomegaly
- Abdominal mass (B-cell lymphoma)
- Signs of SVC obstruction
- Cranial nerve palsies

Investigations, classification, and staging

Investigations
- Full blood count and blood film
- Renal profile and urate/erythrocyte sedimentation rate (ESR)/lactate dehydrogenase (LDH)
- EBV serology and polymerase chain reaction (PCR)
- CXR/chest computed tomography (CT)/baseline positron emission tomography (PET)
- Abdominal ultrasound (US)/CT
- Lymph node biopsy
- Bone marrow aspirate and trephine
- Diagnostic lumbar puncture

Classification
Based on morphology, immunochemistry, and cytogenetics.

Immunohistochemistry
- Pre-B- and T-lymphoblastic lymphoma are terminal deoxynucleotidyl transferase (TDT) positive and express CD19, CD79a (B markers), and cytoplasmic CD3 (T marker).
- BL and DLBCL are TDT negative and express CD 19, CD20, CD79a, often surface immunoglobulin and CD10.
- Anaplastic lymphoma may express T-cell markers and CD30 and Alk 1 in 80% which confers a better prognosis.

Cytogenetics
In all cases of BL, C-MYC at 8q24 is translocated to proximity with an immunoglobulin enhancer. The t (8;14) (q24;q32) is seen in 80% and t(2;8)(p11;q24) and t(8;22) (q24;q11) are less common.
Translocations of ALK and NPM, t(2;5)(p23;q35), and t(1;2)(q25;p23) are present in anaplastic lymphoma.

Staging
In view of the high incidence of extranodal disease, Murphy staging is more appropriate than Ann Arbor for paediatric NHL. Recently a new international paediatric NHL staging system has been proposed:

- Stage I: single tumour excluding mediastinum and abdomen.
- Stage II: single extranodal tumour with regional nodes, two or more nodal areas on the same side of diaphragm, or completely resectable primary GI tumours with or without mesenteric nodes.
- Stage III: two or more extranodal tumours, two or more nodal areas on both sides of diaphragm, intra-abdominal or retroperitoneal disease, paraspinal or epidural tumour, single bone lesion with concomitant extranodal, or non-regional nodal disease.
- Stage IV; involving CNS, bone marrow, or both.

Management

Supportive care
- Prevention of tumour lysis is particularly important in abdominal B-NHL and T-NHL

Curative therapy: risk directed protocols
Multiagent chemotherapy directed by histological subtype is very effective for NHL in childhood. Broadly four different 'disease specific' approaches are used.

Mature B-cell lymphoma. B-NHL has a very high proliferative index and a propensity for CNS involvement. In localized disease (stage I and II), less intensive regimens such as COPAD (cyclophosphamide, vincristine, prednisolone, and doxorubicin) or COMP (cyclophosphamide, vincristine, methotrexate, and prednisone) are curative in almost all patients. For high-risk disease, especially with CNS involvement, CHOP-based (cyclophosphamide, hydroxydaunorubicin (doxorubicin), Oncovin® (vincristine), and prednisone-based) regimens with additional high-dose methotrexate and intensive intrathecal chemotherapy are highly effective giving long-term survival rates of 80%. High-dose cytosine and etoposide are also of value in higher risk groups. It is important to note that cranial irradiation is not required even if there is CNS involvement. The interim results of the ongoing COG (Children's Oncology Group)/European international B-NHL suggest that the addition of rituximab to standard chemotherapy improves EFS in high-risk patients.
Relapse of B-NHL is often rapid and rarely curable. Second-line regimens with rituximab and high-dose therapy, antibody directed radiotherapy, and double bone marrow transplant are being investigated. In those who respond to further therapy, allogeneic BMT is recommended, but there is no evidence of a graft-versus-lymphoma effect.

Lymphoblastic lymphoma. T-lymphoblastic lymphoma is treated similarly to ALL. Comparison of data from the BFM (Berlin-Frankfurt-Munster) and Medical Research Council (MRC) suggest that use of a block of four cycles of high dose methotrexate optimizes systemic and CNS control. Maintenance treatment is required, though several groups are trialling whether the duration of this could be reduced. Cranial radiation is reserved for those with CNS disease at diagnosis. Stage 3 T-NHL has over 90% EFS with BFM chemotherapy. Achieving a second remission in patients with relapsed disease is difficult and patients who achieve a second remission are treated with allogeneic transplantation. Some results suggest that there may be an allogenic graft-versus-lymphoma effect.
B-lymphoblastic lymphoma is optimally treated as ALL with full maintenance chemotherapy. Outcomes are as for B-cell precursor ALL.

New agents such as bortezimab and nelarabine are being investigated in relapsed lymphoblastic lymphoma and patients with high-risk disease.

Anaplastic large cell lymphoma (ALCL). Optimal therapy for ALCL is less well defined than its commoner counterparts. Most regimens rely on B-NHL type therapy. The risk of CNS disease is less than that seen in other NHLs and CNS relapse can be prevented with moderate dose systemic methotrexate. Overall five-year EFS rates of 65–75% are reported. Patients with recurrent disease are considered for transplantation. Brentuximab vedotin and crizotinib (ALK-TKI) are shown to be active in relapsed disease and are currently under evaluation.

EBV driven lymphoproliferative disorder (LPD). This should be staged as for other NHLs. In X-linked proliferative syndrome, disease should be cytoreduced with low-dose chemotherapy and/or rituximab. This should be followed by BMT from an unaffected donor, to restore sufficient immunity to prevent further recurrences.

Where LPD arises in the context of immune suppression, therapy is guided by staging and cytogenetics. Limited stage disease without marrow involvement may respond to withdrawal of immune suppression and/or rituximab. Rapid development of bulky disease, marrow involvement, or clonal cytogenetics are indications for consideration of full B-NHL therapy.

Hodgkin lymphoma

This is the most common childhood cancer in 15–19 year olds. For treatment purposes, these are classified as classical (90–95%) and nodular lymphocyte-predominant (5–10%) HL.

Aetiology

The known risk factors include EBV and immunosuppression. Less than 5% patients have a family history of HL.

Clinical features

- Painless lymphadenopathy (80%), usually cervical, supraclavicular, or axillary.
- Mediastinal disease presenting with cough, dyspnoea, dysphagia, stridor, or SVC obstruction.
- B symptoms (fever >38.0°C, drenching night sweats, and weight loss of ≥10% within six months before diagnosis).
- Hepatosplenomegaly in advanced disease.

Investigations, staging, and risk groups

Investigations are similar to NHL. Excisional biopsy is often needed for biopsy. Diagnostic PET scan is essential to decide risk-adapted treatment approaches. Bone marrow examination is indicated only for stage III–IV disease or if full blood count (FBC) is abnormal.

Staging is according to the Cotswolds modification of Ann Arbor staging.

Patients are broadly categorized into low-, intermediate-, and high-risk groups; but there is no uniform system of prognostic classification. A new childhood Hodgkin lymphoma prognostic score is being prospectively evaluated.

Management

Classical HL

Patients with low risk disease (IA–IIA) are treated with combination chemotherapy (usually up to four cycles) followed by response-adapted modified involved-field/ involved-site radiotherapy. Intermediate-risk disease (bulky stage IA–IIA, IB–IIB, IIIA, IVA) is treated with chemotherapy followed by modified involved-field radiotherapy whereas high-risk disease (IIIB and IVB) is treated with high intensity chemotherapy. In Europe, OEPA (vincristine, etoposide, prednisone, doxorubicin) is the commonly used regimen for low-risk and OEPA with COPDac (cyclophosphamide, vincristine, prednisone, dacarbazine) for intermediate- and high-risk disease. Radiotherapy dose is lower than that used in adults (e.g. the Euronet-PHL C1 study used 19.8Gy in 11 fractions with a boost of 10Gy in five fractions to PET-positive areas). The five-year EFS is >90% with low-risk, 85% for intermediate-risk, and >80% with high-risk disease.

Patients with refractory and early relapse (<12 months after completion of initial treatment) are treated with high-dose chemotherapy followed by autologous stem cell transplantation, which is curative in approximately 50% of patients. Patients with late relapse of low-risk disease previously treated with chemotherapy alone can be treated with standard chemotherapy followed by involved-field radiotherapy.

Nodular lymphocyte-predominant HL (nLPHL)

nLPHL, which has an indolent clinical course, is CD20-positive and CD15-negative (in contrast to classical HL). Patients with completely excised IA disease may be observed (estimated 50-month PFS of 67%). Patients with stage I–IIA disease without a complete excision are treated with low-intensity chemotherapy (usually without anthracycline) with or without involved-site radiotherapy. Older children (>16 years) and young adults may be considered for involved-site radiotherapy alone. The reported five-year OS is almost 100% with EFS ranging from 70% to 90%. Patients with stage III–IV disease or B symptoms are treated similarly to those with classical HL. As this histology is CD20-positive, rituximab (anti-CD20) containing chemotherapy regimens are being increasingly used in children with advanced nLPHL.

Further reading

Cairo MS, Pinkerton R. Childhood, adolescent and young adult non-Hodgkin lymphoma: state of the science. *Br J Haematol* 2016; 173(4):507–30.

Mauz-Körholz C, Metzger ML, Kelly KM, et al. Pediatric Hodgkin lymphoma. *J Clin Oncol* 2015; 33(27):2975–85.

14.3 Paediatric central nervous system tumours

Introduction
CNS tumours are the most common group of solid tumours in childhood and comprise 20–25% of all childhood neoplasms (about 400 cases per year in the UK). The incidence of CNS tumours is about 3.3 cases per 100,000 children.

Classification/types of tumours
The WHO classification of CNS tumours can be found in the further reading section (p. 420).

Aetiology and biology
The only proven environmental aetiological association is ionizing radiation. Fewer than 10% are associated with an inherited syndrome.

Clinical presentation
Brain tumours in childhood frequently present with hydrocephalus due to blockage of cerebrospinal fluid (CSF) flow, for example, by obstruction at the level of the fourth ventricle or the aqueduct, leading to symptoms and signs of raised intracranial pressure such as headache and vomiting. Unsteadiness and visual difficulties are also common. The range of presenting symptoms is, however, protean and many children present with features such as educational and behavioural difficulties, seizures, focal weakness, increased head circumference, growth and endocrine abnormalities and others.

General principles of management
The management of CNS tumours in childhood requires a dedicated multidisciplinary team (MDT) of professionals dealing with the patient's management, psychosocial problems, side effects of treatment, and other important issues.

Imaging
CT is often the initial investigation leading to diagnosis and usually reveals the presence of the tumour and frequently evidence of hydrocephalus with ventricular dilatation. Magnetic resonance imaging (MRI) is essential prior to any surgical intervention. Advanced MRI techniques such tractography, magnetic resonance spectroscopy (MRS), and functional imaging are increasingly incorporated in the clinical management.

Surgery
Surgery provides tumour for histological diagnosis, either from tumour resection or by open or closed (stereotactic) biopsy. For patients presenting with hydrocephalus, surgical removal of the tumour or CSF diversion techniques such as insertion of a shunt or an external ventricular drain or by an endoscopic third ventriculostomy are needed to relieve intracranial pressure.

For several tumour types such as hemispheric low-grade gliomas, surgery alone is curative and for malignant tumours such as high-grade glioma, medulloblastoma, and ependymoma, many studies have shown a correlation between the degree of resection and survival.

Perioperative mortality is now less than 1%. This is attributable to factors such as the use of dexamethasone, improved paediatric intensive care units (PICU) and high dependency unit (HDU) facilities, and improved surgical technique.

Tumours are usually resected using the Cavitron ultrasonic surgical aspirator (CUSA) to gently and steadily remove the tumour. In addition, neuronavigation has become a standard of care. This links the digital data from the patient's MRI or CT scan images with a neuronavigation pointer so that the surgeon is able to define intraoperative anatomy and orientation. The use of endoscopy for procedures within the third and lateral ventricles has also become routine. Intraoperative MRI is being gradually introduced and is likely to become standard practice.

Radiotherapy
Radiotherapy has a vital role in treatment of several tumour types and is curative for lesions such as medulloblastoma, germinoma, and ependymoma. It is, however, especially in young children, associated with long-term side effects, such as neuropsychological damage, learning difficulties, and abnormalities of growth and endocrine function. Such sequelae occur particularly when whole CNS radiotherapy is used or when radiotherapy is given locally to midline structures or to the whole brain. Although the late effects of radiotherapy are greatest in young children, there is clear recent evidence that difficulties with learning and short-term memory affect even adults. Modern radiotherapy is delivered using high-precision techniques such as intensity-modulated radiotherapy (IMRT), tomotherapy, volumetric modulated arc therapy (VMAT), or proton beam therapy.

Chemotherapy
Chemotherapy has been used to attempt to improve survival but also to try to reduce the radiotherapy dose or volume and delay radiotherapy. The commonly used agents include classical alkylators, platinum derivatives, and others such as etoposide.

Chemotherapy clearly has a role in the treatment of medulloblastoma and CNS germ cell tumours but also in low-grade gliomas where it often has benefit in delaying or avoiding radiotherapy.

Regional intrathecal therapy, widely used in leukaemia and lymphoma, offers promise and may be particularly beneficial for young patients with disseminating tumours such as medulloblastoma as a way of replacing or reducing radiotherapy. Encouraging results were noted in the German HIT SKK 92 study in which IT methotrexate was added to systemic chemotherapy in the treatment of infantile medulloblastoma. A number of other intrathecal agents have been explored in phase 1/2 studies.

Individual tumour types
Low-grade gliomas
Low-grade gliomas make up about 30–40% of childhood brain tumours. Most occur in the first decade of life with the most common age of onset at six to nine years. There is a male predominance and an association with neurofibromatosis type I (NF1).

The great majority of low-grade gliomas in childhood are pilocytic astrocytomas (WHO grade I). Others include diffuse astrocytomas, oligoastrocytomas, and oligodendrogliomas. A variant of the pilocytic astrocytoma is the pilomyxoid astrocytoma (WHO grade II) which tends to occur in younger children, often affects the optic pathway/hypothalamus, and has a poorer prognosis.

The most common location is the cerebellar hemisphere followed by the cerebral hemispheres, and then the optic pathway. Leptomeningeal dissemination may occur in up to 5% of cases.

Optic pathway gliomas (OPG) may involve the optic nerves, the chiasm, the hypothalamus, and optic radiations and may extend into adjacent structures. They represent at least 5% of childhood brain tumours and 60–70% occur in the first five years of life. Around 35% of patients with optic pathway glioma have NF1 and around 15% of NF1 patients will develop OPGs. Most OPGs are pilocytic astrocytomas; pilomyxoid and diffuse astrocytomas are less common.

Clinical presentation
The pattern of clinical presentation is related to the location of the tumour. Cerebellar astrocytomas usually present with hydrocephalus. OPGs may present with raised intracranial pressure, altered vision, squint, cranial nerve abnormalities, diencephalic syndrome, or occasionally with symptoms suggestive of hypothalamic or endocrine dysfunction. For tumours of the optic nerve the diagnosis is made radiologically without the need for biopsy, although biopsy is generally indicated for chiasmatic tumours.

Treatment
Standard treatment for most tumours is an attempt at complete surgical excision. This is achievable in the majority of both cerebral and cerebellar hemispheric tumours and in these cases the surgery is usually curative (>90% survival).

In other locations, total excision is generally not possible and the management of low-grade gliomas after biopsy only or incomplete resection is dependent on tumour location, age, severity of neurological symptoms, and risk to neighbouring structures, (e.g. optic pathway and hypothalamus). Stable disease, sometimes for prolonged periods, is often seen after biopsy or incomplete resection, and therefore some patients may be observed only, with serial imaging.

For OPGs, indications to start treatment include severely affected vision bilaterally in which there is a significant threat to remaining vision, progressive visual loss, severe or progressive neurological dysfunction, documented progression of tumour radiologically, or diencephalic syndrome.

If treatment is necessary, radiotherapy (total 54Gy) has been the standard therapy for many years. However, there is now an established role for chemotherapy in low-grade gliomas. It is the treatment of choice in younger children (<8–10 years old) in whom the use of radiotherapy may be delayed or avoided; in patients with neurofibromatosis in whom radiotherapy is associated with an increased risk of second tumours; in those patients whose tumours progress after radiotherapy; and in those with leptomeningeal dissemination. The established first-line combination is vincristine and carboplatin, with weekly vinblastine and combined bevacizumab and irinotecan used as second- and third-line treatments.

Supratentorial high-grade gliomas
They constitute 5–10% of childhood brain tumours outside the brainstem. Median age at diagnosis is nine to ten years. Histologically, the main entities are glioblastoma multiforme (WHO IV), anaplastic astrocytoma (WHO III), and anaplastic oligoastrocytoma, and oligodendroglioma (WHO III). Excluding brainstem tumours, around 25% occur in the (thalamus, hypothalamus, and third ventricle), 15% occur in the cerebellum, and the rest in the cerebral hemispheres.

Clinical presentation
The pattern of presentation and duration of symptoms before diagnosis is more dependent on location than on histological grade. MRI is likely to show a heterogeneous space-occupying lesion with diffuse margins, contrast enhancement, and surrounding oedema.

Management
Gross or near-total resection (>90%) together with tumour grade (III–IV) are the principal prognostic factors in children. Radiation therapy to a dose of 54–59.5Gy to the tumour bed is given postoperatively. There is no convincing evidence that the use of chemotherapy has been associated with an improvement in survival which ranges from 0% to 40%. The current UK treatment guidelines do, however, incorporate the use of temozolamide that has been shown to be of benefit in a subpopulation of adults.

Brainstem gliomas
Tumours of the midbrain, pons, and medulla account for around 10% of CNS tumours in children. The commonest radiological pattern on MRI (brainstem lesions are poorly defined on CT scan) is that of the diffuse intrinsic pontine glioma (DIPG), characterized by mutation of H3 K27M. It is probably useful to consider brainstem tumours as either diffusely infiltrating tumours or focal tumours. Until recently, there has been reluctance to biopsy these lesions but it is now known that within the spectrum of diffuse lesions, gliomas of all grades occur (WHO I–IV) although it would appear that lower grades make up only about one-fourth of biopsied cases. Focal tumours are particularly associated other histologies including primitive neuroectodermal tumours (PNET), ependymoma, and atypical teratoid rhabdoid tumour (ATRT). Focal tumours at the very top (tectum) and bottom (cervicomedullary junction) are most likely to be low-grade gliomas.

Clinical presentation
These tumours commonly present with cranial nerve abnormalities, ataxia, or limb weakness. The history is usually short, although longer symptom duration may suggest lower grade histology.

Treatment
Surgical resection should be performed for tumours at the cervicomedullary junction and dorsally exophytic tumours, and may be considered for other focal tumours. There is no role for surgery in the cases of indolent tectal plate tumours that are usually low-grade tumours and need to be observed only. Other low-grade tumours demonstrated at surgery may also be observed.

For DIPGs, surgery has no place in management, and radiotherapy, which offers palliation, remains the mainstay of therapy. Median survival times for DIPGs are about 12 months with around 5% survival at two years.

Medulloblastoma
Medulloblastoma is the most common malignant brain tumour in childhood, accounting for 15–20% of all

childhood primary CNS neoplasms. The large majority occur within the first decade of life with a peak incidence at five years. There is a 2:1 male to female ratio. By definition, medulloblastoma arises in the posterior fossa, usually from the cerebellar vermis in the roof of the fourth ventricle, although a proportion may arise in a cerebellar hemisphere. Metastatic spread occurs in up to 35% of cases at diagnosis.

Histologically, the majority of medulloblastomas (about 80%) are described as classical phenotype. Other histological types include desmoplastic/nodular medulloblastoma and medulloblastoma with extensive nodularity, both predominantly occurring in very young children, and anaplastic and large cell medulloblastoma that are both associated with a poorer outcome than with the classical phenotype.

Recent research has shown a number of types of medulloblastoma associated with distinct molecular characteristics. At present four subgroups of medulloblastoma are recognized. Group 1 tumours (15–20%) are characterized by mutations of the Wnt/Wingless (Wnt) signalling pathway and clearly have a good prognosis. Wnt tumours are diagnosed on the basis of expression of β-catenin expression on immunohistochemistry and by monosomy 6 or mutation analysis. Group 2 tumours (~20%) are associated with a disordered Sonic hedgehog (SHH) pathway and have an intermediate prognosis. Group 3 tumours (~30%) are associated with amplification of the MYC oncogene and large cell/anaplastic histology and are associated with an adverse outcome. Group 4 medulloblastoma are the most common (~40%) but least well-defined group with a generally good outcome.

Clinical presentation
The majority of patients with medulloblastoma present with signs and symptoms of raised intracranial pressure due to hydrocephalus. Other presenting features include ataxia due to cerebellar involvement and diplopia, cranial nerve palsies, and long tract signs as a result of pressure on, or infiltration of, the brainstem. Occasionally, patients may present with manifestations of spinal metastases such as back pain or lower limb weakness.

Treatment
Staging should include MRI of the head and spine, and postoperative MRI of the head and a lumbar puncture to examine for residual disease and CSF infiltration respectively.

The therapeutic approach for medulloblastoma consists of complete or near complete surgical resection followed by postoperative craniospinal radiotherapy (CSRT) followed by chemotherapy. Standard-risk patients are those aged at least three to five years of age with no evidence of metastatic spread, and with <1.5cm^2 of post-surgical residual disease. In these patients a CSRT dose of 23.4Gy is used with a boost to the posterior fossa or tumour bed (total tumour dose 54Gy). For high-risk cases (e.g. metastatic disease) the CSRT dose is around 36Gy, again with a tumour boost.

Both standard and high-risk cases are given post radiation chemotherapy, with the most widely used regimen consisting of eight courses of a combination of cisplatin, CCNU (lomustine) or cyclophosphamide, and vincristine (or modifications thereof).

Survival is around 75–80% for standard-risk patients and around 50% for those with metastatic disease.

Atypical teratoid rhabdoid tumour
ATRTs are rare embryonal tumours, arising most commonly in infancy and young children. Tumours arise throughout the CNS, more commonly in the infratentorial compartment. They are highly malignant tumours and around one-third are metastatic at diagnosis.

Loss of the gene SMARCB1 is the main event leading to ATRT development. Loss of immuno-histochemical staining for INI 1, the SMARCB1 gene product, allows rapid identification of these tumours. Furthermore, patients with ATRT may have germline mutations of SMARCB1 which are associated with a particularly poor outcome.

Treatment and prognosis
The prognosis for ATRT is generally very poor with historically around 20% of patients surviving. Recently improved biological and clinical information together with refinement of treatment based on clinical trials may, however, be associated with improved outcome.

There is a clear benefit for patients who undergo a complete resection. ATRT is generally a radiosensitive tumour although the use of radiotherapy particularly craniospinal radiotherapy is naturally tempered by the occurrence of ATRT in very young children and the risk of associated severe neuropsychological and other sequelae. All protocols for ATRT use chemotherapy including anthracyclines and alkylating agents, with most protocols including intrathecal treatment. In addition there is some evidence to support the use of myeloablative chemotherapy with stem cell rescue that is particularly used where radiotherapy is deemed inappropriate.

Other embryonal tumours
Until recently, the majority of embryonal tumours not diagnosed as either medulloblastoma or ATRT were included in the diagnostic category of CNS-PNET. These included pinealoblastoma, now clearly a distinct entity. Several groups, however, have shown that despite similar histological appearances, tumours diagnosed as CNS-PNET displayed highly heterogeneous DNA methylation and genomic patterns that related to other pediatric brain tumour types, e.g. ATRT, glioblastoma, or ependymoma.

Furthermore, new genomic and epigenetic information together with a re-evaluation of the histological aspects of embryonal tumours resulted in the term CNS-PNET being removed from the 2016 WHO classification of CNS tumours. Instead the classification refers to the following diagnoses within the overarching embryonal group: ETMR (embryonal tumours with multilayered rosettes) C19MC-altered, ETMR NOS (not otherwise specified), medulloepithelioma, CNS neuroblastoma, CNS ganglioneuroblastoma, and CNS embryonal tumour NOS.

ETMR is now recognized as containing the three histological variants ETANTR, ependymoblastoma, and medulloepithelioma. In 2016, Sturm et al. (2016) proposed four new CNS tumour entities, designated: CNS neuroblastoma with FOXR2 activation, CNS Ewing sarcoma family tumour with CIC alteration, CNS high-grade neuroepithelial tumour with MN1 alteration, and CNS high-grade neuroepithelial tumour with BCOR alteration.

Clinical presentation
These 'other' embryonal tumours are rare and usually arise in the cerebral cortex. They usually present with symptoms and signs associated with the mass effect of the tumour including headaches, seizures, and hemiplegia.

Pineoblastoma usually presents with symptoms and signs of hydrocephalus and sometimes with Parinaud's syndrome. Non-pineal tumours are usually large at presentation with around half being >5cm in diameter at diagnosis.

Treatment

It is clear, that where there is any diagnostic doubt based on histology, tumours should be subject to diagnostic testing using methylation array and genomic analysis. Staging investigations are similar to those for medulloblastoma. At present, these tumours are treated as for high-risk medulloblastoma although clearly more work is required to refine treatment according to the individual disease entity.

Several studies have shown an improved outcome for patients with pineoblastomas with survival of around 65–70% compared with those with non-pineal tumours where the prognosis is poor, e.g. around 20–30% survival for ETMR.

Ependymoma

Ependymomas arise from the ependymal lining of the ventricles or central canal of the spinal cord. Ninety per cent are intracranial of which around 65% arise in the posterior fossa from the fourth ventricle. They make up about 6–10% of childhood brain tumours and tend to occur in younger children under the age of seven.

There now appears to be no clear prognostic implications of the two traditional histological subtypes (classic and anaplastic). Instead, as with other CNS tumours, ependymoma consists of a number of molecularly defined molecular subtypes with prognostic significance. Grade I myxopapillary and subependymal ependymomas occur rarely in children.

Clinical presentation

As with most other CNS tumours in childhood, the presenting features principally reflect tumour location. MRI will show a tumour in the ventricular system or less commonly periventricularly. Calcification, haemorrhage, and cysts are common and most ependymomas will show a degree of gadolinium enhancement. Leptomeningeal dissemination occurs in up to 10% of cases at diagnosis.

Treatment

One of the more significant and consistent prognostic factors in ependymoma is the extent of surgical resection. Every attempt should be made to achieve a complete resection although this may be difficult, particularly with fourth ventricular lesions. A postoperative MRI should be performed within 72 hours of surgery and if there is residual disease the original neurosurgeon should be involved in a decision as to whether second-look surgery is feasible. A lumbar puncture performed 15 days after surgery to assess CSF for malignant cells is mandatory.

Local radiation therapy is standard postoperative treatment. The usual dose is 54Gy, although there is interest in using higher doses of radiation. Craniospinal radiotherapy has ceased to be indicated except in metastatic cases. The role of chemotherapy has been the subject of numerous trials and for older children and adults there appears to be no benefit to date, although chemotherapy will continue to be investigated in future clinical trials. There does appear to be a role for chemotherapy in infants when chemotherapy has been used to delay giving radiotherapy and in some to avoid radiotherapy

completely. Most recurrences are local. Five-year overall survival rates for ependymoma are about 65%.

Germ cell tumours

Intracranial germ cell tumours (GCTs) are a rare (around 3% of childhood CNS tumours) and heterogeneous group of tumours that share a common cellular origin with their extracranial counterparts, the primordial germ cell.

GCTs include benign teratoma and the malignant subtypes, namely germinoma, embryonal carcinoma, yolk-sac tumour, and choriocarcinoma. Non-germinomatous malignant types are characterized by the secretion of tumour markers detected in both blood and CSF; for yolk-sac tumour—alpha-fetoprotein (AFP); and for choriocarcinoma—beta human chorionic gonadotropin (hCG). For yolk-sac tumours a high level of AFP is an adverse prognostic factor.

GCTs mainly arise in the suprasellar region or the pineal area or metachronously in both areas. Malignant types have a propensity to spread locally within the ventricular system with a small proportion of cases metastasizing distally within the CNS.

Clinical presentation

The duration of symptoms prior to diagnosis is variable and relates to tumour location and the rate of tumour growth. Suprasellar tumours typically present with endocrine abnormalities such as diabetes insipidus, hypopituitarism, and visual impairment including visual field defects. Pineal lesions generally present with a short history, with the majority associated with acute hydrocephalus due to cerebral aqueduct obstruction. Visual changes, particularly Parinaud's syndrome, are also common.

Treatment

For treatment purposes, the malignant GCTs are subdivided into either germinoma or non-germinomatous types (also referred to as secreting GCTs).

Patients need complete staging with MRI of the whole CNS axis, lumbar CSF examination for both tumour markers and malignant cells, and also blood sampling for markers. Localized germinomas are treated with chemotherapy followed by whole ventricular radiotherapy (24Gy) with a tumour bed boost (16Gy). Metastatic germinoma is treated with CSRT. The prognosis for germinoma is excellent, with survival of at least 90%.

Non-germinomatous malignant GCTs are more challenging and have a less favourable outcome than germinoma. Standard treatment consists of platinum and ifosfamide-based chemotherapy followed by local radiotherapy for non-metastatic disease. Although surgery is not necessarily required, it is clear that prognosis is related to the degree of residual tumour after treatment. In this respect, surgical excision before radiotherapy should generally be undertaken in patients with significant residual disease after chemotherapy. OS for non-germinomatous malignant GCTs is around 70%.

Craniopharyngioma

Craniopharyngiomas are the commonest tumour in the pituitary area in children. In childhood the peak age of onset is between five and ten years. Despite being classified as low-grade tumours (WHO grade I) and being slow growing, they may often have a very 'malignant' course because of their invasive nature, their tendency to recur locally, and their ability to cause very significant visual, pituitary, and hypothalamic morbidity.

Clinical presentation
Childhood craniopharyngiomas may present with endocrine symptoms (short stature and delayed puberty), raised intracranial pressure (due to hydrocephalus), visual dysfunction (e.g. visual field defects), and behavioural problems. CT and MRI scans are helpful in making a radiological diagnosis, typically showing a mixed solid and cystic tumour with calcification.

Treatment
Complete excision if feasible (around 50%) is the definite treatment. In patients with disease not suitable for resection, particularly when the risk of damage to the hypothalamus is high, partial resection followed by radiotherapy is the accepted standard approach in the UK. In very young patients (e.g. <5 years old), a period of close observation with conservative management may be followed before radiotherapy will usually become necessary. No role for chemotherapy has been proven for craniopharyngiomas. For recurrent craniopharyngiomas after radiotherapy there may be a role for surgery or intracystic instillation of chemotherapeutic agents or radioisotopes.

Intramedullary spinal tumours
Intrinsic spinal cord tumours in childhood are rare, comprising <5% of CNS tumours in childhood. Seventy per cent of them are astrocytomas (mostly low grade), 10% ependymomas, and the rest comprise other glial tumours such as oligodendrogliomas, gangliogliomas, and PNETs. Leptomeningeal spread often accompanies higher grade tumours. Histologically these tumours are indistinguishable from their intracranial counterparts.

Clinical presentation
Spinal tumours in children most often present with persistent back pain, abnormal gait, and neurological deficits in the lower or upper limbs. Abdominal pains may complicate the picture in younger children and bladder and bowel dysfunction may be present.

Treatment
A histological diagnosis is always necessary. Ependymomas are often amenable to complete resection. Complete removal of astrocytomas is achieved much less often (<50%) because of difficulties finding a clear cleavage plane. Consideration of chemotherapy or radiotherapy is given as for intracranial counterparts although the total dose of radiotherapy achievable is limited by spinal cord tolerance. The prognosis for these tumours varies but is mostly poorer than for their intracranial counterparts and morbidity is often significant.

Infant tumours
A third of all childhood brain tumours will occur in infants <3 years old. Tumour types include low-grade (predominantly midline) gliomas, high-grade gliomas, ependymomas, medulloblastomas, ATRT, choroid plexus carcinoma (CPC), and teratoma.

Tumour types such as ATRT and CPC are predominantly tumours of 'infants', and are particularly challenging to treat, with a poor prognosis.

There is, however, evidence that the biology and natural history of 'infant tumours' may differ from their counterparts in older children. For example, the outlook

for high-grade glioma in infants appears better than in individuals >3–5 years of age.

Clinical presentation
Brain tumours occurring in babies <6 months old are termed congenital tumours and indeed some of them are discovered on antenatal scans. Common presentations thereafter are with increasing head circumference, visual abnormalities (particularly roving nystagmus or squint), delayed acquisition or regression of developmental milestones, seizures, or abnormal behaviour. Classical symptoms and signs of raised intracranial pressure may be obscured by the inability of the infant to self-report and the ability of the head to expand.

Management
Infant tumours have generally been considered separately from the older age groups principally because the side effects of treatment, particularly radiotherapy, are greatest in very young children. This necessitates different approaches to therapy, which generally aim to delay or avoid the use of radiation therapy, particularly to the whole CNS or supratentorial structures.

Previously a number of 'baby brain' chemotherapy protocols were developed internationally where all infants were given the same treatment regimens irrespective of the histology, to delay or avoid radiotherapy and improve the often dismal prognosis. More recently disease specific infant protocols are being developed.

The increased ability to deliver precise conformal radiotherapy has led to renewed recent interest in using posterior fossa radiotherapy in upfront strategies for very young children, particularly for posterior fossa tumours such as medulloblastoma and ependymoma.

Late effects
Main late effects include neuropsychological impairment with cognitive defects, short-term memory loss, learning, and behavioural difficulties. More specific abnormalities include growth and endocrine dysfunction, and motor defects and visual impairment.

The aetiology of late effects is frequently multifactorial, and may be due to the effect of the tumour itself, including the effect of hydrocephalus, or be related to treatment. Chemotherapy may lead to specific late effects such as infertility, hearing loss, and nephrotoxicity.

However, the most important factor predisposing to severe late effects, particularly neuropsychological impairment, is the use of radiation therapy. It is clear that these adverse effects are most marked in very young children, aged <5–7 years old, in whom the brain is particularly immature.

Further reading
Louis DN, Perry A, Reifenberger G, von Deimling A, Figarella-Branger D, et al. The 2016 World Health Organization Classification of Tumors of the Central Nervous System: a summary. *Acta Neuropathol* 2016 Jun; 131(6):803–20.

Sturm D, Orr BA, Toprak UH, et al. New brain tumor entities emerge from molecular classification of CNS-PNETs. *Cell* 2016 Feb 25; 164(5):1060–72.

14.4 Paediatric solid tumours and kidney tumours

Solid tumours

Children with solid tumours require multidisciplinary care from paediatric oncologists, radiologists, histopathologists, pharmacists, chemotherapy-trained nurses, radiotherapists, and surgeons. All children with suspected cancer should be referred to a paediatric oncology centre for diagnostic work-up and treatment. Decision making should take place in a multidisciplinary setting. Useful websites to connect to international treatment programmes are given at the end of the chapter in 'Internet resources' (p. 424).

Where possible all children should be treated in a clinical trial. Children should have access to paediatric intensive care, and the paediatric specialties such as endocrinology, nephrology, ophthalmology, and audiology. Painful procedures and the placing of central lines should be done under general anaesthesia. For imaging, sedation may be adequate and young infants may be able to be fed and wrapped if left in a safe position.

Chemotherapy guidelines should be carefully adhered to. Weight, age, and surface area define how the dose is prescribed. Many chemotherapy agents need to be administered with hydration fluids to reduce toxicity, and careful adjustment of total fluid load and electrolytes is required.

Follow-up after treatment should be assured for a minimum of five years with guidance from a specialist in late effects. In addition, the supportive care of children who have become myelosuppressed as a result of chemotherapy is vital. Particularly crucial is the early treatment with antibiotics of children susceptible to severe infections when neutropenic. This care tends to be delivered in local hospitals close to the patient.

Kidney tumours

Kidney tumours account for 6–8% of childhood cancer. The most common form of kidney tumour is Wilms' tumour named after Max Wilms, a German surgeon. Wilms' tumour was the first tumour to be found to be sensitive to radiotherapy and to the first chemotherapeutic agents, vincristine and actinomycin D, which were discovered in the 1950s. A rarer form of kidney tumour, which occurs in very young children, called mesoblastic nephroma, is benign. This is genetically different from Wilms' tumour. Wilms' tumour sometimes develops from nephrogenic rests which can be difficult to distinguish pathologically from Wilms' tumour.

Clear cell sarcoma is a rare form of kidney tumour occurring usually in older children—this used to be called 'bone metastasizing Wilms' tumour'. Rhabdoid tumours can also occur in the kidney as well as in the brain and other organs.

Diagnosis and staging

Children with Wilms' tumour often present with an abdominal mass which has been found incidentally by the carer. Children are often well and asymptomatic.

In a quarter of cases the child may present with haematuria. If the tumour has bled, pressure on the capsule of the kidney may cause pain and there may be a fall in haemoglobin, and in severe cases an increase in the girth of the abdomen may result in respiratory difficulties.

Investigations

The first investigations include urinanalysis, full blood count, ultrasound of the abdomen, and CXR, as Wilms' tumour may metastasize to the lung. If a kidney mass is confirmed on ultrasound, further imaging of the primary tumour with MRI or CT scan is necessary. The chest should be imaged with spiral CT scan to detect smaller lung metastases.

Biopsy

The diagnosis should be confirmed by histological examination following biopsy of the tumour. This can be done as a percutaneous core needle biopsy or open biopsy under general anaesthesia. FNA is a useful tool in resource challenged nations and can be diagnostic; however, the architecture of the tumour is lost. Tumour material should always be sent fresh to paediatric pathologists.

Histopathology, cytogenetics, and molecular biology

Wilms' tumour is commonly a triphasic tumour consisting of blastemal, stromal, and tubular elements. Some tumours are predominantly blastemal in composition and some may contain areas of anaplasia or diffuse anaplasia which increases the risk status of the disease. Cytogenetics will often show abnormalities of the WT1 (Wilms' tumour 1) tumour suppressor gene which can also be found using molecular biological techniques exposing the presence of an abnormal WT1 transcript. WT1, however, has no prognostic importance and other molecular markers have been identified such as the loss of heterozygosity of chromosome 16q and 1p, gain of chromosome 1q, and presence of the NMYC oncogene in anaplastic Wilms' tumours.

Treatment

Treatment consists of a combination of chemotherapy and surgery, the extent of which is defined by both stage and pathology. In North America primary surgery is preferred to permit surgical staging. In Europe, preoperative chemotherapy is preferred and imaging is used to identify image-defined risk factors (IDRFs). Initially the diagnosis of Wilms' tumour, whether metastatic (stage IV) or non-metastatic (stages I–III) and uni- or bilateral (stage V), is sufficient to start treatment. Unilateral non-metastatic tumours receive a short course of preoperative chemotherapy according to the current International Society of Paediatric Oncology (SIOP) Wilms' tumour protocol using a combination of two drugs, vincristine and actinomycin D. For metastatic disease, three drugs may be used as primary therapy with the addition of doxorubicin.

Non-metastatic unilateral disease

In the case of unilateral, non-metastatic disease, surgery is currently performed at week 5, allowing for full histopathological examination of the resected specimen. Postoperative treatment is guided by the histopathological and surgical stage. The postoperative chemotherapy regimen depends on whether or not anaplasia or excessive blastema, a poor prognostic factor, is found on careful histopathological examination, and will consist of further vincristine/actinomycin D chemotherapy or three drugs with the addition of doxorubicin or escalation to intensified treatment postoperatively. The surgical stage of the tumour is described as: stage I—complete resection; stage II—resection but with microscopical residual disease; and stage III—resection leaving macroscopic residual or nodal disease. In the latter case flank radiotherapy will be required.

Bilateral Wilms' tumour
In the case of bilateral Wilms' tumour there is usually an individualized treatment programme with an emphasis on delayed nephrectomy with nephron sparing surgery and postoperative treatment according to the highest staged tumour. Given that these tumours are rare, discussion in a local and national MDT with a renal tumour panel is advisable.

Metastatic Wilms' tumour
In the case of metastatic Wilms' tumour, clearance of lung disease, which may involve surgical metastatectomy, is aimed at by week 7. Postoperative chemotherapy with three agents, and where appropriate additional lung radiotherapy, is given. Radiotherapy is also given to the area of the primary tumour if it is surgical stage III or there is high-risk histology (anaplasia and blastemal type Wilms tumour). A radiotherapy dose of 12–15Gy is used which gives few sequelae to the lungs and is relatively well tolerated by the kidney.

Follow-up
Follow-up is with regular CXR and abdominal ultrasound. All children who have received doxorubicin should have an echocardiogram at six months after ending treatment and, if normal, every five years lifelong.

Prognostic factors and survival
Prognosis and survival are dependent on appropriate treatment, stage, and histopathology. Higher stage, presence of blastemal Wilms' tumour, or anaplasia confers a poorer prognosis. Overall survival at five years ranges from 70% for stage IV tumours to >95% for stage I disease and risk categories and directed treatment continue to be refined in the current SIOP trial. New molecular prognostic markers are now emerging, e.g. the combined presence of LOH 16q and 1p are being used to stratify patients for therapy in the North American trials.

14.5 Sarcomas

Introduction
Whereas the majority of childhood solid tumours are embryonal in nature and carcinomas are extremely rare, sarcomas do occur at all ages and in most parts of the body. The most common sarcoma occurring in children is rhabdomyosarcoma which accounts for 25% of sarcomas. Rhabdomyosarcoma arises from striated muscle elements, while older children may develop clear cell sarcoma of the kidney, Ewing sarcoma of bone and soft tissue, as well as osteosarcoma.

There are also rarer forms of sarcoma occurring in the liver, embryonal sarcoma, and smooth muscle leiomyosarcoma. We will deal here with the most common form of childhood sarcoma, rhabdomyosarcoma, which occurs in two main forms: embryonal and alveolar. Embryonal rhabdomyosarcoma is the most common type and carries a better prognosis.

Diagnosis and staging
Presentation
Presentation is a function of the organ of origin of the tumour and includes pain, visible swelling, palpable mass, lump, proptosis, airway obstruction, visible protrusion/bleeding of tumour through nasal, anal, oral, or vaginal orifices, urinary retention, or symptoms of raised intracranial pressure. In the rare case of widespread medullary metastatic alveolar rhabdomyosarcoma, presenting symptoms may mimic those of leukaemia. The presenting mass may be regional lymph node disease and careful examination of the area of lymph drainage to that region is essential. It is particularly important, when inguinal nodes are found, to examine and image the whole leg including the foot, as well as palpating the foot carefully. The extent of nodal involvement is an important prognostic factor and in uncertain cases lymph node biopsy is necessary, before initiating treatment.

Investigations
Cross-sectional imaging of the primary tumour as well as all areas of regional lymph node drainage should be obtained if possible with gadolinium contrasted MRI. Complete staging includes CXR, spiral CT scan of the chest, technetium bone scan, bilateral bone marrow aspirates, and trephine biopsies. There is no specific serum tumour marker for rhabdomyosarcoma; however, the full blood count will give an indication of bleeding into the tumour or bone marrow invasion. A high level of serum LDH, above the normal for age, is a non-specific marker of high cellular turnover and a very high level may indicate a poorer prognosis. Serum urea and creatinine and liver function tests will guide on the general well-being of the child and any organ failure due to compression. Children with fever should have appropriate cultures and an infectious disease screen. Abdominal ultrasound is useful in assessing liver, kidney, and bladder function. In prostatic or bladder rhabdomyosarcoma, cystourethroscopic examination under general anaesthesia, both at diagnosis and before surgery, is useful. Diagnostic work-up, staging, stabilizing the child, and optimizing organ function should be completed before treatment. Exceptions are where there is spinal cord compression or airway obstruction which demands urgent surgical and chemotherapy reduction. In these cases, full staging can be done after the start of chemotherapy.

Biopsy
Tru-cut or open biopsy needs to be planned so that the biopsy scar and trajectory can be excised at the time of definitive surgery. Freshly obtained biopsy material is needed for immunohistochemistry and biology. Frozen

sections at the time of surgery, for diagnostic purposes, are not useful.

Histopathology and molecular biology
The differential diagnosis between embryonal and alveolar rhabdomyosarcoma can be made from morphology and immunohistochemistry in most cases. Molecular biological techniques can be used to detect the abnormal PAX3 (Paired Box 3, a family of transcription factors) or PAX7 (Paired Box 7) fusion transcript which distinguish the alveolar subtypes.

Prognostic factors and survival
The location of the tumour in the head and neck (parameningeal) or limbs, alveolar pathology, size >5cm, advanced stage, and age >10 years are poor prognostic factors.

Treatment
The current European Paediatric Soft tissue Sarcoma Study Group (EpSSG) trial treats children in four categories; low, intermediate, high, and very high risk. The treatment is with multiagent chemotherapy and local surgery if feasible. Children who have unresectable tumours or parameningeal tumours will require radiotherapy, and discussion of proton therapy may be appropriate. The role of maintenance chemotherapy in rhabdomyosarcoma has shown increases in long-term survival and hence is also recommended.

14.6 Neuroblastoma

Introduction
Neuroblastoma is a malignant tumour of neural crest cells and commonly occurs in the midline or in the adrenal glands. Differentiation into benign ganglioneuroma can occur. Some tumours are mixed ganglioneuroblastomas. If they are inter-mixed they carry a good prognosis; but if there are nodules of undifferentiated neuroblastoma, called nodular ganglioneuroblastoma, they carry a poor prognosis. Age has always been a clear prognostic factor in neuroblastoma, with young age conferring a better prognosis. Older children and adolescents tend to have more indolent but prognostically poor disease, whereas infants, even with stage 4 disease, have a good prognosis if treated appropriately.

Neuroblastoma was the first solid tumour in paediatric practice to have treatment stratified according to molecular markers. Tumours carrying multiple copies of the Myc-N oncogene tend to be aggressive and metastasize. They initially respond well to treatment, but recur early, developing multidrug resistance and making therapy for relapse extremely difficult.

Diagnosis and staging
Infants may present with stage 4 S disease (S stands for special) where a relatively small primary tumour metastasizes to the liver, skin, and occasionally bone marrow. The liver may be diffusely infiltrated and become large enough to fill the abdominal cavity. This can compromise respiration and may be accompanied by intravascular coagulopathy.

Infants and children may also present with signs of spinal cord compression. An urgent MRI scan of the spine should be performed and chemotherapy initiated the same day, even before biopsy, if the imaging is typical. A rare subgroup of patients present with opsoclonus myoclonus (dancing eye syndrome). These children require whole body MRI scanning to exclude neuroblastoma. Ultrasound of the abdomen may show an adrenal primary tumour and aid diagnosis. Most neuroblastomas secrete catecholamine metabolites HVA (homovanillic acid) and VMA (vanillylmandelic acid). A spot urine test for VMA can aid diagnosis. Staging uses an isotope scan with MIBG (metaiodobenzylguanidine) as well as bone marrow aspirates and trephine biopsies. Imaging of the primary tumour should be with MRI. Neuroblastoma rarely metastasizes to the lungs and so CT scan of the chest is not necessary. If the MIBG scan is positive at the primary tumour site, a bone scan is not necessary. If the primary tumour does not take up MIBG, a CT scan of the head with bony windows is advised to exclude bony metastases of the skull and base of skull. Bone scan is adequate for the rest of the body.

Biopsy
Wherever possible, core needle or open biopsy under general anaesthetic should be performed. Fresh tissue should be analysed for immunohistochemistry and Myc-N amplification as well as other structural chromosomal abnormalities such as 1p deletion, 17q gain, 11q deletion, etc.

The International Neuroblastoma Risk Grouping (INRG) has put together data from thousands of patients treated by different national and international groups and has developed criteria to divide patients into low-, intermediate-, and high-risk groups. In order to group the patients successfully, age at diagnosis, operability defined by the presence (L2) or absence (L1) of image-defined risk factors, histopathology, cytogenetics, and molecular biology all need to be considered. Myc-N amplified patients at any stage or age are considered high risk (exceptions may be made for young children with resected stage 1 tumours). Patients <18 months of age carry a better prognosis than those >18 months. An infant with an isolated congenital adrenal tumour carries an excellent prognosis and may require no treatment. A child with a tumour carrying any cytogenetic structural abnormality will have an intermediate prognosis. Survival ranges from <20% to >90% depending on all of these factors. Adolescents carry the worst prognosis and congenital low stage tumours have the best prognosis. The majority of children present with stage 4 disease and are high risk.

Treatment
Treatment should be according to a clinical trial. All children with high-risk disease require induction chemotherapy, surgery to the primary tumour, high-dose chemotherapy with stem cell rescue, radiotherapy to

the preoperative site of the primary tumour, and differentiation therapy with 13 cis-retinoic acid. In Europe treatment protocols are driven by the SIOPEN (Europe neuroblastoma) group and contacts can be found on the SIOPEN-R-NET website listed under 'Internet resources' at the end of this chapter. The UK Neuroblastoma Society website also carries useful information. The study open currently is investigating the role of immunotherapy

in improving survival with anti-GD2, a target of GD2 present on neuroblastoma cells.

Follow-up

Follow-up should take all the side effects of therapy into consideration. After therapy for high-risk disease, hearing loss, kidney problems, and infertility are the most common.

14.7 Other paediatric tumours and Langerhans cell histiocytosis

Extracranial germ cell tumours

In neonates, sacrococcygeal teratomas must be recognized; they can be diagnosed prenatally and affected children may need to be delivered by Caesarean section to prevent complications. These are benign tumours but need to be removed before the age of two months to prevent degeneration to malignancy. The coccyx must be removed in its entirety to prevent recurrence. AFP and β-hCG are serum markers of malignant germ cell tumours. However, the serum levels of AFP are raised from birth to the age of 12 months and so levels in children with tumours must be compared with normal levels for age.

Liver tumours

In young children hepatoblastoma (HB) is the most common primary liver malignancy. HB usually secretes AFP but the levels must be compared with normal levels for age. HBs are staged by the PRE-TEXT system (PRE-Treatment EXTent of disease), with MRI imaging of liver and spiral CT of chest. Treatment and management can be found on the SIOPEL website, the International Society of Paediatric Oncology epithelial liver tumour treatment strategy group (see 'Internet resources').

Langerhans cell histiocytosis

Langerhans cell histiocytosis is a neoplastic disorder affecting CD1a positive dendritic Langerhans cells. Patients present with a wide variety of symptoms, the most common being lytic bony lesions in the skull. In young children the presentation can mimic leukaemia. Another common presenting feature is an eczematous skin rash, stubborn cradle cap, and failure to thrive due to gut involvement. Bone marrow involvement is rare. The spectrum of disease presentation is wide and this can result in delays to diagnosis. For most infants and children disease is confined to a single site, e.g. skin or bone, but for others there is multisite involvement including specialized areas, e.g. CNS, involving the pituitary gland and causing diabetes insipidus. Accurate staging investigations are needed at presentation to confirm whether disease is single or multisystem as this governs therapy. Most Langerhans cell histiocytosis will respond to low-dose chemotherapy with steroids and vinblastine treatment. Cytarabine is reserved for more advanced or resistant disease. Prognosis is usually very good ranging from 75% to 95% depending on response to therapy. Younger children may present with chronic disease which recurs throughout childhood in an indolent manner. Advances in molecular genetics have identified a BRAF fusion gene and BRAF inhibitors are now available and subject to clinical trials.

14. 8 Internet resources

Children's Cancer and Leukaemia group: http://www.cclg.org.uk
Cure4Kids, St. Jude Children's Research Hospital Department of Global Pediatric Medicine: https://www.cure4kids.org/ums/home/
International Society of Paediatric Oncology European Neuroblastoma Research Network, https://www.siopen-r-net.org/

SIOP, de International Society of Paediatric Oncology: http://www.siop.nl/
SIOPEL Group, http://siopel.org/

Oncological emergencies and acute oncology

Chapter contents

15.1 Oncological emergencies and acute oncology

Introduction

Recently the specialty of acute oncology with a clinical service to support patients and coordinate the care of those presenting with oncological emergencies has been developed. Patients who present with oncological emergencies often have a unique set of clinical problems, many of them iatrogenic, and can benefit from specialist advice from teams who are expert in the management of such conditions. Cancer treatments are developing and diversifying from standard cytotoxic chemotherapeutic drugs to targeted agents and immunological therapies. These introduce new toxicities such as dermatological problems, hypertension, and autoimmune phenomena. The management of the problem will vary depending on the underlying process and specific advice related to the causative agent will be required.

The development of an Acute Oncology Service (AOS) is to establish a safe, supportive, and patient-centred service with the aim of improving outcome and reducing morbidity and mortality. Aspects of good practice could include a dedicated telephone helpline which is staffed by trained and experienced personnel, such as specialist nurses, for 24 hours per day, seven days per week to triage patients to appropriate services. Good communication and liaison with emergency departments and shared guidelines on the management of life-threatening conditions such as febrile neutropenic sepsis will improve care and outcomes. Access to treatment protocols, often on-line, advising on the presentation, investigation, and management of common acute problems and emergencies can be of use to those seeing patients with acute oncological problems. However, this should be backed up with early and timely 'hands on' senior medical review by experienced oncologists. Other developments have included dedicated assessment units for cancer patients receiving active treatment who become acutely unwell and training of nurse specialists who can provide timely assessment and treatment. Clinical pathways have been developed to provide prompt and vital front-line assessment and treatments such as intravenous antibiotics in suspected neutropenic sepsis instead of waiting for medical review.

Finally, acute oncology teams may be able to engage and interact to provide advice and help to acute and emergency physicians who are assessing and diagnosing patients admitted to hospital with new or suspected cancers presenting as malignancy of unknown origin. Their expertise can provide valuable aid to these teams in the correct and appropriate selection of tests and investigations. Such interventions may secure an earlier definitive diagnosis and avoid unnecessary interventions.

15.2 Tumour lysis syndrome

Aetiology

Tumour lysis syndrome (TLS) is a constellation of metabolic disturbances resulting from the initiation of anticancer therapy and the subsequent destruction of malignant cells.

It is characterized by hyperkalaemia, followed by hyperuricaemia, hyperphosphataemia, hypocalcaemia, and acute renal impairment. TLS usually becomes evident 12–72 hours after starting cancer treatment. It is most commonly seen in malignancies that have a large tumour bulk, a high proliferative rate, and are highly sensitive to therapy. Examples include acute lymphoblastic leukaemia (ALL), high-grade non-Hogkin lymphoma (NHL), etc.

TLS has also been reported after steroids, monoclonal antibodies, hormonal agents, bisphosphonates, radiotherapy, intrathecal chemotherapy, and tumour embolization procedures.

Hyperkalaemia and hyperphosphataemia are the immediate consequences of cell lysis and the release of these ions. Purine nucleic acids are metabolized to uric acid. The kidney is the major route of excretion for potassium, phosphate, and uric acid, and uric acid crystallization in the kidney tubules is a major cause of the acute renal failure that is part of TLS. Hypocalcaemia occurs because hyperphosphataemia leads to calcium phosphate precipitation and deposition in crystal form in soft tissues. Deposition of calcium in the kidneys (nephrocalcinosis) can cause acute renal failure.

Clinical features

This condition may present with non-specific symptoms due to metabolic disturbances. These include nausea, vomiting, malaise, confusion, oliguria, and anorexia. Symptoms of hyperkalaemia include paraesthesiae, weakness, chest pain, and palpitations. Marked hypocalcaemia can manifest with paraesthesiae, tetany, and myopathy. High uric acid levels may result in arthralgia and sometimes frank gout. Evidence of fluid overload, such as shortness of breath and oedema, can develop as a result of renal failure.

Diagnosis

Blood tests will show metabolic acidosis. Hyperkalaemia is usually the first metabolic abnormality that appears. An electrocardiogram may show the characteristic changes of hyperkalaemia or lengthening of the QT interval as a result of hypocalcaemia. Urine pH needs to be monitored as an acidic pH will further encourage uric acid deposition in the renal tubules. Laboratory definition of TLS is based on threshold and percentage changes (generally 25% from baseline) of calcium, phosphorus, potassium, and uric acid. Clinical tumour lysis syndrome is defined by the presence of renal impairment, seizures, arrhythmias, or sudden death.

Treatment

Prompt recognition and supportive care is the mainstay of treatment. Patients with TLS need continuous cardiac rhythm monitoring and reassessment of electrolyte levels every four to six hours. If metabolic disturbances do not respond to initial acute management, haemodialysis must be considered. Aggressive rehydration is required to maintain urine output, aid excretion of metabolites, and prevent uric acid deposition.

Hyperkalaemia and hyperphosphataemia can be managed initially with short-term measures such as insulin and dextrose infusions until more definitive treatment is in place, such as potassium exchange resins, phosphate binders, or haemodialysis. Hypocalcaemia should not be corrected until phosphate levels have normalized to prevent further calcium deposition, unless there is evidence of neuromuscular irritability.

Rasburicase, a recombinant form of urate oxidase, converts uric acid to water soluble allantoin and therefore can rapidly lower blood uric acid levels. It is the preferred treatment of hyperuricaemia in established TLS (0.2mg/kg/day) but is contraindicated in patients with glucose-6-phosphate dehydrogenase deficiency. In those patients, or if rasburicase is not available, allopurinol (300mg daily) can be used instead. Urinary alkalinization with intravenous bicarbonate or acetazolamide is controversial and requires very close monitoring as it can worsen hypocalcaemia. Diuretics are usually not a key part of early management as the patient is likely to be volume depleted on presentation.

Persistent hyperkalaemia, hyperphosphataemia, hyperuricaemia, uraemia, and symptomatic hypocalcaemia are all indications for haemodialysis or continuous haemofiltration. Haemodialysis is preferred to peritoneal dialysis as uric acid and phosphate clearance is better. Critical care support may be required.

Prevention

An important part of the management of this potentially lethal syndrome is to recognize those at risk before they begin cytotoxic therapy and initiate prophylactic measures.

Patients at low or intermediate risk for TLS should be carefully assessed for dehydration, and prophylactic allopurinol, ideally beginning up to three days before chemotherapy, should be considered. Unlike rasburicase, allopurinol can prevent uric acid formation but will not lower already elevated uric acid levels. Patients at high risk for TLS should receive 24–48 hours of pre-hydration before therapy and up to 72 hours of hydration after therapy. Prophylactic rasburicase should be strongly considered, especially if hyperuricaemia already exists. These patients should be monitored very closely, with laboratory and clinical assessments three to four times daily. If there is any evidence of tumour lysis syndrome before therapy is started, and it is safe to do so, cytotoxic agents should be withheld until this is corrected.

Further reading

Coiffier B, Altman A, Pui CH, et al. Guidelines for the management of paediatric and adult tumor lysis syndrome: an evidence based review. *J Clin Oncol* 2008; 26(16):2767–78.

Sarno J. Prevention and management of tumor lysis syndrome in adults with malignancy. *J Adv Pract Oncol* 2013; 4(2):101–6.

15.3   Hypercalcaemia

Aetiology

Hypercalcaemia occurs in up to 30% of cancer patients at some stage in their disease. It is most commonly seen in breast, renal, and non-small cell cancers of the lung, as well as lymphomas and multiple myeloma.

There are two main mechanisms that contribute to a rise in calcium levels in cancer. The first, and most common, is the secretion of parathyroid hormone-related peptide (PTHrP) by the tumour cells, termed humoral hypercalcaemia of malignancy. PTHrP simulates many of the actions of PTH such as stimulation of osteoclasts, calcium reabsorption from the distal renal tubules, and increased intestinal uptake of calcium. The effects of PTHrP may be systemic in patients with high serum PTHrP levels, or limited to the local tissues. PTHrP production is more often found with solid tumours such as renal cell carcinoma, breast adenocarcinoma, and squamous cancers of the aerodigestive tract.

Local osteolytic hypercalcaemia due to a marked increase in osteoclastic activity in proximity to malignant cells in the marrow or bone space is the second main cause. In multiple myeloma and other haematological malignancies, this is often mediated by secreted cytokines such as tumour necrosis factor, interleukins 1 and 6, and macrophage inflammatory factor 1. These cytokines can stimulate macrophages to differentiate into osteoclasts causing increased bone resorption and release of calcium.

Rarely, vitamin D overproduction or production of vitamin D analogues, including calcitriol, by tumour cells contribute to hypercalcaemia in malignancy. This third mechanism is more common in Hodgkin lymphoma (HL), NHL, and adult T-cell lymphoma.

Clinical features

The early symptoms of hypercalcaemia are vague and non-specific; these include anorexia, nausea and vomiting, constipation, non-specific abdominal pain, fatigue, muscle weakness, and confusion. Polyuria and polydipsia are more specific early symptoms of increasing calcium levels. Patients tend to be dehydrated. As calcium levels rise further, there may be neurological manifestations such as decreased consciousness level, hallucinations, and psychosis. Renal function will also deteriorate.

Diagnosis

High ionized calcium levels, corrected for calcium bound to albumin, can be measured in a peripheral blood sample. Renal function, alkaline phosphatase, and PTH levels should also be evaluated simultaneously as inappropriately high PTH levels suggest coexisting hyperparathyroidism. An electrocardiogram may show signs of hypercalcaemia such as shortening of the QT interval or ventricular arrhythmias.

PTHrP levels can be measured to assess the mechanism of hypercalcaemia but are not essential for a diagnosis of hypercalcaemia of malignancy. High PTHrP levels have been reported, however, to be associated with a poorer response to bisphosphonate therapy and a higher risk of recurrent hypercalcaemia and so PTHrP levels may be useful in guiding treatment.

Treatment

Hypercalcaemic patients are usually profoundly hypovolaemic and the first step in management is aggressive rehydration with intravenous saline, as appropriate to the individual patient's cardiovascular status. Sources of calcium should be eliminated, as should medications such as vitamin D and thiazide diuretics, which could increase calcium levels. Loop diuretics should be avoided in the early stages of treatment as they can exacerbate renal hypoperfusion as a result of hypovolaemia and further impair renal calcium excretion.

Once the patient is adequately hydrated, bisphosphonates are the first-line agents for normalizing calcium levels. Intravenous pamidronate or zolendronic acid effectively inhibit osteoclast activity and restore normocalcaemia within five days in 80% of patients. Zolendronic acid is the more potent bisphosphonate but the clinical relevance of this is uncertain. As it is also more nephrotoxic than pamidronate, the dose must be adjusted according to creatinine clearance as indicated in the package insert information.

Denosumab, a monoclonal antibody targeting receptor activator of nuclear factor-κ B ligand (RANKL) is a potent osteoclast inhibitor. It was more effective than zolendronic acid in preventing hypercalcaemia in patients with metastatic breast cancer. Also, weekly denosumab treatment can restore normocalcaemia in up to 80% of patients with bisphosphonate-refractory hypercalcaemia.

Life-threatening hypercalcaemia can be treated with intravenous calcitonin which causes a rapid but unsustained fall in calcium levels. Haemodialysis may be ultimately needed especially when severe hypercalcaemia is accompanied by renal failure or congestive cardiac failure.

Hypercalcaemia that is caused by elevated vitamin D levels, as occurs in HL and other types of lymphomas, can sometimes be effectively treated with corticosteroids.

Ultimately, appropriate treatment of the underlying tumour can help control recurrent hypercalcaemia.

15.4 Hyponatraemia

Aetiology

Hyponatraemia, defined as a serum sodium concentration of <136mmol/l, is a common finding in hospitalized patients with or without cancer.

Sodium and body fluid balance is under the control of the antidiuretic hormone (ADH) secreted from the posterior pituitary. The osmolality of the blood is tightly maintained at around 285mOsm/kg. If the osmolality increases, ADH secretion increases. It binds to receptors in the collecting ducts of the kidney and stimulates the production and insertion of aquaporins into the collecting duct membrane, increasing water reabsorption with a consequent fall in osmolality. Reduced serum osmolality has the opposite effect on ADH secretion.

Hyponatraemia in cancer patients is due to a variety of reasons. Chemotherapeutic agents such as cyclophosphamide, cisplatin, and vincristine are known to stimulate ADH release. Chemotherapy-induced nausea and vomiting increase ADH production while simultaneously increasing enteral sodium loss. Abdominal radiotherapy and analgesics such as morphine and carbamazepine also promote ADH secretion. In addition, aggressive hydration to prevent the sequelae of anticancer treatment may exacerbate hyponatraemia. Interferon, monoclonal antibodies, and other therapies targeting immune function have also been shown to cause hyponatraemia.

In addition to increased central ADH secretion as a result of malignancy or treatment, around 30% of cases of hyponatraemia in an oncological setting are caused by ectopic ADH secretion from tumour cells, also known as SIADH (syndrome of inappropriate antidiuretic hormone). The patient is euvolaemic and has an inappropriately high urine osmolality and sodium excretion in the setting of hyponatraemia and low plasma osmolality. The commonest cancer by far associated with SIADH is small cell lung cancer (SCLC), but it has been reported in many other types of cancers.

It should also be kept in mind that all the conventional causes of hyponatraemia, such as that secondary to cardiac or hepatic failure or medications such as diuretics, often occur in cancer patients. Particular attention in that regard should be paid to adrenal insufficiency in patients with adrenal metastases or recurrent glucocorticoid treatments, and to nephrotic syndrome in patients receiving anti-angiogenic agents.

Clinical features

Symptoms of hyponatraemia are vague and become more severe as the degree of sodium loss increases or with faster rates of serum sodium decline. Mild hyponatraemia or more severe hyponatraemia of slow onset may be asymptomatic. At lower serum sodium levels, patients may present with headache, anorexia, depression, behavioural changes, lethargy, and mild nausea. Serum sodium levels <115mmol/l may result in psychosis, confusion, coma, respiratory arrest, brainstem herniation, and death.

Diagnosis

A diagnosis of hyponatraemia can be easily made on a venous or arterial blood sample. The volume status of the patient must then be assessed to diagnose the possible cause of the hyponatraemia. Hypervolaemic patients may be overloaded with fluid as a result of renal, liver, or cardiac failure. Hypovolaemic patients may have lost sodium through vomiting or diarrhoea or through the kidneys as a result of aggressive diuresis, adrenal insufficiency, or nephropathy. Cerebral salt wasting may occur as part of central nervous system (CNS) malignancy or after neurosurgery. If the patient is euvolaemic, a diagnosis of SIADH may be made, using paired serum and urine samples.

Treatment

Hyponatraemia associated with malignancy is best treated by treating the underlying cause. A study has shown that 80% of cases of hyponatraemia associated with SCLC resolved within three weeks of beginning chemotherapy. If, however, the malignancy is not amenable to treatment, or drugs that may contribute to the hyponatraemia cannot be stopped, other strategies should be used.

The first-line treatment for euvolaemic patients with hyponatraemia is fluid restriction to 1,000–1,200ml per day. If this is unsuccessful, demeclocycline, a tetracycline antibiotic, may be used (600–1,200mg daily oral in three to four doses initially followed by maintenance of 600–900mg daily). It acts on the collecting tubule to induce nephrogenic diabetes insipidus but it may take up to three weeks for a detectable response to become evident. Possible side effects include photosensitivity, nephrotoxicity, and gastrointestinal (GI) intolerance. In severe hyponatraemia, infusion of hypertonic saline with close monitoring may be appropriate. Increasing the serum sodium level too rapidly carries a risk of cerebral dehydration and central pontine demyelination. Caution should be taken to limit rises in serum sodium levels to no more than 1mmol/l per hour initially and not more than 10mmol/l in the first 24 hours of the infusion.

Vasopressin receptor antagonists, which directly act on ADH receptors in the kidney and increase water excretion whilst sparing electrolytes, are useful for hyponatraemia due to SIADH. Tolvaptan (15mg once daily orally and increased up to 30–60mg if required) has been licensed in Europe. It should be used with caution however in patients with renal or hepatic impairment or those with inadequate fluid intake.

15.5 Hyperkalaemia

Aetiology
Hyperkalaemia in oncology patients often occurs in the context of renal failure or as part of tumour lysis syndrome (see Section 15.2, 'Tumour lysis syndrome'). There exist multiple possible causes of acute kidney injury in cancer patients.

Pre-renal causes of renal impairment include:
- Hyperviscosity in haematological malignancies
- Neutropenic or non-neutropenic sepsis with accompanying hypovolaemia and vasodilatation
- Hyperuricaemia
- Hypercalcaemia
- Nephrotoxic agents such as cisplatin, contrast media, antibiotics, and non-steroidal anti-inflammatory drugs (NSAIDs) directly damage the kidneys and impair function.

Renal function may also be compromised by:
- Direct tumour invasion
- Radiation nephritis
- Renal infections

Urinary tract obstruction by intrinsic or extrinsic malignancy is the commonest post-renal cause of impairment in this setting. Hyperkalaemia may also occur as a result of multiple transfusions of packed red blood cells. Rarer causes in cancer patients include adrenocortical insufficiency and treatment with low-molecular-weight heparins.

High levels of serum potassium prevent repolarization of cardiac and skeletal muscle. Treatment is essential to prevent cardiac arrhythmias, respiratory arrest, and death.

Clinical features
Hyperkalaemia is often asymptomatic. Symptoms that may occur include paraesthesiae, weakness, chest pain, and palpitations.

Investigation
Renal function should be checked simultaneously with serum potassium estimation. Uric acid, calcium, and phosphate levels and an arterial blood gas measurement will help diagnose tumour lysis syndrome if this is suspected. An electrocardiogram may show the classical signs of hyperkalaemia, namely tented T waves, flattened P waves, and widening of the QRS complex. At high potassium concentrations, the QRS complex may appear as a sinusoidal wave.

Treatment
The first priority is to protect the cardiac action potential and prevent arrhythmias. If any changes are apparent on the electrocardiogram, an intravenous bolus of 10% calcium gluconate, which acts as a cardioprotectant, must be given. Short-term effective measures may be employed to lower serum potassium levels. An infusion of short-acting insulin and 10% dextrose will drive potassium into cells and this effect can be supported with salbutamol nebulizers. Potassium excretion needs to be increased to provide a more long-term correction of hyperkalaemia. Diuretics that increase potassium excretion may be used in a patient with normal renal function. Otherwise, a cation exchange resin may be given orally or rectally. In severe hyperkalaemia or hyperkalaemia-resistant to conservative intervention, haemodialysis may become necessary.

15.6   Hypoglycaemia

Introduction

In guidelines published by the American Diabetic Association, the threshold for hypoglycaemia is set at a blood glucose of <3.9mmol/l, but a recent study suggested that 3.1mmol/l would be a more relevant threshold clinically. Hypoglycaemia in oncology patients may be secondary to insulin secretion by neuroendocrine tumours such as insulinomas, or rarely non-islet cell tumours such as bronchial carcinoids or gastrointestinal stromal tumours (GISTs). Other tumours, mostly retroperitoneal and mediastinal malignant mesenchymal tumours, can secrete peptides that stimulate glucose consumption such as insulin-like growth factors (IGF) 1 or 2 which bind IGF receptors and cause hypoglycaemia. Primary or secondary adrenal insufficiency due to adrenal or pituitary tumours should also be considered as well as massive hepatic tumour load. Hypoglycaemia in oncology patients with concomitant diabetes may be due to decreasing antidiabetes treatment requirements in the setting of cachexia, poor appetite, and weight loss.

Clinical features

Adrenergic symptoms usually precede glycopenic symptoms in hypoglycaemia. The sympathetic nervous system has been shown to respond to the absolute level of glucose in the blood. Sympathetic stimulation manifests as sweating, shaking, anxiety, hunger, and palpitations. Glycopenic symptoms reflect the decrease in the amount of glucose available to the brain and include confusion, hallucinations, irritability, coma, and eventually death.

Patients who are recurrently hypoglycaemic may become physiologically unaware of falling blood glucose levels and do not suffer any adrenergic symptoms to alert them to the impending glycopenia.

Blood glucose can be rapidly checked on a blood glucose meter but these estimations may be inaccurate at very low measurements. If hypoglycaemia is suspected, a blood sample should be tested in the laboratory for insulin and glucose levels. Simultaneous C-peptide levels will distinguish between exogenous and endogenous hyperinsulinaemia. The diagnosis of hypoglycaemia can be further proved by reversal of symptoms on administration of glucose and restoration of normal blood glucose levels. A short synacthen test can diagnose primary adrenal insufficiency. Plasma cortisol and adrenocorticotropic hormone (ACTH) levels may suggest a diagnosis of secondary adrenal insufficiency, which can be confirmed with ACTH stimulation tests.

Treatment

The aim of treatment in the short term is to restore blood glucose levels as quickly as possible to prevent any permanent glycopenic damage. This can be achieved by oral intake of sugary foods and drink, or if the patient is unconscious, with intravenous 5–20% dextrose solution. Additionally, glucagon can be administered intramuscularly or subcutaneously, an option particularly appropriate in situations where rapid intra-venous access is not available. A more long-term strategy then must be considered to prevent the recurrence of hypoglycaemia.

15.7   Hyperuricaemia

Introduction

Hyperuricaemia can be isolated or part of tumour lysis syndrome. Isolated hyperuricaemia is often asymptomatic. Chronically hyperuricaemia may result in crystal deposition in joints, causing painful arthralgia, and under the skin as painless gouty tophi. Deposition of uric acid or its metabolites in the kidney tubules may cause renal impairment with accompanying oliguria and fluid overload. The clinical features of acute hyperuricaemia are similar to TLS.

Aggressive hydration appropriate to renal and cardiovascular function should be attempted aiming for a urine output of at least 80–100ml/hour. If the patient is euvolaemic and there is no evidence of renal failure, diuretics may be used to sustain urine output. Urinary alkalinization to encourage solubility of uric acid in the urine is no longer recommended as it promotes xanthine crystal deposition in the renal tubules. Hyperuricaemic patients at low risk of developing tumour lysis syndrome may be managed with hydration and careful monitoring alone.

Management of patients at higher risk of tumour lysis syndrome is discussed earlier (p. 426).

15.8 Febrile neutropenia

Introduction
The diagnosis of febrile neutropenia (FN) requires that the following two criteria are met:
- A single oral temperature measurement of 38.3°C or higher, or two measurements of >38°C ≥1 hour apart.
- A neutrophil count of <0.5 x 10^9/L or a neutrophil count of <1 x 10^9/L with a projected decrease to <0.5 x 10^9/L over the next 48 hours.

It should be noted that the degree of fever necessary for the diagnosis of FN varies across guidelines from a single oral temperature >38°C to >38.5°C.

Most recent reports of causes of bacteraemia in neutropenic patients show approximately equal contributions from Gram-negative and Gram-positive organisms. In situations other than bone marrow transplantation, the risk of FN varies greatly between chemotherapy regimens.

Patients may present with fever alone or with features of systemic infection or rarely, septic shock.

Assessment
Initial assessment includes a clinical examination to identify the potential site of infection. Whereas inspection of the perineum is important, rectal examination is contraindicated in the setting of profound neutropenia as it is thought that it can promote bacteraemia by pathogenic gut bacteria.

Full blood counts and biochemistry along with two sets of blood cultures from different sites is recommended. In the presence of a venous access catheter, cultures should be taken both from the catheter and a peripheral site. Bacteraemia is documented in approximately 20% of cases of uncomplicated FN. A urine culture and a chest radiograph are also recommended, although their diagnostic yield is typically low in the absence of localizing signs. The presence of diarrhoea should prompt examination of a stool sample for clostridium difficile toxin.

Treatment
FN requires urgent treatment. Delayed antibiotic administration leads to increased mortality in septic shock and, although randomized trial data are lacking, many guidelines recommend that the first dose of empirical antibiotics should be administered within 60 minutes of presentation to hospital.

Risk stratification
The Multinational Association for Supportive Care in Cancer (MASCC) system is useful to identify patients at low risk of complications from FN. Using this scoring system, a score ≥21 identifies patients at low risk of complications (risk of serious complications ~6%, mortality <1%). The parameters used to calculate the score include burden of illness (score of 5 for mild or 3 for moderate symptoms, systolic blood pressure (BP) >90 (score 5), no chronic obstructive pulmonary disease (score 4), solid tumour or haematological malignancy with no prior fungal infection (score 4), no dehydration (score 3), outpatient at presentation (3), and age <60 years (score 2).

The availability of the risk stratification tools leads to two main treatment strategies:
- Uniform initial treatment of all patients with high-risk protocols and consideration of treatment de-escalation after 24–48 hours in low-risk patients.

- Upfront treatment de-escalation in low-risk patients, usually involving oral antibiotics and/or outpatient treatment.

Empirical antibiotic treatment of high-risk FN
Current guidelines recommend initial antibiotic monotherapy for most patients presenting with FN. Monotherapy with an extended spectrum antipseudomonal agent is the initial treatment and avoids the use of an aminoglycoside with the attendant nephrotoxicity. Suitable agents include: piperacillin/tazobactam (4.5g IV, three to four times daily), imipenem/cilastatin (500mg IV, four times daily), meropenem (1g IV, three times daily), cefepime (2g IV, three times daily), and ceftazidime (2g IV, three times daily). It should be noted that ceftazidime has limited activity against Gram-positive organisms and that cefepime was inferior to piperacillin/tazobactam in a randomized trial.

While initial monotherapy has similar efficacy to aminoglycoside-containing combinations, the addition of an aminoglycoside to an extended spectrum β-lactam is considered for medically unstable patients and in institutions with frequent isolation of multiresistant organisms. Once daily aminoglycoside dosing (e.g. gentamicin 5–7mg/kg) is less nephrotoxic and ototoxic than schedules utilizing more frequent dosing. An alternative strategy is the combination of an extended-spectrum penicillin such as piperacillin with a quinolone such as ciprofloxacin.

Due to the increasing frequency of fulminant Gram-positive infections, the empirical addition of vancomycin is also increasing in selected patients with intravenous catheter associated infections or soft tissue infections, especially in areas with a high frequency of MRSA (methicillin resistant *Staphylococcus aureus*) colonization, presence of septic shock, or in the presence of Gram-positive cocci grown in blood cultures before susceptibility information becomes available.

Rapid stabilization is critical in the patient with septic shock. Apart from a combination of an antipseudomonal agent, aminoglycoside, and vancomycin, supportive measures include high-flow oxygen, intravenous fluids, and vasopressor support. Stress dose corticosteroids (e.g. hydrocortisone IV 50mg, four times daily) have been shown to improve survival but the role of activated protein C products is controversial. Invasive haemodynamic monitoring and nursing in a high-dependency unit environment may be necessary.

Changes in initial treatment in non-responding patients
The median time to resolution of fever in patients receiving appropriate initial antibiotic treatment is five days. Therefore, a change of antibiotic regimen in a clinically stable patient based solely on the persistence of fever is not indicated. However, new physical examination findings, signs of clinical instability, and radiographic or blood culture results should prompt re-evaluation of the antibiotic regimen being used. Repeating blood cultures after 48 hours if the patient is still febrile is a reasonable strategy.

If the patient is being treated with monotherapy, clinical deterioration should prompt the addition of an aminoglycoside and vancomycin. In the presence of signs suggesting a GI tract infection, the addition of metronidazole (500mg IV, four times daily) is recommended. The presence of mucosal or cutaneous lesions suggestive of herpes simplex virus (HSV) should prompt treatment with acyclovir (5mg/kg IV, three times daily). If *Pneumocystis jiroveci* infection is suspected, treatment with high-dose trimethoprim/sulfamethoxazole (120mg/kg IV in two to four divided doses) is indicated. Close liaison with a microbiologist or infectious disease specialist is invaluable in ensuring that appropriate regimens are utilized.

Even though fungal infections are uncommon in FN of less than seven days' duration, empirical antifungal therapy should be considered if fever persists for four to seven days. Although fluconazole has proven utility as a prophylactic agent, its lack of activity against filamentous fungi makes it unsuitable for empirical antifungal treatment of FN. Options for empirical antifungal treatment include liposomal amphotericin B, voriconazole, posaconazole, and caspofungin

Proven bacteraemia necessitates continuation of intravenous treatment for at least seven to ten days and up to 21 days for complicated intra-abdominal infections. If *S. aureus* is isolated from the blood cultures, transoesophageal echocardiogram can help determine the duration of intravenous treatment. In the absence of valvular vegetations, a 14-day course is considered sufficient; their presence should lead to treatment prolongation for up to four to six weeks.

Changes in initial treatment in responding patients

Antibiotic treatment should generally continue until the neutropenia improves (neutrophil count >0.5 x 10^9/L) and the patient has been afebrile for 24 hours. Patients identified as at low risk for complications can be switched to oral treatment (usually a combination of amoxicillin-clavulanate and ciprofloxacin) after 24–48 hours of intravenous antibiotics and considered for early discharge from hospital. Patients who become afebrile but remain persistently neutropenic should generally remain on oral antibiotics until the neutrophil count is >0.5 x 10^9/L. However, de-escalation to prophylactic doses can be considered.

Empirical antibiotic treatment of low-risk FN

A selected group of low-risk patients with a MASCC score ≥21 with an anticipated duration of neutropenia for <7 days can be treated with oral antibiotics only. For such patients, a combination of ciprofloxacin (750mg, two times daily) and amoxicillin-clavulanate (625mg, three times daily) appears to be efficacious with very low complication rates. A recent randomized trial showed that once daily oral moxifloxacin (400mg) was as effective as the combination above with the added convenience of reduced pill burden. Before discharge, patients should undergo a short period of observation (2–24 hours) to ensure that there is no rapid clinical deterioration and that they can tolerate the oral regimen without nausea or vomiting. Close telephone and face-to-face follow-up is advised for timely intervention if complications occur. An alternative option is daily outpatient intravenous treatment. Although once daily ceftriaxone is frequently used in this setting, it should be noted that many *Pseudomonas* strains exhibit high levels of resistance.

Prevention

Antibiotic prophylaxis has been used as a means to prevent FN. Fluoroquinolones such as ciprofloxacin are the commonest used prophylactic agents and have been shown to decrease infection-related and all-cause mortality in hospitalized neutropenic patients with predominantly haematological malignancies. Currently, most, but not all, professional guidelines do not recommend routine prophylactic antibiotic use in patients with non-haematological malignancies.

Antifungal prophylaxis is not routinely recommended to reduce the risk of invasive fungal infections during neutropenia. However, prophylaxis with fluconazole or posaconazole is recommended for patients undergoing bone marrow transplantation or intensive chemotherapy for acute leukaemias. Routine prophylaxis against HSV, cytomegalovirus (CMV), and *P. jiroveci* is indicated for the above group of patients and for patients receiving alemtuzumab. Patients with chronic hepatitis B or C virus infection should receive prophylactic antiviral treatment if they are to receive anti-CD20 monoclonal antibodies or bone marrow transplantation.

Isolation and the use of high-efficiency particulate air (HEPA) filtration are not necessary for the majority of patients with short-lived neutropenia but are of proven benefit in the setting of bone marrow transplantation.

Secondary prevention after an episode of FN begins with an assessment of the therapeutic goals. If treatment is given with curative intent, it is reasonable to attempt to maintain dose intensity through the use of CSFs (see 'Colony stimulating factors' in Chapter 16, p. 477) and prophylactic antibiotics. For palliative treatments however a reduction in the chemotherapy dose is often more appropriate.

Internet resources

NCCN Clinical Practice Guidelines in Oncology. Febrile neutropenia: https://www.nccn.org/professionals/physician_gls/default.aspx

NICE Neutropenic sepsis: prevention and management of neutropenic sepsis in cancer patients—available at: http://www.nice.org.uk/guidance/cg151

15.9 Catheter associated infections

Introduction

Vascular access devices (VADs) are frequently used in cancer patients to ensure prolonged intravenous access for treatment delivery. Catheters with an external component are simpler to insert and include peripherally inserted central catheters (PICCs) and tunnelled catheters such as the Hickman or Groshong designs. Completely implanted devices are accessed percutaneously; their main advantages are durability and a low device profile.

Infection is the most serious complication associated with the presence of a VAD. Infection rates are lower with completely implanted devices compared to tunnelled lines.

The main causative agents are Gram-positive cocci, mostly coagulase-negative staphylococci and *S. aureus*. Early post-insertion infections follow the pattern of postoperative cellulitis, whereas later infections are mostly related to colonization of the catheter tunnel or hub. The incidence of Gram-negative infections, including those caused by *pseudomonas aeruginosa* and *tenotrophomonas maltophilia*, is rising.

Catheter related infections can be subdivided into:

- Exit site infections
- Tunnel or port infections
- Septic thrombophlebitis
- Catheter associated bacteraemia

Exit site infections may be associated with purulent discharge. However, in immunosuppressed or neutropenic patients, signs of infection may be minimal and difficult to differentiate from sterile inflammation. Pyrexia or rigors following catheter manipulation are strongly suggestive of catheter associated bloodstream infection.

Diagnosis

The diagnostic evaluation of the febrile neutropenic patient is described in section 15.8, 'Febrile neutropenia'. Swabs taken from the exit site as well as blood cultures obtained from both a peripheral site and all catheter lumens are essential.

Treatment

Initial antibiotic treatment of catheter related infections should include vancomycin to provide adequate cover against Gram-positive cocci including MRSA. Most uncomplicated exit site infections can be treated successfully without necessitating catheter removal.

In contrast, tunnel or port infections are difficult to eradicate using only antibiotics and catheter removal is often necessary. Immediate catheter removal is advised if fungi or non-tuberculous mycobacteria are isolated in blood cultures as well as in the presence of clinical instability or septic thrombophlebitis. Opinion is divided as to whether immediate catheter removal is necessary in infections with bacillus species, *Acinetobacter*, *P. aeruginosa*, *S. maltophilia*, enterococci, or *S. aureus*. If an attempt is made to treat the infection with the catheter in situ, repeat blood cultures after 48–72 hours of antibiotic treatment can assist decision making. If blood cultures remain positive or recurrent bacteraemia with the same organism occurs, catheter removal is recommended.

Prevention

Meticulous attention to aseptic techniques when accessing the catheter is paramount in preventing VAD-associated infections. The Dacron cuff of Hickman and Groshong catheters acts as a barrier to propagation of skin organisms and reduces infection rates compared with short-term catheters.

Further reading

Hentrich M, Schalk E, Schmidt-Hieber M, et al. Central venous catheter-related infections in hematology and oncology: 2012 updated guidelines on diagnosis, management and prevention by the Infectious Disease Working Party of the German Society of Hematology and Medical Oncology. *Ann Oncol* 2014; 25(5):936–47.

15.10 Nausea, vomiting, and diarrhoea

See Chapter 17, 'Palliative care' (p. 482).

15.11 Vascular complications

Extravasation

Aetiology
Extravasation is the accidental infiltration into surrounding subcutaneous tissues of a drug that has been administered by the intravascular route either by peripheral cannulation or central venous access device (CVAD).

Clinical features
It is essential the extravasation is recognized and treated urgently. The degree of damage will be dependent on the type of drug. Indications that extravasation has occurred include:
- Increased resistance when administering intravenous drugs
- Lack of blood flow back into the cannula (or CVAD)
- Change in tissue appearance around the infusion site such as redness or blanching
- Pain, swelling, or oedema around the infusion site

Treatment and prevention
Treatment will depend on the classification of the cytotoxic drug:
- Exfoliant/irritant—drug capable of causing inflammation and irritation including shedding of skin but less likely to cause tissue breakdown or tissue death.
- Vesicant—drug capable of causing pain and inflammation as above but also underlying tissue death and necrosis. This can be further classified as anthracycline (e.g. doxorubicin) or non-anthracycline (e.g. vinca alkaloid) related.

Local guidelines should be in place for the management of extravasation, and extravasation of a vesicant should be treated as a medical emergency. Units which administer cytotoxic chemotherapy should have extravasation kits readily available for such incidents.

The basic management should include stopping the infusion immediately and aspirating as much of the drug as possible, leaving the cannula in situ if it is in a peripheral site. Consideration should be given to pain control and elevation of the affected limb.

For non-vesicants, a cold compress should be applied to the affected area for 20 minutes up to four times daily for 24–48 hours. For vesicants or extravasation of large quantities of irritant drugs, the advice of an experienced plastic surgeon must be sought urgently. Local treatment with hyaluronidase and a saline flush out should be considered. For situations where extravasation of an anthracycline is involved, prescription of intravenous dexrazoxane should be considered. As dexrazoxane is itself a cytotoxic drug, appropriate monitoring should take place.

Venous thromboembolism

Aetiology
Venous thromboembolism (VTE), which encompasses both deep venous thrombosis (DVT) and pulmonary embolism (PE), occurs in up to 20% of cancer patients. It seems to be particularly high for pancreatic, ovarian, and brain primaries, whereas renal, lung, gastric, and haematological cancers are also associated with above-average risk. The development of metastatic disease markedly influences the risk of VTE as evidenced by reports of 5–20-fold increased risk compared with patients with localized disease.

High risks of VTE have been reported with the use of thalidomide and lenalidomide-based combinations in the treatment of multiple myeloma, with a risk of VTE of up to 4–6% per treatment cycle. Angiogenesis-targeting agents, including both monoclonal antibodies and tyrosine kinase inhibitors have also been shown to increase the risk of VTE as well as causing arterial thromboembolism and bleeding.

Clinical features
Most DVTs affect the lower limbs where they usually present with pain, tenderness, erythema, and oedema. A difference in calf circumference of >3cm is strongly predictive of DVT whereas Homan's sign (calf tenderness on ankle dorsiflexion) is neither sensitive nor specific. Swelling of the whole leg can be a sign of pelvic or femoral DVT.

Approximately 10% of DVTs affect the upper limb, where they present with similar symptoms. The frequency of upper limb DVT appears to be increasing, probably reflecting the increasing use of central venous catheters.

The clinical features of PE vary depending on the extent of thrombosis and the underlying lung function. Moderate and large PE commonly causes dyspnoea, pleuritic chest pain, cough, and haemoptysis. Massive PE is a frequent cause of circulatory collapse and cardiac arrest. The commonest clinical signs of PE are hypoxia, tachypnoea, and tachycardia; a pleural rub may be audible if pulmonary infarction develops. Massive PE causes signs of acute right ventricular failure with hypotension, distended jugular veins, loud P2, S3, or S4 gallop and a pansystolic murmur of acute tricuspid regurgitation.

Most VTE events however are asymptomatic. This is supported by studies of DVT development in the postoperative setting that have shown that only a small proportion of the ultrasound-detected cases were clinically apparent. Similarly, whereas it is thought that almost all PEs are the consequence of a lower limb or pelvic DVT, clinically apparent DVT is present in only 20% of cases. In addition, the clinical use of multidetector high resolution computed tomography (CT) scanning for staging and response assessment purposes in cancer patients has resulted in increased detection of PE in otherwise asymptomatic patients.

Diagnosis
The use of D-dimer testing as a screening tool before imaging studies is not recommended in patients with malignancy. Duplex ultrasonography is the investigation of choice for suspected DVT. It has high sensitivity (>90%) and specificity (>95%) for femoral or popliteal DVT, particularly if assessment of venous compressibility is carried out. However, the accuracy of the test is lower for calf or pelvic vein DVT. Repeat examination a week later is recommended if the clinical suspicion of DVT is moderate or high but the initial ultrasonography is negative.

CT with intravenous contrast administration is the preferred method for diagnosing thrombi in the pelvic veins or the inferior vena cava (IVC). Catheter-associated DVT can be diagnosed with contrast administration via the catheter ('linogram'). However, it should be kept in mind that neither clot inside the catheter, nor the presence of a fibrin sheath constitutes a DVT.

CT pulmonary angiogram (CTPA) is the investigation of choice for diagnosing PE. In addition to demonstrating any emboli, it allows evaluation of the lung parenchyma and mediastinal structures revealing any additional or alternative pathology. The PIOPED II trial showed that multidetector CT had a sensitivity of 83% and specificity of 96% for the diagnosis of PE. The positive predictive value was 96% when the clinical probability, derived by the Wells' score, was concordant with the scan result. However, a negative CTPA could not reliably exclude PE when the clinical probability was high, as the negative predictive value in that setting was only 60%. Most of the CT scanners used in that study were four-slice machines; whether modern 16- or 64-slice scanners that have shown increased sensitivity in detecting sub-segmental PEs can overcome these limitations, is not yet clear.

V/Q scan is associated with less radiation exposure and is an alternative to CTPA, particularly when renal insufficiency precludes intravenous contrast administration and in pregnant patients. However, it has lower sensitivity and specificity than CTPA and is non-diagnostic when the clinical probability is discordant with the scan results or when the scan shows an intermediate or low probability of PE. Invasive pulmonary angiography, while still considered the 'gold standard' for diagnosing PE, is rarely used clinically.

Treatment

An incidental PE requires the same treatment as clinically apparent PE. Low-molecular-weight heparin (LMWH) is the preferred anticoagulation modality in patients with cancer and VTE. The choice of the specific LMWH (e.g. enoxaparin 1.5mg/kg SC once daily, tinzaparin 175U/kg SC once daily, dalteparin 200U/kg SC once daily) is usually dependent on institutional preference; there is no evidence to suggest that one is more effective or safer than the other. Studies have confirmed the equivalence of LMWH and unfractionated heparin (UFH) in the initial (first five to ten days) treatment of VTE. However, the former is much easier to administer and does not require routine monitoring of coagulation parameters. Fondaparinux, a factor Xa inhibitor, is also recommended as an alternative to LMWH.

Warfarin can be used for the chronic treatment of VTE if patient preference or cost issues dictate it. However, an initial period of heparin therapy for at least five to seven days and until the international normalized ratio (INR) has been >2 for at least 48 hours is recommended. A target INR of 2–3 is reasonable in this setting. Warfarin is subject to many pharmacokinetic interactions and concomitant medications, including chemotherapy, can affect drug levels, necessitating frequent INR monitoring to ensure efficacy and safety. Novel oral anticoagulants such as rivaroxaban and apixaban have been shown to be safe and effective in the management of VTE and PE in unselected patient populations.

The optimum duration of anticoagulant therapy is not defined. Generally, treatment for at least three to six months is recommended for DVT and six to 12 months for PE. Indefinite treatment should be considered for selected patients such as those with metastatic disease or patients on chemotherapy. The presence of residual thrombus or elevated D-dimer levels after an initial period of anticoagulation may help inform this decision but definitive guidance is presently lacking.

Contraindications to anticoagulant therapy in cancer patients include recent major surgery, recent intracranial bleed, active major bleeding, thrombocytopenia, and platelet or coagulation abnormalities. Placement of an IVC filter should be considered in this situation.

Failure of anticoagulation treatment is defined as extension of a known DVT/PE or development of a new DVT/PE while on treatment. In the first instance measurement of INR, activated partial thromboplastin time (APTT), and anti-Xa activity is recommended to ensure adequate drug exposure. Therapeutic manoeuvres include placement of an IVC filter, switching from warfarin to LMWH, increasing the dose of LMWH, moving to a twice-daily schedule of LMWH administration, or switching to a factor Xa inhibitor.

Removal of the catheter, if feasible, is the preferred option for catheter-related DVT. Anticoagulation with LMWH is recommended while the catheter is still in situ and for one to three months afterwards. A small pilot study has demonstrated the feasibility of a strategy of dalteparin and warfarin administration without removing the catheter.

Catheter-directed or intravenous thrombolytic therapy is an option for the treatment of massive PE causing haemodynamic compromise. Thrombolysis has been shown to significantly reduce the risk of death or recurrent PE in these patients compared with heparin treatment alone. However, careful consideration of the risks and benefits of the procedure is important as the risk of major bleeding approaches 15%. There is no evidence to suggest that catheter-directed thrombolysis (with catheter placement in the pulmonary artery) is superior to intravenous thrombolysis or that one agent (e.g. streptokinase, alteplase, reteplase) is superior to another. Surgical or percutaneous transcatheter embolectomy is an option in massive PE when thrombolysis is contraindicated. Thrombolysis should also be considered for patients with massive or non-resolving ileofemoral DVT threatening limb viability.

Prevention

Prophylactic treatment is recommended for all hospitalized patients with cancer, unless there are specific contraindications to anticoagulant use. The recommendation is based on the results of multiple randomized trials that have shown a reduction in VTE events with prophylactic LMWH. However, patients with cancer constituted only a small minority of the enrolled subjects. Suitable options include enoxaparin 40mg SC once daily, dalteparin 5,000U SC once daily, or UFH 5,000U SC once daily.

Patients undergoing surgery require VTE prophylaxis perioperatively. Mechanical devices alone appear to be insufficient and LMWH or UFH should be added for at least seven to ten days following major surgery. Randomized studies have shown that extending prophylactic treatment with LMWH for four weeks following major abdominal or pelvic surgery for cancer is more effective at preventing VTE than a seven-day course.

Routine VTE prophylaxis is not currently recommended for ambulatory cancer patients receiving chemotherapy. Prophylactic treatment, preferably with LMWH but also with low-dose aspirin if LMWH is contraindicated, should be considered for patients receiving thalidomide or lenalidomide based combinations for multiple myeloma in view of the extremely high incidence of VTE in this setting.

Further reading
Lyman G, Bohlke K, Khorana A, et al. Venous thromboembolism prophylaxis and treatment in patients with cancer: American Society of Clinical Oncology Clinical Practice Guideline Update 2014. *J Clin Oncol* 2015; 33(6):654–6.

Internet resources
NCCN Clinical Practice Guidelines in Oncology. Venous thromboembolism. Cancer-associated venous thromboembolic disease—available at: https://www.nccn.org/professionals/physician_gls/default.aspx

15.12 Stridor and airway obstruction

Aetiology
Stridor is a high-pitched musical breathing sound predominantly heard on inspiration. It results from turbulent, partially obstructed airflow in the upper extrathoracic airways and the intrathoracic trachea and major bronchi.

Malignant causes of stridor can be subdivided into extrinsic and intrinsic. Extrinsic causes include:

- Direct invasion, usually by primary pulmonary and oesophageal neoplasms or aggressive thyroid carcinomas.
- Involvement of the airways by enlarged lymph nodes in tumours such as lymphomas.
- Involvement by metastases from a distant site. Metastases that directly invade the major airways most commonly originate from renal, colon, breast, or melanoma primaries and account for 2–5% of all lung metastases.
- Intrinsic obstruction is usually due to bulky primary tumours originating from the hypopharynx, larynx, trachea, or proximal large bronchi.

Clinical features
Supraglottic lesions cause inspiratory stridor whereas glottic and subglottic tumours cause biphasic stridor with both an inspiratory and an expiratory component. Intrathoracic lesions can cause a predominantly expiratory stridor that can easily be confused with wheezing.

Depending on the severity of obstruction there may be signs of respiratory compromise such as dyspnoea, tachypnoea, and cyanosis. Physical examination may reveal clues as to the likely aetiology with thyroid masses, gross cervical lymphadenopathy, clubbing, or pleural effusions.

Diagnosis
The diagnosis of stridor is clinical. Patients who present with severe respiratory compromise require emergency management of their airway. Fibreoptic-assisted intubation in this setting provides both immediate relief and diagnostic information.

Pulse oximetry and arterial blood gas analysis aid in the initial evaluation of the patient. CT scan will delineate extent of lesion. Spirometry with flow-volume loops can help differentiate between extrathoracic and intrathoracic obstruction. Rigid bronchoscopy may facilitate therapeutic interventions and provide tissue for histological diagnosis.

Treatment
Initial treatment depends on the severity of obstruction. Severe respiratory compromise necessitates emergency intubation or tracheostomy. Helium–oxygen gas mixtures (Heliox®) or non-invasive positive pressure ventilation can aid in the stabilization of the acutely unwell patient. High-dose dexamethasone (16mg daily) can help reduce peritumoural oedema and partially relieve the obstruction.

Definitive treatment depends on the diagnosis and extent of disease. Urgent surgery is the preferred option for resectable primary tracheal tumours. A variety of techniques can be used for unresectable endoluminal tumours. Endobronchial techniques, implemented during (rigid) bronchoscopy, include:

- Debulking techniques aiming at tissue destruction (endoluminal resection, Nd:YAG laser vaporization, argon laser coagulation, cryotherapy, brachytherapy with 125I or 192Ir or photodynamic therapy)
- Dilatation using balloons or bougies
- Endoluminal stent insertion

External beam radiotherapy is widely available and is usually the first treatment option for airway obstruction from relatively chemotherapy-resistant tumours such as non-small cell lung cancer (NSCLC). Radiotherapy can initially exacerbate peritumoural oedema and therefore corticosteroid premedication is advisable. Initial chemotherapy is advised for chemotherapy-sensitive tumours such as SCLC or lymphomas; the role of radiotherapy is limited in these situations.

Further reading
Theodore PR. Emergent management of malignancy-related acute airway obstruction. *Emerg Med Clin North Am* 2009; 27(2):231–41.

15.13 Superior vena cava obstruction

Aetiology
Malignancy accounts for approximately 80% of cases of superior vena cava (SVC) obstruction. Lung cancer is the commonest cause and is implicated in almost 75% of cases, with NSCLC causing twice as many cases as SCLC. Rarer causes include lymphomas (~10%), metastatic disease, germ cell tumours, teratomas, thymomas, and mesotheliomas.

Clinical features
Obstruction of the SVC leads to extensive collateral venous circulation redirecting blood flow to the azygos vein or the inferior vena cava. This collateral network develops over a period of several weeks and may result in improvement of symptoms and signs.

The commonest symptoms are dyspnoea (60%) and various degrees of facial or limb oedema (40–80%). Other complaints include cough (20–50%), chest pain (15%), headache (10%), or dizziness or syncope (10%).

The classic physical finding is of fixed engorgement of the neck and chest wall veins (50–60%) with visible cutaneous collaterals, plethora (20%), and cyanosis (20%). Papilloedema can be a late development. Rare but potentially life-threatening presentations include cerebral or upper respiratory tract oedema and cardiac compression. Respiratory compromise is rarely the result of SVC obstruction per se; it usually reflects direct involvement of the major airways by the malignant process.

Diagnosis
The diagnosis is usually evident clinically and subsequent investigations aim to establish the underlying cause, as 60% of cases of SVC obstruction occur without a prior diagnosis of malignancy.

The chest radiograph is abnormal in >85% of cases with superior mediastinal widening and pleural effusion being the commonest findings. CT with intravenous contrast material provides anatomical information and allows the examination of other critical structures such as the trachea and spinal canal. Depending on the distribution of the disease, histological confirmation can be provided by sputum or pleural fluid cytology, and lymph node (enlarged supraclavicular or neck nodes are frequently seen on ultrasound) or mediastinal mass biopsy (either CT-guided or at bronchoscopy). The diagnostic yield of these procedures is in the order of 50–75%. Mediastinoscopy has a higher diagnostic yield (>90%) and it seems to be safe in the hands of an experienced operator.

Prognosis
There are no data to suggest that the presence of SVC obstruction adversely affects prognosis beyond the obvious staging implications.

Treatment
Management aims both at the relief of symptoms and treating the underlying cause. The presence of significant cerebral oedema or cardiovascular compromise leading to hypotension and recurrent syncope are indications for urgent management.

Medical management
Elevation of the patient's head to reduce hydrostatic pressure is a useful therapeutic manoeuvre. Corticosteroids (e.g. dexamethasone 8–16mg daily) are frequently prescribed but there are limited data to support their efficacy except for patients with steroid-sensitive tumours such as lymphomas and thymomas or those treated with radiotherapy.

Stent insertion
Stent placement can result in immediate symptomatic relief while diagnostic investigations are carried out with a very low rate of immediate complications. It is the preferred initial option for most cases of malignant SVC obstruction, with the exception of very chemotherapy sensitive tumours such as lymphomas, germ cell tumours, and SCLC.

Radiotherapy and chemotherapy
The use of radiotherapy or chemotherapy requires a histological diagnosis. Radiotherapy provides symptomatic relief in 60–80% of patients with NSCLC or SCLC; improvement is usually noted within 72 hours. In fit patients without distant metastases, SVC stent followed by radical radiotherapy with or without chemotherapy is the appropriate treatment. In the palliative setting, 20Gy in five fractions or 30Gy in ten fractions are frequently used. Systemic chemotherapy can result in rapid relief of symptoms in chemotherapy-sensitive tumours. Reported rates of complete symptomatic relief range from 40% to 80% for patients with lymphoma or SCLC.

Anticoagulation and thrombolysis
Thrombolytic therapy can be used in the setting of extensive associated thrombosis. The benefit of either short- or long-term anticoagulation is uncertain.

15.14 Gastrointestinal obstruction

Aetiology

Intestinal obstruction in cancer patients can be mechanical or functional. Upper GI obstruction is usually mechanical in origin due to luminal involvement or compression by oesophagogastric or pancreatic neoplasms. Twenty-five per cent of patients with unresectable pancreatic tumours eventually develop gastroduodenal obstruction.

Although obstruction may result from primary small bowel tumours, it is more commonly due to peritoneal metastases from ovarian, gastric, or colorectal primaries. These three tumour sites account for approximately 75% of cases of malignant mechanical small bowel obstruction. Melanoma can cause luminal metastases with obstruction due to intussusception. Primary colorectal tumours account for the vast majority of mechanical large bowel obstruction.

Constipation is a common cause of non-mechanical obstruction. It can be secondary to chemotherapeutic agents such as vinca alkaloids, medications such as opioids, anticholinergicdrugs, and HT3 antagonists, or dehydration and electrolyte abnormalities such as hypercalcaemia.

Colonic and rectal tumours are the main causes of mechanical large bowel obstruction. Other causes of bowel obstruction include late radiation enteritis with stricture formation which predominantly affects the small bowel and autonomic denervation by the tumour (Ogilvie's syndrome).

Clinical features

Upper GI obstruction at the level of the pylorus presents with large volume projectile vomiting soon after eating. Typically, bile is absent and in complete obstruction severe dehydration ensues. A succussion splash may be elicited.

Mechanical small bowel obstruction presents with colicky abdominal pain and tenderness, vomiting, constipation, and abdominal distention. Bowel sounds are characteristically high-pitched and hyperactive. Paralytic ileus is associated with diffuse and typically non-colicky pain as well as absent bowel sounds. Large bowel obstruction produces similar symptoms and signs, although it tends to develop more gradually. Vomiting may be faeculent and an obstructing colonic primary may be palpable. Complete bowel obstruction results in an empty rectum on rectal examination.

Diagnosis

CT of the abdomen and pelvis, which is more sensitive and specific than plain radiographs, is the investigation of choice.

Treatment

Treatment depends on the level of obstruction and the general condition of the patient. As a rule, patients with bowel obstruction are dehydrated and therefore intravenous fluid administration is indicated.

Nasogastric tube placement can help decompress the stomach in upper GI obstruction. Resectable tumours are best managed by definitive surgery. Palliative procedures can include endoscopic stent placement, gastroduodenal bypass, or feeding tube placement.

For the management of small bowel obstruction see Chapter 17, 'Palliative care' (p. 482).

Further reading

Bosscher MR, van Leeuwen BL, Hoekstra HJ. Surgical emergencies in oncology. *Cancer Treat Rev* 2014; 40(8):1028–36.

15.15 Urinary tract obstruction

Aetiology

Advancing pelvic or abdominal malignancy causes obstruction via direct invasion or extrinsic compression of the ureters. Cervical, colorectal, ovarian, or prostate cancers can invade the urinary tract locally whilst retroperitoneal malignancies such as sarcoma encroach on the ureters from the outside. Malignant abdominal lymphadenopathy may also compress the ureters extrinsically.

Ureteral obstruction secondary to malignancy confers a poor prognosis, with a median survival of three months, which must be taken into account when exploring treatment options.

Clinical features

Urinary tract obstruction secondary to malignancy often has a more insidious presentation than the acute urinary obstruction that occurs with urinary tract infection or benign prostatic hypertrophy. Patients may present with obstruction of only one ureter and gradually deteriorating renal function. Symptoms are vague such as lethargy, nausea, vomiting, and abdominal or flank discomfort. If the obstruction develops more rapidly, patients may present with considerable abdominal distension and discomfort accompanied by nausea. In some cases, symptoms of superadded urinary tract infection may be the only indication of underlying obstruction.

Diagnosis

Localization of the obstruction and the resulting dilatation of the proximal urinary tract can be confirmed by ultrasound examination. More detailed imaging of the abdomen and pelvis by CT or magnetic resonance imaging (MRI) will illustrate the cause of the obstruction and the extent of underlying malignant disease. Urine microscopy and culture will accurately diagnose any urinary tract infection. It is important that renal function is also considered as this may alter subsequent management.

Treatment

The variable success rates of the management options available, the generally poor prognosis, and the lack of evidence that intervention actually improves quality of life in the palliative setting make good communication and involvement of the patient in decision making of paramount importance.

Decompression of ureteral obstruction is necessary to prevent hydronephrosis, renal failure, and urinary tract infections. It can be achieved using percutaneous insertion of a nephrostomy tube into the renal pelvis or ureteral stenting.

Relief of ureteral obstruction by percutaneous nephrostomy under ultrasound guidance is an expeditious method of treating urinary tract obstruction with very high initial technical success rates. However, frequent complications include recurrent urinary tract infections and tube dislodgement necessitating repeat procedures and readmission to hospital. Nephrostomies can be well suited to some patient groups such as those with intractable flank pain or obstructive pyelonephritis.

Stent insertion can be accomplished by retrograde or anterograde techniques. The latter generally require prior nephrostomy tube insertion; conversion of nephrostomy to anterograde stenting is successful in ~50% of cases. Factors predicting successful ureteric stent placement are an intrinsic ureteric abnormality rather than extrinsic compression and a short (<3cm) obstructed segment. Late stent failure is attributed to ureteral peristaltic dysfunction, irritation of the urothelium, and stent encrustation. Ureteral obstruction at the pelvic brim and direct invasion of the urothelium at the time of stent placement are highly predictive of stent failure. Drug-eluting and more rigid stents are being developed to provide further interventional options. Patients with ureteral stents often report ongoing lower urinary tract symptoms, pelvic or flank discomfort, and elective stent exchange at approximately six-monthly intervals is required. Studies have shown, however, that there is no significant difference in quality of life from ureteral stent insertion or percutaneous nephrostomy.

Medical therapy may also add symptomatic relief in the treatment of obstruction. The role of prostaglandins, angiotensin II, and calcium channel blockers in urothelial spasm is currently being investigated. Transdermal oxybutynin has few systemic anticholinergic side effects but may help relieve lower urinary tract symptoms. Analgesia remains an important part of symptom control regardless of whether any mechanical intervention takes place.

Further reading

Liberman D, McCormack M. Renal and urologic problems: management of ureteric obstruction. *Curr Opin Support Palliat Care* 2012; 6(3):316–21.

15.16 Thrombocytopenia and disseminated intravascular coagulation

Introduction

Thrombocytopenia generally results from decreased platelet production in the bone marrow or increased peripheral destruction or sequestration. In patients with cancer it is most often secondary to widespread marrow infiltration by haematological malignancies or solid tumours.

Treatment-induced thrombocytopenia is graded using the Common Terminology Criteria for Adverse Events (CTCAE v. 4.0) as follows:

- Grade 1: <LLN (lower limit of normal)—75 x 10^9/L
- Grade 2: <75—50 x 10^9/L
- Grade 3: <50—25 x 10^9/L
- Grade 4: <25 x 10^9/L

Immune-mediated platelet destruction is seen in chronic lymphocytic leukaemia and lymphomas and has been rarely associated with solid organ tumours such as breast, lung, or GI cancer as a paraneoplastic phenomenon.

Treatment with unfractionated or low-molecular-weight heparin is common in patients with malignancy. Rarely (in 1–3% of exposed patients) it is associated with the development of antibodies against platelet factor 4 (PF4)–heparin complexes and subsequently heparin-induced thrombocytopenia (HIT).

It should also be noted that massive red blood cell transfusion may cause or exacerbate thrombocytopenia due to loss of platelet viability in stored blood.

Non-immunological platelet destruction occurs in the setting of disseminated intravascular coagulation (DIC) complicating advanced malignancy, usually with adenocarcinomas of the GI tract, pancreas, lung, breast, or prostate and acute promyelocytic leukaemia (APL). Haemolytic uraemic syndrome and microangiopathic haemolytic anaemia with development of thrombocytopenia has been reported after treatment with mitomycin C.

Clinical features

Although bleeding time can be prolonged when the platelet count drops below 100 x 10^9/L, clinical episodes of bleeding do not seem to increase until the platelet count drops below 50 x 10^9/L. Minor trauma can lead to excessive bleeding when the platelet count is 20–50 x 10^9/L, whereas spontaneous bleeding generally does not occur unless the platelet count is <20 x 10^9/L. Even with platelet counts <10 x 10^9/L, a substantial proportion of patients remains asymptomatic.

Thrombocytopenia causes a characteristic pattern of bleeding with prominent petechiae and small ecchymoses as well as mucosal bleeding (epistaxis, GI bleeding, and haematuria). Haemarthroses and soft tissue haematomas are rare and suggest a coexisting coagulopathy.

DIC is characterized by simultaneous bleeding and thrombotic diatheses. Patients may present with a combination of thrombocytopenic patterns of bleeding and venous or arterial thrombosis as well as features of non-bacterial endocarditis. Similarly, HIT may present with clinical signs of both bleeding and thrombosis; necrotic lesions at injecting sites commonly occur.

Diagnosis

A full blood count and coagulation studies prothrombin time (PT) and APTT are usually adequate for the patient with a solid tumour and extensive bone marrow involvement or recent cytotoxic chemotherapy. A peripheral blood smear, bone marrow examination, and detailed platelet function studies are indicated if the cause of the thrombocytopenia is uncertain.

DIC is characteristically associated with prolonged PT and APTT, increased levels of thrombin degradation products, low levels of fibrinogen, thrombocytopenia, and schistocytes on the blood film.

If HIT is suspected, its pre-test probability can be calculated based on the platelet nadir, the timing of thrombocytopenia development, the presence of thrombosis, and the absence of other causes of low platelets (the '4Ts' test). If the pre-test probability of HIT is moderate or high, enzyme-linked immunoassay testing for HIT antibodies is recommended. Because of low specificity, testing is not recommended if the pre-test probability is low.

Treatment

Platelet transfusion has been the mainstay of thrombocytopenia management in patients with malignancy. Active bleeding in the setting of thrombocytopenia necessitates transfusion, although there is little evidence on which to base recommendations regarding optimum platelet target levels.

Medications that impair platelet function such as aspirin, clopidogrel, and NSAIDs should be discontinued once thrombocytopenia develops and the need for prophylactic LMWH in hospitalized patients is reassessed.

Guidelines from the British Committee for Standards in Haematology and the American Society of Clinical Oncology (ASCO) recommend prophylactic platelet transfusion for platelet counts <10 x 10^9/L. A higher threshold of 20 x 10^9/L should be adopted in patients with sepsis, coagulopathy, rapid fall in platelet count, or in the setting of APL. ASCO recommends a threshold of 20 x 10^9/L for patients receiving aggressive therapy for bladder tumours and those with necrotic tumours because of an increased risk of bleeding.

Platelet transfusion should be used to bring the platelet count above 50 x 10^9/L before invasive procedures such as lumbar puncture, biopsy, or indwelling line insertion. However, experienced practitioners can perform these procedures safely even in patients with severe thrombocytopenia. A platelet count of >100 x 10^9/L is recommended before ophthalmological or intracranial surgery.

Platelet transfusions are contraindicated, except in the presence of life-threatening haemorrhage, for patients with thrombotic thrombocytopenic purpura or HIT as there is an increased risk of thrombotic complications.

Furthermore, platelet transfusion will be ineffective in immune-mediated platelet destruction. The latter, when it occurs as a paraneoplastic syndrome, may respond to splenectomy or high-dose corticosteroids. Thrombopoietin receptor agonists such as eltrombopag and romiplostim may be considered in refractory immune-mediated cases.

Tranexamic acid has been shown to reduce platelet requirements during consolidation therapy for acute myeloid leukaemia and is also a useful adjunct to platelet transfusions in patients with mucosal bleeding.

Treatment of DIC is directed towards the underlying cause if feasible. Infection is a common precipitating factor and broad-spectrum antibiotics are indicated. Cryoprecipitate or fresh frozen plasma is administered to correct the clotting abnormality whereas platelet transfusion is relatively contraindicated.

Treatment of HIT involves discontinuation of the heparin product and alternative anticoagulation with preferably a direct thrombin inhibitor (e.g. bivalirudin or argatroban) or, alternatively, a factor Xa inhibitor (danaparoid) until platelet recovery. If the pre-test probability of HIT is moderate or high, the above treatments should be instituted immediately without waiting for the results of antibody testing. HIT is a prothrombotic state and anticoagulation with warfarin is recommended for at least four weeks after resolution of the thrombocytopenia.

The development of thrombopoietic growth factors is the subject of intense research efforts and has the potential to ameliorate cancer associated thrombocytopenia and reduce the need for platelet transfusions. Further along clinical development is interleukin-11 (oprelvekin) which is licensed in the USA for the prevention of thrombocytopenia and reduction in need for platelet transfusions in patients receiving myelosuppressive chemotherapy for non-myeloid malignancies.

Further reading

Feinstein DI. Disseminated intravascular coagulation in patients with solid tumors. *Oncol (Williston Park)* 2015; 29(2):96–102.

Schiffer CA, Anderson K, Bennett C, et al. Platelet transfusion for patients with cancer: clinical practice guidelines of the American Society of Clinical Oncology. *J Clin Oncol* 2001; 19(5):1519–38.

15.17 Gastrointestinal bleeding

Introduction

Acute GI bleeding as an oncological emergency usually occurs in the setting of advanced, incurable disease and may be a terminal event. It is commonly the result of direct involvement of luminal blood vessels by tumour. Other potential mechanisms include rupture of highly vascularized tumours such as GIST or variceal bleeding in the setting of extensive hepatic disease and portal hypertension.

GI bleeding may be compounded by coagulopathy. Clotting factor abnormalities, thrombocytopenia, and DIC are often present in advanced malignancy, especially with extensive hepatic metastases.

GI bleeding may also be a consequence of anticancer treatments. Most cytotoxic chemotherapy agents cause a degree of myelosuppression, and thrombocytopenia is especially pronounced with drugs such as carboplatin or gemcitabine. Novel compounds targeting cancer angiogenesis such as bevacizumab have a distinct toxicity

profile that includes both bleeding and thrombotic events. Furthermore, the increasing use of indwelling vascular access devices as well as the easier diagnosis of venous thromboembolism afforded by modern imaging techniques result in an increasing proportion of cancer patients being treated with antiplatelet or anticoagulant agents.

Clinical features

Common presentations include haematemesis, melaena, and fresh bleeding per rectum (haematochezia). Loss of large blood volumes leads to hypovolaemic shock presenting with lethargy, excessive sweating, pale, cool, and clammy extremities, and prolonged capillary refill. Tachycardia, hypotension, and decreased urinary output are usually present.

Diagnosis

The diagnosis of major acute GI bleeding is clinical. Further investigations depend on the clinical situation and generally aim to assess either the severity of bleeding or the potential site of origin, determined by upper or lower GI endoscopy, CT, or angiography in selected cases.

Treatment

Treatment is guided by an initial assessment of the severity of bleeding and the overall patient prognosis.

If it is thought that the bleeding represents a terminal event, active resuscitation measures are inappropriate. The patient should be preferably nursed in a single room. Sedation with midazolam and diamorphine is helpful for alleviating pain, anxiety, and distress. Dark towels should be used to cover areas of active bleeding as this has been shown to reduce patient and relative distress.

Immediate fluid resuscitation using crystalloid or colloid solutions is the initial management if active treatment is deemed appropriate. Blood transfusions are used to maintain adequate haemoglobin levels and platelet and coagulation abnormalities are corrected with platelet, fresh frozen plasma, or prothrombin complex concentrate infusions.

Endoscopy can be used as both a diagnostic and therapeutic procedure. GI bleeding originating from relatively immobile structures, such as the rectum or the oesophagus, can be effectively controlled in many instances with palliative radiotherapy. Palliative surgery also has a role in removing a troublesome primary even in the presence of metastatic disease.

Further reading

Heller SJ, Tokar JL, Nguyen MT, et al. Management of bleeding GI tumors. *Gastrointest Endosc* 2010; 72(4):817–24.

15.18 Genitourinary bleeding

Introduction

Eighty per cent of bladder cancers present with painless gross haematuria. Renal and ureteric tumours are also associated with macroscopic haematuria. Postmenopausal vaginal bleeding is the commonest presenting feature of endometrial malignancy. Vaginal bleeding may also result from other tumours such as cervical cancer and rarer malignancies such as invasive trophoblastic disease.

In addition, oncology patients may develop haemorrhagic cystitis as a result of infection or treatment. Those undergoing chemotherapy are more prone to develop infective interstitial cystitis. Haemorrhagic cystitis may become a dose-limiting toxicity in cyclophosphamide or ifosfamide chemotherapy and is particularly noted in the paediatric population. Acrolein, a metabolite of these nitrogen mustard-derived alkylators, is toxic to the urothelium and is the direct causative agent.

Pelvic radiotherapy may also cause acute haemorrhagic cystitis after treatment, but symptoms may develop up to months and years later. Endarteritis results in mucosal ischaemia, ulceration, and bleeding.

Alternatively, genitourinary bleeding in an oncology patient can be a reflection of bone marrow depression or dysfunction and a bleeding diathesis as a result of the primary disease or of treatment.

Clinical features

Painless gross haematuria is the commonest presentation of bladder carcinoma. The haematuria can be complicated by clot retention and urinary incontinence. Haemorrhagic cystitis presents with symptoms of bladder irritation such as urgency, frequency, dysuria, and suprapubic discomfort. There may be microscopic or gross haematuria.

Postmenopausal bleeding due to endometrial malignancy is painless and is often the only symptom. Unlike bladder carcinoma, however, only about 20% of postmenopausal bleeding represents uterine cancer. Cervical malignancy typically causes postcoital bleeding which may be accompanied by vaginal discomfort and abnormal vaginal discharge.

Diagnosis

The method of diagnosis is dependent on the suspected cause of bleeding. All patients should have blood counts, clotting screens, and renal function evaluated. Cystoscopy is the key investigation for suspected bladder carcinoma but it contributes very little to the management of haemorrhagic cystitis. All patients with haematuria should also have a renal and urinary tract ultrasound unless there is a clear precipitant, for example, recent cyclophosphamide therapy. If infective haemorrhagic cystitis is suspected, urine cultures are indicated.

Suspected endometrial carcinoma is diagnosed by hysteroscopy and endometrial biopsy. Cervical carcinoma is evident on cervical smear samples and colposcopy and endocervical biopsy. For evaluation of more widespread cervical or endometrial disease, pelvic MRI, positron emission tomography (PET) scan, or staging CT is appropriate.

Treatment

Treatment is dependent on the severity of genitourinary haemorrhage. Significant bleeding must be treated with fluids, blood transfusions, platelets, and clotting factors as required to stabilize the patient. Large volume frank haematuria and clot retention may be treated with three-way large-bore catheterization and irrigation. Intravenous hydration also helps to prevent clots reforming. If the haematuria persists, cystoscopy with diathermy of identified bleeding points may be helpful. Diffuse haemorrhage may be stopped by injecting intravesical therapy such as prostaglandins, alum, or 1% silver nitrate whilst closely monitoring renal function. Intravesical formalin is toxic and its use is reserved for severe haemorrhagic cystitis. Palliative radiotherapy may be effective in controlling bleeding from an advanced bladder or renal cancer. Intractable haematuria may require surgical intervention.

Prophylactic treatment to prevent haemorrhagic cystitis as a result of cyclophosphamide therapy is recommended. Mesna is a compound that binds the acrolein metabolite of cyclophosphamide and its related compounds, thus reducing their urotoxicity. It is routinely administered with cyclophosphamide therapy. Pentosan polysulfate sodium is also known to decrease the risk of haemorrhagic cystitis, though its mode of action is less clear.

Vaginal bleeding is usually less profuse and so can be conservatively managed. As with haematuria, all patients should have a blood counts, clotting screen, and evaluation of renal function. Treatment is often the definitive treatment of the underlying cause. Tranexamic acid (1g three times daily) and vaginal packing are useful adjunctive therapies. Bleeding in advanced disease where the aim is palliation may be treated with pelvic radiotherapy.

Gonadotropin-releasing hormone analogues, progestins, and the oral contraceptive pill can be used to decrease the severity of menorrhagia in premenopausal patients with significant thrombocytopenias and bleeding diatheses such as those undergoing intensive treatment for leukaemias.

15.19 Cardiorespiratory

Introduction
Cardiac arrest in a cancer patient may be an unexpected event related to potentially reversible causes or the end result of irreversible functional decline in the setting of extensively metastatic disease. There is no evidence to suggest that the pathophysiology and clinical features of cardiac arrest differ in the presence of malignancy and the diagnostic and treatment algorithms are the same as for the general population. Overall survival-to-discharge rates for hospitalized patients with cancer who undergo cardiopulmonary resuscitation are comparable to those of unselected hospitalized patients.

Decision not to resuscitate
Whereas resuscitation may be appropriate in the presence of a reversible precipitant, it is clearly inappropriate in many patients with end-stage disease. Careful and sensitive discussion of end-of-life issues with patients and their families and timely institution of 'do not attempt resuscitation' (DNAR) orders can help prevent inappropriate interventions at the terminal disease phase.

15.20 Cardiac tamponade

Introduction
Pericardial involvement by the tumour is the commonest cause of effusion and tamponade. However, other causes include acute inflammatory or chronic effusive post-radiotherapy pericarditis and drug toxicity. Chemotherapeutic agents that are known to cause pericarditis, and occasionally tamponade, include the anthracyclines, bleomycin, cyclophosphamide, cytarabine, and all-transretinoic acid (ATRA).

Clinical features
Malignant pericardial effusion almost always occurs in the setting of previously diagnosed advanced malignancy. The presence of pericardial effusion may be associated with relatively non-specific symptoms of dyspnoea, cough, chest pain, and oedema. The development of tamponade depends to a great extent on the rate of accumulation of pericardial fluid and the underlying cardiac function; large volumes of pericardial fluid can be tolerated if the rate of accumulation is slow.

Tamponade presents with the clinical features of cardiogenic shock:
- Dyspnoea
- Orthopnoea
- Excessive sweating (diaphoresis)
- Low blood pressure
- Tachycardia
- Signs of low cardiac output (peripheral vasoconstriction, clammy extremities, and poor capillary refill)
- The neck veins are distended, cardiac sounds are muffled, and there is pulsus paradoxus

Diagnosis
A pericardial effusion in an asymptomatic patient can be detected on chest radiograph as an enlarged globular cardiac silhouette. Asymptomatic effusions are also commonly visualized on routine CT scans.

In tamponade, the electrocardiogram usually shows low voltage complexes and electrical alterans but these findings lack sensitivity and specificity. The investigation of choice is two-dimensional echocardiography to confirm the presence of pericardial fluid and its haemodynamic effects. This should be done as an emergency, within minutes, as tamponade causing cardiogenic shock can be rapidly fatal.

Treatment
Medical management
Emergency bedside pericardiocentesis, preferably under echocardiographic guidance, can be life-saving when patients are acutely haemodynamically compromised. Under local anaesthaetic, a needle is inserted at either side of the xiphoid process, at a 45° angle, aiming towards the left scapula. Removal of as little as 50ml of pericardial fluid can result in haemodynamic improvement.

Surgical management
Simple pericardiocentesis is associated with very high recurrence rates and, therefore, definitive surgical management is indicated. Various surgical techniques, such as partial pericardiectomy or 'pericardial window', percutaneous balloon pericardiostomy, and pericardial sclerotherapy, have been described. However, the procedure of choice appears to be subxiphoid pericardiostomy. A review of the clinical experience with this technique showed very low procedural morbidity and mortality with a pericardial effusion recurrence rate of 3.5%.

Further reading
Refaat MM, Katz WE. Neoplastic pericardial effusion. *Clin Cardiol* 2011; 34(10):593–8.

15.21 Pleural effusion

Introduction

Malignant pleural effusion (MPE) is common in advanced malignancy and can be the initial manifestation of cancer in 10–50% of cases. The commonest primary sites include lung (35%), breast (25%), lymphoma (10%), and ovary (either malignant or reactive as in the case of ovarian fibroma—Meig's syndrome). Malignant pleural mesothelioma (MPM) is accompanied by MPE in up to 90% of cases. MPE of unknown primary accounts for approximately 10% of cases.

Clinical features

Dyspnoea is the commonest presenting symptom, followed by cough and pleuritic chest pain. Up to 25% of patients are asymptomatic on presentation, the pleural effusion being an incidental finding on physical examination or the chest radiograph.

Physical findings include decreased expansion and breath sounds in the affected hemithorax with diminution of vocal resonance and tactile fremitus. Mediastinal structure displacement towards the contralateral side can occur with massive effusions, unless there is associated pulmonary collapse.

Diagnosis

CT of the chest can identify fluid loculations and associated parenchymal masses as well as mediastinal or hilar lymphadenopathy. Subsequent interventions, as detailed here, usually aim at both diagnosing the cause of the effusion and providing symptomatic relief.

Thoracentesis is usually the first diagnostic procedure. Typically, MPEs fulfil Light's criteria for an exudate (fluid to serum protein ratio >0.5, fluid to serum LDH ratio >0.6, and fluid LDH level >2/3 the upper limit of normal serum values). Frequently the fluid is haemorrhagic or blood-tinged and in up to one-third of cases acidic; the latter is associated with poorer prognosis. As much fluid as possible should be sent for cytological examination. Initial cytology is positive in approximately 50% of MPEs.

If initial cytology is negative, further diagnostic options include either repeat thoracentesis or thoracoscopy. Video-assisted thoracoscopic surgery (VATS) has a diagnostic yield that approaches 100% in malignant pleural involvement.

Treatment

The management of MPE depends on the fitness of the patient and the overall disease prognosis, with lung primaries or mesothelioma being associated with worse outcomes than breast or ovarian primaries.

Observation is a reasonable treatment strategy for patients who are asymptomatic or if there is no recurrence of the MPE following initial thoracentesis. Chemotherapy for sensitive tumours such as lymphomas or breast or ovarian carcinomas can result in resolution of the MPE; repeated thoracentesis may be required until satisfactory disease response occurs.

Patients with very poor life expectancy can be managed by repeated thoracentesis alone. It must be noted though, that the one-month recurrence rate after aspiration alone approaches 100%.

For the majority of patients, however, definitive management of the MPE is required. Intercostal tube insertion, under ultrasound guidance, is the recommended initial procedure. There is randomized evidence that small-bore (10–14F) tube insertion is as effective as traditional large-bore tubes and is associated with less patient discomfort. Following intercostal tube insertion, drainage of pleural fluid should proceed in a controlled fashion, approximately 500ml/hour, to minimize the risk of re-expansion pulmonary oedema. Once the effusion is drained and lung re-expansion is confirmed, pleurodesis should be performed. Even if only partial pleural apposition can be achieved, an attempt at pleurodesis is still worthwhile. Talc, administered as a slurry through the chest tube, is more effective and less expensive than bleomycin and is usually preferred. As an alternative to intercostal tube insertion, thoracoscopy with talc poudrage insufflation can be used. An advantage of thoracoscopy is the ability to directly inspect the pleural cavity and perform targeted biopsies.

If lung re-expansion does not occur following drainage, the preferred option is usually insertion of an indwelling pleural catheter (IPC). This provides symptomatic relief in >90% of patients and obviates the need for repeated hospital attendances for aspiration. In rare cases, other surgical procedures such as pleuroperitoneal shunting or pleurectomy/decortication can be attempted; the latter can form part of multimodality MPM management.

Further reading

Davies HE, Davies RJ, Davies CW. Management of pleural infection in adults: British Thoracic Society Pleural Disease Guideline 2010. *Thorax* 2010; 65(Suppl. 2):ii41–53.

15.22 Brain metastases and raised intracranial pressure

Introduction

Both primary and metastatic malignancies can cause raised intracranial pressure (ICP). Metastases are a much more common cause of brain lesions causing raised ICP than primary brain tumours, usually astrocytomas. Lung cancer is the most common cancer to metastasize to the brain, closely followed by melanoma, renal cell carcinoma, and breast cancer. Eighty-five per cent of metastases are to the cerebrum and are often located at the watershed between the white and grey matter as a result of haematogenous spread. In some cases, cerebral metastases are the first sign of disseminated malignancy of unknown primary.

Clinical features

The classic description is of a headache that is worse in the morning and on performing the Valsalva manoeuvre. This may be accompanied by nausea and vomiting, also more common in the morning. The subtle development of intracranial malignancy, however, means that only about half of patients report headaches as a presenting symptom. Other generalized symptoms include lethargy, weight loss, confusion, and seizures. Focal neurological signs such as gait disturbance, motor weakness, diplopia, and personality changes may develop depending on the site of the malignancy. Diplopia can be due to focal neural compression or a false localizing sign of cranial nerve VI palsy.

Diagnosis

The most sensitive and specific imaging modality for cerebral malignancy with or without raised ICP is MRI. Contrast-enhanced, fluid-attenuated inversion recovery (FLAIR), and diffusion-weighted sequences aid in lesion characterization. CT, even with contrast, is less sensitive, especially for posterior fossa lesions.

If the intracerebral lesion is the first manifestation of malignancy, further staging, typically with a CT of the thorax, abdomen, and pelvis is necessary. In some cases, stereotactic biopsy of the brain lesion may be necessary to establish a diagnosis.

Treatment

Initial treatment is dexamethasone, 8-16mg/day, unless a primary brain lymphoma is suspected. Hypertonic saline or mannitol can be used in steroid-refractory raised ICP and in some cases emergency neurosurgery, usually for shunt placement, is needed. In patients presenting with seizures, a non-enzyme inducing anti-epileptic such as levetiracetam or sodium valproate is indicated.

Definitive treatment depends on the extent of intra- and extracranial disease and the patient's fitness status and response to steroids. For patients with a limited number of brain metastases, relatively small volume extracranial disease, available systemic treatment options, and good performance status, focal therapy should be considered. This may take the form of surgical excision or stereotactic radiotherapy (SRS). The role of whole brain radiotherapy (WBRT) as an adjunct to focal therapy is still a matter of debate. WBRT improves local control and decreases the risk of neurological death; however, it contributes to cognitive dysfunction and it does not have any significant impact on overall survival (OS).

Patients unsuitable for focal therapy are most commonly treated with WBRT which improves symptoms and modestly prolongs OS. Standard doses are either 30Gy in ten fractions or 20Gy in five fractions. Higher doses or more prolonged regimens have not shown superior effects on OS, neurological impairment, or symptom control. The addition of an SRS boost after WBRT may improve local control and OS for patients with a single lesion. However, with the move towards a preference for focal therapy first, a strategy of WBRT with SRS boost is becoming less appealing.

Prognosis

Metastatic cerebral disease often occurs in the setting of disseminated malignancy and untreated brain metastases give a median OS of one to two months. Studies in the era of WBRT alone reported median OS of six to eight months whereas oligometastatic lesions that are amenable to surgery or SRS have a slightly better prognosis with a median OS of 10–16 months.

15.23 Spinal cord compression

Introduction

Malignant spinal cord compression (MSCC) is a well-recognized oncological emergency. It is estimated to occur in 2.5–6% of patients with malignancy. Nearly two-thirds of cases are due to breast, lung, and prostate cancer. Rarer malignancies with relatively high rates of MSCC include melanoma, lymphoma, multiple myeloma, and renal and thyroid cancers. Most cases of MSCC are due to vertebral body metastases, most commonly in the thoracic spine, followed by the lumbar and cervical segments. Indirect venous or arterial obstruction by malignancy can also result in compression from the resulting cord oedema. More than 80% of patients with metastases to the spine have lesions that involve more than one vertebral body.

Diagnosis

Localized vertebral or radicular pain is a presenting symptom of spinal cord compression in >90% of cases. This pain is not from the cord compression per se but rather from involvement of the vertebral structures and nerve roots at the level of compression. Other common symptoms are gait disturbance, sphincter disturbance, and motor weakness. Physical signs of neuronal compression such as spastic paraparesis and a sensory level may be present. Compression of the cauda equina at the lower lumbar spine may present with only subtle lower motor neurone signs, perineal sensory changes, and sphincter dysfunction. Permanent neurological dysfunction may quickly develop once symptoms of MSCC become obvious. Therefore, it is important to maintain a high index of suspicion for MSCC in oncology patients with back pain and any neurological symptoms. Eighty per cent of cases are in patients already diagnosed with malignancy. There may be compression simultaneously at several levels from multiple metastatic deposits.

Urgent MRI of the whole spine, performed within 24 hours of presentation, is the modality of choice for detecting spinal cord or cauda equina compression. If this is contraindicated or unavailable, CT myelography is an alternative.

Treatment

The presence of neurological signs raising suspicion of MSCC should prompt initiation of corticosteroid treatment even before the MRI scan results become available. Dexamethasone, at a typical dose of 16mg/day in divided doses, is the steroid of choice.

Definitive treatment of MSCC is with either spinal surgery or radiotherapy and all patients should have access to spinal specialists so that appropriate treatment is given without delay. The choice of intervention depends on the patient's frailty, extent of metastatic disease, and systemic treatment options. Emergency transfer to neurosurgical or radiotherapy centres of very frail patients or those with complete para- or tetraplegia lasting >24 hours is generally not appropriate. All other patients with suspected or confirmed MSCC should have access to definitive treatment before they lose the ability to walk, ideally within 24 hours of presentation. Neurosurgical decompression with spine stabilization has been reported to result in improved functional outcomes for selected patients. Ideal candidates for neurosurgery are patients with good performance status, life expectancy >3 months, residual distal motor and sensory function,

and a single level of compression. Additionally, neurosurgery should be considered in cases of mechanical spine instability. In patients with complete paralysis lasting >24 hours, neurosurgery is usually indicated only for spinal instability causing intractable pain.

Patients not suitable for neurosurgery should be offered radiotherapy (8Gy single or 20Gy in five fractions). Postoperative fractionated radiotherapy should also be offered to patients undergoing surgery for their MSCC, except very frail patients with limited life expectancy and those with complete paralysis lasting >24 hours and no pain.

Following definitive treatment, gradual mobilization guided by pain and neurological deficits, rehabilitation, and gradual tapering of dexamethasone should be instituted.

Prognosis

Development of spinal cord compression confers a poor prognosis, with a median OS of three months irrespective of therapy. Factors that influence outcome include rate of symptom development, neurological impairment at diagnosis, tumour type, availability of systemic treatment options, and response to therapy.

Further reading

Loblaw DA, Mitera G, Ford M, Laperriere NJ. A 2011 updated systematic review and clinical practice guideline for the management of malignant extradural spinal cord compression. *Int J Radiat Oncol Biol Phys* 2012; 84(2):312–17.

15.24 Impending and pathological fractures

Introduction

Metastatic disease in the bones could lead to pathological fracture. Once >50% of the cortex has been destroyed, there is an 80% chance of pathological fracture especially if the lesion is lytic and in a weight-bearing bone. Although long bone metastases are more consequential clinically, the commonest sites of pathological fracture are the ribs and the vertebrae.

The solid cancers that metastasize to bone most commonly are breast and prostate cancer. Renal, thyroid, and lung cancers also commonly present with skeletal disease. Lytic skeletal destruction is common in myeloma. Bone pain or pathological fracture may be the presenting feature of bone sarcomas.

Clinical features

Both impending and completed pathological fractures may present with bone pain at the involved site. A number of pain and neurological syndromes may also occur depending on the site of cortical destruction; for example, cranial nerve palsies, neuralgia, and headache may occur secondary to base of skull metastases.

Vertebral pathological fractures may present with symptoms of spinal cord or conus medullaris compression as well as with pain. Spinal metastases are most common in the thoracic region, followed by the lumbar region, with cervical spine involvement being uncommon. Bone pain over the site of the fracture is also very common and is characteristically worse at night or with manoeuvres that increase intradural pressure, such as coughing.

Diagnosis

The likelihood of pathological fracture increases with the amount of cortical destruction. Plain radiographs of the affected bone can aid diagnosis of a metastatic deposit but alone are an unreliable guide to the probability of pathological fracture or to indicate optimal timing of intervention. Various scoring systems have been developed to aid patient selection for prophylactic intervention; the one used most commonly is that published by Mirels (Table 15.24.1) which encompasses the site and type of lesion, the severity of symptoms, and the maximum degree of cortical damage on plain radiographs.

Table 15.24.1 Mirels' scoring system for metastatic bone disease

Variable	Score		
	1	2	3
Site	Upper limb	Lower limb	Peritrochanteric
Pain	Mild	Moderate	Functional
Lesion	Blastic	Mixed	Lytic
Size*	<1/3	1/3–2/3	>2/3

*Indicates maximal cortical destruction as seen on plain X-ray in any view.

Reproduced with permission from Mirels, H. Metastatic Disease in Long Bones A Proposed Scoring System for Diagnosing Impending Pathologic Fractures. *Clin Orthopaed Related Res* 1989; 249:256–64. Copyright © 1989, Wolters Kluwer Health, Inc.

Treatment

The management of patients with impending or completed pathological fractures requires multidisciplinary input. In particular the abnormal local bone environment and its effects on healing, the extent of other metastatic involvement, and the likely life expectancy of the patient need to be taken into account.

The union rate for pathological long bone fractures may be <35% and healing, when it occurs, is often delayed. Therefore, prediction of impending long bone fractures and rigid fixation are particularly important. Patients with a Mirels score of 8 should be referred for prophylactic fixation. This may be even more pertinent for patients with primary tumours that are radioresistant, (e.g. renal cell carcinoma) and for patients with primary tumours typically associated with a prolonged survival when there are only bone metastases such as breast or prostate cancer. The extent of orthopaedic intervention (e.g. joint replacement and arthroplasty or nailing only) is typically determined by patient comorbidities and life expectancy. When a bone sarcoma is suspected as the cause of a pathological fracture, discussion with or referral to an experienced sarcoma centre before intervention is of paramount importance.

Spinal surgery to repair pathological fractures, stabilize the spine, and restore neurological function in spinal cord compression has been shown to affect morbidity dramatically, but no trial has yet reliably shown it to be better than radiotherapy. Surgery is recommended as the preferred initial approach in patients with a single level of cord compression and limited skeletal metastases in the spine. Other factors favouring a surgical approach are neurological deficit of <24 hours, duration, radioresistant histology, progressive neurological deficit despite radiotherapy, spinal instability secondary to fracture, and life expectancy of >3 months.

In recent years, balloon kyphoplasty and vertebroplasty have been increasingly used to treat painful vertebral fractures in a minimally invasive fashion. Although significant pain improvement has been consistently reported, the place of such techniques in relation to surgery and radiotherapy is a subject of ongoing debate.

External beam radiotherapy used as single fraction of 8Gy remains the option when surgey is not an option. Radiotherapy is also commonly used as an adjunct to or instead of surgery in impending or completed fractures; 20–30Gy in five to ten fractions are usually administered. Stereotactic radiotherapy and bone seeking radionuclides may be used in oligometastatic disease and prostate cancer respectively.

Prevention of further skeletal events is important. Many trials have shown significant improvement in morbidity with long-term bisphosphonate therapy, although few studies have evaluated the usefulness of bisphosphonates for metastatic cancers other than multiple myeloma, breast, and prostate cancer. Zolendronic acid is generally considered equally effective as pamidronate and has the advantage of a shorter infusion time. Ibandronate is also being studied as an alternative. There are no clear data to indicate when it is best to initiate bisphosphonate treatment, the most appropriate intervals between treatments, and the duration of treatment. Denosumab, a RANKL-targeting monoclonal antibody has recently been shown to be more effective than zolendronic acid in preventing skeletal-related events (pathological fractures, need for radiotherapy, cord compression) in patients with solid tumours and is rapidly replacing bisphosphonates as the treatment of choice.

Further reading

Coleman R. Clinical features of metastatic bone disease and risk of skeletal morbidity. *Clin Cancer Res* 2006; 12(20 Pt 2):6243s–9s.

Mirels H. Metastatic disease in long bones. A proposed scoring system for diagnosing impending pathologic fractures. *Clin Orthop Relat Res* 1989 Dec; 249:256–64.

Scolaro JA, Lackman RD. Surgical management of metastatic long bone fractures: principles and techniques. *J Am Acad Orthop Surg* 2014; 22(2):90–100.

15.25 Immunotherapy-related emergencies

Introduction

Patients receiving antibodies targeting cytotoxic T-lymphocyte-associated protein 4 (CTLA4) (ipilimumab), programmed cell death protein I (PD-1) (nivolumab and pembrolizumab), and programmed death ligands (PDLs) (collectively called immune checkpoint inhibitors) develop numerous toxicities, some of which will present as medical emergencies. Toxicities can be infusion reactions or immune-related adverse events (iRAEs). Prompt recognition of these complications is important. Principles of management include immediate cessation of the immunotherapy and treatment with immunosuppressants or immune modulating drugs. This following section summarizes common iRAEs.

Skin toxicity

Skin toxicity is the most common iRAE and occurs in up to 45% patients receiving ipilimumab and one-third receiving anti-PD-1. This is the first reaction to occur and in the majority of cases toxicity is minimal (grade 1–2), which does not require any treatment modification.

Grade 3–4 skin reaction occurs in 3–5% of patients. A grading of skin toxicity is:

- Grade 1: macules or papules involving <10% of body surface area (BSA)
- Grade 2: macules or papules involving 10–30% of BSA; limiting instrumental activities of daily living
- Grade 3: macules or papules involving >30% of body surface area; limiting self-care
- Grade 4: papulopustular rash with life-threatening superinfection; Stevens–Johnson syndrome, toxic epidermal necrolysis (TEN), and bullous dermatitis involving >30% of BSA and requiring intensive care

Treatment

- In patients with grade 3–4 toxicity, immunotherapy should be discontinued immediately.
- Supportive treatment includes topical emollients, potent topical steroids, and oral antihistamines.
- Patients with grade 3 reaction are started on oral prednisolone 0.5–1mg/kg daily once daily for three days followed by tapering over one to two months. If

reaction is severe, intravenous (methyl) prednisolone 0.5–1mg/kg may be an initial option followed by conversion to oral prednisolone.

- Patients with grade 4 reaction are admitted immediately and urgent dermatology review is sought. Specific treatment includes intravenous (methyl) prednisolone 1–2mg/kg daily which is tapered when skin reaction resolves to grade 1.

Gastrointestinal toxicity

Gastrointestinal toxicity is the second reaction to occur. It is common with anti-CTLA4 and less common with anti-PD-1 and antiPDL-1. It is the most common (25–50%) and most severe iRAE associated with anti-CTLA4. Symptoms can arise during or even several months after treatment with ipilimumab.

- Clinical symptoms include diarrhoea, abdominal pain, fever, vomiting, and mouth or anal ulcerations.
- Investigations include stool analysis to exclude infection and flexible sigmoidoscopy or colonoscopy with biopsy to confirm anti-CTLA4 induced enterocolitis.
- Patients with grade 1 (<4 liquid stools per day) toxicity persisting for >14 days or grade 2 (4–6 liquid stool per day or abdominal pain or haematochezia or nocturnal episodes) toxicity persisting for >3 days, should be started on non-enteric-coated prednisolone 0.5–1 mg even without endoscopic confirmation and anti-CTLA4 treatment discontinued.
- Patients with grade 3–4 toxicity (≥7 liquid stools per day or life threatening) need urgent hospital admission and isolation, until infection is ruled out. Patients should have gastroenterology consultation, endoscopic confirmation of diagnosis, and CT scan of abdomen and pelvis, if clinically indicated. Anti-CTLA4 should be discontinued and the patient started on intravenous (methyl) prednisolone 1–2mg/kg. If there is no improvement within 48 hours or worsening, patients should be considered for infliximab 5mg/kg, unless there are contraindications (perforation, hepatitis, sepsis, tuberculosis, etc). If there are persistent symptoms, patients may need a second dose of infliximab, a fortnight later.
- Steroid can be generally tapered over two to four weeks in grade 3 and four to eight weeks in grade 4 reaction.
- Patients treated with steroid or immunosuppressive drugs treatment for more than four weeks or with infliximab should be considered for pneumocystis prophylaxis.

Hepatotoxicity

Approximately 5–10% patients develop hepatoxicity with a single agent immunotherapy (1–2% grade 3) and 25–30% with a combination (15% grade ≥3). Hepatitis is often asymptomatic with biochemical changes only. If patients develop hepatitis during immunotherapy, other causes including medications and infections (bacterial and viral) should be ruled out. Liver biopsy is often helpful in deriving a diagnosis of immune-related-hepatitis. With appropriate treatment, hepatitis usually resolves within four to six weeks.

- In patients with prolonged grade 2 hepatitis, oral prednisolone 1mg/kg is given and when toxicity improves to grade 1, steroid is tapered and immunotherapy continued. However, if there is no improvement or

worsening, steroid dose should be increased to 2mg/kg and immunotherapy permanently discontinued.

- In grade 3–4 toxicity, immunotherapy is permanently discontinued and patients should be stated on methylprednisolone 1–2mg/kg. If there is no response within two to three days, mycophenolate mofetil 1,000mg twice daily is added and an opinion from hepatologist should be obtained. Third-line options of immunosuppressants are antithymocyte globulin and tacrolimus.

Endocrinopathies

Thyroid

- Even though both hypo- and hyperthyroidism can occur, patients seldom present as an emergency with grade 3–4 toxicity.
- Patients with hypothyroidism are treated with thyroid hormone replacement.
- In patients with symptomatic hyperthyroidism, immunotherapy should be temporarily withheld until recovery and treated with beta-blockers.

Hypophysitis

- Hypophysitis occurs with anti-CTLA4 alone or in combination with anti-PD-1/PDL-1.
- Patients presents with headache and visual disturbance due to an enlarged pituitary gland.
- MRI shows pituitary swelling or enlargement.
- Biochemically it is characterized by simultaneous decrease in the blood levels of thyroid stimulating hormone (TSH), ACTH, and/or follicle stimulating hormone/luteinizing hormone (FSH/LH).
- Immunotherapy is interrupted in all patients with grade ≥2 toxicity and hormone replacement treatment is started.
- Patients with severe headache and visual disturbance should be started on intravenous (methyl) prednisolone 1mg/kg after sending bloods for pituitary function tests. Patients with headache without visual symptoms are started on oral prednisolone 0.5–1mg/kg with a view to treat with intravenous steroid if there is no improvement within 48 hours.
- Most patients need life-long hormone replacement therapy.

Pneumonitis

Acute interstitial pneumonitis/diffuse alveolar damage syndrome is an acute life-threatening emergency. Pneumonitis is more common when anti-PD-1/PDL-1 agents are combined with anti-CTLA4 (incidence up to 30%). The median time of onset is 2.8 months. Pneumonitis is usually grade <2 (72%) and resolves after drug withholding or immunosuppressants. Radiological features include ground glass opacities and interstitial pneumonia-like pattern.

- Grade 1 (asymptomatic with radiological changes): consider delay of treatment and monitor symptoms.
- Grade 2 (new symptoms of dyspnoea, cough, or chest pain): withhold immunotherapy and if there is suspicion of infection antibiotics are started. If there is no infection or no improvement with antibiotics within 48 hours, start oral prednisolone 1mg/kg. If symptoms persist more than 72 hours after steroids, treat as grade 3–4.

Box 15.25.1 Summary of recommendations for immune-related toxicities

Immune-related skin toxicity
- For grade 1–2 skin AEs, continue (at least one week) with ICPis. Start topical emollients, antihistamines in the case of pruritus and/or topical (mild strength) corticosteroid creams. Reinitiate ICPi when ≤ grade 1.
- For grade 3 skin AEs, interrupt ICPi and start immediate treatment with topical emollients, antihistamines, and high strength corticosteroid creams.
- For grade 4 skin AEs, discontinue ICPi (permanently), consider admitting patient and always consult dermatologist immediately. Start i.v. corticosteroids (1–2 mg/kg (methyl)prednisone) and taper based on response of AE.

Immune-related endocrinopathies
- In symptomatic hyperthyroidism patients, usually grade 1 or 2, interrupt ICPi, start beta-blocker therapy (propranolol or atenolol/metoprolol). Restart ICPi when asymptomatic.
- In the case of hypothyroidism, rarely >grade 2, start HRT depending on the severity (50–100mcg/day). Increase the dose until TSH is normal. In the case of inflammation of the thyroid gland, start prednisone orally 1mg/kg. Taper based on recovery of clinical symptoms. Consider interruption of ICPi treatment when symptomatic.
- In the case of hypophysitis (rarely >grade 2), when headache, diplopia, or other neurological symptoms are present, start (methyl)prednisone 1mg/kg orally and taper over two to four weeks. Start HRT depending on the affected hormonal axis (levothyroxine, hydrocortisol, testosterone).
- In patients with type I DM grade 3–4 (ketoacidotic (sub)coma), admit to hospital immediately and start treatment of new-onset type I DM. Role of corticosteroids in preventing complete loss of insulin producing cells is unknown and not recommended.

Immune-related hepatotoxicity
- For grade 2 hepatitis, withhold ICPi and monitor AST/ALT levels closely (one to two times per week). When no improvement over one week, start (methyl)prednisone 0.5–1mg/kg. Taper over several weeks under close monitoring of AST/ALT and bilirubin.
- For grade 3 hepatitis, discontinue ICPi and immediately start with (methyl)prednisone 1–2mg/kg. When no improvement in two to three days, add MMF (1,000mg three times daily). Taper immunosuppression over four to six weeks under close monitoring of AST/ALT and bilirubin.
- For grade 4 hepatitis, permanently discontinue ICPi, admit patient to the hospital, and initiate (methyl)prednisone 2mg/kg i.v. Add MMF if no improvement is observed within two to three days. Consult hepatologist if no improvement under double immunosuppression. Other immunosuppressive drugs to consider are ATG and tacrolimus. Consult or refer patient to an experienced centre. Taper over six weeks under close monitoring of liver tests.

Gastrointestinal hepatotoxicity
- In patients with non-severe diarrhoea (grade 1), ICPi can be continued. Treatment with antidiarrhoeal medication (e.g. loperamide) should be prescribed.
- In grade 2 diarrhoea, ICPi should be interrupted and the patient should start with corticosteroids depending on the severity and other symptoms (either budesonide or oral corticosteroids 1mg/kg). In the case of no improvement within three to five days, colonoscopy should be carried out and, in the case of colitis, infliximab 5mg/kg should be administered.
- In patients with severe diarrhoea (grade 3–4), permanently discontinue ICPi. Admit patient to the hospital and initiate (methyl)prednisone 2mg/kg i.v. Add MMF if improvement is observed within two to three days. Consult a hepatologist if no improvement under double immunosuppression. Other immunosuppressive drugs to consider are ATG and tacrolimus. Consult or refer patient to an experienced centre. Taper over six weeks under close monitoring of liver tests.

Immune-related pneumonitis
- In grade 1 and 2 pneumonitis, interrupt ICPi therapy, try to rule out infection, and start with prednisone 1–2mg/kg orally. Taper over four to six weeks.
- In grade 3 and 4 pneumonitis, discontinue ICPi permanently, admit the patient to the hospital, even ICU if necessary, and immediately start high-dose (methyl)prednisone 2–4mg/kg i.v. Add infliximab, MMF, or cyclophosphamide in the case of deterioration under steroids. Taper over a period of four to six weeks.

Neurological toxicity
- In the case of mild neurological AEs, withhold ICPi and perform work-up (MRI scan, lumbar puncture) to define nature of neurotoxicity. In the case of deterioration or severe neurological symptoms, admit the patient and start (methyl)prednisone 1–2mg/kg orally or i.v. In the case of Guillain–Barre or myasthenia-like symptoms, consider adding plasmapheresis or i.v. Ig.

Cardiac toxicity
- When a myocarditis is suspected, admit the patient and immediately start high-dose (methyl)prednisone 1–2mg/kg. In the case of deterioration, consider adding another immunosuppressive drug (MMF or tacrolimus).

Rheumatological toxicity
- For mild arthralgia, start NSAIDs, and in the case of no improvement, consider low-dose steroids (10–20mg prednisone). In the case of severe polyarthritis, refer patient to or consult a rheumatologist and start prednisone 1mg/kg. Sometimes infliximab or another anti-TNFα drug is required for improvement of arthritis.

Renal toxicity
- In case of nephritis, rule out other causes of renal failure first. Interrupt or permanently discontinue ICPi depending on the severity of the renal insufficiency. Stop other nephrotoxic drugs. Start (methyl)prednisone 1–2mg/kg. Consider renal biopsy to confirm diagnosis.

AE adverse event; ALT alanine transaminase; AST aspartate transaminase; ATG antithymocyte globulin; DM diabetes mellitus; HRT hormone replacement therapy; ICPi immune checkpoint inhibitor; ICU intensive care unit; Ig immunoglobulin; i.v. intravenous; MMF mycophenolate mofetil; MRI magnetic resonance imaging; NSAID non-steroidal anti-inflammatory drug; TNFα tumour necrosis factor alpha; TSH thyroid-stimulating hormone.

- Grade 1–2: steroids tapered over four to six weeks and immunotherapy re-introduced when daily dose of steroid is equivalent of 10mg of oral prednisone or less.
- Grade 3–4 (severe new symptoms, new or worsening hypoxia, acute respiratory distress syndrome): immunotherapy permanently discontinued and admit patient for intravenous (methyl) prednisolone 2–4mg/kg, intravenous empirical antibiotics, respiratory review, high-resolution CT, and bronchoscopy. Bronchoscopy is indicated to rule out infection before starting steroids. However, if infection can not be assessed, empirical antibiotics should be started along with steroids.
- If grade 3–4 pneumonitis does not improve within 48 hours, add infliximab 5mg/kg or mycophenolate mofetil.

- With clinical improvement steroid can be tapered over six weeks or more.

Rare toxicities

Rarely immune-related neurological, ocular, cardiac, and rheumatological toxicities can occur. Prompt recognition of toxicities and assessment of severity are important. Discontinuation of immunotherapy and steroids are the first-line treatment. A summary of European Society of Medical Oncology (ESMO) recommendation for immune-related toxicities are in Box 15.25.1.

Further reading

Haanen JBAG, Carbonnel F, Robert C, et al. Management of toxicities from immunotherapy: ESMO Clinical Practice Guidelines for diagnosis, treatment and follow-up. *Ann Oncol* 2017; 28(suppl. 4):iv119–42.

Chapter 16

Special situations in oncology

Chapter contents

16.1 Teenage and young adult malignancies

Introduction
The importance of recognizing teenage and young adult (TYA), or adolescent and young adult (AYA) malignancies has now been recognized worldwide. The definition of the age range varies from 13–24 years in the UK, 15–39 in the USA, and combinations of ranges within the 13–39-year age range in other parts of the world. This group of malignancies present specific challenges in diagnosis, treatment, recruitment to clinical trials, and survival. In addition they have particular social, educational, developmental, and psychological needs which, if not addressed, have long-term consequences for the patient and their family.

As with paediatric malignancies, survivors of young adult cancers may also be left with significant medical late effects which need to be recognized and managed (see section 16.6, 'Late effects').

Traditionally these patients have been treated either within a paediatric or adult facility with little account taken of the type of tumour, e.g. a paediatric tumour in an adult, or developmental stage of the patient. These issues and how they may affect outcome are discussed here.

Incidence/epidemiology
The incidence of malignancy in the UK is:
- 14.4 per 100,000 in those 15–19
- 22.6 per 100,000 in those 20–24 (35.2 in USA)
- 54.7 per 100,000 in those 25–29 (USA)
- 83.3 per 100,000 in those 30–34 (USA)
- 128.9 per 100,000 in those 35–39 (USA)

Those aged 14–24 years account for 0.5% of all cancer registrations in the UK. In a study from the north west of England the incidence was 174 cases per million with a male to female ratio of 1.22:1. In the same study the incidence was found to be increasing, particularly for bone tumours, testicular tumours, thyroid cancer, and malignant melanoma. The incidence was also found to be increasing in those aged 15–39 in the SEER (Surveillance, Epidemiology, and End Results) studies (USA).

Cancer is the most frequent natural cause of death in this age group, second only to accidents.

The incidence of specific types of cancers also changes across this age group. In 15–19-year-olds the most frequent malignancies are lymphomas, leukaemias, and carcinomas (especially thyroid and nasopharyngeal). For the 20–24-year-olds lymphomas remained the most common malignancy but with carcinomas (especially cervix, thyroid, and breast) and germ cell tumours as next commonest. Osteosarcomas and germ cell tumours peak at this age. Beyond age 25 other adult cancers such as breast and colorectal become more frequent.

Aetiology
The median age of diagnosis of cancer in the general population is 70 years. The majority of those cancers are related to specific risk factors such as smoking. At the other end of the scale, the majority of paediatric malignancies are thought to be developmental in origin. TYA malignancies fall between these two extremes and may represent a late developmental malignancy or an early adult malignancy due to other factors such as genetic, although less than 5% are thought to be related to a genetic factor. Other environmental factors involved in some cancers such as HPV (human papilloma virus), EBV (Epstein–Barr virus), HIV (human immunodeficiency virus), and ultraviolet light.

The rise in melanoma in the 20–24-year-olds is also greatest in those from more affluent backgrounds, especially in the northern half of the UK. The suggestion is that those with fairer skin types with early sun exposure overseas are at an increased risk of development of melanoma in their 20s.

Clinical features
The clinical features in TYAs are similar to those seen in other age groups with the same malignancies but are often not recognized as such due to the rarity of TYA malignancy. This contributes to significant delays in diagnosis.

Diagnosis and delays
Diagnosis of TYA malignancy follows the pathways for other paediatric or adult cancers. This may mean referral to a paediatric centre or to an adult cancer specialist for a particular body site. Referrals may come from a general practitioner or via an emergency department. Studies have shown that these patients experience significant delays in diagnosis with a mean time from symptom to diagnosis of 16 weeks and a maximum of 192 weeks in one study. Delays in diagnosis were worse for those with no health insurance and varied according to type of malignancy (Martin et al. 2007). Delays were longest for thyroid cancer and sarcomas.

The reasons for delays in this age group include
- Rarity of TYA malignancy
- Lack of knowledge of specific rare TYA malignancies such as sarcomas
- Lack of education and awareness of patients and medical practitioners
- Possible embarrassment of young adults in discovering an abnormal lump, e.g. testicular or breast
- Lack of screening for some cancers that are screened at older ages such as cervix
- In some countries problems with lack of health insurance in this age group which falls between parental cover and adult cover as they are often in full-time education without health insurance

Clinical trials
Traditionally there is a high recruitment to clinical trials for children but trial recruitment is lowest in the adolescent and young adult population when compared with either children or older adults. This is partly due to the rarity of the cancers concerned but also to the fact that these patients are treated in a wide range of settings. Many fall between different groups of physicians who may not be able to provide available trials. There are now efforts to try to minimize this effect by extending the age of paediatric trials in tumours which occur in the young adult, e.g. sarcoma. One study reported the results of a study of TYA trial recruitment and the barriers to recruiting young adults. Their findings were supported by noting an increase in recruitment when trials were designed with this age group in mind (not limiting to under/over 16 or 18) followed by a fall when these trials closed and were not replaced with a follow on or alternative trial. Another way to improve trial recruitment is to establish a specific TYA team to ensure no trial is unavailable locally to a given TYA patient with an adult or paediatric malignancy.

Place of care

In the USA it has been suggested that all these patients be treated in a paediatric oncology hospital to standardize care as adolescents have a better outcome if treated in specialist units. It is recommended that a paediatric oncologist be involved in the discussion of the care of a young adult cancer patient. In the UK, the Teenage Cancer Trust has set up a series of specialist units across the country which help centralize care for this age group. The National Institute for Health and Clinical Excellence (NICE) has published a document giving guidance on the care of children and young adults to provide a focus for specialized care in the UK.

Psychological support

Young adults are at a vulnerable stage of development and treatment for cancer has been shown to have a detrimental long-term psychological impact in many patients. Over 90% report significant stress at some point in the treatment. Up to 15% report symptoms of post-traumatic stress disorder, which is also observed in the patients' mothers. Over the longer term there is an increased risk (although low for some) of many types of mental illness from depression to psychosis. Appropriate support should be offered to patients and their families to try to prevent some of these conditions occurring later on. This is also the age group where many psychiatric disorders first present so careful consideration to understanding all elements of a young person's mental health is essential.

Risk-taking behaviour is also at its greatest in this age group and can affect drug compliance as well as coping mechanisms. Medical professionals (psychologists, nurses, doctors, counsellors) with experience in communicating with and treatment of adolescents will help to reduce the adverse effects these may have.

Body image and fertility

Sexual identity and future fertility are important considerations for the young adult. Loss of hair or a limb will significantly affect body image at an age when this is especially significant. The type of cancer or its treatment may also affect future fertility but this is not universal so specific knowledge is required for each patient (see section 16.5, 'Fertility and cancer').

Education

The majority of TYA patients will be in full time education at the time of diagnosis. Taking a break from studying can add significantly to the psychological burden of cancer at this age. If treatment is lengthy or affects the ability to study in the longer term, this can also result in difficulties reintegrating into society or obtaining a job. TYA centres should be able to support young people to continue their education or consider an alternative if they are no longer able to cope with their previous studies or work. Providing them with life skills in educational or work placed reintegration is essential. Confidence is often lost as they go through treatment and there may be other long-lasting problems (e.g. fatigue, reduced short-term memory) that compound the difficulties. It is important to retain as much normality as possible during treatment and many young people prefer to focus on the educational challenge alongside their peers rather than on their cancer.

Late effects

Following the initial success of treating children's cancers in the 1980s it was subsequently realized that there were significant long-term effects from the treatment. These late effects are also important in the young adult who would expect to have many years of life ahead of them and are considered in section 16.6, 'Late effects'.

Clinical outcome

Survival in TYA cancers has improved over the past 30 years but not in line with improvements for children and older adults.

• Survival for all TYA malignancies overall from 1978–97 was 73% in a European study, which was comparable with the USA.
• Survival was higher in Northern Europe (78%) and lower in Eastern Europe (57%).

In a UK study the mortality rate was 23% higher for males compared with females. Mortality increased in all malignancies with increasing age from 13 to 29.

Trials are ongoing to examine whether these malignancies are better treated with adult, paediatric, or novel protocols. There is some evidence that treatment of acute lymphoblastic leukemia (ALL) with a paediatric protocol improves survival. For malignancies which are not as common as ALL it will take considerable time and multinational efforts to evaluate best practice in TYA cancers.

Transition

Patients in this age group are at a critical stage of development between childhood and independent adulthood. Their ongoing care necessitates an understanding of the transition between these stages. There must be clear communication between different medical teams and agreement about the future care and follow-up of an individual. This can be facilitated by multidisciplinary teams from paediatric, TYA, and adult services as well as joint clinics to facilitate knowledge and experience.

Terminal care and bereavement

Unfortunately, many young adults with cancer will not survive and this will have an enormous impact on their families and friends. Young people, like children, will often choose to spend their final days at home or in a non-hospital environment such as a hospice or teenage cancer unit. Family support at this time, as with the rest of the young adult's treatment, is essential. Liaison with community services is an important part of this process although it can be problematic as some services will consider them as children and others as adults. We need to advocate for their specific needs in a setting most appropriate for them and their families.

Further reading

Albritton K, Bleyer WA. The management of cancer in the older adolescent. *Eur J Cancer* 2003; 39:2584–99.

Bhatia S, Yasui Y, Robinson L, et al. High risk of second neoplasms continues with extended follow up of childhood Hodgkin's disease: report from the late effects study group. *J Clin Oncol* 2003; 21(23):4386–94.

Guidance on Cancer Services—Improving outcomes in Children and Young People with Cancer. August 2005. Available from www.nice.org.uk

Martin S, Ulrich C, Munsell M, et al. Delays in cancer diagnosis in underinsured young adults and older adolescents. *The Oncologist* 2007; 12:816–24.

Royal College of Physicians, Royal College of Radiologists, Royal College of Obstetricians and Gynaecologists. The effects of cancer treatment on reproductive functions: guidance on management. Report of a working party. November 2007.

16.2 Cancer in older people

Epidemiology
The incidence of cancer increases markedly with increasing age, with half of cancers in the UK arising in those aged >70 years. In the USA, 54% of cancer diagnoses and 70% of deaths from cancer occur in those aged >65. For a man aged 65, life expectancy is now 18.6 years, and for a woman 21.1 years so that long-term survival after successful cancer treatment may be obtained.

The most prevalent cancers in older adults are prostate, lung, colorectal, and breast. There is some evidence that the biology of certain cancers differs in older adults as compared with younger patients. For example, breast cancer diagnosed in older women is more likely to be lower grade and hormone receptor-positive compared with those in younger women. Conversely, thyroid cancer in older patients tends to be more aggressive and carry a worse prognosis. Access to treatment is often poorer in the elderly and treatment outcomes overall are significantly worse than in younger age groups. An increasing proportion of oncologists' practice is concerned with the management of elderly patients and it is important to recognize that this group of patients cannot be considered as a homogeneous group, as there are very wide variations in health and function between people of the same age.

Factors affecting access to treatment
Elderly patients are less likely than their younger counterparts to receive standard oncological treatment, a statistic that may only in part reflect appropriate selection for treatment. Many factors may be significant in determining whether elderly patients receive the same treatment as those in the younger age group.

It is known that fewer diagnoses are made and less treatment undertaken in the elderly group than in younger patients although there is no clear evidence that outcome of treatment is affected by age per se. Older patients are more likely to present at a more advanced stage, are less likely to be referred by primary care physicians, and are excluded from many screening programmes which have an upper age limit in the UK of 74 years.

Impaired mobility, lack of social support, and problems with transport may restrict access to hospital and must be taken into account particularly when the chosen management requires daily or frequent visits to hospital for treatment, monitoring, and assessment. Social support is of critical importance. As many as 30% or more elderly cancer patients may live alone, and up to 40% do not have children living near enough to help them.

It is important to recognize that in this population patient preferences regarding the acceptability of treatment may differ from those of clinicians. A study of mental attitudes in the elderly to cancer treatment have shown that some feel that treatment would not be worthwhile for them but that many are anxious to prolong good quality life for as long as possible.

Decision making in the elderly
As with younger patients, treatment decisions in the older oncology patient must balance the potential to benefit from treatment with potential harms of treatment. This is often a delicate balance particularly in an older population where comorbidities, poorer functional reserve, and competing risks on mortality may modify both the potential gains and costs of treatment.

A number of factors must be taken into account when determining the most appropriate management strategy remembering that there may be very considerable differences in treatment possibilities between patients of similar age.

Older patients continue to be under-represented in clinical trials and few trials specifically address optimum treatment strategies in older cancer patients. Between 2001 and 2011 <10% of patients enrolled onto National Cancer Institute (NCI) trials were aged >75 despite this age group making up almost one-third of cancer diagnoses. There is therefore a relatively poor evidence base on which to make decisions about cancer treatment in the elderly, with recommendations often based on a highly selected subgroup of older patients within existing trials (who are likely to be unrepresentative of those encountered in every day clinical practice) or extrapolation of the evidence base obtained for younger patient groups.

Factors affecting choice of treatment
Comorbidities
Whilst it is important to recognize that older oncology patients comprise a heterogeneous population, the likelihood of significant comorbidity such as hypertension, diabetes, or chronic kidney disease increases with increasing age. Cancer patients with comorbidities are at an increased risk of toxicity from treatment. Geriatric syndromes such as dementia, falls, osteoporosis, incontinence, and polypharmacy can also impact the ability to tolerate treatment. Polypharmacy is of particular relevance when considering systemic treatment, increasing the risk of drug interactions which have the potential to both reduce treatment efficacy and increase toxicity.

Even in the fit and healthy elderly patient, reduced organ function that occurs with ageing such as reduced renal function, reduced gastrointestinal (GI) motility, and increased ventricular stiffness may impact functional reserve. Vascular disease and diabetes can impair healing affecting recovery after surgery.

Patient selection
The Karnofsky/ECOG (Eastern Cooperative Oncology Group) scales for performance status (PS) alone are not sensitive enough tools to be useful in this patient group and are a poor reflection of physiological status and reserve. A Comprehensive Geriatric Assessment (CGA) is recommended by the International Society of Geriatric Oncology prior to making treatment decisions. This multidomain assessment considers functional status, fatigue, comorbidity, cognition, mental health status, social support, nutrition, and the presence of geriatric syndromes. Using such scales, treatment decisions can be made on the basis of physiological, functional, and psychosocial capabilities rather than chronological age. Models to predict the risk of chemotherapy related toxicity have been suggested (such as the Chemotherapy Risk Assessment Scale for High Age Patients (CRASH)); however these have yet to be validated on an individual patient basis.

Management of older oncology patients

There is good evidence that appropriately selected older patients can obtain the same benefits from standard treatment approaches as their younger counterparts with acceptable tolerability. Chronological age alone should not affect management approach.

Chemotherapy

There is no direct evidence that chemotherapy is less effective in the treatment of cancer than in younger patients. However, dose reductions which may be necessary due to toxicity and poor haemopoietic tolerance, may lead to reduced efficacy.

Alterations in drug metabolism, distribution and excretion, decreased bone marrow reserves, decreased activity of the CP450 liver enzymes, and decreased glomerular filtration rate may all contribute to increased chemotherapy toxicity seen in older patients. The Cockcroft formula (see Chapter 2, pp. 36, 46) which incorporates an age function may be used to estimate renal capacity and has been shown to provide a good estimation of glomerular filtration rate in elderly cancer patients. Polypharmacy may also alter the pharmacokinetic and pharmacodynamics of chemo-therapeutic agents and increase drug interactions and risk of adverse reactions.

Older patients are particularly susceptible to anthracycline toxicity due to comorbidities such as hypertension, diabetes mellitus, and impaired cardiac function.

Bleomycin lung toxicity is seen more frequently in the elderly and mucositis may be more marked. Elderly patients may also be more susceptible to complications from GI side effects such as vomiting and diarrhoea due to an increased risk of dehydration and renal impairment.

Appropriate supportive care during treatment and use of granulocyte colony stimulating factor (G-CSF) can help to maintain drug intensity. Alternative dosing schedules may be appropriate; for example weekly paclitaxel is associated with less grade 3 neuropathy and neutropenia compared with a three-weekly schedule in patients aged >75 years. Oral agents are often favoured by patients and they have the advantages of convenience and ease of administration. However, there is a risk of poor compliance particularly in the context of cognitive impairment and polypharmacy both of which are more likely with increasing age. Metronomic therapy may represent an attractive option in patients who are unsuitable for standard chemotherapy. Where single agent chemotherapy agents have shown a benefit, such as in the metastatic breast cancer setting, these regimens may represent a better tolerated option than combination regimens.

Targeted agents

Most of the evidence for the use of targeted agents in the elderly is extrapolated from larger trials in which older patients represent a small proportion of total participants. Whilst there is no evidence to suggest reduced benefit in older adults, greater toxicity is seen with targeted agents, mandating careful selection and monitoring for adverse effects. Specific risks of certain targeted agents become more pertinent in the older population, for example cardiac dysfunction for HER2 targeted agents, vascular risk factors for vascular endothelial growth factor (VEGF) inhibitors and diarrhoea with agents targeted at the epidermal growth factor receptor (EGFR) which may be less well tolerated in the elderly due to dehydration and consequent renal impairment.

Immunotherapy

Immunotherapy is being increasingly proven to improve clinical outcome patients with advanced malignancies. Even though there are concerns regarding immunosenescence and its impact on the efficacy and toxicities, there is no evidence that immunotherapy is either less effective or more toxic in elderly. A meta-analysis of nine randomized trials of check point inhibitors reported no difference in survival between those <65 years and those ≥65 years.

Surgery

With accurate selection of elderly patients and adequate perioperative care, outcomes following surgery are similar to those seen in younger patients. There is evidence that elderly patients who survive the first year after surgery have the same cancer-related survival as younger patients. Shortened recovery times following surgery, and improved healing rates may be achieved through the use of laparoscopic surgery which will also help to minimize the risk of complications such as venous thrombosis and embolism. CGA can help identify patients at risk of postoperative complications and increased length of stay.

Radiotherapy

The effect of the ageing process on normal tissue tolerance to radiation is unclear. In whole brain radiotherapy age is the most significant predictor of neurotoxicity.

Specific considerations relating to the ability of elderly patients to tolerate radiotherapy include co-morbidities such as Parkinson's disease that may make it difficult to maintain the precision of radiotherapy or osteoarthritis and kyphoscoliosis which may make maintaining treatment position difficult.

Treatment interruptions and incomplete treatment adversely affect radiotherapy outcomes. The increasing use of hypofractionated treatment regimens delivered over a shorter overall time period may help overcome the fatigue and difficulty with transport that may pose particular problems for the elderly with conventional fractionations. The use of increasingly conformal radiotherapy may reduce normal tissue side effects with particular benefit in this group. Single fraction radiotherapy treatment for palliation of troublesome symptoms is effective and generally well tolerated even in the frail elderly patient.

Management of common cancers in the elderly

Prostate cancer

Prostate cancer incidence increases with age with a median age at diagnosis of 66 years. Over half of new cases in the UK are diagnosed in men aged >70 years. A task force of the International Society of Geriatric Oncology (SIOG) has recently made the following recommendation for the management of prostate cancer in men aged >70 years:

General principles of management
- Fit patients should be managed similarly to younger patients.
- Initial assessment should include health status screening using the G8 tool followed by a further assessment depending on the score.

Management of localized (T1–3N0M0) disease
- Fit older men with a life expectancy >10 years should receive the same standard treatment as younger men.

- Patients with low to intermediate risk may benefit from active surveillance and watchful waiting.
- Radical prostatectomy: studies suggest well selected older men may benefit, as elderly patients generally have larger and higher-grade tumours. Minimally invasive surgery may be associated with higher postoperative complications compared with open surgery.
- External beam radiotherapy: hypofractionated regimens (20 fractions over four weeks) may be preferred. Addition of androgen deprivation therapy (ADT) does not benefit patients with high-risk disease and moderate to severe morbidities.
- Brachytherapy: survival benefit in older men is unknown.
- ADT alone may be considered in older men with co-morbidities precluding active treatment or life expectancy <10 years.

Management of advanced disease
- ADT with six cycles of docetaxel is the first-line treatment for advanced/metastatic disease in fit men. Consider evaluating bone mineral density prior to commencing long-term ADT. Intermittent ADT is an option in those with significant side effects from hormonal therapy.
- Abiraterone and enzulutamide are appropriate first-line treatment.
- Radium-223 is an option for patients who fail androgen receptor targeted agents and taxanes.

Colorectal cancer
The median age at diagnosis for colorectal cancer is 69 years, with peak incidence between 65 and 74 years. A summary of the SIOG recommendations for the management of colorectal cancer in patients >70 years of age is as follows:

Management of early disease
- Surgical management is similar to management of younger patients.
- Adjuvant chemotherapy: indications are the same as for younger patients in appropriate older patients. Fluorouracil (5-FU)/capecitabine monotherapy is recommended for patients aged >70 years in whom there is no clear benefit from the addition of oxaliplatin.

Management of metastatic disease
- Older patients with a good performance status gain a survival benefit from palliative chemotherapy.
- The addition of oxaliplatin or irinotecan to 5-FU/capecitabine improves response rates but does not improve progression-free survival (PFS) or overall survival (OS). Monotherapy should be considered particularly in older adults with poorer PS or comorbidities.
- The addition of bevazucimab to capecitabine improves survival in patients over 70 years, and is an alternative to combination chemotherapy with bevazucimab. The risk of arterial thromboembolic events may be increased in older age groups.
- Highly selected older patients included in clinical trials appear to derive the same benefit from cetuximab as younger patients in terms of PFS.

Breast cancer
A summary of the SIOG and European Society of Breast Cancer Specialists (EUSOMA) recommendations for the management of breast cancer in patients >70 years of age is as follows:

- There is no strong evidence to support routine screening in women older than 70 years.
- Surgical management should be similar management to younger patients.
- Radiotherapy treatment is similar to younger patients. Hypofractionated radiation regimens offer similar outcome.
- Primary endocrine treatment (tamoxifen or aromatase inhibitor) is the treatment option for frail individuals with localized oestrogen receptor (ER)-positive tumours who have a limited life expectancy (<2–3 years) and metastatic ER-positive disease.
- Adjuvant hormone therapy is similar to younger patients. Hormones may be omitted for patients with small tumours (pT1aN0) and significant comorbidities.
- Four cycles of anthracycline-based chemotherapy is the preferred option for node-positive, hormone-negative disease. Addition of taxanes for high-risk disease is considered individually based on weighing appropriate benefits and risks.
- For HER2 positive disease, adjuvant transtuzumab is considered if there are no cardiac contraindications.
- Patients with metastatic ER-negative or hormone-refractory disease are considered for single agent or combination oral chemotherapy. HER2 targeted therapy with or without chemotherapy is appropriate for HER2-positive ER-negative disease whereas in HER2-positive ER-positive disease, HER2 targeted therapy with endocrine treatment is appropriate.
- Elderly men with breast cancer should be treated using guidelines for postmenopausal breast cancer.

Non-small cell lung cancer (NSCLC)
The median age at diagnosis of NSCLC is 70 years. The following is a summary of principles of management of elderly with NSCLC.

Early stage disease
- Limited resections particularly video-assisted thoracoscopic surgery is appropriate. Pneumonectomy and systematic mediastinal lymphadenectomy are associated with higher mortality and therefore not recommended.
- Stereotactic ablative body radiotherapy is the preferred alternative to conventional radiotherapy for patients who are not fit for surgery
- For patients aged 70–80 years, the benefit of adjuvant chemotherapy is similar to younger patients and therefore should be offered to fit elderly. Benefit of adjuvant chemotherapy for patients over 80 years is not known.
- Adjuvant radiotherapy is not recommended as there is no clear benefit.

Locally advanced disease
- Radical chemoradiotherapy therapy is an option for fit patients with no significant comorbidities. Carboplatin based doublets are usually well tolerated. A randomized study showed that up to 12 months of anti-PD-L1 antibody durvalumab in patients without progression after chemoradiotherapy improved survival.
- Frail patients may be considered for palliative radiotherapy or single agent chemotherapy.

Advanced/metastatic disease
- Patients should have tumour assessment of somatic mutations (EGFR, ALK (anaplastic lymphoma kinase), BRAF) and for expression of PD-L1.
- EGFR-TKI are the first-line treatment for patients with EGFR mutated tumours.
- Patients with staining for PD-L1 in at least 50% of tumour cells, should be considered for pembrolizumab monotherapy or a combination of pembrolizumab with chemotherapy, if rapidly progressive disease. Patients with EGFR wild-type tumours and <50% PD-L1 expression on tumour cells are considered for carboplatin based doublets if fit, or single agent chemotherapy.

Conclusion

Treatment in this age group must be individualized on the basis of information about the likely biological behaviour of the tumour, taking account of the available treatments and any comorbid factors in the patient which would alter the cost–benefit ratio. In particular, attention should be paid to conducting trials of new agents and approaches which do not exclude this group in which cancer is commonest. Particular attention should be paid to prevention and early diagnosis of disease so that simpler treatment approaches such as limited surgery may be used.

Further reading

Balducci L, Colloca G, Cesari M, et al. Assessment and treatment of elderly patients with cancer. *Surg Oncol* 2010; 19:117–23.

Biganzoli L, Lichtman S, Michel JP, et al. Oral single agent chemotherapy in older patients with solid tumours: A position paper from the International Society of Geriatric Oncology (SIOG). *Eur J Cancer* 2015; 51(17):2491–500.

Biganzoli L, Wildiers H, Oakman C et al. Management of elderly patients with breast cancer: updated recommendations of the International Society of Geriatric Oncology (SIOG) and European Society of Breast Cancer Specialists (EUSOMA). *Lancet Oncol* 2012; 13(4):148–60.

Droz J, Albrand G, Gillessen S, et al. Management of prostate cancer in elderly patients: recommendation of a task force of the International Society of Geriatric Oncology. *Eur Urol* 2017—available at: http://dx.doi.org/10.1016/j.eururo.2016.12.025

Elias R, Giobbie-Hurder A, McCleary NJ, Ott P, Hodi FS, Rahma O. Efficacy of PD-1 and PD-L1 inhibitors in older adults: a meta-analysis. *J Immunother Cancer* 2018 April 4; 6(1):26.

Gajra A, Jatoi A. Non small cell lung cancer in elderly patients: a discussion of treatment options. *J Clin Oncol* 2014; 24:2562–9.

Kelly CM, Poer DG, Lichtman SM. Targeted therapy in older patients with solid tumours. *J Clin Oncol* 2014; 32(24):235–46.

Korc-Grodzicki B, Downey R, Shahrokni A, et al. Surgical considerations in older adults with cancer. *J Clin Oncol* 2014; 32(24):2647–53.

McCleary N, Dotan E, Browner I. Refining the chemotherapy approach for older patients with colon cancer. *J Clin Oncol* 2014; 32(24):2570–80.

Naeim A, Aapro M, Subbarao R, et al. Supportive care considerations for older adults with cancer. *J Clin Oncol* 2014; 32(24):2627–34.

Pallis A, Gridelli C, Wedding E, et al. Management of elderly patients with NSCLC; updated expert's opinion paper: EORTC elderly task force, lung cancer group and international society for geriatric oncology. *Ann Oncol* 2014; 25(7):1270–83.

Papamichael D, Audisio R, Glimelius B, et al. Treatment of colorectal cancer in older patietns: International Society of Geriatric Oncology (SIOG) consensus recommendations 2013. *Ann Oncol* 2015; 26(3):463–76.

Smith G, Smith B. Radiation treatment in older patients: a framework for clinical decision making. *J Clin Oncol* 2014; 201(24):2669–78.

Wildiers H, Heeren P, Puts M. International Society of Geriatric Oncology consensus on geriatric assessment in older patients with cancer. *J Clin Oncol* 2014; 32(24):2595–603.

Internet resources

International Society of Geriatric Oncology: http://www.siog.org

National Comprehensive Cancer Network: http://www.nccn.org

16.3 Cancer in pregnant women

Epidemiology

The incidence of pregnancy-associated cancer is low, complicating 1:1,000 gestations. However the tendency to delay pregnancy to later reproductive age, as well as the age-dependent increase in the incidence of malignancy, are likely to result in higher incidences of gestational cancer in the next decades. Cancer is the second leading cause of death among women of reproductive age in Western countries. The diagnosis of cancer during pregnancy poses challenging dilemmas for patient, family, and physicians. Invasive carcinomas of the uterine cervix, breast, and melanomas are the malignancies most commonly encountered during pregnancy, followed by lymphomas, leukaemias, genitourinary, and GI tract cancers (Table 16.3.1).

The parameters that modulate the risk of development of cancer during pregnancy are the genetic and environmental factors that define the risk of cancer in the age-matched general population. Hallmarks of pregnancy-associated cancer that are distinct from cancer affecting non-pregnant women are:

- Earlier diagnosis of cervical cancer due to frequent gynaecological examinations, and later diagnosis of most other solid tumours, mostly due to symptom/sign misinterpretation as physiological changes due to pregnancy. Frequent occurrence of poorly differentiated, hormone receptor negative, HER2-overexpressing

Table 16.3.1 Cancer incidence in pregnancy

Malignancy	Incidence per 100,000 pregnancies
Cervical cancer	10–1,000
Breast cancer	10–40
Melanoma	15–100
Lymphomas	10–50
Leukaemias	1–2
Gastrointestinal cancer	5–10
Ovarian cancer	1–10

breast adenocarcinomas, occasionally with genetic background (BRCA1/2 mutations).
- Predominance of high-grade histology among gestational lymphomas.
- Uncommon metastatic spread seen for some malignancies (lymphomas, GI tract cancer).
- Predominance of rectal primaries in gestational colorectal cancer.

Interaction of pregnancy with cancer

Most available data show that pregnancy causes a diagnostic delay of three to seven months, resulting in presentation of cancer at more advanced stages. However, pregnancy has not been associated with adverse maternal prognosis in comparison to non-pregnant patients when matched for stage and age. Only a few gestational melanoma series pointed to decreased maternal survival. Accordingly, current evidence does not establish a significant detrimental effect of pregnancy on the prognosis of cancer patients.

The impact of cancer on pregnancy varies with the stage, site, and bulk of tumour. Published cases show that birth of healthy infants is achieved in three-quarters of patients, with a small increase in the rate of still birth, low birth weight, premature delivery, and myelosuppression. Absolute indication for chemotherapy/abdominal radiotherapy administration during the first trimester, poor maternal life expectancy, poor maternal general condition due to metastatic disease, or presence of locally advanced invasive cervical cancer usually necessitate pregnancy termination and antineoplastic therapy. Metastases to placenta and foetus are extremely rare; malignant melanoma, cancer of unknown primary, lung cancer, and breast cancer being the tumours most often responsible. Placental histological examination should always be done and if there is placental involvement, neonates should be considered high risk and be carefully monitored.

Modifications of investigations and treatment

Physical examination, including examination of the pelvis, rectum, skin, breasts, and lymph nodes, should be thorough. Most biopsy or cytological procedures can be safely performed during pregnancy under local anaesthesia, though the histopathologist should be informed about the presence of pregnancy to avoid false positive results. Foetal radiation exposure at doses >10–20cGy should be avoided, especially during the first trimester (organogenesis) and second trimester (continuing development of eyes, teeth, brain). Estimated foetal average doses per radiographic examinations are shown in Table 16.3.2. Radiographic and staging procedures should offer all necessary and relevant information for

Table 16.3.2 Estimated average foetal dose (mGy) per radiographic examination

Chest X-ray	<0.005
Abdominal/pelvic X-ray	2–2.5
Chest CT	0.2
Abdominal CT	20
Mammography	0.1–1
Thoracic spine X-ray	0.1

assigning a treatment plan while minimizing the risk of untoward effects for mother and foetus. Chest X-ray (CXR) and ultrasound of thorax, abdomen/pelvis, and breasts are safe to perform. Magnetic resonance imaging (MRI) of the brain, or abdomen/pelvis is both sensitive and safe, though gadolinium enhancement should be avoided during the first trimester. Radioisotope scans, abdominopelvic computed tomography (CT)) and 18-FDG-PET (18-fluorodeoxyglucose-positron emission tomography) scans should be avoided. With modern surgical and anaesthetic techniques, surgery can be safely performed throughout pregnancy, with only a slightly increased risk of foetal loss (3–10%) seen for abdominal operations during the first trimester. Oesophagogastroscopy, bronchoscopy, lumbar puncture, and bone marrow aspiration/biopsy are quite safe and should be done when clinically indicated, with appropriate caution to avoid excessive use of intravenous sedatives and opioid drugs. Pulse oximetry monitoring should be implemented to avoid maternal/foetal hypoxia.

Radiation exposure during organogenesis (weeks 2–8) can cause abortion or congenital malformations at a threshold dose of 10cGy, while doses above 10–20cGy during weeks 8–25 may result in mental retardation. Moreover, prenatal radiation has been linked to second tumours during childhood or later adult life. However, radiation therapy is not absolutely contraindicated during pregnancy, if the distance of radiation fields from the uterus is such as to keep foetal exposure below 10–20cGy (e.g. of head, neck, extremities, and chest). This is especially true with appropriate medical/medical physics expertise, or after the 25th week of pregnancy.

Pharmacokinetic effects of pregnancy on cytotoxic drugs are not known, but administration of chemotherapy seems to be feasible after the first trimester. Chemotherapy during the first trimester has been associated with a 17–25% risk of malformations or foetal death and should be avoided. Absolute indication for chemotherapeutic treatment during the first trimester usually necessitates pregnancy termination. Antimetabolites and alkylators seem to have the most potent teratogenic effect, while vinca alkaloids, anthracyclines, and cyclophosphamide have been less often incriminated in causing malformations. Chemotherapy may be administered during the second and third trimesters relatively safely, with a 5–7% incidence of intrauterine growth retardation, premature delivery, or myelosuppression and a 3–5% incidence of foetal death. After administration of chemotherapy, postponement of delivery for two to three weeks allows for placental drug elimination from the foetus and resolution of maternal and foetal myelosuppression. There are no data on the impact of novel targeted therapies (small molecule inhibitors, antibodies) on pregnancy. Current evidence does not seem to show an increased risk of neurocognitive disorders, second cancers, sexual malfunction, or impaired reproductive ability in humans exposed to chemotherapy in utero. Cancer chemotherapy is incompatible with breastfeeding.

Specific cancer management

Cervical cancer

The majority of pregnant patients are asymptomatic, diagnosed by abnormal cytology at early stages of disease

(80% IA–IIA). Atypical cytological findings are common during pregnancy and should be interpreted with caution. Colposcopic examination with biopsy of suspicious lesions should be performed when cervical pathology is suspected. Conization, or loop excision, is associated with increased risks of bleeding, abortion, premature delivery, and residual disease. It is safe to manage cervical intraepithelial neoplasia with follow-up by cytology and colposcopy until delivery. Radical treatment of invasive cervical cancer cannot be performed with preservation of foetal life. Second- or third-trimester pregnant patients with stage IA disease may be amenable to treatment deferral until delivery, followed by radical hysterectomy. For patients in the first or second trimester of pregnancy and invasive cervical cancer (stage IB–IVA), pregnancy termination and immediate therapy is traditionally advised. Third-trimester pregnant patients with invasive disease may opt for deferral of therapy and week 32–36 delivery, as retrospective case series have not shown an adverse impact on prognosis. In such a setting, neoadjuvant chemotherapy for stage IB–IVA disease may be given during the second and third trimesters of pregnancy so as to buy time for delivery of a viable foetus and enable postpartum radical treatment.

Breast cancer

In contrast to other tumours, gestational breast cancer is defined as a tumour diagnosed during pregnancy and up to 12 months postpartum. Delayed diagnosis ranges from two to 15 months and may be seen in up to 78% of pregnant patients who develop breast tumours. Fine needle aspiration (FNA) or core needle biopsy and in dubious cases, an open surgical biopsy, establish the diagnosis. For lactating women, stopping milk production with ice packs, breast binding, and bromocryptine one week prior to biopsy reduces the risk of haematoma and fistula. The majority of tumours are high-grade malignancies, with axillary nodal involvement seen in 60–90% and hormone-negative status in 40–70% of pregnant patients. Recent data suggest that pregnancy does not modify the natural course of breast cancer, nor does it adversely affect patient outcome, despite high circulating oestrogen levels. Modified radical mastectomy with axillary node dissection is the treatment of choice for patients with stage I–II and selected stage III breast cancer patients during the first two trimesters of pregnancy. Patients with localized disease diagnosed in the third trimester may be managed with breast-conserving surgery and postpartum breast irradiation. Patients requiring adjuvant chemotherapy can relatively safely have it administered after the first trimester. CMF (cyclophosphamide, methotrexate, fluorouracil) or anthracycline-based regimens (AC, CAF) have been administered with only 1.3% risk of malformations after week 12. The administration of hormonal therapy and trastuzumab should be avoided throughout gestation. Patients with metastatic disease may be managed preferably with palliative combination chemotherapy (AC, CAF) rather than newer agents (taxanes, vinorelbine) beyond the first trimester of pregnancy. Recent data from a case–control study with matched non-pregnant breast cancer patients, showed no statistical difference in disease-free survival, recurrence, or OS.

Melanoma

A diagnostic delay has been demonstrated in several reviews, resulting in disease presentation with thicker primary lesions and nodal metastases, without any difference observed in site, ulceration, vascular invasion, or distant spread. Excisional biopsy is warranted for diagnosis and assessment of risk factors with thorough physical examination and laboratory work-up. Superficial spreading melanoma accounts for 74% of gestational cases, followed by nodular melanoma (16%). Wide surgical excision with 1–3cm margins according to the thickness of the primary is the treatment of choice for localized melanomas. Regional lymphadenectomy of involved nodes should be performed and although interferon has been safely administered in pregnant women with viral hepatitis, myeloma, and haematological disorders, adjuvant regimens for resected high-risk melanoma employ higher doses and should be avoided. Management of metastatic melanoma is at best palliative. There is no experience of the use of modern immunotherapy, i.e. vemurafenib or ipilimumab.

Lymphomas

The median age of pregnant patients at diagnosis of Hodgkin disease (HD) is 32 years, while that of patients with non-Hodgkin lymphomas (NHL) is 37–42. Recent data show that at presentation stage I–II HD is seen in 70% of both pregnant and non-pregnant women; there is no diagnostic delay during gestation. In contrast, pregnant women present with stage III–IV NHL in 70–80% of cases, with >40% experiencing a diagnostic delay >30 days. Combination chemotherapy is imperative as most HD and NHL patients need treatment with curative intent. When the diagnosis is made in the first trimester, pregnancy termination with prompt institution of chemotherapy is advisable, especially in the presence of B symptoms, bulky stage I–II disease, advanced stage III–IV disease, or evidence of a fulminant course of the lymphoma. In the absence of these or if the mother refuses abortion, single-agent vinblastine may be given or treatment may be deferred until the second trimester. During the second and third trimesters, the relative safety of chemotherapy administration has been demonstrated in several retrospective series, for both mother and foetus. ABVD (doxorubicin (Adriamycin®), bleomycin, vinblastine, dacarbazine) is preferred for HD and CHOP for most high-grade NHL in pregnant women. Alternatively, third trimester pregnant patients may be managed expectantly with 32–35th week delivery and postpartum chemotherapy.

Limited-field supradiaphragmatic radiotherapy has been advocated for stage IA lymphocyte predominant HD, but most physicians would defer any ionizing radiation therapy until after delivery. Rituximab administration during pregnancy is not advised due to lack of safety data. The rare patients with low-grade lymphomas may be managed expectantly, receive second or third trimester single-agent chemotherapy, or limited-field radiotherapy, according to preferences and expertise.

Further reading

Cardonick E, Iacobucci A. Use of chemotherapy during human pregnancy. *Lancet Oncol* 2004; 5:283–91.

Dotters-Katz S, McNeil M, Limmer J, Kuller J. Cancer and pregnancy: the clinician's perspective. *Obstet Gynecol Surv* 2014; 69(5):277–86.

Kal HB, Struikmans H. Radiotherapy during pregnancy: fact and fiction. *Lancet Oncol* 2005; 6:328–33.

Nicklas A, Baker M. Imaging strategies in pregnant cancer patients. *Semin Oncol* 2000; 27:623–32.

Pavlidis N, Pecattori F, Lofts F, Greco AF. Cancer of unknown primary during pregnancy: an exceptionally rare coexistence. *Anticancer Res* 2015; 35:575–9.

Pavlidis NA, Pentheroudakis G. The pregnant mother with breast cancer: diagnostic and therapeutic management. *Cancer Treat Rev* 2005; 31(6):439–47.

Pentheroudakis G, Pavlidis N. Cancer and pregnancy: poena magna, not anymore. *Eur J Cancer* 2006; 42:126–40.

Internet resources

ESMO Clinical Recommendations on Cancer, Fertility and Pregnancy: http://www.esmo.org

Motherisk: http://www.sickkids.ca/Motherisk/index.html

International network on cancer, infertility and pregnancy: https://www.cancerinpregnancy.org/

16.4 Cancer of unknown primary site

Introduction

Cancer of unknown primary (CUP) is an enigmatic disease entity encompassing heterogeneous malignancies without an identifiable primary after an adequate diagnostic work-up. It presents a unique natural history that is characterized by early dissemination, aggressive clinical course, unpredictable metastatic pattern, and dismal prognosis. In the early 1990s, CUP accounted for 3–5% of all malignancies and ranked among the top ten most frequent tumours. In the current era, the diagnostic advances mainly in immunohistochemistry staining and radiology have decreased the prevalence of patients with CUP to 1–2%.

Definition

The definition of CUP was initially controversial as some experts mandated a histologically proven biopsy and some others based their diagnosis on clinical findings without histological confirmation. The latter approach was quickly abandoned as the clinical perspective could not differentiate benign and malignant lesions. Currently, CUP is applied to a group of metastatic tumours without an identified anatomical primary after a standardized diagnostic work-up including a detailed medical history, thorough physical exam, basic blood and biochemical analyses, and CT scans of thorax, abdomen, and pelvis. Further investigations are guided by the clinical presentation as detailed later in this section.

Pathology

The first step in the diagnosis of CUP is based on the morphological features of the tumour and categorizes patients accordingly into carcinomas (approximately 90%), lymphomas, melanomas, and sarcomas. Among carcinomas, well to moderately differentiated adenocarcinomas (60%), poorly differentiated adenocarcinomas (30%), squamous cell carcinomas, and undifferentiated carcinomas are relatively rare (each about 5%). If morphology is entirely unclear, the primary approach consists of identifying the tumour lineage according to immunohistochemical staining patterns including (1) pan-cytokeratin and/or EMA antibodies for detecting carcinomas; (2) CLA and/or CD45RB antibodies for identifying lymphomas; (3) S100, HMB45, and/or Melan-A for detecting melanomas; and (4) vimentin, desmin, SMA, myoD1, CD34, KIT, and/or CD99 for identifying sarcomas. Adenocarcinomas are further classified into four broad diagnostic categories based on the expression of the two cytokeratins CK7 and CK20.

Clinical presentation and management

Patients with CUP are traditionally categorized into two prognostic subsets according to their clinicopathological features. The minority of patients (15–20%) who present a constellation of clinical and pathological findings that are highly suggestive of a specific primary culprit belong to a favourable prognostic subset and are treated according to the potential primary equivalent. The majority of patients (80–85%) present disseminated disease that does not fit any of the favourable subsets and are characterized by chemoresistance and dismal prognosis (median OS duration of 3–11 months, 1-year OS of 25–40%, and five-year OS of 3–15%).

Favourable subsets

Women with adenocarcinoma involving only axillary lymph nodes

Women with adenocarcinomas involving only axillary lymph nodes are usually in their fifties presenting with normal breast examination and lymph node enlargement isolated to one axillary area. Histopathology shows mainly an invasive ductal adenocarcinoma. Breast imaging including breast MRI is highly recommended for primary tumour identification. The treatment of these patients is similar to stage II/III breast cancer patients. The management plan includes loco-regional control and systemic treatment according to the breast cancer treatment guidelines. If the breast MRI is negative, mastectomy or breast irradiation is not recommended. If the breast MRI is positive, mastectomy or radiotherapy provides loco-regional control in 75–85% of cases. Patients with N1 disease can be treated with axillary dissection followed by axillary radiotherapy upfront whereas those with N2 disease are proposed neoadjuvant systemic treatments.

Women with papillary adenocarcinoma of the peritoneal cavity

Women with papillary adenocarcinoma of the peritoneal cavity are usually in their sixties and present commonly with ascites and peritoneal masses without evidence of primary tumour in the ovaries. An exploratory laparoscopy is often recommended for primary identification. In the absence of an identified primary, these patients are treated similarly to those with International Federation of Gynecology and Obstetrics (FIGO) stage III ovarian cancer with optimal surgical debulking and (neo)-adjuvant taxane/platinum-based chemotherapy.

Squamous cell carcinoma involving cervical or supraclavicular lymph nodes

Patients with squamous cell carcinoma involving cervical or supraclavicular lymph nodes are most commonly males in the sixth decade of age. The main clinical feature is cervical and/or supraclavicular lymphadenopathy of squamous histology without a primary detectable site. These patients are recommended to undergo FDG-PET/CT scan for primary identification especially those with supraclavicular nodal metastases in whom hidden primary lung cancer is highly probable. These patients should be treated similarly to locally advanced head and neck cancer with surgery and radiotherapy. Radiotherapy following surgery has been reported to decrease the risk of locoregional relapse and improve survival. Chemotherapy should be considered in patients with N2 or N3 disease.

Poorly differentiated neuroendocrine carcinomas
Patients with poorly differentiated neuroendocrine carcinomas are commonly asymptomatic and present rapidly growing tumours with disseminated metastases. The recommended systemic chemotherapy with platinum plus etoposide yields a response rate, complete response, and long-term survival rate of 50–70%, 25%, and 10–15%.

Men with osteoblastic bone metastases and elevated PSA with adenocarcinoma histology
These patients present solitary or multiple blastic bone metastases, an increased serum prostate-specific antigen (PSA), and a biopsy-proven adenocarcinoma of various differentiations, and staining for PSA and androgen receptor. Bone scan and CT scans are helpful imaging investigations. These patients are managed similarly to metastatic prostate cancer and treated accordingly.

Isolated inguinal lymphadenopathy from squamous cell carcinoma
Isolated inguinal lymphadenopathy from squamous cell carcinoma is a rare subset in which primary tumours of the genital (vulva, vagina, cervix, penis, or scrotum) and anorectal areas should always be ruled out. Nodal dissection with local radiotherapy is the treatment of choice in most cases. Long-term survivors have been observed.

Patients with a single metastatic site
A rare subset of CUP patients presented with a solitary site of metastases in lymph nodes or splanchnic organs. An FDG-PET scan is recommended in these settings. These tumours are treated locally using resection and/or radiotherapy ± systemic chemotherapy.

Adenocarcinoma with a colon-cancer profile (CK20+, CK7–, CDX2+)
Patients with adenocarcinoma presenting a colon-cancer profile are mostly women in their fifties, presenting abdominal masses, peritoneal surfaces and liver involvement, and ascites. A colonoscopy is recommended especially in patients with abdominal symptoms or a positive faecal occult blood test but is commonly normal. These patients should be treated according to the colorectal cancer guidelines.

Squamous cell CUP of the pelvis, abdomen, and retroperitoneum
Patients with squamous cell CUP of the pelvis, abdomen, and retroperitoneum are most commonly females between 50 and 70 years of age. Once the diagnosis is anticipated, a thorough physical exam focusing on rectal and pelvic examinations should be performed. Patients should undergo a colposcopy and anoscopy especially in those with relevant signs and symptoms. The current guidelines recommend a platinum doublet (paclitaxel/platin or gemcitabine/platin) similarly to the poor

prognostic subsets of CUP. The effective treatments for patients with squamous cell cancers of known primary may be useful in treating those with squamous cell CUP of the abdomen, pelvis, and retroperitoneum.

Renal cell CUP
Patients with renal cell CUP have a median age of 64 years and most commonly present clear cell renal cell carcinoma, followed by papillary and unspecified pathology. Targeted therapies such as sunitinib and pazopanib achieved a response rate of 40–50%, median PFS of 8.5 months, and median OS of 6–16 months. This entity should be managed according to the updated renal cell carcinoma treatment guidelines.

Unfavourable subsets
The majority of the patients with unfavourable prognostic subsets present predominantly liver metastases. Liver CUP is the most commonly encountered entity in the unfavourable CUP subset (3–40%). Patients usually present in the seventh decade of life with enlarged palpable liver on physical examination and abnormalities of liver function tests. Imaging identifies multiple liver metastases as well as other metastatic lesions to other organs. Histologically, adenocarcinoma of various differentiation is the usual diagnosis. Investigations including CT scan, endoscopies, and epithelial tumour markers are not usually helpful in detecting the primary site. The most frequent histological subtype in this subgroup is adenocarcinoma (in 64% of patients), followed by undifferentiated carcinoma (20%), neuroendocrine (9%), and squamous cell carcinoma (3%). Other poor prognostic entities include malignant ascites of unknown origin with non-papillary serous adenocarcinoma histology, multiple brain metastases of unknown primary, and multiple metastatic bone lesions of unknown primary.

These patients have chemoresistant tumours with response rates of 10–40% and are generally suboptimally treated according to the individual oncologist's best guess of a primary tumour type. Currently, platinum-based regimens are recommended for younger patients with good PS whereas older patients with poor PS are managed with supportive care.

Advances in the management of CUP
The advances in the molecular diagnostic work-up, notably CUP classifiers, have increased the primary site identification rate and may help in recognizing atypical presentation among patients who often benefit from site-specific therapy. As a result, there is an overall trend favouring the treatment of CUP patients according to the suggested primary. The available literature is discordant between randomized and non-randomized trials comparing empirical CUP regimens and site-specific therapies but a recent meta-analysis has shown a trend favouring the latter approach. Certainly, oncologists should weigh in the input of additional tests to the clinical picture and pathology investigations in establishing a clinically meaningful diagnosis before performing additional investigations.

Further reading
Greco FA. Molecular diagnosis of the tissue of origin in cancer of unknown primary site: useful in patient management. *Curr Treat Options Oncol* 2013; 14(4):634–42.

Overby A, Duval L, Ladekarl M, Laursen BE, Donskov F. Carcinoma of unknown primary site (CUP) with metastatic renal-cell carcinoma (mRCC) histologic and immunohistochemical characteristics (CUP-mRCC): results from consecutive patients treated with targeted therapy and review of literature. *Clin Genitourin Cancer* 2019 Feb; 17(1):e32–7.

Pavlidis N. Forty years' experience of treating cancer of unknown primary. *Acta Oncol* 2007; 46(5):592–601.

Pavlidis N, Briasoulis E, Hainsworth J, et al. Diagnostic and therapeutic management of cancer of an unknown primary. *Eur J Cancer* 2003; 39(14):1990–2005.

Pavlidis N, Pentheroudakis G. Cancer of unknown primary site. *Lancet* 2012; 14(379):1428–35.

Pentheroudakis G, Briasoulis E, Pavlidis N. Cancer of unknown primary site: missing primary or missing biology? *Oncologist* 2007; 12(4):418–25.

Rassy E, Assi T, Pavlidis N. Exploring the biological hallmarks of cancer of unknown primary: where do we stand today? *Br J Cancer* 2020 Feb; 11:1–9.

Rassy EE, Kattan J, Pavlidis N. A new entity of abdominal squamous cell carcinoma of unknown primary. *Eur J Clin Invest* 2019 Mar 25; 49:e13111.

Rassy E, Pavlidis N. Progress in refining the clinical management of cancer of unknown primary in the molecular era. *Nat Rev Clin Oncol* 2020; 17(9):541–55.

Rassy EE, Pavlidis N. The current evidence for a biomarker-based approach in cancer of unknown primary. *Cancer Treat Rev* 2018 Jun; 67:21–8.

16.5 Fertility and cancer

Introduction

Although the average age of a patient with cancer is over 60, approximately 4% of cancers occur in those aged 15–40. These patients may still want to complete a family and yet their treatment could have a significant effect on their fertility. This section concerns the risks and strategies available for managing infertility related to cancer.

Significance

Infertility as a consequence of cancer or its treatment remains a significant issue for young people who have not yet completed their families. The risk depends on the gender of the patient and the type of therapy administered as well as the type of cancer. A UK working party has developed guidelines to highlight possible management strategies and risks of infertility with different cancer treatments. Its importance has been recognized by the formation of new specialist services under the title of oncofertility. There are organizations in the UK and USA which promote inter-specialty working to improve the fertility outcome for patients who have needed oncology treatment.

Overall the fertility of childhood cancer survivors compared with their siblings is 0.76 for men and 0.93 for women. In a study which examined birth of children to those aged up to 35 years, the probability of fathering a child as a cancer survivor (63%) was similar to that of the general population (64%). Carrying a pregnancy to full term was, however, significantly different for female cancer survivors (66%) compared with the general population (79%).

Patients require information about their risks of infertility, possible options, and risks to future pregnancy as part of the discussions about their cancer treatment. Some hospitals provide an acute fertility service linked to the oncology service.

Male infertility

- Infertility in men commonly occurs after alkylating agents or radiotherapy to the gonadal region or after total body irradiation for conditioning for stem cell transplant. For this reason all men who are capable of producing sperm should be offered sperm banking. Sperm production is rarely effective under the age of 13 but semen should be examined if the patient is capable of ejaculation. Research is ongoing into the use of testicular tissue obtained before treatment in pre-pubescent boys. Sperm aspiration may be considered for those unable to ejaculate.

- Some men will regain their fertility. This can occur up to four years after treatment is completed. It is possible to have semen reassessed for sperm production and quality.

- Retrograde ejaculation can occur in men who have had bilateral retroperitoneal lymph node dissection.

- Testosterone production may be impaired if the patient has received gonadal radiotherapy. This should be assessed after treatment is completed.

Female infertility

- Premature ovarian failure may occur in response to pelvic (or spinal) radiotherapy or certain (but not all) chemotherapy agents. The risk of menopause is associated with the type of therapy rather than the type of cancer. The highest risk for women is those aged 21–25 who had radiotherapy below the diaphragm combined with alkylating agents. High-dose treatments (including total body irradiation) and alkylating agents will usually render a woman infertile. Even in those cases where fertility is preserved after treatment, the timing of the menopause is likely to be several years earlier than in their peers.

- Some women do retain their fertility so it is important to continue contraception until a decision is made about future fertility or pregnancy.

- Fibrosis of the uterus (often associated with impaired blood supply) can occur following pelvic radiotherapy and can cause growth restriction (less than 2.5kg birthweight), placental complications, and a greater risk of midterm miscarriage. Such pregnancies should be closely monitored with regular ultrasound examination.

- Fertility sparing surgery should now be considered (where possible) in ovarian germ cell tumours. In one study, 83% who had fertility sparing surgery plus combination chemotherapy had restored menstrual function. Of 61 survivors who had fertility sparing surgery, 24 went on to have a total of 37 children between them. There were no increased risks of congenital abnormalities.

Female fertility strategies

- Ovarian suppression with LHRH (leutinizing hormone-releasing hormone) agonists such as zoladex with hormone replacement therapy (HRT) (for non-oestrogen containing tumours) or hormonal treatment (for oestrogen sensitive tumours) may preserve fertility for some women. Outcomes vary in different studies but it is worth considering when time to treatment is limited.

- Frozen embryos can be stored but the women need to be able to defer her treatment for an IVF (in vitro fertilization) cycle and egg retrieval. This may not be possible for some malignancies, e.g. acute leukaemias. For this option the woman needs to have a long-term partner and if the partner later withdraws consent, the embryos must be destroyed.

- Oocyte removal after an IVF cycle has been tried but again requires the delay of an IVF cycle and is currently far less successful than a frozen embryo in producing a full-term pregnancy.

- Freezing or vitrification (slow freezing) of an immature egg has improved and in other patients has up to a 5% successful pregnancy rate in experienced centres.

- Research has been undertaken in freezing a strip of ovary and there have been some case reports which suggest that this can be successful. However, as some women retain their fertility despite intensive treatment and no fertility intervention, it is not possible to state whether these few cases are due to the re-implanted ovarian tissue. In addition there are cases where the cancer has recurred after re-implantation so histological analysis is essential in a parallel specimen even when ovarian metastases seem unlikely, e.g. leukaemia, Ewing sarcoma. It is offered in some centres and review of tissue to exclude metastases is essential before reimplantation.

- Other options include surrogacy, egg donation, and adoption.

Risks for the offspring of survivors
Women are most concerned not only about retaining their fertility but also about the risks to their future children of congenital abnormalities or cancer. Several large studies have shown no increased risks of congenital abnormalities after chemotherapy or radiotherapy, nor of cancer in the offspring unless there was an underlying genetic predisposition, e.g. with Li–Fraumeni or retinoblastoma.

Timing of future pregnancy
Young women diagnosed with cancer will often ask when they can become pregnant and whether it would affect the risk of cancer returning. In general, patients are advised to wait at least two years from diagnosis (particularly breast cancer patients) as this represents the time within which recurrence is most likely. With the exception of high-risk (node positive, local recurrence, and over 35 years) breast cancer there has been no increased incidence of breast cancer at the time of pregnancy. This has also been shown for melanoma.

This may be complicated by patients being on long-term adjuvant treatment such as tamoxifen. Evidence to date suggests this can be paused in order to plan a pregnancy but the data for other drugs such as imatinib in chronic myeloid leukaemia (CML) or gastrointestinal stromal tumour (GIST) is less clear. Open discussions in those cases are essential.

Monitoring in future pregnancy
Ultrasound to monitor growth and placental blood flow is recommended for those who have had uterine radiation.

In those patients who received anthracyclines during treatment or mediastinal radiation, pregnancy may place an additional strain on cardiac output and cardiac assessment with an echocardiogram is recommended before and during pregnancy.

Those treated for Wilms' tumour who have had a nephrectomy should also have their renal function and blood pressure measured throughout the pregnancy.

Internet resources
British Fertility Society. British Oncofertility network: https://britishfertilitysociety.org.uk/special-interest-groups/fertility-preservation-uk/

The Royal College of Physicians, The Royal College of Radiologist, The Royal College of Obstetricians and Gynaecologists. The effect of cancer treatment on reproductive functions. Guidelines on management. Report of a working party (includes patient information (UK))—available at: https://www.rcr.ac.uk/system/files/publication/field_publication_files/Cancer-fertility_effects_Jan08.pdf

16.6 Late effects

Introduction
The long-term effects of cancer can affect the medical, psychological, and social wellbeing of an individual and their carers. This section concerns the medical effects; infertility and other aspects of cancer survivorship are discussed elsewhere.

Medical late effects
Late effects are dependent upon the original cancer, its treatment, family genetics, and the developmental stage of the individual when treated for cancer.

Lessons learned from paediatrics
The median age of diagnosis of cancer in the general population is 70 years but the most significant increase in survival rates in the past 40 years has been in the area of paediatric oncology. Many of these young people were treated in the context of a clinical trial so that initial survivorship data was gained from paediatric patients. The medical sequelae of cancer treatment as a child have profound consequences given the current average life expectancy. The medical consequences may include development of a second malignancy, infertility, and potentially abnormalities within any organ system of the body. These are described here but it should be noted that paediatric treatment regimens have now been modified to minimize or prevent some sequelae such as deafness or second malignancies in the paediatric and young adult setting.

Second malignancy
The risk of second malignancy is increased with combinations of chemotherapy and radiotherapy. The increased risk of breast cancer in patients treated with mantle radiotherapy for Hodgkin disease has led to the omission

of radiotherapy for most of these patients. The cumulative incidence of any second malignancy increased from 10.6% at 20 years to 26.3% at 30 years following treatment for Hodgkin disease.

In survivors of non-Hodgkin lymphoma, the overall risk of second malignancy was raised (RR 1.3). Specifically there was a significantly increased risk of leukaemia (RR 8.8, 95% CI 5.1–14.1) and lung cancer (RR 1.6, 95% CI 1.1–1.6). The relative risk of second malignancy was greatest with younger age at time of diagnosis and decreased with older age at the time of treatment. The risk of leukaemia was associated with chemotherapy treatment, regardless of whether or not radiotherapy was given. Lung cancer risk was associated with radiotherapy. The 15-year cumulative risk of a second malignancy was 11.2% overall, with the greatest number of cases with lung cancer (2.8%), leukaemia (1.5%), colorectal (1.5%), and breast cancer (1.2%). The cumulative risk was worse for men and those first treated after 50 years of age.

Infertility

Infertility as a consequence of cancer or its treatment remains a significant issue for young people who have not yet completed their families and is discussed in detail in section 16.5, 'Fertility and cancer'.

Osteoporosis and osteonecrosis

Bone growth is affected by steroids given to support chemotherapy or as part of the regimen, or by chemotherapy or radiotherapy treatment itself. Osteopaenia occurs frequently at the end of treatment with combination chemotherapy and, for some, bone recovery will be permanently affected. An extreme example of this is in ER positive breast cancer where patients may have chemotherapy followed by an aromatase inhibitor. The hormonal treatment compounds the osteoporotic effect of the chemotherapy and calcium supplementation or bisphosphonates may be required to prevent fractures. In childhood survivors, 16.7% were found to have significant and 36% moderate bone mineral density deficits following cancer treatment. Endocrine dysfunction was found to be responsible for many cases, highlighting the importance of endocrine follow-up.

Osteonecrosis (avascular necrosis) is a known complication of treatment for leukaemia, lymphoma, or bone marrow transplantation and is thought to be due to high-dose steroids. It tends to occur most in weight-bearing bones and arthroplasty of the hip joint may be needed in up to 20% patients with femoral head osteonecrosis, although conservative measures such as analgesia, physiotherapy, and rest are tried first. Given that many of these patients are young, the joints are likely to require further replacements throughout life.

Neurological

Neurological damage may occur either centrally to the brain itself or to the peripheral nerves depending on the tumour and treatment given. The risk of neurocognitive deficit is greatest amongst survivors of ALL and central nervous system (CNS) tumours. Many of these patients are treated at a young age so that the impact of neurocognitive impairment reduces their chance of further education or employment. Neurocognitive impairment has now also been reported in survivors of childhood cancer who were treated with chemotherapy alone and planning additional neuropsychological and educational support should be built into any paediatric programme.

For those with CNS tumours, cranial radiotherapy is given sometimes in combination with chemotherapy which can produce combined peripheral and central neurological deficits.

The treatment of ALL previously used cranial radiotherapy to prevent or treat CNS disease but there has been a move towards using intrathecal methotrexate and high-dose chemotherapy to reduce neurocognitive impairment.

Certain chemotherapeutic agents, such as platinums and vinca alkaloids, are known to be neurotoxic. The risk is greater with increasing age, particularly over the age of 50 and unless specifically tested during treatment, the damage may be permanent and debilitating.

Adult patients suffer greater neurological side effects and sequelae from cranial radiotherapy with neurotoxic chemotherapy. Alternative chemotherapy or biological therapies may reduce this in the future.

Cardiological

Cardiac toxicity may take several forms following treatment, including cardiac failure, arrhythmias, and increased risk of myocardial infarction. The major risk factors are mediastinal or left chest wall radiotherapy, anthracyclines, and vincristine. Asymptomatic arrhythmias are common. Cardiac failure is associated with the use of anthracyclines in children but occurs rarely in adults if the doses are restricted.

Children treated with anthracyclines have reduced left ventricular wall thickness and reduced left ventricular function which may continue to deteriorate many years after treatment. This can lead to congestive cardiac failure. Treatment with angiotensin converting enzyme inhibitors has been shown to improve left ventricular function in the short term but did not prove effective in symptomatic patients in the longer term.

In a British cohort study of Hodgkin survivors compared with aged matched controls, supradiaphragmatic radiotherapy, treatment before age 55, anthracyclines and vincristine were all associated with an increased risk of death from myocardial infarction (standardized mortality ratio (SMR) of 2.5 overall). The greatest risk was for those who received supradiaphragmatic radiotherapy with vincristine but no anthracyclines (SMR 14.8, 95% CI 4.8–34.5). The chemotherapy regimen with doxorubicin, bleomycin, vinblastine, and dacarbazine was associated with a SMR of 9.5 (95% CI 3.5–20.6).

A screening study of 294 Hodgkin disease survivors who had received at least 35Gy radiotherapy to the mediastinum showed that 21.4% had abnormal left ventricular function at rest and 14% developed perfusion defects on scintigraphy during physical stress. Almost 10% of the patients had had a myocardial infarction during a median follow-up of 6.5 years and two patients had died as a result. Of the 40 patients who underwent angiography as a result of the screening, 55% had significant coronary artery stenosis, 22.5% had less than 50% stenosis, and the remainder had no stenosis.

Recent targeted treatments also lead to cardiac complications such as cardiac failure, hypertension, and arrhythmias. Monitoring for these during and after treatment is essential.

Pulmonary

Long-term pulmonary toxicities include fibrosis (from radiotherapy or bleomycin), pneumonitis (radiotherapy, gemcitabine), asymptomatic abnormalities of lung function tests (radiotherapy and combination chemotherapy), or lung cancer (especially after radiotherapy and chemotherapy). Patients given hemi-thorax radiotherapy for metastatic Wilms' tumours in childhood are at particular risk. The long-term consequences of asymptomatic lung function test abnormalities are currently unknown.

Endocrine

Endocrine abnormalities may occur in those who have received radiotherapy close to the pituitary or thyroid, including those who have had total body irradiation as part of marrow or stem cell transplant. Abnormalities do not occur immediately after treatment so they should be screened for starting at least one-year post treatment or earlier if there are symptoms. Abnormalities of gonadal dysfunction are discussed in section 16.5, 'Fertility and cancer'. Hormonal replacement may be necessary for these patients if not contraindicated by their cancer type.

Chronic health conditions

In addition to specific toxicities, the overall health of an individual is likely to be affected after treatment for cancer. Chronic health conditions, especially those graded as severe by common terminology criteria for adverse events, are significantly higher in survivors compared with siblings or controls. In a study of childhood survivors, chronic health conditions occurred in almost all patients, with 27.5% experiencing severe or life-threatening health effects. Multiple chronic conditions were also more frequent, with 37.6% experiencing at least two, and 23.8% at least three significant comorbidities.

Follow-up

Many centres run late effects clinics to monitor for these and other sequelae of cancer treatment. Ahmad et al. (2016) provided a guideline for follow-up and post treatment screening in survivors of childhood and young adult cancers.

Causes of death after cancer treatment

The main cause of death following a diagnosis of cancer is the cancer itself even after surviving five years from diagnosis. This was confirmed in a childhood cancer survivor study of 20,227 patients who had survived five years from diagnosis. Overall the survivors had a 10.8 times excess mortality compared with age- and sex-matched controls. 67% of deaths were due to recurrence. After recurrence the greatest risk of death was from a second malignancy followed by cardiac then pulmonary problems. The standardized mortality ratio was 19.4 for second malignancy, 8.2 for cardiac death, and 9.2 for pulmonary death, with other causes at 3.3. The risk of death was greatest for women, those diagnosed before age five, and those with an initial diagnosis of leukaemia or CNS tumour. Second malignancies reflect not only risks from treatments for cancer but also individual underlying genetic factors. Other risks, especially cardiac and pulmonary, more greatly reflect treatments given as detailed in relevant chapter headings. It is hoped that many of the treatment related complications may reduce as treatments are changed to try to minimize late effects. This is particularly the case in Hodgkin disease.

In patients treated for Hodgkin disease who do not relapse with their disease, second malignancy is the most common cause of death followed by cardiovascular disease. After 15 years post diagnosis 64% deaths were from second malignancy and 21% from cardiac disease. Given the recent change in treatment to reduce mediastinal radiotherapy both these could be expected to reduce in the future.

Health behaviours

Given that cancer survivors are at increased risk of second malignancy, cardiac, and other medical problems, it is important to encourage them to live a healthy lifestyle after their treatment is over. Smoking, exercise, and reducing risk-taking behaviours, such as alcohol consumption or substance abuse, all contribute to future health. A review of health behaviours of childhood cancer survivors showed that they were less likely to be smokers or to plan to take up smoking than their peers. Binge drinking and heavy drinking were lower in incidence than age-matched controls. However continued cancer screening, dental care, and follow-up clinics were attended less than deemed optimal. Eating balanced meals and exercising for greater than one hour a week occurred in approximately 75% of survivors. Education to minimize future health problems should be a priority in long-term survivorship care.

Treatment summaries and care plans

Many centres produce a treatment summary giving the doses of chemotherapy and radiotherapy administered during treatment and guidelines for further follow-up based on the risks of not only recurrence but also the secondary medical late effects. These have been shown to reduce patient anxiety and admission to hospital for chronic conditions.

Further reading

Ahmad SS, Reinius MA, Hatcher H, et al. Anticancer chemotherapy in teenagers and young adults: managing long term side effects. *BMJ* 2016; 354:i4567.

Kenzik KM, Kvale EA, Rocque GB, et al. Treatment summaries and follow-up care instructions for cancer survivors: improving survivor self-efficacy and health care utilization. *Oncologist* 2016 Jul; 21(7):817–24.

Van Leeuwen FE, Ng AK. Long term risk of second malignancy and cardiovascular disease after Hodgkin lymphoma treatment. *Hematology Ann Soc Hematol Educ Program* 2016 Dec 2; 2016(1):323–30.

Internet resources

SEER Cancer Statistics Review, 1975–2005 (includes survival data): http://seer.cancer.gov/csr/1975_2005/

16.7 Cancer survivorship

Introduction

The term cancer survivorship has many meanings depending on geography, job description, and if you are a patient or a relative. In the context of this book it is meant to describe the medical, psychological, and social consequences of a diagnosis of cancer. More recently this is thought to be the time from diagnosis recognizing that the diagnosis itself has significant consequences for the patient and their family.

In the UK the Cancer Reform Strategy included survivorship issues. In the USA the National Action Plan for Cancer Survivorship has been developed to tackle these.

The long-term medical effects of cancer survivorship and their follow-up have been discussed elsewhere throughout the book. This section concerns the psychological, social, and economic issues which can significantly contribute to a patient's quality of life (QoL) after a diagnosis of cancer. It also touches on the effects on their immediate family.

Prevalence

In the UK the estimated numbers of people living after a cancer diagnosis range from 1 to 1.5 million. With increasing cancer incidence and survival it is thought that this will rise to represent 1.5–2.5% of the adult population.

In the USA over 11 million people were living with a diagnosis of cancer in 2004, representing about 4% of the population. The five-year survival for children diagnosed with cancer is now 79% and for adult cancers is 64%.

The survival rates reflect not only the primary diagnosis but also the availability of healthcare provision, but are increasing in most areas of the world.

Lessons learned from paediatrics

Given the dependence of children upon their parents and the developmental needs of a growing child some of their psychosocial survivorship issues are different to those of adults. In addition, the families of children treated for cancer are significantly affected and many parents of childhood survivors suffer long-lasting psychological and social consequences even when the clinical outcome has been good.

Psychological

Following a diagnosis with cancer patients and their families make psychological adjustments to cope with the treatment and potential outcome. Stress is, not surprisingly, very common and occurs in over 95% patients. The majority of these will have anxiety and mild depression which may not require treatment. However some will have more significant psychological symptoms and needs including depression, post-traumatic stress disorder, suicidal ideation, and various psychoses.

Most psychological studies have been undertaken in patients with breast cancer, haematological malignancy, or childhood cancers. More recently those with colorectal cancer and prostate cancer have been included in such studies due to their improved survival. Men with prostate cancer are also undergoing androgen deprivation for many years even when the disease is advanced.

- There is conflicting evidence about the impact of psychological wellbeing and its affect on outcome in breast cancer. A meta-analysis has, however, shown that stress-related psychosocial factors were associated with a worse prognosis in cancer patients.

- In breast cancer patients with stage IIA–IIIB disease, psychological intervention in addition to health assessment improved survival over health assessment alone (HR 0.44; P=0.016) at a median of 11 years after diagnosis, even when known predictors of prognosis were taken into account.

- In survivors of childhood cancer there is a greater degree of some aspects of psychological distress in the parents than in the patient themselves. Parents were more concerned about their child's health and thought more often of the cancer and its diagnosis than the patient.

- Post-traumatic stress disorder (PTSD) has been described in survivors of childhood cancer and non-Hodgkin lymphoma specifically. The incidence varies from <5% to 80% depending on the type of cancer, age at diagnosis, and degree of PTSD. In one USA study of non-Hodgkin lymphoma survivors ten years after diagnosis only 8% fulfilled all criteria for PTSD, although 39% showed some signs of PTSD. PTSD was associated with treatment intensity, problems with employment or insurance, less social support, and negative appraisals of life threat.

- In survivors of childhood cancer, features of post-traumatic stress (PTS) (intrusion, avoidance, and arousal) have been recorded in approximately up to 12% of parents more than five years after their child's diagnosis. These features occurred in up to 30% of parents within the first three months of diagnosis and fathers were as affected as mothers. Levels of anxiety and depression were also 1.8–2.01 times those of parents with healthy children even after five years since diagnosis.

- Suicidal ideation and previous attempts at suicide have been shown to be present in up to 12.83% of childhood cancer survivors. Standardized mortality ratios for suicide deaths in cancer patients are in the order of 1.35–2.9 compared with the general population. Risk factors include male sex, older age, higher disease stage, poor prognosis, poor performance status, alcoholism, other psychiatric illness, fatigue, pain, loss of function, and previous or family history of suicide attempts. Lack of family or social support also correlates with increased suicide risk.

Relationships

The long-term impact of a cancer diagnosis on the ability to form lasting relationships is of particular concern in those treated as young adults who have not yet formed strong bonds with a partner. On average, cancer survivors are less likely to be married and have a higher incidence of divorce than their peers but there is also more positive evidence. In one study of germ cell survivors, there were more single women among survivors than control but the married survivors reported better relationships with their partners than their age matched controls.

Social consequences

On average, cancer survivors have a lower income than their age matched control. They are more likely to have difficulties obtaining life and health insurance or a mortgage after surviving cancer. In the USA a significantly reduced proportion of cancer survivors have health insurance.

Treatment summaries and care plans

It has become the standard of care to provide cancer patients (and their families) with a summary of their planned, or completed, treatment along with a care plan which documents and signposts people to help with other care they may need. This is especially important at the end of treatment when many patients may now be discharged to self-supported management programmes without regular oncology follow-up, e.g. low-risk breast cancer. The key factors necessary for self-supported management are the facts of expected late effects (including psychological), signposting to services that would help in each case, and a contact number if there are concerns

that are not being addressed by those services or for an unexpected complication.

Further reading

Earle C. Failing to plan is planning to fail: Improving the quality of care with survivorship care plans. *J Clin Oncol* 2006; 24: 5112–16.

Ganz P. *Cancer Survivorship: Today and Tomorrow*. Springer Press, 2007.

Rowland J. Foreword: looking beyond cure: pediatric cancer as a model. *J Pediatr Psychol* 2005; 30 (1):1–3.

Internet resources

ASCO Cancer treatment and survival care plans: http://www.cancer.net/survivorship/follow-care-after-cancer-treatment/asco-cancer-treatment-and-survivorship-care-plans

Livestrong Foundation: https://www.livestrong.org/

SEER Cancer Statistics Review, 1975–2005 (includes survival data): http://seer.cancer.gov/csr/1975_2005/

16.8 Travel

Introduction

For people who have cancer, travelling may raise a number of issues, such as whether they are fit to travel, how to get travel insurance, vaccinations, and other preventive measures, and getting help abroad if needed. This section aims to give an overview of the travel-associated issues for cancer patients.

Pre-travel preparation

The pre-travel preparations of an immunosuppressed person should include contacting their clinicians to assess the current status of the medical status and the medications needed.

The doctor should assess whether the disease or its treatments contraindicate or decrease the effectiveness of any disease prevention measures such as vaccinations and malaria chemoprophylaxis recommended for the proposed travel.

The doctor must consider whether any of the disease prevention measures present a risk for the underlying medical condition. Any specific health hazards at the destination that would be likely to exacerbate the underlying illness or be more severe in an immunocompromised traveller must be considered with any interventions which would mitigate such a risk.

All patients intending to travel are advised to have a medical consultation at least four to eight weeks before to assess the need for any vaccination and/or malarial chemoprophylaxis as well as to order any other medical items the traveller may require. Patients who intend to be away for a long time may also need to think about regular appointments such as dental and gynaecological check-ups.

Issues associated with mode of travel

Air travel

The health problems of air travel are associated with hypoxia, gas expansion, cabin humidity, dehydration, motion sickness, exposure to infection, and risk of deep vein thrombosis (DVT). For people with cancer, air travel may

normally be contraindicated in the following situations due to the effects of disease itself, treatment, or commonly associated medical comorbidities:

- When there are features of increased intracranial pressure or within 24 hours of a seizure.
- After recent surgery where trapped air or gas may be present—abdominal or GI surgery, craniofacial or ocular surgery, and brain surgery.
- If there is breathlessness at rest, unresolved pneumothorax, or major haemoptysis.
- If the person has angina or chest pain at rest.

Fitness to air travel

Prolonged air flight can lead to an increased risk of oxygen desaturation due to the progressive fall in cabin PO_2 and acute mountain sickness, which usually occurs 6–18 hours after exposure to altitudes of >7,000 feet (2,130 metres). Hence a pre-flight assessment is necessary in cancer patients with respiratory or cardiovascular symptoms.

Anaemia is common in oncology patients and should be corrected prior to travel. Lung cancer per se is not a contraindication to fly. People with a baseline SpO_2 >95% or SpO_2 of 92–95% with no risk factors (see later in this section) do not require supplemental oxygen. However, those with SpO_2 92–95% with at least one risk factor need a proper evaluation to assess the need for supplemental oxygen during the flight. The risk factors include hypercapnia, FEV1 (forced expiratory volume in 1 second) <50% predicted, lung cancer, restrictive lung disease involving the parenchyma (fibrosis,) abnormalities of the chest wall (kyphoscoliosis) or respiratory muscles, previous history of ventilator support, cerebrovascular or cardiac disease, and discharge <6 weeks previously for an exacerbation of chronic lung or cardiac disease. Those with SpO_2 of <92% generally need in-flight oxygen supplementation.

One practical method to assess fitness to fly is to see whether the person can walk 50 yards/metres at a normal pace or climb one flight of stairs without severe dyspnoea. If this can be accomplished, it is likely that most people will tolerate the normal aircraft environment.

The hypoxic challenge test is used to determine which patients require in-flight oxygen for air travel. It uses an oxygen–nitrogen mix to simulate the cabin environment. If it results in a PaO_2 of <6.6kPa or SpO_2<85%, medical oxygen is indicated at 2l/min. Oxygen must be booked with the airline in advance.

A number of guidelines are available for assessment for fitness for air travel (see 'Internet resources').

Deep vein thrombosis

Cancer patients have an increased risk of venous thromboembolism (VTE), and the risk is likely to increase further with air travel. Other risk factors for DVT include previous DVT or pulmonary embolism (PE), history of DVT or PE in a close family member, and recent surgery or trauma particularly to the abdomen, pelvic region, or legs. Tamoxifen is also known to increase the risk of VTE.

The results of the World Health Organization (WHO) Research into Global Hazards of Travel (WRIGHT) study have shown that the risk of VTE approximately doubles after a long-haul flight (>4 hours). The risk increases with the duration of the travel and with multiple flights within a short period. However, the additional risk posed for cancer patients is unknown.

All cancer patients with active disease and/or with any of the other risk factors are advised to seek medical advice regarding prevention of DVT during air travel.

General measures such as avoiding dehydration, moving around the cabin during long flights to reduce the period of immobility (e.g. regular trips to the bathroom every two to three hours), calf muscle exercise (most airline cabin leaflets explain this), and wearing loose and comfortable clothes and leg stockings can reduce the risk of thrombosis. It is also advised to avoid excessive alcohol or sleeping tablets. A recent systematic review suggested that travellers on flights of <6 hours and with no known risk factors may not need any DVT prophylaxis. However, patients with known risk factors and/or on flights of >6 hours need risk-based DVT prophylaxis.

There are no evidence-based guidelines on specific DVT prophylaxis. Current evidence suggests no benefit from prophylactic aspirin. In cancer patients with a history of DVT or PE or a perceived high risk of VTE, a single injection of low-molecular-weight heparin (enoxaparin 1,000IU per 10kg of body weight) two to four hours before departure may be considered, especially for flights >4–6 hours.

Travel by sea

The most common health problems due to sea travel are respiratory tract infections, injuries, motion sickness, and GI illnesses. Outbreaks of infection can be a particular problem in immunosuppressed cancer patients.

Before travel it is important to get a letter from the treating physician detailing medical conditions, treatment, and prescription doses.

Specific measures include vaccinations, including influenza and destination-specific vaccinations, and other prophylactic measures (e.g. malaria chemoprophylaxis)

Medical kit for a traveller

The medical kit should contain basic medicines to treatment common illnesses, first-aid articles, and other specific drugs and items (e.g. syringes) which the individual needs. A physician's letter stating the medical conditions and treatment, details of medications, and prescribed doses is necessary as it may be required to clear customs. Regulations for controlled drugs can be obtained by contacting the embassy of the relevant country.

Disability and travel

Physical disability is not a contraindication for travel for an otherwise healthy person. Since there are specific airline regulations, necessary information should be obtained in advance and wheelchairs or other aids booked with the airport authority.

Patients who are unable to look after their own needs during the flight need an escort as the cabin crew is not permitted to provide such a service.

Internet resources

General travel advice

British Foreign Office Safety Information for Travellers: http://www.fco.gov.uk/travel

Centers for Disease control and prevention: Yellow Book—available at http://wwwnc.cdc.gov/travel/

Frontier Medical: http://www.frontiermedical.co.uk/

Health Advice for Travellers from the UK Departments of Health: https://webarchive.nationalarchives.gov.uk/20130103031035/http://www.nhs.uk/nhsengland/Healthcareabroad/pages/Healthcareabroad.aspx

International Association for Assistance for Travellers: http://www.iamat.org/

International Society of Travel Medicine (ISTM): http://www.istm.org

Mobility International: http://www.miusa.org/

National Travel Health Network and Centre (NaTHNaC): http://www.nathnac.org/

Royal Society for the Prevention of Accidents: https://www.rospa.com/

Travel Medicine and Vaccination Centres (TMVC) (Australia): https://tmvc.com/

World Health Organization International Travel: http://www.who.int/ith/

Fitness to fly

British Airways: https://www.britishairways.com/health/docs/before/airtravel_guide.pdf

British Thoracic Society: http://www.brit-thoracic.org.uk/

International Civil Aviation Organizations: http://icao.int

UK Civil Aviation Authority: https://www.caa.co.uk/home/

Sea travel

International Council of Cruise Lines: https://cruising.org/about-the-industry/policy-priorities/Public%20Health%20and%20Medical

International Maritime Health Association: http://www.imha.net/

16.9   Insurance

Travel insurance

Obtaining travel insurance with appropriate cover for cancer patients has become increasingly difficult. This may reflect the increasing cost of healthcare and the different standards of care worldwide. Cancer patients therefore have to shop around or get advice from an insurance broker (see 'Internet resources'). Several insurance companies have been established recently that specialize in offering insurance to cancer patients (see 'Internet resources'). However obtaining travel insurance, particularly during treatment, can be expensive or may not even be possible.

The cost of an insurance premium depends on the destination of travel and on the healthcare system of destination.

Reciprocal arrangements between countries

It is important to seek information on possible reciprocal healthcare arrangements between the country of residence and the destination country. To be eligible for treatment under such an arrangement, it is important to obtain the necessary documentation from the country of residence prior to travel. When a reciprocal arrangement does not exist, or does not cover all the possible health risks, it is important to obtain the necessary special insurance.

Residents of the UK travelling to the Europe can obtain a European Health Insurance card (see 'Internet resources') which covers any medical treatment due to an accident or illness within the European Economic Area and Switzerland. This also covers chronic or pre-existing illness treatments which would normally be covered by the state. However, the EHIC alone may not always be sufficient. The UK also has reciprocal healthcare arrangement with non-EEA countries details of which can be found on the NHS website (see 'Internet resources').

Life insurance and mortgages

Life insurance is usually needed to take out a mortgage. Cancer survivors, especially children and young adults, can be in a difficult position due to either refused insurance cover or an offer of insurance under specific conditions. Most often it also involves paying a high premium.

Approaching a large insurance company or an independent financial adviser can be useful in finding appropriate life insurance cover. Every case will be considered individually based on the prior cancer, its treatment, and the time elapsed since treatment.

Driving and car insurance

Most cancer patients can continue to drive without any problem. In the UK, the Driver and Vehicle Licensing Authority (DVLA) should be notified in the following situations:
- Tumours of the CNS (primary and secondary).
- Treatment or weakness preventing normal daily activities.
- Medications which are likely to affect safe driving.

In these situations, patients are advised not drive with immediate effect and to inform the DVLA, who will then send the patient a medical questionnaire and get relevant information from the doctor, if necessary, before making a decision about fitness to drive.

Car and motor cycle

In patients with brain tumours, driving restrictions depend on the grade, site (supra- or infratentorial), and treatment. In the UK the following driving restrictions may apply for supratentorial tumours:
- Pituitary tumours: can drive on recovery after transphenoidal surgery, six months off driving after craniotomy.
- WHO grade I meningioma: six months off driving after craniotomy, one month after stereotactic radiosurgery and may drive on completion of fractionated radiotherapy.
- WHO grade II meningioma and WHO grade I–II gliomas: one year off driving from the date of completion of treatment.
- WHO grade III meningioma, WHO grade III–IV glioma and metastatic brain tumour: two years off driving after completion of treatment.
- Completely excised solitary metastasis: may be considered for licensing one year after completion of treatment provided there is no evidence of local or systemic spread.
- In patients who suffer fits as part of their illness, one year free from fits (with or without medication) must pass before driving can be resumed.
- Relicensing will take into account any residual neurological or visual deficit.

Large goods vehicle and passenger carrying vehicle

Diagnosis of a brain tumour, except of a benign tumour, leads to a permanent refusal or revocation of a licence to drive in the UK. Permission to drive after treatment of a grade I or grade II meningioma may be considered five years after surgery and is made after individual assessment.

Motor insurance

Insurance companies cannot refuse cover based on a time-restricted licence. However, they can increase the premium or policy excess due to the new disability or condition. Patients have to disclose the details of the medical condition as soon as possible to their motor insurance company. Further details on motor insurance are available from the Cancer Help website (see 'Internet resources').

Internet resources

Driver and Vehicle Licensing Authority (DVLA): www.dft.gov.uk/dvla

European Health Insurance card: http://www.ehic.org/

Macmillan Cancer support provides details on travel insurance and travel advice: http://www.macmillan.org.uk/

NHS—Travelling outside the European Economic Area (EEA): http://www.nhs.uk/NHSEngland/Healthcareabroad/Pages/NonEEAcountries.aspx

Insurance companies and information

A detailed list of insurance companies for UK residents is available from: http://www.macmillan.org.uk

Cancer Research UK. Cancer Help: http://www.cancerhelp.org.uk

Medi TravelCover Ltd: http://www.insurecancer.com/

World First Travel Insurance: http://www.world-first.co.uk

16.10 Vaccination

Introduction

Cancer and its treatment result in varying degrees of immunosuppression. The highest degree of immunosuppression is seen after haematopoietic stem cell transplantation (HSCT), in active leukaemia and lymphoma, in active generalized malignancies, and during chemotherapy. Immunosuppression will persist after chemotherapy for leukaemia and lymphoma for 6–12 months, three months after chemotherapy for other cancers, and two years after stem cell transplantation (SCT).

For the purposes of vaccination and immunization, the following groups of patients are considered as immunosuppressed:

- Patients receiving chemotherapy and up to six months after chemotherapy.
- Patients who had treatment for leukaemia and lymphoma in the previous two years.
- Patients after allogeneic HSCT, not on immunosuppressant drugs, for two years after transplant.
- Patients after autologous HSCT for one year post-transplant

Vaccines

Killed vaccines

Indications for inactivated vaccines (Table 16.10.1) in cancer patients are the same as for the general population. Killed vaccine can also be administered during cancer treatment. However, due to weakened body immunity, these may be less effective than in the general population.

Routine vaccinations in cancer patients are modified based on their individual risk for any particular infection. Patients with chronic cardiovascular and/or respiratory conditions or diabetes mellitus are at high risk of influenza and hence need annual vaccination. Patients with absent spleen function (e.g. after splenectomy or with asplenia) are recommended to have haemophilus influenza type b (Hib), meningococcal (conjugate C or quadrivalent conjugate vaccine), and pneumococcal vaccine (with booster every five years) in addition to the influenza vaccine. Patients who are likely to need blood products are advised to have hepatitis B vaccine along with other routine vaccines. Malaria can be severe in splenectomized patients which necessitates special precautions (see 'Malaria chemoprophylaxis', p. 471).

Live vaccines

Administration of live vaccines in immunosuppressed patients can lead to a high risk of severe complications due to the live organisms in the vaccine. Hence live vaccines (Table 16.10.1) are contraindicated in all cancer patients who had total body radiotherapy or chemotherapy (including high dose) in the past six months. Live vaccines should also be avoided for three months after steroid therapy (received a dose of >2mg/kg prednisolone equivalent for >1 week) and HSCT patients within two years of transplant, with evidence of graft vs. host disease (GVHD) and ongoing immunosuppression. Live vaccines may be avoided for the rest of life in lymphoma, leukaemia, and HIV-related cancer. Safety of live vaccine during immunotherapy is unknown and therefore not recommended. Anti-TNF (tumour necrosis factor) antibodies can reactivate latent tuberculosis and predispose to infections and therefore live vaccines should be used carefully.

Vaccination of family members

In the UK, all vaccines are given by injection and hence cancer patients are not at risk of getting an infection from a vaccinated family member, even after live vaccine. However, in some countries, some live vaccines are given orally (e.g. oral polio) or nasally (e.g. intranasal influenza). After oral polio vaccine, a person can shed the viruses from their bowel for up to three weeks after the vaccination which rarely may be infective. Hence these vaccines are contraindicated for family members of immunocompromised cancer patients. Intranasal and smallpox vaccines also pose a similar risk. It is also important to avoid contact with anyone outside the family who has recently had a live vaccine by mouth.

Live vaccines which are less likely to be transmitted (measles, mumps, rubella (MMR), yellow fever, oral

Table 16.10.1 Types of vaccines and immunization

Live vaccines	Killed vaccines	Passive immunization
Measles, mumps, and rubella (MMR)	Tetanus/diphtheria	Measles
Oral polio	Killed polio	Hepatitis A and B
Bacillus Calmette–Guérin (BCG)	Hepatitis A and B	Varicella
Varicella	Hib	Rabies
Varicella zoster	Meningococcal polysaccharide and conjugate	
Salmonella typhi Ty21a	Salmonella Typhim Vi®	
Intranasal—influenza	Parenteral—influenza	
	Pneumococcal polysaccharide	
	Human papilloma virus (HPV)	
	Rabies	
	Yellow fever	
	Oral cholera	
	Swine flu (H1N1)	

salmonella, and varicella) may be administered to family members. If the varicella vaccine recipient develops a rash, direct contact with the immunocompromised cancer patient should be avoided until the rash resolves.

Family members should receive all other recommended vaccines to reduce the risk of exposure of the immunocompromised patient. Immunization recommendations differ in different countries.

Travel vaccination
Principles of travel vaccination in cancer patients
Indications for vaccination in cancer patients are similar to those for non-immunocompromised people. However, a number of exceptions occur.

Cancer patients should have vaccinations several months prior to travel to allow for serological evaluation and additional booster doses if needed.

Passive immunization should be used if available and emergency travel presents a potential high-risk situation (e.g. hepatitis A immunoglobulin).

To obtain an optimal immunological response, cancer patients should be vaccinated during periods of no or low immunosuppression.

Cancer patients are likely to have less immunoresponse to vaccination and any response can be shortlived.

The vaccination needs of cancer patients during travel depend on the destination(s). Inactivated vaccines such as hepatitis A and B, inactivated polio, Japanese encephalitis, meningococcal polysaccharide and conjugate, typhim Vi®, and rabies vaccines are safe if needed. Table 16.10.2 gives recommendations for individual travel vaccines.

Revaccination
After HSCT, recipients lose immunological memory of previous exposure to infectious agents and vaccines. Hence all patients who have had high-dose chemotherapy and a stem cell transplant need revaccination six months after treatment. The recommended vaccinations in this group include diphtheria/tetanus toxoid, pertussis vaccine, Hib conjugate, inactivated influenza and polio vaccine, live attenuated MMR, pneumococcal, and other vaccines.

The Advisory Committee on Immunization Practices (ACIP) suggest that patients vaccinated while on chemotherapy should be considered unimmunized and be revaccinated. An adequate immune response usually occurs 3–12 months after cessation of chemotherapy. There are no definite recommendations on revaccination with live or inactivated vaccines for individuals vaccinated prior to undergoing treatment with immunosuppressive therapy. The options are booster dose and individualized vaccination based on serological testing for antibody.

Passive immunization
Passive immunization with immunoglobulins, if available, should be considered prior to emergency travel to countries with a high risk of infection or when travelling to an area at high risk of disease when live vaccines are contraindicated. Immunoglobulins are available for measles, hepatitis A and B, rabies, and varicella. Passive immunization should also be considered for immunosuppressed patients exposed to these infections.

Table 16.10.2 Recommendations on individual vaccines for immunosuppressed patients

Vaccine	Recommendation
Tetanus	Routine booster for all
Diphtheria	Indicated if antibody titre is <0.1IU/ml or last injection >10 years prior to travel
Influenza	Annually; recommended for family members as well; appropriate influenza vaccine if travelling to the opposite hemisphere
Pneumococcal	Before travel
Hepatitis B	Check for serology to exclude prior to chronic infection prior to vaccination. Indicated in those with new sexual partners while travelling and those likely to need blood products or medical procedures (including injections) during travel. After three doses, anti-Hbs titre is measured and re-vaccinate if titre is <10mIU/ml
Hepatitis A	Indicated when travelling to high-risk destinations. At least two doses, six months apart are needed. If less than six months prior to travel, intramuscular immunoglobulin, which offers protection for three to six months
Inactivated polio	Consider if travelling to a destination with a polio outbreak (e.g. Haiti, Dominican Republic, Philippines) or with circulating wild-type polioviruses. Recommend a booster dose if >10 years after previous dose
Meningococcal	Indicated when travelling to destinations with known outbreaks, meningitis belt of sub-Saharan Africa and travelling to Saudi Arabia for Muslim pilgrimages
Salmonella	Indicated when travelling to endemic areas. Inactivated vaccine (Typhim Vi®) is the choice in immunocompromised patients
Rabies	Indicated if intense contact with animals is expected or in those who plan to be far from medical care. An adequate response after vaccination (antibody titre >0.5IU/ml) is unlikely in immunocompromised patients and hence immunoglobulin is advised after all risk exposures
Japanese encephalitis	When travelling to endemic Asian destinations
Swine flu (H1N1)	Recommended for cancer patients and family members
Papilloma virus vaccine	Indication same as general population, i.e. girls and young women
Inactivated typhoid vaccine	Advised during prolonged trip to Indian subcontinent

Table 16.10.3 Summary of recommendations for vaccination in cancer patients

During and within six months of chemotherapy/total body irradiation	Routine vaccines: • Live vaccines are contraindicated • Killed vaccines are recommended. According to national guidelines: Give killed vaccines >2 weeks before start of chemotherapy or total body radiotherapy. Some vaccines (e.g. varicella zoster) need to be given at least one to three months prior to undergoing immunosuppressive treatments. If vaccines cannot be given during this time scale, they should be given when the neutrophil and lymphocyte count is >1.0 x 10^9/L • Travel vaccines and chemoprophylaxis: Live vaccines are contraindicated; consider passive immunization if urgent travel is contemplated Killed vaccines are recommended as indicated based on the destination(s) Malaria chemoprophylaxis is advised if indicated
Six months after chemotherapy/total body irradiation	• All vaccines can be given provided there is no active cancer • Routine and travel vaccinations as indicated
Bone marrow and STC patients	• Revaccination: All patients should receive vaccination for tetanus, diphtheria, polio, Hib two doses at fourth and twelfth month), pneumococcal, influenza (seasonal, can start after six months), hepatitis A and hepatitis B 12 months after transplantation • Travel vaccination: Live vaccines if indicated can be considered if patients are not on immunosuppressant drugs, have no active disease, and are at least 24 months after transplantation. Otherwise passive immunization should be considered
Vaccination of family members of cancer patients	Oral polio, intranasal influenza, and smallpox vaccines are contraindicated in family members of the cancer patients with immunosuppression to prevent cross infection

Timing and administration of vaccines

It is preferable to administer vaccines at least two weeks before the start of chemotherapy or SCT, during maintenance chemotherapy (for acute lymphatic leukaemia), or when the peripheral neutrophil and lymphocyte counts are >1.0 x 10^9/L. Revaccination can be deferred until completion of treatment and immune recovery (Table 16.10.3).

Inactivated vaccines do not generally interfere with other vaccines and can therefore be given with other vaccines or separately at any time.

Live vaccines are given simultaneously and if they cannot be given on the same day should be separated by an interval of at least four weeks.

A number of combination vaccines are available now which are convenient for travellers.

Assessment of success of vaccination

Measurement, if available, of antibody titres following immunization is helpful to assess the need for booster doses. A four-fold increase in the antibody titre is generally considered as evidence of seroconversion. The specific titres for seroprotection depend on the individual vaccines. In immunocompromised patients the immunological response is often partial and of short duration.

Malaria chemoprophylaxis

Cancer patients travelling to malaria-endemic areas should receive malaria chemoprophylaxis and advice on avoiding mosquito bites. Appropriate clinical assessment should be performed to address the potential possibilities of:
• Malaria chemoprophylaxis drugs interacting with treatment of cancer.
• Risk of acquiring serious malarial infection in certain subgroups (e.g. after splenectomy).
• Impact of malaria infection and its treatment on the course of malignancy.

Enteric infections

• Enteric infections can be severe in immunocompromised cancer patients. These infections can be either water- or food-borne.
• To avoid water-borne infections, patients are advised to avoid swallowing water during swimming and to avoid swimming in possibly contaminated water.
• Frequent and thorough hand washing is the best way to prevent gastroenteritis.

Further reading

Askling HH, Dalm VASH. The medically immunocompromised adult traveler and pre-travel counseling: status quo 2014. *Travel Med Infect disease* 2014; 12:219–28.

Ljungman P. Vaccination of immunocompromised patients. *Clin Microbiol Infect* 2012; 18 (Suppl. 5):93–9.

Internet resources

Advisory Committee on Immunization Practices (ACIP): https://www.cdc.gov/vaccines/acip/index.html

UK Immunisation against infectious disease: the Green Book—available from: https://www.gov.uk/government/collections/immunisation

16.11 Lifestyle choices after cancer

Introduction

Through a combination of earlier detection and enhanced treatments, the chance of surviving cancer is improving significantly. As a result, the number of cancer survivors in the UK is growing by 3% per annum. By 2040, it is forecast that there will be over three million people living with the consequences of cancer and its therapies. This includes over a quarter of people over 65 years. Unfortunately, people living with and beyond cancer (PLWBC) are often troubled with acute and long-term physical and psychological adverse effects. This section reviews the evidence that lifestyle and self-help strategies can help diminish many of the adverse effects of treatments, maximize the probability of long-term control, and in some cases improve OS. Although lifestyle should be considered as a whole, for ease of explanation the research evidence has been categorized separately into:

- Adiposity and weight gain
- Diet and dietary supplements
- Alcohol
- Smoking
- Physical activity and other helpful lifestyle factors

Adiposity and weight gain

Weight gain during and after adjuvant cancer treatments is becoming an increasing concern. Patients who are overweight or obese during and after cancer treatments have a higher risk of infection, thromboembolism, delayed wound healing, cardiac impairment, and side effects such as hot flushes, joint pains, lymphoedema, urinary incontinence, erectile dysfunction, and diabetes. Numerous studies have also linked obesity not only with a greater risk of cancer but also with a greater risk of relapse and worse OS after successful cancer treatments. Obese women who also had other unhealthy habits such as high alcohol intake or smoking had the greatest risk. Likewise women who gained more than $0.5kg/m^2$ at one year post treatment did worse. Despite this evidence, women in the UK are rarely told to avoid weight gain during chemotherapy. Fortunately, intervention programmes are usually successful.

The mechanisms of risks for obesity include overeating and alterations in cytokine and sex hormone levels:

- Overeating high calorific foods, particularly those rich in sugar and fat content, is known to increase the risk of metabolic syndrome (abdominal obesity, high triglyceride levels, and hyperglycaemia). After colon cancer, individuals who eat these foods have a significantly increased chance of dying or relapsing. An excess of refined sugars leads to a higher risk of diabetes and heart disease but it also leads to insulin resistance and higher insulin-like growth factor (IGF) levels which, in laboratory studies have been shown to promote proliferation and dedifferentiation and block apoptosis of cancer cells. Clinically there is a link to a higher risk of cancer and progression.

- Leptin is a multifunctional neuroendocrine cytokine generated primarily from fat cells so there is a direct correlation between amount of body fat and circulating blood levels. Leptin promotes proliferation and markers of metastasis, and reduces markers of apoptosis and adhesion. High serum levels are linked to higher serum insulin, IGF-1, and higher expression of cycloxidase 2.

- Sex hormones: oestrogen levels are raised in the serum of obese women. This increases IGF levels which are known to stimulate abnormal growth and inhibit apoptosis in oestrogen sensitive cell lines. In postmenopausal women, adiposity increases bioavailable oestrogen and can increase the aromatase enzyme found in fat cells. Fortunately, oestrogen levels reduce following weight reduction programmes and following a diet low in fat and high in fibre as a consequence of higher urinary excretion of estrogen. Progesterone tends to be lower in overweight women particularly in the premenopausal setting. This is thought to be caused by androgenic inhibition of ovulation. Progesterone has multiple effects but exerts its protective role on cancer by counteracting the effects of endogenous oestrogen by promoting synthesis of IGF binding protein.

Diet

Independent of overeating, the quality of foods consumed has been linked with cancer incidence as well as a number of degenerative chronic illnesses. Cohort studies have linked polyphenol rich foods, such as leafy green and cruciferous vegetables, colourful fruits, and flavanoid rich foods, such as pulses and legumes, with a lower risk of prostate cancer. Regular tea drinkers have a significantly lower incidence of breast, prostate, ovarian, and oesophageal cancers. Higher intake of curcumin and other spices is associated with a lower level of colon cancer and high polyphenol rich foods are linked to lower risks of pancreatic, ovarian, and skin cancers.

The benefits of a healthy diet, however, do not stop after a diagnosis of cancer. Women with early breast cancer taking higher than the recommended '5 a day' fruits and vegetable have been found to lower their risk of recurrence by one-third especially if combined with physical activity. A large randomized controlled trial (RCT) found that women who were randomly assigned to receive healthy dietary guidelines had a lower relapse rate compared with controls, especially those experiencing hot flushes. Other trials have reported lower breast cancer recurrence among regular green tea drinkers or consumers of foods rich in dietary lignans, isoflavones, and flavanones. Women with adequate versus low serum carotenoid levels have lower breast cancer relapse rates. Individuals with a higher lutein and zeaxanthin intake (from leafy green vegetables) treated for skin cancer have a reduced the rate of new cancer formation. Diets rich in polyphenols (herbs, berries, spices), carotenoids (carrots, kale), and isoflavones (soy based foods) slow the rate of PSA progression or relapse in men with prostate cancer. Survivors of colon and ovarian cancer with a high intake of fruit, vegetables, poultry, and fish had lower relapse rates.

Food supplements

Cancer survivors are attracted to the potential health benefits of food supplements with over 70% reporting regular intake. The majority of studies to date have evaluated extracted chemicals such as vitamins and minerals. Unfortunately, most of these have shown no benefit or were actually linked to an increased risk of cancer unless there was a pre-existing micronutrient deficiency to be corrected. For example, the CARET study found that beta carotene and retinol increased the risk of lung cancer. Likewise, the ATBC study found that alpha vitamin E and beta carotene increased lung cancer risk. In a subsequent analysis, men with low pre-intervention plasma levels of beta-carotene had a lower prostate cancer risk following supplementation, whereas those with high levels had a higher risk. This u-shaped distribution of risk was also observed in the EPIC study with those whose diets were deficient in folate and those with the highest folate intake both having the highest cancer risk. Two other Scandinavian studies demonstrated a higher cancer risk following vitamin B supplementation. In the HPFS, men who took zinc (more than 100mg/day) were more than twice as likely to develop advanced prostate cancer. The SELECT study showed an increased prostate cancer incidence with vitamin E and selenium supplements and a study from Australia showed that individuals who took beta carotene and vitamin E supplements had a higher rate of new skin cancer formation.

Despite some initial encouragement from laboratory studies and small evaluations of extracted phytochemicals, subsequent RCTs of lycopene, soy extracts, saw palmetto, or genistein given on their own have not demonstrated a benefit for either prostate cancer or benign prostatic hypertrophy or breast cancer.

More recently, scientific attention has turned towards the evaluation of concentrated wholefoods, particularly those rich in polyphenols and other healthy phytochemicals. A wide range of foods contain these natural chemicals, particularly herbs, spices, green vegetables, teas, and colourful fruits. Pomegranate extract, rich in ellagic acid, broccoli, rich in isothiocyanate (ITC) and its metabolite sulforaphane, curcumin, which gives turmeric its yellow colour, and green tea rich in epigallocatechin gallate (EGCG) have all demonstrated anticancer effects in laboratory and small clinical studies.

The largest clinical trial evaluating the health benefits of these foods was the National Cancer Research Network Pomi-T study which combined four phytochemical rich foods. It found a statistically significant 64% reduction in the median PSA progression rate compared to placebo and reported an impact on mens' decisions to remain off androgen deprivation therapies, making it clinically relevant. Further studies are underway to evaluate its impact for other stages of prostate cancer and other cancers.

Alcohol

The Million Women Study found statistically significant increased risks for a number of cancers in those who regularly consumed alcohol. Another study reported that >1 drink a day specifically increased the risk of breast cancer, but up to one drink was not associated with an increased risk. The risk of alcohol appears to be worse if women have a family history of breast disease, especially if they start drinking as a teenager. Men who drank heavily doubled their risk of high-grade prostate cancers compared to other men, although there was no difference in the incidence of low-grade cancers. There is also evidence that alcohol intake increases the risk of relapse following radical treatments for head and neck cancer. Two cohort studies reported an increased risk of contralateral breast cancer with more than four to seven alcoholic beverages a week, especially if subjects

were overweight or smoked. On the other hand, another study demonstrated no survival disadvantage of drinking alcohol before or after breast cancer diagnosis. Furthermore, a Swedish study actually demonstrated a slight advantage with one glass of wine equivalent per day after diagnosis, a finding supported by a University of Cambridge study reporting that women who drank three and a half small glasses of wine a week were 10% more likely to survive. The intensity rather than total amount appears to be important, as a study of women showed no increased mortality with total alcohol intake but those drinking intensely (more than three drinks on the day of consumption) had worse outcomes.

Smoking

Patients who smoke around the time of surgery increase their risk of thromboembolic events, poor wound healing, and infection. During radiotherapy smokers have an increased risk of acute mucositis, acute skin reactions, xerostomia, long-term fibrosis, breast pain, erectile dysfunction, incontinence, and proctitis. There is convincing data to suggest that individuals who continue to smoke after cancer treatments have worse cancer outcomes. This is thought to be related to the continued exposure to carcinogens causing further DNA damage, as well as a direct impact on cellular function, by inhibiting apoptosis and stimulating proliferation. Studies of patients with small cell lung cancer and head and neck cancer showed that the risk of a second lung cancer is higher and OS lower among those did not quit. Cohort studies have reported similar findings for non-epithelial cancers including breast, bowel, prostate, colorectal, and ovarian cancer.

Physical activity after cancer

A physically active lifestyle improves well-being by reducing many of the common adverse effects that plague individuals after cancer and its treatments. Numerous studies have tested the feasibility and benefits of exercise rehabilitation programmes in cancer survivors. A number of RCTs and two large meta-analyses of exercise interventions showed a statistically significant benefit for a number of troublesome symptoms, particularly fatigue, mood, anxiety and depression, muscle power, hand grip, exercise capacity, and overall QoL. The evidence for intervention programmes is particularly robust for fatigue, psychological distress, body constitution, cardiac function, joint pains, pelvic symptoms, lymphoedema, bone mineral density, and thromboembolism.

Cancer related fatigue (CRF): is reported by 60–96% of patients after surgery, during chemotherapy and radiotherapy, and whilst they remain on long-term hormones or biological therapies. It prevents people returning to normal activities of daily living, and affects overall QoL and cognitive function. Supervised exercise programmes, on their own or combined with cognitive behavioural therapy (CBT) have been shown to improve CRF.

Psychological distress: common and often unrecognized after cancer, as well as being distressing, has also been shown to reduce survival. Group exercise classes, especially if combined with relaxation, mindfulness, and healthy eating programmes, have been shown to help alleviate mood and especially reduce anxiety and fear of relapse.

Body constitution, cardiac function, and unwelcome weight gain: exercise programmes, especially if combined with nutritional counselling, not only reduce the risk of unwelcome weight gain but also have significant benefits for lean mass indices, bone mineral density, cardiopulmonary function, muscle strength, general fitness, and walking distance. In particular, men with prostate cancer have significantly less weight gain, hot flushes, and mood changes related to androgen deprivation and recommendations for a 12-week programme have been incorporated in the latest UK National Institute for Health and Care Excellence (NICE) prostate guidelines.

Joint pains: are common after cancer but several cohort studies link exercise with a lower incidence of arthritis. An exercise intervention study from New York reported significant and specific reduction in arthralgia amongst women with breast cancer taking an aromatase inhibitor. The benefits of exercise are likely to be enhanced by other lifestyle factors such as diet supplementation with polyphenol rich foods. This is being investigated in the ongoing UK arthro-T study.

Pelvic symptoms: pelvic floor exercises have demonstrated an improvement in pelvic symptoms such as urinary and rectal urgency and erectile dysfunction but need to be continued for the long term. Benefits often do not start until after 12 weeks of intervention so patients need strong encouragement to persevere with appropriate verbal advice supplemented by written information sheets. Men who exercise during and after radiotherapy have a lower risk of pelvic symptoms.

Lymphoedema: the incidence of upper limb lymphoedema is decreasing with advances in surgery. Management includes advice to avoid secondary infection, and use of massage and compression garments. Studies have linked general exercise and weight reduction programmes with improvements. An intervention study of weight lifting reported significant reductions in lymphoedema flares requiring acute intervention.

Bone mineral density (BMD): accelerated bone loss, brought on by a premature menopause after chemotherapy, surgery, or hormone therapy, has been reported after treatment for a number of cancers. Fortunately, a number of intervention studies have linked regular physical activity with a reduction in the risk of bone mineral loss. Exercise also helped preserve bone mineral density even when bisphosphonates have been prescribed. It is particularly helpful if combined with other factors which help preserve bone health such as a low animal, high plant protein diet or high vegetables, fruit, and soy fruit diets.

Thromboembolism: DVT and PE remain a significant risk for patients with malignancy. Although strategies such as compression stockings, warfarin, and low molecular weight heparin are essential, early mobilization and exercise remain practical additional aids in reducing this life-threatening complication.

Evidence that physical activity improves survival and reduces relapse rates

Regular physical activity is a significant factor for the risk of cancer development. Although evidence from RCTs is lacking, there is emerging evidence that exercise may slow the progression of some cancers, reduce the probability of relapse, and reduce the risk of overall death from cancer. The most comprehensive ongoing study of physical activity and outcome is the CHALLENGE study (Colon Health and Lifelong Exercise Change) whose end points include disease-free survival, QoL, health-related fitness, and biomarkers.

Most other published evidence originates from retrospective analyses or prospective cohort studies. A recent meta-analysis from the National Cancer Institute reviewed 45 observational studies and reported that between two to five hours physical activity a week was linked to a significant reduction in cancer relapse rates; in some trials this was up to 60%. The strongest evidence was demonstrated for breast cancer, the next strongest for colorectal cancer, and then prostate cancer.

Mechanisms of the potential anticancer effects of exercise

The most likely mechanism involves growth factors such as IGF-1 and insulin-like growth factor binding proteins (IGFBPs) relating to the central role of these proteins in the regulation of cell growth inhibition, apoptosis, and angiogenesis. Exercise reduces IGF-1 levels and increases the levels of IGFBP3. Exercise has also been shown to impact on gene expression. Among the genes more highly expressed in men who exercise were BRCA1 and BRCA2, both of which are involved in DNA repair processes. Neuropeptide cytokines, which decrease after exercise, include vasoactive intestinal protein (VIP) and leptin, both of which have cancer promoting properties in laboratory studies. Patients with breast and prostate cancers have been found to have higher VIP titres compared with individuals who regularly exercise. The reduction in leptin levels may be a direct effect or an indirect effect from a reduction in adiposity after exercise. Female sex hormones, particularly relevant for cancers of breast, ovaries, and uterus, reduce after exercise. In men, the clinical benefits of exercise cannot be explained by sex hormone levels, as these tend to be higher in fitter men. Other chemical changes include NK cell cytolytic activity which modulates apoptotic pathways through an influence on p53. The messenger protein irisin is released from muscle into the serum after vigorous exercise which among other health benefits, enhances the effect of chemotherapy.

Incorporating healthy living and exercise programmes into mainstream cancer management

Macmillan Cancer Relief has produced a series of helpful booklets and web-based patient information materials designed to inform and motivate individuals to exercise and eat well as part of its 'Move More and Living Well' programmes. The Cancernet.co.uk and Macmillan.org websites have links to help search for local exercise facilities by postcode, which can aid health professionals when counselling patients. Several supervised pilot schemes have been started throughout the UK with the aim of incorporating exercise programmes into standard oncology practice. The National Exercise Referral Scheme exists for other chronic conditions such as cardiac rehabilitation, obesity, and lower back pain, and the national standards to expand the scheme to include cancer rehabilitation were written and accepted in 2010 by the governing body, SkillsActive. The Wright Foundation has now developed training courses for exercise professionals using these standards.

Summary

With the publication of more and more lifestyle related research there is justifiably increased interest in the management of patients living with and beyond cancer. There are increasingly strong data to support the development of supervised rehabilitation and self-help intervention programmes during or after anticancer therapies, to reduce acute and late risks and consequences of treatments, and improve outcomes. These programmes, if integrated into the main stream management of cancer patients, are likely to have multiple other benefits, including empowering patients and their carers, ensuring greater autonomy, and reducing the increasing burden on healthcare providers.

Further reading
Thomas R, Davies N. Cancer—the roles of exercise in prevention and progression. *Nutr Food Sci* 2007; 37:319–28.
Thomas R, Davies N. Lifestyle during and after cancer treatments. *Clin Oncol* 2007; 19:616–27.

Thomas R, Williams M, Bellamy P, et al. A double blind, placebo controlled randomised trial (RCT) evaluating the effect of a polyphenol rich whole food supplement on PSA progression in men with prostate cancer—The UK National Cancer Research Network (NCRN) Pomi-T study. *J Clin Oncol* 2013; 31(Suppl): Abstr. 5008.

Internet resources
Cancernet-UK: http://www.cancernet.co.uk
Forefront fitness, Cambridge UK: http://www.forefrontfitness.co.uk
MacMillan Cancer Support: http://www.macmillan.org.uk
National Institute for Health and Care Excellence: http://www.nice.org.uk
Wright Foundation Cancer Rehabilitation course: http://www.wrightfoundation.com

16.12 Complementary therapies

Introduction
Complementary therapy is an umbrella term for a heterogeneous array of interventions which are not part of mainstream medicine. Table 16.12.1 provides an overview of some of the most popular modalities. Even though the treatments differ in many respects, they have in common certain assumptions regularly made for them by their proponents:
- The interventions are holistic.
- They are natural and hence safe.
- They are highly individualized and patient-centred.
- They maximize the self-healing properties of the human body.

Essentially, these are claims which require evidence. Many complementary therapies are furthermore characterized by the fact that they have a long history of usage and, in most countries, constitute part of private medicine.

The reason why complementary therapy is an important topic in oncology seems obvious: at least one-third of all cancer patients use some type of complementary therapy. Exact figures for prevalence of use depend on a range of factors, including, for instance, the definition of what constitutes a complementary therapy. Many patients do not volunteer information about their use of complementary medicine. A thorough medical history should therefore include questions about this issue.

The reasons why so many cancer patients try complementary therapies are diverse and include:
- Desperation
- Hope for a cure
- Incessant media-hype
- The wish to leave no stone unturned
- Irresponsible marketing of some interested parties
- The fact that many patients can afford the extra cost

Disappointment with conventional oncology is, contrary to what is often argued, not a prominent reason; only very few cancer patients forfeit conventional for complementary treatments.

Table 16.12.1 Some of the most important complementary therapies used in oncology

Therapy	Description
Acupuncture	Insertion of a needle into the skin and underlying tissues in special sites, known as points, for therapeutic or preventive purposes
Aromatherapy	The use of plant essences for medicinal purposes
Biofeedback	The use of apparatus to monitor, amplify, and feedback information on physiological responses so that a patient can learn to regulate these responses. It is a form of psychophysiological self-regulation
Chiropractic	A system of healthcare which is based on the belief that the nervous system is the most important determinant of health and that most diseases are caused by spinal subluxations which respond to spinal manipulation
Herbal medicine	The medical use of preparations that contain exclusively plant material
Hypnotherapy	The induction of a trance-like state to facilitate the relaxation of the conscious mind and make use of enhanced suggestibility to treat psychological and medical conditions and effect behavioural changes
Massage	A method of manipulating the soft tissue of whole body areas using pressure and traction
Osteopathy	Form of manual therapy involving massage, mobilization, and spinal manipulation
Reflexology	The use of manual pressure on reflex zones usually on the soles of the feet to prevent or treat illness
Relaxation therapy	Techniques for eliciting the 'relaxation response' of the autonomic nervous system

In order to assess complementary therapies, it is helpful to differentiate between: 1) interventions claimed to change the natural history of the disease, e.g. 'curative treatments'; 2) preventative measures; and 3) supportive or palliative approaches. This section addresses these three areas in turn, asking which complementary therapies demonstrably generate more good than harm based on the evidence of rigorous clinical trials and systematic reviews of such studies.

Curative treatments

It is in this area where patients' interest is keenest. A sizeable part of cancer patients' reason for trying complementary therapies is their claim to change the natural history of the disease, i.e. offer a cure, a reduction of tumour burden, or a prolongation of life (e.g. Trevena and Reeder 2005). A simple Google search (accessed in December 2015) for 'cancer, alternative medicine' generated 5.6 million hits. Patients are thus bombarded with promises that this or that alternative remedy will cure their cancer, and the daily press does its share in promoting the myth that 'alternative cancer cures' exist.

Evaluating the evidence for such claims is, however, a sobering task indeed. Data from clinical trials are available for numerous different modalities, but in no case is it convincing or even promising (Table 16.12.2).

In fact, the concept of an 'alternative cancer cure' turns out to be inherently absurd. It presupposes that reasonably good evidence exists suggesting that a treatment is effective yet nevertheless rejected by the conventional oncological community for the sole reason of not originating from conventional medicine. Even though this type of conspiracy theory is very much alive in the field of complementary medicine (it might even be a precondition for selling quackery to unsuspecting, vulnerable patients), there is no evidence at all that oncologists behave in this way. Clinicians would be generally delighted to add another effective curative method to the existing therapeutic options. Thus 'alternative cancer cures' is and will remain a contradiction in terms.

Preventative measures

Several 'natural' approaches have shown considerable promise in reducing the risks of certain cancers. Modalities with encouraging evidence include:
- Regular consumption of allium vegetables (e.g. garlic)
- Regular consumption of green tea

Table 16.12.2 Selection of treatments that have been tested as 'alternative cancer cures'

Aloe vera	Melatonin
Asian mixtures	Mistletoe
Beta glucan	PC-SPES
Di Bella therapy	Reishi
Essiac	Shark cartilage
Gerson	Support group therapy
Hydrazine sulphate	Thymus extracts
Laetrile	Ukrain
Macrobiotic	'714-x'

- Regular consumption of tomato-based products (lycopene)
- Regular exercise

Arguably all of these approaches are entirely mainstream lifestyles or nutritional habits based on the evidence from conventional epidemiological and other research. Even if we initially considered them to be complementary therapies, they would rapidly become conventional cancer prevention, once the evidence is promising.

Supportive and palliative care during chemotherapy

In this area, complementary therapies might have an important role to play. Many of the modalities have the potential to increase well-being and QoL of cancer patients by alleviating the symptoms of the disease or by reducing the adverse effects of conventional treatments.

For instance, several complementary therapies have been shown to reduce cancer pain:
- Exercise (arguably a conventional intervention)
- Hypnotherapy
- Massage
- Reflexology

Other complementary treatments alleviate other symptoms:
- Acupuncture and acupressure reduce nausea and vomiting after chemotherapy.
- Aromatherapy improves psychological well-being of cancer patients.
- Music therapy enhances QoL and mood of cancer patients.
- Specific relaxation programs reduce fatigue and improve QoL of cancer patients.

One could argue that the level of proof does not need to be as high for palliation as for curative treatments. If a dying cancer patient feels simply better after an aromatherapy massage, for instance, few clinicians would insist on irrefutable evidence before administering it. On the other hand, we have to note that the trial evidence for these treatments may be promising but it is usually far from compelling. Many studies are designed such that cause and effect remain unclear. Furthermore, conventional methods of care do, of course, also generate benefit, and it is still unclear whether orthodox or heterodox approaches yield greater effect sizes or is better value for money.

Integrative medicine

In recent years, the term 'integrative (or integrated) medicine' has received some attention. In oncology, it means integrating complementary with conventional therapies in cancer palliation and supportive care. It seems obvious that this only makes sense for evidence-based complementary therapies. Once they are supported by solid evidence, they would automatically become part of mainstream healthcare; arguably 'integrative medicine' should therefore be a superfluous replication of evidence-based medicine. But this is not what is currently happening in clinical practice: regrettably 'integrated medicine' turns out to provide little more than a smoke-screen for smuggling bogus treatments into clinical routine. It is self-evident that this development is not an improvement and not in the best interest of cancer patients.

Conclusion

Complementary therapies are popular with cancer patients. Oncologists should therefore know the essentials about them. The evidence is vastly different depending on whether we are dealing with alleged cancer 'cures', prevention, or supportive/palliative care. Alternative cancer 'cures' turn out to be a contradiction in terms. The most important role of the oncological team in this setting may well be to show empathy and prevent serious harm. Some 'natural' therapies have shown promise in cancer prevention. It is, however, debatable whether these are complementary or conventional approaches. In the area of supportive/palliative care, complementary therapies could find a truly beneficial role. Several of the modalities in question can improve the QoL of cancer patients either through alleviating some of the symptoms of the disease or through reducing the adverse effects of the treatment.

Further reading

Ernst E. Integrated medicine. *J Intern Med* 2012; 271(1):25–8.

Ernst E, Cassileth BR. The prevalence of complementary/alternative medicine in cancer: a systematic review. *Cancer* 1998; 83:777–82.

Ernst E, Pittler MH, Wider B, et al. *Complementary Therapies for Pain Management*. Edinburgh: Mosby/Elsevier, 2007.

Ernst E, Pittler MH, Wider B, Boddy K. *The Desktop Guide to Complementary and Alternative Medicine*. 2nd edn. Edinburgh: Mosby/Elsevier, 2006.

Marchand L. Integrative and complementary therapies for patients with advanced cancer. *Ann Palliat Med* 2014; 3(3):160–71.

Milazzo S, Lejeune S, Ernst E. Laetrile for cancer: a systematic review of the clinical evidence. *Supp Care Cancer* 2007; 15:583–95.

Trevena J, Reeder A. Perceptions of New Zealand adults about complementary and alternative therapies for cancer treatment. *N Z Med J* 2005; 16:U1787.

Ernst E, Smith K. *More Harm than Good?: the moral maze of complementary and alternative medicine*. New York: Springer, 2018.

Internet resources

PDQ Cancer Information Service. Complementary and alternative medicine—available from: http://www.ncbi.nlm.nih.gov/books/NBK82221/

16.13 Supportive care during chemotherapy

Nausea and vomiting

This may occur in up to 70% of patients receiving cancer chemotherapy and is of three types:

- Acute nausea and vomiting within the first 12–24 hours after chemotherapy.
- Delayed nausea and vomiting occurring up to five days after chemotherapy.
- Anticipatory nausea and vomiting which is a conditioned response because the patient expects to experience nausea and vomiting.
- Drugs vary in their emetogenic potential as shown in Table 16.13.1.
- Appropriate antiemetic regimens for each group are shown in Table 16.13.2.

Myelosuppression

Myelosuppression is a potentially serious consequence of cancer chemotherapy. Chemotherapy-induced febrile neutropenia often leads to hospital admission for administration of parenteral antibiotics and has a considerable impact on QoL. It is also a major cause of treatment delays and dose reductions which may result in poorer tumour control rates.

Colony stimulating factors

Recombinant human G-CSF or granulocyte-macrophage colony stimulating factors (GM-CSFs) can be used to reduce the incidence, severity, and duration of neutropenia and its associated complications and to support dose-dense and dose-intense chemotherapy regimens. The risk of febrile neutropenia (FN) is related to chemotherapy regimen, dose intensity, and individual patient factors. International guidelines advocate routine G-CSF support as primary prophylaxis in patients with solid tumours and lymphomas, where the risk of FN is estimated to be >20%. Chemotherapy regimens commonly associated with high risk (>20%) of FN are listed in Table 16.13.3. Where patients are receiving a chemotherapy regimen associated with an intermediate risk of FN (10–20%), primary prophylaxis with G-CSF should be considered if other risk factors are present. Factors associated with increased risk of FN are age >65 years, advanced stage of disease, previous episodes, and lack of antibiotic prophylaxis. Previous chemotherapy, use of high-intensity regimens, and diagnosis of haematological

Table 16.13.1 Emetogenic potential of various drugs

Highly emetic treatment (>90%)	Cisplatin
	Cyclophosphamide (high dose)
	Dacarbazine
	Streptozocin
	Anthracycline/cyclophosphamide combination
Moderately emetic regimens (>30–90% risk)	Carboplatin
	Cyclophosphamide (low/intermediate doses)
	Doxorubicin
	Epirubicin
	Ifosfamide
	Irinotecan
	Oxaliplatin
Low-risk emetic treatment (10–30% risk)	Fluorouracil
	Taxanes
	Etoposide
	Gemcitabine
	Methotrexate
	Mitomycin
	Topotecan
Minimal risk emetic treatment (<10% risk)	Bleomycin
	Vinca alkaloids

Table 16.13.2 First-line antiemetic therapy for chemotherapy

Chemotherapy	Antiemetic
Highly emetic regimens	NK1 receptor antagonist (aprepitant 125mg oral day 1, 80mg oral days 2–3, or fosprepitant 125mg IV day 1)
	Dexamethasone 12mg oral/IV day 1, 8mg oral days 2–3 or days 2–4
	5HT3 receptor antagonist day1 (ondansetron 8mg oral BD or 0.25mg/kg IV BD or granisetron 2mg oral or 1mg IV or palonosetron 0.5mg oral or 0.25mg IV or dolasetron 100mg oral or tropisetron 5mg oral/IV or ramosetron 0.3mg IV)
	Or
	Combined NK1 receptor antagonist and 5HT3 receptor antagonist NEPA (300mg netupitant and 0.5mg palonsetron)
	Dexamethasone 12mg oral/IV day 1, 8mg oral days 2–3 or days 2–4
Moderately emetic regimens	Dexamethasone 8mg oral/IV day 1, 8mg oral days 2–3
	5HT3 receptor antagonist day 1 (ondansetron 8mg oral BD or 0.25mg/kg IV BD or granisetron 2mg oral or 1mg IV or palonosetron 0.5mg oral or 0.25mg IV)
	+/− NK1 receptor antagonist (aprepitant 125mg oral day 1, 80mg oral days 2–3, or fosprepitant 125mg IV day1)
Low emetic regimen	Dexamethasone 8mg oral or IV day 1

malignancies also increase the risk of FN. It is also recommended that G-CSF is used as a supportive treatment in dose-dense or dose-intense chemotherapy strategies.

Therapeutic use of G-CSF in patients with FN reduces the duration of hospitalization and neutropenia but does not improve survival. G-CSF is not indicated routinely for patients with uncomplicated FN who have not received prophylactic G-CSF and use should be limited to those patients who are not responding to appropriate antibiotic management and in the presence of severe sepsis. Following an episode of FN, G-CSF should be used as secondary prophylaxis.

The available preparations including biosimilars are considered to be equally effective. Pegfilgrastim has the advantage of once per cycle administration compared with filgrastim and lenograstim which are administered as daily injections and there is some evidence that some patients receive suboptimal dosing with daily G-CSFs. European Society for Medical Oncology guidelines suggest administration of G-CSF 24–72 hours after chemotherapy continuing until recovery of neutrophil counts. Doses of filgrastim used are 5mcg/kg by daily subcutaneous injections starting on day 2 for up to 14 days or absolute neutrophil count of 10×10^9/L and of pegfilgrastim 100mcg/kg on day 2 of each cycle as a single subcutaneous injection. The commonest adverse effect seen with G-CSFs is bone pain (20–30%) which usually responds to simple analgesia.

Erythropoietin

Maintenance of good haemoglobin levels is important for patients with cancer both for general well-being and to ensure efficacy of treatment. A target haemoglobin level of 12g/dl is recommended. Studies of erythropoiesis stimulating agents (ESAs) in patients receiving chemotherapy have shown that ESAs reduce the need for blood transfusion and may improve QoL. Epoietin alpha, beta, and darbepoietin are equally effective and can be used in patients for whom blood transfusion is contraindicated or where there is symptomatic anaemia. However, these agents increase the risk of thromboembolic events and there is strong evidence that ESAs are associated with increased mortality. Therefore the potential benefits of ESAs as supportive therapy for

anaemia should be carefully weighed against the risks on an individual patient basis.

Mouth care

Mucositis is a troublesome side effect of neutropenia and may be exacerbated by secondary infection and trauma. Chemotherapy agents which may cause oral mucositis include cyclophosphamide, doxorubicin, methotrexate, taxanes, irinotecan, and 5-flourouracil. Patients should be advised to avoid spirits and spices. Good mouth care is essential with use of a soft toothbrush and mouthwashes with saline, 0.15% benzydiamine three-hourly, or chlorhexidine. Soluble aspirin or paracetamol may help pain. Protective gels such as Orobase® or Gelclair® may be used. Oral candidal infections may be treated with topical nystatin 100,000 units four times daily after food or in the immune suppressed patient with oral fluconazole 50–100mg daily for 14 days. Herpetic ulcers may be treated with topical acyclovir 5% cream five times a day for five days, or widespread infection with oral acyclovir 400mg five times a day for five days.

Preventing hair loss

Use of scalp cooling with a cold cap can reduce blood flow to the scalp and therefore dose of chemotherapy to the hair follicles. It should not be used if there is a risk of scalp metastasis or for haematological malignancies and it is only effective for some chemotherapy schedules such as single agent anthracyclines, regimens including Adriamycin® or epirubicin in combination with other cytotoxic drugs which cause minimal hair loss, and the taxanes. It must be applied at least 30 minutes before administration of chemotherapy and remain in place for 60–90 minutes after completion. It may cause discomfort or headaches.

Preservation of fertility during chemotherapy

(See section 16.5, 'Fertility and cancer'.)

There is as yet no means of preventing the gonadal toxicity of chemotherapy in men, and sperm storage before treatment starts is the only option. Gonadal toxicity of chemotherapy occurs in up to 60% of girls and women. The risk of premature ovarian failure increases with

Table 16.13.3 Common chemotherapy regimens associated with high risk of febrile neutropenia (>/20%)

Malignancy	Regimen
Breast cancer	AC followed by docetaxel
	Docetaxel followed by AC
	FEC followed by docetaxel
	Doxorubicin/docetaxel
	Doxorubicin/paclitaxel
	TAC
	Docetaxel + trastuzumab
Non-small cell lung cancer	Docetaxel/carboplatin
	Etoposide/cisplatin
	Cisplatin/vinorelbine/cetuximab
Small cell lung cancer	ACE
	Topotecan
	ICE
	VIDE
Ovarian cancer	Docetaxel
	Paclitaxel
	Topotecan
Urothelial cancer	Paclitaxel/carboplatin
	MVAC
	Doxorubicin/gemcitabine
Germ cell tumours	BOP followed by VIP-B46
	VeIP
	TIP
	BEP
Gastric cancer	LVFU
	LVFU-cisplatin
	LVFU-irinotecan
	DCF
	TC
	TCF
	ECF
Other cancers	TIC (head and neck cancer)
	MAID (sarcoma)
	Paclitaxel/cisplatin (cervical cancer)
Hodgkin disease	BEACOPP
Non-Hodgkin disease	DHAP
	ESHAP
	R-ESHAP as salvage after prior rituximab
	CHOP-21
	HyperCVAD + rituximab
	ICE/R-ICE
	Stanford V*
	MOPPEB-VCAD
	FC
	FCR

* Routine use of G-CSF is not recommended due to increased risk of bleomycin toxicity.

increasing age, and with cumulative drug dose. Options for preservation of fertility include IVF and embryo cryopreservation, unfertilized ova cryopreservation, or use of gonadotrophin releasing hormone (GnRH) agonists. The first two options necessitate delay in starting treatment, whereas hormonal treatment can start immediately.

Goserelin 3.6mg is given subcutaneously, one week before chemotherapy and then four-weekly throughout the course of treatment. Side effects are minimal with only a small decrease in bone mineral density. The mode of action is uncertain. There may be a direct effect on the ovary, or it may break the cycle of follicle depletion with chemotherapy followed by a rise in follicle stimulating hormone (FSH) and consequent accelerated recruitment of more follicles with further damage.

LHRH analogues given during treatment can decrease the rate of ovarian failure. Using the agent goserelin, various groups have shown a reduction in premature ovarian failure from approximately 55% to 11% as indicated by return of menses and FSH level of <40IU/l within 12 months of the last cycle of chemotherapy.

In survivors of childhood cancer there is an 8% risk of premature ovarian failure before the age of 40 compared with an incidence of <1% in the general population. Several large clinical trials of goserelin are recently completed or are still continuing, including the German ZORO trial and the SWOG S0230 phase 3 trial of LHRH analogue administration during chemotherapy to reduce ovarian failure following chemotherapy in early stage or receptor-negative breast cancer. There is some evidence that use of goserelin may also decrease recurrence rate and death from recurrence in breast cancer.

Bone modifying agents in the supportive care of cancer patients

The role of bone modifying agents in the treatment of bone metastases

Bone metastases are common in cancer patients, occurring most frequently in breast, prostate, lung, thyroid, and renal cancers and in multiple myeloma. When tumour cells metastasize to bone they interact with the bone microenvironment resulting in a disturbance of the balance between new bone formation and bone resorption. Tumour cells release cytokines and growth factors which stimulate osteoblasts to produce receptor activator of nuclear factor kappa B ligand (RANKL). Osteoclasts are activated by RANKL resulting in the breakdown of the bone matrix and release of bone derived factors that can lead to further growth and proliferation of tumour cells.

Bone metastases cause significant pain, morbidity, and reduce QoL. Complications from bone metastases are often described as 'skeletal related events' (SREs) typically defined as pathological fracture, need for radiotherapy or surgery, metastatic spinal cord compression, and hypercalcaemia.

There is good evidence that morbidity from bone metastases can be reduced by treatment with bone modifying agents. Bisphosphonates selectively concentrate in bone and are potent inhibitors of osteoclastic activity and directly induce apoptosis of osteoclasts. The bisphosphonates zolendronate, pamidronate, and ibandronate reduce the risk of SREs in breast cancer patients with bone metastases by 15% (RR 0.85, 95% CI 0.77–0.94), delay the time to first SRE, and improve bone pain. In prostate cancer zolendronate is the only bisphosphonate shown to reduce skeletal complications, reducing the incidence of SREs by 36% (HR 0.64) and delaying time to first SRE. The benefit appears to be in castrate resistance disease only. Denosumab is a fully human monoclonal antibody to RANKL and has been shown to be superior to zolendronate in reducing and

Table 16.13.4 Bone modifying agents used in the supportive care of cancer patients

Recommended dose and frequency of administration	Prescribing notes
Prevention of skeletal-related events in metastatic bone disease:	
Zolendronate 4mg over 15 minutes every 3–4 weeks	Reduce dose if CrCl <60ml/min. Avoid CrCl <30ml/min
Pamidronate[1] 90mg IV over 90–120 minutes twice every 3–4 weeks	Infusion rate should not exceed four hours in renal impairment or multiple myeloma, avoid if CrCl <30ml/min
Ibandronate[2] 50mg oral daily or 6mg IV over 1–2 hours every 3–4 weeks	Reduce dose if CrCl <50ml/min
Denosumab 120mg SC every 4 weeks	Should be administered with calcium supplement 500mg and vitamin D 400IU daily, no dose adjustment required in renal failure
Prevention of bone loss:[3]	As above.
Zolendronate 4mg over 15 minutes every 3–4 weeks	
Pamidronate 90mg IV over 90 minutes every 3–4 weeks	
Denosumab 50mg SC every six months	

1. Only licensed in breast cancer and multiple myeloma.

2. Only licensed in breast cancer.

3. Alternative dose intervals (e.g. every 12 weeks) are currently being investigated in clinical trials.

delaying skeletal complications in both breast and prostate cancer. Data from other cancers are more limited but both zolendronate and denosumab have been shown to reduce skeletal complications from bone metastases in other cancers including lung, renal, and thyroid cancer.

No survival benefit has been seen with either bisphosphonates or denosumab in patients with metastatic bone disease. There may however be an emerging role for bisphosphonate therapy in early stage cancer, to prevent or delay bone metastases. In pre-clinical studies bisphosphonates have been found to have direct and indirect antitumour effects. A recent meta-analysis of individual patient data by the Early Breast Cancer Trialists' Collaborative Group found that in postmenopausal women adjuvant bisphosphonate use reduced the risk of bone and distant recurrences and reduced mortality. Two randomized controlled trials investigating whether zolendronate can prevent the development of bone metastases in early prostate cancer have been negative; however other trials addressing this issue are ongoing.

Side effects of bone modifying agents include acute phase reactions (such as transient fever), renal dysfunction, hypocalcaemia, and GI upset with oral bisphosphonates. Osteonecrosis of the jaw (ONJ) is a rare but serious complication of treatment with bisphosphonates seen in 0.7–2% of patients. Risk is increased in those with a history of dental surgery, dental trauma, and poor oral hygiene. The recommended doses and frequency of administration of bone modifying agents are shown in Table 16.13.4.

The role of bone modifying agents in bone health

Many of the treatments commonly used to treat cancer have effects on reproductive hormones which can result in accelerated bone loss. Other risk factors for osteoporosis may also be seen more commonly in cancer patients including increasing age, smoking, excess alcohol, and vitamin D deficiency.

Premature menopause secondary to chemotherapy carries the greatest risk for bone loss, 7.7 times that seen with the natural menopause. Chemotherapy agents associated with a high risk of ovarian failure include alkylating agents, platinums, and anthracyclines. Aromatase inhibitors (AIs) are used in the treatment of ER-positive breast cancer, either alone in postmenopausal women or with a GnRH in premenopausal women. AIs accelerate bone loss and an increased incidence of fractures is seen in women taking an AI compared to those taking tamoxifen. Although tamoxifen has a favourable effect on BMD in postmenopausal women it increases bone loss in premenopausal women. Long-term androgen deprivation therapy (ADT) with orchidectomy or GnRH agonist or antagonist is used in the management of advanced prostate cancer. The risk of osteoporosis in these patients increases steadily with the duration of ADT and the relative increase in fracture risk is reported to be 21–54%. Use of glucocorticoids (>3 months) is also a risk factor for secondary osteoporosis.

The National Comprehensive Cancer Network (NCCN) recommends assessment of bone health in all patients receiving treatment that lowers sex hormones. Assessment of BMD can be made by dual X-ray absorptiometry (DXA) scan of the hip and spine and predicts for osteoporotic fracture risk. Each standard deviation decrease in BMD increases fracture risk approximately twofold. The WHO Fracture Risk Assessment tool (FRAX) combines BMD and clinical risk factors to provide an estimate of ten-year fracture risk.

Treatment with bone modifying agents can prevent or mitigate the damaging effects of treatment on bone health. In breast cancer bisphosphonates have been shown to prevent bone loss in premenopausal women receiving adjuvant chemotherapy or treatment with a GnRH plus tamoxifen or an AI. In women receiving AIs both bisphosphonates and denosumab can reduce bone loss, but only denosumab has been shown to reduce fracture risk in this setting. Oestrogen therapy may be an option in chemotherapy induced menopause to manage menopausal symptoms and to reduce bone loss but should not be used in either ER positive or negative breast cancer due to an increased risk of breast cancer recurrence. In prostate cancer, treatment with bisphosphonates and denosumab has been shown to increase BMD and reduce fracture risk in men receiving ADT.

Further reading

Aapro M, Bohlius J, Cameron D et al. 2010 update of EORTC guidelines for the use of granulocyte-colony stimulating factor to reduce the incidence of chemotherapy-induced febrile neutropenia in adult patients with lymphopro-liferative disorders and solid tumours. *Eur J Cancer* 2011; 47:8–32.

Coleman R, Body JJ, Aapro M et al. Bone health in cancer patients: ESMO Clinical Practice Guidelines. *Ann Oncol* 2014; 25 (S3):124–137

Tonia T, Mettler A, Robert N et al. Erythropoietin or darbepoetin for patients with cancer. *Cochrane Datab Syst Rev* 2012; 12:CD003407.

Internet resources

FRAX tool: http://www.shef.ac.uk/FRAX/

International Osteoporosis Foundation: http://www.iofbonehealth.org

National Comprehensive Cancer Network: http://www.nccn.org

NIH. Goserelin acetate study for ovarian function in patients with primary breast cancer: http://clinicaltrials.gov/ct2/show/NCT00429403

482

Chapter 17

Palliative care

Chapter contents

17.1 Pain management

Incidence of pain

According to a systematic review of the literature, pain prevalence ranges from 33% in patients after curative treatment to 59% in patients on anticancer treatment and to 64% in patients with metastatic, advanced, or terminal phase disease. No difference in pain prevalence was found between patients undergoing anticancer treatment and those in an advanced or terminal phase of the disease.

Despite published guidelines and educational programmes on the assessment and treatment of cancer-related pain, in any stage of oncological disease, unrelieved pain continues to be a substantial worldwide public health concern in patients with either solid or haematological malignancies. Cancer-related pain may be presented as a major issue of healthcare systems worldwide if we consider that the incidence of cancer was 12,667,470 new cases in 2008 and, based on projections, it will be >15 million in 2020.

Assessment

The comprehensive pain assessment should focus on the type and quality of pain; pain history (e.g. onset, duration, course); pain intensity (i.e. pain experienced at rest, with movement); location; referral pattern; radiation of pain; impact of pain (i.e. interference with activities such as work, sleep, and interpersonal interactions); the associated factors that exacerbate or relieve the pain; current pain management plan; patient's response to current therapy; prior pain therapies; breakthrough or episodic pain inadequately managed with existing pain regimen; important psychosocial factors (e.g. patient distress, family/caregiver and other support, psychiatric history, risk factors for undertreatment of pain); and other special issues relating to pain (e.g. meaning of pain for patient and family/caregiver; cultural beliefs toward pain, pain expression, and treatment; spiritual or religious considerations and existential suffering). Finally, the patient's goals and expectations of pain management should be discussed, including level of comfort and function, with family/caregivers included.

Pharmacological interventions

In general, cancer pain management should be focused on the three-step World Health Organization (WHO) analgesic ladder for cancer pain relief (Figure 17.1.1). According to WHO guidelines, opioid analgesics are the mainstay of analgesic therapy and are classified according to their ability to control pain from mild to mild/moderate to moderate/severe intensity. This strategy should, however, be integrated with other methods, as appropriate, of cancer pain control. These include chemotherapy or other anticancer therapies, radiotherapy, palliative surgery, physiotherapy, occupational therapy, anaesthetic interventions, psychosocial care, and any other care, which adds to pain relief. It can be more appropriate with some patients to miss step two of the ladder and simply prescribe low-dose step three (strong opioid) which can mean fewer drug changes. In specialist units, following the WHO ladder will relieve up to 80% of cancer pain.

Step one: Non-opioid analgesia

The most common non-opioid analgesic used is paracetamol, usually prescribed 1g four times daily. The side effects of paracetamol are minimal and it is generally effective in mild pain. As paracetamol works differently from opioids, it is usual to continue it even on the second and third steps of the analgesic ladder. Non-steroidal anti-inflammatory drugs (NSAIDs) are an alternative or addition to paracetamol at each step.

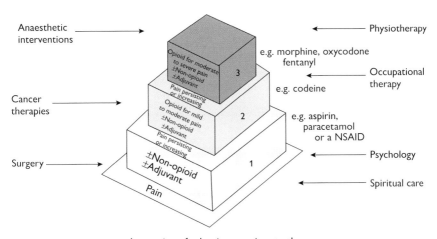

Fig. 17.1.1 World Health Organization analgesic ladder for cancer pain relief.
Adapted with permission from 'WHO Guidelines for the Pharmacological and Radiotherapeutic Management of Cancer Pain in Adults and Adolescents'. Geneva: World Health Organization; © 2018. Available from: https://www.ncbi.nlm.nih.gov/books/NBK537492/.

Step two: Weak opioid

The most commonly used weak opioid is codeine. This has a potency of approximately one-tenth of morphine. It often exists in combination with paracetamol; co-deine 60mg/paracetamol 1g prescribed four times daily. Although other weak opioids are available, there is no evidence to suggest any benefit over codeine. Codeine remains the weak opioid of choice in stage two of the analgesic ladder. Tramadol is another weak opioid, which is often prescribed; however, this can cause confusion in elderly patients.

The use of drugs of the second step of the WHO ladder has several controversial aspects. The first criti-cism concerns the absence of a definitive proof of effi-cacy of weak opioids: in a meta-analysis of data reported from clinical randomized controlled trials, no significant difference was found in effectiveness between non-opioid analgesics alone, and the combination of these with weak opioids. The available studies do not demon-strate a clear difference in the effectiveness of the drugs between the first and the second step.

A recent experience by Bandieri et al. (2016) analyzed the efficacy of low-dose morphine versus weak opi-oids such as tramadol, or codeine in fixed combination with paracetamol. The study was conducted among 240 Italian cancer patients randomly assigned to receive ei-ther low-dose oral morphine or a weak opioid for 28 days. The primary outcome (number of responder pa-tients) occurred in 88.2% of the low-dose morphine and in 57.7% of the weak-opioid group. The percentage of responders (88% vs. 57.7%) was higher in the low-dose morphine group, as early as one week. Furthermore, the general condition of patients, based on the Edmonton Symptom Assessment System overall symptom score, was better in the morphine group. Adverse effects were similar in both groups. No differences in the intensity and frequency of opioid-related symptoms were observed between the two groups. This study does not support the use of tramadol versus low-dose morphine and rep-resents a simplified approach to increase patient access to strong (and low-cost) opioids at an earlier stage in the disease trajectory, improving overall pain control.

Step three: Strong opioids

These should be prescribed at low doses and titrated as described in the following section. Patients often have preconceptions regarding strong opioids and thus they should be counselled fully regarding their use and any concerns explored.

Strong opioid titration

An immediate release strong opioid should be prescribed orally on a regular basis, typically four-hourly.

Normal-release morphine has a short half-life and is indicated: during the titration phase; for treating break through pain (BTP) episodes; and for treating predictable episodes of acute pain in patients on regular analgesics (administration should take place 20–30 minutes before the predictable episode of acute pain). Intravenous titra-tion is indicated in patients with severe pain.

Breakthrough (rescue) analgesia, at the same dose as the regular dose, should also be available. The 'breakthrough dose' is usually equivalent to +10% to 15% of the total daily dose. If more than four 'rescue doses' per day are ne-cessary, the baseline opioid treatment with a slow-release formulation must be adapted. Opioids with a rapid onset and short duration are preferred as rescue medications.

After a period of 48–72 hours the daily analgesic dose can be calculated.

Following the titration period, slow-release opioids are indicated.

Strong opioids

Morphine
- Remains the gold standard opioid.
- Available by oral route or by injection (subcutaneous, intramuscular, intravenous).
- Half-life of 2–3.5 hours.
- Duration of analgesia four to six hours.
- Metabolized to M-6-G (morphine-6-glucuronide) that is active and M-3-G (morphine-3-glucuronide), which is not analgesic but is thought to cause neuroexcitation.
- Metabolites are eliminated by the kidney and accumu-late in renal insufficiency.
- Starting dose from 2.5–10mg (orally, four times daily) depending on patient.
- Commonly available preparations: sustained release (SR), e.g. MST Continus® (lasts 12 hours), immediate release, e.g. Sevredol® (tablets) or Oramorph® (liquid).

Diamorphine (diacetylmorphine)
- Pro-drug of morphine but more soluble.
- Only available in UK and Canada.
- Potency ratio 3:1 with oral morphine.
- Generally only available as a parenteral preparation.

Oxycodone
- Semi-synthetic opioid.
- Metabolized in the liver and excreted in the urine.
- Fewer hallucinations, less confusion/itch than morphine.
- Oral preparations are immediate release (oxynorm) and sustained release (oxycontin) in UK.
- Injection (oxynorm) also available.

Hydromorphone
- Available in oral or injectable form.
- Common preparations: sustained release, Palladone® SR (lasts 12 hours); immediate release, Palladone®.

Fentanyl
- Short half-life when used sublingually or intravenous or subcutaneous.
- Transdermal patches available for cancer pain deliver 12–100mcg/h over three days.
- Transmucosal, buccal, and nasal preparations are be-coming available and may be beneficial in breakthrough pain.
- Elimination half-life after patch removal is almost 24 hours, compared with 3–4 hours after IV injection.
- May take 48 hours to reach steady state when first applied.
- Patches used only for stable pain.
- Breakthrough opioid should be used at appropriate dose.
- Relatively safer in renal failure than renally excreted drugs such as morphine.

Alfentanil
- Injection or buccal spray only, short half-life.
- Like fentanyl—often used perioperatively, however becoming more commonly used in palliative care.
- Relatively safe in renal failure.

Buprenorphine
- Opioid with agonist and antagonist action—effects are only partly reversed by opioid antagonist naloxone.
- Exists in the UK as transdermal patches.
- Relatively safe in renal failure.

Methadone
- N-methyl-D-aspartate acid (NMDA) antagonist—useful in neuropathic pain.
- Plasma half-life 24 hours on average.
- Duration of analgesia often only four to eight hours.
- Can take 5–28 days to reach steady state.
- More potent by oral route than subcutaneous.
- Morphine equivalent dose varies according to prior morphine dose—when using methadone, specialist advice is advised.
- Potentially of use in renal failure.

Transdermal buprenorphine
New transmucosal buccal and nasal fentanyl preparations are the latest additions to the opioid armamentarium.

Choice of strong opioid
In general, morphine is the strong opioid of choice. The greatest amount of evidence exists for morphine; therefore unless a specific reason exists, this should be prescribed in preference to other opioids. It is available in both oral and parenteral preparations. Most palliative care patients respond well to titrated oral morphine:
- For frail/elderly patients, consider a lower starting dose of opioid.
- Seek specialist advice if the patient is in moderate to severe pain with frequent use of breakthrough medication, i.e. more than three doses in 24 hours.

A small number of patients may need to be changed to another opioid if:
- Oral route is not available.
- Pain is responding but the patient has persistent intolerable side effects.
- Moderate to severe liver or renal impairment.
- Poor compliance with oral medication.
- Complex pain where adjuvant analgesics/other pain treatments must be considered.

Transdermal opioids
If a transdermal route is indicated, fentanyl or buprenorphine patches may be of use. Transdermal opioids are only indicated when the pain is stable and are not advised in the acute pain setting. A transdermal fentanyl patch of 12mcg/h equates to a daily morphine dose of approximately 40mg, so caution is advised.

Opioid toxicity
Opioid toxicity can carry a 50% mortality rate in its severe form, and it is therefore important to identify early. Opioid toxicity can occur when the patient has reached the maximum tolerated dose of a specific opioid. It can also be caused by dehydration, with an accumulation of opioid metabolites. Toxicity can occur with any opioid and has a spectrum of clinical features.

Many patients develop adverse effects such as constipation, nausea/vomiting, urinary retention, pruritus, and central nervous system (CNS) toxicity (drowsiness, cognitive impairment, confusion, hallucinations, myoclonic jerks, and opioid-induced hyperalgaesia/allodynia).

Clinical features of opioid toxicity
- Pseudo-hallucinations—shadows at the peripheries of the field of vision.
- Myoclonic jerks—rapid involuntary jerks of muscle groups.
- Cognitive impairment—can range from mild to severe. Often confused with distress or terminal agitation.
- Hallucinations—both auditory and visual hallucinations may occur and may be frightening for the patient.
- Intractable nausea.

Management of opioid toxicity
- Early recognition is important as it can often be reversed easily.
- Several strategies have been recommended to manage opioid-related toxicity. These include switching from one opioid to another opioid agonist, hydration, and reducing the opioid dose. Reducing the opioid dose is an option if pain is well controlled and the toxicity is minimal. A combination of rotating to an alternative opioid and hydration is often effective.
- Step 1: Hydration:
  - If oral intake is limited, parenteral hydration may need to be started. The rationale for hydration is that it can correct delirium caused by dehydration and renal impairment which, in turn, causes metabolites to accumulate.
- Step 2: Opioid reduction.
- Step 3: Opioid rotation (see following section).
- Step 4: Treat symptoms (consider anticipatory prescribing).

When a patient is opioid toxic, but still has not attained sufficient analgesia, general reassessment of pain, biochemistry (urea and electrolytes and corrected calcium in particular), and general drug review should be the first step. Once this has been done, if the patient still has insufficient analgesia and is opioid toxic, a switch to another opioid may be indicated.

Management of opioid side effects
Sometimes, the reduction of the opioid dose may reduce the incidence and/or severity of adverse events. This may be achieved by using a coanalgesic or an alternative approach such as a nerve block or radiotherapy (RT). Other strategies include the continued use of antiemetics for nausea, laxatives for constipation, major tranquilizers for confusion, and psychostimulants for drowsiness. However, as just reported, some of the side effects may be caused by accumulation of toxic metabolites and switching to another opioid agonist and/or another route may allow titration to adequate analgesia without the same disabling effects. This is especially true for symptoms of CNS toxicity such as opioid-induced hyperalgesia/allodynia and myoclonic jerks. Dose reduction or opioid switching is a potentially effective way to manage delirium, hallucination, myoclonus, and hyperalgesia. For opioid-related constipation there is a strong recommendation routinely to prescribe laxatives for prophylaxis and management of opioid-induced constipation. For the other treatment of opioid-induced constipation, see section 17.4, 'Constipation'.

Metoclopramide and antidopaminergic drugs are the drugs most frequently used for treatment of low-grade opioid-related nausea/vomiting.

Opioid switching

If the situation exists where toxicity occurs but adequate analgesia is not achieved, then, assuming a history of opioid responsiveness, the ceiling dose of that particular opioid has been reached and a switch to another opioid is indicated. There is little evidence to support the use of any particular opioid over another. Oxycodone or hydromorphone are alternative opioids, which may be used if morphine toxicity exists. When converting from one opioid to another it is usual to calculate the total daily dose of morphine—morphine equivalent daily dose (MEDD). In general the equi-analgesic dose is calculated, and then this figure is reduced further, usually by one-third. This should be done with specialist guidance in the complex situation of opioid toxicity.

Adjuvant analgesics

Adjuvant analgesics are drugs whose primary function is not analgesia but which can have an analgesic effect (Table 17.1.1). Examples include anti-inflammatory, anticonvulsive, and antidepressant medications. In neuropathic pain, amitriptyline or gabapentin are commonly used. These should be started at low doses and titrated to reach the desired effect. As sedation may occur, it is helpful to commence treatment at night, as any sedation should then be less pronounced.

Non-steroidal anti-inflammatory drugs

NSAIDs are particularly useful analgesics and are usually prescribed for metastatic bone pain, although they are also used for other indications. Co-prescription of a proton pump inhibitor is advised to reduce the incidence of gastrointestinal (GI) side ffects. While interesting preclinical data support the role of the COX-2 inhibitors, particularly in malignant bone pain (antiangiogenesis role), clinical superiority remains unclear. For practical purposes, etirocoxib can be used for patients at high risk of GI side effects.

Breakthrough pain

Defined as a transient exacerbation of pain which occurs either spontaneously or in relation to a specific trigger (incident pain) in someone who has mainly stable or adequately relieved background pain.

A systematic literature review shows that there is no widely accepted definition and classification system or any well validated assessment tools for cancer-related

BTP and the setting of care. These findings could explain why a wide range (19–95%) of prevalence is reported.

Available pharmacological treatment options include oral transmucosal, buccal, oral immediate-release morphine sulfate (IRMS) or nasal, subcutaneous, or intravenous opioids; however, there are few randomized controlled trials. Intravenous opioids, buccal, sublingual, and intranasal fentanyl drug delivery have a shorter onset of analgesic activity in treating BTP episodes than oral morphine.

How to start

- Prescribe immediate release morphine at 1/10th to 1/6th of the regular 24 hour dose, as required.
- Assess 30–60 minutes after a breakthrough dose.
- Immediate release formulation of opioids must be used to treat exacerbations of controlled background pain, especially in the outpatient setting.
- If pain persists give a second dose as required.
- If pain is still not controlled seek advice.
- Change breakthrough dose if regular dose altered.

Movement or incident related predictable pain

- Can be difficult to manage; a dose of short-acting opioid before moving or when pain occurs may help. Immediate release oral morphine is appropriate to treat predictable episodes of BTP (pain on moving, on swallowing, etc.) when administered at least 20 minutes before such potential pain triggers. If pain is short-lived and the patient develops excessive drowsiness seek specialist advice.

Neuropathic pain

Malignant neuropathic pain remains a significant clinical challenge and the reasons are two-fold. Firstly, it is one of the most common symptoms in patients with cancer and some studies have suggested that 50% of all difficult to manage cancer pain is neuropathic. It is often complex to manage and may respond poorly to standard analgesics so specialist advice should be sought early. Neuropathic pain is commonly found in conjunction with other types of pain. Secondly, neuropathic pain can be poorly responsive to opioids because higher doses of opioids are often required, increasing the likelihood of unacceptable side effects which limit dose escalation.

Table 17.1.1 Adjuvant analgesics

Drug	Dosage	Indications	Side effects
NSAIDs (COX-2 inhibitors can be used if high risk of GI side effects)	e.g. diclofenac 50mg TDS orally, 100mg OD per rectum	Bone metastases, hepatic pain, inflammatory pain, soft tissue infiltration	Gastric irritation, headache, fluid retention. Use with caution in renal impairment
Steroids	e.g. dexamethasone 8–16mg daily, best used in the morning. Titrate down to the lowest dose which controls pain	Raised intracranial pressure, nerve compression, soft tissue infiltration, hepatic pain	Hyperglycaemia, cushingoid appearance, confusion, gastric irritation if used with a NSAID
Gabapentin	100–300mg (nocte). Titrate to 600mg three times daily. Higher doses may be needed	Nerve pain of any cause	Mild sedation, confusion, tremor
Amitriptyline	Starting dose 25mg (nocte). In elderly start at 10mg	Nerve pain of any cause	Sedation, dizziness, confusion, dry mouth, constipation, urinary retention. Avoid in cardiac disease
Carbamazepine	Starting dose 100–200mg (nocte)	Nerve pain of any cause	Vertigo, sedation, constipation, rash

Adjuvant analgesics are an important part of the neuropathic pain armamentarium. Most commonly used adjuvant analgesics have a number needed to treat of about three (NNT=3). This means that of every three patients treated, one is likely to get pain relief. The choice of adjuvant analgesic is based on an individual's predicted sensitivity to a specific side-effect profile, e.g. postural hypotension with amitriptyline and the usefulness of the adjuvant in dealing with more than one symptom, e.g. duloxetine for neuropathic pain and depression.

Assessment

Pain in a dermatomal or neuro-anatomical area, combined with a history of a disease or a lesion that might affect the nervous system, might suggest the possibility of neuropathic pain. This should be confirmed by clinical examination or detailed imaging.

Sensory descriptors associated with neuropathic pain include burning, tingling, pins and needles, shooting, and numbness. They are not diagnostic, however.

Confirm altered sensation in the area of pain by comparing responses with the non-painful contralateral or adjacent area of the body:

- Allodynia—painful response to light touch, e.g. stroking the skin with a finger or cotton wool.
- Hypoaesthesia—an area of reduced sensation to non-painful or painful stimuli.
- Hyperalgesia—an exaggerated pain response to stimulus, e.g. a lowered pin prick threshold.
- Altered thermal threshold to cold or hot (e.g. reduced or exaggerated response to a cold metal spoon, or a hot cup of tea).

Principles of adjuvant analgesic use

Antidepressants and anticonvulsants are first-line adjuvant analgesics for the treatment of cancer-related neuropathic pain. These drugs can be helpful for patients whose pain is only partially responsive to opioids. The use of adjuvant analgesics in the cancer population is often based on guidelines or experience derived from data for the treatment of pain not caused by cancer (non-malignant pain).

- Effective use is predicated on an assessment that clarifies the nature of the pain as most adjuvant analgesics are more likely to be effective in the management of neuropathic pain.
- As with opioids, response to adjuvant analgesics may vary according to the type/cause of neuropathic pain and the individual patient.
- Drug selection may be in influenced by other symptoms and comorbidities. For example, a sedating drug may be useful in a patient in whom insomnia is a problem.
- Patient education should emphasize the trial and error nature of the treatment so patients do not get discouraged.
- Doses should be increased until the analgesic effect is achieved, adverse effects become unmanageable, or the conventional maximal dose is reached.

Anticonvulsants

- Currently gabapentin and pregabalin are commonly used as adjuvant analgesics on the basis of easier titration.

- Frequently used as an adjuvant analgesic in combination with an opioid for the neuropathic component of the pain.

Anticonvulsants examples

Gabapentin—starting dose 100–300mg nightly, increase to 900–3600mg daily in divided doses two to three times a day. Dose increments of 50–100% every three days. Slower titration for the elderly or medically frail. Dose adjustment required for those with renal insufficiency.

Pregabalin—starting dose 50mg three times a day, increase to 100mg three times a day. Slower titration for the elderly or medically frail. Dose adjustment required for those with renal insufficiency. Pregabalin is more efficiently absorbed through the GI tract than gabapentin. May increase further to a maximum dose of 600mg in divided doses two to three times a day.

When switching from gabapentin to pregabalin—the following would be reasonable:

- Replace gabapentin 300mg three times a day with pregabalin 100mg twice a day.
- Replace gabapentin 600mg, 900mg, and 1,200mg three times a day with pregabalin 200mg twice a day.
- The dose of pregabalin can be further increased depending on response and tolerability to a maximum of 300mg twice a day.

Antidepressants

- A Cochrane review provided a valuable summary of the current evidence for the use of antidepressants in nonmalignant neuropathic pain.
- Analgesic effectiveness is not dependent on its antidepressant activity. Effective analgesic dose: (1) may be lower than that required to treat depression; and (2) the onset of analgesic relief may occur earlier than antidepressive effects.
- Frequently used as an adjuvant analgesic in combination with an opioid for the neuropathic component of the pain.
- Check for drug interactions with special regard to serotonergic medications due to risk of serotonin syndrome.
- Tricyclic antidepressants (e.g. amitriptyline, imipramine, nortriptyline, desipramine).
- Start with low dose and increase every three to five days if tolerated (e.g. nortriptyline and desipramine starting dose 10–25mg nightly, increase to 50–150mg nightly). The tertiary amines (i.e. amitriptyline, imipramine) may be more efficacious but secondary amines (i.e. nortriptyline, desipramine) are better tolerated. Anticholinergic adverse effects such as sedation, dryness of mouth, and urinary hesitancy are more likely to occur with amitriptyline and imipramine.
- Other examples:
  - Duloxetine—starting dose 20–30mg daily, increase to 60–120mg daily.
  - Venlafaxine—starting dose 37.5mg daily, increase to 75–225mg daily.

Ketamine

- The NMDA receptors within the spinal cord have been shown to have a significant role in the pathophysiology of neuropathic pain. Ketamine is an NMDA antagonist which has been studied in neuropathic pain and evidence exists for its use, either orally or parenterally.

It can be useful in neuropathic pain where there are clinical indicators of central wind-up such as pain on light touch and increased pain to any painful stimulus. In addition, if opioid doses are escalating with reduced response, ketamine may be considered to achieve renewed opioid response.

Topical agents
* Act locally and may be used as an adjuvant analgesic in combination with an opioid, antidepressant, and/or an anticonvulsant.
* Topical agent example: lidocaine patch—5%—apply daily to the painful site. There is minimal systemic absorption. There is supporting evidence advocating the use of topical lidocaine in patients with post-herpetic neuralgia and patients with localized peripheral neuropathic pain. It is available either as a patch or as a topical gel. Lidocaine patches have been used in cancer-related neuropathic pain where allodynia (sensitivity to light touch) exists.

Corticosteroids
* Consider dexamethasone (due to less mineralocorticoid effect).
* Long half-life of these drugs allows for once daily dosing, preferably in the morning due to their stimulating effect and to prevent night-time insomnia.
* Useful in the acute management of a pain crisis when neural structures or bones are involved.
* Long-term adverse effects are significant.

Neuropathic cancer pain—treatment strategy
The commonly used drugs in cancer-related neuropathic pain have been studied extensively in non-malignant neuropathic pain. It is reasonable to extrapolate these findings to neuropathic cancer pain.

A suggested treatment strategy, which is based on a combination of available evidence and clinical experience in the UK, is as follows.

All steps are in conjunction with the WHO analgesic ladder. Titrate individual drugs to desired effect:
* Start amitriptyline. If patient is already taking amitriptyline, then,
* Add in or replace amitriptyline with either gabapentin or pregabalin.
* Trial of ketamine—either orally or via parenteral route.
* Anaesthetic interventions, e.g. nerve block, epidural, or intrathecal.

Cancer-induced bone pain
Cancer-induced bone pain (CIBP) is a major cause of morbidity in patients with cancer. Up to 85% of patients with bone metastases have pain and CIBP is a common cause of hospital or hospice admission. Commonly occurring malignancies such as cancers of the breast and prostate frequently metastasize to bone. In addition, advances in treatment have led to patients living longer with advanced cancer and developing symptoms of bone metastases.

Palliative radiotherapy remains the most effective anticancer treatment for CIBP. Systematic reviews show 41% of patients achieve 50% pain relief within four weeks of treatment. While this is an excellent response for any analgesic method, for individual patients, other methods may be required.

Treatment of CIBP
The treatment of CIBP involves a combination of analgesia (according to the WHO ladder), NSAIDs, and appropriate short-acting opioids.
* Rest pain responds well to conventional analgesic regimens.
* CIBP is often worsened by movement-related pain.
* Movement-related CIBP often responds poorly to opioid analgesia because it can be sudden and of short duration. This means that opioid-related adverse effects will be more common.
* Use short-acting oral opioids (fentanyl lozenges, alfentanil spray) before movement. Short-acting opioids briefly increase analgesic levels during movement so minimizing unwanted opioid side effects at rest.

Bisphosphonates
Bisphosphonates (BPs) have been shown to be effective in reducing the incidence of skeletal events and time to skeletal events. There is sufficient evidence supporting the analgesic efficacy of BPs in patients with bone pain due to bone metastases from solid tumours and multiple myeloma. However, the prescription of BPs should not be considered as an alternative to analgesic treatment and their administration should be started after preventive dental measures. After the first IV infusion of BPs, pain can appear or its intensity increase, and the use of analgesics such as paracetamol or a basal analgesic dose increase is necessary.

Denosumab
Denosumab, a targeted RANK ligand inhibitor, is a new therapy for the prevention of skeletal-related events (SREs). Three prominent clinical trials were conducted to establish the efficacy of denosumab. In two of three trials, denosumab was found to delay the time to first SRE significantly, more than zoledronic acid in patients with breast or castration-resistant prostate cancer with bone metastasis. The third trial found denosumab to be non-inferior to zoledronic acid in patients with metastases from solid tumours, excluding breast and prostate solid tumours.

The integrated analysis of pain outcomes, presented only in the form of an abstract, found a superiority of denosumab when compared with zoledronic acid in delay time to moderate/severe pain occurrence and in reducing analgesic use. The prescription of denosumab should be started after preventive dental measures.

Anaesthetic interventions
In the majority of cases, cancer pain can be controlled using conventional analgesics. The WHO ladder can be thought of as the central pillar of analgesic management, but additional therapies such as radiotherapy and chemotherapy, surgery, physiotherapy, and transcutaneous electrical nerve stimulation (TENS) can be used alongside the WHO ladder.

If, however, standard systemic analgesia has been either ineffective or side effects have prevented adequate doses being reached, anaesthetic interventions may be necessary. Anaesthetic interventions are often regarded as step four of the WHO ladder but can be implemented at any stage of the ladder as clinical need dictates.

Methods include regional nerve blocks (commonly coeliac plexus block for upper abdominal pain) and neuro-destructive blocks. The latter are often reserved

Table 17.1.2 Factors affecting choice of neuraxial analgesia

Epidural	Intrathecal (spinal)
Prognosis	
Short-term use only—where prognosis is limited	Long-term use—both external or implantable pumps can be used
As a trial of analgesia prior to intrathecal	
Other treatment planned, e.g. radiotherapy	
Procedure	
Usually local anaesthetic ± sedation	Sedation or general anaesthetic usually required
Fixation may be difficult	Deep fixation when inserted
Catheters may migrate to intrathecal space—potential for overdose	Catheters can only migrate back to epidural space
Drug distribution may be limited if there is epidural tumour or radiotherapy scarring	Drug distribution is determined by lipid solubility and spreads within cerebrospinal fluid
Catheters short-term use only	Catheters designed for long-term use
Drug dose	
One-tenth of systemic dose	One-hundredth of systemic dose

for cases when other measures have failed. Neuraxial analgesia (epidural and intrathecal—also known as spinal) is often used in the management of malignant pelvic pain (Table 17.1.2).

Whether or not an anaesthetic intervention is indicated is influenced by:

- Underlying pain and pathology
- Patients' expectations
- Prognosis
- Required duration of analgesia
- Availability of specialist staff

If the choice of route is appropriate and the technique undertaken and managed by trained staff, neuraxial analgesia can provide effective analgesia. Often a trial of epidural analgesia is done to determine the effect. If this is successful, intrathecal analgesia may follow on from this. Intrathecal catheters are often tunnelled subcutaneously to reduce the risk of infection and dislodgement. A trial of an external pump is usually done before an implantable pump is inserted.

Choice of drug

Usually a combination of local anaesthetic (levobupivicaine) and strong opioid (morphine or diamorphine) is effective. For intrathecal administration, opioid doses are usually in the region of one-hundredth of the systemic dose. This allows much smaller doses to be administered, minimizing side effects and toxicity.

Clonidine, ketamine, and midazolam can also be delivered via the intrathecal route.

Non-pharmacological interventions

Non-pharmacological interventions are an important adjunct in the management of cancer pain with a very low risk of side effects. TENS, acupuncture, relaxation techniques, and massage may all be of benefit. Appropriate review and intervention by both physiotherapists and occupational therapists may improve pain through rehabilitation and functional aids.

Further reading

Bandieri E, Romero M, Ripamonti CI, et al. Randomized trial of low-dose morphine versus weak opioids in moderate cancer pain. *J Clin Oncol* 2016; 34(5):436–42.

Dworkin RH, O'Connor AB, Backonja M, et al. Pharmacologic management of neuropathic pain: evidence-based recommendations. *Pain* 2007; 132:237–51.

Finnerup NB, Otto M, McQuay HJ, et al. Algorithm for neuropathic pain treatment: an evidence based proposal. *Pain* 2005; 118:289–305.

Mercadante S, Radbruch I, Caraceni A, et al. Episodic breakthrough pain: consensus conference of an export working group of the European Association for Palliative Care. *Cancer* 2002; 94:832–9.

Ripamonti CI, Santini D, Maranzano E et al. Management of cancer pain: ESMO Clinical Practice Guidelines. *Ann Oncol* 2012 Oct; 23(Suppl. 7):vii139–54.

17.2 Nausea and vomiting

Introduction

The most common symptoms in advanced cancer, nausea, and vomiting, can be difficult to palliate unless treatment is directed in a logical and specific way. To this end an understanding of the pathophysiology of nausea and vomiting is required (Figure 17.2.1).

Vomiting is the result of stimulation of the vomiting centre. The vomiting centre is not an anatomical area per se but rather acts as a coordinating centre for various neurogenic inputs.

Knowledge of the pathophysiology of nausea and vomiting, in combination with history and examination findings, will assist in recognizing the pathway affected. The receptors in this specific pathway should then be targeted by the appropriate antiemetic (Figure 17.2.2).

Clinical approach

History: Key points

- Nature of vomits, e.g. bile stained vomiting may suggest a more proximal cause and help to rule out gastric outlet obstruction; faecally stained vomit suggests a more distal cause or the presence of a fistula between the large and small bowel.
- Volume of vomits—large volume may suggest gastric stasis or bowel obstruction.
- Timing of vomiting—early morning vomiting may be a sign of raised intracranial pressure (brain tumours, cerebral metastases, or meningeal carcinomatosis). Vomiting late in the day may be due to bowel obstruction.
- Query triggering/alleviating factors.
- Frequency of vomiting (high frequency can lead to dehydration).
- Vomiting related to movement may suggest an inner ear cause.

Examination: Key points

- Assess for hydration state.
- Abdominal examination; including careful observation looking for peristalsis, testing for a succussion splash, auscultation.
- Rectal examination—to exclude constipation.

Investigations

Investigations are tailored to the individual and may include the following:

- Plasma urea and electrolytes, glucose
- Serum corrected calcium—hypercalcaemia commonly causes constipation
- Abdominal X-ray—presence of air-fluid levels suggests obstruction

Possible causes of nausea and vomiting in cancer

- Bowel obstruction—secondary to underlying disease or constipation
- Chemotherapy
- Radiotherapy
- Pain
- Drug-induced, e.g. opioids, antibiotics

- Electrolyte imbalance, e.g. uraemia, hypercalcaemia, severe hyponatraemia
- Paraneoplastic causes
- Vestibular dysfunction
- Gastric stasis-related, such as with ascites, hepatomegaly, paraneoplastic neuropathy, opioid-induced, malignant bowel obstruction, etc.
- Brain metastases or meningeal carcinomatosis
- Psychological factors, e.g. anxiety, anticipatory emesis in patients undergoing chemotherapy

Management

- There are two therapeutic approaches. One is empirical; starting with one drug and if unsuccessful adding or rotating to another. The second is aetiological; that is management tailored to the suspected cause and/or likely receptors involved in generating nausea and/or vomiting.
- Use appropriate non-pharmacological measures.
- Identify the specific pathway(s) involved and receptors.
- Use the most potent drug for the pathway identified (Table 17.2.1).
- Use the most appropriate route of administration.
- In established nausea and vomiting, parenteral administration is needed in the initial stages—to ensure drug absorption.
- Titrate the dose and monitor clinical effect.
- If symptoms do not improve, consider additional antiemetics, use another antiemetic or coadjuvant drugs (e.g. corticosteroids)
- In malignant bowel obstruction, unlike chemotherapy-induced nausea and vomiting, there is no evidence that combining antiemetics improves responses over monotherapy, although this needs formal research confirmation.

Non-pharmacological measures

Remove any nausea stimuli from the environment.

- Use palatable food and drinks.
- Offer frequent small amounts of food and drink.
- Cognitive therapy may be helpful in anticipatory nausea.
- TENS can enhance pharmacological measures.
- Acupuncture/acupressure: thought to work peripherally and centrally by stimulating small myelinated nerves, and by causing release of natural endogenous opioids and neurotransmitters, e.g. serotonin. Most common points used are P6 and ST36.

First-line antiemetics

Haloperidol

- Antipsychotic.
- Acts on the dopamine (D2) receptors in the chemoreceptor trigger zone.
- Effective in nausea and vomiting associated with drugs and metabolic disturbance such as morphine, hypercalcaemia, renal failure, etc.
- Dose: usually 1.5mg at night by mouth which can be increased to 3mg if needed.

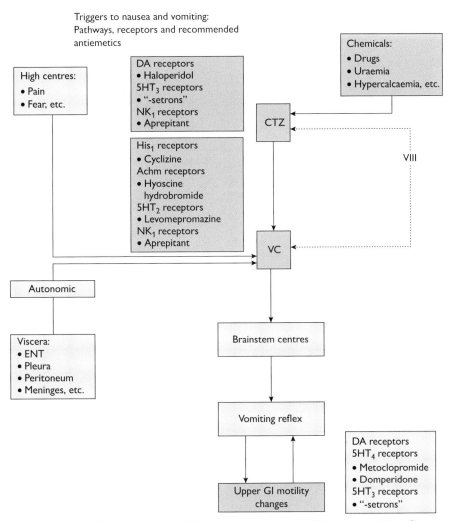

Fig. 17.2.1 Pathophysiology of nausea and vomiting. CTZ, chemoreceptor trigger zone; ENT, ear, nose, and throat; GI, gastrointestinal; VC, vomiting centres.

- Long half-life so a single daily dose is usually sufficient. Parenteral doses are usually between 2.5 and 5mg subcutaneously over 24 hours.
- Extrapyramidal effects (including tardive dyskinesia), hypotension (peripheral alpha blocker), weak antimuscarinic and antihistaminic effects including sedation at high doses (generally >20mg daily), neuroleptic malignant syndrome.

Cyclizine
- Antihistamine.
- Acts on the H1 receptors in the cerebral cortex, vomiting centre, and inner ear.
- Antiemetic of choice in mechanical bowel obstruction and motion sickness.
- Effective in nausea associated with cerebral irritation, e.g. cerebral metastases (in conjunction with dexamethasone). Usual dose is 25–50mg three times daily (p.o.).

- Can be given parenterally, 75–150mg over 24 hours.
- Can cause sedation.

Metoclopramide
- Prokinetic.
- Acts mainly on 5-HT4 and D2 receptors and is effective in gastric stasis.
- Has been shown to be beneficial in incomplete bowel obstruction (functional bowel obstruction, peristaltic failure) but should be avoided in cases of complete obstruction as colic may occur.
- In early satiety associated with delayed gastric emptying, metoclopramide is usually effective (gastritis, gastric stasis).
- Dose: usually 10mg four times daily (p.o.) but can also be given parenterally 40–80mg over 24 hours.
- Adverse effects: extrapyramidal, acute dystonic reactions and oculogyric crisis, restlessness, diarrhoea, colic, neuroleptic malignant syndrome.

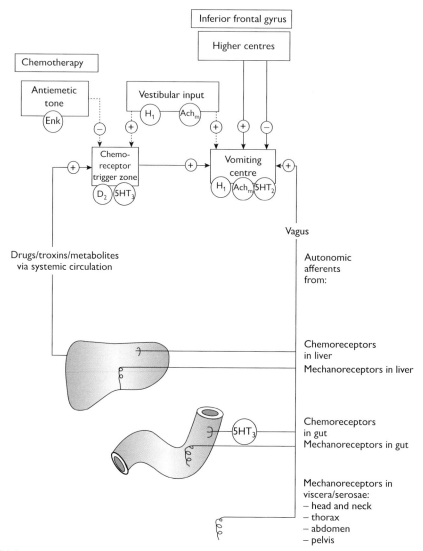

Fig. 17.2.2 Receptors involved in nausea and vomiting.
Reproduced with permission from Cherny N, et al. *Oxford Textbook of Palliative Medicine*, 5th edn. Copyright © 2015, Oxford University Press. doi: 10.1093/med/9780199656097.001.0001.

Table 17.2.1 Common causes of nausea and vomiting and first-line treatments

Cause of nausea and vomiting	Treatment: first-line antiemetic
Chemotherapy	Granisetron 1mg bd p.o. Dexamethasone 4–8mg od p.o. Metoclopramide 20mg qds p.o.
Radiotherapy	Granisetron 1mg bd p.o. Haloperidol 1.5mg o.d. or bd. p.o.
Raised intracranial pressure	Cyclizine 50mg tds p.o.
Delayed gastric emptying	Metoclopramide 10–20mg qds p.o. *or* domperiodone 10–20mg qds p.o.
Drug induced	Haloperidol 1.5mg od or bd p.o.
Metabolic, e.g. uraemia or hypercalcaemia	Haloperidol 1.5mg od or bd p.o.

bd twice daily; p.o. by mouth; od once daily; qds once a day; tds three times daily.

- Domperidone is an alternative to metoclopramide, which has less central activity and therefore is less likely to cause extrapyramidal side effects.

5-HT3 antagonists
- For example, ondansetron, granisetron, palonosetron, dolasetron, tropisetron.
- 5-HT3-receptor antagonist.
- Very useful in nausea and vomiting secondary to chemo- or radiotherapy, in association with dexamethasone or other drugs (such as NK1 receptor antagonist drugs) according to chemotherapy schedule.
- Adverse effects: headache, constipation, sedation and fatigue, rarely extrapyramidal symptoms, dystonic reaction.

Second-line antiemetics

Levomepromazine
- Broad spectrum; acts on Ach, H1, 5-HT2, and D2 receptors.
- Effective in most cases of nausea and vomiting.
- Can cause sedation so in general it is started at low doses and increased as needed.
- Usual dose is 6.25–25mg subcutaneously per 24 hours.
- An oral preparation is available (6mg tablet) administered once per day, usually at night.

Dexamethasone
- No specific receptor affinity.
- Mechanism of action is unclear. It is often used in addition to first-line antiemetics.

- Dose 4–8mg once daily (p.o.) with equivalent doses parenterally (often given as a single daily dose)
- Adverse effects: agitation, insomnia, euphoria, increased appetite, fluid retention, dyspepsia, raised blood sugar, myopathy.

Cannabinoids
Cannabis-based medications may be useful for treating refractory chemotherapy-induced nausea and vomiting, which has not responded to established antiemetics. There are over 300 compounds in marijuana.
- Nabilone is the only licensed cannabinoid in UK—second-line treatment of nausea and vomiting secondary to cytotoxic chemotherapy.
- Adverse effects: sedation, psychomimetic—agitation, intoxication, clumsiness, dizziness, dry mouth, lowered blood pressure, increased heart rate.
- However, methodological limitations of the trials limit our conclusions and further research reflecting current chemotherapy regimens and newer antiemetic drugs is likely to modify these conclusions.
- Evidence still remains poor.

Further reading
Roila F, Molassiotis A, Herrstedt J, et al. 2016 MASCC and ESMO guideline update for the prevention of chemotherapy- and radiotherapy-induced nausea and vomiting and of nausea and vomiting in advanced cancer patients. *Ann Oncol* 2016; 27(Suppl. 5):v119–33.

Smith LA, Azariah F, Lavender VT, et al. Cannabinoids for nausea and vomiting in adults with cancer receiving chemotherapy. *Cochrane Database Syst Rev* 2015 Nov 12;(11):CD009464.

17.3 Malignant bowel obstruction

Introduction
Malignant bowel obstruction (MBO) is a common complication in patients with abdominal or pelvic cancers (e.g. those arising from colon, ovary, and stomach). Treatment depends on various factors from level of obstruction to underlying disease. MBO can be a clinical challenge and surgery, if appropriate, is the treatment of choice. Often surgery is not appropriate due to poor clinical condition and thus conservative management is the mainstay of treatment in these cases.

Clinical approach: Key points
The clinical approach is very much dependent on the level of the obstruction. However the following symptoms and signs are often present:
- Abdominal pain: frequently colicky in character prior to vomiting.
- Nausea: usually relieved to varying degrees after a vomit.
- Vomiting: this is often bile stained if the obstruction is proximal. If the obstruction is distal it is more likely to be faecally stained.
- Constipation: if complete obstruction is present, the patient is unable to pass flatus. In the early stages of constipation, diarrhoea can occur.
- Abdominal distension.
- Succussion splash.
- Increased bowel sounds (borborygmi) often 'tinkling' in nature.

Investigations
- Plasma urea and electrolytes: patients often uraemic.
- Abdominal X-rays show dilated loops of bowel and can assist in locating the level of the obstruction.
- CT of abdomen is useful to determine if there are multiple levels of obstruction, which would normally preclude surgery.

Management
Palliative surgery can reverse malignant bowel obstruction. The type of obstruction (partial vs. complete) and method of surgical treatment (bypass vs. resection and re-anastomosis) have no significant effect on the outcome.

Poor prognostic factors that preclude a surgical approach include:

- Intestinal motility problems due to diffuse intraperitoneal carcinomatosis
- Patients over 65, particularly if cachectic
- Ascites requiring frequent paracentesis
- Advanced cachexia
- Previous radiotherapy of the abdomen or pelvis
- Palpable intra-abdominal masses and liver involvement
- Distant metastases, pleural effusion, or pulmonary metastases
- Multiple partial bowel obstructions with prolonged passage time on radiographic examination

• Poor general performance status

While, if possible, surgery is the treatment of choice, in most cases treatment is conservative.

Pharmacological symptomatic treatment (Figure 17.3.1) should be used in inoperable patients with the following aims:

• To relieve continuous abdominal pain and intestinal colic.
• To reduce vomiting to an acceptable level for the patient (e.g. one to two times in 24 hours) without the use of a nasogastric tube.
• To relieve nausea.
• To achieve hospital discharge, and to allow for home/hospice care.

Analgesics

The administration of analgesics, mainly strong opioids, according to the WHO guidelines, allows adequate pain relief in most patients. The dose of opioids should be titrated against the effect and most usually be administered parenterally.

If colic persists despite the use of an opioid, hyoscine butylbromide or hyoscine hydrobromide should also be administered in association.

Nausea and vomiting

Nausea and vomiting can be managed using two different pharmacological approaches:

• Administration of drugs that reduce GI secretions such as anticholinergics (hyoscine hydrobromide, hyoscine butylbromide, glycopyrrolate) and/or somatostatin analogues (octreotide).

• Administration of antiemetics acting on the central nervous system, alone or in association with drugs to reduce GI secretions.

Steroids

Several authors recommend the use of corticosteroids to manage the symptoms of bowel obstruction because they can reduce peritumour inflammatory edema and improve intestinal motility. To date, no controlled clinical trials have been carried out and the various administration routes and dosing of these medications have not been standardized.

• Dexamethasone is the usual prescribed steroid in MBO.
• Doses range of 8–16mg per day, administered parenterally (usually subcutaneously) to ensure absorption.

Somatostatin analogue (octreotide)

• Octreotide is a synthetic analogue of somatostatin. Somatostatin and its analogues have been shown to inhibit the release and activity of GI hormones, modulate GI function by reducing gastric acid secretion, slow intestinal motility, decrease bile flow, increase mucous production, and reduce splanchnic blood flow.
• Dose: the recommended starting dose is 0.3mg/day subcutaneously. The dose can be titrated upward until symptom control is achieved, usually at 0.6–0.9mg/day.
• Sustained release formulation of octreotide is administered intramuscularly once every four weeks (20mg) (equates to a dose of approx. 1mg per day).

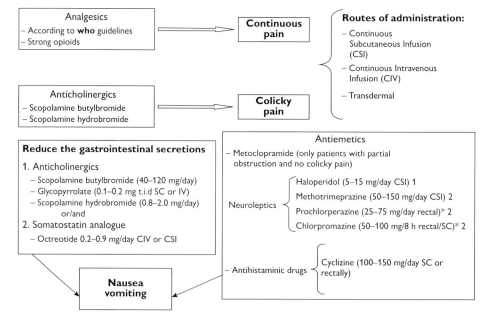

1 butyrophenones   2 phenothiazines   * Skin irritation when administered subcutaneous (SC)

Fig. 17.3.1 Pharmacological approach in the management of malignant bowel obstruction.
Reproduced with permission from Ripamonti I, Easson AM, Gerdes H. Management of malignant bowel obstruction. *Eur J of Cancer* 2008; 44(8):1105–15. Copyright © 2008, Elsevier Ltd.

Antinauseants
- Incomplete obstruction: metoclopramide is the antiemetic of choice providing there is no colic present. Metoclopramide is both an antidopaminergic antiemetic and a GI prokinetic agent.
- Complete obstruction: haloperidol is an effective antidopaminergic antiemetic. It can be combined with scopolamine and an opioid in the same solution for simpler administration parenterally. A standard dosing regimen is: haloperidol, 1mg IV/SC q 6–8 hours.
- Scopolamine butylbromide, also known as hyoscine butylbromide, decreases tone and peristalsis in smooth muscle, decreases the secretions in the GI tract, and lessens the resulting pain. Scopolamine butylbromide is preferred over atropine and scopolamine hydrobromide as it is much less lipid soluble, does not penetrate the blood–brain barrier, and produces fewer adverse effects (e.g. somnolence and hallucinations) when administered in combination with opioids. Dry mouth is reported to be the most significant adverse effect, but patients tolerate it by sucking ice cubes and drinking small sips of water. Standard dosing regimens include:
  - Scopolamine 0.1–0.4mg SC q 6 hours or scopolamine 0.1mg/hour SC/IV continuous infusion.
- Glycopyrrolate can be used with similar effects and properties. It is a quaternary ammonium anticholinergic agent that also has limited lipid solubility and less risk of both central nervous system and ocular effects. The onset of its action is 35–45 minutes when given subcutaneously and one minute when given intravenously. Glycopyrrolate cannot be mixed with diazepam, methylprednisolone, dexamethasone, dimenhydrinate, or phenobarbital. A common dosing range is:
  - Glycopyrrolate 0.2–0.4 mg SC q 6 hours or 0.02mg/hour continuous infusion.

Venting gastrostomy
- When obstructive symptoms cannot be controlled with medications, percutaneous gastrostomy is believed to be a more effective and acceptable alternative to the prolonged use of a nasogastric tube.
- Useful in proximal GI obstruction.
- Inserted relatively easily by endoscopy.

- Often better tolerated than nasogastric tubes and complications are far less frequent.

Nasogastric intubation and intravenous fluids
Nasogastric suction decompresses the stomach and/or intestine; intravenous fluids correct fluid and electrolyte imbalance. Both of these techniques can be employed before surgery or while a decision is being made. Because a nasogastric tube often becomes occluded and requires flushing and/or replacement, it is not a realistic long-term solution. During long-term drainage, the tube interferes with coughing to clear pulmonary secretions and may be associated with nasal cartilage erosion, otitis media, aspiration pneumonia, esophagitis, and bleeding. This treatment can also create considerable discomfort in patients who are already distressed by previous anticancer and surgical therapies. Consider long-term use of a nasogastric tube only when pharmacological therapy for symptom control is ineffective or when gastrostomy cannot be carried out.

Malignant bowel obstruction: a strategy
A multifaceted approach is often needed. Parenteral drug administration (usually subcutaneous) is usually needed to ensure absorption.
- Pain: is managed according to the WHO analgesic ladder. Patients will often require strong opioids.
- Nausea and vomiting: in incomplete obstruction, metoclopramide can be used. If complete obstruction develops, cyclizine is the antiemetic of choice.
- Steroids can be beneficial to control nausea, and reduce gut wall oedema and extrinsic compression. This may assist in resolution of an incomplete obstruction.
- Nasogastric tube: consider this on an individual basis.
- Octreotide: helpful in reducing intestinal secretions and may be beneficial in patients with vomiting as a symptom.

Further reading
Ripamonti C. Malignant bowel obstruction. In Ripamonti C, Bruera E, (eds). *Gastrointestinal Symptoms in Advanced Cancer Patients*. Oxford: Oxford University Press, 2002:235.
Ripamonti C, Eassonc AM, Gerdsed H. Management of malignant bowel obstruction. *Eur J Cancer* 2008; 44:1105–15.

17.4 Constipation

Introduction
Constipation is a common cause of morbidity in palliative care patients. Some studies suggest that up to 50% of cancer patients will develop constipation and up to 95% of patients who are taking opioids if not treated prophylactically.

Causes
- Poor oral intake or dehydration.
- Malnutrition: autonomic neuropathy related to the anorexia/cachexia/asthenia syndrome of advanced cancer.
- Drugs: primarily opioids, anticholinergic drugs, diuretics, iron, etc.
- Decreased mobility leading to decreased frequency of peristalsis.
- Dehydration and subsequent electrolyte abnormalities, e.g. hypercalcaemia, hypokalaemia.

- It can also be the due to intestinal obstruction secondary to the underlying malignancy.
- Neurological—spinal cord compression will leave the anocolic reflex intact—thus rectal intervention will stimulate bowel emptying. In cauda equina lesions the colon will be lax.

Complications of constipation
- Abdominal pain and aggravation of cancer pain in patients with abdominal or retroperitoneal malignancy.
- Abdominal distension and discomfort.
- Nausea and vomiting.
- Overflow diarrhoea.
- Haemorrhoids and anal fissures.
- Bowel pseudo-obstruction.
- Urinary retention.

Clinical approach: Key points

- Suspect constipation in any patient with advanced cancer presenting with, amongst other symptoms, one or more of the following: irregular bowel movements, diarrhoea, nausea and vomiting, abdominal discomfort, and bowel obstruction.
- Perform a digital rectal examination.
- Occasionally a plain abdominal radiograph may assist in the diagnosis.
- A 'constipation score' is occasionally very helpful in assessing constipation.

Management

Prevention

General measures:
- Encourage generous fluid intake (8–10 glasses/day).
- Large amounts of dietary fibre are often poorly tolerated by debilitated patients and should only be increased gradually.
- Encourage exercise as tolerated.
- When starting a patient on an opioid, start laxatives simultaneously. Start with a bowel stimulant and a stool softener, e.g. senna 1–2 tabs + docusate 100mg bid p.o. Doses can be titrated upwards so as to achieve a bowel movement regularly (every one to two days).
- If patients find it difficult to swallow tablets/capsules, senna and docusate come in liquid forms. (Lactulose, 30ml tid, is an alternative.)
- If patient is unable to achieve a bowel movement within three days, administer a fleet enema or bisacodyl suppository rectally on day three.
- Commonly used doses are:
  - Senna 2–4 tabs bid, up to qid if necessary; or
  - Docusate 240mg tid, up to qid if necessary.

Treatment of established constipation (with or without faecal impaction)

- Requires the use of enemas and/or suppositories.

- Administer a fleet enema or a bisacodyl suppository. Repeat if unsuccessful.
- If still unsuccessful, administer an oil retention enema followed by a soapsuds enema several hours later. (Caution: debilitated, frail patients may poorly tolerate soapsuds enemas. A high fleet is an alternative in these patients.)
- If the impaction appears to be in the proximal colon, magnesium citrate, up to 250 ml p.o., may be tried.
- Manual disimpaction is seldom necessary.

Opioid induced constipation

- Constipation has been reported in 50–95%, with the highest incidence observed in patients receiving opioids. Prophylactic use of laxatives is required at the time of initiating opioids.
- Titrate laxatives based on stool consistency and frequency
- If unsuccessful, give suppository every three days based on stool consistency
- If suppository unsuccessful, give fleet enema or micro enema
- If still no success, give high mineral oil retention enema; after at least four to six hours, follow with a soap suds enema.
- Consider naloxegol in the management of opioid-induced constipation in adult patients with chronic non-cancer pain.
- Dosing: 25mg once daily; if not tolerated, reduce to 12.5mg once daily.

Further reading

Chey WD, Webster L, Sostek M, et al. Naloxegol for opioid-induced constipation in patients with non-cancer pain. *N Engl J Med* 2014 Jun 19; 370(25):2387–96.

Pereira J, Otfinowski PB, Hagen N, Bruera E, et al. *Alberta Hospice Palliative Care Resource Manual.* 2nd edn. Alberta: Alberta Cancer Foundation, 2001.

17.5 Diarrhoea

Introduction

Diarrhoea is much less common than constipation in patients with advanced disease, affecting less than 10% of patients with cancer admitted to hospital or palliative care units.

Common causes

- Drugs: laxatives, antibiotics, antacids, chemotherapy (5-fluorouracil, irinotecan, tyrosine kinase inhibitors (TKIs), etc.)
- Diet
- Tumour
- Colon or rectum, pelvi pancreatic (islet cell) carcinoid
- Fistula
- Radiotherapy
- Intestinal obstruction (including faecal impaction)
- Concurrent disease, such as inflammatory bowel disease

- Malabsorption: pancreatic carcinoma, gastrectomy, ileal resection, colectomy
- Infection (e.g. *Clostridium difficile*).

Clinical approach: Key points

- The underlying cause should be investigated, but relief is generally achieved with non-specific antidiarrhoeal agents.
- History: particularly recent bowel habit and medication.
- Examination: should include rectal exam.
- Abdominal X-ray: may show obstruction or toxic colon.
- Electrolytes: dehydration may be present.
- The most common cause of diarrhoea in patients with advanced disease is use of laxatives. Patients may use laxatives erratically; some wait until they become constipated and then use high doses of laxatives, with resultant rebound diarrhoea.

- Among elderly patients constipation with faecal impaction and overflow accounts for over half the cases of diarrhoea.

Management

Supportive
Rehydrate as appropriate. Oral hydration is preferred.

Loperamide
Reduces secretion of digestive agents into the bowel. Approximately 50 times more potent than codeine for treatment of diarrhoea. Dose usually 4mg (four times daily). This can be reduced to twice daily dosing once diarrhoea has responded to treatment.

Octreotide
Useful in severe diarrhoea. It is given via subcutaneous infusion in doses of 200–1200mcg per 24 hours.

The usual indication is a high effluent volume from a stoma.

Antibiotics
If an infective cause has been identified, appropriate antibacterial treatment is indicated.

Opioids (other)
Act by reducing peristalsis in the gut. Loperamide should be used in preference to opioids as first-line treatment. If the patient requires opioid analgesics this may negate the need for any additional antidiarrhoea agents. Also consider codeine (10–60mg every four hours). Codeine may cause central effects, but these are rare with loperamide.

17.6 Hiccups

Introduction
Hiccups are a reflex spasm of the diaphragm causing sudden movement of the glottis. Hiccups lasting more than 48 hours are not uncommon in patients with advanced disease and can be very distressing and exhausting. They can affect a patient's daily living and social functioning.

Most studies were uncontrolled, underpowered, and lacked comprehensive data and therefore recommendations for any treatments are made cautiously. Treatment of intractable and persistent hiccup is based on patients' and clinicians' preferences until more evidence from randomized controlled trials is available.

Pharmacological treatment should take into account the potential side effects and risks of medication.

Assessment
- Careful assessment is required to identify the cause.
- Consider severity, duration, and impact on a patient's quality of life.
- Causes include:
  - Gastric stasis and distension (the most common cause)
  - Gastroesophageal reflux
  - Metabolic disturbances (e.g. uraemia, hypercalcaemia, magnesium deficiency)
  - Infection
  - Irritation of diaphragm or phrenic nerve
  - Hepatic disease/hepatomegaly
  - Cerebral causes (e.g. tumour, metastases)
  - Damage to phrenic nerve over its course from skull to diaphragm, e.g. shingles, pressure from mediastinal tumours
  - Steroids
  - Electrolyte imbalance (e.g. hyponatraemia, uraemia)

Management
- Depends on treating the underlying cause.

- Treat reversible causes.
- Hiccups often stop spontaneously.
- Treatment is only required if hiccups are persistent.

Gastric distension and gastro-oesophageal reflux disease (GORD)
- Prokinetic drugs such as metoclopramide (10mg qds p.o.). Dimethicone, which is an antifoaming agent which eases flatulence and distension (Asilone® 5ml four times daily), can be effective. Also consider domperidone.
- Treat any gastroesophageal reflux with a proton pump inhibitor.
- Smooth muscle relaxants.
- Baclofen and nifedipine may also be effective and act by relaxing smooth muscle. Baclofen (5mg three times daily p.o.) or nifedipine can be used either PRN (5mg) or regularly (5mg three times daily).

Central hiccup reflex suppression
- Chlorpromazine is often effective but should only be used when other measures have failed due to its sedating side effects. Usual dose (12.5–25mg daily).
- Levomepromazine oral 3–6mg at bed time (now used as an alternative to chlorpromazine).

Other considerations
Dexamethasone oral 4–8mg in the morning may reduce compression/irritation if the patient has a hepatic, mediastinal, or cerebral disease/tumour. Stop if no benefit after a week.

In severe intractable hiccups if the patient becomes exhausted, a trial of midazolam by continuous subcutaneous infusion may be appropriate.

Internet resources
NHS Choices. Hiccups—available at: http://www.nhs.uk/conditions/Hiccup/Pages/Introduction.aspx

17.7 Depression

Introduction

Depression is common in patients with advanced cancer, occurring four times more frequently than it does in the general population. It is often underdiagnosed in patients with cancer and antidepressants are used fairly infrequently. Depression is often easily treated and this can improve quality of life and also physical symptoms such as pain.

There are many reasons why depression is under-diagnosed and undertreated. It is often assumed that patients with advanced malignancy will be depressed. It is reasonable to assume that patients will have a low mood at times, but persistent low mood warrants further assessment. There may be stigma associated with depression and this can result in patients being reluctant to commence treatment.

Clinicians may also be less likely to diagnose depression. This can be due to lack of experience or even prejudice. Clinical depression can and does frequently exist and is a real clinical problem that should be considered as important as other symptoms.

Diagnosis

In the physically well patient, the main symptoms used to diagnose depression are poor appetite, weight loss, and fatigue. These are less reliable in patients with advanced cancer as the symptoms can often be due to the underlying cancer.

Psychological indicators for the presence of depression are:

* Profound feelings of worthlessness
* Profound feelings of guilt
* Profound anhedonia (no pleasure)
* Profound thoughts of 'wishing to die soon'
* Profound feelings of hopelessness

Suicidal ideation

It is impossible to diagnose depression if there is cognitive impairment present. In particular hypoactive delirium is often misdiagnosed as depression and therefore it is essential to ensure the patient has no cognitive impairment before assessing for depression.

The Endicott Criteria (Table 17.7.1) are a modified version of the DSM (Diagnostic and Statistical Manual of Mental Disorders) criteria, which replaces symptoms which may be attributable to cancer (Endicott 1984).

The Hospital Anxiety and Depression Scales (HADS) were designed to assist in diagnosing anxiety and depression. It has been shown to be effective at diagnosing depression in patients with advanced cancer. This has a maximum score of 42 (encompassing both anxiety and depression scores). A combined anxiety and depression score of 20 or above makes a diagnosis of depression highly likely.

Diagnostic and screening tools for depression commonly used in the general population are often not very helpful in patients with advanced cancer. It has been suggested that asking a patient the simple question 'are you depressed?' can be a useful screening—but not a diagnostic—tool. However, the term 'depression' means different things in different cultures and thus should be interpreted with caution.

Table 17.7.1 Endicott criteria for diagnosing depression in advanced cancer

1	Depressed mood, subjective or observed
2	Marked diminished interest or pleasure in most activities, most of the day
3	Fearful or depressed appearance
4	Social withdrawal or decreased talkativeness
5	Psychomotor agitation or retardation
6	Brooding, self-pity, or pessimism
7	Feelings of worthlessness, or excessive or inappropriate guilt
8	Mood is non-reactive to environmental events
9	Recurrent thoughts of death or suicide

For a diagnosis of depression to be present, five out of nine symptoms must be present most of the time, most days over a two-week period.

Source: data from Endicott J. Measurement of Depression in Patients With Cancer. *Cancer* 1984; 53 (Suppl 10):2243–9. 1984, American Cancer Society.

Principles of management

* Look for any past psychiatric disorders.
* Look for clinical conditions that may mimic depression and treat these (metabolic, endocrine, other drugs or polipharmacy/interaction, review medication, screen for dementia).
* Look for drug abuse, alcoholism, other.
* Symptom assessment (e.g. Edmonton Symptoms Assessment Scale or ESAS).
* Investigate social, spiritual, and cultural issues.
* In mild depression, psychological support can be as effective as medication.
* Adequate pain control may significantly improve depressive symptoms.
* Spiritual distress may be a component of depression, or distinct from it.
* Consider supportive psychotherapy or cognitive behavioural therapy.
* Patients with severe depression and/or suicidal ideation should be referred to psychological medicine/psychiatry for assessment.

Drug treatments

Selective serotonin reuptake inhibitors (SSRIs) are better tolerated and are safer in overdose than other classes of antidepressants and so are often considered first line. Notes about specific SSRIs are given below.

* Sertraline (25–50mg/day p.o. until 100mg): this may be a useful SSRI if there has been a recent cardiac event.
* Citalopram/escitalopram (20mg/day until 40mg/day p.o.). It is useful for agitated depression/anxiety and relatively safe if the patient is at risk of seizures. There is a risk of QT prolongation and drug interactions.
* Fluoxetine (10mg/day p.o. am, until 2mg). It is long acting and offers low risk of withdrawal effects. It has many drug interactions so it may not be suitable in palliative care patients.

Mirtazapine
- Noradrenaline and specific serotonin antagonist (NaSSA).
- Dose: 15mg daily, increased to 45mg daily if needed. Paradoxically, lower doses can be more sedating.
- May be effective in nausea (action on the 5-HT3 receptor).
- Appetite stimulant and sedative, particularly at lower doses.
- Well tolerated in the elderly and patients with heart failure.

Venlafabxine
- Serotonin–noradrenergic reuptake inhibitor (SNRI).
- Effective in depression with lack of noradrenergic drive.
- Starting dose 75mg daily.

Once an antidepressant is chosen it is important to start at a therapeutic dose and monitor response. If a patient does not begin responding within four weeks of treatment it is appropriate to change to another class of antidepressant, either an SNRI (venlafaxine) or a NaSSA (mirtazapine).

Unfortunately, there is a delay of two to four weeks in the onset of the antidepressant effect of these drugs. In patients with a short life expectancy or with severe depression this period may be too long. Where a rapid antidepressant effect is desired, psychostimulants can be very useful.

Psychostimulants, e.g. methylphenidate
These drugs have been used successfully in the treatment of depression in cancer patients. They have a rapid onset of action and are especially useful in patients with severe psychomotor slowing. Other benefits include:
- Energizing effect: improved appetite; and reduced opioid-induced sedation.
- Potential side effects include:
  - Anxiety
  - Insomnia and nightmares
  - Psychosis, paranoia.
  - Tolerance and physical dependence occur with prolonged use.

When initiating a psychostimulant therapy, a test dose is advised. It can be given at 8am and the patient reassessed one to two hours later. If side effects occur after the test dose (psychomotor agitation, hallucinations), discontinue the psychostimulants.

Methylphenidate
- Test dose: 5mg p.o. at 8am
- Starting dose: 10mg p.o. at 8am and 5mg p.o. at noon
- Avoid psychostimulants after noon to prevent insomnia
- The dose may need to be increased gradually over many days to weeks

Further reading
Block SD. Assessing and managing depression in the terminally ill patient. ACP-ASIM End-of-Life Care Consensus Panel. American College of Physicians—American Society of Internal Medicine. *Ann Intern Med* 2000; 132:209–18.

Endicott J. Measurement of depression in patients with cancer. *Cancer* 1984; 53(Suppl. 10):2243–8.

Laird BJ, Mitchell J. The assessment and management of depression in the terminally ill. *Eur J Palliat Care* 2005; 12:4.

Ostuzzi G, Matcham F, Dauchy S, et al. Antidepressants for the treatment of depression in people with cancer. *Cochrane Database Syst Rev* 2018; 4(4):CD011006.

Pereira J, Otfinowski PB, Hagen N, Bruera E, et al. *Alberta Hospice Palliative Care Resource Manual*. 2nd edn. Alberta: Alberta Cancer Foundation, 2001.

Rayner L, Price A, Evans A, et al. Antidepressants for the treatment of depression in palliative care: systemic review and meta-analysis. *Palliat Med* 2011; 25(1):36–51.

Rozans M, Dreisbach A, Lertora JJ, et al. Palliative uses of methylphenidate in patients with cancer: a review. *J Clin Oncol* 2002; 20:335–9.

Vodermaier A, Millman, R. D. Accuracy of the Hospital Anxiety and Depression Scale as a screening tool in cancer patients: a systematic review and meta-analysis. *Support Care Cancer* 2011; 19(12):1899–908.

Wasteson E, Brenne E, Higginson I. et al. Depression assessment and classification in palliative cancer patients: a systematic literature review. *Palliat Med* 2009; 23(8):739–53.

17.8 Delirium

Introduction
Delirium is the most common neuropsychiatric syndrome in patients with advanced cancer and tends to occur in individuals with underlying comorbid conditions who encounter additional acute insults. Delirium is associated with significant morbidity and mortality. The early diagnosis of delirium is critical for the appropriate management and prevention of severe distress in patients, their families, and medical staff; however, delirium is frequently missed or misdiagnosed as worsening pain, depression, or anxiety. It is important to be able to distinguish between dementia and delirium. Both can be due to a number of underlying conditions, but dementia is usually chronic and irreversible. It is possible to have an acute delirium on a background of a dementing illness.

Cardinal features that distinguish delirium from dementia in palliative care patients:

- Delirium: sudden onset, altered level of consciousness, clouded sensorium, occasionally reversible

- Dementia: gradual onset, unimpaired level of consciousness, chronic

There are many subtypes of delirium ranging from pseudodelirium to hypoactive delirium and the classical manic delirium. The underlying pathophysiology is unclear although various theories have been postulated. From a clinical point of view it is often best to determine the likely causes.

Causes
On multivariate analysis, one small prospective study in 145 oncology admissions found the following five risk factors for the development of delirium: advanced age, cognitive impairment, low albumin, bone metastases, and haematological malignancy. However, often a specific cause remains unidentified. Predisposing factors increase a patient's baseline susceptibility for developing delirium. Examples are pre-existing cognitive impairment, such as dementia, and reduced sensory input because of poor vision or deafness.

Drug-induced delirium

The most commonly implicated medications are opioids (see 'Opioid toxicity', p. 485), corticosteroids, benzodiazepines, and anticholinergic. Delirium can occur with all known opioid agonists that are used in cancer pain management, including morphine, hydromorphone, oxycodone, fentanyl, and methadone.

Diagnosis of delirium

Evaluation

Clinical features of delirium

Early diagnosis is important, because this enables not only earlier treatment but also provision of education and support to the patient and family.

An essential feature for the clinical diagnosis of delirium of the DSM-IV-TR criteria is a disturbance of consciousness. Non-core clinical features of delirium include sleep–wake cycle disturbance, altered psychomotor activity, and emotional lability. Patients may exhibit prodromal features including anxiety, restlessness, irritability, disorientation, and sleep disturbances. Patients may have disorganized thinking and disjointed unintelligible speech. The altered perceptions that may occur include misperceptions, illusions, delusions, and hallucinations. Clinical features include neurological motor abnormalities: tremor, asterixis, myoclonus, and tone and reflex changes. Dysgraphia may also occur. Other neurological abnormalities that may be present include constructional apraxia, dysnomia, and aphasia. Generalized slowing of the electroencephalogram is a classic finding.

Delirium assessment tools

Delirium is frequently underdiagnosed in the clinical setting, even by experienced physicians and nurses. A brief description of three delirium assessment tools used in clinical practice follows:

CAM

- The Confusion Assessment Method (CAM) is based on the DSM-III-R criteria. Although it is a brief, four-item diagnostic algorithm that takes <5 minutes to administer, it does require training in its use. It has recently been validated in the palliative care setting.

MDAS

- The Memorial Delirium Assessment Scale (MDAS) is a ten-item, four-point, clinician-rated instrument (possible range, 0–30). It was originally designed to measure severity but can be used as a diagnostic tool using a cutoff total MDAS score ≥7 of 30. This is a validated instrument. The objective cognitive testing items (items 2, 3, and 4) should be completed first because this achieves a higher rate of completion and allows assessment time for the more observational or subjective items.

NuDESC

- The Nursing Delirium Screening Scale (NuDESC) is an observational five-item scale (possible range, 0–10) that includes the four items of the Confusion Rating Scale (CRS) and an additional assessment of psychomotor retardation. Each symptom (disorientation, inappropriate behaviour, inappropriate communication, illusions, or hallucinations, as well as psychomotor retardation) is rated 0–2 according to its presence and severity. It is a low burden tool that takes <2 minutes to complete, and can be used for screening and monitoring delirium severity. The NuDESC has been validated and is reported to have a sensitivity of 85.7% and a specificity of 86.8%.

Table 17.8.1 Confusion assessment method

1	*Acute onset and fluctuating course*
	Evidence of a change in the patient's mental status from its baseline. Does this fluctuate during the day?
2	*Inattention*
	Does the patient have difficulty focusing attention?
3	*Disorganized thinking*
	Is the patient's thinking incoherent, have an illogical flow, or rambling?
4	*Altered level of consciousness*
	This can range from a coma to a hyperalert state

To diagnose delirium features 1 and 2 plus either 3 or 4 are required to be present.

Further clinical assessment

The assessment of delirium also includes the investigation of all potential precipitating factors for the delirium episode in order to identify reversible causes. Medication history for both new and continuing drugs should be reviewed. Predisposing factors that increase the patient's baseline susceptibility for developing delirium may also be identified, such as pre-existing cognitive impairment or reduced sensory input with poor vision or deafness. Urinary retention and constipation may aggravate agitation, especially in the elderly (Table 17.8.1).

Treatment of delirium

The multimodal management of delirium includes non-pharmacological and environment management strategies, in addition to neuroleptic and other medications, while simultaneously identifying and treating underlying causes when appropriate. Comprehensive management should involve a multidisciplinary team. The patient's delirium severity and response to treatment need to be monitored regularly.

Treatment of underlying causes

Because 50% of delirium episodes in advanced cancer are reversible, possible contributors to delirium should be appropriately treated. For drug-induced delirium, all implicated medications should be discontinued or undergo a dose reduction if cessation of the implicated medication is not possible.

Pharmacological treatment

Haloperidol has the advantage of versatile routes of administration: oral, SC, IM, and IV It is rarely sedating. Because the average oral bioavailability of haloperidol is approximately 60%, parenteral doses are about twice as potent as oral doses.

Clinical guidelines recommend starting haloperidol doses of 0.5–2mg, with varying frequency and routes of administration. Most studies to date report dose ranges of 2–10mg/day. However, further research in the form of randomized, double blind, placebo-controlled trials is needed in the advanced cancer population to determine appropriate dosing schedules for all delirium subtypes.

Dosing in case of agitation/hallucinations

Start haloperidol 1mg p.o./SC q8–12h and 1mg q1h p.o./SC prn for agitation. If the agitation/hallucinations are severe, higher doses of haloperidol are indicated, e.g. haloperidol 2mg q6–8h SC/p.o. with breakthrough orders of 2mg q1h SC/p.o. To bring severe agitation rapidly under control, it may be necessary to give haloperidol more frequently initially, e.g. haloperidol 2mg q30 minutes SC/p.o. PRN in the first few hours and thereafter q1h prn. It is appropriate to bring an agitated delirium under control rapidly to prevent patient, family, and staff distress.

If symptoms persist, or worsen, the dose of haloperidol can be increased up to a maximum of 20–30mg/day.

Always assess for the possible occurrence of extrapyramidal adverse effects or other adverse effects.

If symptoms persist after 36–48 hours despite optimal haloperidol doses, an alternative drug, perhaps more sedating, needs to be offered, e.g. methotrimoprazine. Starting doses are 6.25–12.5mg SC/p.o. q8–12h. This drug can be sedating and the family needs to be informed of this. Breakthrough doses for agitation/hallucinations can also be ordered, e.g. methotrimoprazine 6.25mg or 12.5mg q1h p.o. or SC PRN.

Sedation with midazolam for uncontrolled agitation is very rarely required. When indicated, start a continuous subcutaneous infusion at 1mg/hour and titrate up to 4mg/hour.

More recently, atypical antipsychotics, such as olanzapine, risperidone, quetiapine, and aripiprazole, have been used in the management of delirium in patients with cancer.

Olanzapine has a common side effect of sedation, which may be potentially beneficial in a hyperalert, hyperaroused patient with delirium. The parenteral olanzapine preparation for IM injection has been well tolerated, with no injection site toxicity when administered by the SC route in some units.

Pitfalls
- Not recognizing the presence of delirium.
- Diagnosing a hypoactive delirium as depression and treating inappropriately with antidepressants.
- Interpreting agitation and the accompanying moaning and grimacing of a delirium as a direct indication of poor pain control and responding by increasing opioid doses.

In many cases opioids are the cause of delirium and by giving more opioids, one aggravates the situation.
- Not discontinuing drugs that could be causing or aggravating the delirium.
- Occasionally delirium is superimposed on pre-existing dementia. Some medications that are used for symptom control in advanced disease may unmask a pre-existing cognitive problem that was previously unrecognized by the patient's family.
- Urinary retention and constipation in cognitively impaired patients are not uncommon and can increase agitated behaviour because of discomfort and inability to communicate the source of discomfort. Catheterization or disimpaction will probably not resolve the delirium but may decrease the agitation.

Further reading
Brajtman S, Wright D, Hogan DB, Allard P, et al. Developing guidelines on the assessment and treatment of delirium in older adults at the end of life. *Can Geriatr J.* 2011 Jun;14(2):40–50.

Bush SH, Bruera E. The assessment and management of delirium in cancer patients. *Oncologist* 2009 Oct; 14(10):1039–49.

Harris D. Delirium in advanced disease. *Postgrad Med J* 2007 Aug; 83(982):525–8.

Inouye SK, van Dyck CH, Alessi CA, et al. Clarifying confusion: the confusion assessment method. A new method for detection of delirium. *Ann Intern Med* 1990; 113:941–8.

Lawlor PG, Bush SH. Delirium in patients with cancer: assessment, impact, mechanisms and management. *Nat Rev Clin Oncol* 2015 Feb; 12(2):77–92.

Logan J. Recognising and managing delirium in patients receiving palliative and end of life care. *Nurs Stand* 2018 Nov 1; 33(8):63–8.

Park M, Unutzer J. Geriatric depression in primary care. *Can Geriatr J* 2011 Jun; 14(2):40–50.

Pereira J, Otfinowski PB, Hagen N, Bruera E, et al. *Alberta Hospice Palliative Care Resource Manual.* 2nd edn. Alberta: Alberta Cancer Foundation, 2001.

17.9 Oral care

Introduction
Oral care is an extremely important aspect of care for the cancer patient. Mouth care is a frequently neglected but crucial aspect of palliative care in all settings. It maintains self-esteem, comfort, and the person's ability to communicate, socialize, and enjoy food and drinks. Mouth care should be part of daily routine patient care and intervention should be instigated early to prevent more serious problems and treatment complications. Cancer treatments, drugs, dehydration, and localized disease all affect the normal function of the oral cavity.

Stomatitis and xerostomia
Stomatitis
Stomatitis is characterized by an inflamed oral mucosa that can range from mild inflammation to ulceration that can bleed or become infected. There are many possible causes of stomatitis.

Causes: infection, medication (cytotoxic agents, TKI, etc.), radiotherapy, poor mouth hygiene, poorly fitting dentures, trauma, blood disorders.

Treatment of stomatitis
1 Provide regular mouth care.

2 Treating symptoms:
- Analgesia: soluble paracetamol and/or aspirin used as a mouthwash with xylocaine 2% provides topical relief. If systemic analgesia is required, consider common guideline on pain management.
- Oral infections: treat candidiasis or thrush with nystatin, fluconazole, or ketoconazole. Oral medications should be swallowed as the thrush infection may extend into the oesophagus.
- Herpes simplex; consider acyclovir.
- Bacterial infection: treat with antibiotics.
- First-line antimicrobial therapy should be commenced with treatment directed at the likely causal organism.
- Good oral hygiene will minimize the risk of infection and will aid resolution.

Xerostomia
Xerostomia, or dry mouth, is a very common complaint in patients with advanced cancer. In most cases it can be managed adequately with oral sips of water. It may be due to:
- Opioids
- Other drugs, e.g. anticholinergics

- Dehydration
- Radiation

Treatment of xerostomia
- General measures such as regular oral hygiene, frequent swabbing with moist sponge swabs.
- Saliva substitutes such as oral-balance gel.
- Pilocarpine 5mg p.o. qid. It has been shown to be useful in radiotherapy-induced xerostomia. It is contraindicated in chronic obstructive airway disease, congestive heart failure, glaucoma, acute iritis, and hypotension.
- Treat xerostomia by addressing the cause when possible (e.g. rehydration, antibiotics).
- Provide artificial saliva products if useful.

- Encourage frequent sips of water, ice chips, or popsicles.

Further reading

Clarkson JE, Worthington HV, Furness S, McCabe M, Khalid T, et al. Interventions for treating oral mucositis for patients with cancer receiving treatment. *Cochrane Database Syst Rev* 2010; 2010(8):CD001973.

Pereira J, Otfinowski PB, Hagen N, Bruera E, et al. *Alberta Hospice Palliative Care Resource Manual.* 2nd edn. Alberta: Alberta Cancer Foundation, 2001.

Internet resources

NHS Scotland. Scottish Palliative Care Guidelines: http://www.palliativecareguidelines.scot.nhs.uk/guidelines/symptom-control/Mouth-Care.aspx

17.10 Cancer-related fatigue

Introduction

Cancer-related fatigue is a distressing, persistent, subjective sense of physical, emotional, and/or cognitive tiredness or exhaustion related to cancer or cancer treatment that is not proportional to recent activity and interferes with usual functioning.

Fatigue is rarely an isolated symptom and most commonly occurs with other symptoms, such as pain, emotional distress, anaemia, and sleep disturbances, in symptom clusters.

Fatigue is a subjective experience that should be systematically assessed using patient self-reports and other sources of data.

Fatigue should be screened, assessed, and managed according to clinical practice guidelines.

All patients should be screened using age-appropriate measures for fatigue at their initial visit, at regular intervals during and following cancer treatment, and as clinically indicated.

Fatigue should be recognized, evaluated, monitored, documented, and treated promptly for all age groups, at all stages of disease, prior to, during, and following treatment.

Patients and families should be informed that management of fatigue is an integral part of total health care and that fatigue can persist following treatment.

Epidemiology

- Prevalence varies from 39% to 90%.
- Increases in prevalence as disease progresses.
- Patients are more likely to have fatigue when undergoing cancer treatment.

Assessment

- Explore the person's experience and understanding of fatigue.
- Acknowledge and validate the reality and significance of the symptoms.
- Be aware that patients may have multi-morbidities impacting on fatigue, e.g. cardiac/respiratory disease, renal or hepatic impairment, malignancy, hypothyroidism, hypogonadism, adrenal insufficiency, neurological conditions.

Management

A combination of person-centred approaches in partnership with the individual using the multidisciplinary team will be required to maximize potential.

Treat potentially reversible factors if appropriate, e.g. blood transfusions may be helpful for some patients. Other symptoms and comorbidities should be managed, and all medications reviewed.

Non-pharmacological management

- Diary—an activity/fatigue diary may help to identify precipitants and timing of symptoms.
- Energy conservation/restoration.
- Consider a self-management plan to set priorities and delegate tasks.
- Pace activities and attend to one activity at a time.
- Schedule activities at times of peak energy and conserve energy for valued activities.
- Eliminate non-essential activities.
- Occupational therapy referral for advice on minimizing energy expenditure and appropriate aids/equipment.
- Physical activity and exercise.
- An appropriate level of exercise can reduce fatigue and should be recommended.
- Consider physiotherapy referral to ensure exercises are tailored to individual needs particularly for those patients who have advanced disease or are experiencing effects of treatments, e.g. anaemia, osteoporosis/bone metastases, falls.
- Psychosocial interventions.

Pharmacological management

- Consider psychostimulants (methylphenidate) after ruling out other causes of fatigue.
- Consider corticosteroids (prednisone or dexamethasone).
- Treat for pain, emotional distress, and anaemia as indicated.
- Optimize treatment for sleep dysfunction and comorbidities.

Further reading

Berger AM, Mooney K, Alvarez-Perez A, et al. Cancer-related fatigue, version 2.2015. *J Natl Compr Cancer Netw.* 2015 Aug; 13(8):1012–39.

Internet resources

NHS Scotland. Scottish Palliative Care Guidelines: http://www.palliativecareguidelines.scot.nhs.uk/guidelines/symptom-control/weakness-fatigue.aspx

17.11 Cancer cachexia

Introduction

Cachexia is physical wasting with loss of skeletal and visceral muscle mass and is very common among patients with cancer. It is now recognized that cancer cachexia is a triad of the following:

- Weight loss >10%
- Reduced food intake (<1500kcal/day)
- Systemic inflammation (CRP >10mg/l)

Many patients with cancer lose the desire to eat (anorexia), which contributes to cachexia. Cachexia can also occur independently from anorexia, as pro-inflammatory cytokines and tumour-derived factors directly lead to muscle proteolysis. Cachexia leads to asthenia (weakness), hypoalbuminemia, emaciation, immune system impairment, metabolic dysfunction, and autonomic failure. Asthenia is a syndrome of fatigue (physical and mental) and generalized weakness. Anorexia, asthenia, and cachexia will often coexist in the cancer patient.

Cachexia results in the loss of both lean and fatty tissue. It is associated with psychological distress, altered body image, and reduced physical function. Cancer-related cachexia has been associated with failure of anticancer treatment, increased treatment toxicity, delayed treatment initiation, early treatment termination, shorter survival, and psychosocial distress.

Epidemiology

Epidemiology is difficult to determine due to lack of consistent definitions. Approximately 50% of cancer patients will lose weight and 20% will die directly as a result of cachexia. Cachexia is more common in tumours of the GI tract and lung than in breast or prostate cancer. Cachexia increases in prevalence towards the end of life.

Cachexia is a complex condition that is a combination of anorexia and an altered metabolism. When anorexia exists as a sole entity, nutritional supports may allow some weight gain. However as anorexia commonly exists as a component of cachexia, treatment is less straightforward.

Pathophysiology

All the following are thought to be implicated in the underlying mechanisms of cachexia:

- Systemic inflammation resulting from tumour–host interaction—fat reserves utilized in the acute phase response.
- Tumour producing 'pro-cachectic factors' which cause protein and fat degradation.
- Negative nitrogen balance in cancer cachexia results in wasting of skeletal muscle.
- Hypermetabolism results from activation of neuro-endocrine pathways.
- Altered protein metabolism.
- Lack of physical activity may exacerbate muscle wasting.

Assessment

The assessment is much more than the patient's calorific intake versus their body weight. It is worth considering if recording the patient's weight is necessary as this may result in increasing anxiety regarding their weight loss. A nutritional assessment needs to be holistic and acknowledge the emotional, social, cognitive, and biochemical aspects of nutrition and diet. Each assessment should be individualized taking the patient's condition and stage of illness into consideration.

- Look for any reversible problems that may exacerbate anorexia including pain, breathlessness, depression, ascites, nausea and vomiting, constipation, dysphagia, heartburn, gastritis, anxiety, and medication.
- Oral problems: such as dry mouth, ill-fitting dentures, ulcers, candidiasis.
- Odours: cooking smells, incontinence, fungating lesions and fistulae can contribute to anorexia.
- Delayed gastric emptying (for example, due to local disease, autonomic neuropathy) causing early satiety and vomiting of undigested foods.
- Ask the patient and the caregiver about their perspectives on weight, body image, nutrition, and dietary intake.

Treatments

Reversible causes should be identified and treated, e.g. treat psychological distress. Use enzyme supplements where needed (e.g. in pancreatic cancer).

Nutritional support: supplements containing at least 1.5kcal/ml are effective in preventing further weight loss.

Pharmacological management

Corticosteroids

- Established role in short-term improvement of appetite. Rapid effect but tends to decrease after three to four weeks.
- May also help to reduce nausea, improve energy, and general feeling of wellbeing. However, there is often no significant effect on nutritional status.
- Starting dose: oral dexamethasone 4mg or prednisolone 30mg (given in the morning).
- Consider need for gastric protection, such as H2 receptor blocker or proton pump inhibitor.
- Prescribe for one week and if helpful, reduce gradually to lowest effective dose. If no effect, stop.
- Assess and review dose regularly.
- Side effects: fluid retention, candidiasis, myopathy, insomnia, gastritis, and steroid-induced diabetes.

Progestogens

- May stimulate appetite and weight gain in patients with cancer.
- May take a few weeks to take effect but benefit is more prolonged than steroids.
- More appropriate for patients with a longer prognosis.
- Megestrol acetate: starting dose 160mg/daily and then after two to three weeks assess and review. For appetite stimulation, lower doses are as effective as higher doses but for weight gain there does appear to be more of a dose–response relationship. There is no evidence for an optimal dose but the maximum dose is 800mg daily. Reduce dose gradually if it has been used for more than three weeks (adrenal suppression).
- Side effects: nausea, fluid retention, and increased risk of thromboembolism.

Fish oils
- There is evidence that some patients respond but further characterization of responders is required.

Cannabinoids
- Although cannabinoid-based interventions (e.g. dronabinol, cannabis) have some demonstrated efficacy for treating chemotherapy-induced nausea and vomiting and AIDS-related anorexia, the data to support cannabinoid-based interventions for treating anorexia/cachexia in patients with cancer are very limited.

A combination therapy approach may yield the best possible outcomes for patients with cancer cachexia.

Further reading
Fearon KC. Cancer cachexia: developing multimodal therapy for a multidimensional problem. *Eur J Cancer* 2008; 44:1124–32.
Levy M, Smith T, Alvarez-Perez A, et al. Palliative Care Version 1. *J Natl Compr Cancer Netw* 2016 Jan; 14(1):82–113.

17.12 Breathlessness

Introduction
Breathlessness is the subjective experience of discomfort in breathing that consists of qualitatively distinct sensations that vary in intensity. It can be very distressing for patients and is very subjective. It can occur in cancer due either to direct effects of the tumour or indirect effects. Breathlessness is a common symptom for patients with advanced cancer, chronic obstructive pulmonary disease (COPD), lung fibrosis, and heart failure. It can be associated with any combination of physiological, psychological, social, and spiritual factors. The impact and distress caused by breathlessness is often underestimated.

Epidemiology
It varies in prevalence from 40% to 80% and can occur at any stage of the cancer illness. It commonly occurs in lung, lymphoma, head and neck, genitourinary, and breast cancer.

Pathophysiology
Normally, breathing is maintained by a physiological pathway controlled by the respiratory centre in the brainstem. Various factors including oxygen and carbon dioxide levels, lung mechanoreceptors, and arterial chemoreceptors all help regulate respiration. In cancer, distortion of mechanoreceptors (through disease), fatigue, muscle weakness, disease bulk, and anxiety can all impede the normal breathing process. Usually oxygen levels are maintained in cancer patients who are breathless.

Common causes
- Lung metastases
- Primary tumour site, e.g. lung
- Coexisting conditions, e.g. COPD
- Pulmonary thromboembolism
- Pleural effusions
- Anaemia
- Increased intra-abdominal pressure, e.g. ascites
- Anxiety
- Cachexia resulting in muscle weakness
- Cardiac failure

Assessment
- Undertake a holistic assessment using a multiprofessional approach.
- Ask the patient to rate symptom severity and assess the level of associated distress/anxiety.
- Explore the patient's understanding of the reasons for breathlessness, fears, and impact on functional abilities and quality of life.
- Clarify pattern of breathlessness, precipitating/alleviating factors, and associated symptoms.
- Look for any potentially reversible causes of breathlessness, such as infection, pleural effusion, anaemia, arrhythmia, pulmonary embolism, bronchospasm, or hypoxia (check oxygen saturation levels using pulse oximeter).
- Determine if treatment of the underlying disease is appropriate.

Last day of life
Oxygen can improve breathlessness, but only if the patient is hypoxic. If oxygen is needed for symptom control, nasal prongs may be better tolerated than a mask.

A fan (either on a table or handheld) should be tried, and a more upright position can help.

Management
General principles
As breathlessness can be very distressing for patients, it is important to reassure both patients and family members. A multidisciplinary approach is often needed with physiotherapists available to offer techniques for managing dyspnoea. Advice on breathing exercises, management of anxiety attacks, posture, and expectoration can often be beneficial.

A stream of air, either from a fan or through an open window, will often provide symptomatic relief.

Correct reversible causes
- Treat respiratory infections with antimicrobial treatment.
- Manage coexisting disease (e.g. COPD, cardiac failure) in the usual manner.
- Treat anaemia.

Cancer-specific treatment
- Radiotherapy to large tumour bulk.
- Endobronchial disease can be treated by stenting or removed by laser treatment.
- Lymphangitis carcinomatosis can be treated with high-dose steroids (dexamethasone 16mg orally or subcutaneously, or prednisolone 60mg orally).

Drainage of effusions
- Drainage of large pleural effusions may lead to relief of symptoms. If they recur consider pleurodesis.
- If symptomatic, drain pericardial effusions.

Oxygen therapy
- Hypoxic respiratory drive usually only occurs when SaO_2 <90%. In cases where SaO_2 is >90%, oxygen is less likely to be of any benefit.
- Short-burst oxygen therapy (intermittent use of oxygen for the relief of dyspnoea either before or after exercise) may be useful in some cases. Each case must be assessed on an individual basis and the response monitored.
- Ambulatory oxygen therapy (use of oxygen during exercise or activities of daily living) may be of use in those who desaturate on exertion.
- In those patients with COPD, assessment should be made on an individual basis.

Opioids
- The exact mechanism of effect in dyspnoea is unclear but opioids may work in several ways. They reduce pain, cough, the ventilator reaction to hypercapnia, and also pre- and post-cardiac load.
- There is no inherent benefit of one opioid over another in managing dyspnoea. The opioid most commonly used is morphine. This is usually commenced orally at a dose of 5mg four times daily and the effect subsequently assessed. This can be titrated upwards as effect dictates. If the patient is already taking opioids for pain it may be that the opioid dose prescribed to be given as required can be increased by 25–50% to be used as needed for dyspnoea.
- Respiratory depression is very rare, provided treatment of opioid naive patients is commenced with low doses and titrated upwards slowly.

Benzodiazepines
May relieve anxiety and panic associated with severe breathlessness, but are less effective than opioids

for breathlessness and should be a third-line treatment for patients with symptoms unresponsive to non-drug measures and opioids. The following can be considered:
- Lorazepam (scored tablet) sublingual 500mg, given four to six hourly as required.
- Diazepam oral 2–5mg at night, if there is continuous distressing anxiety.
- Midazolam subcutaneously 2–5mg, given four to six hourly as required, if oral or sublingual routes are not available.

Further reading
Cachia E, Ahmedzai SH. Breathlessness in cancer patients. *Eur J Cancer* 2008; 44:1116–23.
Chan KS, Tse DMV, Sham MMK, Thorsen AB. Palliative medicine in malignant respiratory diseases. In Hanks G, Cherny NI, Christakis NA, Fallon M, Kaasa S, Portenoy RK (eds). *Oxford Textbook of Palliative Medicine*. 4th edn. Oxford: Oxford University Press, 2010.
Simon ST, Bausewein C, Schildmann E, Higginson IJ, Magnussen H, Scheve C, Ramsenthaler C. Episodic breathlessness in patients with advanced disease: A systematic review. *J Pain Sympt Manag* 2013; 45(3):561–78.
Simon ST, Higginson IJ, Booth S, et al. Benzodiazepines for the relief of breathlessness in advanced malignant and non-malignant diseases in adults C. *Cochrane Database Syst Rev* 2016 Oct 20; 10:CD007354.
Spathis A, Davies HE, Booth S. *Respiratory Disease: From Advanced Disease to Bereavement*. 5th edn. New York: Oxford University Press, 2011.
Twycross R, Wilcock A. *Palliative Care Formulary (PCF4)*. 4th edn. Nottingham: palliativedrugs.com, 2011.
Twycross R., Wilcock, A, Stark Toller C. *Symptom Management in Advanced Cancer*. 4th edn. Nottingham: Palliativedrugs.com, 2009.

17.13 Cough

Introduction
Cough is a forced expulsive manoeuvre usually against a closed glottis, which is associated with a characteristic sound. It usually has a protective function in maintaining patency and cleanliness of the airways.

The impact of cough on patients and relatives is often underestimated. Patients may need symptomatic treatment when cough is persistent, distressing, or affecting sleep and/or quality of life. An assessment of the pattern and character of the patient's cough is essential to optimize treatment. Acute cough is defined as duration of <3 weeks, subacute as three to eight weeks, chronic as >8 weeks.

Although cough is a normal physiological mechanism, it is more common in malignant disease. There are a number of causes, which can be due to the underlying malignancy or due to coexisting non-malignant conditions (Table 17.13.1).

Management
- Depends on the type of cough and underlying cause.
- If stridor is present, seek specialist advice. Give high-dose steroids in divided doses: dexamethasone 16mg orally or subcutaneously, or prednisolone 60mg orally.

- Consider treating any potentially reversible causes.
- Optimize current therapy (non-drug management and medication); in particular, ensure adequate analgesia as pain may inhibit effective coughing.
- Acknowledge fear and anxieties, and provide supportive care. Offer written information and verbal explanation.

Table 17.13.1 Common causes of cough

Malignant	Non-malignant
Airway obstruction	Infection (acute or chronic)
Lymphangitis	Chronic obstructive pulmonary disease (COPD)
Pulmonary metastases	Asthma
Radiotherapy related pneumonitis	Recurrent aspiration
Pleural effusions	Drug related, e.g. ACE inhibitors
Hilar disease affecting vocal cord	

- Consider referral to physiotherapy services if difficulty in expectorating retained secretions.
- Agree a self-management plan.

General principles
- Physiotherapy will aid expectoration.
- Repositioning (lying on same side as pleural effusion) may palliate cough.
- Treat any underlying infection.
- Drain pleural effusions if thought to be causal.
- Treat stridor secondary to central airway tumour with steroids.
- Remove any drugs thought to be causing the cough.
- In patients who are generally weak and unable to cough, repositioning, suction and the use of drugs to manage respiratory secretions are advised.

Expectorants
- Stimulate cough reflex or reduce viscosity of mucus aiding expectoration, e.g. nebulized saline.

Cough suppressants (antitussives)
- Most potent are opioids.
- Work on opioid receptors centrally (cough centre) and in the airways.
- Usually start with codeine linctus (unless taking strong opioid for another reason).
- If ineffective, use strong opioids.
- Morphine (monitor for side effects including opioid toxicity):
  - Opioid naive—2mg orally, four to six hourly if required (six to eight hourly if frail or elderly).
  - Already on morphine—continue and use the existing immediate-release breakthrough analgesic

dose (oral if able or subcutaneous equivalent) for the relief of cough. A maximum of six doses can be taken in 24 hours for all indications (pain, breathlessness, and cough). Titrate both regular and breakthrough doses as required.
- Nebulized local anaesthetics may be helpful in endobronchial malignancy.

Key points
- Non-drug management techniques that help patients and families cope are essential. Using a self-management plan can help with symptom relief.
- As the illness progresses, medication to relieve cough may become more necessary.
- Starting opioids at a low dose and titrating carefully is safe and does not cause respiratory depression in patients with cancer, airways obstruction, or heart failure.

Further reading
Gibson PG, Ryan NM. Cough pharmacotherapy: current and future status. *Expert Opin Pharmacother* 2011; 12(11):1745–55.

Marks S, Rosielle DA. Opioids for cough #199. *J Palliative Med* 2010; 13(6):769–70.

Wee B. Chronic cough. *Curr Opin Support Palliative Care* 2008; 2(2):105–09.

Wee B, Browning J, Adams A, Benson D, Howard P, Klepping G, Molassiotis A, Taylor D. Management of chronic cough in patients receiving palliative care: review of evidence and recommendations by a task group of the Association for Palliative Medicine of Great Britain and Ireland. *Palliative Med* 2012; 26(6):780–7.

Internet resources
NHS Scotland. Scottish Palliative Care Guidelines: http://www.palliativecareguidelines.scot.nhs.uk/guidelines/symptom-control/Cough.aspx

17.14 Haemoptysis

Introduction
One-third of patients with lung cancer experience haemoptysis and 3% suffer fatal bleeds, often without warning. Death is generally due to suffocation and not exsanguination. Massive haemoptysis is most likely with squamous cell carcinoma, especially if it causes cavitations with necrosis of vessels within the tumour bed. Metastatic lung cancers can also bleed, most commonly with breast, colorectal, renal, or melanoma primary tumours. Chest infection and pulmonary embolism may also present with haemoptysis in cancer patients. Haemoptysis may have been the presenting symptom in the cancer patient and can be worrying for the patient and family.

There is a paucity of evidence-based treatment recommendations for haemoptysis in the literature.

Assessment
Assess whether it is severe acute bleeding which is life threatening, or more controllable with specific measures. If the latter, discuss management with appropriate specialist.

Also assess whether bleeding is due to local effects (such as blood vessel invasion) or to systemic effects of disease (such as disseminated intravascular coagulopathy).

Review the need for drugs that increase risk of bleeding, e.g. low-molecular-weight heparin, aspirin, warfarin, dexamethasone, NSAIDs.

Management
Anticipatory planning
- If significant bleeding can be anticipated, it is usually best to discuss the possibility with the patient and their family.
- Ensure caregivers at home have an emergency contact number.
- An anticipatory care plan is helpful. This includes having sedative medication prescribed for use if needed.
- If the patient is at home, discuss options for sedation and enquire if carers feel able to administer this medication.
- Discuss resuscitation; document and communicate resuscitation status.

Mild haemoptysis
- Patient should be reassured.
- Maintain the airway.

- If the bleeding site is known, lay the patient on the bleeding side to reduce effect on the other lung.
- Use oxygen and suction as required.
- Exclude or treat infection or pulmonary thromboembolism (PTE) if appropriate.
- Cough suppressant may be helpful.
- Tranexamic acid.
- Radiotherapy can give full control of bleeding in 85% of patients with lung bleeding.
- Nebulized adrenaline (1ml of 1 in 1,000 in 4ml normal saline qds.)
- Epinephrine diluted to 5ml in 0.9% N saline and nebulized up to four times a day.

Massive haemoptysis

Massive haemoptysis (>200ml of blood in 24 hours) should be considered an emergency. Studies suggest this is usually more prevalent in non-malignant disease than lung cancer.

Sedative medication for use in massive terminal hemorrhage:

- If the patient is distressed, a rapidly acting benzodiazepine is indicated.

- The aim of such treatment is not to make the patient unconscious but to sedate to appropriate levels to relieve distress.
- The route of administration guides the choice of drug:
  - Intravenous (IV) access available: midazolam 10mg IV or diazepam 10mg IV.
  - Intramuscular (IM) injection: midazolam 10mg can be given into a large muscle such as deltoid, gluteal.
  - Rectal route or via a stoma: diazepam rectal solution 10mg.

After the event

- Offer debriefing to team and family.
- Ongoing support as necessary for relatives and staff members.
- Disposal of clinical waste appropriately.

Further reading

Anwar D, Schaad N, Mazzocato C. Treatment of haemoptysis in palliative care patients. *Eur J Palliative Care* 2003; 10(4):137–9.

Doyle D, Hanks G, Cherny N, Calman K (eds). *Oxford Textbook of Palliative Medicine*. 3rd edn. Oxford: Oxford University Press, 2004.

Twycross R, Wilcock A. *Symptom Management in Advanced Cancer: Haemoptysis*. Oxford: Radcliffe Medical Press, 2001:239–42.

17.15 Symptom clusters

Introduction

Although the aforementioned symptoms are discussed individually, in the cancer patient these symptoms rarely exist in isolation. A symptom cluster has been defined as 'three or more concurrent symptoms that are related to each other'. Relationship does not imply causality or a common underlying mechanism. There has been increasing interest in symptoms with a common underlying pathophysiology.

Patients with cancer often have multiple concurrent symptoms. Some of the common symptoms, such as pain and fatigue, occur together or have been correlated in terms of intensity. Recently, interest in the symptom management of cancer patients has shifted from individual symptoms to symptom clusters. However, few studies have used multivariate data reduction techniques to explore the underlying dimensions of symptoms experienced by cancer patients.

At present, a firm evidence base, which defines clearly specific symptom clusters, is lacking. Studies have shown that fatigue, pain, and drowsiness tend to occur together. Other clusters suggested include poor appetite, nausea, anxiety, and low mood. It has also been demonstrated that pain, fatigue, low mood, and function may cluster together.

Currently there is a lack of consistently validated symptom clusters and work in this field is ongoing. Nevertheless, clinical experience would support the dictum that symptoms often coexist.

It is important, therefore, to note that in the optimal symptom management of the cancer patient, treating a single symptom in isolation may not achieve resolution. The approach should be adopted where several symptoms are treated in unison, e.g. the patient who has pain and depression should be treated for both. By addressing several symptoms at once, the individual symptoms may respond better to treatment.

Further reading

Chen ML, Tseng HC. Symptom clusters in cancer patients. *Support Care Cancer* 2006; 14:825.

Chow E, Fan G, Hadi S, et al. Symptom clusters in cancer patients with brain metastases. *Clin Oncol* 2008; 20:76–82.

Dodd M, Miaskowski C, Paul S. Symptom clusters and their effect on the functional status of patients with cancer. *Oncol Nurs Forum* 2001; 28:465–70.

17.16 End of life care

Introduction

End of life care of the cancer patient can be one of the most rewarding aspects of care. It can also be the most challenging, as it is the end of the cancer journey for the patient, the family, and the health professionals involved in their care. It is important that care at this stage is tailored to the patient and the family. As death approaches there will be increased physical and psychological needs. Greater nursing needs and increased symptoms often necessitate 'intensive' care. The physician should accept that the primary illness is no longer the priority and the focus of care should move to physical and psychological symptom control. Patient and family anxiety is often high so a thoughtful, sensitive approach is needed. Dying patients may wish to prepare for death and to help prepare family members to go on without them. Both patients and families benefit from education on the dying process. Families should be guided through their anticipatory grief, and arrangements should be made to ensure that the patient's and family's needs and goals regarding the dying process are respected. Planning to ensure continuing care and referrals to appropriate care is important. Arrangements should be available to ensure that the patient does not die alone unless that is the patient's preference.

Recognition of end of life

Perhaps one of the most difficult aspects is to recognize, and subsequently acknowledge, that someone has entered the terminal phase of their illness. If the oncologist has cared for the patient for a considerable length of time it can be challenging to decide that treatment should be stopped or that further active treatment is unlikely to confer a benefit. Clinicians should discuss the prognosis with patients and their families clearly and consistently to help them develop realistic expectations. Assessment and confirmation of understanding of prognosis is important and may guide treatment decisions. Information about the natural history of the specific tumour and the realistic outcomes of any intervention should be included in the discussion. Decisions are best made following consultation with the patient, family, and members of the oncology team. It is important that the realization that the patient is dying is understood and accepted by all involved parties. Only then can care be directed towards patient comfort and family support, as the primary aim. Social and spiritual support and resource management interventions should be provided to ensure a safe end of life care environment, a competent primary caregiver, and access to necessary medications and treatments. Providers must be sensitive to cultural values that may influence the best way for this information to be presented and discussed.

Signs of dying

The following signs and symptoms (in the context of the patient's disease state) are suggestive that the patient is dying:
- Usually bedbound or immobile
- Difficulty managing medication
- Confusion
- Marked generalized weakness
- Drowsy or comatose
- Poor appetite and decreased fluid intake

General principles of end of life care

The general principles of end of life care are as follows:
- Discontinue any inappropriate interventions. This includes blood tests, antibiotics, and intravenous fluids or parenteral nutrition.
- Document that the patient is not to receive cardiopulmonary resuscitation. Ensure that any implantable defibrillators have been deactivated.
- Stop any inappropriate nursing interventions. Regular observations of vital signs should be stopped. Blood glucose monitoring should be undertaken if clinically indicated. Patients should only be repositioned for comfort rather than on a routine basis.
- Required medications (analgesics and anxiolytics) should be given by syringe driver and this should be started within four hours of prescribing.
- Assess that communication is not an issue, particularly if English is not the first language. Interpreters may be needed.
- Assess insight of condition of patient (if patient requests this) and family.
- Assess any religious/spiritual needs and involve appropriate clergy at patient's request.
- Give appropriate information to relevant hospital professionals and general practice.
- Ensure that the plan of care (if the Liverpool Care Pathway for the Dying Patient (LCP) is being utilized explain the nature of this) has been understood.
- Following death, the patient's body should be managed according to local policy. Any religious requirements should be adhered to.
- The GP should be informed of the patient's death.
- Appropriate information regarding arranging a funeral and death registration should be given to the family in written format.
- Information on bereavement support should be given to the family.

Principles of drug use in end of life care

- Use the minimum amount of medications to treat the patient and ease distress and pain.
- Use of parenteral routes of medication—as condition deteriorates and conscious level decreases, the ability to swallow effectively declines. Medication should change to parenteral routes. A subcutaneous infusion via syringe driver is preferred.
- Assess pain and other symptoms regularly.
- Continue with medications even if the patient is in a coma as pain and other symptoms may be present and cause distress, indicated through non-verbal means.
- Often other drugs can be administered parenterally in combination with the strong opioid. This should be checked on an individual basis.
- Stop non-essential medications, e.g. those for hypertension, diabetes, etc. as the potential benefit is likely to be very low, but the evidence in literature on this topic is very poor.

Specific symptom control

Pain

Pain should be managed according to the basic principles of the WHO analgesic ladder. Thorough assessment of pain through history and examination should be followed by appropriate treatment. Analgesic requirements may increase so regular review of pain should be undertaken. Particular care should be taken of the unconscious patient as they will not be able to complain of pain but pain may still exist.

- Convert oral analgesia (usually a strong opioid) to a parenteral route (subcutaneous) via syringe driver.
- Opioid conversions should be done as indicated previously.
- Long-acting opioids such as analgesic patches should not be stopped at this stage due to the delay in reaching peak plasma levels.
- Adjuvant analgesics and NSAIDs should still be used when appropriate.
- Pain may also be helped by non-drug measures such as repositioning, TENS, etc.

It is important to note that dying patients in their last weeks of life have several specific requirements. For instance, opioid dose should not be reduced solely for decreased blood pressure, respiration rate, or level of consciousness when opioid is necessary for adequate management of dyspnoea and pain. In fact, opioids can be titrated aggressively for moderate/severe acute/chronic pain.

Dyspnoea

Breathlessness may be due to a number of causes including pre-existing disease and manifestations of malignancy, e.g. lung metastases, pleural effusions, lymphangitis carcinomatosis.

Reversible causes should be treated when appropriate. Use of diuretics (cardiac failure) and bronchodilators (bronchospasm) are indicated where appropriate.

Supportive measures such as positioning, assistance with expectoration, and the use of cool air (via fan or open window) will relieve the sensation of breathlessness.

Oxygen has been shown to be helpful in some patients with dyspnea. Often patients find facemasks restrictive and uncomfortable and nasal cannulae are often preferred. Oxygen can be delivered effectively up to 28% (4L) via this route.

Nebulized saline may help to expectorate secretions if present.

The use of opioids and benzodiazepines in patients with dyspnoea is often helpful. The choice of anxiolytics is often determined by what is the most suitable route of administration, but the speed and duration of action are also important.

As the conscious level deteriorates, changes in the breathing pattern occur. Cheyne–Stokes breathing is frequently observed and consists of alternating periods of rapid breathing followed by spells of apnea.

Noisy respiration may be helped by repositioning the patient and, if substantial secretions are present, use of hyoscine hydrobromide (0.4–0.6mg subcutaneous bolus or up to 2.4mg/24 hours via infusion device). Hyoscine butylbromide (20mg subcutaneous bolus; up to 120mg/24 hours) and glycopyrronium (0.4mg subcutaneous bolus; up to 1.2mg/24 hours) are non-sedating alternatives. Occasionally, gentle suction may be required.

End stage stridor is managed with opioids and anxiolytics, as it is usually too late for corticosteroids.

Anxiety/restlessness

Anxiety and restlessness can be due to angst regarding death and the plethora of accompanying emotions. It can also be due to symptoms and should be managed as a priority. Exploration of fears, discussion, and reassurance should be undertaken in the first instance. Often however, pharmacological interventions are needed to manage this. Even in small doses, drugs can alleviate the symptoms of anxiety without causing sedation. The key to treatment lies in calming the acute state while dealing with the cause, if it is apparent and appropriate. A notable example is the mental clouding, hallucinations, confusion, and restlessness associated with opioid toxicity, which can be eased with haloperidol while the opioid dose is reviewed. In general, choice of drug treatment depends on the likely cause. Doses are titrated up or down to achieve the desired effect, and the situation should be reviewed regularly and often until the acute episode settles.

Low-dose anxiolytics (e.g. benzodiazepines) are usually used in these situations and can be administered concurrently with strong opioids in a syringe driver. In the UK, the commonly used benzodiazepine in this setting is midazolam, usually starting at doses of 5–10mg via subcutaneous syringe driver over 24 hours. As required, doses of one-sixth of the total daily dose should be prescribed concurrently.

Delirium/acute-confusional state

When delirium occurs at the end of life it is often referred to as terminal agitation and can be very distressing for the patient and the family (see Table 17.16.1).

Delirium in patients with advanced cancer and limited life expectancy may shorten prognosis.

It can affect cognition and thus affect the emotional issues that require to be worked through at the end of life. There can be many causes including biochemical disturbance, hypoxia, hepatic and renal failure, cerebral disease, infective sources, and drugs, e.g. steroids or opioids.

Table 17.16.1 Drug treatment for terminal agitation and distress

Drug	Route	Indication	Usual starting dose	Dose range over 24 hours (continuous infusion)
Haloperidol	SC	Delirium	2.5mg	5–30mg
Midazolam	SC	Distress	2.5–5mg	10–80mg
Methotrimeprazine*	SC	Delirium	25mg	25–250mg

*Usually used when standard doses of haloperidol and midazolam have been ineffective.

SC subcutaneous.

Treatment of the underlying source is important but in many cases the cause is unknown and treatment has to be given 'blind'. Use of antipsychotic medications, such as haloperidol, is helpful and can usually be given in a syringe driver with opioids and anxiolytics.

Haloperidol is of particular use in cases of opioid toxicity at the end of life. At this point, switching to another opioid to combat toxicity is not advised. Thus controlling side effects appropriately is the ideal. If the patient is markedly distressed, the use of midazolam for anxiety/distress and haloperidol (to treat psychosis) is the normal practice in the UK. The lowest dose should be used to achieve the desired effect.

In cases of severe terminal agitation where escalating doses of midazolam and haloperidol have been unsuccessful, second-line agents should be used. Methotrimoprazine is helpful and should be titrated to achieve effect. Where terminal agitation exists, frequent review is needed, as this will be a very distressing time for both patients and family members.

Respiratory secretions

As the patient becomes increasingly weak and exhausted, respiratory secretions gather in the posterior pharynx. The sound produced is often referred to as the 'death rattle'. However, this term is best avoided as its use can be distressing for patients and family members.

Marked respiratory secretions at the end of life are present in approximately 50% of deaths. These usually occur when the patient is comatose so that they are often unaware of them. It could be argued that as the patient is unaware of the symptom it is not necessary to treat it. However, family members can find this disturbing and often concerns are expressed that the patients is either choking or drowning. It is accepted practice that respiratory secretions should be treated and antimuscarinic agents such as hyoscine hydrobromide, hyoscine butylbromide, and glycopyrronium are used (Table 17.16.2). There is insufficient evidence to indicated superiority of any one over the other.

In some cases oral pharyngeal suction is needed. This is best used in patients who are comatose as it can be distressing if patients are conscious.

Mouth care

Mouth care is extremely important at the end of life. Patients are likely to be dehydrated and if conscious level is impaired, their oral hygiene and intake may have been compromised. It is important that regular mouth care is undertaken throughout the dying phase. The principles are the same as those discussed previously. The use of mouth swabs soaked in cool water can be used to hydrate the oral mucosa and improve mouth care. Family members can be instructed to do this in addition to healthcare staff.

Fluids and parenteral nutrition

Patients who have undergone intensive hospital treatment may have intravenous fluids and parenteral nutrition in place. As the dying process is acknowledged and the focus of care changes to symptom control, dealing with fluids and parenteral nutrition can be challenging. These are highly visible, intensive treatments and withdrawing them carries much meaning. In these cases, careful, thoughtful discussions with the patient and family members should be undertaken. Concerns are often raised that the patient will starve or be thirsty. Abrupt cessation of these may be perceived as lack of care or abandonment.

In the end of life setting, intravenous fluids and nutritional support are unlikely to provide any benefit.

Decisions regarding the administration of hydration and/or artificial nutrition therapy are independent of the decision about whether to administer palliative sedation. Opinions and practices vary. This variability reflects the heterogeneity of attitudes of involved clinicians, ethicists, patients, families, and local norms of good clinical and ethical practice.

Individual patients, family members, and clinicians may regard the continuation of hydration as a non-burdensome humane supportive intervention that represents (and may actually constitute) one means of reducing suffering. Alternatively, hydration may be viewed as a superfluous impediment to inevitable death that can be appropriately withdrawn, because it does not contribute to patient comfort or the prevailing goals of care.

Often, the patient will request relief of suffering and give no direction regarding hydration and nutrition. Under these circumstances, family members and healthcare providers must work to reach a consensus on what constitutes a morally acceptable plan based on the patient's best interests. If adverse effects of artificial hydration and/or nutrition therapy exacerbate patient suffering, then reduction or withdrawal of artificial hydration/nutrition should be considered.

Psychological aspects of end of life care

Ideally a good death should be free from distress. Symptoms, both physical and psychological, should be addressed appropriately. Whilst we often have at our disposal a variety of drugs to treat physical symptoms, addressing psychosocial aspects can be more challenging. An important psychological issue is patient dignity. Dignity is a triad of honor, self-esteem, and respect, and is a key area that should be addressed in end of life care.

Dignity has been examined in patients who are terminally ill: 46% of patients had some loss of dignity, whilst 7.5% considered loss of dignity a serious issue. In the hospital setting patients were more likely to suffer a loss

Table 17.16.2 Drug treatment for respiratory secretions at the end of life

Drug	Route	Initial dose	Review response after	Dose over 24 hours (continuous infusion)—if initial dose effective
Hyoscine hydrobromide	SC	400mcg	30 minutes	1.2–2mg
Glycopyrronium	SC	200mcg	60 minutes	1.2–2mg
Hyoscine butylbromide	SC	20mg	30 minutes	200mg

SC subcutaneous.

of dignity as opposed to patients in primary care. There does not appear to be any relationship between prognosis and loss of dignity. Patients who feel their dignity has not been compromised are less likely to suffer from depression, anxiety, and even a feeling of hopelessness. Also, as sense of dignity increases, there is an increase in quality of life. In contrast, loss of dignity is positively correlated with a desire for hastened death.

Dignity therapy

The concept of dignity therapy was devised by Chochinov et al. (2002). It builds on the foundations of dignity conserving care, which should occur in the management of every patient. Dignity therapy is based on the concept of generativity with the aim of bringing meaning to the life lost.

Dignity therapy can be undertaken by trained therapists. Through careful discussion, the patient is interviewed about their life and how they feel they would like to be remembered. Areas are explored such as life history, key events, and accomplishments. If the patient wants to impart any specific messages, these can also be documented.

Conversations are recorded and are then transcribed to meaningful narrative form. Following this and after the patient is happy with the end result, the patient is given the finished document. The patient is free to give this to whomever they choose, but these are often given to young ones.

Although dignity therapy is best done by those who have had formal training, it can also be done less formally. Through the use of a question-based format, health professionals or even family members can discuss these issues.

Care should be taken if the patient is very near dying and in particular has cognitive impairment. If records of conversations or thoughts are not recorded accurately, false information may be imparted. In the scenario of end of life there may be no opportunity to address this.

How long?

This question is commonly asked by patients and families and may be a source of anxiety for the health professional who has to answer this. It may be very difficult to estimate and there is a dearth of research within this area. As a result, physicians are often very bad at estimating prognosis. Patients and families will however request this information. If a likely timescale is known, this allows for business and emotional issues to be addressed. It may also be necessary if family members are overseas and wish or are requested by the patient to be seen. It can be very useful for the patient to know how close death is and if this is the patient's wish, it should be discussed.

It is often very difficult to predict death and usually it is best to give estimates in the region of 'days', 'weeks', 'days to weeks', etc. Often a useful predictor is the rate of decline over a set time period. If patients have deteriorated very quickly in a short spell then it is likely that their decline will continue at this rate and death is likely to be sooner. Frequent discussions with patients and more often family members will be of great comfort. Changes such as marked decrease in urine output, deterioration in conscious level, or Cheyne–Stokes breathing are likely to signify that few days are left.

In some cases, if the dying process is slow some patients and families feel it is taking too long. This is a particular issue if families are caring for a patient at home on the basis that they can cope for a short time. This too can be a real challenge to deal with. There should be regular review and discussions with patients and their families. Although these patients may not require much in the way of medical or nursing support (particularly when they are in a coma) they should still have regular review. It is important in these times that families feel supported and not abandoned.

The bitter or angry patient

This is an area which can be very difficult to manage. As a result of the intense psychological stresses the dying patient is under, there may be bitterness and anger. Lack of independence and increased level of care can cause frustration which can lead to anger, often directed at loved ones, causing distress. Delirium may cause anger and should be addressed.

It is important to try to address any issues and in some cases spiritual and psychological support may be required. The physician should explore tactfully any concerns or anxieties and address as many issues as possible. It should be acknowledged that in some cases this may be very difficult or impossible for the doctor to correct. In these cases ongoing support for the patient and family should continue, despite any hostility.

Post-death care

Comprehensive palliative care for the patient's family and caregivers continues after the patient's death. Immediate issues include informing the family (if not present), offering condolences, and providing family time with the body. Additional concerns include ensuring culturally sensitive and respectful treatment of the body, including removal of tubes, drains, lines, and the Foley catheter (unless an autopsy is planned); facilitating funeral arrangements through completion of necessary paperwork; and informing insurance companies and other healthcare professionals of the patient's death. It is often helpful to meet with the family to explain this and answer any questions or address any concerns. Depending on religion or beliefs there may be certain requirements or rituals that should be adhered to and all efforts should be made to deal with these.

Bereavement support should be offered, beginning with a personal visit or telephone call from the patient's primary oncology team. Family members at risk for complicated bereavement or prolonged grief disorder should be identified, and complicated grief should be treated. Children of patients with cancer represent a uniquely at-risk population for psychosocial dysfunction. Bereavement care is often best provided by an experienced hospice team or a skilled mental health care professional. The family may request a debriefing meeting from the medical team and may require assistance in identifying community bereavement resources. A well-supported end of life care experience will facilitate the family's acceptance of appropriate referrals for cancer risk assessment and risk modification.

Conclusion

End of life care is one of the most rewarding aspects of care. It can also be one of the most challenging.

Despite best efforts, in some cases patients do not have a good death. In these cases it is important to remember that we may not be able to fix all symptoms but we should continue to offer our support and be there for the patient and family at this distressing time.

Further reading

Adam J. ABC of palliative care. The last 48 hours. *BMJ* 1997; 315:1600–3.

Cherny NI; ESMO Guidelines Working Group. ESMO Clinical Practice Guidelines for the management of refractory symptoms at the end of life and the use of palliative sedation. *Ann Oncol* 2014 Sep; 25(Suppl. 3):iii143–52.

Chochinov HM, Hack T, Hassard T, et al. Dignity in the terminally ill: a cross-sectional, cohort study. *Lancet* 2002; 360:2026–30.

Fallon M, Hanks G. *ABC of Palliative Care*, 2nd edn. Oxford: Blackwell Publishing, 2006.

Levy M, Smith T, Alvarez-Perez A, et al. Palliative Care Version 1.2016. *J Natl Compr Cancer Netw* 2016 Jan; 14(1):82–113.

Clinical management of cancers—flowcharts

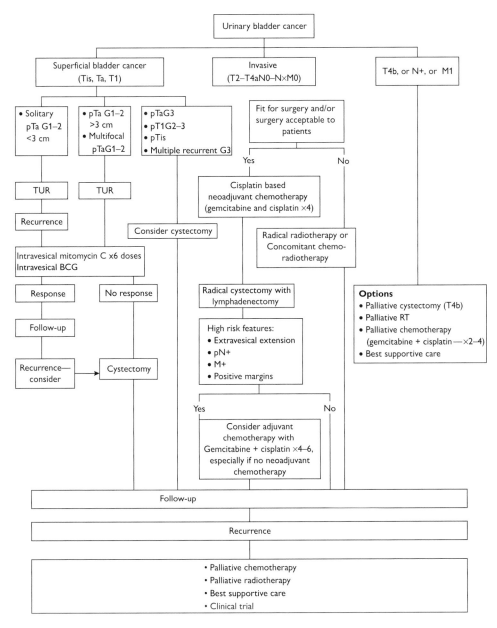

Fig. 18.1 Bladder cancer.

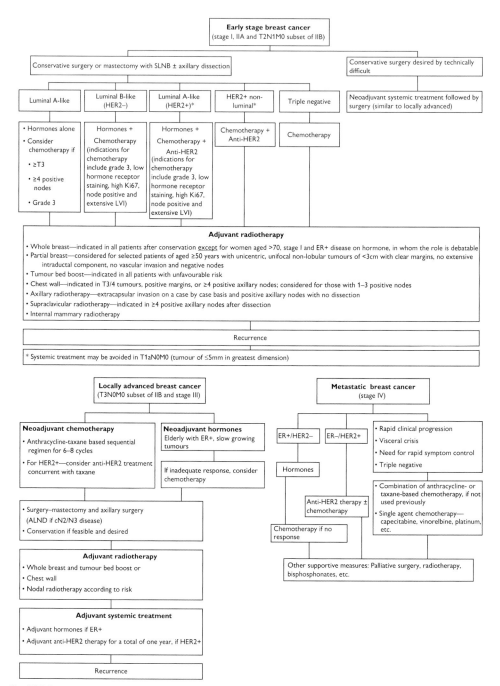

Fig. 18.2 Breast cancer.

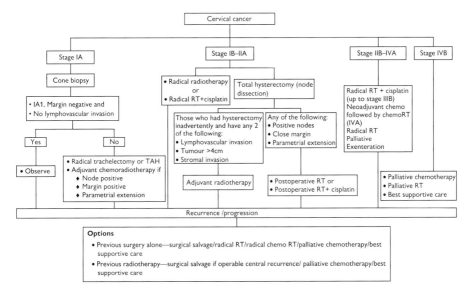

Fig. 18.3 Cervical cancer.

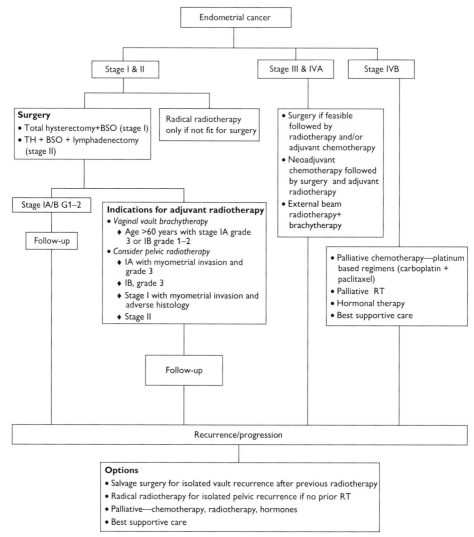

Fig. 18.4 Endometrial cancer.

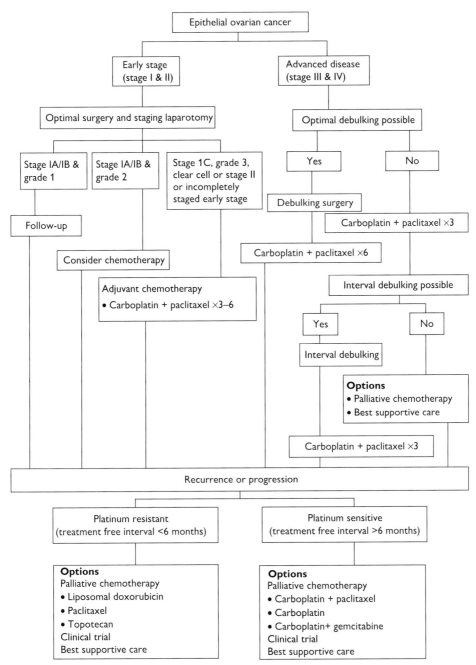

Fig. 18.5 Epithelial ovarian cancer.

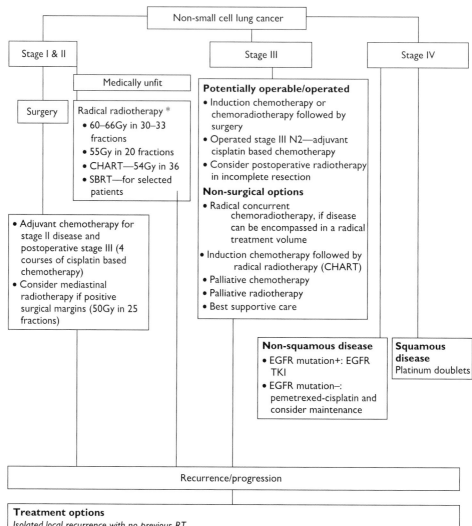

Fig. 18.6a NSCLC.

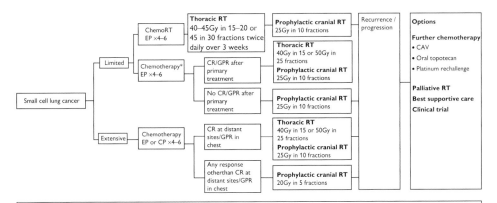

* Very limited disease (T1–2N0–1M0)—if staging does not show any mediastinal nodes, surgery followed by 4 cycles of EP and PCI if appropriate is justified

Fig. 18.6b SCLC.

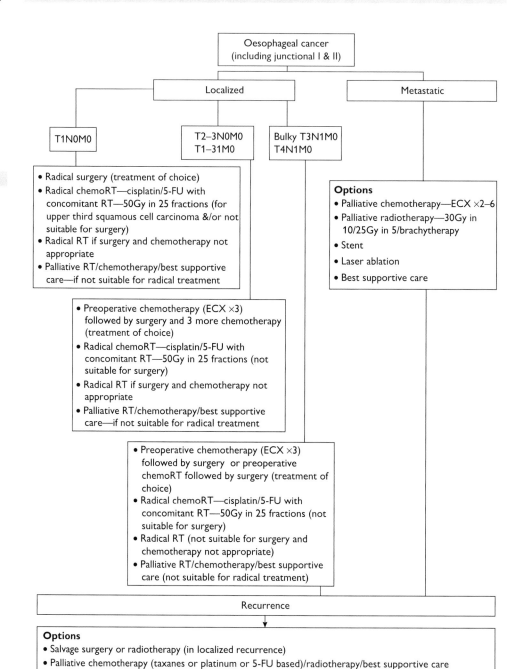

Fig. 18.7 Oesophageal cancer.

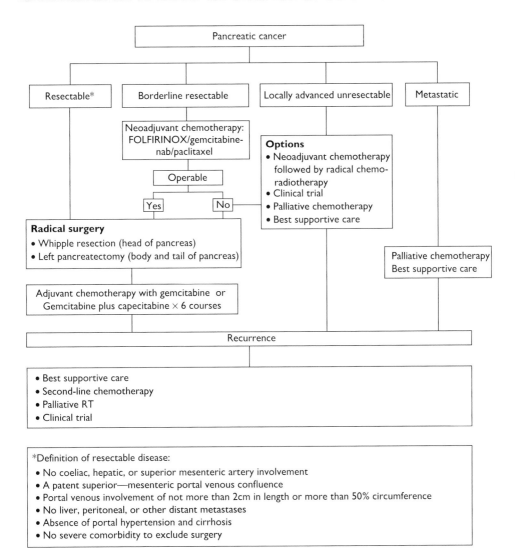

Pancreatic cancer

Resectable*

Borderline resectable

Locally advanced unresectable

Metastatic

Neoadjuvant chemotherapy: FOLFIRINOX/gemcitabine-nab/paclitaxel

Operable

Yes   No

Options
- Neoadjuvant chemotherapy followed by radical chemo-radiotherapy
- Clinical trial
- Palliative chemotherapy
- Best supportive care

Radical surgery
- Whipple resection (head of pancreas)
- Left pancreatectomy (body and tail of pancreas)

Palliative chemotherapy
Best supportive care

Adjuvant chemotherapy with gemcitabine or Gemcitabine plus capecitabine × 6 courses

Recurrence

- Best supportive care
- Second-line chemotherapy
- Palliative RT
- Clinical trial

*Definition of resectable disease:
- No coeliac, hepatic, or superior mesenteric artery involvement
- A patent superior—mesenteric portal venous confluence
- Portal venous involvement of not more than 2cm in length or more than 50% circumference
- No liver, peritoneal, or other distant metastases
- Absence of portal hypertension and cirrhosis
- No severe comorbidity to exclude surgery

Fig. 18.8 Pancreatic cancer.

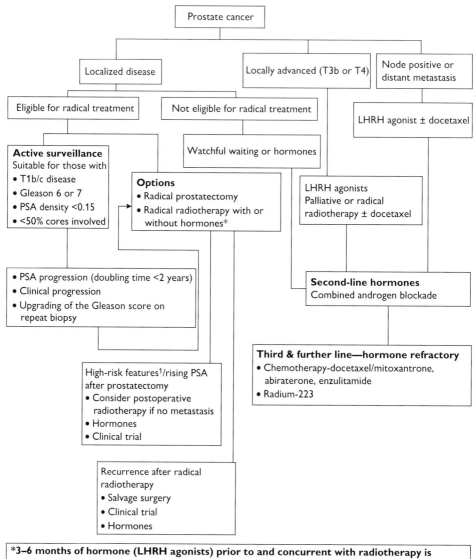

Fig. 18.9 Prostate cancer.

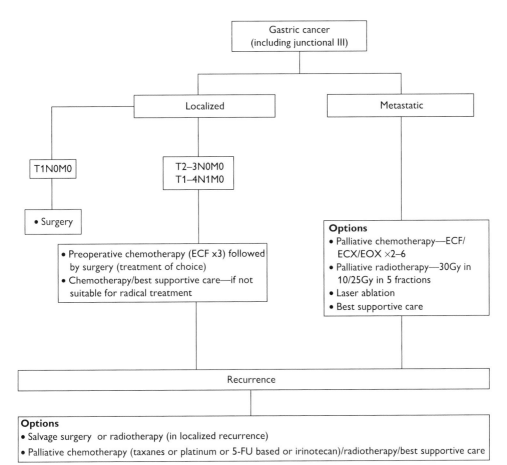

Gastric cancer
(including junctional III)

Localized

Metastatic

T1N0M0

T2–3N0M0
T1–4N1M0

• Surgery

Options
• Palliative chemotherapy—ECF/
  ECX/EOX ×2–6
• Palliative radiotherapy—30Gy in
  10/25Gy in 5 fractions
• Laser ablation
• Best supportive care

• Preoperative chemotherapy (ECF x3) followed
  by surgery (treatment of choice)
• Chemotherapy/best supportive care—if not
  suitable for radical treatment

Recurrence

Options
• Salvage surgery or radiotherapy (in localized recurrence)
• Palliative chemotherapy (taxanes or platinum or 5-FU based or irinotecan)/radiotherapy/best supportive care

Fig. 18.10 Stomach cancer.

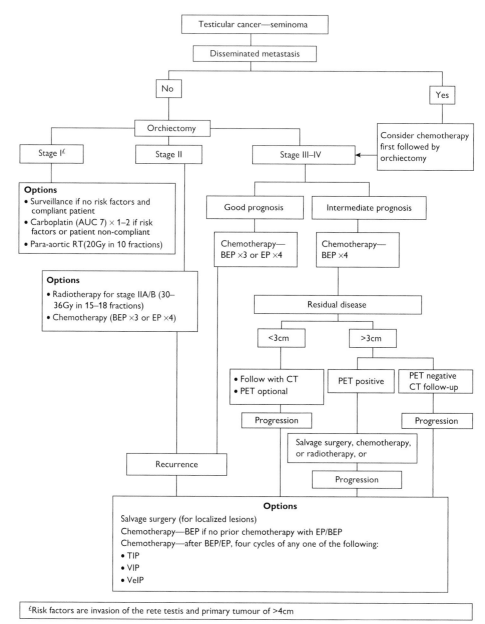

Fig. 18.11a Testicular tumour: seminoma.

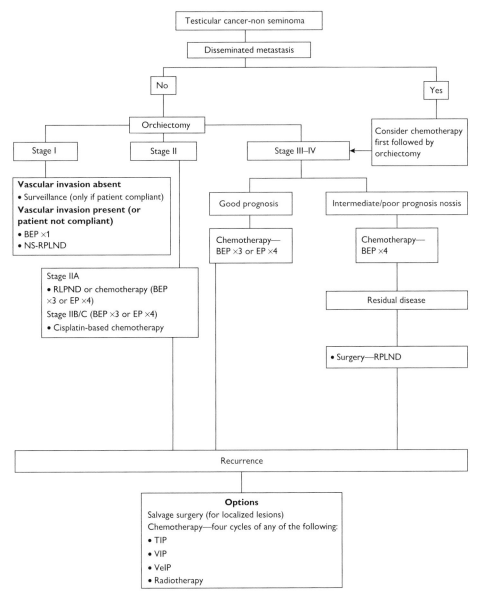

Fig. 18.11b Testicular tumour: non-seminoma.

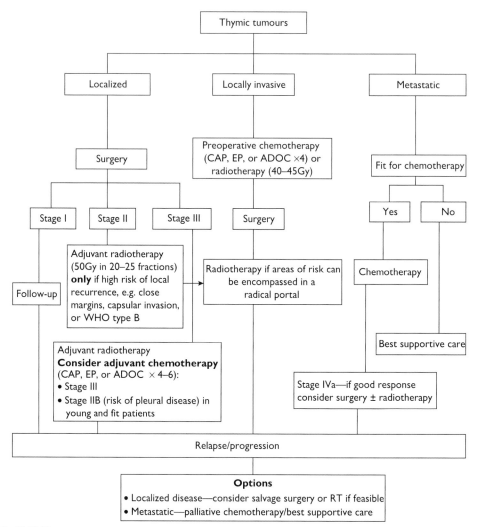

Fig. 18.12 Thymoma.

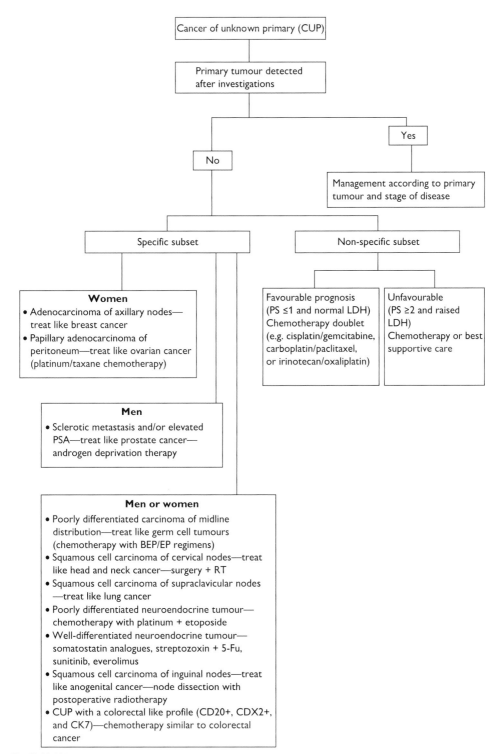

Fig. 18.13 Unknown primary.

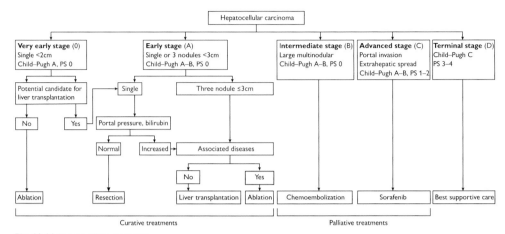

Fig. 18.14 Hepatocellular carcinoma.

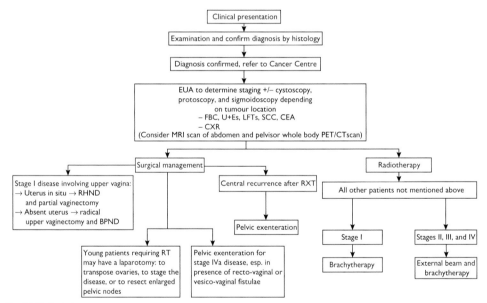

Fig. 18.15 Vaginal cancer.

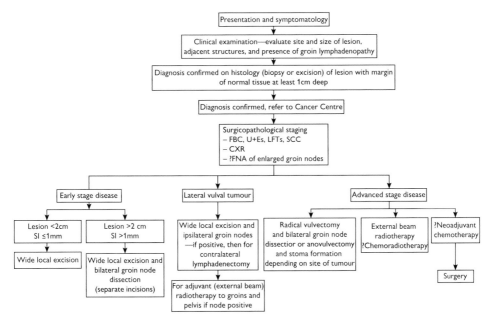

Fig. 18.16 Vulval cancer.

Appendix 1

Systemic therapy regimens

Tumours of head and neck

Cisplatin–5-fluorouracil
- Cisplatin 80–100mg/m^2 IV infusion Day 1
- 5-FU 1g/m^2 24-hour infusion Days 1–5
- 3-week cycle

Docetaxel
- 75 mg/m^2 IV every 21 days

Tumours of nervous system

Temozolomide
Concomitant
- 75mg/m^2 for 42 days starting on the first day of radiotherapy. Give 1 hour prior to radiotherapy and morning at weekend

Adjuvant and palliative
- 150mg/m^2 first course and if well tolerated increase to 200mg/m^2 for a total of 6 courses. 4-week cycle

PCV
- Procarbazine 100mg/m^2 oral Days 1–10
- CCNU 100mg/m^2 oral Day 1
- Vincristine 1.4mg/m^2 (max. dose 2mg) IV Day 1
- 6-week cycle

Thoracic tumours

Non-small cell lung cancer
Cisplatin–vinorelbine
- Cisplatin 80mg/m^2 IV Day 1
- Vinorelbine 30mg/m^2 IV Days 1 and 8
- 3-week cycle—adjuvant 4 cycles, palliative 4–6 cycles

Gemcitabine–carboplatin
- Gemcitabine 1000mg/m^2 IV Days 1 and 8
- Carboplatin (AUC 5) IV Day 1
- 3-week cycle, 4–6 cycles

Carboplatin–paclitaxel
- Carboplatin AUC 6 Day 1
- Paclitaxel 225mg/m^2 IV Day 1
- 3- week cycle

Carboplatin – Pemetrexed
- Carboplatin AUC 5 IV Day 1
- Pemetrexed 500 mg/m^2 IV Day 1
- 3-week cycle

Pemetrexed maintenance
- 500mg/m^2 IV Day 1
- 3-week cycle

Docetaxel
- Docetaxel 75mg/m^2 Day 1
- 3-week cycle

Vinorelbine
- Vinorelbine 30mg/m^2 (max 60mg) Days 1, 8—3-week cycle
- Oral vinorelbine 60mg/m^2 Day 1—weekly.
- Increase to 80mg/m^2 if no grade 4 neutropenia after third cycle

Afatinib
- 400 mg OD PO continuously until progression

Crizotinib
- 250 mg BD PO continuously until progression

Erlotinib
- 150 mg OD PO continuously until progression

Gefitinib
- 250 mg OD PO continuously until progression

Small-cell lung cancer
Carboplatin–etoposide
- Carboplatin AUC 5 IV Day 1
- Etoposide 100mg/m^2 IV Days 1–3 (day 2–3 can be substituted with oral etoposide 100mg/m^2 twice daily)
- 3-week cycle

VAC
- Vincristine 1.4mg/m^2 (max 2mg) IV Day 1
- Adriamycin 40mg/m^2 IV Day 1

- Cyclophosphamide 600mg/m^2 Day 1
- 3-week cycle

CAP

- Cyclophosphamide 500 mg/m^2 IV Day 1
- Adriamycin 50 mg/m^2 IV Day 1
- Cisplatin 50 mg/m^2 Day 1
- 3-week cycle

Oral topotecan

- Topotecan 2.3mg/m^2 Days 1–5
- 3-week cycle

Oral etoposide

- Oral etoposide 50mg PO twice daily Days 1–5
- 3-week cycle

Mesothelioma

Cisplatin–pemetrexed

- Cisplatin 75mg/m^2 Day 1 (carboplatin AUC 5)
- Pemetrexed 500mg/m^2 Day 1
- 3-week cycle

Thymoma

- *CAP*
- Cyclophosphamide 500mg/m^2 Day 1
- Adriamycin 50mg/m^2 Day 1
- Cisplatin 50mg/m^2 Day 1
- 3-week cycle

Cisplatin–etoposide

- See above

Breast cancer

AC

- Adriamycin 60mg/m^2 IV Day 1
- Cyclophosphamide 600mg/m^2 IV Day 1
- 3-week cycle for 4–6 cycles

EC

- Epirubicin 90mg/m2 IV Day 1
- Cyclophosphamide 500 mg/m2 IV Day 1
- 3-week cycle for 6 cycles

E-CMF

- Epirubicin 100mg/m^2 Day 1, 3-week cycle for 4 courses followed by 4 cycles of CMF
- Cyclophosphamide 100mg/m^2 PO Days 1–14
- Methotrexate 40mg/m^2 IV (max. 50) Days 1, 8
- 5-FU 600mg/m^2 IV (max. 1g) Days 1, 8
- 4-week cycle

FEC

- 5-FU 600mg/m^2 IV bolus Day 1
- Epirubicin 60mg/m^2 IV bolus Day 1
- Cyclophosphamide 600mg/m^2 IV bolus Day 1
- 3-week cycle for 6 courses

FEC-T

- 3 courses of FEC (100mg/m^2) followed by 3 courses of T (docetaxel)
- Docetaxel 100mg/m^2 IV—3-week cycle

TAC

- Docetaxel 75mg/m^2 IV
- Adriamycin 50mg/m^2 IV
- Cyclophosphamide 500mg/m^2 IV
- 3-week cycle for 6 courses

Docetaxel

- 75mg/m^2 IV infusion Day 1
- 3-week cycle for 6 courses

Capecitabine

- 1000–1250mg/m^2 PO Days 1–14
- 3-week cycle until progression or intolerable toxicity

Vinorelbine

- 25–30mg/m^2 IV (max 60mg) Days 1, 8
- 3-week cycle for 6 courses

Oral vinorelbine

- 60mg/m^2 (increase dose to 80mg/m^2 in second cycle if no neutropenia) Day 1, 8
- 3-week cycle

Paclitaxel

- 175mg/m^2 3-hour infusion Day 1; 3-week cycle or
- 80mg/m^2 1-hour infusion Day 1, 8, 15; 4-week cycle

Hormones

- Tamoxifen 20mg PO daily
- Letrazole 2.5mg PO daily
- Anastrazole 1mg PO daily
- Exemestane 25mg PO daily
- Megesterol 160mg PO daily

Trastuzumab

- Loading dose 8mg/kg 90-minute infusion followed after 3 weeks by 6mg/kg IV infusion—3-week cycle. Total 17 cycles for adjuvant setting and until disease progression for metastatic disease

Trastuzumab–docetaxel

- Trastuzumab followed by 30 minutes to 1-hour observation followed by docetaxel

Capecitabine-Lapatinib

- Capecitabine 1000mg/m2 Days1–14
- Lapatinib 1250 mg OD days 1–14
- 3-week cycle

Cancers of gastrointestinal system

Oesophageal and gastric cancer

Cisplatin–5-fluorouracil
- Cisplatin 100mg/m^2 Day 1
- 5-FU 1000mg/m^2 Days 1–4 IV infusion
- 3-week cycle

Cisplatin – Capecitabine
- Cisplatin 80 mg/m2 IV Day 1
- Capecitabine 1000 mg/m2 IV Day 1–14
- 3-week cycle

ECX
- Epirubicin 50mg/m^2 Day 1
- Cisplatin 60mg/m^2 Day 1
- Capecitabine 625mg/m^2 twice daily Days 1–21
- 3-week cycle

ECF
- Epirubicin 50mg/m^2 Day 1, repeat 3-weekly
- Cisplatin 60mg/m^2 Day 1, repeat 3-weekly
- 5-FU 200mg/m^2 IV 24-hour continuous infusion for 18–24 weeks

EOX
- Epirubicin 50mg/m^2 Day1
- Oxaliplatin 130mg/m^2 Day 1
- Capecitabine 625mg/m^2 Day 1
- 3-week cycle

Docetaxel
- 75 mg/m^2 IV Day 1
- 3-week cycle

Pancreatic cancer

Gemcitabine
- 1000mg/m^2 weekly for 7 weeks followed by 1 week's rest

Folfironox
- 5-fluorouracil 400 mg/m2 IV bolus Day 1 and 2400 mg/m^2 IV over 46 hours
- Folinic acid 400 mg/m^2 IV Day 1
- Irinitecan 180 mg/m^2 IV Day 1
- Oxaliplatin 85mg/m^2 IV Day 1
- 2-week cycle

Biliary tumours

Cisplatin-Gemcitabine
- Cisplatin 25 mg/m^2 Days 1&8
- Gemcitabine 1000mg/m^2 Days 1&8
- 3-week cycle

Hepatocellular carcinoma
- Sorafenib 400 mg BD continuously until progression

Colorectal cancer

Oxaliplatin–5 Fluorouracil/FA
- Oxaliplatin 85mg/m^2 IV infusion Day 1
- 5-FU 400mg/m^2 bolus Days 1 and 2
- 5-FU 600mg/m^2 22-hour infusion Days 1 and 2
- Folinic acid 200mg/m^2 infusion Days 1 and 2
- 2-week cycle

5-Fluorouracil–folinic acid (Mayo regimen)
- 5-FU 425mg/m^2 IV (325mg/m^2 when given with radio-therapy) Days 1–5
- Folinic acid 20mg/m^2 IV Days 1–5
- 4-week cycle

Capecitabine
- Capecitabine 1250mg/m^2 twice daily Days 1–14
- 4-week cycle

Irinotecan
- Irinotecan 300–350mg/m^2 IV Day 1
- 3-week cycle

Capecitabine –irinotecan
- Capecitabine 800 mg/m^2 BD PO Day 1–11
- Irinotecan 180 mg/m^2 IV Day 1
- 2-week cycle

Capecitabine –oxaliplatin
- Capecitabine 1000 mg/m^2 BD PO Day 1–14
- Oxaliplatin 130mg/m^2 IV Day 1
- 3-week cycle

Irinotecan–5-fluorouracil/folinic acid
- Irinotecan 125mg/m^2 IV infusion Day 1
- Folic acid 20mg/m^2 IV bolus Day 1
- 5-FU 500mg/m^2 bolus Day 1
- 3-week cycle
- There are modifications of the above regimen with infusional 5-FU/FA.

Anal cancer

Mitomycin C–5-fluorouracil
- Mitomycin C 10mg/m^2 IV Day 1
- 5-FU 750mg/m^2 24-hour infusion Days 1–5 repeated at week 5

Cancers of genitourinary system

Urinary bladder
Gemcitabine–cisplatin
- Gemcitabine 1000mg/m^2 IV infusion Days 1, 8, and 15
- Cisplatin 70mg/m^2 IV infusion Day 1
- 4-week cycle

MVAC
- Methotrexate 30mg/m^2 IV Days 1, 15, 22
- Vinblastine 3mg/m^2 IV Days 1, 15, 22
- Doxorubicin 30mg/m^2 IV Days 1
- Cisplatin 70mg/m^2 IV infusion Day 1
- 4-week cycle

Testicular cancer
BEP (3-day)
- Bleomycin 30mg Day 2, 8, 15
- Etoposide 120mg/m^2 Days 1–3
- Cisplatin 50mg/m^2 Days 1, 2
- 3-week cycle

BEP (5 day)
- Bleomycin 30mg Days 2, 8, 15
- Etoposide 100mg/m^2 Days 1–5
- Cisplatin 20mg/m^2 Days 1–5
- 3-week cycle

Carboplatin
- AUC 7 Day 1—one course

TIP
- Paclitaxel 175mg/m^2 Day 1
- Ifosfamide 1.2 gm/m^2 Days 2–6 with mesna

- Cisplatin 20mg/m^2 Days 2–6
- 3-week cycle

VIP
- Vinblastine 0.11mg/kg Days 1, 2
- Ifosfamide 1.5 gm/m^2 Days 1–4 with mesna
- Cisplatin 20mg/m^2 Days 1–5
- 3-week cycle

Prostate cancer
Abiraterone – prednisolone
- Abiraterone 1g OD PO daily and Prednisolone 5 mg BD PO continuous

Cabazitaxel – prednisolone
- Cabazitaxel 25 mg/m^2 IV Day 1
- Prednisolone 10 mg PO OD Days 1–21
- 3-week cycle

Docetaxel- prednisolone
- Docetaxel 75 mg/m^2 IV Day 1
- Prednisolone 10 mg PO OD Days 1–21
- 3-week cycle

Enzulatamide
- *160 mg daily continuously*

Mitozantrone–prednisone
Mitozantrone 12mg/m^2 Day 1
- Prednisone 10mg daily
- 3-week cycle

Cancers of female genital system

Cervical cancer
Cisplatin (concurrent with radiotherapy)
- Cisplatin 40mg/m^2 IV weekly for 4–5 courses

Carboplatin-paclitaxel
- Carboplatin AUC 2 Days 1,8 and 15
- Paclitaxel 80 mg/m2 Days 1,8, and 15
- 3-week cycle

Endometrial cancer
Cisplatin–doxorubicin
- Cisplatin 50mg/m^2 IV Day 1
- Doxorubicin 50mg/m^2 Day 1
- 3- week cycle

Paclitaxel–carboplatin
- See 'Epithelial ovarian cancer'

Epithelial ovarian cancer
Paclitaxel–carboplatin
- Paclitaxel 175mg/m^2 3-hour infusion Day 1
- Carboplatin (AUC 5) 1-hour infusion Day 1
- 3-week cycle

Carboplatin
- AUC 7—3-week cycle

Paclitaxel
- 175mg/m^2 Day 1, 3-week cycle *or*
- 90mg/m^2 Day 1, 1-week cycle for 18 weeks

Carboplatin –Liposomal doxorubicin
- *Pegylated liposomal doxorubicin 30 mg/m^2 IV Day 1*
- *Carboplatin AUC 5 IV Day 1*
- *4-week cycle*

Liposomal doxorubicin
- Liposomal doxorubicin 50mg/m^2 IV Day 1
- 4-week cycle

Topotecan
- Topotecan 1.5mg/m^2 Days 1–5
- 3-week cycle

Carboplatin–gemcitabine
- Carboplatin AUC 5 IV
- Gemcitabine 1000mg/m^2 Days 1, 8
- 3-week cycle

Ovarian germ cell tumour
- See 'Testicular cancer'

Malignant melanoma
Dabrafenib
- 150 mg BD PO continuous

Dabrafenib-Trametinib
- Dabrafenib 150 mg BD PO continuous
- Trametinib 2 mg OD PO continuous

Ipilimumab
- 3 mg/mg IV 3-week cycle

Nivolumab – Ipilimumab
- Ipilimumab 3mg/kg with Nivolumab 1 mg/kg once 3 weeks for 4 cycles followed by Nivolumab 3mg/kg once in 2 weeks

Vemurafenib
- 960 mg BD PO continuous

Cutaneous T cell lymphoma
- Bexarotene 300 mg /m^2 daily PO

Basal cell carcinoma
Vismodegib
- 150 mg OD PO continuous

Appendix 2

Radiotherapy fractionation

Please see Tables A2.1–A2.12.

Table A2.1 Tumours of head and neck

Indication	Dose fractionation
T1-T2 glottic cancer	• 50 Gy in 16 fractions (T1 only) • 63 Gy in 28 fractions • 55 Gy in 20 fractions
Stage I/II oropharynx, hypopharynx and non-glottic larynx	• 70 Gy in 25 fractions/ 65-66 Gy in 30 fractions • 66 Gy in 33 fractions or 70 Gy in 35 fractions, 6 fractions per week
Concomitant chemoradiotherapy (stage III-IVb excluding nasopharyngeal)	• 70 Gy in 35 fractions • 65-66 Gy in 30 fractions
Radical radiotherapy (stage III-IVb excluding nasopharyngeal)	• 66 Gy in 33/ 70 Gy in 25 fractions, 6 fractions per week • 65-66 Gy in 30 fractions
Adjuvant (postoperative) radiotherapy	• 60 in 30 fractions with a 6 Gy in 3 fraction boost to high risk sites
Nasopharyngeal cancer	• 70 Gy in 35 fractions/ 70 Gy in 33 fractions/ 65 Gy in 30 fractions
Palliative radiotherapy	• 40 Gy in 10 fractions over 4 weeks as split course • 21 Gy in 3 fractions • 14 Gy in 4 fractions

Table A2.2 Tumours of nervous system

Indication	Dose fractionation
Glioma	
Low grade glioma—radical	• 50.4 Gy in 28 fractions or 54Gy in 30 fractions
Grade III – radical	• 59.4 in 33 fractions or 60 Gy in 30 fractions
Grade IV —radical	• 60Gy in 30 fractions over 5 weeks
High grade glioma—palliative	• 40Gy in 15 fractions (PS0–1), 34 Gy in 10 fractions or 30Gy in 6 fractions over 2 weeks (>70 years or PS 2)
Ependymoma	
Cranial	• 59.4 Gy in 33 fractions
Spinal—localized (low grade)	• 50.4Gy in 28 fractions
Spinal—metastasis to spinal cord	• Craniospinal RT 35Gy in 21 fractions followed by boost to the sites of disease to a total dose of 54 -55.8 Gy in 1.8 Gy fractions
Craniospinal RT—medulloblastoma	• Craniospinal RT 36-39.6 Gy in 20-22 fractions followed by posterior cranial fossa RT 19Gy in 12 fractions
Primary CNS lymphoma	• 40Gy in 20 or 45Gy in 25 fractions
Germinoma	• 24Gy in 15 fractions whole ventricular radiotherapy followed by a boost 16 Gy in 10 fractions
Non-germinoma	• 54 Gy in 30 fractions
Germ cell tumour with CNS dissemination	• 30Gy in 20 fractions to craniospinal axis followed by 25.2Gy in 14 fractions to primary tumour
Pituitary adenoma	• 45Gy in 25 fractions over 5 weeks
Craniopharyngioma	• 50-55Gy in 30-33 fractions over 6-6.5 weeks or 52.2-54 Gy in 27-28 fractions over 5.5weeks
Meningioma	• Grade 1: 50.4-54 Gy in 28-30 fractions or 50-55 Gy in 30-33 fractions • Grade 2: 54-60 Gy in 30 fractions • Grade 3: 60 Gy in 30 fractions
Acoustic neuroma	• 50Gy in 30 fractions
Brain metastasis	
SRS – for Solitary or multiple metastases up to 20 cm^3 with KPS≥70 and controlled extracranial disease	• <20 mm – 24 Gy single dose • 21-30mm – 18 Gy single dose • 31-40mm – 15 Gy single dose
Metastases—multiple	• 30 Gy in 10 fractions (as individually or with SRS) • 20Gy in 5 fractions
Spinal cord compression	
Impending or evolving compression/ postoperative and good PS	• 20Gy in 5 fractions or 30Gy in 10 fractions
Established paraplegia/poor performance status	• 8Gy in 1 fraction or 20 Gy in 5 fractions
Re-treatment	• 8Gy in 1 or 20Gy in 5 fractions (maximum cumulative BED <120 Gy$_2$

Table A2.3 Thoracic tumours

Indication	Dose fractionation
Non-small cell lung cancer	
Stage I-II medically inoperable Radical radiotherapy	• 54Gy in 36 fractions over 12 days (CHART) • 55 Gy in 20 fractions
Medically inoperable ≤5 cm (SABR)	• 54 Gy in 3 fractions over 5-8 days • 60 Gy in 5-8 fractions over 10-20 days
Stage III (with chemotherapy)	• 55 Gy in 20 fractions (concurrent or sequential with chemotherapy) • 60-66 Gy in 30-33 fractions ((concurrent or sequential with chemotherapy) • 54 Gy in 36 fractions treating thrice daily over 12 consecutive days (CHART) (sequential only)
Stage III (RT alone)	• CHART (as above) • 55 Gy in 20 fractions • 66 Gy in 33 fractions
Pancoast's tumour	• 45 Gy in 25 fractions with chemotherapy
Postoperative	• 60Gy in 25–30 fractions • 50Gy in 20–25 fractions
Palliative	• 36–39Gy in 12–13 fractions (36Gy if spinal cord in the field)—PS 0–1 • 30 Gy in 10 fractions / 20Gy in 5 fractions—PS 0–1 • 17Gy in 2 fractions (PS 2) • 10Gy single (PS>2)
Small-cell lung cancer	
Localized	• 50Gy in 25 fractions/40Gy in 15 fractions (sequential chemoradiotherapy) • 45Gy in 30 fractions twice daily over 3 weeks/ 66 Gy in 33 fractions or 40 Gy in15 fractions (concurrent chemoradiotherapy)
Palliative	• 30 Gy in 10 fractions/ 20 Gy in 5 fractions
Prophylactic cranial RT	
Small cell lung cancer	• 20 Gy in 5 fractions/ 30 Gy in 10 fractions/ 25 Gy in10 fractions/ 30 gy in 12fractions
Thymus	
Postoperative	• 50Gy in 25 fractions or 60Gy in 30 fractions
Primary radiotherapy	• 60Gy in 30 fractions
Mesothelioma	
Palliative chest wall	• 20Gy in 5 or 36 Gy in 6 fractions twice per week

Table A2.4 Breast cancer

Indication	Dose fractionation
Whole breast	• 40Gy in 15 fractions • 28-30 Gy in 5 fractions over 5 weeks or 26 Gy in 5 fractions (selected patients with node-negative breast cancer that do not require a boost radiotherapy)
Boost RT	• 16Gy in 8 fractions (with 50Gy whole breast RT) • 10Gy in 5 fractions
Postoperative chest wall	• 40Gy in 15 fractions
Supraclavicular fossa	• 40Gy in 15 fractions

Table A2.5 Cancers of gastrointestinal system

Indication	Dose fractionation
Oesophagus	
Radical chemoradiotherapy	• 50Gy in 25 fractions • 50.4 Gy in 28 fractions
Preoperative chemoradiotherapy	• 41.4 Gy in 23 fractions • 45Gy in 25 fractions
Radical radiotherapy	• 50 Gy in15-16 fractions • 55Gy in 20 fractions • 60 Gy in 30 fractions
Palliative	• 20Gy in 5 or 30Gy in 10 fractions or 40 Gy in 15 fractions
Stomach	
Adjuvant chemoradiotherapy	• 45Gy in 25 fractions
Pancreas	
Radical chemoradiotherapy	• 45–50.4Gy in 25–28 fractions
Palliative	• 30Gy in 10 fractions
Rectal cancer	
Preoperative—short course	• 25Gy in 5 fractions
Preoperative—long course	• 45Gy in 25 fractions • 50.4 Gy in 28 fractions
Postoperative	• 45Gy in 25 fractions • 50.4 Gy in 28 fractions
Palliative	• 30 Gy in 10 fractions • 20-25 Gy in 5 fractions
Anal cancer	
Two-phase radical or adjuvant	• 30.6Gy in 17 fractions followed by 19.8Gy in 11 fractions
One-phase radical Palliative	• 50.4Gy in 28 fractions • 30Gy in 10 or 20 Gy in 5

Table A2.6 Cancers of genitourinary system

Indication	Dose fractionation
Prostate cancer	
Prostate	• 74-78Gy in 37-39 fractions/60Gy in 20 fractions
Nodal irradiation	• 55-60 Gy in 37 fractions
Postoperative	• 66 Gy in 33 fractions • 52.5 Gy in 20 fractions
Palliative	• 21 Gy in 3 fractions on alternate days/ 20 Gy in 5 fractions / 30Gy in 10 fractions
Urinary bladder cancer	
Radical	• 60-64Gy in 30-32 fractions • 52.5-55 Gy in 20 fractions
Palliative	• 21Gy in 3 fractions on alternate days/30-36Gy in 5-6 fractions twice weekly
Testicular cancer	
Seminoma stage I	• 20Gy in 10 fractions
Seminoma stage IIA–B	• 30 Gy in 15 fractions
Testicular carcinoma in situ	• 20Gy in 10 fractions
Palliative	• 20Gy in 5 fractions/30Gy in 10 fractions
Penile cancer	
Radical	• 60-66 Gy in 30-33 fractions to primary and 50.4 Gy in 28 fractions to pelvic and inguinal nodes with boost up to 66 Gy to gross nodes
Adjuvant	• 54 Gy in 25 fractions to inguinal region with boost up to a total of 57 Gy
Palliative	• 30Gy in 10 fractions

Table A2.7 Cancers of female genital system

Indication	Dose fractionation
Cervical cancer	
Stage IB2–IVA	• 45Gy in 25 fractions followed by brachytherapy (LDR 27–30Gy to point A or 90% dose covering 100% of high-risk CTV or HDR 28Gy in 4 fractions) • 50.4Gy in 28 fractions followed by brachytherapy (LDR 22.5–25Gy to point A or HDR 14Gy in 3 fractions
Central tumour boost when brachytherapy not possible	• 15Gy in 8 or 20Gy in 11 (total 65Gy)
Boost to residual tumour	• 5.4Gy in 3 or 10.8Gy in 6 fractions
Adjuvant RT	• 40 Gy in 20 fractions/ 45Gy in 25 fractions/ 50 Gy in 25 fractions/50.4 Gy in 28 fractions
Para-aortic radiotherapy	• 45Gy in 25 fractions
Endometrial cancer	
High-risk	• 46 Gy in 23 fractions/48.6 Gy in 27 fractions followed by HDR 8Gy at 5 mm in 2 fractions
Intermediate-risk	• 21 Gy at 5mm in 3 fractions over 3 weeks
Primary radiotherapy	• 45Gy in 25 fractions/50 Gy in 25 fractions followed by HDR brachytherapy 28 Gy in 4 fractions or 25 Gy in 5 fractions prescribed to the uterine serosa
Primary brachytherapy alone	• 36 Gy in 5 fractions or 37.5 Gy in 6 fractions prescribed to the uterine serosa
Palliative	• 20Gy in 5 fractions/30Gy in 10 fractions
Vaginal cancer	
Radical	• 45–50Gy in 25 fractions followed by HDR brachytherapy (18.75-20 Gy in 5 fractions)
Brachytherapy alone	• 65–70Gy in 2 fractions using LDR or 33Gy in 6 fractions using HDR.
Vulval cancer	
Postoperative	• 45 Gy in 25 fractions or 50 Gy in 25 fractions
Inoperable	• 45 Gy in 25 fractions or 50 Gy in 25 fractions or 50.4 Gy in 28 fractions with concurrent weekly cisplatin. Primary and involved nodes boosed to 60-65 Gy EQD2

Table A2.8 Cancers of skin

Indication	Dose fractionation
Basal cell carcinoma	
Lesion <3cm	• 36Gy in 8 fractions/3 fractions per week
	• 30–32Gy in 4 fractions/1–2 fractions per week
	• 18Gy single fraction
Lesion 3–5cm or nose/pinna/poorly vascular area	• 45Gy in 9 fractions/3 fractions per week
Lesion >5cm	• 50–55Gy in 15-20 fractions/3-4 weeks
	• 60Gy in 30 fractions/6 weeks
Squamous cell carcinoma	
Lesion <5cm	• 45Gy in 9 fractions on alternate days over 3 weeks
	• 45 Gy in 10 fractions over 2-3 weeks
	• 55Gy in 20 fractions over 4 weeks
Lesion >5cm	• 55Gy in 20 fractions over 4 weeks
	• 60Gy in 30 fractions
Brachytherapy (HDR)	• 45Gy in 10 fractions
Postoperative nodal radiotherapy	• 50-60 Gy in 25-30 fractions (boost up to a total of 66 Gy in 33 fractions in the head and neck region if high risk features)
Palliative RT	• 20Gy in 5 fractions
	• 8Gy single
Malignant melanoma	
Adjuvant RT after node dissection	• 48 in 20 fractions
	• 50-60 Gy in 25-30 fractions
Cutaneous T cell lymphoma	• 8Gy in 2 fractions (for patch and plaque)
	• 12Gy in 3 fractions (nodule)
	• 20Gy in 10 fractions (mucosal disease)
	• 30Gy in 15 fractions (lymph node disease)
	• 30Gy in 20 fractions over 5 weeks (total body electrons)
Cutaneous B cell lymphoma	• 15Gy in 5 fractions (indolent)
	• 30Gy in 15 fractions (aggressive)
Kaposi's sarcoma—skin	• 8Gy single or 15Gy in 3 fractions
Kaposi's sarcoma—mucosal	• 20Gy in 10 fractions/2 weeks
Merkel cell carcinoma	• 60-66 Gy in 30-33 fractions/50-55 Gy in 20-25 fractions /40-45 Gy in 15 fractions (radical)
	• 50Gy in 25 fractions (with chemotherapy)
	• 50-60 Gy in 25-30 or 40-45Gy in 15 (adjuvant RT)

Table A2.9 Soft tissue sarcoma

Indication	Dose fractionation
Postoperative	• 50 Gy in 25 fractions followed by a boost of 10 Gy in 5 fractions or 16 Gy in 8 fractions for high risk disease
Preoperative	• 50Gy in 25 fractions
Radical (inoperable)	• 66 Gy in 33 fractions
Retroperitoneal sarcoma	• 50 Gy in 25 fractions • 50.4 Gy in 28 fractions
Desmoid tumour – postoperative	• 56 Gy in 28 fractions
Palliative	• 8 Gy in single fraction • 20-30 Gy in 5-10 fractions • 36-39 Gy in 12-13 fractions • 40 Gy in 15 fractions

Table A2.10 Tumours of haemopoietic system

Indication	Dose fractionation
Hodgkin lymphoma	
Nodular LP	• 30 Gy in 15 fractions
Favourable group	• 20Gy in 10 fractions
Unfavourable group	• 30Gy in 15 fractions
Residual disease in advanced disease	• 30-40 Gy in 15-20 fractions
Palliative	• 30 Gy in 10 fractions/ 20Gy in 5 fractions/ 7-8 Gy single
Non-Hodgkin lymphoma	
Primary RT for low grade	• 24 Gy in 12 fractions
RT after chemotherapy	• 30Gy in 15 fractions
NK/T cell	• 50 Gy in 25 fractions
Palliative	• 20Gy in 5 fractions/30Gy in 10 fractions/ 4 Gy in 2 fractions / 8-10 Gy in 1 fraction
Splenic irradiation	• 10–12Gy in 0.5–1.5Gy 3 times per week
Solitary plasmacytoma	• 40–50Gy in 20-25 fractions

Table A2.11 Palliative radiotherapy

Indication	Dose fractionation
Superior vena caval obstruction	• 20Gy in 5 fractions or 30Gy in 10 fractions
Choroidal metastasis	• 20Gy in 5 fractions
Bone pain	• 8Gy single • 8 Gy single or 20 Gy in 5 fractions (re-irradiation/prevention of pathological fracture/fractured bones and postoperative fixing) • Upper hemibody 6 Gy single for diffuse pain • Lower hemibody 8 Gy single for diffuse pain

Table A2.12 Oligometastatic disease

Indication	Dose fractionation
Bone and lymph node	• 18-24 Gy single or 30-45 Gy in 3 fractions on alternately days (initial treatment) • 30 Gy in 5 fractions given on alternate days (Pelvis-reirradiation) • 20-30 Gy in 2-5 fractions given on alternate days (Spine re-irradiation)
Lung	• 48-54 Gy in 3 fractions given on alternate days • 55-60 Gy in 5 fractions given on alternate days
Liver	• 45-60 Gy in 3 fractions given on alternate days • 50-60 Gy in 5 fractions given on alternate days
Adrenal	• 30-36 Gy in 3 fractions given on alternate days

Internet resource

The Royal College of Radiologists. (2019). *Radiotherapy Dose Fractionation, Third edition.* London, UK: The Royal College of Radiologists. https://www.rcr.ac.uk/system/files/publication/field_publication_files/brfo193_radiotherapy_dose_fractionation_third-edition.pdf

Appendix 3

Glomerular filtration rate

Calculation of glomerular filtration rate

Calculation of glomercular filtration rate (GFR) is a prerequisite before prescription of platinum chemotherapy or other agents likely to cause renal dysfunction. It is calculated by one of the following methods:

1. 24-hour urine collection method
2. Using the Cockcroft-Gault formula

Cockcroft-Gault formula

$$\text{Creatinine clearance} = \frac{(140 - \text{age}) \times \text{weight (kg)} \times A}{\text{Serum creatinine}}$$

$A = 1.04$ in females and 1.23 in males

This method of calculation of GFR is less accurate in:

- Malnourished patients (weight loss of >5kg in the last month)
- Obese patients—needs to be calculated using adjusted ideal body weight
- Patients under 18 years old
- Patients with a rapidly changing creatinine level

Calculation of carboplatin dose (Calvert formula)

- Carboplatin dose = AUC x (GFR+25)

Most protocols use AUC of 5 for measured GFR and 6 for calculated creatinine clearance. 120mL/min is the cap on CrCl as this is the maximum physiological GFR. Carboplatin is not given if GFR is <20mL/min. The calculated GFR should be recalculated before each cycle and if there is >25% change from the baseline calculated GFR, Cr Cl should be measured and dose modified accordingly.

Index

Abbreviations used in the index can be found in the abbreviation list.
Tables, figures and boxes are indicated by an italic *t, f* or *b* following the page number.